W9-CRP-744

Lippincott Williams & Wilkins'

COMPREHENSIVE

Medical Assisting

THIRD EDITION

Lippincott Williams & Wilkins'

COMPREHENSIVE
Medical Assisting

THIRD EDITION

Judy Kronenberger, RN, CMA, MEd

Associate Professor, Medical Assistant Technology
Sinclair Community College
Dayton, Ohio

Laura Southard Durham, BS, CMA

Medical Assisting Technologies Program Coordinator
Forsyth Technical Community College
Winston-Salem, North Carolina

Denise Woodson, MA, MT(ASCP)SC

Academic Coordinator
Health Professions and Nursing
Smarthinking, Inc.
Richmond, Virginia

 Wolters Kluwer | Lippincott Williams & Wilkins
Health

Philadelphia · Baltimore · New York · London
Buenos Aires · Hong Kong · Sydney · Tokyo

Exexutive Editor: John Goucher
Managing Editor: Kevin C. Dietz
Development Editor: Rose Foltz
Senior Marketing Manager: Nancy Bradshaw

Production Editor: Beth Martz
Design Coordinator: Stephen Druding
Compositor: Maryland Composition

Third Edition

Copyright © 2005, 2008 Lippincott Williams & Wilkins, a Wolters Kluwer business.

351 West Camden Street   530 Walnut Street
Baltimore, MD 21201   Philadelphia, PA 19106

Printed in the People's Republic of China

All rights reserved. This book is protected by copyright. No part of this book may be reproduced or transmitted in any form or by any means, including as photocopies or scanned-in or other electronic copies, or utilized by any information storage and retrieval system without written permission from the copyright owner, except for brief quotations embodied in critical articles and reviews. Materials appearing in this book prepared by individuals as part of their official duties as U.S. government employees are not covered by the above-mentioned copyright. To request permission, please contact Lippincott Williams & Wilkins at 530 Walnut Street, Philadelphia, PA 19106, via email at *permissions@lww.com*, or via website at lww.com (products and services).

Library of Congress Cataloging-in-Publication Data

Kronenberger, Judy.
  Lippincott Williams & Wilkins' comprehensive medical assisting. —3rd ed. / Judy Kronenberger, Laura Southard Durham, Denise Woodson.
     p. ; cm.
  Rev. ed. of: Lippincott Williams and Wilkins' comprehensive medical assisting / Elizabeth A. Molle ... [et al.]. 2nd ed. c2005.
  Includes bibliographical references and index.
  ISBN-13: 978-0-7817-7004-0 (alk. paper)
  ISBN-10: 0-7817-7004-1 (alk. paper)
  1. Medical assistants. I. Durham, Laura Southard. II. Woodson, Denise. III. Lippincott Williams and Wilkins' comprehensive medical assisting. IV. Title. V. Title: Comprehensive medical assisting. VI. Title: Lippincott Williams and Wilkins' comprehensive medical assisting.

  [DNLM: 1. Physician Assistants. 2. Clinical Medicine--methods. 3. Medical Secretaries. 4. Practice Management, Medical. W 21.5 K93L 2008]
  R728.8.H66 2008
  610.73'7069--dc22

                                                                                    2007044261

DISCLAIMER

Care has been taken to confirm the accuracy of the information present and to describe generally accepted practices. However, the authors, editors, and publisher are not responsible for errors or omissions or for any consequences from application of the information in this book and make no warranty, expressed or implied, with respect to the currency, completeness, or accuracy of the contents of the publication. Application of this information in a particular situation remains the professional responsibility of the practitioner; the clinical treatments described and recommended may not be considered absolute and universal recommendations.

The authors, editors, and publisher have exerted every effort to ensure that drug selection and dosage set forth in this text are in accordance with the current recommendations and practice at the time of publication. However, in view of ongoing research, changes in government regulations, and the constant flow of information relating to drug therapy and drug reactions, the reader is urged to check the package insert for each drug for any change in indications and dosage and for added warnings and precautions. This is particularly important when the recommended agent is a new or infrequently employed drug.

Some drugs and medical devices presented in this publication have Food and Drug Administration (FDA) clearance for limited use in restricted research settings. It is the responsibility of the health care provider to ascertain the FDA status of each drug or device planned for use in their clinical practice.

To purchase additional copies of this book, call our customer service department at (800) 638-3030 or fax orders to (301) 223-2320. International customers should call (301) 223-2300.

Visit Lippincott Williams & Wilkins on the Internet: *http://www.lww.com*. Lippincott Williams & Wilkins customer service representatives are available from 8:30 am to 6:00 pm, EST.

3 4 5 6 7 8 9 10

CCS0409

Although I owe much gratitude to many people for their support, I have to personally thank my husband Joe for believing in me and providing unconditional love and understanding for the "missed" family events, movies, and general companionship during the completion of this edition of the book. In addition, special thanks and lots of love go to our children including my son Brian and his wife Vanessa, daughters Jennifer and Brittany, and my youngest "captain" Eric. Most of all, I have to thank two special people in my life, Arthur and Victor, who provided "grandma" with lots of much needed laughter and joy as well as plenty of distractions, reminding me that life is short and babies are only little once. Last, but certainly not least, I have to thank the many students that I have had the pleasure to teach over the years who have given me purpose and vision for this book and who continue to teach me new lessons every day.

JUDY KRONENBERGER

This labor of love is dedicated to the people who helped me complete it while trying to meet the demands of everyday life: My amazing daughter Amanda, the reason for everything I do; her husband Brad, my honorary son and good friend; and Gracie who blessed me with the title of "Nana," the most beautiful sound in the world. To the rest of my family who I love with all my heart: My sister Susan and her children, Dana, Laila, Ramsey, who make me so proud to be their Auntie 1; Ellen, my cousin and best friend, the bravest person I know. To my parents, Mamie and Joe, who still guide me through their teachings and inspiration—even from heaven; and to LeRoy who seems to get left behind in a busy life but who owns my heart. To my students who have helped and encouraged me every step of the way and to my fellow authors who have become true friends for life.

LAURA SOUTHARD DURHAM

My dedication is to my husband John, my knight in shining armor, whose love, patience, and support have carried me through this edition and through the other life challenges we have faced at the same time. You are my best friend and the love of my life. I thank my Mother and my sister Jeana for their love and prayers. To Judy and Laura, thanks for your friendship, your encouragement, and for the laughter we have shared.

DENISE WOODSON

Preface

This is an exciting and challenging time to enter the field of medical assisting. You are uniquely poised to function as the most versatile professional in the medical office. As a medical assistant, you will have the opportunity to perform a variety of clinical and administrative skills. The skills you will perform and your job title will vary among offices. This book was written to help you succeed in performing a variety of administrative and clinical medical assisting procedures.

Lippincott Williams & Wilkins' Comprehensive Medical Assisting 3e will define your roles and responsibilities as a professional medical assistant. The book is based on the American Association of Medical Assisting (AAMA) role delineation components for certified medical assistants and the competencies described by the American Medical Technologists (AMT) Registered Medical Assistant Competency Inventory. These roles have evolved and grown over the past decade and will continue to expand to meet the needs of the medical profession.

ORGANIZATION OF THE TEXT

As experienced medical assisting instructors, we understand the complexity of this subject matter can be overwhelming to a new student. Great care and concern were taken to organize this book into a logical and reader-friendly presentation. The book is divided into sections:

- Part I, Introduction to Medical Assisting, consists of one unit. Chapter 1 provides you with a brief history of the medical profession and the practice of medical assisting. Legal and ethical issues governing the medical community and your practice are discussed in Chapter 2. Chapter 3 helps you sharpen your communication skills, and Chapter 4 gives you the tools to deliver effective patient education.
- Part II, The Administrative Medical Assistant, consists of two units. Unit 2 helps you master basic administrative skills and the basics of office management. Unit 3 explores financial management of the medical office.
- Part III, The Clinical Medical Assistant, consists of two units. Unit 4 provides you with critical information regarding aseptic technique and infection control. The basic components of patient assessment, which include conducting the patient interview, obtaining vital signs, and assisting with the physical ex-

amination, are discussed in detail. You will also find an overview of pharmacology as well as information to help you properly prepare and administer medications. The final chapter in this unit will give you the tools to recognize and respond to emergencies in the medical office. Unit 5 focuses on specialty examinations, diagnostic tests, and therapeutic procedures for specific areas of medicine. Each chapter provides you with a brief overview of the system and common disorders associated with it. Then, the common diagnostic and therapeutic procedures are discussed to help you deliver the proper treatment. The last two chapters in this unit focus on duties relating to special populations.

- Part IV, The Clinical Laboratory, introduces you to the physician's office laboratory. The laboratory is one of medicine's most powerful diagnostic tools. This section provides you with detailed information on maintaining a safe laboratory environment that operates in compliance with all state and federal regulations. It offers instructions on collecting and processing specimens and for handling the specimens in a manner that supports accurate testing. It also explains CLIA-waived procedures for analyzing blood, urine, and other body samples and their relationship to clinical symptoms, diseases, and disorders. In addition, you will learn how to document and maintain a quality assurance program to ensure thorough patient care. Finally, the section will cover a quality control protocol for monitoring and evaluating testing procedures, supplies, and equipment that will ensure accuracy in laboratory performance.
- Part V, Career Strategies, helps you make a smooth transition from the classroom environment to the workforce.

Lippincott Williams & Wilkins' Comprehensive Medical Assisting, 3e is packaged with a complimentary CD-ROM to help you prepare for examinations. The CD-ROM contains questions to help you prepare for CMA and RMA certification and four interactive case studies that place you inside actual situations you will encounter in practice.

FEATURES

Our goal is to make this textbook the most student-friendly resource available in the medical assisting field. For students who use English as a second language

(ESL), an ESL learning expert reviewed the entire text to ensure the language is appropriate and understandable to non-native English students.

A variety of key features are included to spark interest and promote comprehension. Most chapters include the following:

- A chapter outline
- Learning objectives and performance objectives
- Chapter competenices—CAAHEP and ABHES
- Key terms
- Key points highlighted throughout the text
- Step-by-step procedure boxes
- Spanish terms and phrases
- Critical thinking challenges
- Checkpoint questions
- Unique information boxes, tables, and displays
- Online resources at the end of each chapter
- Full-color illustrations
- Media Menu, containing information on video clips, animations, and Internet resources

This textbook is fully supported with a robust teaching and learning package, each element of which is designed to help you and your instructor get the most out of the textbook. The resource package includes the following:

- A student study guide to enhance learning and comprehension includes competency evaluation forms for each procedure in the textbook; critical thinking exercises; self-assessment exercises, such as matching and multiple choice; and study and work products.
- A complete instructor's resource kit accompanying the textbook includes suggested classroom activities; chapter quizzes and answer keys; answers to workbook questions; and frequently asked questions about teaching the course, preparing instructional material, and gaining and maintaining accreditation. A CD-ROM with a test generator, image bank, and PowerPoint slides is packaged with the instructor's manual.

As medical assisting instructors, we hope these books exceed your expectations. May your career in medical assisting be challenging and fulfilling!

Judy Kronenberger, RN, CMA, MEd
Laura Southard Durham, BS, CMA
Denise Woodson, MA, MT(ASCP)SC

User's Guide

This User's Guide shows you how to the put the features of *Lippincott Williams & Wilkins' Comprehensive Medical Assisting, 3e* to work for you.

Chapter Opening Elements

Each chapter begins with the following elements, which will help orient you to the material:

Chapter Outline

This serves as your "roadmap" to the chapter content.

Learning Objectives and Performance Objectives

The Learning Objectives list the skills learned in the chapters, and the Performance Objectives detail the competency procedures performed in the chapter.

Competencies – CAAHEP and ABHES

The CAAHEP and ABHES Competencies specific to the chapter are listed in the Chapter Opener.

Key Terms

The key terms that are defined in the chapter are listed for quick reference.

Special Features

Unique chapter features will aid readers' comprehension and retention of information—and spark interest in students and faculty:

Percutaneous transluminal coronary angioplasty (PTCA). (A) A guide is threaded into the coronary artery. (B) A balloon catheter is inserted through the occlusion. (C) The balloon is inflated and deflated until plaque is flattened and the vessel is opened.

Stunning Art Program

More than 300 full-color illustrations and photographs—over 100 of which are new—clarify clinical concepts for the learner.

PROCEDURE 17-2:	Removing Contaminated Gloves *(continued)*
Steps	**Purpose**
4. Holding the soiled glove in the palm of your gloved hand, slip your ungloved fingers under the cuff of the glove you are still wearing, being careful not to touch the outside of the glove.	Skin should touch skin but never the soiled part of the glove.
	Step 4. Slip your free hand under the cuff of the remaining glove.
5. Stretch the glove of the dominant hand up and away from your hand while turning it inside out, with the already removed glove balled up inside.	Turning it inside out ensures that the soiled surfaces of the gloves are enclosed.
	Step 5. Remove the glove by turning it inside out over the previously removed glove.
6. Both gloves should now be removed, with the first glove inside the second glove and the second glove inside out.	
7. Discard both gloves as one unit into a biohazard waste receptacle.	
8. Wash your hands.	Wearing gloves is NOT a substitute for washing your hands!

Procedure Boxes

Breaks procedures down into steps, demonstrating how to perform essential skills properly. Needed equipment and supplies are listed. Rationales are given for each step, ensuring greater understanding.

CHECKPOINT QUESTION
6. What level of disinfection would you use to clean a reusable instrument that comes into contact with the vaginal mucosa, such as a vaginal speculum? Why?

Checkpoint Questions

Review questions appear throughout the chapter to ensure student comprehension of the material learned in the section.

PATIENT EDUCATION
GENETIC DISEASES

The patient's family history can provide you with many teaching opportunities. If a patient indicates that previous members of his or her family had certain diseases, then there may be a genetic link. A genetic disease is noted by a mark on the DNA (genetic material) for a specific illness or disease. The patient receives this mark from either or both parents. Some common examples include some forms of high blood pressure, diabetes, heart disease, obesity, and certain cancers. Examples of less common genetic disorders are Tay-Sachs disease, Marfan syndrome, and Huntington disease. Great strides have been made in genetic testing. This allows the patient to have the DNA examined for potential markers

Patient Education Boxes

Contains in-depth information on topics the student needs to know in order to be a successful medical assistant.

SPANISH TERMINOLOGY

A que se debe su visita?
  Why do you need to see the doctor?
Desde cuando se siente mal?
  How long has this been going on?
Prefiere la cita en la manana o en la tarde?
  Would you prefer morning or afternoon?
Llamo para recordarle su cita.
  I am calling to remind you of your appointment.
Le dare una cita para que vea al Doctor nuevamenta.
  I will give you an appointment to return to see the doctor.
Para su proxima visita, por favor traiga su tarjeta del seguro y todas las medicinas que
  Please bring your

Spanish Terms and Phrases

Assists students communicating with Spanish-speaking patients.

WHAT IF?

What if your patient is offended that you are wearing gloves when drawing a blood specimen?

Sometimes patients become defensive and make statements to the effect that they are "disease free." If this happens to you, reassure the patient by saying that wearing gloves is a standard practice and is used for the protection of the patient also. Use this occasion to teach the patient about standard precautions and the importance of following these guidelines.

What If Boxes

Presents a variety of real-life scenarios that students must be prepared to handle in the medical office. Each situation is clearly defined and explained.

Legal Tip Boxes

Contains important legal information to help the aspiring medical assistant understand the legal implications associated with the profession.

LEGAL TIP
DOCUMENT, DOCUMENT, DOCUMENT!

When a patient does not show up for his appointment, you must make an entry in the chart. Because your physician has a legal contract with the patient, he has an obligation to treat him as long and as often as necessary. If the patient does not report for his scheduled appointments, the patient is breaking the contract. This would be an important factor in a court cases involving a physician being sued for abandonment. The chart is the physician's defense. Being diligent with documentation is not optional.

Example:

Special Features *(continued)*

ETHICAL TIP

Think Before You Speak

As discussed throughout the text, it is illegal and unethical to release patient information without the patient's consent. You may be breaching confidentiality without even realizing it. Consider this: You are a receptionist in a busy OB/GYN practice. A former classmate comes in for a pregnancy test. While you are making her return appointment, she tells you that the test was positive. Later, while having lunch at a nearby restaurant, you see her mother. You congratulate her on her new grandchild and quickly realize that she doesn't know yet. You have just breached the patient's confidentiality.

What if the scenario had been like this: "Hi, Mrs. Roberts. What a coincidence; I just saw Susie this morning." Mrs. Roberts says, "Where did you see her?" You reply, "At work." You have just told Mrs. Roberts that her daughter was at an OB/GYN.

Ethical Tip Boxes

Offers guidelines to help the student learn and abide by the ethical standards set forth by the AAMA.

MEDIA MENU

- **Student CD**
  - **Case Study**
    Clinical Interactive Case Study 3: Dealing with a Sick Patient, Infection Control, and Medication Administration
  - **Video Procedure**
    Procedure 17-1 video clip
  - **CMA/RMA Certification Exam Review**
- **Premium Online Course**
  http://thePoint.lww.com/Kronenberger3e
- **LWW's Medical Assisting Skills DVD**
  - Procedures 17-1, 17-2
- **Internet Resources**

Media Menus

Located at the end of every chapter, the Media Menu contains information on video clips, animations, case studies, and Internet resources that are available to the student.

Chapter Closing Elements

Chapter Summary
Reviews key points from the chapter.

Chapter Summary

- Anthropometric measurements include height and weight. Vital signs include:
  - temperature (T)
  - pulse (P)
  - respirations (R)
  - blood pressure (BP)

- When a patient first visits the medical office, these measurements are recorded as a baseline and used as a comparison for data collected at subsequent visits. These measurements, which provide important data for the physician to use in diagnosing and treating illnesses, are very frequently performed by medical assistants.

Warm Ups for Critical Thinking

1. You are asked to teach a patient, Mr. Stone, how to take his blood pressure at home once in the morning and once at night and record these readings for 1 month. Create a patient education brochure that explains the procedure in understandable terms and design a sheet that Mr. Stone can easily use to record these readings.

2. Ms. Black arrived at the office late for her appointment; she was frantic and explained that she had experienced car trouble on the way to the office, could not find a parking place, and just locked her keys inside her car. How would you expect these events to affect her vital signs? Explain why.

3. What size of cuff would you choose for Mrs. Cooper, an elderly female patient who is 5 feet 3

inches tall and weighs 90 pounds? Why?

4. How would you respond to a patient who asks you to give advice on what type of thermometer to buy for use at home? Would the age of the patient be relevant with regard to the type of thermometer you might suggest?

5. An elderly male patient tells you that he is considering stopping the blood pressure medication the physician ordered at the previous visit. He further explains that he has "read all about this drug on the internet," and he informs you that "it has side effects," although he denies experiencing any at this time. Describe how you would handle this situation.

Answers to Checkpoint Questions

1. Accurately measuring vital signs assists the physician in diagnosing and treating various disorders.

2. Rectal temperature measurements are usually 1° higher than oral measurements because of the vascularity and tightly closed environment of the rectum.

3. A child's body temperature may be slightly higher than an adult's because of the faster metabolism in a child.

4. The electronic, tympanic, and temporal artery thermometers have digital display screens that show the obtained temperature.

5. Measuring a patient's pulse entails assessing and recording the rate (number of heartbeats in 1

minute), rhythm (regular or irregular), and volume (thready, bounding).

6. Contraction of the diaphragm causes negative pressure in the lungs, which respond by filling with inhaled air.

7. During systole, the heart contracts and forces blood out and through the arteries. In diastole, the heart relaxes and fills with blood.

8. The pulse pressure is the difference between the systolic and diastolic blood pressures, and the auscultatory gap is an abrupt, but temporary, end to the tapping sound heard when auscultating the blood pressure.

404

Warm Ups for Critical Thinking
Real-life scenarios that require the student to develop, create, write, or search for more information.

Answers to Checkpoint Questions
Allows students to check their answers to the questions found within each chapter.

Additional Learning Resources

This powerful learning tool also includes:

Live/Advise

- **LiveAdvise Student Tutoring** is available free to students.
- **LiveAdvise Competency Training** gives students the ability to practice CAAHEP and ABHES competencies with a live tutor.

Visit **http://thePoint.lww.com/liveadvise** for more information and to try this free service.

- **LWW's Medical Assisting Skills DVD** covers the most critical medical assisting skills; available for students and for institutional purchase.

- **Student Resource CD** comes with animations, interactive exercises, student quiz bank, competency evaluation forms, and sample video clips from the Medical Assisting Skills Video Series, and more.

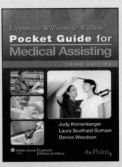

- **Pocket Guide** gives step-by-step coverage of medical assisting procedures in both administrative and clinical settings. The small size, spiral binding and new write on/wipe off paper make it perfect for clinical and office use.

- **thePoint Companion Site** for students comes with a Stedman's English to Spanish audio glossary, student work products, English as a second language resources, interactive math review, and drug administration animations.

- **Interactive Online Course** supports the text and simulates a virtual externship through interactive case studies.

- **Instructor Resource CD-ROM** includes an image bank, test generator, PowerPoint lecture slides, competency evaluation forms, competency correlation grids, and more.

- **Study Guide** comes with competency work products including sample forms for student practice, critical thinking activities, multiple choice, matching exercises, and more.

Acknowledgments

This book would never have been successfully completed without the assistance, persistence, and hard work of many people. First, we would like to thank John Goucher, the Acquisitions Editor, who was there from the beginning to offer support and insight whenever needed. In addition, a special thank you should go to all of the staff of Lippincott Williams & Wilkins for making this book a reality and supporting the education of medical assistants. In particular, we would like to thank Kevin Dietz at LWW for his guidance in making this text a reality. We would also like to thank Rose Foltz for helping us keep the project organized and to ensure the chapter content meets the needs of the students. Additionally, we thank Chris Merillo and Rachelle Detweiler for assisting us with the video shoot.

The authors and staff at LWW thank the administration, staff, and students at Forsyth Technical Community College in Winston-Salem, NC, who provided the location, faces, and skills for the photo and video shoots. Special thanks to Dr. Shari Covitz, Bernie Yevin, Marcia Polanis, Beth Sprinkle, Cindy Nivens, Annette Hedrick, Lisa Hunt, Roberta Allen, Elsie and Chris Pearce, Rick Yokely, Heather Bass and Rhonda Whisenhunt for their tremendous help, support, and encouragement. Many thanks to Donna Bell, Jenifer Gibson and all of the medical assisting students and graduates who offered their time and skills to help get these big jobs done!

We also thank Scott Yingling at MICA Information Systems; Diane Poindexter and Rhea Teague of Novant/Forsyth Medical Group for their help and support in providing skills, materials, and expertise. We thank Amy Semenchuk, Sandra Lehrke, Geri Kale-Smith and Brenda Holzinger for their expertise and help with Chapter 8.

COVERAGE OF CAAHEP ENTRY-LEVEL COMPETENCIES

Competency #	Description	3rd Edition Procedure Number	Competency Practice and Check-Off Available through LiveAdvise (powered by Smarthinking, Inc.)
a. ADMINISTRATIVE COMPETENCIES			
(1)	**Perform Clerical Functions**		
a. (1) (a)	Schedule and manage appointments	6-1 Making an Appointment for a New Patient 6-2 Making an Appointment for an Established Patient	III.A.3.a.1.a - Schedule and manage appointments
a. (1) (b)	Schedule inpatient and outpatient admissions and procedures	6-3 Making an Appointment for a Referral to an Outpatient Facility 6-4 Arranging for Admission to an Inpatient Facility	III.A.3.a.1.b - Schedule inpatient and outpatient admissions and procedures
a. (1) (c)	Organize a patient's medical record	8-1 Establishing, Organizing, and Maintaining a Medical File	
a. (1) (d)	File medical records	8-2 Filing Medical Records	
(2)	**Perform Bookkeeping Procedures**		
a. (2) (a)	Prepare a bank deposit	12-9 Complete a Bank Deposit Slip and Make a Deposit	III.A.3.a.2.a - Prepare a bank deposit
a. (2) (b)	Post entries on a daysheet	12-1 Post Charges on a Daysheet 12-2 Post Payments on a Daysheet 12-5 Post Adjustments to a Daysheet 12-8 Balance a Daysheet	III.A.3.a.2.b - Post entries on a daysheet
a. (2) (c)	Perform accounts receivable procedures	12-1 Post Charges on a Daysheet 12-2 Post Payments on a Daysheet 12-5 Post Adjustments to a Daysheet 12-4 Process Refunds	III.A.3.a.2.c - Perform accounts receivable procedures
a. (2) (d)	Perform billing and collection procedures	12-3 Process a Credit Balance 12-6 Post Collection Agency Payments 12-4 Process Refunds	III.A.3.a.2.e - Post adjustments III.A.3.a.2.i - Post collection agency payments III.A.3.a.2.f - Process a credit balance III.A.3.a.2.g - Process refunds III.A.3.a.2.d - Perform billing and collection procedures
a. (2) (e)	Post adjustments	12-5: Post Adjustments to a Daysheet	III.A.3.a.2.e - Post adjustments
a. (2) (f)	Process credit balance	12-3 Process a Credit Balance	III.A.3.a.2.f - Process a credit balance
a. (2) (g)	Process refunds	12-4 Process Refunds	III.A.3.a.2.g - Process refunds
a. (2) (h)	Post NSF checks	12-7 Process NSF Checks	III.A.3.a.2.h - Post non-sufficient funds (NSF) checks
a. (2) (i)	Post collection agency payments	12-6 Post Collection Agency Payments	III.A.3.a.2.i - Post collection agency payments
(3)	**Process Insurance Claims**		
a. (3) (a)	Apply managed care policies and procedures	13-1 Completing a CMS-1500 Claim Form	
a. (3) (b)	Apply third-party guidelines	15-1 Locating a CPT Code	
a. (3) (c)	Perform procedural coding	15-1 Locating a CPT Code	
a. (3) (d)	Perform diagnostic coding	14-1 Locating a Diagnostic Code	
a. (3) (e)	Complete insurance claim forms	13-1 Completing a CMS-1500 Claim Form	

Competency #	Description	3rd Edition Procedure Number	Competency Practice and Check-Off Available through LiveAdvise (powered by Smarthinking, Inc.)
b. CLINICAL COMPETENCIES			
(1)	**Fundamental Procedures**		
b. (1) (a)	Perform handwashing	17-1 Handwashing for Medical Asepsis	
b. (1) (b)	Wrap items for autoclaving	21-2 Wrapping instruments for sterilization in an autoclave	
b. (1) (c)	Perform sterilization techniques	21-1 Sanitizing Equipment for Disinfection or Sterilization 21-3 Operating an Autoclave	
b. (1) (d)	Dispose of biohazardous materials	17-3 Cleaning Biohazardous Spills All procedures in Chapter 24: Preparing and Administering Medications	
b. (1) (e)	Practice Standard Precautions	17-2 Removing Contaminated Gloves 21-1 Sanitizing Equipment for Disinfection or Sterilization 21-2 Wrapping Instruments for Sterilization in an Autoclave 21-3 Operating an Autoclave 24-1 Administering Oral Medications 24-2 Preparing Injections 24-3 Administering an Intradermal Injection 24-4 Administering a Subcutaneous Injection 24-5 Administering an Intramuscular Injection 24-6 Administering an Intramuscular Injection Using the Z-Track Method 24-7 Applying Transdermal Medications 24-8 Obtaining and Preparing an Intravenous Site 35-2 Assisting With the Pelvic Exam and Pap Smear 35-3 Assisting With the Colposcopy and Cervical Biopsy	
(2)	**Specimen Collection**		
b. (2) (a)	Perform venipuncture	41-1 Obtaining a Blood Specimen by Evacuated Tube or Winged Infusion Set	
b. (2) (b)	Perform capillary puncture	41-2 Obtaining a Blood Specimen by Capillary Puncture	
b. (2) (c)	Obtain specimens for microbiological testing	44-1 Collect a Throat Specimen 44-2 Collecting a Nasopharyngeal Specimen 44-3 Collecting a Wound Specimen 44-4 Collecting a Sputum Specimen 44-5 Collecting a Stool Specimen 44-6 Collecting Blood for Culture 44-7 Collecting Genital Specimens for Culture	
b. (2) (d)	Instruct patients in the collection of a clean-catch and midstream urine specimen	43-1 Obtaining a Clean-Catch Midstream Urine Specimen	III.C.3.b.2.d - Instruct patients in the collection of a clean-catch, mid-stream urine specimen

Competency #	Description	3rd Edition Procedure Number	Competency Practice and Check-Off Available through LiveAdvise (powered by Smarthinking, Inc.)
b. CLINICAL COMPETENCIES			
b. (2) (e)	Instruct patients in the collection of fecal specimens	44-5 Collecting a Stool Specimen	III.C.3.b.2.e - Instruct patients in the collection of a fecal specimen
(3)	**Diagnostic Testing**		
b. (3) (a)	Perform electrocardiography	31-1 Performing a 12-Lead Electrocardiogram 31-2 Applying a Holter Monitor	
b. (3) (b)	Perform respiratory testing	30-1 Instructing a Patient on Using the Peak Flowmeter 30-3 Perform a Pulmonary Function Test	
b. (3) (c)	CLIA Waived Tests:		
b. (3) (c) (i)	Perform urinalysis	43-1 Obtaining a Clean-Catch Midstream Urine Specimen 43-2 Obtaining a 24-Hour Urine Specimen 43-3 Determining Color and Clarity of Urine 43-4 Chemical Reagent Strip Analysis 43-5 Preparing Urine Sediment	III.C.3.b.2.d - Instruct patients in the collection of a clean-catch, mid-stream urine specimen
b. (3) (c) (ii)	Perform hematology testing	42-1 Making a Peripheral Blood Smear 42-2 Staining a Peripheral Blood Smear 42-3 Performing a Hemoglobin Determination 42-4 Performing a Microhematocrit Determination 42-5 Westergren Erythrocyte Sedimentation Rate	
b. (3) (c) (iii)	Perform chemistry testing	45-1 Perform Blood Glucose Testing 45-2 Perform Blood Cholesterol Testing	
b. (3) (c) (iv)	Perform immunology testing	44-12 Mononucleosis Testing 44-14 Rapid Group A Strep Testing	
b. (3) (c) (v)	Perform microbiology testing	44-9 Preparing a Smear for Microscopic Evaluation 44-10 Performing a Gram Stain 44-11 Inoculating a Culture 44-8 Testing Stool Specimen for Occult Blood Guaiac Method 44-12 Mononucleosis Testing 44-13 HCG Pregnancy Test 44-14 Rapid Group A Strep Testing	
(4)	**Patient Care**		
b. (4) (a)	Perform telephone and in-person screening	5-1 Handling Incoming Calls 18-1 Interviewing the Patient to Obtain a Medical History 18-2 Document a Chief Complaint (CC) and Present Illness (PI)	III.C.3.b.4.a - Perform telephone and in-person screening

Competency #	Description	3rd Edition Procedure Number	Competency Practice and Check-Off Available through LiveAdvise (powered by Smarthinking, Inc.)
b. CLINICAL COMPETENCIES			
(4)	**Patient Care**		
b. (4) (b)	Obtain vital signs	19-1 Measuring Weight 19-2 Measuring Height 19-3 Measure Oral Temperature Using a Glass Mercury Thermometer 19-4 Measuring a Rectal Temperature 19-5 Measuring an Axillary Temperature 19-6 Measuring Temperature Using an Electronic Thermometer 19-7 Measuring Temperature Using a Tympanic Thermometer 19-8 Measuring Temperature Using a Temporal Artery Thermometer 19-9 Measuring Radial Pulse 19-10 Measuring Respirations 19-11 Measuring Blood Pressure	
b. (4) (c)	Obtain and record patient history	18-1 Interviewing the Patient to Obtain a Medical History	
b. (4) (d)	Prepare and maintain examination and treatment areas	20-1 Assisting With the Adult Physical Exam	
b. (4) (e)	Prepare patient for and assist with routine and specialty examinations	20-1 Assisting With the Adult Physical Exam 35-2 Assisting With the Pelvic Exam and Pap Smear 35-3 Assisting With the Colposcopy and Cervical Biopsy • Procedures in all of the clinical chapters in which the medical assistant is dealing with a patient	
b. (4) (f)	Prepare patient for and assist with procedures, treatments, and minor office surgeries	22-1 Opening Sterile Surgical Packs 22-2 Using Sterile Transfer Forceps 22-3 Adding Sterile Solution to a Sterile Field 22-4 Performing Hair Removal and Skin Preparation 22-5 Applying Sterile Gloves 22-6 Applying a Sterile Dressing 22-7 Changing an Existing Sterile Dressing 22-8 Assisting with Excisional Surgery 22-9 Assisting with Incision and Drainage (I & D) 22-10 Removing Sutures 22-11 Removing Staples 25-1 Preparing a Patient for an X-Ray 35-2 Assisting With the Pelvic Exam and Pap Smear 35-3 Assisting With the Colposcopy and Cervical Biopsy • Procedures in all of the clinical chapters in which the medical assistant is dealing with a patient	

Competency #	Description	3rd Edition Procedure Number	Competency Practice and Check-Off Available through LiveAdvise (powered by Smarthinking, Inc.)
b. CLINICAL COMPETENCIES			
(4)	**Patient Care**		
b. (4) (g)	Apply pharmacology principles to prepare and administer oral and parenteral (excluding IV) medications	24-1 Administering Oral Medications 24-2 Preparing Injections 24-3 Administering an Intradermal Injection 24-4 Administering a Subcutaneous Injection 24-5 Administering an Intramuscular Injection 24-6 Administering an Intramuscular Injection Using the Z-Track Method 24-7 Applying Transdermal Medications 24-8 Obtaining and Preparing an Intravenous Site	
b. (4) (h)	Maintain medication and immunization records	24-1 Administering Oral Medications 24-2 Preparing Injections 24-3 Administering an Intradermal Injection 24-4 Administering a Subcutaneous Injection 24-5 Administering an Intramuscular Injection 24-6 Administering an Intramuscular Injection Using the Z-Track Method 24-7 Applying Transdermal Medications 24-8 Obtaining and Preparing an Intravenous Site	III.C.3.b.4.h - Maintain medication and immunization records
b. (4) (i)	Screen and follow-up test results	40-1 Screen and Follow-Up Laboratory Results and Document Appropriately	III.C.3.b.4.i - Screen and follow-up test results
c. GENERAL COMPETENCIES			
(1)	**Professional Communications**		
c. (1) (a)	Respond to and initiate written communications	7-1 Composing a Business Letter 7-2 Opening and Sorting Incoming Mail	
c. (1) (b)	Recognize and respond to verbal communications	18-1 Interviewing the Patient to Obtain a Medical History	
c. (1) (c)	Recognize and respond to nonverbal communications	18-1 Interviewing the Patient to Obtain a Medical History	
c. (1) (d)	Demonstrate telephone techniques	5-1 Handling Incoming Calls 5-2 Calling Emergency Medical Services	
(2)	**Legal Concepts**		
c. (2) (a)	Identify and respond to issues of confidentiality		C.2.a - Identify and respond to issues of confidentiality
c. (2) (b)	Perform within legal and ethical boundaries	24-1 Administering Oral Medications 24-2 Preparing Injections 24-3 Administering an Intradermal Injection 24-4 Administering a Subcutaneous Injection 24-5 Administering an Intramuscular Injection	C.2.b - Perform within legal and ethical boundaries

Competency #	Description	3rd Edition Procedure Number	Competency Practice and Check-Off Available through LiveAdvise (powered by Smarthinking, Inc.)
c. GENERAL COMPETENCIES			
(2)	**Legal Concepts**		
		24-6 Administering an Intramuscular Injection Using the Z-Track Method 24-7 Applying Transdermal Medications 24-8 Obtaining and Preparing an Intravenous Site • Procedures in all of the administrative, clinical, and laboratory chapters	
c. (2) (c)	Establish and maintain the medical record	8-1 Preparing a Medical File	
c. (2) (d)	Document appropriately	18-2 Document a Chief Complaint (CC) and Present Illness (PI) 24-1 Administering Oral Medications 24-2 Preparing Injections 24-3 Administering an Intradermal Injection 24-4 Administering a Subcutaneous Injection 24-5 Administering an Intramuscular Injection 24-6 Administering an Intramuscular Injection Using the Z-Track Method 24-7 Applying Transdermal Medications 24-8 Obtaining and Preparing an Intravenous Site 35-1 Instructing the Patient on the Breast Self-Examination 35-2 Assisting With the Pelvic Exam and Pap Smear 35-3 Assisting With the Colposcopy and Cervical Biopsy 40-1 Screen and Follow-Up Laboratory Test Results and Document Appropriately	C.2.d - Document appropriately
c. (2) (e)	Demonstrate knowledge of federal and state health care legislation and regulations	2-1 Monitoring Federal and State Regulations, Changes, and Updates	C.2.e - Demonstrate knowledge of federal and state health care legislation and regulations
(3)	**Patient Instruction**		
c. (3) (a)	Explain general office policies	5-3 Explain General Office Policies	
c. (3) (b)	Instruct individuals according to their needs	4-1 Instruct a Hearing-Impaired Patient by Giving Directions to a Radiology Appointment 35-1 Instructing the Patient on the Breast Self-Examination	C.3.b - Instruct individuals according to their needs
c. (3) (c)	Provide instruction for health maintenance and disease prevention	16-1 Instruct a Patient to Read Food Labels	
c. (3) (d)	Identify community resources	4-2 Locating Community Resources	
(4)	**Operational Functions**		
c. (4) (a)	Perform an inventory of supplies and equipment	12-12 Order Supplies	

Competency #	Description	3rd Edition Procedure Number	Competency Practice and Check-Off Available through LiveAdvise (powered by Smarthinking, Inc.)
c. GENERAL COMPETENCIES			
(4)	**Operational Functions**		
c. (4) (b)	Perform routine maintenance of administrative and clinical equipment	40-3 Perform Routine Maintenance of Glucose Meter 45-3 Perform Routine Maintenance of a Glucose Meter 9-1 Caring for and Maintaining Computer Hardware	
c. (4) (c)	Utilize computer software to maintain office systems	12-3 Process a Credit Balance	C.4.c - Utilize computer software to maintain office systems
c. (4) (d)	Use methods of quality control	10-2 Create a Quality Improvement Program 40-2 Quality Control Monitoring Using a QC Chart	C.4.d - Use methods of quality control

COVERAGE OF ABHES ENTRY-LEVEL COMPETENCIES

Procedure	ABHES Competencies
Procedure 2-1: Monitoring Federal and State Regulations, Changes, and Updates	5.g. Monitor legislation related to current health care issues and practices
Procedure 4-1: Instructing a Hearing-Impaired Patient by Giving Directions to a Radiology Appointment	7.b. Instruct patients with special needs
Procedure 4-2: Locating Community Resources	3.e. Locate resources and information for patients and employers
Procedure 5.1: Handling Incoming Calls	2.e. Use proper telephone techniques
Procedure 5-2: Calling Emergency Medical Services	4.e. Recognize emergencies
Procedure 5-3 Explain General Office Policies	7.a. Orient patients to office policies and procedures
Procedure 6-1: Making an Appointment for a New Patient	3.c. Schedule and monitor appointments
Procedure 6-2: Making an Appointment for an Established Patient	
Procedure 6-3: Making an Appointment for a Referral to an Outpatient Facility	3.g. Schedule inpatient and outpatient admissions
Procedure 6-4: Arranging for Admission to an Inpatient Facility	3.g. Schedule inpatient and outpatient admissions
Procedure 7-1: Composing a Business Letter	2.o. Fundamental writing skills
Procedure 7-2: Opening and Sorting Incoming Mail	
Procedure 8-1: Establishing, Organizing, and Maintaining a Medical File	3.b. Prepare and maintain medical records
Procedure 8-2: Filing Medical Records	3.h. File medical records
Procedure 9-1: Caring for and Maintaining Computer Hardware	6.b. Operate and maintain facilities and perform routine maintenance of administrative and clinical equipment safely
Procedure 9-2: Searching on the Internet	2.n. Application of electronic technology
Procedure 10-1: Create a Procedures Manual	
Procedure 10-2: Create a Quality Improvement Program	5.h. Perform risk management procedures
Procedure 11-1: Evaluate and Manage a Patient's Account	3.l. Perform billing and collection procedures
Procedure 11-2: Composing a Collection Letter	2.o. Fundamental writing skills
Procedure 12-1: Post Charges on a Daysheet	3.k. Post entries on a daysheet
Procedure 12-2: Post Payments on a Daysheet	3.k. Post entries on a daysheet
Procedure 12-3: Process a Credit Balance	3.p. Process credit balance

Procedure	ABHES Competencies
Procedure 12-4: Process Refunds	3.q. Process refunds
Procedure 12-5: Post Adjustments to a Daysheet	3.0. Post adjustments
Procedure 12-6: Post Collection Agency Payments	3.s. Post collection agency payments
Procedure 12-7: Process NSF Checks	3.r. Post NSF funds
Procedure 12-8: Balance a Daysheet	
Procedure 12-9: Complete a Bank Deposit Slip and Make a Deposit	3.i. Prepare a bank statement deposit record
Procedure 12-10: Reconcile a Bank Statement	3.j. Reconcile a bank statement
Procedure 12-11: Maintain a Petty Cash Account	3.n. Establish and maintain a petty cash fund
Procedure 12-12: Order Supplies	6.d. Evaluate and recommend equipment and supplies for practice
Procedure 12-13: Write a Check	3.m. Prepare a check
Procedure 13-1: Completing a CMS-1500 Claim Form	3.w. Complete insurance claim forms
Procedure 14-1: Locating a Diagnostic Code	3.v. Perform diagnostic coding
Procedure 15-1: Locating a CPT Code	
Procedure 16-1: Instruct a Patient to Read Food Labels	7.c. Teach patients methods of health promotion and disease prevention
Procedure 17-1: Handwashing for Medical Asepsis	4.c. Apply principles of aseptic techniques and infection control
Procedure 17-2: Removing Contaminated Gloves	4.c. Apply principles of aseptic techniques and infection control
Procedure 17.3: Cleaning Biohazardous Spills	4.q. Dispose of biohazardous materials
Procedure 18-1: Interviewing the Patient to Obtain a Medical History	4.a. Interview and take patient history; 5.a. Determine needs for documentation and reporting
Procedure 18-2: Document a Chief Complaint (CC) and Present Illness (PI)	4.a. Interview and take patient history; 5.b. Document accurately
Procedure 19-1: Measuring Weight	4.b. Prepare patients for procedures
Procedure 19-2: Measuring Height	4.b. Prepare patients for procedures
Procedure 19-3: Measuring Oral Temperature Using a Glass Mercury Thermometer	4.d. Take vital signs
Procedure 19-4: Measuring a Rectal Temperature	4.d. Take vital signs
Procedure 19-5: Measuring an Axillary Temperature	4.d. Take vital signs

Procedure	ABHES Competencies
Procedure 19-6: Measuring Temperature Using an Electronic Thermometer	4.d. Take vital signs
Procedure 19-7: Measuring Temperature Using a Tympanic Thermometer	4.d. Take vital signs
Procedure 19-8: Measuring Temperature Using a Temporal Artery Thermometer	4.d. Take vital signs
Procedure 19-9: Measuring the Radial Pulse	4.d. Take vital signs
Procedure 19-10: Measuring Respirations	4.d. Take vital signs
Procedure 19-11: Measuring Blood Pressure	4.d. Take vital signs
Procedure 20-1: Assisting with the Adult Physical Examination	4.h. Assist physician with examinations and treatments
Procedure 21-1: Sanitizing Equipment for Disinfection or Sterilization	4.c. Apply principles of aseptic techniques and infection control
Procedure 21-2: Wrapping Instruments for Sterilization in an Autoclave	4.o. Wrap items for autoclaving
Procedure 21-3: Operating an Autoclave	4.p. Perform sterilization techniques
Procedure 22-1: Opening Sterile Surgical Packs	4.c. Apply principles of aseptic techniques and infection control
Procedure 22-2: Using Sterile Transfer Forceps	4.c. Apply principles of aseptic techniques and infection control
Procedure 22-3: Adding Sterile Solution to a Sterile Field	4.c. Apply principles of aseptic techniques and infection control
Procedure 22-4: Performing Hair Removal and Skin Preparation	4.b. Prepare patients for procedures; 4.c. Apply principles of aseptic techniques and infection control
Procedure 22-5: Applying Sterile Gloves	4.c. Apply principles of aseptic techniques and infection control
Procedure 22-6: Applying a Sterile Dressing	4.c. Apply principles of aseptic techniques and infection control
Procedure 22-7: Changing an Existing Sterile Dressing	4.c. Apply principles of aseptic techniques and infection control
Procedure 22-8: Assisting with Excisional Surgery	4.b. Prepare patients for procedures; 4.h. Assist physician with examinations and treatments
Procedure 22-9: Assisting with Incision and Drainage (I & D)	4.b. Prepare patients for procedures; 4.h. Assist physician with examinations and treatments
Procedure 22-10: Removing Sutures	4.b. Prepare patients for procedures; 4.h. Assist physician with examinations and treatments
Procedure 22-11: Removing Staples	4.b. Prepare patients for procedures; 4.h. Assist physician with examinations and treatments
Procedure 24-1: Administering Oral Medications	4.m. Prepare and administer medications as directed by physician; 4.n. Maintain medication records
Procedure 24-2: Preparing Injections	4.m. Prepare and administer medications as directed by physician; 4.n. Maintain medication records

Procedure	ABHES Competencies
Procedure 24-3: Administering an Intradermal Injection	4.b. Prepare patients for procedures; 4.m. Prepare and administer medications as directed by physician; 4.n. Maintain medication records
Procedure 24-4: Administering a Subcutaneous Injection	4.m. Prepare and administer medications as directed by physician; 4.n. Maintain medication records
Procedure 24-5: Administering an Intramuscular Injection	4.b. Prepare patients for procedures; 4.m. Prepare and administer medications as directed by physician; 4.n. Maintain medication records
Procedure 24-6: Administering an Intramuscular Injection Using the Z-Track Method	4.b. Prepare patients for procedures; 4.m. Prepare and administer medications as directed by physician; 4.n. Maintain medication records
Procedure 24-7: Applying Transdermal Medications	4.m. Prepare and administer medications as directed by physician; 4.n. Maintain medication records
Procedure 24-8: Obtaining and Preparing an Intravenous Site	4.b. Prepare patients for procedures; 4.h. Assist physician with examinations and treatments; 4.s. Perform venipuncture
Procedure 25-1: Preparing a Patient for an X-Ray	4.b. Prepare patients for procedures
Procedure 26-1: Administer Oxygen	4.b. Prepare patients for procedures; 4.h. Assist physician with examinations and treatments
Procedure 26-2: Perform Cardiopulmonary Resuscitation (Adult)	4.f. Perform first aid and CPR
Procedure 26-3: Use an Automatic External Defibrillator (AED) (Adult)	4.f. Perform first aid and CPR
Procedure 26-4: Manage a Foreign Body Airway Obstruction (Adult)	4.f. Perform first aid and CPR
Procedure 26-5: Control Bleeding	4.f. Perform first aid and CPR
Procedure 27-1: Applying a Warm or Cold Compress	4.b. Prepare patients for procedures; 4.h. Assist physician with examinations and treatments
Procedure 27-2: Assisting With Therapeutic Soaks	4.b. Prepare patients for procedures; 4.h. Assist physician with examinations and treatments
Procedure 27-3: Applying a Tubular Gauze Bandage	4.b. Prepare patients for procedures; 4.h. Assist physician with examinations and treatments
Procedure 28-1: Apply an Arm Sling	4.b. Prepare patients for procedures; 4.h. Assist physician with examinations and treatments
Procedure 28-2: Apply Cold Packs	4.b. Prepare patients for procedures; 4.h. Assist physician with examinations and treatments
Procedure 28-3: Use a Hot Water Bottle or Commercial Hot Pack	4.b. Prepare patients for procedures; 4.h. Assist physician with examinations and treatments
Procedure 28-4: Measure a Patient for Axillary Crutches	4.b. Prepare patients for procedures; 4.h. Assist physician with examinations and treatments
Procedure 28-5: Instruct a Patient in Various Crutch Gaits	4.b. Prepare patients for procedures; 4.h. Assist physician with examinations and treatments
Procedure 29-1: Measuring Distance Visual Acuity	4.b. Prepare patients for procedures; 4.h. Assist physician with examinations and treatments
Procedure 29-2: Measuring Color Perception	4.b. Prepare patients for procedures; 4.h. Assist physician with examinations and treatments
Procedure 29-3: Instilling Eye Medications	4.b. Prepare patients for procedures; 4.h. Assist physician with examinations and treatments
Procedure 29-4: Irrigating the Eye	4.b. Prepare patients for procedures; 4.h. Assist physician with examinations and treatments

Procedure	ABHES Competencies
Procedure 29-5: Irrigating the Ear	4.b. Prepare patients for procedures; 4.h. Assist physician with examinations and treatments
Procedure 29-6: Audiometry Testing	4.b. Prepare patients for procedures; 4.h. Assist physician with examinations and treatments
Procedure 29-7: Instilling Ear Medication	4.b. Prepare patients for procedures; 4.h. Assist physician with examinations and treatments
Procedure 29-8: Instilling Nasal Medication	4.b. Prepare patients for procedures; 4.h. Assist physician with examinations and treatments
Procedure 30-1: Instructing a Patient on Using the Peak Flowmeter	4.b. Prepare patients for procedures; 4.h. Assist physician with examinations and treatments; 4.ee. Perform respiratory testing; 7.c. Teach patients methods of health promotion and disease prevention
Procedure 30-2: Performing a Nebulized Breathing Treatment	4.b. Prepare patients for procedures; 4.h. Assist physician with examinations and treatments; 4.m. Prepare and administer medications as directed by physician
Procedure 30-3: Perform a Pulmonary Function Test	4.b. Prepare patients for procedures; 4.h. Assist physician with examinations and treatments; 4.ee. Perform respiratory testing
Procedure 31-1: Performing a 12-Lead Electrocardiogram	4.b. Prepare patients for procedures; 4.h. Assist physician with examinations and treatments; 4.dd. Perform electrocardiograms
Procedure 31-2: Applying a Holter Monitor	4.b. Prepare patients for procedures; 4.h. Assist physician with examinations and treatments
Procedure 32-1: Assisting With Colon Procedures	4.b. Prepare patients for procedures; 4.h. Assist physician with examinations and treatments
Procedure 33-1: Assisting With a Lumbar Puncture	4.b. Prepare patients for procedures; 4.h. Assist physician with examinations and treatments
Procedure 34-1: Female Urinary Catheterization	4.b. Prepare patients for procedures; 4.h. Assist physician with examinations and treatments
Procedure 34-2: Male Urinary Catheterization	4.b. Prepare patients for procedures; 4.h. Assist physician with examinations and treatments
Procedure 34-3: Instructing a Male Patient on the Testicular Self-Examination	7.c. Teach patients methods of health promotion and disease prevention
Procedure 35-1: Instructing the Patient on the Breast Self-Examination	7.c. Teach patients methods of health promotion and disease prevention
Procedure 35-2: Assisting With the Pelvic Exam and Pap Smear	4.b. Prepare patients for procedures; 4.h. Assist physician with examinations and treatments
Procedure 35-3: Assisting With the Colposcopy and Cervical Biopsy	4.b. Prepare patients for procedures; 4.h. Assist physician with examinations and treatments
Procedure 36-1: Manage a Patient With a Diabetic Emergency	4.e. Recognize emergencies
Procedure 37-1: Obtaining an Infant's Length and Weight	4.h. Assist physician with examinations and treatments
Procedure 37-2: Obtaining the Head and Chest Circumference	4.h. Assist physician with examinations and treatments
Procedure 37-3: Applying a Urinary Collection Device	4.h. Assist physician with examinations and treatments

Procedure	ABHES Competencies
Procedure 39-1: Caring for a Microscope	10.a.5. Care of microscope
	6.b. Operate and maintain facilities and perform routine maintenance of administrative and clinical equipment safely
	5.b. Document accurately
	4.r. Practice standard precautions
Procedure 40-1: Screen and Follow-Up Laboratory Test Results and Document Appropriately	4.(l) Screen and follow up patient test results; 5.b. Document accurately
Procedure 40-2: Quality Control Monitoring Using a QC Chart	10.c.9. Quality control
	4.i. Use quality control
	5.b. Document accurately
Procedure 40-3: Perform Routine Maintenance of Glucose Meter	6.b. Operate and maintain facilities and perform routine maintenance of administrative and clinical equipment safely
	10.f. OSHA compliance rules and regulations
Procedure 41-1: Obtaining a Blood Specimen by Evacuated Tube or Winged Infusion Set	4.c. Apply principles of aseptic technique and infection control
	10.c.1. Personal protective equipment
	10.c.2.a. Specimen collection: venipuncture
	10.c.9. Quality Control
	10.f. OSHA compliance rules and regulations
	4.q. Dispose of biohazardous materials
	4.r. Practice standard precautions
	4.s. Perform venipuncture
Procedure 41-2: Obtaining a Blood Specimen by Capillary Puncture	4.c. Apply principles of aseptic technique and infection control
	10.c.1. Personal protective equipment
	10.c.2.b. Specimen collection: finger puncture
	10.c.9. Quality Control
	10.f. OSHA compliance rules and regulations
	4.q. Dispose of biohazardous materials
	4.r. Practice standard precautions
	4.t. Perform capillary puncture
Procedure 42-1: Making a Peripheral Blood Smear	4.c. Apply principles of aseptic technique and infection control
	4.z. Perform hematology
	4.j. Collect and process specimens
	10.b.1. Specimen collection
	4.k. Perform CLIA-waived tests that assist with diagnosis and treatment
	4.q. Dispose of biohazardous materials
	4.r. Practice standard precautions
	5.b. Document accurately
	4.i. Use quality control
	10.f. OSHA compliance rules and regulations

Procedure	ABHES Competencies
Procedure 42-2: Staining a Peripheral Blood Smear	4.c. Apply principles of aseptic technique and infection control
	4.z. Perform hematology
	4.j. Collect and process specimens
	10.b.1. Specimen collection
	4.k. Perform CLIA-waived tests that assist with diagnosis and treatment
	4.q. Dispose of biohazardous materials
	4.r. Practice standard precautions
	5.b. Document accurately
	4.i. Use quality control
	10.f. OSHA Compliance rules and regulations
Procedure 42-3: Performing a Hemoglobin Determination	4.c. Apply principles of aseptic technique and infection control
	4.z. Perform hematology
	4.j. Collect and process specimens
	10.b.1. Specimen collection
	4.k. Perform CLIA-waived tests that assist with diagnosis and treatment
	4.q. Dispose of biohazardous materials
	4.r. Practice standard precautions
	5.b. Document accurately
	4.i. Use quality control
	10.f. OSHA compliance rules and regulations
Procedure 42-4: Performing a Microhematocrit Determination	4.c. Apply principles of aseptic technique and infection control
	4.z. Perform hematology
	4.j. Collect and process specimens
	10.b.1. Specimen collection
	4.k. Perform CLIA-waived tests that assist with diagnosis and treatment
	4.q. Dispose of biohazardous materials
	4.r. Practice standard precautions
	5.b. Document accurately
	4.i. Use quality control
	10.f. OSHA compliance rules and regulations
Procedure 42-5: Westergren Erythrocyte Sedimentation Rate	4.z. Perform hematology
	4.c. Apply principles of aseptic technique and infection control
	4.j. Collect and process specimens
	10.b.1. Specimen collection 4.k. Perform CLIA-waived tests that assist with diagnosis and treatment
	4.q. Dispose of biohazardous materials
	4.r. Practice standard precautions
	5.b. Document accurately
	4.i. Use quality control
	10.f. OSHA Compliance rules and regulations

Procedure	ABHES Competencies
Procedure 43-1: Obtaining a Clean-Catch Midstream Urine Specimen	4.w. Instruct patients in the collection of a clean-catch midstream urine specimen
Procedure 43-2: Obtaining a 24-Hour Urine Specimen	4.j. Collect and process specimens
Procedure 43-3: Determining Color and Clarity of Urine	10.b.2. Urinalysis: physical exam
Procedure 43-4: Chemical Reagent Strip Analysis	10.b.3. Urinalysis: chemical analysis
Procedure 43-5: Preparing Urine Sediment	10.b.4. Urinalysis: microscopic exam
Procedure 44-1: Collect a Throat Specimen	4.u. Obtain throat specimen for microbiological testing
	10.f. OSHA compliance rules and regulations
	4.r. Practice standard precautions
	4.k. Perform CLIA-waived tests that assist with diagnosis and treatment
	4.b. Prepare patients for procedures
	4.q. Dispose of biohazardous materials
Procedure 44-2: Collecting a Nasopharyngeal Specimen	4.j. Collect and process specimens
	10.f. OSHA compliance rules and regulations
	4.r. Practice standard precautions
	4.k. Perform CLIA-waived tests that assist with diagnosis and treatment
	4.b. Prepare patients for procedures
	4.q. Dispose of biohazardous materials
Procedure 44-3: Collecting a Wound Specimen	4.v. Perform wound collection procedure for microbiological testing
	10.f. OSHA compliance rules and regulations
	4.r. Practice standard precautions
	4.k. Perform CLIA-waived tests that assist with diagnosis and treatment
	4.b. Prepare patients for procedures
	4.q. Dispose of biohazardous materials
Procedure 44-4: Collecting a Sputum Specimen	4.j. Collect and process specimens
	10.f. OSHA compliance rules and regulations
	4.r. Practice standard precautions
	4.k. Perform CLIA-waived tests that assist with diagnosis and treatment
	4.b. Prepare patients for procedures
	4.q. Dispose of biohazardous materials
Procedure 44-5: Collecting a Stool Specimen	4.x. instruct patient in the collection of fecal specimen
	10.f. OSHA compliance rules and regulations
	4.r. Practice standard precautions
	4.k. Perform CLIA-waived tests that assist with diagnosis and treatment
	4.b. Prepare patients for procedures
	4.q Dispose of biohazardous materials

Procedure	ABHES Competencies
Procedure 44-6: Collecting Blood for Culture	4.j. Collect and process specimens
	10.f. OSHA compliance rules and regulations
	4.r. Practice standard precautions
	4.k. Perform CLIA-waived tests that assist with diagnosis and treatment
	4.b. Prepare patients for procedures
	4.q. Dispose of biohazardous materials
Procedure 44-7: Collecting Genital Specimens for Culture	4.j. Collect and process specimens
	10.f. OSHA compliance rules and regulations
	4.r. Practice standard precautions
	4.k. Perform CLIA-waived tests that assist with diagnosis and treatment
	4.b. Prepare patients for procedures
	4.q. Dispose of biohazardous materials
Procedure 44-8: Testing Stool Specimen for Occult Blood Guaiac Method	4.cc. Perform microbiology testing
	10.f. OSHA compliance rules and regulations
	4.r. Practice standard precautions
	4.k. Perform CLIA-waived tests that assist with diagnosis and treatment
	4.q. Dispose of biohazardous materials
Procedure 44-9: Preparing a Smear for Microscopic Evaluation	4.j. Collect and process specimens
	10.f. OSHA compliance rules and regulations
	4.r. Practice standard precautions
	4.k. Perform CLIA-waived tests that assist with diagnosis and treatment
	4.q. Dispose of biohazardous materials
Procedure 44-10: Performing a Gram Stain	4.cc. Perform microbiology testing
	10.f. OSHA compliance rules and regulations
	4.r. Practice standard precautions
	4.k. Perform CLIA-waived tests that assist with diagnosis and treatment
	4.q. Dispose of biohazardous materials
Procedure 44-11: Inoculating a Culture	4.cc. Perform microbiology testing
	10.f. OSHA compliance rules and regulations
	4.r. Practice standard precautions
	4.k. Perform CLIA-waived tests that assist with diagnosis and treatment
	4.q. Dispose of biohazardous materials
Procedure 44-12: Mononucleosis Testing	4.bb. Perform immunology testing
	10.f. OSHA compliance rules and regulations
	4.r. Practice standard precautions
	4.k. Perform CLIA-waived tests that assist with diagnosis and treatment
	4.q. Dispose of biohazardous materials

Procedure	ABHES Competencies
Procedure 44-13: HCG Pregnancy Test	4.bb. Perform immunology testing
	10.f. OSHA compliance rules and regulations
	4.r. Practice standard precautions
	4.k. Perform CLIA-waived tests that assist with diagnosis and treatment
	4.q. Dispose of biohazardous materials
Procedure 44-14: Rapid Group A Strep Testing	4.bb. Perform immunology testing
	10.f. OSHA compliance rules and regulations
	4.r. Practice standard precautions
	4.k. Perform CLIA-waived tests that assist with diagnosis and treatment
	4.q. Dispose of biohazardous materials
Procedure 45-1: Perform Blood Glucose Testing	4.aa. Perform chemistry testing
	4.k. Perform CLIA-waived tests that assist with diagnosis and treatment
Procedure 45-2: Perform Blood Cholesterol Testing	4.aa. Perform chemistry testing
	4.k. Perform CLIA-waived tests that assist with diagnosis and treatment
Procedure 45-3: Perform Routine Maintenance of a Glucose Meter	6.b. Operate and maintain facilities and equipment safely
Procedure 46-1: Writing a Resume	11.d. Resume writing, interviewing techniques, and follow-up

Contents

Preface   vii
Users Guide   ix
Acknowledgments   xiii

PART I

Introduction to Medical Assisting

Unit One: Understanding the
Profession 3

1. Medicine and Medical Assisting 3
2. Law and Ethics .20
3. Communication Skills 49
4. Patient Education 67

PART II

The Administrative Medical Assistant

Unit Two: Fundamentals of Administrative
Medical Assisting 91

5. The First Contact: Telephone and
   Reception 91
6. Managing Appointments 112
7. Written Communications 131
8. Health Information Management:
   Electronic and Manual 152
9. Computer Applications in the Medical
   Office 178
10. Management of the Medical Office 196

Unit Three: Managing the Finances in the
Practice 221

11. Credit and Collections 221
12. Accounting Responsibilities 232
13. Health Insurance 260
14. Diagnostic Coding 276
15. Outpatient Procedural Coding 292

PART III

The Clinical Medical Assistant

Unit Four: Fundamentals of Clinical
Medical Assisting 311

16. Nutrition and Wellness 311
17. Medical Asepsis and Infection Control . .333
18. Medical History and Patient
    Assessment 356
19. Anthropometric Measurements and
    Vital Signs 371
20. Assisting with the Physical
    Examination 405
21. Sterilization and Surgical Instruments . .425
22. Assisting with Minor Office Surgery 445
23. Pharmacology 480
24. Preparing and Administering
    Medications 493
25. Diagnostic Imaging 532
26. Medical Office Emergencies 546

Unit Five: Clinical Duties Related to
Medical Specialties 575

27. Dermatology .575
28. Orthopedics .598
29. Ophthalmology and Otolaryngology . . .629
30. Pulmonary Medicine 658
31. Cardiology 675
32. Gastroenterology 702
33. Neurology 722
34. Urology 739
35. Obstetrics and Gynecology 759
36. Endocrinology 792
37. Pediatrics 805
38. Geriatrics 834

PART IV

The Clinical Laboratory

Unit Six: Fundamentals of Laboratory
Procedures 857

39. Introduction to the Clinical Laboratory . .857
40. CLIA Compliance and Laboratory
  Safety 873
41. Phlebotomy .896
42. Hematology .926
43. Urinalysis 944
44. Microbiology and Immunology 964
45. Clinical Chemistry 1002

PART V

Career Strategies

Unit Seven: Competing in the Job
Market 1023

46. Making the Transition: Student to
  Employee 1023
47. Comprehensive Final Examination . . .1045

Appendix A   *1053*
Appendix B   *1055*
Appendix C   *1061*
Appendix D   *1062*
Appendix E   *1067*
Appendix F   *1069*
Appendix G   *1078*
Appendix H   *1079*
Appendix I   *1080*
Glossary   *1085*
Index   *1107*

Introduction to Medical Assisting

Understanding the Profession

Welcome! The world of medicine is an exciting and challenging frontier. This unit consists of four chapters that will introduce you to the field of medicine and medical assisting, offer vital help in communication skills, and provide you with information to enable you to educate your patients. In the first chapter, you will learn how medicine has evolved through the years from an era of superstition and magical cures to an age of modern technology. The second chapter introduces you to legal and ethical responsibilities that affect medical professionals. Sometimes, the advances in medicine challenge our laws and ethics. Chapter 3 covers communication skills, and Chapter 4 introduces you to the concepts of patient education. This unit will help you to understand the bond between medicine, law, and ethics, and to communication with patients and co-workers. Let the exploration begin!

Medicine and Medical Assisting

Outline

History Of Medicine
  Ancient Medical History
  Modern Medical History
  Strides in the Prevention of
    Disease Transmission
  Possibilities in Surgery
  Women in Medicine
  Important Discoveries
  Recent Medical History
**The American Health Care
  System**
The Medical Office
Medical Specialties

**The Medical Assisting
  Profession**
  What Is a Medical Assistant?
  Duties of a Medical
    Assistant
**Characteristics Of A
  Professional Medical
  Assistant**
**Members Of The Health Care
  Team**
  Health Care Providers
  The Nursing Profession
  Allied Health Professionals

**The History Of Medical
  Assisting**
Medical Assisting Education
  Medical Assisting Program
    Accreditation
**Medical Assisting
  Certification**
  Certified Medical Assistant
  Registered Medical Assistant
**Medical Assisting And Related
  Allied Health Associations**
  Association Membership
Employment Opportunities

Learning Objectives

Upon successfully completing this chapter, you will be able to:

1. Spell and define the key terms
2. Summarize a brief history of medicine
3. Identify the key founders of medical science
4. Explain the system of health care in the United States

5. Discuss the typical medical office

6. List medical specialties a medical assistant may encounter

7. List settings in which medical assistants may be employed

8. List the duties of a medical assistant

9. Describe the desired characteristics of a medical assistant

10. Identify members of the health care team

11. Explain the pathways of education for medical assistants

12. Discuss the importance of program accreditation

13. Name and describe the two nationally recognized accrediting agencies for medical assisting education programs

14. Explain the benefits and avenues of certification for the medical assistant

15. List the benefits of membership in a professional organization

Key Terms

accreditation
administrative
caduceus
certification

clinical
continuing education units
externship

inpatient
laboratory
medical assistant
multidisciplinary

multiskilled health professional
outpatient
recertification
specialty

Welcome to the field of medicine and to the medical assisting profession! You have selected a fascinating and challenging career, one of the fastest growing specialties in the medical field. The need for the **multiskilled health professional**—an individual with versatile training in the health care field—will continue to grow within the foreseeable future, and you are now a part of this exciting career direction.

To help you understand the significance of the medical knowledge and skills you will receive during your course of study, we begin by taking a chronological look at the history of medicine and then explore the profession of medical assisting.

History of Medicine

Tremendous achievements in the general health, comfort, and well-being of patients have been made just within the past 100 to 150 years, with the greatest advances occurring in the 20th century. The 21st century has brought continued advancement in cancer research, the human genome project, and the eradication of more diseases. It is difficult to imagine health care without antibiotics, x-ray machines, or anesthesia, but these developments are fairly new to medicine. For example, penicillin was not produced in large quantities until World War II, and surgery was performed without anesthesia until the mid 1800s. The possibility of cures for some of the devastating diseases humans face gets closer with every research project, and there are many being conducted. Chances are good that the next great medical discovery will result from stem cell and cord blood research.

Ancient Medical History

The earliest recorded evidence of medical history dates to the early Egyptians. Papyrus records of tuberculosis, pneumonia, and arteriosclerosis are still in existence from 4000 B.C. It is evident that, during this time, the Egyptians performed surgeries, including brain surgery. Fossil remains have shown patients with fractures (broken bones) that were splinted and subsequently healed. Although many cultures practiced primitive forms of surgery, most early practitioners used a combination of religion and superstition to heal ailments. Herbs, roots, and plants were used as medications.

Some of these early medications played a key role in the development of our modern pharmacology. Digitalis, from the common garden plant foxglove, is still in use today for its original purpose of strengthening the heart's action. Opium, from the pods of the poppy plant, is still used to induce stupor and a level of painlessness. Supplemental iron as a method of treating anemia was recognized by the Chinese as early as 2500 B.C. Medical research is constantly uncovering evidence that previously used treatment methods were based on sound theory, and these treatments are being incorporated into our modern arsenal against illness.

More than 1000 years before Christ, Moses was appointed the first public health officer. He wrote rules for sanitation. He stated that all people preparing and serving public food must be neat and clean. In the days long before refrigeration, it became a religious law that only freshly slaughtered animals could be eaten. Moses also required that serving dishes and cooking utensils be washed between customers at public restaurants.

Aesculapius, Greek god of healing and the son of Apollo, had many followers who used massage and exercise to treat patients. This god is also believed to have used the magical powers of a yellow, nonpoisonous serpent to lick the wounds of surgical patients. Aesculapius was often pictured holding the serpent wrapped around his staff or wand; this staff is a symbol of medicine. Another medical symbol is the caduceus, the staff of the Roman god Mercury, shown as a winged staff with two serpents wrapped around it (Fig. 1-1).

Around 400 B.C., Hippocrates practiced medicine and set high behavioral standards for practicing physicians. Hippocrates, called the "Father of Medicine," turned medicine into a science and erased the element of mysticism that it once held. He wrote the Hippocratic Oath, which is still part of medical school graduation ceremonies.

The Greek physician Galen (131–201 A.D.), became known as the "Father of Experimental Physiology." He was the first physician to document a patient's pulse, although he did not know that the pulse was related to the heart. Galen identified many parts of the body. His anatomic findings were mostly incorrect, however, because they were based on the dissection of apes and swine. Postmortem human dissections were illegal and were considered sacrilegious until the Renaissance (1350–1650 A.D.).

The rule of the Roman Empire, from about 200 B.C. until its dissolution several centuries later, brought great strides in public health. Water was brought from clean mountain streams by way of raised aqueducts that were regularly cleaned and maintained; sewers carried wastes away from the cities; and personal cleanliness was encouraged. One Roman physician, Marcus Varro (116–21 B.C.), even suggested that there might be creatures too small to be seen that caused illness. This was 1800 years before the invention of the microscope.

During the Dark Ages (400–800 A.D.) and through the Middle Ages (800–1400 A.D.), few advances were made in the medical field. Medicine was practiced primarily in convents and monasteries and consisted of simply comforting patients rather than trying to find a cure for the illness. The population became more mobile, ranging away from traditional homelands for war, crusades, and exploration. Each venture exposed whole cultures to diseases against which they had no immunity. Cities grew larger but without the Roman technology for maintaining sanitation. Ignorance, crowding, and poor health practices led to the eruption of the bubonic plague, which twice swept through Europe and Asia, killing approximately 20 million people. This deadly disease, the greatest killer in our history, spread from rat fleas to humans, killing approximately half of the known population within a few years.

 CHECKPOINT QUESTION

1. Why were Galen's anatomic findings considered incorrect?

Modern Medical History

The Renaissance was a period of enlightenment in all areas of art, science, and education, and it fostered great strides in medicine. The advent of the printing press and the establishment of great universities made the practice of medicine more accessible to larger numbers of practitioners. Great minds collaborated to advance medical and scientific theories and perform experiments that led to discoveries of enormous benefit in the fight against disease.

During this period, Andreas Vesalius (1514–1564) became known as the "Father of Modern Anatomy." He corrected many of Galen's errors and wrote the first relatively correct anatomy textbook. Soon afterward, William

Figure 1-1 (**A**) Staff of Aesculapius. (**B**) Caduceus.

Harvey identified the pumping action of the heart. He described circulation as a continuous circuit pumped by the heart to carry blood through the body. Harvey studied the action of the heart using dogs, not humans.

The microscope was invented in the mid 1660s by a Dutch lens maker, Anton von Leeuwenhoek. He was the first person to observe bacteria under a lens, although he had no idea of the significance of the microorganisms to human health. His instrument also allowed him to accurately describe a red blood cell.

John Hunter (1728–1793) became known as the "Father of Scientific Surgery." He developed many surgical techniques that are still used today. Hunter also developed and inserted the first artificial feeding tube into a patient in 1778 and was the first to classify teeth in a scientific manner.

In 1796, Edward Jenner, a physician in England, overheard a young milkmaid explain that she could not catch smallpox because she had already had the very mild cowpox caught while milking her cows. Several weeks later, Jenner inoculated a small boy with smallpox crusts. The boy did not contract the disease, and the prevention for smallpox was discovered. Jenner's discovery of the smallpox vaccine led to more emphasis on prevention of disease rather than on cures.

Also during the early 1800s, the importance of the mind as a part of the health care process was becoming a recognized field of medicine. The first extensive work and writing on mental health was published in 1812 by Benjamin Rush, entitled *Medical Inquiries and Observations upon Diseases of the Mind.* He advocated humane treatment of the mentally ill at a time when most were imprisoned, chained, starved, exhibited like animals, or simply killed. Rush's influence began the separate field of study into the working of the mind that became modern psychiatry.

Strides in the Prevention of Disease Transmission

The mid 1880s saw a surge in the study of disease transmission. Louis Pasteur (1822–1895) became famous for his work with bacteria. Pasteur discovered that wine turned sour because of the presence of bacteria. He found that, when the bacteria were eliminated, the wine lasted longer. Pasteur's discovery that bacteria in liquids could be eliminated by heat led to the process known as pasteurization. This finding led to using heat to sterilize surgical instruments. Pasteur has been called the "Father of Bacteriology" for this accomplishment. Pasteur also focused on preventing the transmission of anthrax and discovered the rabies vaccine and was honored with the title "Father of Preventive Medicine" for this work.

In the mid 1880s, Ignaz Semmelweis, a Hungarian physician, noticed that women whose babies were born at home with a midwife in attendance had childbed fever less often than those who delivered in well-respected hospitals with prestigious physicians at the bedside. He was ridiculed by the medical establishment and was fired from his position when he required medical personnel to wash their hands in a solution of chlorinated lime before performing obstetric examinations. He was right, of course, and handwashing is still the most important factor in the fight against disease transmission.

At about the same time, Joseph Lister began to apply antiseptics to wounds to prevent infection. The concept was not clearly understood, but before Lister's practices, as many patients died of infection as died of the primitive surgical techniques of the early part of the century.

In 1928, Sir Alexander Fleming, a bacteriologist, accidentally discovered penicillin when his assistant forgot to wash the Petri dishes Fleming had used for experiments. When he noticed the circles of nongrowth around areas of a certain mold, he was able to extract the prototype for one of our most potent weapons against disease. He won the Nobel Prize in 1945 for this accomplishment.

Possibilities in Surgery

Modern anesthesia was discovered in 1842 by Crawford Williamson Long. The effects of nitrous oxide were known by the mid 1700s, but Long discovered its therapeutic use by accident when he observed a group of chemistry students inhaling it for amusement. Before this time, anesthesia consisted of large doses of alcohol or opium, leather straps for patient restraint, or the unconsciousness resulting from pain. Ether and chloroform came into use at about this time.

Women in Medicine

The 1800s brought the first notable records of the contributions of women to the medical field. Florence Nightingale (1820–1910) was the founder of modern nursing. She set standards and developed educational requirements for nurses (Fig. 1-2).

Elizabeth Blackwell (1821–1910) became the first woman to complete medical school in the United States when she graduated from Geneva Medical College in New York. In 1869, Blackwell established her own medical school in Europe for women only, opening the door for a rapidly expanding role for women in the medical field.

Clara Barton (1821–1912) founded the American Red Cross in 1881 and was its first president. She identified the need for psychological as well as physical support for wounded soldiers in the Civil War.

Marie Curie (1867–1934), a brilliant science student, married Pierre Curie, and together they discovered polonium and radium. Their discovery revolutionized the principles of energy and radioactivity. Marie and Pierre Curie shared the Nobel Prize for chemistry in

Figure 1-2 Florence Nightingale.

1903. Marie continued the research after Pierre's death and again won the Nobel Prize for physics in 1911.

Important Discoveries

X-rays were discovered in 1895 by Wilhelm Konrad Roentgen when he observed that a previously unknown ray generated by a cathode tube could pass through soft tissue and outline underlying structures. Medical diagnosis was revolutionized, earning Roentgen a Nobel Prize in 1901 for his discovery. The therapeutic uses of x-rays were recognized much later.

Jonas Edward Salk and Albert Sabin discovered the vaccines for polio in the 1950s, which led to near eradication of one of the 20th century's greatest killers.

 CHECKPOINT QUESTION

2. How was penicillin discovered?

Recent Medical History

Throughout the next three decades, public health protection improved and advancements continued. Government legislation mandated clean water, and citizens reaped the benefits of preventive medicine and education about health issues.

In the 1980s, advancements in radiology gave doctors ways to see inside a patient with such accuracy that patients no longer had to have exploratory surgery. With computed tomography (CT) scans, radiologists can see tumors, cysts, inflammation, and so on, with cross-sectional slices of the patient's body. Magnetic resonance imaging (MRI) uses a strong magnetic field to realign ions to form an image on a screen. MRI is used to detect internal bleeding, tumors, cysts, and so on. Positron emis-

sion tomography (PET) has further revolutionized radiology. A "map" of the body shows the tissues in which the molecular probe has become concentrated and can be interpreted by nuclear medicine physicians or radiologists in the context of the patient's diagnosis and treatment plan. PET scans are increasingly read alongside CT scans or MRI scans, the combination giving both anatomic and metabolic information (what the structure is and what it is doing). PET is used in clinical oncology, showing tumors and determining areas where cancer has spread or metastasized. Researchers are using these scans in studying the human brain and the heart.

In July 1998, Ryuzo Yanagimachi of the University of Hawaii announced the cloning of mice when 7 of 22 mice were cloned from the cell of a single mouse. In December 1998, researchers from Kinki University in Nara, Japan, cloned 8 calves from a single cell.

In 2006, the final human genome papers were published. After years of work, a team of scientists from both the public and private sectors completed the identification and mapping of human genes. Mapping the sequence of the letters of the human genome that represent the handbook of a human being is a breakthrough that will revolutionize the practice of medicine by paving the way for new drugs and therapies. The achievement is one of the most significant scientific landmarks of all time. Many medicines that can be tailored to an individual's genetic makeup are on the market or in development. New discoveries will continue to expand the parameters of medicine as further research in recombinant DNA, transplantation, immunizations, diagnostic procedures, and so forth push back the boundaries of health care and make today's therapies seem as primitive as those we have just covered. You will be present during this fascinating evolution of health care. Within the next decade, expect to see immunization against or cures for many of the illnesses that continue to plague us.

Your role as a **medical assistant,** the ultimate multi-skilled health care professional, will expand as the need for highly trained, versatile medical personnel keeps pace with the ever-changing practice of medicine. Today, heart bypass surgeries and organ transplants are performed routinely. Researchers continue to search for the cures for cancer, acquired immunodeficiency syndrome, and many other ailments. Scientists are learning more about mutating organisms and ways to fight them. As a medical assistant, you will witness the progress made as you play a key role in caring for patients.

The American Health Care System

The American health care system is complex and has seen many changes in the past few decades. Twenty years ago, a patient had medical insurance that paid a percentage of his or her medical bills. In today's world of managed care, which is discussed in the chapter on health insurance, many patients are a part of a group of covered members of an HMO (health management organization). With this change came new ways of treating patients. The doctor–patient relationship was one of trust and privacy. In a managed care system, patients are treated as outlined by the insurance companies. The purpose of this change was to control health care costs. The government monitors medical finances and controls the Medicare and Medicaid systems through the Centers for Medicare and Medicaid Services (CMS). This government agency was formerly called the Health Care Financing Administra-tion (HFCA). It has been estimated that, by 2013, 60% of patients being seen in the medical office will be over 65 years of age and will be covered under the Medicare system of insurance for the elderly. As technology advanced the capabilities of medical facilities to operate electronically, the government responded with The Health Insurance Portability and Accountability Act of 1996 (HIPAA), which was passed to simplify the administrative process of transmitting insurance claims, receiving payments, and sharing private health information. HIPAA is discussed throughout the text and covered thoroughly in Chapter 8, Electronic Medical Records and Records Management. The need to adhere to the rules and regulations of the government drives the management practices of the **outpatient** medical facility. The allied health care arena has grown quickly. New professions have been added to the health care team, and each one is an important part of a patient's total care. As an allied health student, you have an exciting course of study ahead of you. Soon you will find yourself among a caring and conscientious group of health care professionals.

The Medical Office

Today's medical office is quite different from the office of the past, where patients were treated by their family physician, insurance was filed, and reimbursement was based on a percentage of the cost. Large corporations and hospitals now own many medical clinics, and physicians are their employees. Billing, collections, insurance processing, laboratory procedures, and other tasks performed in the medical office may be outsourced or handled in a central office for the corporation. Medical practices now have the capability to maintain a patient's record without a single piece of paper. Office employees need a general understanding of the many regulations of insurance carriers. Every employee must be computer literate and should understand the legal aspects of the medical office. Although there are many medical specialties, the skills and basic functions of any medical office will be similar. With the new technology and the need

for constant monitoring of regulations and changes, the medical office employee is now expected to acquire a formal education and certification.

The typical medical office employs one or more physicians. To assist with examining and treating patients, the physician may employ physician assistants and/or nurse practitioners. These are the providers, and they need support staff. The goal of any medical practice is to provide quality care while maintaining sound financial practices within the laws and ethics of the medical profession. To achieve this goal, the physician needs a solid team. The administrative staff handles the financial aspects of the practice, and the clinical staff assists the providers with patient care. Both aspects of the office must run smoothly to reach the ultimate goal of the practice. The makeup of the team may differ among specialties. For example, an orthopedist may have an x-ray technologist on staff, or an obstetrician may have an on-site sonographer to perform ultrasounds on mothers-to-be. Regardless of the mix of the team, the medical assistant is an integral part.

The day-to-day operation of a medical office requires all the skills you learn in your curriculum. The patient's health care encounter can be pleasant or unpleasant, depending on the skills and the attitude of the team.

 CHECKPOINT QUESTION

3. What governmental agency monitors medical care finances?

Medical Specialties

After completion of medical school, physicians choose a **specialty**. Some prefer treating patients of all ages and will choose family medicine or internal medicine. Others choose surgery and further specialize in fields like cosmetic surgery or vascular surgery. Table 1-1 lists the most common surgical specialties. Table 1-2 lists specialists who may employ medical assistants.

 CHECKPOINT QUESTION

4. What is the specialty that treats newborn babies?

The Medical Assisting Profession

What Is a Medical Assistant?

A medical assistant is a multiskilled allied health professional, a member of the health care delivery team who performs administrative and clinical procedures. **Clinical** tasks generally involve direct patient care; **administrative** tasks usually focus on office procedures.

TABLE 1-1	Common Surgical Specialties
Surgical Specialty	**Description**
Cardiovascular	Repairs physical dysfunctions of the cardiovascular system
Cosmetic, reconstructive	Restores, repairs, or reconstructs body parts
General	Performs repairs on a variety of body parts
Maxillofacial	Repairs disorders of the face and mouth (a branch of dentistry)
Neurosurgery	Repairs disorders of the nervous system including brain and back surgery
Orthopedic	Corrects deformities and treats disorders of the musculoskeletal system
Thoracic	Repairs organs within the rib cage
Trauma	Limited to correcting traumatic wounds
Vascular	Repairs disorders of blood vessels, usually excluding the heart

Medical assistants are employed in physicians' offices and ambulatory care settings. Salaries, hours, and benefits depend on experience, size of practice or corporation, and geographic salary ranges. Working conditions for medical assistants vary greatly according to state laws regarding the medical assisting profession and the scope of the specialty of employer and job responsibilities.

Duties of a Medical Assistant

The duties of a medical assistant are divided into two categories: administrative and clinical, which includes **laboratory** duties. The ratio of administrative to clinical duties varies with your job description. For example, if you work in a family practice office, you may do mostly clinical work; a psychiatric practice will probably require primarily administrative duties.

Administrative Duties

Performing administrative tasks correctly and in a timely manner will make the office more efficient and productive. Conversely, an office that is not managed correctly can result in loss of business, poor patient service, and loss of revenue. Following is a partial list of standard administrative duties:

- Managing and maintaining the waiting room, office, and examining rooms
- Handling telephone calls
- Using written and oral communication
- Maintaining medical records
- Bookkeeping
- Scheduling appointments
- Ensuring good public relations
- Maintaining office supplies

- Screening sales representatives
- Filing insurance forms
- Processing the payroll
- Arranging patient hospitalizations
- Sorting and filing mail
- Instructing new patients regarding office hours and procedures
- Applying computer concepts to office practices
- Implementing ICD-9 and CPT coding for insurance claims
- Completing medical reports from dictation

Clinical Duties

Clinical responsibilities vary among employers. State laws regarding the scope of practice for medical assistants also differ. In some states, CMAs are not allowed to perform invasive procedures, such as injections or laboratory testing. Most states, however, leave the responsibility for the medical assistant's actions with the physician-employer. American Association of Medical Assistants (AAMA) has outlined the scope of practice for the medical assistant. Following is a partial list of clinical duties:

- Preparing patients for examinations and treatments
- Assisting other health care providers with procedures
- Preparing and sterilizing instruments
- Completing electrocardiograms
- Applying Holter monitors
- Obtaining medical histories
- Administering medications and immunizations
- Obtaining vital signs (blood pressure, pulse, temperature, respirations)
- Obtaining height and weight measurements
- Documenting in the medical record
- Performing eye and ear irrigations
- Recognizing and treating medical emergencies
- Initiating and implementing patient education

TABLE 1-2	Specialists Who Employ Medical Assistants
Surgical Specialty	**Description**
Allergist	Performs tests to determine the basis of allergic reactions to eliminate or counteract the offending allergen
Anesthesiologist	Determines the most appropriate anesthesia during surgery for the patient's situation
Cardiologist	Diagnoses and treats disorders of the cardiovascular system, including the heart, arteries, and veins
Dermatologist	Diagnoses and treats skin disorders, including cosmetic treatments for the reversal of aging
Emergency physician	Usually works in emergency or trauma centers
Endocrinologist	Diagnoses and treats disorders of the endocrine system and its hormone-secreting glands, e.g., diabetes and dwarfism
Epidemiologist	Specializes in epidemics caused by infectious agents; studies toxic agents, air pollution, and other health-related phenomena; and works with sexually transmitted disease control
Family practitioner	Serves a variety of patient age levels, seeing patients for everything from ear infections to school physicals
Gastroenterologist	Diagnoses and treats disorders of the stomach and intestine
Gerontologist	Limits practice to disorders of the aging population and its unique challenges
Gynecologist	Diagnoses and treats disorders of the female reproductive system and may also be an obstetrician or limit the practice to gynecology, including surgery
Hematologist	Diagnoses and treats disorders of the blood and blood-forming organs
Immunologist	Concentrates on the body's immune system and disease incidence, transmission, and prevention
Internist	Limits practice to diagnosis and treatment of disorders of internal organs with medical (drug therapy and lifestyle changes) rather than surgical means
Neonatologist	Limits practice to the care and treatment of infants to about 6 weeks of age
Nephrologist	Diagnoses and treats disorders of the kidneys
Neurologist	Limits practice to the nonsurgical care and treatment of brain and spinal cord disorders
Obstetrician	Limits practice to care and treatment for pregnancy, the postpartum period, and fertility issues
Oncologist	Diagnoses and treats tumors, both benign (noncancerous) and malignant (cancerous)
Ophthalmologist	Diagnoses and treats disorders of the eyes, including surgery (an optometrist monitors and measures patients for corrective lenses, and an optician makes the lenses or dispenses contact lenses)
Orthopedist	Diagnoses and treats disorders of the musculoskeletal system, including surgery and care for fractures
Otorhinolaryngologist	Diagnoses and treats disorders of the ear, nose, and throat
Pathologist	Analyzes tissue samples or specimens from surgery, diagnoses abnormalities, and performs autopsies
Pediatrician	Limits practice to childhood disorders or may be further specialized to early childhood or adolescent period
Podiatrist	Diagnoses and treats disorders of the feet and provides routine care for diabetic patients who may have poor circulation and require extra care
Proctologist	Limits practice to disorders of the colon, rectum, and anus
Psychiatrist	Diagnoses and treats mental disorders
Pulmonologist	Diagnoses and treats disorders of the respiratory system
Radiologist	Interprets x-rays and imaging studies and performs radiation therapy
Rheumatologist	Diagnoses and treats arthritis, gout, and other joint disorders
Surgeon	Performs surgical procedures (see Table 1-1, Common Surgical Specialties)
Urologist	Diagnoses and treats disorders of the urinary system, including the kidneys and bladder, and disorders of the male reproductive system

Laboratory Duties

- Low- and moderate-complexity laboratory tests as determined by the Clinical Laboratory Improvement Amendments (CLIA) of 1988
- Collecting and processing laboratory specimens

 CHECKPOINT QUESTION

5. What are five administrative duties and five clinical or laboratory duties performed by a medical assistant?

Characteristics of a Professional Medical Assistant

Medical assistants play a key role in creating and maintaining a professional image for their employers. Medical assistants must always appear neat and well groomed. Clothing should be clean, pressed, and in good condition. Footwear should be neat, comfortable, and professional. If sneakers are approved by your supervisor, they should be all white. Only minimal makeup and jewelry should be worn. You should wear a watch with a second hand. Fingernails should be clean and at a functional length. If polish is worn, it should be pale or clear.

Medical assistants must be dependable and punctual (Fig. 1-3). Tardiness and frequent absences are not acceptable. If you are not at work, someone must fill in for you. Medical assistants must be flexible and adaptable to meet the constantly changing needs of the office. Weekend and holiday hours may be required in some specialties.

Additional characteristics vital to the profession include the following:

- Excellent written and oral communications skills. You will be required to interact with patients and other health care workers on a professional basis. Only the best spelling and grammar skills are acceptable. (Communication skills are covered in appropriate sections of this text.)
- Maturity. Remaining calm in an emergency or during stressful situations and being able to calm others is a key skill. You must also be able to accept constructive criticism without resentment.
- Accuracy. The physician must be able to trust you to pay close attention to detail because the health and well-being of the patients are at stake. Careless errors could cause harm to the patient and result in legal action against the physician.
- Honesty. If errors are made, they must be admitted, and corrective procedures must be initiated immediately. Covering up errors or blaming others is dishon-

Figure 1-3 Medical assistants play a key role in creating and maintaining a professional image for their employers.

est. So are using office property for personal business, making telephone calls during work time, and falsifying time records. Such practices can ruin your career and are to be strictly avoided.

- Ability to respect patient confidentiality. Few issues in health care can damage your career as profoundly as divulging confidential patient information.
- Empathy. The ability to care deeply for the health and welfare of your patients is the heart of medical assisting.
- Courtesy. Every patient who enters the office must be treated with respect and gracious manners.
- Good interpersonal skills. Tempers may flare in stressful situations; learn to keep yours in check and work well with all levels of interaction.
- Ability to project a positive self-image. If you are confident in your abilities as a professional, this attitude will reflect in all of your relationships.
- Ability to work as a team player. The patient's return to health is the most important objective of the office. Each staff member must work toward this goal.
- Initiative and responsibility. You must be able to move from one task to another quickly and without

direct supervision. The entire team expects each of its members to perform assigned responsibilities.

- Tact and diplomacy. The right word at the right moment can calm and soothe anger, depression, and fear and relieve a potentially unsettling situation.
- High moral and ethical standards. Project for your profession the highest level of professionalism.

 CHECKPOINT QUESTION

6. What are eight characteristics that a professional medical assistant should have?

Members of the Health Care Team

As a medical assistant, you will work with a variety of health care workers. Today's health care team must be **multidisciplinary.** A multidisciplinary team is a group of specialized professionals who are brought together to meet the needs of the patient. Some patients will need the assistance of many individuals, whereas other patients may only need one or two members of the team. The team may be broken into three groups: health care providers, nurses, and allied health care professionals.

Health Care Providers
Physicians

Physicians generally are the team leaders. They are responsible for diagnosing and treating the patient. Minimum education for a physician consists of a 4-year undergraduate degree, often consisting of premedical studies, and 4 years of medical school, followed by a residency program usually concentrating on a certain specialty. The residency program can vary from 2 to 6 years based on the field of study. Physicians must pass a licensure examination for the state in which they wish to practice.

Physician Assistants

Physician assistants (PAs) are specially trained and usually licensed. They work closely with a physician and may perform many of the tasks traditionally done by physicians. What a physician assistant does varies with training, experience, and state law. Their scope of practice corresponds to the supervising physician's practice. In general, a physician assistant will see many of the same types of patients as the physician. The cases handled by physicians are generally the more complicated medical cases or those cases that require care that is not

a routine part of the PA's scope of work. Close consultation between the patient, the PA, and the physician is done for unusual or hard to manage cases. Forty-nine states, the District of Columbia, and Guam have enacted laws that allow PAs to prescribe medications. Their educational levels vary from several months to 2 years, depending on the program and the individual's background in medicine. Most PA programs require a Bachelor's degree and 2 to 4 years of experience in the medical field.

National certification is available through the American Association of Physician Assistants. A physician assistant may also choose to become certified by the National Commission on Certification of PAs (NCCPA) and become a PA-C. This requires the PA to acquire 100 hours of continuing medical education every 2 years and take a recertification exam every 6 years.

Nurse Practitioners

Nurse practitioners (NPs) are trained to diagnose patients and treat illnesses. In most states, NPs can write prescriptions, operate their own offices, and admit patients to hospitals. In other states, NPs work more closely with a physician. NPs are experienced RNs and, in most cases, have a master's degree in nursing with the addition of specialized training as an NP. In some states, NPs are regulated by the Board of Nursing. In five states, they are regulated by the Board of Nursing and the Board of Medicine. There has been a recent collaborative effort by the American Academy of Nurse Practitioners (AANP) to identify the Nurse Practitioners' Primary Care Competencies, which include adult, family, gerontology, pediatrics, and women's health.

The Nursing Profession

Nurses work with physicians and implement various patient care needs in the inpatient or hospital setting. Their job descriptions vary according to their experiences, specialties, and certifications. There are several levels of education in nursing. A Bachelor of Science (BS) degree in nursing requires 4 years of college. A Licensed Practical Nurse (LPN) must complete a 1-year program. A nurse with an Associate in Applied Science (AAS) degree in nursing attends 2 years of college and becomes a Registered Nurse (RN). The nursing profession also monitors the education and provides the means for certification of the Certified Nursing Assistant (CNA I and CNA II). CNAs offer personal care and assist in nursing tasks. CNA programs usually last 4 to 6 weeks.

LEGAL TIP

Although a nurse's training involves inpatient care, some physicians choose to employ nurses in their offices. Some states do not allow nurses working in physician offices to supervise or delegate their authority to unlicensed allied health personnel. However, the medical assistant works under the supervision of the physician, not the nurse. For example, in the North Carolina law regarding this issue, the legislation refers to medical assistants as "unlicensed health care personnel." Medical assistants are certified, not licensed. Certification, by definition, indicates a higher level of competence. The legal issues involving licensure and certification are discussed in Chapter 2.

ETHICAL TIP

It is important that medical assistants represent themselves honestly. Physicians often innocently refer to every employee as the "nurse." It is more accurate to say my assistant, my CMA/RMA, or my clinical assistant. There are documented court cases involving misrepresentation of one's education and credential. Protect yourself by referring to yourself appropriately to patients and co-workers. Do not identify yourself as "Dr. Smith's nurse." When patients refer to you as a nurse, you should correct them. The more your credential is heard by patients and co-workers, the more understood and recognized it will be. You should be proud of your profession and your credential. Let it be known.

Allied Health Professionals

Allied health care professionals make up a large section of the health care team. Box 1-1 lists and describes some of these team members. The educational requirements and responsibilities vary greatly among these professionals. One thing they all have in common is the support of a professional organization. Medical assistants fall into this category.

The History of Medical Assisting

Medical assisting as a separate profession dates from the 1930s. In 1934, Dr. M. Mandl recognized the need for medical professionals who possessed the skills required in an office environment and opened the first

BOX 1-1

ALLIED HEALTH CARE PROFESSIONALS

Chiropractor—Manipulates the musculoskeletal system and spine to relieve symptoms

Dental hygienist—Trained and licensed to work with a dentist by providing preventive care

Electrocardiograph technician—Assists with the performance of diagnostic procedures for cardiac electrical activity

Electroencephalograph technician—Assists with the diagnostic procedures for brain wave activity

Emergency medical technician—Trained in techniques of administering emergency care en route to trauma centers

Health Information technologist—Trained in managing medical records, health care coding, and HIPAA regulations

Histologist—Studies cells and tissues for diagnosis

Infection control officer—Identifies risks of transmission of infection and implements preventive measures

Laboratory technician—Trained in performance of laboratory diagnostic procedures

Medical assistant—Trained in administrative, clinical, and laboratory skills for the medical facility

Medical coder—Assigns appropriate codes to report medical services to third- party payers for reimbursement

Medical office assistant—Trained in the administrative area of the outpatient medical facility

Medical transcriptionist—Trained in administrative skills; produces printed records of dictated medical information

Nuclear medical technician—Specializes in diagnostic procedures using radionuclides (electromagnetic radiation); works in a radiology department

Nutritionist—Addresses dietary needs associated with illness; assists and trains patients with special diets for weight control and supplementation needed for patients undergoing cancer treatment, etc.

Occupational therapist—Evaluates and plans programs to relieve physical and mental barriers that interfere with activities

Paramedic—Trained in advanced rescue and emergency procedures

Pharmacist—Prepares and dispenses medications by the physician's order

Phlebotomist—Collects blood specimens for laboratory procedures by performing venipuncture

(continued)

BOX 1-1 *(continued)*

Physical therapist—Plans and conducts rehabilitation to improve strength and mobility

Psychologist—Trained in methods of psychological assessment and treatment

Radiographer—Works with a radiologist or physician to operate x-ray equipment for diagnosis and treatment

Respiratory therapist—Trained to preserve or improve respiratory function

Risk manager—Identifies and corrects high-risk situations within the health care field

Speech therapist—Treats and prevents speech and language disorders

school for medical assistants in New York City. Although medical assistants were employed before 1934, no formal schooling was available. Office assistants were trained on the job to perform clinical procedures, or nurses were trained to perform administrative procedures. The need for a highly trained professional with a background in administrative and clinical skills led to the formation of an alternative field of allied health care. In 1956, the American Association of Medical Assistants (AAMA), a professional organization for medical assistants, was founded during a meeting of medical assistants in Milwaukee, Wisconsin. The constitution and bylaws adopted by the group were commended by the American Medical Association (AMA), the professional association of licensed physicians. In 1959, Illinois recognized the AAMA as a not-for-profit educational organization. The national office was established in Chicago, with state and local chapters throughout the United States. The AAMA has guided the practice of medical assisting with strong leadership and vision. With its help, the medical assistant has grown into a highly respected and versatile member of the health care team. In 1963, a certification examination for CMA was conducted that would set the standards required for medical assistant education. The first AAMA examinations were given in Kansas, California, and Florida. In the next two decades, the profession grew rapidly. The AMA collaborated in the development of the curriculum and accreditation of educational programs. In 1974, the US Department of Health, Education, and Welfare recognized the AAMA Curriculum Review Board in conjunction with the American Medical Association's Council on Medical Education as an official accrediting agency for medical assisting programs in public and private schools.

In 1991, the Board of Trustees of the AAMA approved the current definition of medical assisting: Medical assisting is an allied health profession whose practitioners function as members of the health care delivery team and per-form administrative and clinical procedures. Medical assistants continue to be vigilant for threats to their right to practice their profession. Each state mandates the actions of allied health professionals. It is the responsibility of medical assistants to be familiar with the laws of the state in which they are working. Membership in the AAMA exceeds 20,000 medical assistants, with more than 400 local chapters in 42 states. A complete history of the AAMA is available at www.aama-ntl.org. Box 1-2 outlines important changes made by the House of Delegates of the AAMA.

 CHECKPOINT QUESTION

7. What prompted the establishment of a school for medical assistants?

Medical Assisting Education

A medical assisting curriculum prepares individuals for entry into the medical assisting profession. Medical assisting programs are found in postsecondary schools, such as private business schools and technical colleges, 2-year colleges, and community colleges. Programs vary in length. Programs of 6 months to a year offer a certificate of graduation or a diploma, and 2-year programs award the graduate an associate degree. The 2-year curriculum usually includes general studies, such as English, mathematics, and computer skills, in addition to the core courses, such as medical terminology and insurance coding. The curriculum in every accredited program must include the skills determined by the accrediting agency. Specific requirements for an accredited program are discussed later.

Accredited programs must include an **externship.** An externship is an educational course offered in the last module or semester during which the student works in the field gaining hands-on experience. It varies in length from 60 to 240 hours. Students are not paid but are awarded credit toward the degree. (See Chapter 46 for more detailed information.) Some schools offer job placement services.

After you finish school, your education should not stop. You should continue to take courses on various related topics. These may include new computer programs, new clinical procedures, new laws and regulations, or pharmaceutical updates. Some employers pay for conferences. In some situations, conference costs may be listed for tax credit when filing your income tax.

Medical Assisting Program Accreditation

In 1995, the AMA House of Delegates voted to require graduation from an accredited medical assisting program for admission to the CMA examination. This change went into effect in January 1998. **Accreditation** is a non-

BOX 1-2

AAMA HOUSE OF DELEGATE CHANGES

- In 1995, the AAMA House of Delegates approved changing the eligibility pathway for candidates of the AAMA certification examination as follows: "Any candidate for the AAMA CMA Certification Exam must be a graduate of a CAAHEP-accredited medical assisting program." Before June 1998, medical assistants who had been employed by a physician for 1 year full-time or 2 years part-time were eligible to sit for the CMA Certification Examination.

- In 2001, AAMA made the decision to grant graduates of ABHES-accredited medical assisting programs immediate eligibility to sit for the CMA examination beginning in January 2002.

- In January 2003, all CMAs employed or seeking employment were required to have current certification to use the CMA credential in connection with employment.

- Effective January 2007, CMAs recertifying by continuing education method must attain 30 credits that are AAMA approved, with 10 recertification points in each content category: general, administrative, and clinical. Prior to 2007, 20 of the 60 CEUs required had to be AAMA approved with 15 recertification points in each content category.

governmental professional peer review process that provides technical assistance and evaluates educational programs for quality based on pre-established academic and administrative standards. Medical assisting program accreditation is based on a school's adherence to the essentials of a sound education and services for students. The skills that medical assistants need to be successful in a job are taught and documented in a competency-based format. Entry level competency is acquired and documented in a competency-based format that includes the specific skill to be mastered, the conditions under which you are to perform the skill (including equipment and supplies needed), and the standard of performance for the skill.

The Commission on Accreditation of Allied Health Education Programs

The Commission on Accreditation of Allied Health Education Programs (CAAHEP), in collaboration with the curriculum review board of the American

Association of Medical Assistants' Endowment, accredits medical assisting programs in both public and private postsecondary institutions throughout the United States. CAAHEP accredits many education programs for the professions included in Box 1-1.

The Accrediting Bureau of Health Education Schools

The Accrediting Bureau of Health Education Schools (ABHES) accredits private postsecondary registered medical assistant (RMA) **certification** through a program review process conducted by the American Medical Technologists (AMT). This body has accredited medical technicians, medical laboratory technicians, and dental technicians since the late 1930s but offered its first medical assisting examination in 1972.

 CHECKPOINT QUESTION

8. What are the two accrediting agencies for medical assisting education programs?

Medical Assisting Certification

The AAMA and the AMT have developed certification examinations that test the knowledge of a graduate and indicate entry level competency. After passing the examination, the person can use the initials CMA (certified medical assistant) or RMA (registered medical assistant) after his or her name.

 WHAT IF?

You are a brand new RMA, and it is your first day in a busy internal medicine practice. You are welcomed and taken to meet your co-worker who is a CMA. She asks, "What is the difference between a CMA and an RMA?" What do you tell her?

A graduate of a CAAHEP- or ABHES-accredited medical assisting program is eligible to sit for the CMA or RMA exam. Someone who has worked in a physician's office can challenge the examination and become an RMA. You must be a member of the American Medical Technologists in order to use the RMA credential. Membership in an organization is not required to take the CMA exam or to use the CMA credential. Together, you could search the Internet for certified medical assistant and registered medical assistant and become familiar with the two credentials, their differences, and their similarities.

Certified Medical Assistant

Graduates of medical assisting programs accredited by CAAHEP or ABHES are immediately eligible to take the CMA Certification Examination of the AAMA. Effective January 2008, the CMA credential was changed to CMA (AAMA). Examinees who pass this test hold the designation CMA (AAMA). The National Board of Medical Examiners, which administers several medical specialty examinations, serves as test consultant for the CMA Certification Examination of the AAMA. Once you pass the examination and become a CMA (AAMA), you are required to recertify every 5 years.

Recertification may be obtained either by taking the examination again or by acquiring 60 continuing education units (CEUs) (see Box 1-3). Proof of current CPR training is also required for recertification.

Registered Medical Assistant

In 1972, the AMT offered the first RMA examination. Graduates from ABHES-accredited medical assisting programs are immediately eligible to take the RMA examination. Medical assistants who have been employed in the profession for a minimum of 5 years, no more than 2 of which may have been as an instructor, are also eligible. Those who pass this examination are designated as RMAs.

Although formal recertification is not required by AMT, members and nonmembers are invited to participate in the STEP program, a continuing education home study program for health care practitioners. AMT keeps a record of earned credit and issues annual reports of STEP activities to program participants. The RMA credential remains current as long as the RMA remains a member of AMT.

 CHECKPOINT QUESTION

9. What is required to maintain current status as a CMA?

Medical Assisting and Related Allied Health Associations

Association Membership

You are not required to join a national organization to work as a medical assistant or to be eligible to take the certification examination. The associations have many benefits, however, for members. These benefits include the following:

- Access to educational seminars
- Access to continuing education units
- Subscription to the professional journals that alert you to new procedures and trends in medicine

---

BOX 1·3

HOW DOES A CMA RECERTIFY BY CONTINUING EDUCATION?

A CMA is recertified by completing 60 continuing education units (CEUs) in a 5-year period. CEUs are awarded for attendance at approved AAMA local and state affiliate meetings classes and seminars, for completion of guided study courses, and by journal articles designed with a post-test that can be submitted for CEU credit. A free transcript of all AAMA-approved CEUs acquired is available to members of AAMA.

As of January 2007, the 60 CEUs must include at least 10 recertification points from programs related to administrative duties, 10 from programs related to clinical duties, and 10 from general medical assisting topics. One CEU is awarded for each hour of training. For example, 1.5 CEUs is equal to 1.5 hours. Also as of 2007, 30 of the 60 CEUs must be AAMA approved.

The other 30 CEUs may come from other educational programs such as OSHA training offered by your employer. A program will be accepted if its subject matter is relevant to the medical assisting profession, but any paperwork associated with these programs, such as a syllabus, a workshop flyer describing the topic, and documentation of formal credit, must be furnished with the application for recertification. Aside from the application, the AAMA provides three documents that serve as useful guidelines for identifying relevant topics. These topics include the Role Delineation Study and the Content Outline for the exam, and the Advanced Practice Guidelines. All three documents are available at the AAMA website.

Whether recertifying by the continuing education or by taking the examination, applicants must furnish proof of current health care provider CPR certification.

Source: http://www.AAMA-ntl.org.

- Access to the annual conventions
- Group insurance plans
- Networking opportunities

For further information on these organizations, visit the websites listed at the end of the chapter. Contact your local chapter or speak with your instructor for the procedure for applying for membership. You can download applications and requirements from the AAMA website (http://www.aama-ntl.org/) and the AMT website (http://www.amt1.com/).

American Association of Medical Assistants

The purpose of the AAMA is to promote the professional identity and stature of its members and the medical assisting profession through education and credentialing. *CMA Today,* which is published and distributed to members of the organization, includes articles of interest to the medical assistant to keep knowledge and skills current. Readers may take post-tests at the end of articles and receive CEUs. Approved continuing education opportunities are available through the national organization, and free transcripts of acquired AAMA approved CEUs are available online to members. Professional benefits, such as insurance, are also made available to AAMA members. Active members are CMAs; associate members are medical assistants who are not yet CMAs; and affiliate members are those interested in medical assisting. Students are encouraged to join and stay active in AAMA. Student members receive a reduced dues rate while in school and for 1 year following graduation. Figure 1-4 displays the insignia of the AAMA.

American Medical Technologists

The AMT and its governing body are set up similarly to the AAMA, with local, state, and national affiliations, opportunities for continuing education, professional benefits, and a professional journal. Members include medical technologists, medical laboratory technicians, medical assistants, dental assistants, office laboratory technicians, phlebotomy technicians, laboratory consultants, and allied health instructors. To join AMT, you need to be certified or registered by meeting educational, professional experience, and examination requirements. Figure 1-5 displays the insignia of the AMT.

Figure 1-4 Insignia commemorating AAMA's 50th anniversary. Courtesy of American Association of Medical Assistants.

Figure 1-5 Insignia of AMT.

Professional Coder Associations

The American Academy of Professional Coders (AAPC) is dedicated to providing the highest standard of professional coding and billing services to employers, clients, and patients. Services to members include discounts on services and products and networking opportunities. AAPC provides a credentialing program that offers examinations to obtain the credential of certified professional coder (CPC).

American Health Information Management Association

The American Health Information Management Association (AHIMA) is a national professional organization dedicated to supporting the medical records or health information specialists. AHIMA administers the examination and awards the certified coding specialist (CCS) and certified coding specialists–physician-based (CCS-P) through testing at a specified time and place.

 CHECKPOINT QUESTION

10. List six benefits of membership in a professional organization.

Employment Opportunities

The medical assisting profession has found its place in the allied health arena. In many areas, credentialed medical assistants are in great demand. Salaries are going up, and employers appreciate the value of the skills a medical assistant possesses. Health care costs are a concern, and health care management consultants tout medical assistants as cost-effective employees in health care today. Because of the flexible, multi-skilled nature of their education, medical assistants can work in a variety of health care settings. Medical assistants work under the direct supervision of a licensed health care provider. They perform many functions. Following are examples of the ambulatory settings

PATIENT EDUCATION
THE HEALTH CARE SYSTEM

As a medical assistant, you play a key role in teaching patients not only about their health, but also about the health care system. Some patients become confused and are overwhelmed by the number and variety of health care workers. You can help by providing the answers to these common questions:

- What is a multidisciplinary team?
- Who will conduct the examination (physician, physician's assistant, or nurse practitioner)?
- What is a medical assistant?
- What do medical assistants do?
- What kind of training is required for medical assistants?
- What does certification or registration mean for a medical assistant?

When patients understand the health care field and know what to expect, they recover more quickly and are more comfortable asking questions about their health.

where a medical assistant may work with a variety of responsibilities:

- Physicians' offices
- Chiropractors' offices
- Podiatrists' offices
- Physical therapy facilities
- Laboratories
- Imaging centers
- Research facilities
- Walk-in clinics
- Ambulatory surgical centers

MEDIA MENU

- **Student CD**
  - **Case Study**
    Interactive Case Study on Conducting Patient Teaching
  - **CMA/RMA Certification Exam Review**
- **Premium Online Course**
  http://thePoint.lww.com/Kronenberger3e
- **Internet Resources**

  LiveAdvise Online Tutoring & Competency Training
  http://thePoint.lww.com/LiveAdvise

  ABHES—Accrediting Bureau of Health Education Schools
  http://www.abhes.org

  AHIMA—American Health Information Management Association
  http://www.ahima.org

  AMT—American Medical Technologists
  http://www.amt1.com

  CAAHEP—Council on Accreditation of Allied Health Education Programs
  http://www.caahep.org

  ABMS—American Board of Medical Specialties
  http://www.abms.org

 CHECKPOINT QUESTION

11. Why is it important that medical assistants are multiskilled?

- Medical history reveals 150 years of progress, with the most amazing strides made in the 20th century.
- Changes in the American health care system brought the necessity for highly trained professionals.
- The health care team works together to deliver quality patient care and remain financially sound.
- A graduate of an accredited medical assisting program can pursue certification or registration, which brings increasing marketability in the health care arena.
- By ensuring that educational levels are constantly enhanced and by continuing to grow professionally, the medical assistant graduate will prepare for the challenge of a lifelong career that is both fascinating and rewarding.

Warm Ups for Critical Thinking

1. Review the list of characteristics for medical assistants. Which characteristics do you already have? How will you acquire the others? Are there additional characteristics that you have that will make you a good medical assistant?

2. Look at the list of physician specialties. Which type of physician would you want to work for and why? Which physician specialties would you least want to work with? Explain your response.

3. Visit www.aama-ntl.org and determine which local chapter you would be a member of. How would membership benefit your career as a medical assistant?

4. How does certification or registration as a medical assistant improve your success in the profession?

5. What is the importance of continuing education?

6. How would you answer the question, "Legally, who is responsible for the actions of a CMA or an RMA as they perform their skills?"

Answers to Checkpoint Questions

1. Galen's anatomic findings were mostly incorrect because they were based on the dissection of apes and swine, not humans.

2. Sir Alexander Fleming saw areas clear of microorganism growth surrounding the mold gathering on the unwashed petri dishes in his lab. He was able to extract the prototype for the first antibiotic.

3. The Centers for Medicaid and Medicare Services (CMS) monitors medical financing.

4. The specialty that treats newborn babies is neonatology.

5. Examples of administrative duties include managing the medical office, handling telephone calls, preparing written communications, bookkeeping, scheduling, filing, and sorting mail. Examples of clinical duties include preparing patients for examinations, collecting and processing urine and blood specimens, completing electrocardiograms, and applying Holter monitors.

6. Professional characteristics include punctuality, dependability, honesty, showing respect for patient confidentiality, courtesy, diplomacy, and having high ethical and moral standards.

7. The first school for medical assistants was established because of the need for a highly trained professional with administrative and clinical skills.

8. The two accrediting agencies are the Council on Accreditation of Allied Health Education Programs (CAAHEP) and the Accrediting Bureau of Health Education Schools (ABHES).

9. To remain current, a CMA who takes the AAMA examination must recertify every 5 years by either taking a certification examination again or acquiring 60 continuing education units.

10. The benefits of membership in a professional organization include: access to educational seminars, access to continuing education units, subscription to the professional journals that alert you to new procedures and trends in medicine, access to the annual conventions, group insurance plans, and networking opportunities.

11. Medical assistants are the most cost-effective employees because they can perform so many different skills.

Outline

The American Legal System
Sources of Law
Branches of the Law
The Rise in Medical Legal
Cases
**Physician–Patient
Relationship**
Rights and Responsibilities of
the Patient and Physician
Contracts
Consent
Releasing Medical Information
Legally Required Disclosures
**Specific Laws and Statutes
that Apply to Health
Professionals**
Medical Practice Acts
Licensure, Certification, and
Registration
Controlled Substances Act
Good Samaritan Act

Basis of Medical Law
Tort Law
Negligence and Malpractice
(Unintentional Torts)
Intentional Torts
The Litigation Process
**Defenses to Professional
Liability Suits**
Medical Records
Statute of Limitations
Assumption of Risk
Res Judicata
Contributory Negligence
Comparative Negligence
**Defense for the Medical
Assistant**
Respondeat Superior or Law of
Agency
Employment and Safety Laws
Civil Rights Act of 1964, Title
VII

Occupational Safety and Health
Act
Other Legal Considerations
Medical Ethics
American Medical Association
(AMA) Code of Ethics
Medical Assistant's Role in
Ethics
American Association of
Medical Assistants Code of
Ethics
Bioethics
American Medical Association
(AMA) Council on Ethical
and Judicial Affairs
Social Policy Issues
**Professional and Ethical
Conduct and Behavior**
**Ethical Issues in Office
Management**

Learning Objectives

*Upon successfully completing this chapter, you
will be able to:*

1. Spell and define the key terms

2. Identify the two branches of the American
legal system

3. List the elements and types of contractual
agreements and describe the difference in
implied and express contracts

4. List four items that must be included in a
contract termination or withdrawal letter

5. List six items that must be included in an
informed consent form and explain who
may sign consent forms

6. List five legally required disclosures that
must be reported to specified authorities

7. Describe the four elements that must be
proven in a medical legal suit

8. Describe four possible defenses against
litigation for the medical professional

9. Explain the theory of respondeat superior, or law of agency, and how it applies
to the medical assistant

10. List ways that a medical assistant can assist in the prevention of a medical malpractice suit

11. Outline the laws regarding employment and safety issues in the medical office

12. List the requirements of the Americans with Disabilities Act relating to the medical office

13. Differentiate between legal issues and ethical issues

14. List the seven American Medical Association principles of ethics

15. List the five ethical principles of ethical and moral conduct outlined by the American Association of Medical Assistants

16. Describe the purpose of the Self-Determination Act

17. List 10 opinions of the American Medical Association's Council pertaining to administrative office procedures

Performance Objectives

Upon successfully completing this chapter, you will be able to:

1. Monitor federal and state health care legislation (Procedure 2-1)

Competencies

CAAHEP

- Identify and respond to issues of confidentiality
- Perform within legal and ethical boundaries
- Document appropriately
- Demonstrate knowledge of federal and state health care legislation and regulations

ABHES

- Determine needs for documentation and reporting
- Use appropriate guidelines when releasing records or information
- Follow established policy in initiating and terminating medical treatment
- Maintain licenses and accreditation
- Monitor legislation related to current health care issues and practices

Key Terms

abandonment	assault	bioethics	breach
advance directive	battery	blood-borne	certification
appeal	bench trial	pathogens	civil law

common law
comparative negligence
confidentiality
consent
contract
contributory negligence
damages
defamation of character
defendant

deposition
durable power of attorney
duress
emancipated minor
ethics
expert witness
expressed consent
expressed contracts
fee splitting
fraud
implied consent

implied contracts
informed consent
intentional tort
legally required disclosure
libel
licensure
litigation
locum tenens
malpractice
negligence
plaintiff

precedents
protocol
registered
res ipsa loquitur
res judicata
respondeat superior
slander
stare decisis
statute of limitations
tort

During your career as a medical assistant, you will be involved in many medical situations with potential legal implications. You must uphold ethical standards to ensure the patient's well-being. Ethics deals with the concept of right and wrong. Laws are written to carry out these concepts. Physicians may be sued for a variety of reasons, including significant clinical errors (e.g., removing the wrong limb, ordering a toxic dose of medication), claims of improperly touching a patient without consent, or failure to properly diagnose or treat a disease. Medicare **fraud** (concealing the truth) and falsifying medical records can also result in a lawsuit. Medical assistants and other health care workers are included in many of the suits brought to court. You may help to prevent many of these claims against your physician and protect yourself by complying with medical laws, keeping abreast of medical trends, and acting in an ethical manner by maintaining a high level of professionalism at all times.

The American Legal System

Our legal system is in place to ensure the rights of all citizens. We depend on the legal system to protect us from the wrongdoings of others. Many potential medical suits prove to be unwarranted and never make it into the court system, but even in the best physician–patient relationships, **litigation** (lawsuits) between patients and physicians may occur. Litigation may result from a single medication error or a mistake that costs a person's life. It is essential that you have a basic understanding of the American legal system to protect yourself, your

patients, and your physician-employer by following the legal guidelines. You must know your legal duties and understand the legal nature of the physician–patient relationship and your role and responsibilities as the physician's agent.

Sources of Law

Laws are rules of conduct that are enforced by appointed authorities. The foundation of our legal system is our rights outlined in the Constitution and the laws established by our Founding Fathers. These traditional laws are known as **common law**.

Common law is based on the theory of **stare decisis**. This term means "the previous decision stands." Judges usually follow these **precedents** (previous court decisions) but sometimes overrule a previous decision, establishing new precedent. Statutes are another source of law. Federal, state, or local legislators make laws or statutes, the police enforce them, and the court system ensures justice. Statutes pertaining to Medicare, Medicaid, and the Food and Drug Administration are common examples in the medical profession.

The third type of law is administrative. These laws are passed by governmental agencies, such as the Internal Revenue Service.

Branches of the Law

The two main branches of the legal system are public law and private or **civil law**.

Public Law

Public law is the branch of law that focuses on issues between the government and its citizens. It can be divided into four subgroups:

1. Criminal law is concerned with issues of citizen welfare and safety. Examples include arson, burglary, murder, and rape. A medical assistant must stay within the boundaries of the profession. Treating patients without the physician's orders could result in a charge of practicing medicine without a license—an act covered under criminal law.
2. Constitutional law is commonly called the law of the land. The United States government has a constitution, and each state has a constitution of its own, laws, and regulations. State laws may be more restrictive than federal laws but may not be more lenient. Two examples of constitutional law are laws on abortion and civil rights.
3. Administrative law is the regulations set forth by governmental agencies. This category includes laws pertaining to the Food and Drug Administration, the Internal Revenue Service, and the Board of Medical Examiners.
4. International law pertains to treaties between countries. Related issues include trade agreements, extradition, boundaries, and international waters.

Private or Civil Law

Private or civil law is the branch of the law that focuses on issues between private citizens. The medical profession is primarily concerned with private law. The subcategories that pertain to the medical profession are contract, commercial, and tort law. Contract and commercial laws concern the rights and obligations of those who enter into contracts, as in a physician–patient relationship. **Tort** law governs the righting of wrongs or injuries suffered by someone because of another person's wrong doing or misdeeds resulting from a **breach** of legal duty. Tort law is the basis of most lawsuits against physicians and health care workers. Other civil law branches include property, inheritance, and corporation law.

 CHECKPOINT QUESTION

1. Which branch of law covers a medical assistant charged with practicing medicine without a license?

The Rise in Medical Legal Cases

Malpractice refers to an action by a professional health care worker that harms a patient. A rise in the amounts of settlement awards has had a negative impact on the cost and coverage of malpractice insurance. With this rise, some physicians have actually changed the scope of their practice to reduce their costs. For example, an obstetrician may choose to limit practice to the care of nonpregnant women to avoid the high cost of malpractice insurance for physicians who deliver babies. In an attempt to protect professionals, legislation designed to limit the amount a jury can award has been introduced in Congress. Legal issues involving the medical field are referred to as medicolegal, which combines the words medical and legal.

A government task force found four primary reasons for the rise in malpractice claims:

1. *Scientific advances.* As new and improved medical technology becomes available, the risks and potential for complications of these procedures escalate, making physicians more vulnerable to litigation.
2. *Unrealistic expectations.* Some patients expect miracle cures and file lawsuits because recovery was not as they hoped or expected, even if the physician is not at fault.
3. *Economic factors.* Some patients view lawsuits as a means to obtain quick cash. (In fact, the number of lawsuits filed has increased during economic recessions.)
4. *Poor communication.* Studies show that when patients do not feel a bond with their physician, they are more likely to sue. Attention to customer service helps develop a good rapport between patients, the provider, and the staff.

Physician–Patient Relationship

Rights and Responsibilities of the Patient and Physician

In any contractual relationship, both parties have certain rights and responsibilities. The rights of the patient include the ability to choose a physician. This right may be limited to a list of participating providers under a patient's insurance plan. Patients have the right to determine whether to begin medical treatment and to set limits on that treatment. The patient also has the right to know in advance what the treatment will consist of, what effect it may have, and what dangers are to be expected. The concept of informed consent is discussed later in the chapter. Patients have the right to privacy. The Health Insurance Portability and Accountability Act of 1996 (HIPAA) outlines specific policies for protecting the privacy of electronic submissions of medical information. HIPAA is discussed at length in Chapter 8, Health Information Management.

Physicians have the right to limit their practice to a certain specialty or a certain location. For example, patients may not expect a physician to treat them at home. Physicians also have the right to refuse service to new patients or existing patients with new problems unless they are on emergency room call, in which case they must continue to treat patients seen during this time. The subject of abandonment is discussed later. Doctors have the right to change their policies or availability as long as they give patients reasonable notice of the change. This can be done through a local newspaper advertisement and/or a letter to each patient. Box 2-1 lists the patient's and physician's responsibilities.

Contracts

A **contract** is an agreement between two or more parties with certain factors agreed on among all parties. The physician–patient relationship is reinforced by the formation of a contract. All contractual agreements have three components:

1. Offer (contract initiation)
2. Acceptance (both parties agree to the terms)
3. Consideration (the exchange of fees for service)

BOX 2-1

RESPONSIBILITIES OF THE PATIENT AND THE PHYSICIAN

Responsibilities of the Patient

- Provide the physician with accurate data about the duration and nature of symptoms
- Provide a complete and accurate medical history to the physician
- Follow the physician's instructions for diet, exercise, medications, and appointments
- Compensate the physician for services rendered

Responsibilities of the Physician

- Respect the patient's confidential information
- Provide reasonable skill, experience, and knowledge in treating the patient
- Continue treating the patient until the contract has been withdrawn or as long as the condition requires treatment
- Inform patients of their condition, treatments, and prognosis
- Give complete and accurate information
- Provide competent coverage during time away from practice
- Obtain informed consent before performing procedures (informed consent is a statement of approval from the patient for the physician to perform a given procedure after the patient has been educated about the risks and benefits of the procedure)
- Caution against unneeded or undesirable treatment or surgery

---

A contract is not valid unless all three elements are present. A contract offer is made when a patient calls the office to request an appointment. The offer is accepted when you make an appointment for the patient. You have formed a contract that implies that for a fee, the physician will do all in his or her power to address the health concerns of the patient.

Certain individuals, such as children and those who are mentally incompetent or temporarily incapacitated, are not legally able to enter contracts. Patients in this category do not have the capacity to enter into a contract, and therefore, decisions about health care should be made by a competent party acting as a health care decision maker for the minor or incompetent person.

The two types of contracts between physicians and patients are implied and expressed.

Implied Contracts

Implied contracts, the most common kind of contract between physicians and patients, are not written but are assumed by the actions of the parties. For example, a patient calls the office and requests to see Dr. Smith for an earache. The patient arrives for the appointment, is seen by the physician, and receives a prescription. It is *implied* that, because the patient came on his own and requested care, that he wants this physician to care for him. The physician's action of accepting the patient for care *implies* that he acknowledges responsibility for his part of the contract. The patient *implies* by accepting the services that he will render payment even if the price was not discussed.

Expressed Contracts

Expressed contracts, either written or oral, consist of specified details. A mutual sharing of responsibilities is always stated in an expressed contract. The agreement you have with your creditors is an expressed contract. These kinds of contracts are not used as often in the medical setting as implied contracts.

 CHECKPOINT QUESTION

2. What action should be taken when a physician makes a change in his services?

Termination or Withdrawal of the Contract

A contract is ideally resolved when the patient is satisfactorily cured of the illness and the physician has been paid for the services. The patient may end the contract at any time, but the physician must follow legal **protocol** to dissolve the contract if the patient still seeks treatment, and the physician wishes to end the relationship.

Patient-Initiated Termination

A patient who chooses to terminate the relationship should notify the physician and give the reasons. You must keep this letter in the medical record. After the receipt of this letter, the physician should then send a letter to the patient stating the following:

- The physician accepts the termination.
- Medical records are available on written request.
- Medical referrals are available if needed.

If the patient verbally asks to end this relationship, the physician should send a letter to the patient documenting the conversation and, again, offering referrals and access to the medical records. Clear documentation is essential.

Physician-Initiated Termination

The physician may find it necessary to end the relationship. A physician may terminate the contract if the patient is noncompliant or does not keep appointments or for personal reasons. The physician must send a letter of withdrawal that includes:

- A statement of intent to terminate the relationship
- The reasons for this action
- The termination date at least 30 days from the date of receipt of the letter
- A statement that the medical records will be transferred to another physician at the patient's request
- A strong recommendation that the patient seek additional medical care as warranted

The letter must be sent by certified mail with a return receipt requested. A copy of the termination letter and the return receipt are placed in the patient's record. Figure 2-1 shows a sample letter of intent to terminate a physician–patient relationship.

Abandonment

If a contract is not properly terminated, the physician can be sued for **abandonment**. Abandonment may be charged if the physician withdraws from the contractual relationship without proper notification while the patient still needs treatment. Physicians must always arrange coverage when absent from the office for vacations, conferences, and so on. Patients may sue for abandonment in any instance that a suitable substitute is not available for care. Coverage may be provided by a **locum tenens**, a substitute physician.

Other examples of abandonment include:

- The physician abruptly and without reasonable notice stops treating a patient whose condition requires additional or continued care.

Amy Fine, MD
Charlotte Family Practice
220 NW 3rd Avenue
Charlotte, NC 25673

August 22, 2008

Regina Dodson
Jones Hill Road
Charlotte, NC 25673

Dear Ms. Dodson:

Due to the fact that you have persistently refused to follow my medical advice and treatment of your diabetes, I will no longer be able to provide medical care to you. Since your condition requires ongoing medical care, you must find another physician as soon as possible. I will be available to you until that time, but no longer than 30 days.

To assist you in continuing to receive care, we will make records available to your new physician as soon as you authorize us to send them.

Sincerely,

Amy Fine, MD

Figure 2-1 Letter of intent to terminate physician–patient relationship.

- The physician fails to see a patient as often as the condition requires or incorrectly advises the patient that further treatment is not needed.

CHECKPOINT QUESTION

3. What five elements must be included in a physician's termination intent letter?

Consent

The law requires that patients must **consent** or agree to being touched, examined, or treated by the physician or agents of the physician involved in the contractual agreement. No treatment may be made without a consent given orally, nonverbally by behavior, or clearly in writing. Patients have the right to appoint a health care surrogate or health care power of attorney who may make health care decisions when the patient is unable to make them. A health care surrogate may be a spouse, a friend, a pastor, or an attorney. A **durable power of attorney** for health care gives the patient's representative the ability to make health care decisions as the health care surrogate. A patient's physician should be aware of the power of attorney agreement, and a copy of the legal documentation should be kept in the office medical record.

Implied Consent

In the typical visit to the physician's office, the patient's actions represent an informal agreement for care to be given. A patient who raises a sleeve to receive an injection implies agreement to the treatment. **Implied consent** also occurs in an emergency. If a patient is in a life-threatening situation and is unable to give verbal permission for treatment, it is implied that the patient would consent to treatment if possible. As soon as possible, informed consent should be signed by either the patient or a family member in this type of situation. When there is no emergency, implied consent should be used only if the procedure poses no significant risk to the patient.

Informed or Expressed Consent

The physician is responsible for obtaining the patient's **informed consent** whenever the treatment involves an invasive procedure such as surgery, use of experimental drugs, potentially dangerous procedures such as stress tests, or any treatment that poses a significant risk to the patient. A federal law discussed later requires that health care providers who administer certain vaccines give the patient a current vaccine information statement (VIS). A VIS provides a standardized way to give objective information about vaccine benefits and adverse events (side effects) to patients. The VIS is available online through the Centers for Disease Control and Prevention (CDC) in 26 languages. The Web address can be found at the end of the chapter.

Informed consent is also referred to as **expressed consent.** Informed consent is based on the patient's right to know every possible benefit, risk, or alternative to the suggested treatment and the possible outcome if no treatment is initiated. The patient must voluntarily give permission and must understand the implications of consenting to the treatment. This requires that the physician and patient communicate in a manner understandable to the patient. Patients can be more active in personal health care decisions when they are educated about and understand their treatment and care.

A consent form must include the following information:

1. Name of the procedure to be performed
2. Name of the physician who will perform the procedure
3. Name of the person administering the anesthesia (if applicable)
4. Any potential risks from the procedure
5. Anticipated result or benefit from the procedure
6. Alternatives to the procedure and their risks

I hereby authorize Dr. _____, and such assistants as may be designated, to perform:

_____
(Name of treatment/procedure)

and any other related procedures or forms of treatment, including appropriate anesthesia, transfusions that they deem necessary for the welfare of:

_____
(Name of patient)

I consent to the administration of anesthesia and/or such drugs as may be necessary. I understand that all anesthetics involve risks of complications, serious injury, or rarely death from both known and unknown causes.

I consent to the examination and retention for educational, scientific and research purposes by the Medical Staff of

_____

of all body fluids, tissues and organs removed during the course of the above treatment/procedure with privilege of ultimate use and disposal resting with said medical staff.

The following has been explained to me and I understand:

A. The nature and character of the proposed treatment/procedure.
B. The anticipated results of the proposed treatment/procedure.
C. The recognized alternative forms of treatment/procedure.
D. The recognized serious possible risks and complications of the treatment/procedure and of the recognized alternative forms of treatment/procedure, including non-treatment.
E. The possible consequences of no treatment.
F. The anticipated date and time of the proposed treatment/procedure.

Additional M.D. comments: _____

_____

My physician has offered to answer all inquiries concerning the proposed treatment/procedure. I understand that I am free to withhold or withdraw consent to the proposed treatment/procedure at any time.

Witness			Signature of Person Giving Consent
Date Signed	Time	☐ A.M. ☐ P.M.	Relationship to patient (if applicable)

☐ Please check if this is a telephone monitored consent.
No treatment will be performed until this consent has been executed. This consent will be permanently filed in the patient's medical record.

Pt. No. _____
Name _____
D.O.B. _____

Gastroenterology Associates
Anytown, PA

Special Consent to Treatment
(Diagnostic & Surgical Procedures, Anesthesia, Medical Treatment & Other Procedures)

Figure 2-2 Sample consent form.

7. Probable effect on the patient's condition if the procedure is not performed
8. Any exclusions that the patient requests
9. Statement indicating that all of the patient's questions or concerns regarding the procedure have been answered
10. Patient's and witnesses' signatures and the date

As the medical assistant, you will frequently be required to witness consent signatures. A sample consent form is seen in Figure 2-2.

The informed consent form supplied for the patient's signature must be in the language that the patient speaks. Most physicians who treat multicultural patients have consent forms available in a variety of languages. Never ask a patient to sign a consent form if he or she:

- Does not understand the procedure
- Has unanswered questions regarding the procedure
- Is unable to read the consent form

Never coerce (force or compel against his or her wishes) a patient into signing a consent form. Figure 2-3 shows a deaf patient, a signing interpreter, and a certified medical assistant (CMA) with a consent form.

Who May Sign a Consent Form

An adult (usually someone over age 18) who is mentally competent and not under the influence of medication or other substances may sign a consent form. Depending on state law a minor may sign a consent form if he or she is:

- In the armed services
- Requesting treatment for communicable diseases (including sexually transmitted diseases)
- Pregnant
- Requesting information regarding birth control, abortion, or drug or alcohol abuse counseling
- Emancipated

An **emancipated minor** is under the age of majority but is either married or self-supporting and is responsible for his or her debts. The age of majority varies from state to state and ranges from 18 to 21 years. Minors may give consent if any one of the above-listed criteria is present.

Legal guardians may also sign consent forms. A legal guardian is appointed by a judge when the court has ruled an individual to be mentally incompetent. Health care surrogates may also sign consent forms. Health care surrogates are discussed later in the chapter.

Figure 2-3 Using an interpreter, the CMA helps this patient understand the procedure.

 CHECKPOINT QUESTION

4. Under what circumstances should a patient never be asked to sign a consent form?

Refusal of Consent

Patients may refuse treatment for any reason. Sometimes, patients make treatment choices based on religious or personal beliefs and preferences. For instance, a Jehovah's Witness may refuse a blood transfusion on religious grounds, or an elderly person may not want to undergo serious surgery because the potential complications may limit future lifestyle options. In this situation, the patient must sign a refusal of consent form indicating that the patient was instructed regarding the potential risks and benefits of the procedure as well as the risks if the procedure is not allowed. If the patient is a minor, the courts may become involved at the request of the physician or hospital and may award consent for the child. In this situation, the physician should follow legal counsel and document the incident carefully. In any instance that the patient refuses treatment, documentation must be made to protect the physician. The physician has a legal right to refuse to perform elective surgery on a patient who refuses to receive blood if needed.

Releasing Medical Information

The medical record is a legal document. Although the medical record itself belongs to the physician, the information belongs to the patient. Patients have the right to their medical information, and they have the right to deny the sharing of this information.

 WHAT IF?

A well-meaning family member asks for information about her mother's condition. What should you say?

Tell the family member that HIPAA's Privacy Rule does not allow you to discuss the patient without his or her permission. No information can be released to anyone—friends, family, media, or insurance companies—without prior written approval from the patient (see Chapter 8).

HIPAA also requires that each patient complete a form that establishes his or her wishes about giving information to family members and friends. If there is a particular family member who brings the patient to the office, the patient may sign a release form giving that person the right to receive information. Many physicians provide the patient with a short progress report including the patient's test results, diagnosis, treatment, and next appointment. A form could be designed for this purpose. This gives the patient the opportunity to share complete and accurate information if they choose.

Requests for medical records are common. Other health care facilities, insurance companies, and patients themselves may need information from the medical chart. Staying within the law when releasing medical information is covered in Chapter 8.

Legally Required Disclosures

Even though patients have the right to limit access to their medical records, health care facilities have a responsibility to report certain events to governmental agencies without the patient's consent, which are referred to as **legally required disclosures**. You and other health care providers must report to the department of public health the situations described in the following sections.

Vital Statistics

All states maintain records of births, deaths, marriages, and divorces. These records include the following:

- Birth certificates.
- Stillbirth reports. Some states have separate stillbirth forms; other states use a regular death certificate.
- Death certificates. These must be signed by a physician. The cause and time of death must be included.

You may assist the physician in completing a death certificate and filing the finished report in the patient's chart.

Medical Examiner's Reports

Each state has laws pertaining to which deaths must be reported to the medical examiner's office. Generally, these include the following:

- Death from an unknown cause
- Death from a suspected criminal or violent act
- Death of a person not attended by a physician at the time of death or for a reasonable period preceding the death
- Death within 24 hours of hospital admission

Infectious or Communicable Diseases

These reports are made to the local health department. The information is used for statistical purposes and for preventing or tracking the spread of these diseases. Although state guidelines vary, there are usually three categories of reports:

- Telephone reports are required for diphtheria, cholera, meningococcal meningitis, and plague, usually within 24 hours of the diagnosis. Telephone reports must always be followed by written reports.
- Written reports are required for hepatitis, leprosy,

malaria, rubeola, polio, rheumatic fever, tetanus, and tuberculosis. Sexually transmitted diseases must also be reported. Notification is usually required within 7 days of the date of discovery.
- Trend reports are made when your office notes an unusually high occurrence of influenza, streptococcal infections, or any other infectious diseases. Box 2-2 is a sample of reportable diseases and their time frames.

BOX 2-2

REPORTABLE CONDITIONS

Chapter 19—Health: Epidemiology
Subchapter 19a—Communicable Disease Control
Section .0100—Reporting of Communicable Diseases
.0101 Reportable Diseases and Conditions
(a) The following named diseases and conditions are declared to be dangerous to the public health and are hereby made reportable within the time period specified after the disease or condition is reasonably suspected to exist:

acquired immune deficiency syndrome (AIDS)—7 days
amebiasis—7 days
anthrax—24 hours
blastomycosis—7 days
botulism—24 hours
brucellosis—7 days
Campylobacter infection—24 hours
chancroid—24 hours
chlamydial infection (laboratory confirmed)—7 days
cholera—24 hours
dengue—7 days
diphtheria—24 hours
E. coli infection—24 hours
encephalitis—7 days
food-borne disease, including but not limited to Clostridium perfringens, Staphylococcal, and Bacillus cereus—24 hours
gonorrhea—24 hours
granuloma inguinale—24 hours
Haemophilus influenzae, invasive disease—24 hours
hepatitis A—24 hours
hepatitis B carriage—7 days
hepatitis non-A, non-B—7 days
human immunodeficiency virus infection (HIV) confirmed—7 days
legionellosis—7 days
leprosy—7 days
leptospirosis—7 days
Lyme disease—7 days

(continued)

BOX 2-2 (continued)

lymphogranuloma venereum—7 days
malaria—7 days
measles (rubeola)—24 hours
meningitis, pneumococcal—7 days
meningitis, viral (aseptic)—7 days
meningococcal disease—24 hours
mucocutaneous lymph node syndrome (Kawasaki syndrome)—7 days
mumps—7 days

Excerpt from the North Carolina Administrative Code Regarding Reporting of Communicable Diseases.

BOX 2-3

VACCINATIONS REQUIRING VACCINE INFORMATION STATEMENTS

Anthrax
Chickenpox
Diphtheria, tetanus, and pertussis
Haemophilus influenzae type b (Hib)
Hepatitis A
Hepatitis B
Influenza
Lyme disease
Measles, mumps, and rubella
Meningococcal
Pneumococcal polysaccharide
Pneumococcal conjugate
Polio

The CDC keeps a watchful eye on the public health. When necessary, the CDC establishes directives for the protection of the public. For example, when the public appeared to be at risk for contracting anthrax in 2001, the CDC mandated that documented anthrax cases be reported immediately. Fax machines and e-mail help facilitate such urgent public health communication.

National Childhood Vaccine Injury Act of 1986

Health care providers who administer certain vaccines and toxoids must report to the US Department of Health and Human Services (DHHS) the occurrence of any side effects listed in the manufacturer's package insert. In addition, health care providers must record in the patient's record the following information:

1. Date the vaccine was administered
2. Lot number and manufacturer of vaccine
3. Any adverse reactions to the vaccine
4. Name, title, and address of the person who administered the vaccine

Box 2-3 lists the vaccines and toxoids covered by the National Childhood Vaccine Injury Act.

Abuse, Neglect, or Maltreatment

Abuse, neglect, or maltreatment of any person who is incapable of self-protection usually falls under this category and may include the elderly or the mentally incompetent. Each state has its own regulations regarding what must be reported. Patient confidentiality rights are waived when the law requires you to report certain conditions.

Abuse is thought to be the second most common cause of death in children under age 5. The Federal Child Abuse Prevention and Treatment Act mandates that threats to a child's physical and mental welfare be reported. Health care workers, teachers, and social workers who report suspected abuse are not identified to the parents and are protected against liability. State laws vary regarding the procedure for reporting abuse. Local regulations should be outlined in the policies and procedures manuals at any outpatient facility. If you suspect a child is being abused, relay your suspicions to the physician. The physician will make the formal report. When authorities receive a report from a health care provider, they follow up by investigating the situa-

PATIENT EDUCATION

LEGALLY REQUIRED DISCLOSURES

Inform patients who have conditions that require legal disclosure about the applicable law. Assure them that you will protect their confidentiality. Educate them about why the disclosure is necessary, who receives the information, what particular forms will be completed, and any anticipated follow-up from the organization. For example, you are required to give the local health department the name, address, and condition of a patient with a sexually transmitted disease. The health department then contacts the patient to acquire the names of the patient's sexual contacts. These contacts are notified and counseled by the health department official. Patients who are educated about these legally required disclosures will better understand and accept the need to file official reports.

tion. For assistance in reporting suspected child abuse, you may call the national 24-hour hotline at 800-4 A CHILD (800-422-4453).

Spousal abuse is a significant problem in this country. Many women and children are trapped in a cycle of abuse. Mothers who are financially dependent on their abusers may see no way out. You should record any information gathered in the patient interview or anything observed in the course of dealing with the patient that may indicate abuse. Report these observations to the physician. Most communities have anonymous safe places for victims of domestic abuse, and you should be familiar with these services. With proper referrals, you may be able to help break the cycle of domestic abuse.

This country is also undergoing a rise in elderly parents being cared for by their adult children who also have the responsibility of raising young children. This phenomenon can cause great stress among caregivers. Abuse of the elderly can be in the form of mistreatment or neglect (not providing appropriate care). You should pay attention to observations and information provided by your elderly patients. If mistreatment is suspected, alert the physician. Support groups for those caring for the elderly are useful in dealing with the challenges of caring for others.

Violent Injuries

Health care providers have the legal duty to report suspected criminal acts. Injuries resulting from weapons, assault, attempted suicide, and rape must be reported to local authorities.

Other Reports

A diagnosis of cancer must be reported to assist in tracking malignancies and identifying environmental carcinogens. Just as the CDC keeps track of all communicable diseases reported, a database of treated tumors is kept in hospitals through a tumor registry. Some states also require that epilepsy (a seizure condition) be reported to local motor vehicle departments. The testing of newborns for phenylketonuria (PKU), which can cause mental retardation, is required in all states. Some states require positive PKU results to be reported to the health department so that close observation and follow-up care are ensured to prevent serious complications for the infant. Infantile hypothyroidism is also a reportable condition in some states.

 CHECKPOINT QUESTION

5. List six situations and conditions you are legally required to report.

Specific Laws and Statutes That Apply to Health Professionals

Medical Practice Acts

Although each state has its own medical practice act, the following elements are usually included:

- Definition of the practice of medicine.
- Requirements that the physician must have graduated from an accredited medical school and residency program and have passed the state medical examination.
- Description of the procedure for **licensure**.
- Description of the conditions for which a license can be suspended or revoked.
- Description of the renewal process for licensure. Most states require the physician to have attended a certain number of continuing education hours.
- Personal requirements necessary to become a licensed physician. Generally, a licensed physician must be a state resident, of good moral character, a US citizen, and 21 years of age or older.

A physician may have his or her license revoked or suspended by the board of medical examiners in most states for a variety of reasons, including certain criminal offenses, unprofessional conduct, fraud, or professional or personal incompetence. Criminal offenses include but are not limited to murder, manslaughter, robbery, and rape. Examples of unprofessional conduct may include invasion of a patient's privacy, excessive use of alcohol or use of illegal drugs, and **fee splitting** (sharing fees for the referral of patients to certain colleagues). Fraud is a common reason for revoking a license. Fraud may include filing false Medicare or Medicaid claims, falsifying medical records, or professional misrepresentation. Examples of misrepresentation or fraud include advertising a medical cure that does not exist, guaranteeing 100% success of a treatment, or falsifying medical credentials. Incompetence is often a hard charge to prove. The three most common examples are insanity, senility, and other documented mental incompetence.

As a medical assistant, it is your responsibility to report illegal or unethical behavior or signs of incompetence in the medical office. See Box 2-10 and think about how you would handle this difficult situation. (We will discuss ethics later in this chapter.)

Licensure, Certification, and Registration

Medical professionals can be licensed, certified, or **registered**. Licensure is regulated by laws, such as medical practice acts and nursing practice acts. If a particular profession is a licensed one, it is mandatory that one maintain a license in each state where he or she works. Each state determines the qualifications and requirements for licensure of a particular profession. A state agency will be responsible for issuing and renewing licenses. Most professionals are licensed to practice their profession according to certain guidelines and are limited to specific duties. For example, nurses are licensed. As mentioned earlier, in North Carolina, the Nursing Practice Act specifically prohibits a nurse from delegating professional authority to unlicensed personnel.

The term registered indicates that a professional has met basic requirements, usually for education, has passed standard testing, and has been approved by a governing body to perform given tasks within a state. X-ray technologists are registered as registered radiologic technologists. A national registry is available to verify a potential employee's status.

Certification is a voluntary process regulated through a professional organization. Standards for certification are set by the organization issuing the certificate. The CMA and registered medical assistant (RMA) credentials are nationally recognized and do not require any action when moving from one state to another. Remember, you must adhere to the laws regarding the CMA or RMA in the state where you work.

As a medical assistant, you are not licensed and therefore not limited to certain duties. The physician-employer has the sole responsibility of setting any limits on the duties of a medical assistant. Although most states do not require certification for employment, employers seek the CMA or RMA because certification indicates the achievement of certain standards of competence. A few states require that you take a test or short course before performing certain clinical duties.

Controlled Substances Act

The Controlled Substances Act of 1970 is a federal law enforced by the Drug Enforcement Agency (DEA). The act regulates the manufacture, distribution, and dispensing of narcotics and nonnarcotic drugs considered to have a high potential for abuse. This act was designed to decrease the illegal use of controlled substances and to prevent substance abuse by medical professionals. The law requires that any physician who dispenses, administers, or prescribes narcotics or other controlled substances be registered with the DEA.

Physicians who maintain a stock of controlled substances in the office for dispensing or administration must use a special triplicate order form available through the DEA. A record of each transaction must be kept and retained for 2 to 3 years. The record must be available for inspection by the DEA at any time. The act requires that all controlled substances be kept in a locked cabinet out of the patients' view and that the keys be kept secure. Theft should be reported immediately to the local police and the nearest DEA office. Prescription pads used for prescribing controlled sub-

stances must remain in a safe place at all times. The Legal Tip box lists steps you can take to keep these prescription pads safe.

This act also requires a physician to return all registration certificates and any unused order forms to the DEA if the practice is closed or sold. Violation of this act is a criminal offense. Penalties range from fines to imprisonment.

LEGAL TIP

PRESCRIPTION PAD SAFETY TIPS

- Keep only one prescription pad in a locked cabinet in the examining room. All other pads should be locked away elsewhere. Do not leave prescription pads unattended.

- Keep a limited supply of pads. It is better to re-order on a regular basis than to overstock.

- Keep track of the number of pads in the office. If a burglary occurs, you will be able to advise the police regarding the number of missing pads.

- Report any prescription pad theft to the police and alert local pharmacies of the theft. If the theft involves the loss of narcotic pads, the Drug Enforcement Agency must be notified.

Good Samaritan Act

As the number of lawsuits against physicians began to rise, physicians feared that giving emergency care to strangers outside the office could lead to malpractice suits. To combat that fear, all states now have Good Samaritan acts. Good Samaritan acts ensure that caregivers are immune from liability suits as long as they give care in good faith and in a manner that a reasonable and prudent person would in a similar situation. Each state has specific guidelines. Some even set standards for various professional levels, such as one set of standards for a physician and another set of standards for emergency medical technicians. Your state's Good Samaritan Act will not protect you if you are grossly negligent or willfully perform negligent acts.

You are not covered by the Good Samaritan Act while you are working as a medical assistant, nor does it cover physicians in the performance of their duties. Liability and malpractice insurance policies are available to protect you in those situations. If you render emergency care and accept compensation for that care, the act does not apply.

The provisions only cover acts outside of the formal practice of the profession.

BASIS OF MEDICAL LAW

Tort Law

A tort is a wrongful act that results in harm for which restitution must be made. The two forms of torts are intentional and unintentional. An allegation of an unintentional tort means that the accuser (the **plaintiff**) believes a mistake has been made; however, the plaintiff believes the caregiver or accused party (the **defendant**) was operating in good faith and did not intend the mistake to occur. Consider the following scenario as an example of an unintentional tort: A medical assistant giving a patient a heat treatment for muscle aches inadvertently burns the arm of the patient because the equipment is faulty. This act was not intentional or malicious, but it caused damage to the patient. About 90% of suits against physicians fall into this category.

Negligence and Malpractice (Unintentional Torts)

Most unintentional torts involve negligence. These are the most common forms of medical malpractice suits.

Negligence is performing an act that a reasonable health care worker or provider would not have done or the omission of an act that a reasonable professional or provider would have done. Failure to take reasonable precautions to prevent harm to a patient is termed **negligence**. If a physician is involved, the term usually used is malpractice. Malpractice is said to have occurred when the patient is harmed by the professional's actions. There are three types of malpractice:

- Malfeasance—incorrect treatment
- Misfeasance—treatment performed incorrectly
- Nonfeasance—treatment delayed or not attempted

In a legal situation, the standard of care determines what a reasonable professional would have done. Standards of care are written by various professional agencies to clarify what the reasonable and prudent physician or health care worker would do in a given situation. For example, a patient comes to an orthopedist's office after falling from a horse and complains of arm pain. The standard of care for orthopedists would require an x-ray of the injured extremity after trauma. Standards of care vary with the level of the professional. A registered nurse is not held to the same standards of care as a physician, and a medical assistant is not expected to perform by the same standards as the registered nurse. Each must practice within the scope of their training. The representing attorney may seek an **expert witness** to state under oath the standards of care for a specific situation. Expert witnesses may be physicians, nurses, physical therapists, or other specialized practitioners who have excellent reputations in their field.

Expert witnesses are always used in malpractice cases, except when the doctrine of **res ipsa loquitur** is tried. This doctrine means "the thing speaks for itself." In other words, it is obvious that the physician's actions or negligence caused the injury. A judge must preapprove the use of this theory in pretrial hearings. An example of a case tried under this doctrine might be a fracture that occurred when the patient fell from an examining table.

For negligence to be proved, the plaintiff's attorney must prove that the following four elements were present: duty, dereliction of duty, direct cause, and damage. The courts place the burden of proof on the plaintiff; the physician is assumed to have given proper care until proven otherwise.

Duty

Duty is present when the patient and the physician have formed a contract. This is usually straightforward and the easiest of the elements to prove. If the patient presented to the physician's office and the physician sees the patient, there is duty.

Dereliction of Duty

The patient must prove that the physician did not meet the standard of care guidelines, either by performing an act inappropriately or by omitting an act.

Direct Cause

The plaintiff must prove that the derelict act directly caused the patient's injury. This can be difficult to prove if the patient has an extensive medical history that may have contributed to the injury.

Damage

The plaintiff must prove that an injury or **damages** occurred. Documentation must be available to prove a diagnosis of an injury or illness.

Jury Awards

There are three types of awards for damages:

1. *Nominal.* Minimal injuries or damages occurred, and compensation is small.
2. *Actual (compensatory).* Money is awarded for the injury, disability, mental suffering, loss of income, or the anticipated future earning loss. This payment is moderate to significant.
3. *Punitive.* Money is awarded to punish the practitioner for reckless or malicious wrongdoing. Punitive damages are the most costly. (Note: A

physician may have committed a medical error, but if the patient suffered no injuries or damages, he or she cannot win the suit. Also, if the outcome was not as expected but the physician cannot be shown to be at fault, the patient will not be compensated.)

 CHECKPOINT QUESTION

6. What four elements must be proved in a negligence suit?

Intentional Torts

An **intentional tort** is an act that takes place with malice and with the intent of causing harm. Intentional torts are the deliberate violation of another person's legal rights. Examples of intentional torts are assault and battery, use of duress, invasion of privacy, defamation of character, fraud, tort of outrage, and undue influence. These are described next.

Assault and Battery

Assault is the unauthorized attempt or threat to touch another person without consent. **Battery** is the actual physical touching of a patient without consent; this includes beating and physical abuse. By law, a conscious adult has the right to refuse medical care. Care given without the patient's consent constitutes assault. An example of battery might be suturing a laceration against the patient's expressed wish.

Duress

If a patient is coerced into an act, the patient can possibly sue for the tort of **duress**. Following is an example in which a patient may be able to sue successfully for assault, battery, and duress. A 22-year-old woman arrives at a pregnancy center. She is receiving public assistance and has five children. Her pregnancy test is positive. The staff persuades her to have an abortion. She signs the consent form, and the abortion is performed. Later she sues, stating that she was verbally coerced into signing the consent form (duress) and that the abortion was performed against her wishes (assault and battery).

Invasion of Privacy

Patients have the right to privacy. Remember, HIPAA regulates the sharing of information. Most offices have patients sign an authorization to release information to their insurance company on their first visit. This covers each return visit unless the insurance carrier changes. Written permission must be obtained from the patient to:

- Release medical records or personal data
- Publish case histories in medical journals
- Make photographs of the patient (exception: suspected cases of abuse or maltreatment)
- Allow observers in examination rooms

For example, a 57-year-old woman is seen in your office for a skin biopsy. Her insurance company calls asking for information regarding the bill and asks for the biopsy report. You give the requested information and then find that the patient never signed a release form. She has a valid case for invasion of privacy.

Defamation of Character

Making malicious or false statements about a person's character or reputation is **defamation of character**. Libel refers to written statements, and **slander** refers to oral statements. For example, a patient asks for a referral to another physician. She states that she has heard, "Dr. Rogers is a good surgeon." You have heard that he has a history of alcoholism. You tell the patient that he is probably not a good choice because of his drinking. That is defamation of his character, and you could be sued for saying it.

Fraud

Fraud is any deceitful act with the intention to conceal the truth, such as:

- Intentionally raising false expectations regarding recovery
- Not properly instructing the patient regarding possible side effects of a procedure
- Filing false insurance claims

Tort of Outrage

Tort of outrage is the intentional infliction of emotional distress. For this tort to be proved, the plaintiff's attorney must show that the physician:

- Intended to inflict emotional distress
- Acted in a manner that is not morally or ethically acceptable
- Caused severe emotional distress

Undue Influence

Improperly persuading another to act in a way contrary to that person's free will is termed undue influence. For instance, preying on the elderly or the mentally incompetent is a common type of undue influence. Unethical practitioners who gain the trust of these persons and persuade them to submit to expensive and unnecessary medical procedures are practicing undue influence.

✓ CHECKPOINT QUESTION

7. What is the difference between assault and battery?

The Litigation Process

The litigation process begins when a patient consults an attorney because he or she believes a health care provider has done wrong or becomes aware of a possible prior injury. The patient's attorney obtains the medical records, which are reviewed by medicolegal consultants. (Such consultants may be nurses or physicians who are considered experts in their field.) Then the plaintiff's attorney files a complaint, a written statement that lists the claim against the physician and the remedy desired, usually monetary compensation.

The defendant and his or her attorney answer the complaint. The discovery phase begins with interrogatories and **depositions**. During this phase, attorneys for both parties gather relevant information.

Next, the trial phase begins. A jury is selected unless the parties agree to a **bench trial**. In a bench trial, the judge hears the case without a jury and renders a verdict (decision or judgment). Opening statements are given, first by the plaintiff's attorney, then by the defendant's attorney. The plaintiff's attorney presents the case. Expert witnesses are called, and the evidence is shown. Examination of the witnesses begins. Direct examination involves questioning by one's own attorney; cross-examination is questioning by the opposing attorney. When the plaintiff's attorney is finished, the defense presents the opposing arguments and evidence. The plaintiff's attorney may cross-examine the defendant's witnesses. Closing arguments are heard. Finally, a verdict is made.

If the defendant is found guilty, damages are awarded. If the defendant is found not guilty, the charges are dismissed. The decision may be appealed to a higher court. An **appeal** is a process by which the higher court reviews the decision of the lower court.

Defenses to Professional Liability Suits

The objective of all court proceedings is to uncover the truth. Many defenses are available to a health care worker who is being sued. These include the medical record, statute of limitations, assumption of risk, res judicata, contributory negligence, and comparative negligence, discussed next.

Medical Records

The best and most solid defense the caregiver has is the medical record. Every item in the record is considered to be a part of a legal document. Juries may believe a medical record regardless of testimony. Juries tend to believe these records because they are tangible items from the actual time the injury occurred. There is a common saying in the medicolegal world: "If it's not in the chart, it did not happen." This means that even negative findings should be listed. For example, instead of saying that the patient's neurologic history is negative, the documentation might say the patient reports no headaches, seizures, one-sided weakness, and so on. Entries in the medical record refresh the memory of the defendant and provide documentation of care. As a medical assistant, you must make sure that all of your documentation is timely, accurate, and legible. (See Chapter 8 for specific information regarding charting practices.)

Statute of Limitations

Each state has a statute that defines the length of time during which a patient may file a suit against a caregiver. When the **statute of limitations** expires, the patient loses the right to file a claim. Generally, the limits vary from 1 to 3 years following the alleged occurrence. Some states use a combination rule. Some states allow 1 to 3 years following the patient's discovery of the occurrence. States vary greatly when an alleged injury involves a minor. The statute may not take effect until the minor reaches the age of majority and then may extend 2 to 3 years past this time. Some states have longer claim periods in wrongful death suits.

Assumption of Risk

In the assumption of risk defense, the physician will claim that the patient was aware of the risks involved before the procedure and fully accepted the potential for damages. For example, a patient is instructed regarding the adverse effects of chemotherapy. The patient fully understands these risks, receives the chemotherapy, and wants to sue for alopecia (hair loss). Alopecia is a given risk with certain forms of chemotherapy. A signed consent form indicating that the patient was informed of all of the risks of a procedure proves this point.

Res Judicata

The doctrine of **res judicata** means "the thing has been decided." Once the suit has been brought against the physician or patient and a settlement has been reached, the losing party may not countersue. If, for instance, the physician sues a patient for not paying bills and the court orders the patient to pay, the patient cannot sue the physician for malpractice. The opposite may occur as well. If the physician is sued for malpractice and loses, he cannot countersue for defamation of character.

Contributory Negligence

With the **contributory negligence** defense, the physician usually admits that negligence has occurred; he or she will claim, however, that the patient aggravated the injury or assisted in making the injury worse. For example, the patient's laceration is stitched with only three sutures when 10 were needed. The physician instructs the patient to limit movement of the arm. The patient plays baseball; the laceration reopens, causing infection; and subsequently, extensive scar tissue forms. Both the patient and the physician contributed to the postoperative damages. Most states do not grant damage awards for contributory negligence. If an award is granted, the courts assess **comparative negligence**.

Comparative Negligence

In comparative negligence, the award of damages is based on a percentage of the contribution to the negligence. If the patient contributed 30% to the damage, the damage award is 30% less than what was granted. In the example in the previous paragraph, the courts may decide that the negligence is shared at 50%. Therefore, if the court assessed damages of $20,000, the physician would be responsible for $10,000.

In the past, contributory negligence, such as a patient not returning for appointments, was seen as absolute defense for the physician. This has changed over the years, however, and many defendants use the defense of comparative negligence, with the responsibility shared between the physician and the patient.

DEFENSE FOR THE MEDICAL ASSISTANT

Respondeat Superior or Law of Agency

The doctrine of **respondeat superior** literally means "let the master answer." This may also be called law of agency. This doctrine implies that physicians are liable for the actions of their employees. The physician is responsible for your actions as a medical assistant as long as your actions are within your scope of practice. Figure 2-4 features a scope-of-practice decision tree designed to help you make such decisions. As a new medical assistant, you can use this tool to guard against overconfidence. If your actions exceed your abilities or training, the physician is not generally responsible for any error that you make. You must understand that you can be sued in this instance and that respondeat superior does not guarantee immunity for your actions.

For example, Mrs. Smith is a chronic complainer, calling your office frequently with minor concerns. Today, she calls complaining of tingling in her arms.

Scope of practice decision making

When faced with a new or unfamiliar procedure, the following thought pattern is suggested:

1) Verbalize the steps involved in the procedure to be performed. Review the scope of practice for your profession. Is this procedure expressly prohibited by any state laws, rules, or regulations?

   NO ⟶ (down)   YES ⟶ STOP

2) Do you personally possess the depth and breadth of knowledge to perform the procedure safely and effectively from formal academic training or on-the-job supervised training?

   YES ⟶ (down)   NO ⟶ STOP

3) Do you personally possess current clinical skills to perform the procedure safely?

   YES ⟶ (down)   NO ⟶ STOP

4) Is the performance of the procedure within the accepted standard of care which would be provided in similar circumstances by reasonable and prudent medical assistants who have similar training and experience?

   YES ⟶ (down)   NO ⟶ STOP

5) Is the performance of the procedure consistent with appropriately established facility/agency policies and procedures?

   YES ⟶ (down)   NO ⟶ STOP

6) Are you prepared to accept the consequences of your action?

   YES ⟶ (down)   NO ⟶ STOP

PERFORM THE PROCEDURE

Figure 2-4 Scope of practice decision-making tree. (Adapted from the Washington State Department of Health, Nursing Care Quality Assurance Commission, "Scope of Practice Decision Tree.")

The physician has left for the day, so you tell Mrs. Smith, "Don't worry about this; take your medication, and call us tomorrow." During the night, a blood vessel in Mrs. Smith's brain bursts. She has a cerebral hemorrhage (bleeding inside the brain) and dies. The family sues. The physician claims that you were instructed not to give advice over the telephone. You are not covered by respondeat superior because you acted outside of your scope of practice.

To protect yourself from situations such as this, have your job description in written form and always practice within its guidelines. Do not perform tasks that you have not been trained to do. Never hesitate to seek clarification from a physician. If you are not sure about something, such as a medication order, ask!

Malpractice insurance is available to allied health care professionals for further protection. Malpractice premiums are inexpensive and afford protection against losing any personal assets if sued. The insurance company would pay damages as assessed by a jury. Of course, as with any insurance policy, there will be conditions of coverage and maximum amounts the company will pay. The Legal Tip box provides some additional advice for preventing lawsuits.

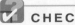

LEGAL TIP
YOU CAN AVOID LITIGATION

- Keep medical records neat and organized. Always document and sign legibly.

- Stay abreast of new laws and medical technology.

- Become a certified or registered medical assistant (CMA or RMA).

- Keep your CPR and first aid certification current.

- Never give any information over the telephone unless you are sure of the caller's identity and you have patient consent.

- Keep the office neat and clean. Make sure that children's toys are clean and in good condition to avoid injuries. Perform safety checks frequently.

- Limit waiting time for patients. If an emergency arises, causing a long wait, explain to the patients in a timely and professional manner.

- Practice good public relations. Always be polite, smile, and show genuine concern for your patients and their families.

CHECKPOINT QUESTION

8. What is the law of agency, and how does it apply to the medical assistant?

Employment and Safety Laws

Civil Rights Act of 1964, Title VII

Title VII of the Civil Rights Act of 1964 protects employees from discrimination in the workplace. The Equal Employment Opportunity Commission (EEOC) enforces the provisions of the act and investigates any possible infractions. Employers may not refuse to hire, limit, segregate or classify, fire, compensate, or provide working conditions and privileges on the basis of race, color, sex, religion, or national origin. This act determines the questions that may be asked in a job interview. For example, a potential employee cannot be asked questions that would reveal age, marital status, religious affiliation, height, weight, or arrest record. It is acceptable, however, to ask if an applicant has ever been convicted of a crime. In the health care setting, employers can require a criminal records check and even drug screening to ensure the safety of the patients. The American Association of Medical Assistants (AAMA) has made recent changes to prohibit convicted felons from taking the CMA examination.

Sexual Harassment

In recent years, Title VII has been expanded to include sexual harassment. Sexual harassment is defined by the EEOC as unwelcome sexual advances or requests for sexual favors in the workplace. The definition includes other verbal or physical conduct of a sexual nature when such conduct is made a condition of an individual's employment, is used as a basis for hiring or promotion, or has the purpose or effect of unreasonably interfering with an individual's work performance. If such behavior creates an intimidating, hostile, or offensive working environment, it is considered sexual harassment. In the past two decades, court decisions have confirmed that this form of harassment is a cause for both criminal prosecution and civil litigation.

In the medical office setting, the office manager must be alert for signs of harassment and should have in place a policy for handling complaints.

Americans with Disabilities Act

Title VII also includes the Americans with Disabilities Act (ADA), which prohibits discrimination against people with substantial disabilities in all employment practices, including job application procedures, hiring, firing, advancement, compensation, training, benefits, and all other privileges of employment. The ADA applies to all employers with 15 or more employees. The law covers those with impairments that limit their major life activities. The statute also protects those with AIDS or HIV-positive status and individuals with a history of mental illness or cancer. ADA also requires that employers provide basic accommodations for disabled employees. Those basic accommodations include extra-wide parking spaces close to the door, ramps or elevators, electric or easily opened doors, bathroom facilities designed for the disabled, an accessible break room, and a work area with counters low enough for a person in a wheelchair.

The ADA also takes safety into consideration. Employers are permitted to establish qualification standards that will exclude individuals who pose a direct threat to others if that risk cannot be lowered to an acceptable level by reasonable accommodations. In the medical field, technical standards are established that outline physical requirements of a certain job. For example, if a particular job requires adequate vision to see the dials on a piece of laboratory equipment, it is unreasonable to expect an employer to hire a person who is sight impaired. The law is designed to protect employees, not to require unreasonable accommodations.

The ADA also requires that all public buildings be accessible to physically challenged people. Following is a partial list of ways the medical office can comply with this act:

- Entrance ramps
- Widened rest rooms to be wheelchair accessible
- Elevated toilet bowls for easier transferring from wheelchairs
- Easy-to-reach elevator buttons
- Braille signs
- Access to special telephone services to communicate with hearing-impaired patients

Occupational Safety and Health Act

Employers must provide safe environments for their employees. In accordance with the Occupational Safety and Health Act of 1970, the Occupational Safety and Health Administration (OSHA) controls and monitors safety for workers. Specific OSHA rules and regulations protect the clinical worker from exposure to **blood-borne pathogens**. Blood-borne pathogens are organisms that can be spread through direct contact with blood or body fluids from an infected person. Universal or standard precautions are designed to protect health care workers from blood and body fluids contaminated with HIV, hepatitis, or any contagious "bugs" by requiring that those in direct contact with patients use protective equipment (e.g., gloves, gowns, face mask). In days past, health care workers felt that they needed protection only from patients with known risk factors (sharing needles, having unprotected sexual intercourse). OSHA's regulations ensure protection from contracting a contagious disease from *any* body fluids handled.

Your medical assisting training will include an extensive study of safety issues and protection against accidental exposure to blood-borne pathogens. Box 2-4 outlines OSHA rules governing all free-standing health care providers. Box 2-5 outlines the laws governing employer and employee rights and responsibilities.

BOX 2-4

OCCUPATIONAL SAFETY AND HEALTH ACT OF 1970 RULES GOVERNING HEALTH CARE PROVIDERS

OSHA defines body fluids as semen, blood, amniotic fluids, vaginal secretions, synovial fluid (from joint spaces), pleural fluid (from the lungs), pericardial fluid (from the heart), cerebrospinal fluid (from the spinal cord), and saliva. OSHA employs inspectors who may conduct inspections and issue citations for violations and recommend penalties. Under specific rules, OSHA requires that health care facilities provide:

- A list of all employees who might be exposed to blood-borne diseases on either a regular or an occasional basis.
- A written exposure control plan that outlines steps to be taken in the event of an employee's accidental exposure to blood-borne pathogens.
- One employee who is responsible for OSHA compliance.
- Availability of protective clothing that fits properly.
- An employee training program in writing and records of sessions and participants.
- Warning labels and signs denoting biohazards (potentially dangerous materials).
- Written guidelines for identifying, containing, and disposing of medical waste, including housecleaning and laundry decontamination.
- Written guidelines and procedures to follow if any employee is exposed to blood or other potentially infectious materials, as well as a policy for reporting incidents of exposure and maintaining records.
- Postexposure evaluation procedures, including follow-up testing of the exposed employee.
- Material safety data sheets (MSDS) listing each ingredient in a product used in the office. Manufacturers provide an MSDS for every product they sell. Information included in the sheets includes any hazards involved or necessary precautions that must be taken when handling materials.
- Hepatitis B vaccine free of charge to employees working with body fluids.

BOX 2-5

LAWS GOVERNING EMPLOYER AND EMPLOYMENT RIGHTS AND RESPONSIBILITIES

FAIR LABOR STANDARDS ACT OF 1939

- Regulates wages and working conditions including:
- Federal minimum wage, overtime compensation, equal pay requirements, child labor, hours, and requirements for record keeping.

Civil Rights Act of 1964, Title VII

- Applies to employers with 15 or more employees for at least 20 weeks of the year.
- Federal regulation forbids discrimination on the basis of race, color, sex, religion, or national origin. Some state laws also prohibit discrimination for sexual orientation, personal appearance, mental health, mental retardation, marital status, parenthood, and political affiliation.

Americans with Disabilities Act of 1990

- Applies to employers with 15 or more employees.
- Prohibits discrimination against individuals with substantial impairments in all employment practices.

Age Discrimination in Employment Act of 1967

- Applies to employers with 15 or more employees.
- Regulates discrimination against workers on the basis of age. Protects those who are 40–65 years of age.

Family and Medical Leave Act of 1993

- Employees are covered after 1 year or 1250 hours of employment over the past 12 months.
- Provides up to 12 weeks per year of unpaid, job-protected leave to eligible employees for certain family and medical reasons.

Immigration Reform and Control Act of 1986

- Applies to employers with four or more employees.
- Prohibits employment of illegal aliens and protects legal aliens from discrimination based on national origin or citizenship.

Other Legal Considerations

The Clinical Laboratory Improvement Amendments (CLIA) of 1988 contain specific rules and regulations regarding laboratory safety.

The Joint Commission on Accreditation of Healthcare Organizations (JCAHO) is a private organization that sets standards for health care administration. Each state also has specific laws regarding patient care, insurance billing, collections, and other such matters.

 CHECKPOINT QUESTION

9. What are blood-borne pathogens? Which government agency governs their control in the medical office?

Medical Ethics

Medical **ethics** are principles of ethical and moral conduct that govern the behavior and conduct of health professionals. These principles define proper medical etiquette, customs, and professional courtesy. Ethics are guidelines specifying right or wrong and are enforced by peer review and professional organizations. Laws are regulations and rules that are enforced by the government. **Bioethics** are issues and problems that affect a patient's life; many bioethical issues have arisen from the advances of modern medicine.

American Medical Association (AMA) Code of Ethics

A code of ethics is a "collective statement from a professional organization that depicts the behavioral expectations for its members. Additionally, a code of ethics allows the organization to set standards by which it may discipline its members." The AMA Code of Ethics states that physicians must recognize and accept their responsibilities for both patients and society. It also states that these are "not laws but standards of conduct by which a physician's professional behavior will be assessed." Box 2-6 outlines the AMA Code of Ethics.

Violations of these AMA principles may result in censure, suspension, or expulsion by the state medical board. Censure, the least punitive action, is a verbal or written reprimand from the association indicating negative findings regarding a specific incident. Suspension is the temporary removal of privileges and association with the organization. Expulsion is a formal discharge from the professional organization and is the maximum punishment. Many of these issues, however, deal with laws and the patient's rights as established by law. When violations of laws are involved, physicians may

BOX 2-6

AMA CODE OF ETHICS

Seven principles in the AMA Code of Ethics state that the physician shall:

1. Practice competent medical care with compassion while respecting human dignity.
2. Remain honest in dealings with patients and colleagues; expose colleagues with character deficiencies or who are incompetent or who engage in fraud or deception.
3. Adhere to all laws, and when needed, be a voice to lawmakers in the best interest of patient care.
4. Respect the rights of patients and other health care professionals; safeguard patient confidentiality (privacy) except within the provisions of the law.
5. Continue appropriate education to remain current; request consultation and obtain the knowledge and skills of other health professionals when needed.
6. Be free to select whom to treat, where to establish a practice, and whom to associate with except in emergency situations.
7. Participate in activities to enhance the community.

lose their license to practice, may be fined, or may be imprisoned. Serious consequences can arise from a breach of this code of ethics.

Medical Assistant's Role in Ethics

As an agent of the physician in the medical office, you are also governed by ethical standards and are responsible for:

- Protecting patient confidentiality
- Following all state and federal laws
- Being honest in all your actions

As a medical assistant, you must apply ethical standards as you perform your duties. You must realize that your personal feelings of right and wrong should be kept separate if they differ from the ethics of your profession. For example, a medical assistant who has a strong opinion against abortion would not be happy working in a medical facility that performs abortions. The care you give patients must be objective, and personal opinions about options must not be shared.

Patient Advocacy

Your primary responsibility as a medical assistant is to be a patient advocate at all times. Advocacy requires that you consider the best interests of the patient above all other concerns. This often means setting aside your own personal beliefs, values, and biases and looking at a given situation in an objective manner. You should never, however, be asked or forced to compromise your own value system.

Patient Confidentiality

Confidentiality of patient information is one of the most important ethical principles to be observed by the medical assistant. As discussed earlier, information obtained in the care of the patient may not be revealed without the permission of the patient unless required by law. Whatever you say to, hear from, or do for a patient is confidential. Patients will reveal some of their innermost thoughts, feelings, and fears. This information is not for public knowledge. Family members, friends, pastors, or others may call the physician's office to inquire about a patient's condition. Many of these calls are made with good intentions; NO INFORMATION, however, should be released to anyone—friends, family, media, or insurance companies—without prior written approval from the patient (see Chapter 8).

Honesty

One of the most important character traits for medical assistants is honesty. We all make mistakes at times; how we handle our mistakes is the indication of our ethical standards. If you make a mistake (e.g., giving the wrong medication), you must immediately report the error to your supervisor and the attending physician. The mark of a true professional is the ability to admit mistakes and take full responsibility for all actions. When speaking to patients concerning medical issues, be honest; give the facts in a straightforward manner. Never offer false expectations or hope. Never minimize or exaggerate the risks or benefits of a procedure. If you do not know the answer to a question, say, "I don't know, but I will find out for you," or refer the question to the physician. Treating the patient with dignity, respect, and honesty in all interactions will build trust in you and your professional abilities.

 CHECKPOINT QUESTION

10. What are the three ethical standards a CMA, as an agent of the physician, should follow?

American Association of Medical Assistants (AAMA) Code of Ethics

Principles

The AAMA has published a set of five principles of ethical and moral conduct that all medical assistants must follow in the practice of the profession. They state that the medical assistant must always strive to:

1. Render services with respect for human dignity
2. Respect patient confidentiality, except when information is required by the law
3. Uphold the honor and high principles set forth by the AAMA
4. Continually improve knowledge and skills for the benefit of patients and the health care team
5. Participate in community services that promote good health and welfare to the general public

These principles are outlined in the AAMA creed seen in the Medical Assistants' Creed. (See Box 2-7.)

In 1999, the AAMA adopted *AAMA's Disciplinary Standards & Procedures for CMAs*. For the first time, a policy was established for sanctions against CMAs who violate the disciplinary standards. Possible sanctions include denial of eligibility for the certification examination, probation, reprimand, temporary revocation of the CMA credential, and permanent revocation of the CMA credential. For more information, see the AAMA website.

Bioethics

Bioethics deals specifically with the moral issues and problems that affect human life. As a result of advances in medicine and research, many situations require moral decisions for which there are no clear answers. Abortion and genetic engineering are examples. The goal is to make the right decision in each specific instance as it applies to an individual's specific circumstances. What may be right for one patient may be wrong for another; that is the foundation of bioethics.

American Medical Association (AMA) Council on Ethical and Judicial Affairs

Because of the broad scope of medical ethics and bioethical issues, the AMA formed a subcommittee to review AMA principles and to interpret them as they apply to everyday clinical situations. This subcommittee is called the Council on Ethical and Judicial Affairs. The council has formulated a series of opinions on various medical and bioethical issues that are intended to provide the physician with guidelines for professional con-

---

BOX 2·7

MEDICAL ASSISTANTS' CREED

The AAMA also has a written a creed for medical assistants. The creed of the AAMA is:

I believe in the principles and purposes of the profession.

I endeavor to be more effective.

I aspire to render greater service.

I protect the confidence entrusted to me.

I am dedicated to the care and well-being of all patients.

I am loyal to my physician-employer.

I am true to the ethics of my profession.

I am strengthened by compassion, courage, and faith.

---

duct and responsibilities. These opinions, most recently revised in 1992, are divided into four general categories:

- Social policy issues
- Relations with colleagues and hospitals
- Administrative office procedures
- Professional rights and responsibilities

The following discussion provides a summary of these opinions along with questions designed to promote your ability to use reasoning to examine difficult ethical issues. These issues are not within the scope of decisions for medical assistants, but you will be faced with their consequences at some time in your career.

Social Policy Issues

The social policy section deals with various issues of societal importance and provides guidelines to aid the physician in making ethical choices. Five common societal topics and the opinion statements from the AMA Council on Ethical and Judicial Affairs follow.

Allocation of Resources

The term *allocate* means to set aside or designate for a purpose. Allocation of resources in the medical profession may refer to many health needs:

- *Organs for transplantation.* Who gets the heart, the college professor or the young recovering addict whose heart was damaged by his lifestyle? Should lifestyle or perceived worth be considered in the decision?
- *Funds for research.* Which disease should receive more funding for research, cancer or AIDS?

- *Funds for health care.* For what should the money be spent, for keeping alive extremely premature infants or making preventive health care available for a greater number of poor children?
- *Hospital beds and professional care.* With hospital care at a premium, who will pay for the indigent? How is it decided which patient is entitled to the last bed in the intensive care unit?

Box 2-8 outlines the judicial council's viewpoints on allocation of limited resources.

Clinical Investigations and Research

Physicians are frequently involved in studying the effectiveness of new procedures and medications, often called clinical investigations or research. New drugs and treatments are tested on animals first and then considered safe for human testing. The council's viewpoint on research investigation of new drugs and procedures states:

- *A physician may participate in clinical research as long as the project is part of a systematic program with controls for patient evaluation during all phases of the re-*

search. At all stages of the testing and at the completion of the study, a protocol must be in place to evaluate the immediate and the long-term effects of the study.
- The goal of the research must be to obtain scientifically valid data. The objectives of the study must be available to the physician and the patient, results must be provided to all participants on request, and the testing must serve a medically sound purpose to provide better patient care.
- Utmost care and respect must be given to patients involved in clinical research. They are entitled to be treated just as any other patient receiving health care.
- Physicians must obtain the patient's permission or consent before enrolling the patient in a research project.
- The patient's decision to participate in the program must be completely voluntary.
- The patient must be advised of any potential risks, side effects, and benefits of participating in the project.
- The patient must be advised that this procedure or drug is experimental. Patients must be made aware that research is not complete, that this is the purpose of the trials, and that the risks and benefits are not fully known at this time.
- The physician and the institution must have a check and balance system in place to ensure that quality care is always given and ethical standards are followed. Documentation of patient education and instruction for following testing guidelines and patient response to the treatment must be ongoing and thorough.

BOX 2-8

AMA COUNCIL ON ETHICAL AND JUDICIAL AFFAIRS VIEWPOINT

- When resources are limited, decisions for allocating health care materials should be based on fair and socially acceptable criteria. Economic or social position should not be a factor in the decision.
- Priority care is given to the person or persons who are more likely to receive the greatest long-term benefit from the treatment. Patients with other disease processes or who are not good candidates for treatment for whatever reason will be less likely to receive treatment than otherwise healthy patients. For instance, a patient with cancer in other sites would not be considered for a liver transplant, whereas a patient whose liver was damaged by trauma but who has no other involvement would probably be a good candidate.
- An individual's societal worth must not be a deciding factor during the decision process. A socially or politically prominent patient should not be considered a better recipient of treatment options than a young mother on welfare.
- Age must not be considered in the decision process. If the age of the patient is not a contraindication for the treatment, all ages should be considered on an even basis for most medical resources.

Obstetric Dilemmas

Advances in technology have created legal and ethical situations that have polarized opinions and are difficult to bring to consensus. Issues such as the beginning of life, genetic testing and engineering, sex determination, the rights of the fetus, ownership of the fertilized egg, and so forth will not be easily answered. The council formulated an opinion regarding obstetric issues as fairly as possible that states the following:

ABORTION. As the law now stands, a physician may perform an abortion as long as state and federal laws are followed regarding the trimester in which it is performed. A physician who does not want to perform abortions cannot be forced to perform the procedure; that physician, however, should refer the patient to other health care professionals who can assist the patient.

GENETIC TESTING. If amniocentesis is performed on a mother and a genetic defect is found, both parents must be told. The parents may request or refuse to have the pregnancy terminated. (Amniocentesis is a procedure in which a needle is inserted in a pregnant woman's abdomen to remove and test amniotic fluid.

Many abnormalities and disorders can be diagnosed early in pregnancy by this procedure.)

ARTIFICIAL INSEMINATION. Artificial insemination involves the insertion of sperm into a woman's vagina for the purpose of conception. The donor may be the husband (artificial insemination by husband [AIH]) or an anonymous donor (artificial insemination by donor [AID]). The council states that both the husband and wife must consent to this procedure. If a donor is used, the sperm must be tested for infectious and genetic disorders. Complete confidentiality for the donor and recipient must be maintained.

 CHECKPOINT QUESTION

11. What is the opinion of the AMA's Council on Ethical and Judicial Affairs regarding abortion?

Stem Cell Research

As we continue to find new technologies, ethical dilemmas continue to emerge. Stem cell research is an ethical issue resulting from our ability to program the immature and undifferentiated cells of a fetus to be muscle, liver, or cardiac cells. The implications of this ability have become a political issue in the last several years. Researchers have found that stem cells taken from the umbilical cord of a newborn are also useful. It is even possible for parents to have the umbilical cord of their infant frozen and stored for use in later years to cure any diseases encountered. Some people believe that the potential to cure such diseases as Parkinson's disease and cystic fibrosis is worth using embryonic stem cells. Others believe that using fetal cells and tissue is immoral. The political debate about government funding of stem cell research continues.

Organ Transplantation

Organ transplantation became a medical option in the mid 1950s, although at that time, there were many problems with rejection of the organs by the recipient's immune system. When this postoperative complication was corrected by antirejection drugs, the practice became more common. Organs are viable (able to support life) for varying lengths of time, but most can be used successfully if transplanted within 24 to 48 hours. An organization in Richmond, Virginia, the United Network of Organ Sharing, coordinates local organ procurement teams that will fly to areas where organs are to be harvested to assist with the surgery if needed and to ensure the integrity of the organ. There are far fewer organs available than are needed, and every year, thousands of patients die who could have lived if an organ had been available.

The use of organs from a baby born without a brain (anencephaly) raises serious ethical issues. The council states that everything must be done for the infant until the determination of death can be made. For infant organs to be transplanted, both parents must consent.

The council's views on transplantation state:

- *The rights of the donor and organ recipient must be treated equally. The imminent death of the donor does not release the medical personnel from observing all rights that every patient is due.*
- *Organ donors must be given every medical opportunity for life. Life support is not removed until the patient is determined to have no brain activity and could not live without artificial support.*
- *Death of the donor must be determined by a physician who is not on the transplant team to avoid a charge of conflict of interest.*
- *Consent (permission) must be received from both the donor, if possible, and recipient before the transplant. Family members may give consent if the donor is unable to do so.*
- *Transplants can be performed only by surgeons who are qualified to perform this complex surgery and who are affiliated with institutions that have adequate facilities for the surgery and postoperative care.* Box 2-9 highlights the Uniform Anatomical Gift Act.

Withholding or Withdrawing Treatment

Physicians have a professional and ethical obligation to promote quality of life, which means sustaining life and relieving suffering. Sometimes, these obligations conflict with a patient's wishes. Patients have the right to refuse medical treatment and to request that life support or life-sustaining treatments be withheld or withdrawn. Withholding treatment means that certain medical treatments may not be initiated. Withdrawing treatment is terminating a treatment that has already begun. In 1991, congress passed the Self-Determination Act, which gave all hospitalized patients the right to make health care decisions on admission to the hospital. These decisions may be referred to as advance directives. Today, everyone is encouraged to participate in his or her own end-of-life decisions. You can go online and complete an advance directive. An **advance directive** is a statement of a person's wishes for medical decisions prior to a critical event. Advance directives may include specific wishes, such as whether a ventilator can be used, whether cardiopulmonary resuscitation (CPR) should be initiated, and whether a feeding tube should be inserted. Just completing an advance directive does not ensure that the patient's wishes will be carried out. It is important to make family members aware of these wishes. The patient's next of kin should keep a copy of the advance directive, and one should be placed in the medical office chart with special notation. Figure 2-5 is a sample of an advance directive.

BOX 2-9

UNIFORM ANATOMICAL GIFT ACT

Many organs can be transplanted, including the liver, kidney, cornea, heart, lung, and skin. To meet the growing need for organs and to allay the concern over donor standards, the National Conference of Commissioners for Uniform State Laws passed legislation known as the Uniform Anatomical Gift Act.

All acts include the following clauses:

- Any mentally competent person over age 18 may donate all or part of his or her body for transplantation or research.
- The donor's wishes supersede any other wishes except when state laws require an autopsy.
- Physicians accepting donor organs in good faith are immune from lawsuits against harvesting organs.
- Death of the donor must be determined by a physician not involved with the transplant team.
- Financial compensation may not be given to the donor or survivors.
- Persons wishing to donate organs can revoke permission or change their minds at any time.

In most states, the Department of Motor Vehicles asks applicants for a driver's license about organ donation and indicates their wishes on their license. In addition, an individual may declare the wish to donate all or parts of the body in a will or any legal document, including a Uniform Donor Card. Organ donors should make their families aware of their wishes to ensure they will be carried out.

CHECKPOINT QUESTION

12. What is an advance directive? How can a patient be sure his or her wishes will be followed?

Professional and Ethical Conduct and Behavior

The council states that all health care professionals are responsible for reporting unethical practices to the appropriate agencies. No health care professional should engage in any act that he or she feels is ethically or morally wrong.

Additionally, the council states:

- A physician must never assist or allow an unlicensed person to practice medicine.

- Hospitals and physicians must work together for the best care for patients. Hospitals should allow physicians staff privileges based on the ability of the physician, educational background, and the needs of the community. (Staff privileges allow physicians to admit their patients to a given hospital.) Issues of a personal nature must never be considered when accepting or declining a physician's application for privileges.
- It is unethical for physicians to admit patients to the hospital or to order excessive treatments for the sole purpose of financial rewards.

Ethical Issues in Office Management

As a medical assistant, you are directly involved in some of the council's guidelines regarding administrative issues. In relation to fees, the council states:

- Financial interests must never come above patient care. Ordering the most expensive tests or not ordering needed tests based on the patient's ability to pay is not acceptable.
- If a physician's office routinely charges patients for canceling appointments within 24 hours of the actual scheduled appointment, a warning must be posted to advise patients of this charge.
- The medical record must never be held against nonpayment of a bill.
- Fees cannot be excessive. They must be based on fair and standard charges for all patients. Guidelines for charges should consider the difficulty and unique nature of the services involved and the use of medical equipment.
- Interest on past due accounts can be charged in accordance with state laws and with prior notification to the patient.
- No fees can be charged for physician referrals or for admitting a patient to the hospital.
- A fee should not be charged to the patient for completing or filing a simple insurance form. If the form is extensive, a minimal fee may be charged.
- Caution must be used with computers to maintain patient confidentiality. If patient data are sent via fax machine, utmost care must be used to ensure that the material is received by only the correct recipient.
- If the physician advertises his or her practice, it must be done with the utmost honesty. Misrepresentation of information is never appropriate.
- If a physician closes the practice or dies, all patients must be notified that the office is closing and must be given instructions for retrieving their medical records. Generally, copies of medical records are transferred to another local physician. The originals are stored as directed by state law. Box 2-10 describes an ethical

ADVANCE DIRECTIVE

UNIFORM ADVANCE DIRECTIVE OF [list name of declarant]

To my family, physician, attorney, and anyone else who may become responsible for my health, welfare, or affairs, I make this declaration while I am of sound mind.

If I should ever become in a terminal state and there is no reasonable expectation of my recovery, I direct that I be allowed to die a natural death and that my life not be prolonged by extraordinary measures. I do, however, ask that medication be mercifully administered to me to alleviate suffering, even though this may shorten my remaining life.

This statement is made after full reflection and is in accordance with my full desires. I want the above provisions carried out to the extent permitted by law. Insofar as they are not legally enforceable, I wish that those to whom this will is addressed will regard themselves as morally bound by this instrument.

If permissible in the jurisdiction in which I may be hospitalized I direct that in the event of a terminal diagnosis, the physicians supervising my care discontinue feeding should the continuation of feeding be judged to result in unduly prolonging a natural death.

If permissible in the jurisdiction in which I may be hospitalized I direct that in the event of a terminal diagnosis, the physicians supervising my care discontinue hydration (water) should the continuation of hydration be judged to result in unduly prolonging a natural death.

I herewith authorize my spouse, if any, or any relative who is related to me within the third degree to effectuate my transfer from any hospital or other health care facility in which I may be receiving care should that facility decline or refuse to effectuate the instructions given herein.

I herewith release any and all hospitals, physicians, and others for myself and for my estate from any liability for complying with this instrument.

Signed:

_____

[list name of declarant]

City of residence: _____

[city of residence]

County of residence: _____

[county of residence]

State of residence: _____

[state of residence]

Social Security Number: _____

[social security number]

Date: _____

_____

Witness

_____

Witness

STATE OF _____

COUNTY OF _____

This day personally appeared before me, the undersigned authority, a Notary Public in and for _____ County, _____ State,

_____   _____

(Witnesses)

who, being first duly sworn, say that they are the subscribing witnesses to the declaration of [list name of declarant], the declarant, signed, sealed, and published and declared the same as and for his declaration, in the presence of both these affiants; and that these affiants, at the request of said declarant, in the presence of each other, and in the presence of said declarant, all present at the same time, signed their names as attesting witnesses to said declaration.

Affiants further say that this affidavit is made at the request of [list name of declarant], declarant, and in his presence, and that [list name of declarant] at the time the declaration was executed, in the opinion of the affiants, of sound mind and memory, and over the age of eighteen years.

Taken, subscribed and sworn to before me by _____(witness) and

_____ (witness) this _____ day of_____, 20_____.

My commission expires: _____

_____ Notary Public

Figure 2-5 Sample advance directive.

issue that might occur in a medical office. Read it carefully. If you were the physician, how would you handle the problem?

It is also your ethical responsibility to stay abreast of any changes in regulations or guidelines regarding health care. The medical field changes often. Procedure 2-1 outlines the steps for monitoring legislation for changes and updates.

BOX 2-10

ETHICAL DILEMMA

How would you handle the following hypothetical situation?

You are the office manager for a well-respected family physician in a small town. He is 70 years old and is starting to show signs of senile dementia. He is forgetful and has even been disoriented and confused a few times. No one else seems to have noticed. Should you report your concerns? If so, to whom?

The AMA Principles of Medical Ethics require that physicians, and medical assistants through the law of agency, report unethical behavior among colleagues. The medical profession is also governed by the patient's right to safety and quality care. It is your ethical responsibility to report the doctor's condition to the administration of the hospital where the physician has privileges or to the state board of medicine. The physician's family should be involved in the situation.

 CHECKPOINT QUESTION

13. What steps should be taken when a physician closes his or her practice?

 MEDIA MENU

- **Student CD**
  - **Case Studies**
    Administrative Interactive Case Study on Maintaining Medical Records and HIPAA; Managing a Medical Office Emergency Clinical Interactive Case Study on Triage in an Emergency Situation, Communication, and Documentation
  - **CMA/RMA Certification Exam Review**
- **Premium Online Course**
  http://thePoint.lww.com/Kronenberger3e
- **Internet Resources**

  LiveAdvise Online Tutoring & Competency Training
  http://thePoint.lww.com/LiveAdvise

  Websites to keep abreast of changes in the medical field:
  Go to your state's home page and click on the link to the state legislature to view pending state legislation.
  Go to The Library of Congress to view federal legislation to be considered in the coming week.
  http://Thomas.loc.gov

  Equal Employment Opportunity Commission
  http://www.eeoc.gov/

  US Department of Labor, Bureau of Labor Statistics
  http://stats.bls.gov

  To complete an advance directive
  http://www.legalzoom.com/

  To download and print a Vaccination Information Statement
  http://www.cdc.gov/nip/publications/VIS/default.htm

español SPANISH TERMINOLOGY

¿Usted entiende la información que acaba de recibir?

Do you understand the information I have given?

¿Usted nos autoriza a llevar a cabo este procedimiento médico?

Do you give us permission to perform this procedure?

Firme aquí, por favor.

Please sign here.

PROCEDURE 2-1: Monitoring Federal and State Regulations, Changes, and Updates

Purpose: To ensure compliance with regulations by keeping abreast of changes and actions affecting medical assisting issues and health care legislation

Equipment: Computer, Internet connection, search engine or website list

Steps	Reasons
1. Using a search engine, input the keywords for your state legislature, OR go to the homepage for your state government. Example: www.nc.gov	The best source for legislative changes is a state's legislative website.
2. Follow links to the legislative branch of your state.	The homepage will give you the appropriate links.
3. Search for such issues as health care finances, allied health professionals, outpatient medical care, Medicare, etc.	These general search words will lead you to information about current or pending legislation.
4. Read and share information from the Centers for Disease Control and Prevention (CDC), Occupational Safety and Health Act (OSHA), your state medical society, and the American Medical Association (AMA).	Information you receive from outside sources will keep you abreast of changes and trends. For example, OSHA informed providers about changes in the regulations for needle disposal.
5. Create and enforce a policy for timely dissemination of information received by fax or e-mail from outside agencies. OSHA and the CDC alert providers of vital information via fax or e-mail.	OSHA and the CDC alert providers of vital information via fax or e-mail.
6. Circulate information gathered to all appropriate employees with an avenue for sharing information. Any information obtained should be shared.	Any information obtained should be shared.
7. Post changes in a designated area of the office.	A break room or time clock area is a good place to display important information.

- The fields of medicine and law are linked in common concern for the patient's health and rights. Increasingly, health care professionals are the object of malpractice lawsuits.
- You can help prevent medical malpractice by acting professionally, maintaining clinical competency, and properly documenting in the medical record. Promoting good public relations between the patient and the health care team can avoid frivolous or unfounded suits and direct attention and energy toward optimum health care.
- Medical ethics and bioethics involve complex issues and controversial topics. There will be no easy or clear-cut answers to questions raised by these issues. As a medical assistant, your first priority must be to act as your patients' advocate, with their best interests and concerns foremost in your actions and interactions. You must always maintain ethical standards and report the unethical behaviors of others.
- Many acts and regulations affect health care organizations and their operations. A medical office must keep current on all legal updates.
- Most states publish a monthly bulletin that reports on new legislation. Every state has a website that will link you to legislative action. Read these on a regular basis.
- Each office should have legal counsel who can assist in interpreting legal issues.

Warm Ups for Critical Thinking

1. An acquaintance who knows you work in the medical field asks you to diagnose her rash. What do you say?
2. A patient owes a big bill at your office. She requests copies of her records. What do you do?
3. You suspect that a new employee in the office is misusing narcotics. What do you do?
4. Mrs. Rodriguez has bone cancer. Her doctor has estimated that she has 6 months to live. Mrs. Rodriguez wants the physician to withhold all medical treatments. She does not want chemotherapy or any life-sustaining measures. Her family disagrees. Should her family have any input into her health care decisions?
5. You are on your lunch hour from your job at a Planned Parenthood clinic. You run into the mother of a friend who happened to be seen earlier that day in your clinic. You say, "Hi, I just saw Heather this morning." Heather's mother says, "Oh, yes? And where did you see her?" What now? Discuss the need to think before you speak where confidentiality is concerned.

Answers to Checkpoint Questions

1. Criminal law deals wih the act of practicing medicine without a license.
2. When a physician changes the scope of his practice, patients should be given advance notice. A letter should be sent to each active patient, or an ad may be placed in a local newspaper.
3. The following elements must be in a physician's termination intent letter: statement of intent, explanation of reasons, termination date, availability of medical records, and a recommendation that the patient seek medical help as needed.
4. Never ask a patient to sign a consent form if the patient does not understand the procedure, has questions about the procedure, or is unable to read the consent form.
5. The six situations or conditions legally requiring disclosure are vital statistics, medical examiner reports, infectious diseases, abuse or maltreatment, violent injuries, and others according to state laws.
6. The four elements that must be proved in a negligence suit are duty, dereliction of duty, direct cause, and damages.
7. Assault is the attempt or threat to touch another person without permission; battery is the actual touching.
8. The law of agency implies that physicians are liable for the actions of their employees. The physician is responsible for your actions as a medical assistant, as long as your actions are within your scope of practice and you practice the standard of care required for your assigned duties and responsibilities.

9. Blood-borne pathogens are organisms that can be spread through direct contact with blood or body fluids from an infected person. OSHA governs their control in the medical office.

10. The three ethical standards the CMA must follow are protecting patient confidentiality, following laws, and being honest.

11. A physician may perform an abortion as long as state and federal laws are followed regarding the trimester in which an abortion may be performed. A physician who does not want to perform abortions cannot be forced to perform the procedure; that physician, however, should refer the patient to other health care professionals who can assist the patient.

12. An advance directive is a statement of a person's wishes for medical decisions prior to a critical event. Letting family know of these wishes and keeping a copy in the medical office chart will help ensure that these wishes are carried out.

13. If a physician closes the practice (or dies), all patients must be notified that the office is closing and must be given instructions for retrieving their medical records.

Communication Skills

Outline

Basic Communication Flow
Forms of Communication
  Verbal Communication
  Nonverbal Communication
Active Listening
Interview Techniques
  Reflecting
  Paraphrasing or Restatement
  Asking for Examples or
    Clarification
  Asking Open-Ended Questions
  Summarizing
  Allowing Silences

Factors Affecting
** Communication**
  Cultural Differences
  Stereotyping and Biased
    Opinions
  Language Barriers
Special Communication
** Challenges**
  Hearing-Impaired Patients
  Sight-Impaired Patients
  Speech Impairments
  Mental Health Illnesses
  Angry or Distressed Patients
  Children

Communicating With a
  Grieving Patient or Family
  Member
Establishing Postive Patient
** Relationships**
  Proper Form of Address
  Professional Distance
Teaching Patients
Professional Communication
  Communicating With Peers
  Communicating With
    Physicians
  Communicating With Other
    Facilities

Learning Objectives

Upon successfully completing this chapter, you will be able to:

1. Spell and define the key terms

2. List two major forms of communication

3. Explain how various components of communication can affect the meaning of verbal messages

4. Define active listening

5. List and describe the six interviewing techniques

6. Give an example of how cultural differences may affect communication

7. Discuss how to handle communication problems caused by language barriers

8. List two methods that you can use to promote communication among hearing-, sight-, and speech-impaired patients

9. Discuss how to handle an angry or distressed patient

10. List five actions that you can take to improve communication with a child

11. Discuss your role in communicating with a grieving patient or family member

12. List the five stages of grief as outline by Elisabeth Kubler-Ross

13. Discuss the key elements of interdisciplinary communication

CAAHEP

- Recognize and respond to verbal communications
- Recognize and respond to nonverbal communications

ABHES

- Be attentive, listen, and learn
- Recognize and respond to verbal and nonverbal communication
- Principles of verbal and nonverbal communication

Key Terms

anacusis	discrimination	messages	presbyacusis
bias	dysphasia	mourning	reflecting
clarification	dysphonia	nonlanguage	stereotyping
cultures	feedback	paralanguage	summarizing
demeanor	grief	paraphrasing	therapeutic

Communication is sending and receiving **messages** (information), verbally or otherwise. Until the message is received accurately, communication has not taken place. The ability to communicate effectively is a crucial skill for medical assistants. In your role, you must accurately and appropriately share information with physicians, other professional staff members, and patients. When communicating with patients, you must be able to receive messages correctly, interpret them, and respond to the sender appropriately. Proper grammar is important! Although you may speak in an informal way with family and friends, you must speak in a professional manner while at work. The medical assistant is usually the first person the patient meets in the medical office. Thus, your positive attitude, pleasant presentation, and use of good communication skills will set the tone for future interactions.

Basic Communication Flow

Communication requires the following elements:

- A message to be sent
- A person to send the message
- A person to receive the message

During the act of communicating, two or more people will alternate roles as sender and receiver as they seek **feedback** (responses) and **clarification** (understanding) regarding the message. The process of message ex-change is like a swing moving back and forth between two people. Figure 3-1 illustrates the flow of communication and its common components.

As a medical assistant, you will primarily be communicating in a therapeutic manner. This means that your communication will focus on conversations regarding pertinent topics relating to office procedures, policies, and patient care. Your other responsibilities for ensuring good communication include the following:

- Clarifying confusing messages
- Validating (confirming) the patient's perceptions
- Adapting messages to the patient's level of understanding
- Asking for feedback to ensure that the messages you sent were received by the patient or other persons as intended

 CHECKPOINT QUESTION

1. What three elements must be present for communication to occur?

Forms of Communication

Verbal Communication

Verbal communication involves an exchange of messages using words or language; it is the most commonly

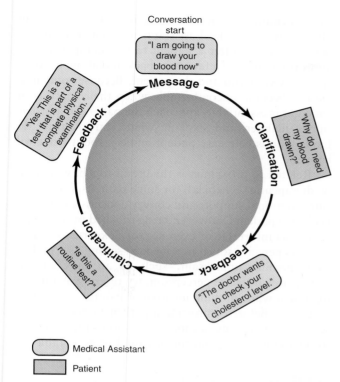

Conversation start
"I am going to draw your blood now"

Message

"Yes. This is a test that is part of a complete physical examination."

Feedback

"Why do I need my blood drawn?"

Clarification

"Is this a routine test?"

Clarification

"The doctor wants to check your cholesterol level."

Feedback

Medical Assistant

Patient

Figure 3-1 Flow of communication.

used form and is usually the initial form of communication. You need good verbal communication skills when performing such tasks as making appointments, providing patient education, making referrals, and sharing information with the physician.

Oral communication is sending or receiving messages using spoken language. As a professional, you should use a pleasant and polite manner of speaking. Use proper English and grammar at all times; lapsing into slang and colloquialisms projects an unprofessional image.

Gear your conversation to the patient's educational level. A well-educated patient may resent your using other than the correct terms, yet a less educated patient may be confused and intimidated by the same phrases. Avoid using elaborate medical terminology if you think it might confuse or frighten a patient. Will this patient understand "myocardial infarction," or should you say heart attack? Do not talk down to the patient, but do phrase your communication appropriately.

Be aware, too, that the meaning of spoken messages may be affected by other components of oral communication, including paralanguage and nonlanguage sounds. The cliché that it's not what you say but how you say it is true. Research shows that the primary message is transmitted more by the way it is said than by the words that are used. This refers to paralanguage. **Paralanguage** includes voice tone, quality, volume, pitch, and range. **Nonlanguage** sounds include laugh-

ing, sobbing, sighing, grunting, and so on. Other nonlanguage clues to understanding can be found in a speaker's grammatical structure, pronunciation, and general articulation, which can indicate regional or cultural background and level of education. Knowing this information can help you adapt responses and explanations to the patient's level of understanding.

Written communication uses written language to exchange messages. The ability to write clearly, concisely, and accurately is important in the health care profession (see Chapter 7). Typically, patients receive oral instructions first, as you or the physician explain key points of concern. These verbal instructions are then reinforced with written instructions (Box 3-1).

If the instructions, oral or written, are not clear, the patient may misinterpret them. This misunderstanding can hinder treatment and recovery and possibly even require the patient to be admitted to the hospital. Here is an example of an unclear instruction: "Return to the office if you don't feel better." This provides the patient with no details. Clearer instructions would state, "If your fever and sore throat are not better in 24 hours, call the office to schedule a revisit." Even the most clearly outlined instructions can be misunderstood, particularly by those with deficient hearing or reading abilities. As a medical assistant, you are responsible for asking questions to verify that the patient has correctly understood the information. To verify that the patient understood these instructions, a good question to ask would be, "When should you call the office if you don't feel better?"

 CHECKPOINT QUESTION

2. List five examples of paralanguage.

Nonverbal Communication

Nonverbal communication—exchanging messages without using words—is sometimes called body language. Body language includes several types of behaviors, such as kinesics, proxemics, and the use of touch. Kinesics refers to body movements, including facial expressions, gestures, and eye movements. A patient's face can sometimes reveal inner feelings, such as sadness, happiness, fear, or anger, that may not be mentioned explicitly during a conversation. Gestures also carry various meanings. For instance, shrugging the shoulders can mean simple lack of interest or hopeless resignation. Eyes can often hint at what a person may be thinking or feeling. For example, a patient whose eyes wander away from you while you are talking may be impatient, lack interest, or not understand what you are saying.

BOX 3-1

EXAMPLE OF WRITTEN DISCHARGE INSTRUCTIONS

Main Street Pediatric Group
343 Main Street, Suite 609
King, NC 27021

Instructions for Otitis Media

Your child has an ear infection. It is easily treated with antibiotics. Get the prescription filled immediately. The first dose should be given as soon as you arrive home. Read the attached information on the antibiotic.

Here are some other important things to remember:

- Ear infections are not contagious.
- Symptoms usually resolve within 24 hours of beginning antibiotics. It is very important to make sure your child takes all of the prescription.
- If the pain persists for more than 48 hours, call the office.
- If you see any blood in the ear canal, call the office.

Make an appointment for a follow-up visit in 2 weeks.

_____   _____
Patient's signature   Physician's signature

Nonverbal communication may more accurately reflect a person's true feelings and attitude than verbal communication. In other words, people may say one thing but show a completely different response with their body language. For example, if the patient says, "The pain in my foot is not too bad," but the patient's face shows pain with each step, the nonverbal clues demonstrate an inconsistent message. Many patients mask their feelings, so you must learn to read their actions and nonverbal clues in addition to what they tell you. Be aware that patients are also acutely attuned to your facial and nonverbal reactions. Responding with an expression of disgust or shaking your head in a negative way can jeopardize communication and rapport between you and the patient.

How and where individuals physically place themselves in relation to others can affect communication as well. Proxemics refers to spatial relationships or physical proximity tolerated by humans. Generally, the area within a 3-foot radius around a person is considered personal space and is not to be invaded by strangers, although this area varies among individuals and people of

various **cultures** (societies). To deliver care to a patient, physicians and medical assistants must enter a patient's personal space. After a patient task is completed, it is appropriate to take a few steps back and allow for more space between you and the patient. Because some individuals become uncomfortable when their space is invaded, it is essential to approach the patient in a professional manner and explain what you plan to do. Explanations help ease patient anxiety about what will happen.

Related to proxemics is the use of touch, which can be **therapeutic** (beneficial) for some patients. It can indicate emotional support and convey concern and feeling. For some patients, however, being touched by a stranger is an uncomfortable or even negative experience. Many patients perceive touch in a medical setting as a prelude to something unpleasant, such as an injection. To change this negative perception, try offering a comforting touch when nothing invasive or painful is imminent (Fig. 3-2). Before comforting a patient by touching, assess the patient's **demeanor** (expressions and behavior) for clues indicating that touch would be acceptable.

Active Listening

Active listening is important to ensure that messages are correctly received and interpreted. Failure to do so can result in poor patient care. To listen actively, you must give your full attention to the patient with whom you are speaking. Interruptions should be kept to a minimum. You need to focus not only on what is being said, but also on what is being conveyed through paralanguage, body language, and other aspects of communication. Occasionally, a patient's verbal messages may seem to conflict with the nonverbal messages. For example, a patient who is wringing his hands while telling you that everything is fine is sending conflicting signals that require further exploration. If a patient's verbal response

Figure 3-2 Therapeutic touch conveys caring and concern.

does not correspond to your observations, convey your concern to the physician.

Active listening is a skill that develops with practice. To test your listening ability, try the following exercise. Ask another student to speak continuously for 1 to 2 minutes while you listen. (The student should discuss a topic with which you are unfamiliar.) When he or she finishes, wait silently for the same amount of time. Then try to repeat the message. If you have trouble doing this exercise, you need to practice listening.

Interview Techniques

As a medical assistant, you are typically responsible for gathering initial information and updating existing information about the patients. This task is accomplished by interviewing the patient. The interview will consist of you asking certain questions and then interpreting the patient's responses. The initial interview includes many areas. The key areas are the patient's medical and family history, a brief review of the body systems, and a social history. Table 3-1 has sample questions that you may ask in each of these areas. The main goal is to ob-

tain accurate and pertinent information. The interview for an established patient, however, is much different. First, you should review the chart to look at the patient's health problems. Make a list of questions regarding the pertinent medical problems. Reconfirm medication usage and any specific treatments the patient is supposed to be doing.

To conduct either type of interview, you must use effective techniques: listen actively, ask the appropriate questions, and record the answers. During the interview, you must demonstrate professionalism. Begin by introducing yourself (Fig. 3-3). Always conduct the interview in a private area. Know what questions you need to ask and in what order to ask them before you begin the interview. Be organized. It is also helpful to have an extra pen. And most important, do not answer phone calls or attend to other distractions until you have finished the interview. Last, when you leave the room, let patients know who will be in to see them and the approximate time, for example, "Dr. Sanchez will be in to see you in about 10 minutes."

The six interviewing techniques are reflecting, paraphrasing, clarification, asking open-ended questions, summarizing, and allowing silences.

TABLE 3-1	Initial Patient Interview Components
Area	**Sample Questions**
Past medical history	Any previous hospitalizations? If so, when?
	Any previous surgeries? If so, when?
	Any chronic problems (e.g., asthma, diabetes, heart condition)?
	Any past pregnancies? Any complications?
	Any miscarriages, stillbirths, or abortions?
Family history	Age and health of parents?
	If deceased, what was the cause and at what age did they die?
	Age and health of siblings?
	Are there any genetic disorders?
Body system review	General questions regarding all body systems: cardiovascular, pulmonary, integumentary, musculoskeletal, neurologic, sensory, gastrointestinal, endocrine, immune, urologic, and reproductive
Social history	Alcohol use?
	Smoking?
	Drug use?
	Hobbies?
	Education?
	Employment?
Medications	What do you take? When? How much?
	Any vitamins or herbal supplements?

Figure 3-3 Begin the interview by introducing yourself.

Reflecting

Reflecting is repeating what you have heard the patient say, using open-ended statements. With this technique, you do not complete a sentence but leave it up to the patient to do so. For example, you might say, "Mrs. Rivera, you were saying that when your back hurts you . . . ." Reflection encourages the patient to make further comments. It also can help bring the patient back to the subject if the conversation begins to drift. (Reflecting is a useful tool, but be careful not to overuse it, because some patients find it annoying to have their words constantly parroted back.)

Paraphrasing or Restatement

Paraphrasing or restatement means repeating what you have heard, using your own words or phrases. Paraphrasing can help verify that you have accurately understood what was said. It also allows patients the opportunity to clarify their thoughts or statements. Typically, a paraphrased statement begins with "You are saying that . . . ," or "It sounds as if . . . ," followed by the rephrased content.

Asking for Examples or Clarification

If you are confused about some of the information you have received, ask the patient to give an example of the situation being described. For instance, "Can you describe one of these dizzy spells?" The patient's example should help you better understand what the patient is saying. It also may give you an insight into how the patient perceives the situation.

Asking Open-Ended Questions

The best way to obtain specific information is to ask open-ended questions that require the patient to formulate an answer and elaborate on the response. Open-ended questions usually begin with what, when, or how. For example, "What medications did you take this morning?" "When did you stop taking your medication?" "How did you get that large bruise on your arm?" Be careful about asking "why" questions, because they can often sound judgmental or accusing. For example, asking "Why did you do that?" or "Why didn't you follow the directions?" may imply to patients that you have already made a negative value judgment about their behavior, and they could become defensive and uncooperative. Instead, you might ask, "What part of the instructions did you not understand?" or "How can we help you follow these instructions?"

Avoid closed-ended questions that allow the patient to answer with one word, such as yes or no. For example, suppose you ask the patient, "Are you taking your medications?" The patient can easily say yes but may not be taking all of them. However, suppose you ask, "What medications do you take every day?" The patient's answer will give you a clearer understanding of whether the patient is taking the correct medications.

Summarizing

Briefly reviewing the information you have obtained, or **summarizing**, gives the patient another chance to clarify statements or correct misinformation. This technique can also help you organize complex information or events in sequential order. For example, if the patient has been feeling dizzy and stumbling a lot, you might summarize by saying, "You told me that you have been feeling dizzy for the past 3 days and that you frequently stumble as you are walking."

Allowing Silences

Periods of silence sometimes occur during the interview. These can be beneficial. Some people are uncomfortable with prolonged silences and feel a need to break the silence with words in an effort to jump-start a stalled conversation. Silences are natural parts of conversations and can give patients time to formulate their thoughts, reconstruct events, evaluate their feelings, or assess what has already been said. During moments of silence, gather your thoughts and formulate any additional questions that you may have.

 CHECKPOINT QUESTION

3. What are the six interviewing techniques?

Factors Affecting Communication

Sometimes, despite your best efforts, others may not receive your message accurately. A common occurrence that causes messages to be misinterpreted is the use of a cliché. For example, suppose you are teaching a patient to use crutches and she is having difficulty managing them. A cliché comment may be, "Don't worry. Rome wasn't built in a day. This takes time." The cliché is innocent and not meant to be demeaning, but the patient may misinterpret it to mean that she is slow, ancient. A more positive message would be, "I can see that you are making progress. Let's try walking down the hallway."

Here are some reasons for miscommunication:

1. The message may have been unclear or inappropriate to the situation. For example, "I have scheduled you for a PET scan in radiology tomorrow at 8 AM" Keep in mind that most of your patients do not understand medical abbreviations and terms. Since positron emission tomography (PET) is a newer technology, they may confuse it with computed tomography (CT). Also, where is radiology? A better message would be, "The doctor wants you to have a test done tomorrow. It is called a PET scan; here is a brochure that explains it. Go to the second floor of the outpatient center on Main Street. Do you know how to get there?"

2. The person receiving the message may have been distracted, anxious, or confused. A common cause of distraction is pain. For example, teaching a patient how to use crutches cannot be done if the patient's ankle or knee still hurts. The concentration will be on the pain, not on what you are saying. Patients who have just received positive news can also be anxious to contact loved ones. This is commonly seen with patients who have just been told that they are pregnant. The patient's focus is on calling family members and not on your conversation.

3. Environmental elements, such as noise or interruptions, may also distort messages. Environmental noises from staff lounges or break rooms can easily be overheard. Keep the doors to these areas closed. Cleaning staff should not be vacuuming or emptying trash while patients are present.

In addition to these three items, other factors may affect communication. They are discussed next.

Cultural Differences

The way a person perceives situations and other people is greatly influenced by cultural, social, and religious beliefs or firmly held convictions. Personal values (principles or ideals) are commonly developed from these same beliefs. As a medical assistant, you will interact with people from varied ethnic backgrounds and cultural origins who bring with them beliefs and values that may differ from your own. Understanding those differences can aid communication and thereby improve patient care (Table 3-2). It is very important that you not form preconceived ideas about a given culture. Remember that each of your patients is unique and that their health care needs differ.

Some cultures may be offended by the types of intensely personal questions necessary for a medical history and may perceive them as an inexcusable invasion of privacy. If this occurs, your physician may be required to intervene to allay the patient's concerns.

Looking someone else directly in the eyes, or eye contact, is also perceived differently by people of various backgrounds. Eye contact occurs more often among friends and family members than among acquaintances or strangers. In the United States, someone who maintains good eye contact is usually perceived as being honest, believable, and concerned. In contrast, in some Asian and Mideastern cultures, direct eye contact is perceived as sexually suggestive or disrespectful. In other cultures, lack of eye contact or casting the eyes downward is a sign of respect.

In addition to cultural differences in values, many differences occur among individuals. Some people are just more reserved or shy than others and may feel less comfortable in medical settings. To help avoid miscommunication and offending patients, you must be sensitive to these differences in all of your patient interactions.

Stereotyping and Biased Opinions

Medical assisting deals with people of different ages, races, and sexual orientation. Sometimes, your values may be in stark contrast to those held by a patient, but you should not let your personal values or **biases** (opinions) affect your communication or treatment of a patient. All patients must be treated fairly, respectfully, and with dignity, regardless of their cultural, social, or personal values. To treat them in any other fashion is **discrimination**.

Stereotyping is holding an opinion of all members of a particular culture, race, religion, age group, or other group based on oversimplified or negative characterizations. It is a form of prejudice. Examples of negative stereotypes include "All old people are frail and senile" and "Those people are always dirty and never bathe." Stereotyping and prejudice are deterrents to establishing therapeutic relationships because they do not allow for patients' individuality and can prevent quality care from being given to everyone on an equal basis.

TABLE 3-2	Cultural Factors That Affect Patient Care[a]		
Cultural Group	**Family**	**Folk and Traditional Health Care**	**Common Health Problems**
White	Nuclear family is highly valued Elderly family members may live in a nursing home when they can no longer care for themselves	Self-diagnosis of illnesses Use of over-the-counter drugs, especially vitamins and analgesics Dieting, especially fad diets Extensive use of exercise and exercise facilities	Cardiovascular disease Gastrointestinal disease Some forms of cancer Motor vehicle accidents Suicide Mental illness Substance abuse
African American	Close and supportive extended-family relationships Strong kinship ties with nonblood relatives from church or organizational and social groups Family unity, loyalty, and cooperation are important. Frequently matriarchal	Varies extensively and may include spiritualists, herb doctors, root doctors, conjurers, skilled elder family members, voodoo, faith healing	Hypertension Sickle cell anemia Skin disorders; inflammation of hair follicles, various types of dermatitis and excessive growth of scar tissue (keloids) Lactose enzyme deficiency resulting in poor toleration of milk products High rate of tuberculosis Diabetes mellitus Higher infant mortality rate than in the white population
Asian	Welfare of the family is valued above the individual person Extended families are common A person's lineage (ancestors) is respected Sharing among family members is expected	Theoretical basis in Taoism, which seeks balance in all things Good health is achieved through proper balance between yin (feminine, negative, dark, cold) and yang (masculine, positive, light, warm) An imbalance in energy is caused by an improper diet or strong emotions Diseases and food are classified as hot or cold, and a proper balance between them will promote wellness (e.g., treat a cold disease with hot foods) Many Asian health care systems use herbs, diet, and application of hot or cold therapy Many Asians believe some points on the body are on the meridians, or energy pathways; if the energy flow is out of balance, treatment of the pathways may be necessary to restore the energy equilibrium *Acumassage:* Manipulation of points along the energy pathways *Acupressure:* Technique for compressing the energy pathway points *Acupuncture:* Insertion of fine needles into the body at energy pathway points	Tuberculosis Communicable diseases Malnutrition Suicide Various forms of mental illness Lactose enzyme deficiency

(continued)

TABLE **3-2**	**Cultural Factors That Affect Patient Care**[a] *(continued)*		
Cultural Group	**Family**	**Folk and Traditional Health Care**	**Common Health Problems**
Hispanic, Mexican American	Familial role is important *Compadrazgo:* Special bond between a child's parents and grandparents Family is the primary unit of society	*Curanderas(os):* Folk healers who base treatments on humoral pathology: basic functions of the body are controlled by four body fluids, or humors—blood, hot and wet; yellow bile, hot and dry; black bile, cold and dry; and phlegm, cold and wet. The secret of good health is to balance hot and cold within the body; therefore, most foods, beverages, herbs, and medications are classified as hot (caliente) or cold (fresco, frio); a cold disease will be cured with a hot treatment	Diabetes mellitus and its complications Problems of poverty, such as poor nutrition, inadequate medical care, and poor prenatal care Lactose enzyme deficiency
Hispanic, Puerto Rican	*Compadrazgo:* similar to Mexican-American culture	Similar to that of other Spanish-speaking cultures	Parasitic diseases, such as dysentery, malaria, filariasis, hookworms Lactose enzyme deficiency
Native American	Families large and extended Grandparents are official and symbolic leaders and decision makers A child's namesake may assume equal parenting authority with biological parents	Medicine men (shamans) are frequently consulted Heavy use of herbs and psychological treatments, ceremonies, fasting, meditation, heat, and massage	Alcoholism Suicide Tuberculosis Malnutrition Communicable diseases Higher maternal and infant mortality rates than in most of the population Diabetes mellitus Hypertension Gallbladder disease

Reprinted with permission from Taylor C, Lillis C, LeMone P. Fundamentals of Nursing, 2nd ed. Philadelphia: Lippincott-Raven, 1996:122–125.

[a] The beliefs and practices vary within each group, and no assumptions should be based on a patient's cultural background alone. The factors in this table are merely a guide to some commonly observed and documented cultural factors.

As a health care professional, you are expected to treat all patients impartially, to guard against discriminatory practices, remain nonjudgmental, avoid stereotypes, and have a professional demeanor. By doing so, you communicate to patients that you accept human differences and that quality health care will be provided to all those who seek it.

Let's suppose Ms. Henry arrives with her 3-year-old daughter for a checkup. The mother says, "I think she has gotten head lice from someone at the shelter." Which response would be most appropriate? "Don't worry about it. The shelter is full of people with lice. Do you know anyone with lice?" or "I will mention to the doctor that you are concerned that she may have lice. Is anyone else in your family being treated for lice?" The latter response demonstrates appropriate caring and concern. It also begins the dialogue for determining additional people who may need to be checked, which is key to preventing community outbreaks. The first response communicates stereotyping of a particular lifestyle and prevents collection of additional data.

Language Barriers

Effective communication depends on the use of language, but some patients cannot speak or understand English well enough for good communication. Because it is crucial for you to give and receive accurate information, you will need to use an interpreter to help bridge any language barriers. A staff person might serve as the interpreter, or an English-speaking member of the patient's family may be able to help. In either case, be sure the interpreter fully understands what you are saying. In the absence of a reliable interpreter, a phrase book of common medical questions with lists of possible answers may be of help. If your area has a large population of non–English-speaking patients, your office should be equipped with an appropriate phrase book. (See Appendix B for a list of key health care phrases in English and Spanish.)

When choosing an interpreter, try to find someone of the same sex as the patient because certain cultures prohibit members of the opposite sex (even family members) from discussing personal issues about the body. Some cultures follow religious guidelines dictating how members of the opposite sex should interact with each other.

Use the following suggestions for communicating with non–English-speaking patients:

1. Do not shout. Raising your voice will not increase their understanding.
2. Demonstrate or pantomime as needed. Gestures are usually relatively universal.
3. If you are using an interpreter, speak directly to the patient, with the interpreter in your line of vision, so that the patient can read your facial expressions.
4. Speak slowly with simple sentences and phrases that require simple answers. The patient may comprehend some simple English.
5. Avoid slang; it may not translate well.
6. Avoid distractions and provide a relaxed, quiet interview space.
7. Learn some basic phrases of the most common language used in your area. Patients appreciate your effort.

Special Communication Challenges

Many situations present special communication challenges. For instance, hearing- or sight-impaired patients, young children, patients with limited understanding, those who are too ill or sedated to comprehend, and those who are frightened or anxious require particular attention. In each instance, you will need to assess the situation and the patient's ability to comprehend. In some cases, a responsible family member will be with the patient and can be included in the communication process. Never exclude the patient from the exchange, but do ensure that all needed information is communicated, whether you obtain the information through questions about the patient's condition or you give instructions for further care. Patients must feel that they are part of the process even if their condition requires involvement by family members or other caregivers.

Hearing-Impaired Patients

There are many forms of hearing impairments. Impairments can vary from a partial loss to **anacusis**, complete hearing loss. The two types of impairments are conductive and sensorineural. Conductive hearing loss is caused by interference with sound in the external canal or the middle or inner ear. Sensorineural hearing loss is caused by lesions or problems with either nerves or the cochlea. The cochlea is a coiled tubular structure that turns vibrations into sounds. Most patients with anacusis are adept with communicating through sign language, interpreters, or other tools. However, patients with **presbyacusis**, a common hearing impairment in older patients, often have a more difficult time communicating and tend to be in denial about their hearing abilities. Patients with presbyacusis benefit from hearing aids and other amplification devices.

To communicate with patients who have trouble hearing what you are saying, you need tact, diplomacy, and patience. These suggestions may help.

1. Touch the patient gently to gain his or her attention.
2. Talk directly face-to-face with the patient, not at an angle and certainly not with your back turned.
3. Turn to the most prominent light so that your face is illuminated.
4. Lower the pitch of your voice, since higher pitches are frequently lost with nerve impairment, but speak distinctly and with force. In most instances, shouting does not help and will only distort what might be heard.
5. Use note pads or demonstration as needed.
6. Pictograms are very helpful and should be readily available. A pictogram is a flash card that shows basic medical terms (Fig. 3-4).
7. Use short sentences with short words. Enunciate clearly, but do not exaggerate your facial movements.
8. Eliminate all distractions. Extraneous noises may confuse the patient.

If you need to call a hearing-impaired patient, keep in mind that patients can make and receive calls using a special telephone with a service called converse communication center, which uses a system called telecommunication device for the deaf (TDD) or a text telephone (TTY). If your office has either of these types of phones, you call the patient and type in your message. The patient reads your message and types a response. If your office does not have one of these phones, your local telephone company can communicate with TDD/TTY users and nonusers. Check your telephone directory for more information. Most hospitals have TDD/TTY phones available.

 CHECKPOINT QUESTION

4. How does the TDD system work?

Sight-Impaired Patients

Sight impairments range from complete blindness to blurred vision. The changes in vision tend to be slow and progressive. Some common medical conditions that can cause visual impairment include cataracts, glaucoma, macular degeneration, retinal detachment, hyperopia (farsightedness), myopia (nearsightedness), nyctalopia (night blindness), retinopathy, strabismus, and presbyopia. Patients who cannot see lose valuable information from nonverbal communication. To improve communication with a sight-impaired patient, try these suggestions.

1. Identify yourself by name each time the patient comes into the office.
2. Do not raise your voice; the patient is not hearing impaired.
3. Let the patient know exactly what you will be doing at all times, and alert him or her before touching.

 WHAT IF?

A patient is hearing impaired, and you cannot communicate with him to explain the procedure you are about to perform. What should you do?

If the patient does not understand the procedure, he or she is not *informed*. Legally, you have not met your responsibilities to obtain informed consent if the patient does not understand the information you are trying to convey. If the patient cannot provide his or her own assistance, it is the legal responsibility of the physician and his agents to provide the means for effective communication (see Chapter 2 for more information about informed consent).

Most community colleges offer courses in sign language. The Internet offers a site for the deaf community that will direct you to resources in your area. The American Sign Language alphabet chart is available online. It can be printed out for use with hearing-impaired patients. Handspeak is another website that provides a visual language dictionary. These websites are listed at the end of this chapter.

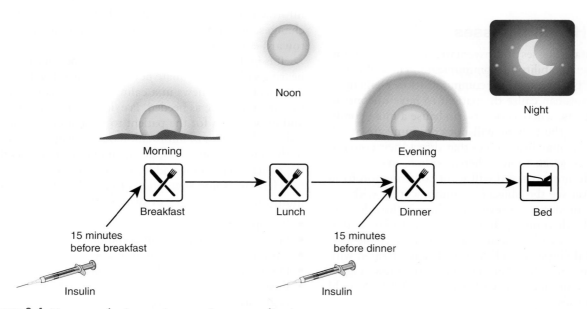

Figure 3-4 Pictogram for instructing a patient on medication route.

4. Orient the patient spatially by having him or her touch the table, the chair, the counter, and so forth.

5. Assist the patient by offering your arm and escorting him or her to the interview room.

6. Tell the patient when you are leaving the room and knock before entering.

7. Explain the sounds of machines to be used in the examination (e.g., buzzing, whirring) and what each machine will do.

Speech Impairments

Speech impairments can come from a variety of medical conditions. The medical term for difficulty with speech is **dysphasia**. Dysphasia is usually the result of a neurologic problem. A common neurologic condition that can result in dysphasia is a stroke. **Dysphonia** is a voice impairment that is caused by a physical condition, such as oral surgery, cancer of the tongue or voice box, or cleft palate. Stuttering is another medical condition that can impair the patient's ability to communicate.

Here are some suggestions to help you communicate with a patient who has a speech impediment:

- Allow such patients time to gather their thoughts.
- Allow plenty of time for them to communicate.
- Do not rush conversations.
- Offer a note pad to write questions.
- Discuss with the physician the potential benefits for getting a speech therapist referral for the patient.

 CHECKPOINT QUESTION

5. What is the difference between dysphasia and dysphonia?

Mental Health Illnesses

Many mental illnesses and psychiatric disorders can impair a patient's ability to communicate. These illnesses produce a broad range of communication challenges. Some illnesses can cause the patient to have uncontrollable outbursts, whereas others can cause a mute condition in which the patient will not communicate at all. Some patients may hear voices that direct their communication to a given topic, whereas others may see objects that do not exist and will want confirmation from you that you see the objects. Communicating with patients with moderate to severe psychiatric disorders requires in-depth training. It is important to stress that not all patients with mental illnesses will be challenges. Most mental illnesses can be controlled and treated with medications and other therapies. Here are a few suggestions for communicating with patients who have mild mental illnesses.

- Tell the patient what to expect and when things will happen.
- Keep conversations focused and professional.
- Do not force or demand answers from patients who are withdrawn or mute.
- If you feel unsafe communicating with a given patient, speak to either your supervisor or the physician regarding your concerns.
- Do not confirm hearing voices or seeing nonexistent objects.
- Orient the patient to reality as appropriate.

Patients with a history of substance abuse, alcoholism, and other addictions can also present a communication challenge. Patients may have euphoria and communicate with a flight of ideas. Or they may demonstrate aggression and agitation while they are withdrawing from the addiction. Your responsibility in communicating with patients who have any of these conditions is to identify the reasons for today's visit and follow your regular assessment duties. It is not the role of the medical assistant to recommend treatments or counseling for these patients. Your communication should be professional, nonjudgmental, and encouraging when appropriate.

Angry or Distressed Patients

Patients' emotions can run the spectrum from polite and cordial to angry and upset. There are numerous reasons for the latter. Prolonged waiting times, financial issues, and illness can spark untoward emotions. At some time in our lives, we all have had a cold, felt terrible, and snapped angrily at an innocent bystander. The key to communicating with upset patients is to prevent an escalation of the problem (Box 3-2). Keep your patients informed about waiting times, billing and insurance changes, and other office policies that might trigger untoward emotions.

It is understandable that patients will become upset on hearing sad or unfortunate news about their health. Most patients take sad news in a calm manner. It is important to offer assistance as needed. Provide written instructions and information for the patient to read later. This material should consist of information on the diagnosis, causes of the illness, treatment options, and phone numbers that the patient may call for additional information.

Here are some suggestions that will help you communicate with an angry or distressed patient.

- Be supportive.
- Be open and honest in all communication.
- Do not provide false reassurances.
- Do not belittle the problem or concern.
- Ensure your own safety if the angry patient becomes aggressive or threatening.

BOX 3-2

CASE SCENARIO: COMMUNICATING WITH A PATIENT WHO IS UPSET

Mr. Hunt, an elderly, long-time patient, calls the office and asks to speak to the doctor. When you inquire about the nature of his call, he begins to get louder and more upset.

Note: When patients ask to speak directly to the doctor, it is usually because they don't understand the workings of the office. Let the patient know that it is your job to screen the doctor's calls.

Mr. Hunt: "I just got this bill in the mail, and it says that I owe Dr. Smith $152.00. He is crazy if he thinks I'm paying this."

Note: Patients will say things they regret later. You may want to just let this one go.

Medical Assistant (MA): "I would be glad to help you with this, Mr. Hunt. Please hold while I look at your account."

Note: Putting the patient on hold may calm him down.

Mr. Hunt: "I'm not holding on very long."

Note: You can assure him that you will be right back.

MA: "I see that your balance is $152.00, Mr. Hunt, but you may make arrangements to pay this over several months."

Note: Giving the patient options may calm him down.

Mr. Hunt: "I'm not paying it at all because Dr. Smith didn't help me. I'm no better."

Note: A statement like this is upsetting, but you must remain professional.

MA: "I'm so sorry you are not feeling better, but Dr. Smith performed a service that you agreed to pay for. I will be happy to make you another appointment to come in and talk with him about a different course of treatment."

Note: Be firm but kind. Hopefully being firm will let the patient know who is in charge, but kindness will help defuse the anger.

Mr. Hunt: "I'll make an appointment, but I am not paying until I talk to the doctor."

Note: Again, you must not show your own feelings.

MA: "I will make a note of that on your account, and we can see you tomorrow at 9:30. Is that all right?"

Note: Documenting the patient's call will alert anyone working with the account. You would not want to add fuel to the flame by sending him another bill right away or making a collection call.

Mr. Hunt: "I'll be there, but you can tell that doctor that I'll have a thing or two to say to him."

Note: Document the conversation in the chart and be sure that the physician knows what to expect during the visit.

MA: "I hope we can resolve this, Mr. Hunt. We will see you tomorrow."

Note: You must remain calm and in control of the conversation.

Children

Levels of comprehension vary greatly during childhood, and therefore, communication needs must be tailored to the specific child's needs. The following suggestions will help facilitate communication:

1. Children are responsive to eye-level contact. Either raise them to your height or lower yourself to theirs (Fig. 3-5).
2. Keep your voice low-pitched and gentle.
3. Make your movements slow and keep them visible. Tell children when you need to touch them.
4. Rephrase your questions until you are sure that the child understands.
5. Be prepared for the child to return to a lower developmental level for comfort during an illness. For example, a child may revert to thumb sucking during a stressful event.
6. Use play to phrase your questions and to gain the child's cooperation. (For example, if the child appears shy and does not want to talk, start by asking the child how a stuffed animal feels today. "How

Figure 3-5 The medical assistant communicates at the child's eye level.

does teddy feel today?" Follow up on the child's answer with "And how do you feel?" Offering to take the teddy's temperature first may lessen any fear of thermometers.)

7. Allow the child to express fear, to cry, and so on.

8. Many adolescents resent authority. During the interview, some teenagers may not want a parent in the room. Assess the situation before including the parent.

9. Never show shock or judgment when dealing with adolescents; this will immediately close communication.

Communicating With a Grieving Patient or Family Member

Occasionally, you will need to support patients who are in **grief** or great sadness caused by a loss. Grieving starts when a person experiences a significant loss, such as the loss of a loved one through death or the end of a relationship, a body part, or personal health. Grief includes such emotional responses as anger, sadness, and depression, and each emotion may trigger certain behaviors. For example, anger may result in outbursts, sadness may cause crying, and depression may lead to unusual quietness or isolation.

Dr. Elisabeth Kubler-Ross identified five distinct stages in the human grieving process. In her book *On Death and Dying*, she lists these stages that follow the realization that a person has a terminal illness: denial, anger, bargaining, depression, and acceptance. Dr. Kubler-Ross believed that these stages are also found in those experiencing change. Box 3-3 outlines these stages with examples. These stages may spread over months or years. It is possible to go through stages more than once. Sometimes, the collective signs of grief are referred to as **mourning**.

In medical settings, expect to see grief displayed in many ways. Know, too, that several factors can influence how a patient demonstrates grief and that different cultures and individuals demonstrate their grief in a variety of ways, ranging from stoic, impassive responses to loud, prolonged wailing and fainting. Other responses may reflect religious beliefs about the meaning of death. Grieving is a unique and personal process. There is no set time period for grieving, and there is no "right" way to grieve. It is very important to remember that everyone grieves in their way at their own pace.

Grieving patients may want to talk about their feelings and review events. Terminally ill patients may want to discuss their fears of dying and concerns for surviving loved ones. Many times, it is too difficult to discuss dying with family members. Dying patients may want to spare their family's feelings. To support grieving patients, allow time for them to express themselves and actively listen to what they say. When appropriate, con-

---

> ### BOX 3-3
>
> ### THE FIVE STAGES OF GRIEVING AS IDENTIFIED BY ELISABETH KUBLER-ROSS
>
> | Mechanism | Quote |
> |---|---|
> | Denial | "The doctor must have read the test wrong." "I don't have cancer; I feel fine." |
> | Anger | "I hate the doctor." "This is a terrible place." |
> | Bargaining | "God, I will be the best person I can be if you take away this disease." |
> | Depression | "I don't care if I live anymore." |
> | Acceptance | "I understand that I have terminal disease and am going to die." |

sider using touch to convey your understanding. If patients' concerns stem from a lack of understanding about their condition, provide pertinent education for them and for their caregivers (if appropriate). You should also become familiar with available community resources, such as grief or other counseling services and hospice care, so you can assist the patient and physician when these services are necessary.

It is normal for you to feel sad when a patient dies. It is important that your communication focuses on empathy, not sympathy. Many psychologists describe sympathy as feeling *for* someone and empathy as feeling *with* someone. In the health care setting, empathy means trying to understand what patients are feeling so you can help them. Empathy can help you recognize a patient's fear and discomfort so you can do everything possible to provide support and reassurance. Sympathy, or pitying your patient, may compromise your professional distance and cause you to become personally involved. Box 3-4 offers suggestions for helping grieving patients.

 CHECKPOINT QUESTION

6. What are the five stages of grieving?

Establishing Positive Patient Relationships

Your approach to patients conveys a message about who you are and how you feel about yourself and your profession. Medical assistants can be role models, earning the trust and admiration of patients. To establish

BOX 3-4

COMMUNICATING WITH A GRIEVING FAMILY MEMBER OR PATIENT

Patients and families faced with great loss can be helped through a variety of community resources. Hospice is national program that offers support to patients and family members dealing with a loss. Hospice deals with all types of medical conditions and with people of all ages. The earlier the patient is introduced to a hospice program, the more beneficial. Hospice does have a palliative component. Hospice staff and volunteer grief counselors are trained to answer the questions, acknowledge the fears and anger, ease the transition, and offer respite for caregivers. A patient must never be forced to use hospice or other community resources. Grieving is an individual experience. Your local hospital may also have grief counselors or social workers who can help your patients. Other community resources may be available. The knowledgeable medical assistant will, with the physician's permission, direct the patient and the family to the proper organization.

and maintain positive relationships with patients, speak respectfully and exhibit an appropriate demeanor during all interactions.

Proper Form of Address

The way you address patients provides clues about your attitude and how you will likely provide care. When greeting patients, use a proper form of address, for example, "Good morning, Mr. Jones!" or "How are you feeling, Mrs. Smith?" This type of address shows respect and sets a professional tone. In contrast, calling patients by pet names, such as sweetie, granny, gramps, or honey, can offend the person. These terms denigrate the individual's dignity and put the interaction on a personal, not professional, level. Always call patients by their last name unless and until they instruct you otherwise. Some people are bothered or offended by being addressed by their first names; others prefer it. When patients indicate a preference or ask you specifically to use their first name, document this in the chart so others will know.

Other inappropriate forms of address include referring to the patient as a medical condition, such as "the gallbladder in room 2" or "the broken arm in the waiting room." Patients often come to the medical office feeling anxious, so they may be particularly sensitive to everything they see and hear (or overhear). Referring to

the patient as a medical condition sends the message that the staff values the patient as nothing more than an illness, which can lead to heightened anxiety.

Professional Distance

How people interact with each other is influenced by the level of emotional involvement between them. For instance, communication between a husband and wife is more intimate than the personal level of communication between friends or the social level of communication between acquaintances. In the health care setting, you must establish an appropriate level of communication to be effective. You should not become too personally involved with patients because doing so may jeopardize your ability to be objective. It is easy to become overattached, especially to elderly patients who are lonely. For example, do not offer to drive patients to appointments, pick up prescriptions, or do their grocery shopping. Keeping a professional distance allows you to deal objectively with patients while creating a therapeutic environment. To keep this distance, avoid revealing intimate information about yourself (e.g., marital woes, financial troubles, family conflict) that might shift the dynamics of the relationship to a more personal level. Small talk may put a patient at ease, and you may need to distract a patient who is going through an unpleasant treatment or procedure, but be careful to choose general topics and keep the conversation light. Often, in an attempt to comfort a patient, we might say, "My grandmother was diagnosed with cancer too, but she is fine; it's not a big deal. You will be okay too." Every situation is different. The patient may misinterpret this to mean that you don't think that his or her diagnosis of cancer is a big deal. But at that moment, it is a very big deal to the patient!

Teaching Patients

One of the fundamental communication skills you will need is the ability to teach patients about their medical conditions. (See Chapter 4.) Teaching patients might involve something as relatively simple as explaining how often they should take a medication or instructing a newly diagnosed diabetic patient about self-injection. The guidelines listed below incorporate such key communication skills as interviewing and active listening. Follow these to provide effective patient education.

1. Be knowledgeable about current medical issues, discoveries, and trends.
2. Be aware of special services available in your area.
3. Have pertinent handouts or information sheets available.
4. Allow enough teaching time so that you are not interrupted or rushed.
5. Find a quiet room away from the main office flow if at all possible.

6. Give information in a clear, concise, sequential manner; provide written instructions as a follow-up.
7. Allow the patient time to process this new information.
8. Encourage the patient to ask questions.
9. Ask open-ended questions in a way that will allow you to know whether the patient understands the material.
10. Invite the patient to call the office with additional questions that may arise.

Professional Communication

Communicating With Peers

Communication among your peers must remain professional and appropriate throughout the workday. Discussions of non–work-related topics should be kept to a minimum and occur only during designated break times. It is not appropriate to discuss last night's TV shows, family issues, shopping lists, and so on in front of patients. Excessive laughing, high-pitched voice tones, and whispering can produce an unprofessional atmosphere.

During your career, you may come across a situation that requires communication with your supervisor about another peer's actions. Your communication must always be honest and accurate when reporting facts to a supervisor. Embellishing or hiding information can result in termination of your employment.

An excellent way to promote communication among your peers is to become active in your local professional organization. Your involvement at the local level can spread to national exposure. Involvement in local community organizations and support groups is also beneficial to promoting you and your profession.

Communicating With Physicians

Physicians and other health care practitioners will rely on you to communicate pertinent information to patients in a timely manner to provide quality care. Your communication must always be professional. The physician should always be addressed as doctor unless he specifies otherwise. The use of inappropriate terms is never acceptable. When possible, the correct medical terminology should be used. If you are unsure of the correct medical term, however, explain the condition rather than use a term that you do not understand. For example, if a patient comes into the office with a chief complaint of difficulty urinating, simply say, "Mr. Bowen is complaining of trouble urinating." Never use a slang expression, such as "He is having trouble peeing."

Do not feel intimidated when speaking to a physician. Speak slowly and confidently and you will develop a professional rapport. Be honest. It is better to say, "I am not sure what to do with this specimen" than to assume and make a mistake.

Remember, there is a time and place for everything. The physician may be the biggest jokester or sports fan in the office, but it is not appropriate to draw on these topics in front of patients or family members.

Communicating With Other Facilities

The medical administrative staff often makes referrals to other facilities or physicians. Box 3-5 has examples of various referrals you might make. No matter who you are contacting, follow these key points:

- Maintain patient confidentiality. Make sure you have appropriate patient consent.
- Observe all legal requirements for dispensing patient data.
- Use caution with fax machines, e-mail, and other electronic devices. Make sure the intended receiver is the one who gets the communication.
- Provide only the facts. Do not relay suspicions or assumptions.
- Always be nonjudgmental.
- Confirm that the message was received and that the referral will be handled.

BOX 3-5

TYPES OF REFERRALS

Numerous types of referrals can be made. Here are some of the most common examples:

Cardiac rehabilitation
Diabetes education
Dietitian
Home care services
Laboratory studies
Occupational therapy
Physician specialties (cardiologist, pulmonologist, podiatrist)
Physical therapy
Psychotherapy
Radiology
Social worker
Speech therapy

ETHICAL TIP

All patient communication is confidential. Patient information is sometimes discussed unintentionally, however. To avoid breaching confidentiality, follow these guidelines:

- Do not discuss patients' problems in public places, such as elevators or parking lots. A patient's friends or family members might overhear your conversation and misinterpret what is said.
- Keep the glass window between the waiting room and the reception desk closed.
- Watch the volume of your voice.
- When calling co-workers over the office intercom, do not use a patient's name or reveal other information. Avoid saying something like, "Bob Smith is on the phone and wants to know if his strep throat culture came back." Instead, say "There's a patient on line 1."
- Before going home, destroy any slips of paper in your uniform pockets that contain patient information (e.g., reminder notes from verbal reports).

español
SPANISH TERMINOLOGY

Hable despacio, por favor.
  Please speak slowly.
Sí, hablo español un poco.
  Yes, I speak Spanish a little.
No, no comprendo.
  No, I don't understand.
¿Comprende?
  Do you understand?
¿Cuándo?
  When?
¿Qué clase?
  What kind?
¿Porqué?
  Why?
¿Cuántos?
  How many?
¿Qué, Qué tal?
  What?
¿En qué puedo ayudarlo?
  What can I help you with?
¿Dígame porque esta aquí?
  Tell me why you are here?
¿Cómo?
  How?

MEDIA MENU

- **Student CD**
  - **Case Studies**
    Administrative Interactive Case Studies on Maintaining Medical Records and HIPAA; Conducting Patient Teaching
    Clinical Interactive Case Studies on Triage in an Emergency Situation, Communication and Documentation; Vital Signs, Patient Education, and Refusal of Treatment; and Dealing with a Sick Patient, Infection Control, and Medication Administration
  - **CMA/RMA Certification Exam Review**
- **Premium Online Course**
  http://thePoint.lww.com/Kronenberger3e
- **Internet Resources**

  LiveAdvise Online Tutoring & Competency Training
  http://thePoint.lww.com/LiveAdvise

  National Institute of Deafness and Other Communication Disorders
  http://www.nidcd.nih.gov/

  National Association for the Deaf
  http://www.nad.org/

  American Speech-Language-Hearing Association
  http://www.asha.org/

  Hearing, Speech and Deafness Center
  http://www.hsdc.org/

  National Hospice and Palliative Care Organization
  http://www.nhpco.org/

  Handspeak: American Sign Language Online Dictionary
  http://www.handspeak.com.

- Communication is a complex and dynamic process involving the sending and receiving of messages. It includes verbal and nonverbal forms of expression and is influenced by personal and societal values, individual beliefs, and cultural orientation.
- In the medical practice, important aspects of patient communication are interviewing and active listening.
- You will need to overcome many communication challenges to communicate with all patients. These challenges include patients with hearing, sight, and speech impairments.
- Children, angry or distressed patients, and patients with mental illnesses can also present a challenge to communication.
- To communicate effectively, you must understand the various factors that can affect the exchange of messages and use the communication techniques that are most appropriate for each individual situation.

Warm Ups for Critical Thinking

1. Dr. Hedrick has just told a patient that she has breast cancer. The words "breast cancer" can spark many emotions and fears. Write three sample questions that you could ask the patient to promote open communication about her feelings.

2. Dr. Yevin has just discharged a patient with specific instructions for crutch walking. How would you determine the patient's understanding of these instructions? Can nonverbal clues help you determine whether the patient is confused?

3. A mother brings in her 3-year-old child for a checkup. The child refuses to open her mouth so the doctor can examine her throat. How would you go about communicating the importance of this? What if the child was 6 years old?

4. A patient arrives in your office demanding to see the physician immediately. He is yelling and obviously very angry. The doctor is with another patient. Write three statements that you could say that might help the situation. Write three statements that would escalate the situation.

5. List five local resources that can assist a grieving patient or family member. Include the name of the agency, type of help that it offers, any special information, and its phone number.

Answers to Checkpoint Questions

1. For communication to occur, these three elements must be present: a message to be sent, a person to send the message, and a person to receive the message.

2. Voice tone, quality, volume, pitch, and range are five examples of paralanguage.

3. When interviewing patients, you can use six different techniques. These include reflecting, paraphrasing or restatement, asking for examples or clarification, asking open-ended questions, summarizing, and allowing silences.

4. The caller types their message, and the patient reads the message and types a response.

5. Dysphasia is difficulty with speech. Dysphonia is a voice impairment.

6. The five stages of grieving are denial, anger, bargaining, depression, and acceptance.

Patient Education

Outline

The Patient Education Process
Assessment
Planning
Implementation
Evaluation
Documentation
Conditions Needed for Patient Education
Maslow's Hierarchy of Needs
Environment
Equipment
Knowledge
Resources

Factors that Can Hinder Education
Existing Illnesses
Communication Barriers
Age
Educational Background
Physical Impairments
Other Factors
Teaching Specific Health Care Topics
Preventive Medicine
Lifestyle Changes
Medications

Alternative Medicine
Stress Management
Patient Teaching Plans
Developing a Plan
Selecting and Adapting
Teaching Material
Developing Your Own Material
Locating Community
Resources and
Disseminating Information

Learning Objectives

Upon successfully completing this chapter, you will be able to:

1. Spell and define the key terms

2. Explain the medical assistant's role in patient education

3. Define the five steps in the patient education process

4. Identify five conditions that are needed for patient education to occur

5. Explain Maslow's hierarchy of human needs

6. List five factors that may hinder patient education and at least two methods to compensate for each of these factors

7. Discuss five preventive medicine guidelines that you should teach your patients

8. Explain the kinds of information that should be included in patient teaching about medication therapy

9. Explain your role in teaching patients about alternative medicine therapies

10. List and explain relaxation techniques that you and patients can learn to help with stress management

11. Describe how to prepare a teaching plan

12. List potential sources of patient education materials

13. Locate community resources and list ways of organizing and disseminating information

Competencies

CAAHEP

- Instruct individuals according to their needs
- Identify community resources

ABHES

- Instruct patients with special needs
- Be impartial and show empathy when dealing with patients
- Adapt what is said to the recipients' level of comprehension

Key Terms

alternative	documentation	learning objectives	planning
assessment	evaluation	noncompliance	psychomotor
disseminates	implementation	placebo	stress

In the current health care climate of short hospital stays, patients seen in the medical office typically have acute conditions requiring intensive and extensive education from their health care provider. This will be one of your most challenging and rewarding roles as a medical assistant. Of course, you will not be responsible for teaching patients everything they need to know about health care. Patient education is performed under the direction of the physician. The amount and types of education that you will be expected to do will vary greatly from office to office. This chapter will give you the foundation needed for providing patient education.

The Patient Education Process

Patient education involves more than telling patients which medications they need to take or which lifestyle behaviors they need to change and expecting them to follow these instructions blindly. To educate patients effectively, you need to help them accept their illness, involve them in the process of gaining knowledge, and provide positive reinforcement. Ultimately, that knowledge should lead to a change in behavior or attitudes.

The process of patient education involves five major steps:

- Assessment
- Planning
- Implementation
- Evaluation
- Documentation

These five steps collectively produce the teaching plan. The plan may be formally written as the process is occurring or may be documented after the event. You must follow all these steps to achieve effective patient education.

Assessment

Before you begin to teach, you must assess your feelings and attitudes about the patient and the topic to be taught. Sometime in your career as a medical assistant, you may encounter situations or patients that make you feel uncomfortable. Your role as an educator, however, requires that you set aside your own personal feelings and life experiences to instruct the patient objectively and to the best of your ability. Always consider how your responses and actions will affect the patient, and be sure to treat each patient impartially.

Assessment requires gathering information about the patient's present health care needs and abilities.

In addition to knowing the present health care needs, you must also look at these other areas:

- Past medical and surgical conditions
- Current understanding and acceptance of health problems
- Needs for additional information
- Feelings about their health care status
- Factors that may hinder learning (covered in detail later in the chapter)

You may obtain this information from a number of sources. The most comprehensive source will be the medical record. The patient's medical record consists of all information regarding current diagnoses, treatments, medications, past medical history, and a variety of other documentation. Some medical records have a problem list on the inside cover. This will provide you with a snapshot of the patient and save you time from reading the entire document. Other sources of information will be the physician, family members, significant others, and other members of the health care team. When you have collected all of the assessment data, you are ready to start the next step of the education process: planning.

 CHECKPOINT QUESTION

1. What is the purpose of the assessment step during patient education?

Planning

Planning involves using the information you have gathered during the assessment phase to determine how you will approach the patient's learning needs. If possible, involve the patient in this part of the process. Learning goals and objectives that are established with input from the patient are most meaningful. A patient's learning goal is what the patient and educator want to be the outcome of the program. The patient's **learning objectives** include procedures or tasks that will be discussed or performed at various points in the program to help achieve the goal. Make certain the objectives you establish are specific for each individual patient and are measurable in some manner. If the objectives are measurable, you will be able to evaluate when or whether the patient successfully completed them.

For example, consider a patient who needs to limit his fluid intake. Which of the following objectives is more specific and would allow you to evaluate the patient's progress? (1) The patient understands why he should limit his fluid intake, or (2) the patient is able to prepare a schedule for daily fluid intake and explain why it is important that he limit his fluids. The second objective is more specific and not only evaluates the patient's understanding but also requires the patient to demonstrate understanding. Having patients prepare their own schedule gets them involved in their health care. It allows them to customize the schedule to fit their lifestyle, which is likely to increase compliance.

Implementation

After you establish the need for patient teaching and agree on the goals and objectives, you begin implementation. **Implementation** is the process used to perform the actual teaching. The teaching usually is carried out in several steps. Box 4-1 presents some commonly used teaching strategies. For example, you may start by telling the patient how to use crutches, followed by a demonstration, and finally, the patient may do a return demonstration. Patients also benefit from the use of teaching aids (drawings, charts, graphs, pamphlets) that they can take home and use as reference material. You

---

BOX 4-1

IMPLEMENTATION STRATEGIES

Implementing the learning process should be individualized to the patient's best method of comprehension and retention. These may include:

1. *Lecture and demonstration.* This method presents the information in the most basic form but requires no patient participation for reinforcement and retention.
2. *Role playing and demonstration.* The patient watches you perform a medical procedure, then performs it to ensure understanding. Information is more likely to be recalled if the patient actively participates in the process.
3. *Discussion.* This two-way exchange of information and ideas works well for lifestyle changes (e.g., making dietary changes to lower cholesterol) rather than for medical procedures.
4. *Audiovisual material.* Audiocassettes or videos can often be taken home and reviewed by the patient and family members as needed. This allows for reinforcement of teachings and provides both visual and auditory stimulation.
5. *Printed material and programmed instructions.* All information should be discussed with the patient to clarify points and to elicit questions before assuming that the instructions are understood.

can also use videos and audiocassettes to supplement the implementation process.

Miscommunication or misinterpretation can lead to serious complications or injury. For example, assume you are teaching a patient to use crutches. It is very important that you stress to the patient that the crutch must not press directly into the axillary area. (There should be a two-finger distance between the crutch and the armpit.) If the patient does not comprehend the dangers of nerve damage to the axillary area from pressing the crutch into the armpit, a serious complication to the patient could occur. Miscommunication about medications can have fatal consequences. The implementation stage may occur once or over a longer period. The disease process and the patient's ability to comprehend information will dictate the length of teaching. For example, teaching a patient about diabetes takes place over multiple sessions. The first session may focus on what diabetes is, while subsequent teachings may include topics such as diet, foot care, glucose monitoring, and insulin injection.

After implementation of a given skill or knowledge, you must determine whether your teaching was effective. This step is called evaluation.

Evaluation

Is the patient progressing? Did the teaching plan work? Does the plan need any changes? These are a few of the questions you may ask yourself when you begin to evaluate. **Evaluation** is the process that indicates how well patients are adapting or applying new information to their lives.

In the medical setting, where contact with patients is limited, part of the evaluation may have to be done by patients at home. For example, if office visits for direct observation are not scheduled, patients will be responsible for telephoning and reporting their status. In other words, can patients do the task they were taught, or are they having troubles? If they voice concern or appear unclear about their instructions, you should either redirect them on the phone or schedule them for an office appointment.

During the evaluation, you may discover **noncompliance**. Noncompliance is the patient's inability or refusal to follow a prescribed order. After determining that the given order is not being followed, your first step is to determine why the order is not being followed. It may be a misunderstanding. For example, a patient who is to take a certain medication twice a day may be taking it only twice a week because that is what he or she thought you said. If the noncompliance is because the patient refuses to follow these orders, however, you must notify the physician. Remember that the patient has the right to refuse medical treatment unless the patient is determined to be mentally incompetent. The physician will determine the next appropriate action in these cases.

Evaluation is an ongoing process, so you should expect to update and modify your plan periodically.

 CHECKPOINT QUESTION

2. What is the purpose of evaluation during patient education?

 WHAT IF?

You are instructing a 60-year-old gentleman in the use of a Holter monitor (an ambulatory heart monitor) when he tells you that he has not been taking his heart medication because it makes him feel tired. You have heard Dr. Jones tell other patients that this particular medication can cause fatigue at first, but that the patient should keep taking it, and after several weeks, he will have more energy. Should you give the patient this information?

As long as you are sure that your information is correct, you should share this with the patient. The patient then says that he still does not want to take the medication, but he asks that you not to tell the doctor because he may get angry. Since the patient needs this medication for a serious problem, the doctor must be notified. A doctor cannot force a patient to take his medication, but he may be able to convince him to take the medication. Perhaps the patient could try another medication that may not have the same effect. Remember to document the details of the encounter in the patient's chart.

Documentation

Documentation includes the recording of all teachings that have occurred. It should consist of the following information:

- Date and time of teaching.
- What information was taught, e.g., "Diabetes foot care was discussed. It consisted of the proper method for toenail cutting and regular examination by a podiatrist."
- How the information was taught, e.g., "ADA [American Diabetes Association] foot care video shown to the patient."
- Evaluation of teaching. For example, "Patient verbalized the need to make an appointment with a podiatrist."
- Any additional teaching planned, e.g., "Patient will return on Monday to the office with his wife for glucose monitoring instructions."

Box 4-2 has a charting example for patient education.

BOX 4-2

CHARTING EXAMPLE

11/27/07

Patient arrived in the office for teaching on the glucose meter; brought meter from home. Following steps were demonstrated by me: calibration of meter strips, battery change, finger sticks, strip insertion into machine, use of the patient logbook. Normal BGM ranges were reviewed along with the treatment of low blood sugar. Pt returned demonstration without problem. Reviewed glucose meter instructions manual with pt. Pt instructed to bring logbook to each MD appointment.—Margaret Blackwell, CMA

Your signature implies that you performed the teaching. If this is untrue or if another staff member assisted you in teaching, make sure that information is clearly noted. Also include the names of any interpreters who were used. You must also document all telephone conversations (e.g., "I spoke with this patient via the telephone today, and he said he is testing his blood sugar every morning without problems.").

Documentation is essential because, from a legal viewpoint, procedures are only considered to have been done if they are recorded. Documentation should become second nature to you as you interact with patients each day. A complete and accurate medical record indicates good care and attention to detail.

LEGAL TIP

ALWAYS REMEMBER TO DOCUMENT YOUR ACTIONS

There is a common saying in health care: "If it is not in the chart, it did not happen." In a court of law, the medical record is a health care professional's best defense. Always take special care to succinctly and accurately record every interaction with a patient and to give patients their instructions in writing. When patients receive a new diagnosis, provide educational materials about their disorder and direct them to appropriate websites. Document any instructions, information, or written materials given to the patient.

Conditions Needed for Patient Education

Learning is the process of acquiring knowledge, wisdom, or skills through study or instruction. This process does not occur without certain conditions. Learning cannot occur without motivation or a perceived need to learn. For example, suppose you want to teach a patient about the need to adopt a low-sodium diet because of hypertension. Patients who feel that hypertension is not a problem, however, will not be motivated to learn the diet because they have not accepted the need for the teaching. For such patients to be taught, the following steps must occur:

1. The patient must accept that the hypertension has to be managed.
2. The patient must accept that there is a correlation between high sodium intake and hypertension.
3. The patient must accept and be willing to make this dietary change.

Only if these steps have occurred can teaching begin. In addition to patient motivation, basic human needs must be met first.

Maslow's Hierarchy of Needs

Abraham Maslow, an American psychiatrist, recognized that people are motivated by needs and that certain basic needs must be met before people can progress to higher needs, such as taking personal responsibility for their health (self-actualization). Maslow arranged human needs in the form of a pyramid, with basic needs at the bottom and the higher needs at the top (Fig. 4-1). The patient progresses upward, fulfilling different levels of needs toward the highest level, which results in a state of health and well-being. In your responsibility as an educator, you need to be aware that patients must have the basic needs satisfied before they are willing or able to learn to take care of their own health. Not everyone will

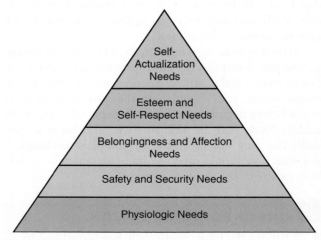

Figure 4-1 Maslow's hierarchy pyramid.

start at the bottom of the pyramid. Some patients will never reach the top, while others may be at the top and slide backward as a result of unfortunate circumstances.

Physiologic needs are air, water, food, rest, and comfort. If these basic needs are unmet, the patient cannot begin the process. Everyone has a different tolerance and expectation for these needs. For example, one person may expect that their food is served over three meals with full courses, while another person may accept that they will have one meal a day from a soup kitchen. If the patient perceives that these needs are met, we need to accept that and not judge the situation.

Safety and security needs include a safe environment and freedom from fear and anxiety. Patients are susceptible to fear and anxiety that accompany many medical conditions. For example, patients diagnosed with cancer may be so frightened that they are unable to think of anything but dying. Patients who have undergone some sort of trauma or disaster (hurricane, fire, motor vehicle accident) may place the need to feel safe above all other needs.

Affection needs, or the need for love and belonging, are essential for feeling connected and important to others. A sense of love or belonging can often be a powerful motivation for patients to try to regain good health.

Esteem needs involve our need to feel self-worth. Esteem can be self-generated, or it can come from those who admire us. If others value us or if we value ourselves, we are more likely to strive to maintain good health. Patients who lack self-esteem are less likely to want or accept education that targets improving their health. Thus, they will not see this as important information and will not be motivated to learn.

Self-actualization is the pinnacle of the pyramid, at which a person has satisfied all the other basic needs and feels personal responsibility and control over his or her own life. Self-actualized patients will strive to control their state of wellness by following all health directives and may even help others to achieve wellness. Not all patients will reach this level. Patients who have met this level will be ready to learn a multitude of health care skills and will strive to follow preventive health care maintenance guidelines.

After determining where on the pyramid the patient is, you can determine the appropriateness of education. For example, if the patient has not met the basic physiologic needs, you should help the patient meet these needs before beginning to teach. Patients who are in the middle levels may be able to focus and learn certain skills but may not be ready for complex teachings. If possible, you should involve family members or significant others in the teaching process.

✔ CHECKPOINT QUESTION

3. What are the basic physiologic needs outlined in Maslow's pyramid?

Environment

The environment where you teach must be conducive to learning. The room should be quiet and well lit and have limited distractions. It is not appropriate to teach patients a skill in a hallway, waiting room, or other high-traffic area. These areas produce distractions and prohibit confidentiality.

For patients to acquire knowledge, they must feel relaxed and comfortable. For example, it would be inappropriate to attempt to teach a patient who is sitting on an examination table with the stirrups in place. She will not feel comfortable. Reset the stirrups and direct the patient to dress and have a seat in a chair. If the patient had a procedure done in the room and bloody dressings or suture equipment is still present, clean the area and then return for teaching.

Equipment

A common type of education is teaching patients to perform a **psychomotor** skill. A psychomotor skill requires the participant to physically perform a task. Some examples include crutch walking, glucose monitoring, eye drop instillation, and dressing changes. The equipment for the skill must be present and functional. If possible, the equipment should be from the patient's home or be the exact replica of it.

The steps to teach a psychomotor skill are as follows:

1. Demonstrate the entire skill.
2. Demonstrate the skill step by step, explaining each step as you complete it.
3. Have the patient demonstrate the skill with your help.
4. Have the patient demonstrate the skill without your help.

Provide positive reinforcement throughout the steps. Always provide written step-by-step instructions. Always include instructions from the manufacturer for use and maintenance of any equipment.

Knowledge

The person teaching the skill must have a solid knowledge of the material. Imagine how difficult it would be to learn to ski from an instructor who did not know how to put skis on. The same is true in medical assisting. If you are not comfortable or do not feel knowledgeable about the topic, ask for help before starting to teach a patient. Be reassured that you do not have to be an expert on the topic, but you do need to feel comfortable with the information. If you start teaching a given topic and the patient asks you a question that you are not able to answer, state that you are not sure about that specific piece but you will get the answer. Then, either research the answer or ask for help from another health care professional. Never guess or imply that you know something that you do not know.

Resources

For patient education to be effective, it must consist of multiple techniques or approaches. The more techniques that are used, the more the patient will learn and retain. The three ways that we can learn are through hearing, seeing, and touch. If you can apply at least two of these senses in your teaching, your patient will be more stimulated to learn and will remember more information. For example, if you were teaching a patient about the dangers of smoking, which of the following would be more effective: (1) giving the patient a pamphlet that explains the dangers of smoking along with statistical data, or (2) showing a patient a diagram of what a nonsmoker's lung looks like versus a smoker's and providing the patient with pamphlets about local smoking cessation programs? The teaching in the second approach would be more beneficial. The patient sees the dangers of smoking and receives a brochure that contains practical hands-on information.

Fortunately, there is a wealth of information available for patient education. Tools to help teach patients include audiocassettes, compact discs, food labels, Internet and websites, manikins, models (heart, lungs), plastic food settings, pamphlets, and videos.

In addition to the five conditions already discussed, these factors will be necessary for the patient to learn:

- Family or significant others should be present if the information is complex or if it will require their assistance. Family members are essential if the patient is confused or unreliable.
- Patients should be wearing any sensory devices that they need (glasses, hearing aids).
- Qualified interpreters should be present if needed.
- Written instructions and materials should be prepared.

Factors That Can Hinder Education

Many factors or circumstances can hinder learning. It is important to recognize these factors and intervene as appropriate. In certain cases, teaching may have to be delayed, or your teaching plan may have to be revised.

Existing Illnesses

The type of illness that patients have will play a large role in their ability and willingness to learn. Generally, patients with acute short-term illnesses will be moti-

vated to learn a skill that will accelerate healing. Examples of short-term illnesses are orthopedic injuries (uncomplicated fractures, sprains), colds, and viruses.

These are six examples of illnesses or conditions that will affect learning:

- *Any illness in which the patient has moderate to severe pain.* Examples of these illnesses include neuropathies, bone cancer, kidney stones, and recent surgical procedures. The patient's pain level must reach a tolerable stage before teaching can start and the patient can concentrate on learning.
- *Any illness or condition with a poor prognosis or limited rehabilitation potential.* Examples include progressive neurologic disorders, certain cancers, and large traumatic events. It is important that you assess such patients' readiness to learn and their level of acceptance of their illness before you proceed with your teaching.
- *Any illness or condition that results in weakness and general malaise as a primary symptom.* Examples include gastrointestinal disorders that cause vomiting and diarrhea, anemia, Lyme disease, and recent blood transfusion. For these patients, teaching should be limited to the essential information and expanded on as the patient regains strength.
- *Any illness or condition that impairs the patient's mental health or cognitive abilities.* Examples of these conditions include brain tumors, Alzheimer's disease, substance abuse, and psychiatric disorders. In these patients, education should be provided to patients at their ability level. Family members or significant others should be brought in to complement the learning process.
- *Any patient who has more than one chronic illness.* For example, patients with diabetes often have cardiac, renal, and integumentary complications. In patients with multiple system failures, it is important to prioritize the learning needs. Focus your education on the main problem and work from there.
- *Any illness or condition that results in respiratory distress or difficult breathing.* Examples of these conditions include chronic obstructive pulmonary disease, pneumonias, lung cancer, and asthma. The priority goal is first to establish optimal oxygenation for the patient. Once this is met, you can begin teaching. These patients tend to become exhausted easily during acute exacerbations of their illnesses. Keep the teaching time short and to the point and expand teachings as their activity tolerance allows.

CHECKPOINT QUESTION

4. List six types of conditions or illnesses that may hinder your ability to educate patients effectively.

Communication Barriers

Effective communication skills are essential for patient education. Any barriers to communication must be resolved before you can start teaching the patient. If an interpreter is needed for language translation or for hearing-impaired patients, schedule a time convenient to all parties. (See Chapter 3.)

Age

The age of the patient plays a very important part in the amount and type of education that you can do. Small children need to be educated at an age-appropriate level (Fig. 4-2). For example, it would be inappropriate to teach a 2-year-old child how to assemble an asthma nebulizer. The parent or caregiver must be taught. It would be appropriate, however, to explain to the 2-year-old child that the nebulizer is not a toy and that it contains medication. Safety education is a prime teaching focus for small children and their parents. Box 4-3 presents some tips for communicating with and teaching children.

As children mature at different speeds, you should assess what information this child can handle and what information should not be shared with the child. Communication with the parents is essential. They know the child's developmental stage. For example, a 7-year-old child who has just been diagnosed with diabetes needs to know the signs and symptoms of low blood sugar and how to treat it. The child may not be ready, however, to learn about the long-term complications (e.g., blindness, renal failure). It is important to teach the child that the disease must be well controlled to prevent future problems, but not to the extent that the child develops fear.

The challenge in teaching adults is that they often have multiple responsibilities to their children, spouses, or aging parents. Obligations at work, school, church, and other activities may also limit their free time. These

Figure 4-2 Establishing rapport with the child.

> ### BOX 4-3
>
> ## TIPS FOR TEACHING CHILDREN
>
> Children require special communication skills and different teaching strategies. Here are a few tips to help you:
>
> - Encourage the child to be part of the teaching process.
> - Speak directly to the child.
> - Avoid confusing medical terms.
> - Avoid using baby language.
> - Teach only age-appropriate information.
> - Discuss with the parents the child's knowledge base about the illness and any feelings the parent may have regarding what they want the child to know. (This should not be done in front of the child.)
> - Demonstrate skills on stuffed animals or dolls.

obligations and responsibilities can interfere with willingness to learn and attentiveness. Your teaching may have to occur in short sessions over long periods. This age group may benefit from electronic resources that they can access on their own time schedule.

Elderly patients can be a challenge to teach for a variety of reasons. These reasons include confusion, lack of interest, and overall poor health. Some older patients, however, can be the most attentive and curious learners. It is fairly common for this age group to address items that they have heard on the news. For example, a patient may hear an advertisement for a new medication for arthritis and request clarification from you regarding its effectiveness.

✓ CHECKPOINT QUESTION

5. What is the primary teaching focus for small children and their parents?

Educational Background

Most initial health assessment forms ask patients what level of education they have obtained. This information may help you to determine the patient's ability to read. Caution is essential because graduation alone does not guarantee that the patient can read. You will need to use your tact and diplomacy to evaluate the situation.

Patients who have completed some college courses, however, are likely to be interested in preventive health care. Patients with an educational background in health care will still need the same attention and teaching from you. Do not assume that, since the patient is a nurse or a physician, you can skip teaching a skill. Their specialty may be in an unrelated area.

Physical Impairments

Numerous physical impairments may hinder learning. For example, patients with severe arthritis in their hands may have difficulty performing certain psychomotor skills, like giving themselves insulin. An occupational therapist is the best resource to assist you. Speak to the physician to obtain the proper referrals.

Other Factors

Other factors may hinder your ability to teach patients. The patient's culture may affect willingness to learn or the family's involvement in learning. Patients with financial troubles may not be ready to focus on learning new skills or knowledge. It is important that you assess the patient's readiness to learn and either try to remove or work around any obstacles that may be present.

Teaching Specific Health Care Topics

Your role in patient education will vary greatly. The topics that you will teach will depend on the patient, type of medical office, and physician's preferences. Staying well is a topic often discussed in the exam room. Medical assistants provide information and support about nutrition, exercise, and wellness. These topics are discussed in Chapter 16, Nutrition and Wellness. Next are some other topics commonly taught by medical assistants.

Preventive Medicine

Preventing health problems is the key to living a long, healthy life. But the advantages to good preventive medicine extend much further. There are huge economic benefits to preventing illnesses. Millions of people are hospitalized each year. Caring for sick patients at home costs Medicare billions of dollars annually. These statistics affect everyone. They lead to higher taxes, higher health care insurance premiums, and limited programs for low-income families.

These are some commonly recommended preventive health care tips that you should teach all of your patients:

- Regular physical examinations for all age groups
- Annual flu and regular pneumonia vaccinations
- Adult immunizations for tetanus and hepatitis B
- Childhood immunizations
- Regular dental examinations
- Monthly breast self-examinations for women and regular physician examinations

- Cancer Screening to include:
  - Mammograms
  - Colonoscopy
  - Annual Pap tests
  - Prostate-specific antigen blood tests for all men, along with need for regular digital rectal examinations

The frequency and age at which these procedures will be recommended to patients vary with the patient's medical history and genetics and the physician's preference. Some insurance will pay for these procedures, while others will not pay unless the procedure is deemed diagnostic. Many hospitals and clinics offer free preventive screenings to patients. Your office should have a list of which free screenings are available. Public health departments may also have this information available for your patients. Most providers and insurance coverage base the frequency and type of testing on the guidelines set forth by the American Cancer Society.

Your role as a medical assistant is to promote preventive screenings. The physician you work with will instruct you in his or her recommendations for these tests.

Another large part of preventive medicine is teaching safety tips. Preventable injuries can arise from bicycle and car accidents, poisoning, fires, choking, falls, drownings, firearms, and lawn mowers. Toys can lead to injuries when they are broken or used by a child of an inappropriate age. The American Academy of Pediatrics (AAP) offers injury prevention tips for parents and health care providers. While working as a medical assistant, you will find valuable teaching tips to give to parents from their website. The AAP also provides numerous educational materials that can be mailed to physician offices and given to your patients.

According to the American Academy of Orthopaedic Surgeons (AAOS), falls cause 90% of the hip fractures that occur each year in the United States. By 2050, the AAOS estimates that the number of hip fractures per year will reach 650,000. Hip fractures require long hospitalizations and often rehabilitation in a nursing home. Most falls occur at home and are preventable. Fall prevention tips should be taught to all older patients or any patient who has a problem with maintaining balance or uses an ambulation device (cane, walker). Here are some tips that you can use to teach fall prevention:

- Encourage patients to remove all scatter rugs in their home. Remind patients to keep hallways clutter free.
- Instruct the patient to ensure adequate lighting in all rooms and hallways.
- Encourage the patient to avoid steps. Encourage one-floor living.
- Ensure that the patient has well-soled shoes or sneakers. Advise the patient to avoid wearing heels.
- Instruct the patient to place nonskid surfaces in bathtubs or purchase a shower chair.

- Instruct the patient to install handrails or grab bars in hallways and stairwells.
- Advise patients taking medications that lower their blood pressure to stand up slowly and get their balance, and then begin to walk.
- Advise patients to have regular eye examinations and have their glasses adjusted as needed.
- Encourage patients to have a plan for power outages and severe storms.

Lifestyle Changes

In addition to instructing patients, in many cases, you will be asking them to make changes in their lifestyle. Change is difficult for anyone. It is easier to continue doing what you have always done. Some patients view illness as strong motivation to follow the physician's orders. Others are resistant to eating less and moving more to lose extra pounds or beginning a walking program to help their arthritis. You can help with the difficult process of change. Encouragement and close follow-up are effective ways to keep a patient on the right track. When a patient sees results from his changes, he is encouraged and wants to continue. Eventually, the changes become habits, and the patient has been successful in making a lifestyle change that will probably add years to his life. Giving up foods you love, pushing yourself to work hard, and resisting addictions are difficult and a continuous battle. Patients should be reminded to strive for small successes at first, monitor their progress weekly, and take one day at a time.

ETHICAL TIP

Be Supportive, Not Judgmental

Even with your best efforts, some patients do not follow the doctor's orders. It is hard to understand a lung cancer patient who is still smoking or a patient with high cholesterol levels who continues to eat fried food. As a health care professional, you should never judge a patient or offer your personal opinions. Avoid showing negative feelings or distaste for patients or their actions. Provide patients with as much information, support, and encouragement as possible. People respond to positive reinforcement, and your interest and concern may be just what they need to help them make difficult lifestyle changes.

CHECKPOINT QUESTION

6. Which patients should you teach fall prevention tips?

Medications

With the increasing number of medications available, the possibilities for teaching patients in this area are virtually endless. Pharmaceutical companies offer in-depth medication information for health care providers and patients concerning the chemical makeup of the drug, physiologic reactions in the body, prescribed dosage and route, and possible side effects. This information comes from the pharmaceutical companies either by mail or from the sales support team. In addition, some of this information will come in package inserts. If this information is not available, the patient may not understand the importance of the medication therapy, and this could lead to noncompliance, drug interactions, or other serious side effects. You may be responsible for gathering the information needed and preparing teaching materials for your patients to help prevent such complications.

When preparing a medication therapy teaching tool, you must consider such factors as the patient's financial abilities, social or cultural demands, physical disabilities, and age. Be sure to include the following information in any teaching:

- Medication name (generic or brand)
- Dosage
- Route
- What the medication is for
- Why the medication must be taken as prescribed
- Possible changes in bodily functions (e.g., colored urine)
- Possible side effects
- Other medications, such as over-the-counter drugs, herbal supplements, and so on, that might interfere with the action of the medication
- Foods or liquids to be avoided
- Activities to be avoided
- Telephone number to call for any questions or concerns

Figure 4-3 shows a medication therapy teaching tool that incorporates all of these elements.

Medication teaching should also include any over-the-counter medications or herbal supplements the patient is taking. This information should consist of the same items listed above. Many patients have the misconception that over-the-counter medications (e.g., aspirin, ibuprofen, cough syrup) are 100% safe and no dangers are associated with them. Some of these medications may interact with their prescribed medications.

After assessing patients' understanding of all of their medications, you may find that scheduling is a prime concern. For example, the patient may be taking several types of medications at different times of the day or week. Before developing a medication schedule, evaluate the patient's daily routine to see how adhering to the

Figure 4-3 Medication therapy teaching tool.

schedule may affect the patient's lifestyle. For instance, you might ask the patient:

- How late do you sleep each morning?
- What time do you go to bed?
- When do you usually eat?

Once you have collected this information, you can create a scheduling tool to serve as a reminder to the patient about what medications to take when. Pillboxes can also help to remind patients to take their medication. Pillboxes are plastic containers prelabeled with the days of the week and times. You may instruct the patient in how to fill them. Pillboxes are sold in most pharmacies.

Another patient education area that falls under the category of medication therapy includes how to administer medications—orally, vaginally, rectally, and so on. This information will be taught in the clinical part of your curriculum. A patient's medication regimen should be reviewed at each visit to be sure the patient is taking the right medication in the right way. For more patient teaching information regarding safe and effective use of medications, you can contact the National Council on Patient Information and Education (NCPIE), a nonprofit organization, at 666 Eleventh Street, NW, Suite 810, Washington, DC 20001. NCPIE can provide you with literature and referrals to other sources.

Alternative Medicine

Many ancient remedies that were once considered voodoo and dismissed by Western medicine have proven to be beneficial. Billions are spent yearly on **alternative** medicine, and surveys have shown that about 51% of all Americans have used some form of unconventional medicine. In 1998, a federal agency was created to evaluate and monitor alternative medicine therapies. That agency, the National Center for Complementary and Alternative Medicine (NCCAM), also conducts clinical trials and training programs for practitioners of alternative medicine.

There are numerous types of alternative medicine therapies. Following is a discussion of four of the most common therapies.

Acupuncture

Acupuncture is one of the oldest forms of Chinese medicine. Acupuncture works on the principle that there are 2000 acupuncture points in the human body. These 2000 points are connected throughout the body by 12 pathways called meridians. The meridians conduct energy, or qi, in the body when they are triggered. The trigger comes in the form of a needle. When the meridian is stimulated, it prompts the brain to release certain chemicals and hormones.

Acupuncture is primarily used to treat addictions, fibromyalgia, osteoarthritis, asthma, and chronic back pain. It is sometimes used in treating children with attention-deficit/hyperactivity disorder.

In 1996, the Food and Drug Administration (FDA) required that all acupuncture needles be labeled for single use. Training and legal requirements vary among states.

Acupressure

Acupressure is similar to acupuncture, except that it does not use needles. The practitioner applies pressure to the meridians through direct touch. This method has shown great success in treating nausea and vomiting associated with chemotherapy. Some hospitals and clinics offer acupressure on an outpatient basis to cancer patients. Studies have shown that acupressure may help alleviate chronic pains and may even boost the immune system. Requirements for licensure and training vary among states.

Hypnosis

Hypnosis is portrayed on television as a magical method for reaching the inner workings of the brain. There is proof, however, that when conducted properly, it may provide some health care benefits. It is primarily used for weight reduction, for treatment of obsessive-compulsive disorders, and for smoking cessation. Hypnosis can be used for pain control and relaxation. Patients with anxiety disorders can be taught to do self-hypnosis. The training requirements vary greatly from state to state, and in most areas, licensure is not required.

Yoga

Yoga has proved to be very beneficial for relieving stress and improving flexibility. Yoga consists of a comprehensive discipline of physical exercise, posture, breathing exercises, and meditation. There are a variety of types of yoga. Iyengar consists of motionless poses that emphasize posture and form. Once this method is learned, patients are able to practice this at home. This method may help patients who are recovering from injuries. Bikram consists of 26 poses that are conducted at 100°F. This method promotes muscle relaxation and stretching. Perspiration is thought to help cleanse the body of various toxins. Sivananda is a five-step system that focuses on breathing exercises, relaxation, diet, and meditation.

Herbal Supplements

The use of herbal supplements is a multibillion-dollar business in the United States. The general public views herbal supplements as "natural," and hence safe. This is a misconception. Herbal supplements, vitamins, and similar substances are not regulated by the FDA. The patient or consumer must understand that, because there has been no formal government testing or approval of these substances, their dosages, side effects, interactions, and possible benefits are unclear. A classic example of an herbal supplement that has been shown to have dangerous side effects is ephedrine. This supplement was once thought to be the weight-loss miracle. It can, however, cause heart attacks and strokes. The FDA issued many warnings about ephedrine's dangers and potential for abuse; in 2004, the FDA banned dietary supplements containing ephedra in the United States.

Furthermore, since these products are not regulated, there is no guarantee that what the label claims is in the bottle is actually there. The quality and the purity of the herbal supplements have shown to vary greatly from manufacturer to manufacturer. Patients should be advised to purchase only supplements that are stamped with a US Pharmacopeia bar code. This bar code means that the manufacture site has met certain standards for distribution but does not mean that the supplement has been tested for health care benefits. Box 4-4 provides some general teaching tips for any patient using an herbal supplement.

Some of these substances have evolved through folklore, various cultures, or clinical research. In some cases, there is an element of **placebo** action involved. Placebo is the power of believing that something will make you better when there is no chemical reaction that warrants such improvement. Other supplements actually have scientific studies to document their effects. Table 4-1 lists some commonly used herbal supplements and their reported benefits.

Your role as a medical assistant is to assess whether patients are using any alternative therapies. Your assessment should include the length of time they have used these treatments and any side effects or benefits that the patient has noted, and you should report such informa-

---

BOX 4-4

GENERAL TEACHING TIPS FOR HERBAL SUPPLEMENTS

Here are a few general teaching points on herbal supplements:

- Explain to patients the importance of always telling the physician or other health care provider about any herbal supplements that they are taking.
- Explain to patients that the fact that a product is "natural" does not mean it is safe. A good example is mushrooms. All mushrooms are natural, but some are very poisonous.
- Teach patients the importance of looking for the USP (United States Pharmacopeia) label. Teach patients to look for expiration dates on all supplements.
- Advise patients not to ask health store clerks for information on supplements but to speak to physicians or pharmacists.
- Advise patients to distrust advertisements that use words like magical or breakthrough or that claim to detoxify the whole body.
- Instruct patients to stop taking all herbal supplements at least 2 weeks prior to surgery and to tell their surgeon what supplements they have been using and how long. (Some supplements can increase bleeding time.)
- Warn diabetic patients that many supplements will interfere with blood sugar levels.
- Advise parents to avoid giving herbal supplements to their children unless approved by a physician.
- Advise pregnant or breast-feeding patients to consult with a pharmacist or physician before taking any supplements.

---

tion to the physician. Patients should be advised to verify the training and credentials of the practitioner they are using and to ascertain that the practitioner is appropriately licensed. Patients should be encouraged to look at the National Center for Complementary and Alternative Medicine (NCCAM) website for safety updates and for more detailed information about alternative medicine. You should never recommend that a patient start taking herbal supplements or other alternative medicine therapies without a physician's approval.

CHECKPOINT QUESTION

7. What is a placebo?

TABLE **4-1.** Herbal Supplements[a]	
Supplement	**Reported Benefits**
Alfalfa	Relief from arthritis pain; strength
Anise	Relief of dry cough; treatment of flatulence
Black cohosh root	Relief of premenstrual symptoms; rheumatoid arthritis
Chamomile	Treatment of migraines, gastric cramps
Cholestin	Lowers cholesterol and triglycerides
Echinacea	Treatment of colds; stimulates immune system; attacks viruses
Garlic	Treatment of colds; diuretic; prevention of cardiac diseases
Ginkgo	Increased blood flow to brain; treatment of Alzheimer's disease
Ginseng	Mood elevator, antihypertensive
Glucosamine	Treats arthritis symptoms; improves joint mobility
Kava	Treatment of anxiety, restlessness; tranquilizer
Licorice	Soothes coughs, treats chronic fatigue syndrome
St. John's wort	Treats depression, premenstrual symptoms; antiviral

[a] This box lists some commonly used herbal supplements and their reported benefits. Research is an ongoing process to document these findings. Some of these herbal supplements may have side effects or may interact with prescribed medications.

Stress Management

Everyone is affected by an illness or injury at some time. Along with this often comes stress. **Stress** can come from forces such as fear, anger, anxiety, crisis, and joy. Stress may produce physiologic changes as well as psychological effects. When faced with illness or injury, a patient usually must confront:

- Physical pain
- Inability to perform self-care
- Stress of treatments, procedures, and possible hospitalization
- Changes in role identity and self-image
- Loss of control and independence
- Changes in relationships with friends and family

Patients with chronic conditions may need more time to adjust than patients with acute illnesses. If patients are able to deal with stress factors, they are more likely to adapt and adjust to lifestyle changes.

Many other causes besides illness or injury can place patients under stress. The best way to cope with stress is by living a healthy lifestyle. When the body is healthy, it can handle stress more easily. Unfortunately, most of the reasons that hinder learning are the same factors that hinder patients' ability to comply with patient education. Patients who are not capable of coping with stress on their own or with the help of instruction provided by the medical office staff may need professional counseling.

Positive and Negative Stress

Two types of stress affect all of us daily: positive stress and negative stress. Positive stress motivates individuals to work efficiently and perform to the best of their abilities. Examples of positive stress include working on a challenging new job or assignment, getting married, and giving a speech or performance. In fact, many people work best under positive stress. Under positive stress, the brain releases chemicals that increase the heart rate and breathing capacity. The body also releases stored glucose that gives an energy boost. Once the job (or wedding) is over, though, time must be taken to relax and prepare for the next project. If relaxation techniques are not incorporated into the daily routine, positive stress can become negative stress.

Negative stress is the inability to relax after a stressful encounter. Left unchecked, it can lead to such physiologic responses as:

- Headache
- Nausea, diarrhea
- Sweating palms
- Insomnia
- Malaise
- Rapid heart rate

Long-term physical effects of unrelieved stress include increases in blood pressure, glucose levels, metabolism, intraocular pressure, and finally exhaustion. There is also an increased risk of heart attack, stroke, diabetes, certain cancers, and immune system failure. If the stress is not relieved, patients will progress to higher anxiety levels and will require all of their energy and attention to focus solely on the problem at hand. Most mental and physical activity will be directed at relief of the stress to avoid the ultimate anxiety level known as panic—a sudden, overwhelming state of anxiety or terror.

It may be difficult to escape completely from stress-causing factors, but management of them is possible. For a patient suffering from the physiologic effects of negative stress, you can offer the following coping strategies:

- Encourage patients to attempt to reduce stressors, but emphasize that it is not possible to remove all stressors. Warn them to avoid attempting to make everything perfect; perfectionism adds its own stress.
- Encourage patients to organize and limit activities as needed.
- Try to lessen patients' fear of failure so they just do the best they can.
- When patients are feeling anxious, encourage them to talk to someone about their problems and let off steam.

Any one of these tips may help patients to regain control over stressors. In addition, a number of relaxation techniques described in the following sections may help.

Psychological Defense Mechanisms

Humans employ the use of defense mechanisms to cope with the painful and difficult problems life can bring. Freud's unconscious awareness theory says that we unconsciously avoid conflict and situations that cause us feelings of anxiety. Patients can use defense mechanisms to hide from or ignore their problems, especially those resulting from illness. We all use defense mechanisms from time to time, but psychologists say that the key to good mental health is to face our real conflicts and problems. You may encounter patients who are using such mechanisms to hide their true feelings. You must keep this possibility in mind as you attempt to understand and help patients. Table 4-2 outlines some common defense mechanisms.

Relaxation Techniques

Patients can use any of several types of relaxation techniques. To determine what works best for them, they must first consider how much time they have and what type of relaxation they need. Next are three examples of relaxation techniques.

Breathing Techniques

Breathing exercises can be done anywhere. Most people are shallow breathers and need to be instructed on deep-breathing techniques. To perform these breathing exercises, the patient should sit up straight with hands placed on the stomach and take a deep breath in through the

nose, feeling the hands being pushed away by the stomach. (This may feel awkward because most people do just the opposite.) The patient holds the breath for a few seconds and then exhales through pursed lips as the hands are felt being pulled in. This exercise allows for good control of the rate of exhalation. Sometimes, getting the oxygen flowing through the body at a faster rate is all that is needed to relieve boredom, tension, and stress.

Visualization

Visualization is a relaxation technique that involves allowing the mind to wander and the imagination to run free and focus on positive and relaxing situations. It is similar to daydreaming. It can "remove" the patient from a stressful situation and put him or her in a place where, if nothing else, the mind can relax. Instruct the patient to find a quiet place, close the eyes, and then visualize a soothing scene. Sometimes, background music helps. Remind the patient that it is important to choose appropriate times for this daydreaming technique. For example, it would be dangerous to use this technique when driving a car or operating heavy equipment.

Physical Exercise

There is no better tranquilizer than physical exercise. Walking at least 30 minutes 3 times a week is a great stress reliever. Most people who exercise regularly say that it helps them reduce tension, relax, and rest better at night. Exercise is discussed in Chapter 16.

 PATIENT EDUCATION

SELF-RELAXATION TECHNIQUES

Here are examples of self-relaxation techniques for you and your patients.

Sit with both feet on the floor, place your hands in your lap, and close your eyes. Visualize yourself standing at the top of a staircase with six steps. Now imagine that you are going down each step very slowly. With each step down, your body becomes more relaxed. When you feel completely relaxed for a minute or so, imagine going back up the steps. With each step up, you feel more alert and ready to take on the world. It takes practice, but after awhile, the process can be done in the time it takes to take a bathroom break. You will be refreshed and ready to sail through the rest of the day.

In a sitting position, concentrate on relaxing the muscles in your body. Beginning with the top of your head and moving down, concentrate on relaxing your shoulders, your arms, your hips, your legs, etc. Try this technique when you are having trouble getting to sleep or you're anxiously sitting in the dentist's chair.

TABLE 4-2	Common Defense Mechanisms	
Defense Mechanism	**Explanation**	**Example**
Denial	Refusing to acknowledge an unpleasant fact of life in order to delay facing it. Allowing yourself to believe that the problem does not exist.	A parent of a teen ignores or trivializes physical signs of drug abuse.
Displacement	Taking out your anger and frustration on someone other than the person responsible for the bad feelings.	A medical assistant is angry with her physician-employer. Later, she yells at her husband when he asks about dinner.
Intellectualization	Analyzing a difficult situation to try to make sense of it.	A daughter spends hours researching Alzheimer's disease after her mother's diagnosis.
Projection	Blaming others for your unacceptable qualities.	A medical assisting graduate blames her teachers when she has trouble finding a job because of poor personal work history.
Rationalization	Using excuses for unacceptable behavior.	A patient says it is alright for him to smoke because he has a high-stress job.
Regression	Behaving in an immature way when faced with difficulty.	A patient pouts when she has to wait because the doctor has been called to the hospital.
Repression	Blocking out bad memories.	An abused wife remembers only "the good times" when she thinks about leaving her abuser.
Sublimation	Changing unwanted aggressive or sexual drives by finding an outlet through creative mental work.	A recovering abuser volunteers at a shelter and counsels abused spouses.
Withdrawal	Physically or emotionally pulling away from difficult situations.	A child sits alone on the playground because he is not as good at kickball as the others.

Patient Teaching Plans

Developing a Plan

Because medical assistants are usually allotted only minimal time for patient teaching, you may often find yourself teaching without a written plan. To ensure that teaching is done logically, always use the education process to help you formulate a plan in your mind. Also remember to document in the patient's record whatever teaching you perform and the patient's response.

Many facilities use preprinted teaching plans for common problem areas, such as "Controlling Diabetes," "Living With Multiple Sclerosis," and "Coping With Hearing Loss." Although these save time, they are not individualized to the patient. If you use preprinted teaching plans, be sure to adapt them to your particular patient's learning needs and abilities.

If preprinted plans are not an option, consult teaching plan resource books, which contain the necessary information in outline form. You can take the plans from these sources and transfer them as needed to your facility-approved teaching plan format, adding your own comments to fit the patient's needs.

All teaching plans, no matter what the design, should contain the following elements:

- *Learning goal.* A description of what the patient should learn from implementation of the teaching plan.
- *Material to be covered.* All major topics to be discussed.
- *Learning objectives.* Steps or procedures the patient must understand or demonstrate to accomplish the learning goal.
- *Evaluation.* Appraisal of the patient's progress.
- *Comments.* Remarks concerning circumstances that may be preventing successful completion of the objectives.

Teaching plans must also include an area for documenting when the information was presented to the patient and when the patient successfully completed each objective. Figure 4-4 is an example of a teaching plan.

Teaching Plan: 32-year-old female with Iron Deficiency Anemia
Patient Learning Goal: Increase patient's knowledge of Iron Deficiency Anemia, its complications and treatments
Material to be Covered: Description of disorder, complications, diet, medications, procedures

Learning Objectives Comments	Teaching Methods/Tools	Procedure Explained/Demonstrated Date/Initial	PT Demonstrated/ Objectives Met Date/Initial
1. Patient describes what happens when body's demand for oxygen is not met. a. oxygen and hgb concentration decrease b. signs/symptoms of anemia c. anemia occurs only after body stores of iron are depleted	Instruction		
2. Patient describes complications caused by decrease of oxygen concentration a. chronic fatigue b. dyspnea c. inability to concentrate, think d. decrease in tissue repair e. increase of infection f. increase in heart rate	Instruction		
3. Patient discusses importance of diet in prevention of iron deficiency anemia a. including iron-rich foods in diet (beef, poultry, green vegetables) b. including foods that contain ascorbic acid to assist in absorbing iron in body (fruits) c. importance of limiting large meals if fatigued; stress importance of several small meals	Instruction/Video: "Your Diet: Why It Is Important"		
4. Patient describes prescribed medication, its purpose, dosage, route, and side effects	Instruction/Pamphlet: *Taking Your Iron Supplements*		
5. Patient aware of importance of follow-up appointments for evaluation of prescribed plan of treatment	Instruction/Appointment slip with next scheduled appointment		

Figure 4-4 Teaching plan.

Selecting and Adapting Teaching Material

An enormous amount of teaching material is available. Although the physician or institution may select much of the material you will use, you may be responsible for selecting some teaching aids. Assess your patients' general level of understanding to choose materials appropriately. When using preprinted material, consider the format, headings, illustrations, vocabulary, and writing style for overall clarity and readability. Also, ensure that the information provided on commercial materials is truthful and in agreement with the policies and procedures of your facility. A good rule of thumb is to use commercial material only from nationally recognized organizations or government agencies.

Many patient education textbooks are available from your clinic library. If you do not have access to a library, you can order most texts from local bookstores or through the Internet. Many of these sources list addresses for other patient education materials available from companies or associations. These materials commonly include printed items as well as videos, audiocassettes, and compact discs. Use commercially prepared materials to start a patient teaching library in the physician's office so you will have information at your fingertips when needed.

Developing Your Own Material

Sometimes, you may need to create your own teaching materials. Review available resources and teaching aids, and adapt the information to benefit your patients. When developing teaching material, remember to do the following:

- Indicate the objective of the information.
- Personalize the information so the patient wants to learn.
- Make sure information is clear and well organized.
- Use lists and outlines, which are easier to read and remember than paragraphs.
- Avoid medical jargon as much as possible.
- Focus on the key points.
- Select appropriate printing type.
- Use diagrams that are simple, clear, and well labeled.
- Include the names and telephone numbers of people or organizations that patients can call with further questions or concerns.

After patients have been using the material for a while, periodically evaluate its effectiveness and modify your teaching plan as needed.

Not all of the patient teaching materials you create will have to be in print form. Patients must be motivated to read, but many will be more receptive to audiovisual instruction. Take advantage of any opportunity to develop teaching materials in other media.

 CHECKPOINT QUESTION

8. List the elements of a written teaching plan.

Locating Community Resources and Disseminating Information

Patients have access to many services that sometimes they do not even realize are available. Many communities have a central agency that coordinates and **disseminates** or distributes information about many or all community resources. If this is not the case in your area, you will want to gather the information and create an information sheet for patients to take home. The patient and his family can then examine the resources, decide if they want to participate, and contact the appropriate community resource. Support groups not only provide assistance for patients and their families in coping with illness, but they also give the patient an opportunity to meet and exchange ideas with others who are experiencing the same issues such as Alzheimer disease, cancer, and diabetes.

Most local telephone directories include a section that outlines the agencies and resources available through the city and state. Information for patients who need financial assistance or assistance with transportation would be found in a telephone directory. The Internet is an excellent resource for local, state, and national agencies that provide information, support, and services to patients. Box 4-5

lists some of the agencies that might be available in your area. For information about local support, the websites of these agencies are listed as well.

 MEDIA MENU

- **Student CD**
  - **Case Studies**
    Administrative Interactive Case Study on Conducting Patient Teaching
    Clinical Interactive Case Study on Patient Interviewing, Education and Confidentiality, and Specimen Handling
  - **CMA/RMA Certification Exam Review**
- **Premium Online Course**
  http://thePoint.lww.com/Kronenberger3e
- **Internet Resources**

  LiveAdvise Online Tutoring & Competency Training
  http://thePoint.lww.com/LiveAdvise

  American Academy of Pediatrics
  www.aap.org

  American Cancer Society
  www.cancer.org

  American Heart Association
  www.americanheart.org

  American Lung Association
  www.lungusa.org

  Food and Drug Administration
  www.fda.gov

  National Center for Complementary and Alternative Medicine
  www.nccam.nih.gov

  National Council on Patient Information and Education
  www.talkaboutrx.org

BOX 4-5

COMMUNITY RESOURCES

Council on Aging; www.ncoa.org
American Red Cross; www.redcross.org
Hospice; www.hospicefoundation.org
American Cancer Society; www.acscsn.org
American Heart Association;
  www.americanheart.org
Civic organizations
Public health department
Social services
Home health agencies

Various support groups can be located in the telephone directory or local newspaper. Cancer centers would have information about the support they offer.

---

español SPANISH TERMINOLOGY

Tres veces al día.
  Three times a day
Antes/después de las comidas
  Before/after meals
Al acostarse
  At bedtime
Tómela con la comida.
  Take this with food.
Dele la medicina cada cuatro horas.
  Give him the medicine every 4 hours.

PROCEDURE 4-1: **Instructing a Hearing-Impaired Patient by Giving Directions to a Radiology Appointment**

Purpose: To convey necessary information to a patient with hearing difficulties
Equipment: Patient's chart, internet, printer, paper

Steps	Reasons
1. Using the patient's chart, identify the patient's communication barrier and assess the tools needed.	The patient's level of hearing will determine whether you should speak louder, hand write your instructions, or use a sign language interpreter.
2. Using an online map service, print out a map of the specific route.	The Internet is a good resource for obtaining door-to-door travel directions.
3. Use the suggestions listed in Chapter 3 for communicating with the hearing-impaired to explain the appointment and directions to the patient.	It is important to follow certain suggestions for the best chance at successful communication when the patient has hearing difficulties.
4. In a well-lit area and facing the patient, speak clearly and in a low tone.	These actions are recommended for successful communications with the hearing impaired.
5. Be sure that the patient understands.	Through nonverbal or written communication, you can assess the patient's level of understanding.

PROCEDURE 4-2:   Locating Community Resources

Purpose: To assist patients to identify and obtain assistance from available community resources
Equipment: Computer with Internet access

Steps	Reasons

1. Assess the patient's needs. Does he or she need:
  a. Education
  b. Someone to talk to
  c. Financial information
  d. Support groups
  e. Home health needs
	You must know what resources the patient needs. If there are several, organize the information to avoid confusion.

2. Be prepared with materials already on hand. Create a resource for patients using Word or an Excel sheet, for example.	With each resource located, place the information in a manual so that you will have general information about the resources available to patients.
3. Check the local telephone book for local and state resources.	Most telephone directories include a section for local, county, and state resources. It is difficult for some patients to sort all of the information out.
4. Check for websites for the city and/or county in which the patient lives.	Many patients do not have access to a computer, but phone numbers can be obtained from websites.

Step 4: Check websites for information.

Steps	Reasons
5. Disseminate the information to patients at their level of understanding.	Remember that communication is not effective unless it is understood.
6. Give the patient the contact information in writing.	Instructions for patients should be in writing to avoid any confusion or memory loss.
7. Document your actions and the information you gave the patient.	If it's not in the chart, it did not happen.
8. Instruct the patient to contact the office if there is any difficulty.	Always make sure the patient knows how to contact you. This is good customer service.

- Your role in teaching depends on the clinical setting in which you work. Never pass up an opportunity to teach.
- Encourage patients to ask questions.
- Periodically check to ensure that your teaching has been effective.
- Do not overstep your role as a medical assistant. The teaching you provide should clarify and complement information provided by the physician.
- A well-planned patient education program helps ensure that patients receive the high-quality health care they deserve.

Warm Ups for Critical Thinking

1. Look at the Maslow's hierarchy pyramid. What level are you on? What steps can you take to reach the self-actualization level? If you are at that level, what steps can you take to ensure that you remain there?

2. Review the list of information that you should teach patients about their medications. Choose two medications, herbal supplements, or vitamins that you have taken. (The medication can be over-the-counter or prescribed.) Using all available resources, write the information for these two medications or supplements.

3. Review the material on fall prevention and preventing childhood injuries. Make a checklist of at least 10 safety tips for both groups. Take your list and visit an elderly family member, friend, or neighbor's home. Review these tips with the person. Inspect the home for safety. What improvements or recommendations were you able to provide?

4. Make a list of preprinted educational materials that every office should have. What professional organizations (e.g., American Heart Association, American Cancer Society) could help provide these materials?

5. From information found at the American Cancer Society's website, develop a patient education information sheet for the current guidelines for breast cancer screening.

Answers to Checkpoint Questions

1. The purpose of the assessment step in teaching patients is to allow you to gather information about the patient's health care needs and abilities.

2. The purpose of the evaluation step in teaching patients is to allow you to determine how well patients are adapting or applying the new information to their lives.

3. The basic physiologic needs are air, food, water, rest, and comfort.

4. Six types of conditions or illnesses that may hinder patients' ability to learn effectively are illnesses with moderate to severe pain; illnesses with a poor prognosis or limited rehabilitation; illnesses resulting in weakness or general malaise as a primary symptom; illnesses that impair the patient's mental health or cognitive ability; more than one chronic illness; and illnesses that result in respiratory distress or difficulty in breathing.

5. The primary teaching focus for small children and their parents is safety and injury prevention.

6. Any patient who has trouble maintaining balance or uses an ambulation device should be taught fall prevention tips.

7. Placebo is the power of believing that something will make you better when there is no chemical reaction that warrants such improvement.

8. The elements necessary for a written teaching plan are: learning goals, the material to be covered, learning objectives, evaluation, comments, and documentation.

UNDERSTANDING THE PROFESSION (Chapters 1–4)

1. You are a CMA in a busy OB/GYN practice. You have been asked to orient a high school student who was hired to help up front and in medical records in the afternoons. She wants a career in health care but is unsure if she would be happier in a doctor's office or a hospital. She is debating between becoming a CMA or a CNA but is confused about the difference. She asks for your help in deciding what profession to choose. After hearing about medical assisting, she decides to take the path to become a CMA.

   A. What do the acronyms CNA and CMA stand for? (knowledge)

   B. How would you describe a typical day for a medical assistant? (comprehension)

   C. What path would you suggest she take to achieve her goal of becoming a medical assistant? (application)

   D. Compare the skills of a medical assistant to those of nursing assistant in a hospital setting. (analysis)

   E. What if the co-worker says that she will go through a program, but she doesn't plan to get certified? (synthesis)

   F. How would you reassure your co-worker that she has chosen an exciting and rewarding profession? (evaluation)

2. You work for a neurologist who asks you to construct a letter of withdrawal for Mrs. Jane Johnson. He states that she has been noncompliant and has missed three appointments in a row, and he wants to discharge her from the practice. Since Mrs. Johnson has a seizure disorder, she will need ongoing care.

   A. Does the doctor have the right to discharge a patient? (knowledge)

   B. What are the necessary components of the letter? (comprehension)

   C. How would the letter need to be sent? (application)

   D. What statement would need to be made so that the patient will not be abandoned in the legal sense? (analysis)

   E. What documents would need to be placed in the patient's record? Why? (synthesis)

   F. Why is it important for physicians to have this right? (evaluation)

3. You work in a pediatric practice. A mother brings her 6-month-old son in for a routine checkup. The child has a visible lump on the right side of his head, just above his ear. The mother states that the child fell off a twin bed when she was changing his diaper. After examining the child, the physician asks you to instruct the mother in safety and also have her watch the baby closely for the next few days for signs of concussion.

   A. What resources might be available to you? (knowledge)

   B. How might you evaluate the mother's barriers to communication and understanding? (comprehension)

   C. What method of instruction would you use for this situation? (application)

   D. What would your teaching plan need to include? (analysis)

   E. What measures should be taken if the child's injuries were consistent with possible abuse? (synthesis)

   F. Why is patient education important? (evaluation)

PART

II

The
Administrative
Medical
Assistant

TWO

Fundamentals of Administrative Medical Assisting

A well-run medical office requires that everyone works together as a team. Unit Two consists of six chapters that address administrative duties performed in the medical office. These duties include telephone and reception, appointment management, written communications, health information management, computer use, and medical office management. Some of these duties are shared with clinical personnel. This unit will help you to perform these duties whether you work in the front desk area or in the clinical area.

CHAPTER 5

The First Contact: Telephone and Reception

Outline

Professional Image
Importance of a Good Attitude
The Medical Assistant as a Role Model
Courtesy and Diplomacy in the Medical Office
First Impressions
Reception
The Role of a Receptionist
Duties and Responsibilities of the Receptionist

Ergonomic Concerns for the Receptionist
The Waiting Room Environment
The End of the Patient Visit
Telephone
Importance of the Telephone in the Medical Office
Basic Guidelines for Telephone Use

Routine Incoming Calls
Challenging Incoming Calls
Triaging Incoming Calls
Taking Messages
Outgoing Calls
Services and Special Features

Learning Objectives

Upon successfully completing this chapter, you will be able to:

1. Spell and define the key terms

2. Explain the importance of displaying a professional image to all patients

3. List six duties of the medical office receptionist

4. List four sources from which messages can be retrieved

5. Discuss various steps that can be taken to promote good ergonomics

6. Describe the basic guidelines for waiting room environments

7. Describe the proper method for maintaining infection control standards in the waiting room

8. Discuss the five basic guidelines for telephone use

9. Describe the types of incoming telephone calls received by the medical office

10. Discuss how to identify and handle callers with medical emergencies

11. Describe how to triage incoming calls

12. List the information that should be given to an emergency medical service dispatcher

13. Describe the types of telephone services and special features

Performance Objectives

Upon successfully completing this chapter, you will be able to:

1. Handle incoming calls (Procedure 5-1)

2. Call Emergency Medical Services (Procedure 5-2)

3. Explain general office policies (Procedure 5-3)

Competencies

CAAHEP

- Demonstrate telephone techniques
- Explain general office policies
- Instruct individuals according to their needs.

ABHES

- Use proper telephone technique
- Orient patients to office policies and procedures
- Adapt what is said to the recipient's level of comprehension
- Perform basic administrative medical assisting functions

Key Terms

attitude	diplomacy	ergonomic	teletypewriter (TTY)
closed captioning	emergency medical service (EMS)	receptionist	triage
diction			

As a medical assistant, you are the patient's primary contact with the physician. In certain situations, the patient may spend more time with you than with the physician. Your interaction with the patient sets the tone for the visit and directly influences the patient's perception of the office and the quality of care the patient will receive. Therefore, it is vital that you project a caring and competent professional image at all times. You will have various responsibilities and duties when working as a receptionist. These duties will vary among physician offices. Proper telephone etiquette and use is an essential skill for all medical assistants. You must be able to handle incoming and outgoing calls correctly and efficiently.

The Health Insurance Portability and Accountability Act (HIPAA), which is discussed throughout this text, requires all health care settings to ensure privacy and security of patient information. HIPAA's Privacy Rule affects every area of the office. In waiting areas where conversations can be overheard or information can be seen by patients, you must take precautions to protect patient confidentiality.

Professional Image

Importance of a Good Attitude

An **attitude** is a state of mind or feeling regarding some matter. It can be either positive or negative. Attitudes can be formed by past or present experiences; they can be transmitted from one person to another. How you feel influences how you act; thus, your attitude shapes your behavior. You transmit your attitude to others through your behavior, thereby influencing their attitudes and behaviors.

The medical assistant must be able to transmit a positive attitude to the patient. This requires acceptance of the patient as a unique individual who has the right to be treated with dignity and compassion in a nonjudgmental manner. Ask yourself how you would feel in a similar situation and how you would want to be treated. By demonstrating empathy, interest, and concern, you tell the patient that he or she is important to you and that you care. This exerts a positive influence on the patient's own attitude, behavior, and response.

For example, let's assume that you are working as a receptionist in a busy family practice office. It is the peak of the flu and cold season. Which of the following interactions between the medical assistant and the patient transmits a positive attitude to the patient:

- "I know you feel terrible, Mr. Smith, but so does everyone else in the waiting room. It's the flu season. Just have a seat, and the doctor will see you shortly."
- "I'm sorry you don't feel well. Do you feel well enough to sit in the waiting room for about 10 minutes? The doctor will be ready to see you then."

The second interaction shows the patient that you care about how he feels and reassures him that he will be seen by the physician shortly. In the first interaction, the attitude that was transmitted made Mr. Smith feel like just another sick patient. Your positive attitude will influence the patient's attitude, behavior, and response.

The Medical Assistant as a Role Model

Another way in which you as a medical assistant influence the patient's perception of the medical office is your personal appearance. Good health and good grooming present a positive image to the patient. Taking care of yourself by eating well, exercising regularly, and getting enough rest is important not only for your appearance but also for your job performance. If you are tired or sluggish, you cannot give good patient care.

Pay particular attention to your personal hygiene to avoid offending your patients. A person who is ill is often acutely sensitive to odors, even those normally considered pleasant. A daily bath or shower is essential, followed by an unscented deodorant. Keep your hair clean and styled. Good oral hygiene is important, and during the day you should avoid foods that may give an offensive odor. Keep your fingernails clean and trimmed, with clear or neutral polish. Long nails polished with vivid colors are not appropriate for the medical office. Natural nail tips must be less than a quarter inch long, according to the Centers for Disease Control and Prevention (CDC). Artificial nails may increase the potential for infection transmission to you and your patients. The CDC recommendation is for health care providers not to wear artificial nails if high-risk patient care is required. If you wear makeup, keep it natural and apply it lightly. Do not wear perfume, cologne, scented lotion, hair spray, or the like.

Most offices have a dress code. Whether you wear a uniform or street clothes, they should be clean, neat, pressed, and in good repair (Fig. 5-1). Wrinkles, missing buttons, split seams, torn hems, and stains project a negative image. Always wear clean, polished shoes. Stockings should be full length, of a neutral shade, and free from runs and holes. Jewelry such as dangling earrings, large rings, long chains, and ornate or multiple bracelets are not appropriate in the health care environment.

Courtesy and Diplomacy in the Medical Office

Being a medical assistant requires excellent human relations skills. In the course of a day, you will interact with a variety of personalities in a variety of situations, and

Figure 5-1 The properly dressed medical assistant presents a professional and positive image to patients.

you must be able to maintain a positive professional attitude regardless of how difficult the encounter may be. For example, you may have to interact with a person who has done domestic violence to a patient. It is important that you treat him or her with the same courtesy and respect that you offer all patients. Courtesy and diplomacy are fundamental to successful human relations.

Courtesy is based on sensitivity to the needs and feelings of others and demands that everyone be treated with respect and dignity. It is disrespectful to refer to physicians by first name or title only. Always use the title and last name. It is permissible to call a physician by his or her first name outside of clinical areas if the physician so requests. Be courteous to your co-workers as well as your employer and your patients. Do not borrow supplies or use someone else's desk without asking permission. Always knock before entering an office, even if the door is open.

Diplomacy is the art of handling people with tact and genuine concern. Use diplomacy in difficult situations. Patients may be curious about other patients; family members may want to know what the doctor said to the patient—such questions must be met with a polite refusal to disclose confidential information. Pain, worry, and waiting can make a patient unreasonable or irritable. You must exercise self-control and understanding and maintain your professional attitude. Never argue with a patient. Try to calm the patient and communicate your desire to help. Table 5-1 lists three common problems with patients and the diplomatic way to control each situation.

First Impressions

First impressions are lasting. Remember, you have only one chance to make a first impression on patients and other health care professionals. The patient's perception of the medical office is based in part on the impression you make. A negative perception can adversely affect the patient's health. A positive perception contributes to a successful doctor–patient relationship. Patients who feel positive about their relationship with health care providers are likely to follow treatment regimens.

Physician offices must operate as a business to remain financially sound. Patients want, expect, and deserve excellent customer service. Those who are not satisfied with their service may opt to leave the practice. Loss of patients will result in loss of revenue for the practice. As a medical assistant, you play a key role in promoting a positive image for the physician's practice. It has been said that patients who have a negative experience will tell eight people. This can have a spiraling effect on your practice.

 CHECKPOINT QUESTION

1. What are four ways that you can demonstrate a professional image to patients?

Reception

The Role of a Receptionist

The role of receptionist will vary greatly among offices. According to the 10th edition of *Merriam-Webster's Collegiate Dictionary*, a **receptionist** is a person employed to greet telephone callers, visitors, patients, or clients. In certain physician offices, the receptionist may be a non–medically trained professional whose primary task is to greet patients, alert staff members when patients are present, and serve as a telephone operator. This situation is generally found in large, multiphysician practices. If you are working in this type of setting, your role as a medical assistant will be to provide coverage while the receptionist is on break or at lunch.

In other office settings, however, you may work as the receptionist. These offices may also have multiple physicians but choose to have a medically trained person as the receptionist. No matter which type of office you work in, you will need to know and be able to assume the duties and responsibilities of a receptionist.

Duties and Responsibilities of the Receptionist

The duties of the receptionist begin long before the first appointment of the day. Most offices have the receptionist arrive at least 30 minutes prior to the first ap-

TABLE 5-1 Diplomatic Solutions to Common Challenges		
Common Problem	**Example of What to Say**	**Example of What Not to Say**
Prolonged Waiting Time		
"My appointment was for 9:30, and it is now 10:00. When am I going to be seen?"	"The doctor will see you in about 30 minutes." "We have had some emergencies. Would you like to wait or reschedule your visit?"	"It's flu season. Everyone is sick. Please sit down." "We'll get to you when we get to you."
Patient Confidentiality		
"I am worried about my neighbor. He was seen here yesterday and sent to the hospital by ambulance. What happened?"	"We appreciate your concern, but it is against federal privacy rules to give you confidential patient information."	"He was having some chest pain, but he is fine now." "Yes, we sent him by ambulance because he was very sick."
Patient Discomfort		
"I am in a lot of pain. I want to see the doctor now!"	"I can see that you are in pain. Please have a seat for 1 minute. I will find a room for you to lie down in."	"You are going to have to wait your turn. There are three patients ahead of you."
"I have been vomiting all day. I can't sit in the waiting room. I need to be seen now!"	"Please come with me. Here is a basin." Escort the patient to the restroom or assess patient's need for assistance.	"I can see that you are sick. You'll still have to wait your turn. Here is a trash can."

pointment. Your first task will be to prepare the office for patient arrivals.

Prepare the Office

As receptionist, you are responsible for preparing the office for patients and for other employee arrivals. These tasks should be done first:

- Unlock doors as appropriate.
- Disengage the alarm system.
- Turn on appropriate lights.
- Turn on computers, printers, copiers, and other electronic devices.
- If the office uses a drop box to leave specimens for evening pickups, check the box to ensure that the specimens were taken.

After those five tasks are done, do a systematic check of the office. The reception area should be clean and tidy. The reception desk should be free from clutter with confidential material safely out of sight Restock your desk with necessary forms and office supplies before patients arrive. In smaller offices, you may be responsible for checking the examination rooms.

This process should not take long. The office should never be left messy or in disarray at the end of the day. Stocking of supplies and cleaning and disinfecting exam-

ination rooms should be done before the staff leaves at night. The office should be left in a professional manner.

Retrieve Messages

Another responsibility you may have as a receptionist is to retrieve messages that were left while the office was closed. All physician offices have a method for communicating with their patients after hours. Most offices leave a greeting message on their main incoming line that directs patients to call a given number (answering service) for acute medical problems. Usually, this message also instructs patients to leave nonemergency messages on the voice mail.

Messages may be obtained from four sources:

- Answering service
- Voice mail system
- Electronic mail
- Facsimile machine

No matter how a message has been sent, however, all information must be treated confidentially and handled according to HIPAA regulations. The Privacy Rule of HIPAA requires that you avoid inadvertently revealing electronically shared medical information. Box 5-1 provides suggestions to help you adhere to HIPAA's Privacy Rule.

BOX 5-1

SUGGESTIONS FOR ADHERING TO HIPAA'S PRIVACY RULE

1. Design office furniture to provide the most privacy around the front desk.
2. Keep monitors, fax machines, patient charts, etc. out of the sight of those at the front desk and in the waiting room.
3. Talk to patients about their private and protected health information in as private an area as possible.
4. Keep reception window closed when possible.
5. Be mindful that your conversations with co-workers can be heard by patients and others in the area.

Messages should be checked as soon as the office opens, at midday, after breaks, and periodically throughout the day. After retrieving the messages, forward them to the appropriate staff for resolution.

Answering Service

Answering services receive calls from patients, hospital staff, and other physicians and communicate the emergency messages to the physician, generally by beeper. Other messages are left for the office staff to obtain the following morning. Examples of messages that could be left here are:

- Patients calling the office for a sick appointment (not an emergency) (such as an earache, flulike symptoms)
- Calls from hospitals or skilled nursing facilities about changes in patient status (new wounds or bed sores, patient falls without injury)

Voice Mail Systems

A voice mailbox is a type of answering machine in which the caller can leave a detailed message. You will need to know the security access code to obtain messages. After you obtain the messages, delete them from the recorder unless otherwise directed by office policy. Examples of messages that could be left here are:

- Patients wishing to change or cancel their appointment
- Patients requesting prescription refills
- Family members or patients calling to ask for additional information or clarification about their medical care or test results

Electronic Mail

The computer is a vital link for physicians to communicate with all health care professionals. E-mail messages are sent from other physicians, professional organizations, and hospital personnel. Some physician offices provide patients with their e-mail address. Examples of messages left here are:

- Memos from professional organizations
- Pharmaceutical representatives' updates or announcements
- Medical staff meeting minutes, announcements from hospital administration
- Upcoming continuing education courses for physicians
- Insurance representatives regarding billing issues

 LEGAL TIP

GUIDELINES FOR HANDLING ELECTRONICALLY SHARED INFORMATION

Federal law requires you to protect medical information.

- When a patient e-mails a provider, the communication should be documented just as any other exchange with the patient.
- Print the e-mail or cut and paste it into the patient's electronic chart.
- Delete the e-mail from the computer.
- Document any actions that were taken, instructions given, etc.
- Place the copy in the patient's chart or cut and paste it into the patient's electronic chart.
- Make sure only the people who need the information have access to it.
- Keep fax machines out of the public eye.
- Retrieve faxes promptly as they are received.
- Check to be sure you can read the fax. If the print on the fax is not clear, request a hard copy from the sender.
- Use plain paper in the fax machine to avoid fading with age as some forms of paper will do.

Facsimile Machines

All physician offices have a fax machine. The most common messages left here are:

- Patient referrals
- Consultation reports
- Laboratory and radiology reports

 CHECKPOINT QUESTION

2. What four locations should you retrieve messages from?

Prepare the Charts

Your next duty will be to gather charts. Gather the charts of all of the patients scheduled to be seen for the day and put them in order by appointment. Review each chart to ensure that it is complete and up to date. Check that adequate clinical data sheets are available for the doctor to record any notes. Test results received since the patient's last appointment and any other new information are placed in the front of the chart for the doctor's review. Make up a chart for each new patient and have the appropriate registration forms ready for the patient to complete. Once the charts are prepared, they are usually kept at the reception desk and given to the doctor or clinical assistant as the patient arrives, although some doctors prefer to have all charts on their desk at the start of the day. (See Chapter 8.)

Welcome Patients and Visitors

Make every attempt to greet patients personally and by name, e.g., "Good morning, Ms. Misko." A smile and cheerful greeting promote a positive image and make the patient feel welcome. Try to remember something personal about each patient, such as hobbies, pets, or special interests about which you can ask. Sometimes, you will not be at your desk when a patient arrives. Check the waiting room for new arrivals upon your return. Many offices install a bell or chime on the door and post a sign requesting patients to check in with the receptionist. Even if you cannot greet them immediately, acknowledge them with a smile and a nod until you can help them. You would not let someone walk into your home without greeting them immediately. If it is your responsibility to greet patients, you should make this a top priority.

Register and Orient Patients

Patients who are new to the office will have to complete a registration form, also called a patient information sheet. On this form, the patient provides name, address, and telephone number; the name, address, and telephone number of the insurance company or other party responsible for payment; employer names and addresses; marital status; spouse's name; social security number; and name of the person who referred the patient. Some information sheets include questions about medical history. In some cases, you may complete the form while interviewing the patient. Most offices have the patients fill in these forms and ask for your help if questions arise.

After registration, orient the patient to the office. Brochures that give the names of the doctor and staff, office hours, and telephone numbers are helpful. Explain any pertinent office policies or procedures, such as billing procedures, how to make or cancel appointments, and parking. Ask if the patient has any questions. Procedure 5-3 outlines the steps for explaining office policies to a new patient. Tell the patient where the water fountain and restrooms are, but caution the patient against using the restroom without checking with you to determine whether a urine specimen is needed. Urine specimens are generally needed for pregnant patients, patients with lower back or abdominal pain or back injuries, and patients being seen for drug or pre-employment health examinations. At the appropriate time, you may be responsible for taking patients to the examination room unless another health care worker escorts the patients.

Manage Waiting Time

Patients expect to be seen at the appointed time. They have allotted time in their schedule to see the doctor and do not want to be kept waiting. One of the major complaints of patients is the length of time they must wait to see the physician. Be sure to tell the patients if the doctor is behind schedule. If you expect the wait to be 30 minutes or more past the scheduled time, offer waiting patients some choices. Some choose to leave and come back in an hour, and some choose to reschedule the appointment for another time. Be honest with waiting patients. Tell them why there is a delay. If the provider has been called away for an emergency, patients will respect his dedication and appreciate the fact that if they need their doctor in an emergency, he will be there for them.

Ergonomic Concerns for the Receptionist

For most of the day you will be sitting at your desk performing these tasks. Occasional lifting of delivery boxes, paper supplies, and so on is required. The duties of the receptionist require you to twist from your primary desk to other areas to reach for files or to answer the telephone. These actions can lead to back injuries and other musculoskeletal disorders. Medical professionals are at high risk for such injuries. Having a good **ergonomic** workstation and good body mechanics, however, can prevent most injuries.

An ergonomic workstation is designed specifically to prevent injuries and often results in increased employee satisfaction and work efficiency. The Occupational Safety and Health Administration (OSHA) has many recommendations for preventing such injuries. Here are some other suggestions to prevent injuries:

- Keep items that you must lift at waist level when possible. Keep the load close to the body. Bend at your hips.

N

- Instruct delivery people to place packages in locations that will not require movement.
- Carry only small loads of paper. Make additional trips as needed.
- Place items that you frequently use within easy reach. Moves from side to side are safer than twisting to a desk behind you. Avoiding storing charts above chest level to limit reaching over your head. Use a step stool to reach high shelves instead of stretching.
- Telephones with headsets will keep your head upright and allow your shoulders to relax. If you use a stationary phone, a long handset cord can reduce muscle strain. Do not rest the telephone on your shoulder while talking, since this causes neck and back injuries.

 CHECKPOINT QUESTION

3. What is the purpose of having an ergonomic workstation?

The Waiting Room Environment
General Guidelines for Waiting Rooms

The reception area should be designed for the comfort, safety, and enjoyment of all patients. It should be kept clean and uncluttered, with the furniture arranged to allow ample room for walking. A coat rack and umbrella stand should be present. Restrooms and a water fountain should be easily accessible.

Furniture should be aesthetically pleasing, comfortable, and durable. Chairs are preferable to sofas because most people find sharing a sofa with strangers uncomfortable. Chairs allow patients to maintain a degree of privacy and personal space. There should be a variety of soft chairs and firm chairs and chairs with and without arms. Some patients find it hard to stand up from a soft chair; others prefer the comfort. Some need chair arms to push themselves up, and others are more comfortable without chair arms.

A low-key color scheme is advisable. Muted pastels are preferable to bright primary colors, although the latter work well in pediatric offices (Fig. 5-2). Lighting should be bright but not harsh. The room should be well ventilated and kept at a comfortable temperature. Many offices provide soothing background music.

Landscapes, waterscapes, and floral and animal pictures make better wall décor than abstract art. Lamps and plants can add interest to corners. Keep plants in good condition, and remove any dead leaves. An office with dead or dying plants does not project a comforting image.

A good selection of reading material should be available. Have a variety of current magazines that are ap-

Figure 5-2 Children will respond to a doctor's visit more positively if the office is decorated for them.

propriate for your patients. The doctor's professional journals should not be included. The reception area is a good place to set out patient education materials.

Some offices provide television for patients who prefer not to read. Most patients find television relaxing and entertaining, but other patients find it annoying. Television can serve as an education tool. Here are a few tips that you should follow regarding television:

- The volume should be set to allow a group of people to hear the television but not at a distracting volume for the whole waiting room.
- A simple sign placed on the television, "Please do not touch the controls; see the receptionist for channel changes" will prevent patients from selecting inappropriate programs.
- Only family-oriented programs should be shown. It is acceptable to select a news channel. No shows with violence, strong language, or sexual content should be on. Soap operas are not suitable for medical office waiting rooms.
- Some offices leave the television off unless a patient asks to have it on.
- Patients with hearing impairments must be offered the option of **closed captioning** if they choose to watch television. (Closed captioning is the translation of the spoken word into a written format. Most televisions have this capability under their options menu.)

You should check the waiting room several times during the day to make sure it is clean and tidy. Also check the entrance, hallways, and stairs. These areas too must be well lighted and maintained. Liability is a concern if patients slip on ice or snow coming into the office. Remember, the patient's privacy must be protected in the reception and waiting areas of the office as well (see Box 5-1).

PATIENT EDUCATION

TELEVISION AS A TEACHING TOOL

A television in the reception area can entertain patients while they wait for an appointment, but it can also be a patient education tool. By using a television in conjunction with a VCR, you can play a variety of educational videos. Here are some points to keep in mind:

- Be sure all videos have been previewed by the physician.
- Select videos that are geared toward the specialty of the practice (e.g., a video about heart attacks is appropriate for a cardiologist's office but not for a dermatologist's office).
- Carefully assess the graphic nature of certain videos. (A picture of the birth of a child may interest you, but it might be too much for some patients.)
- Keep in mind the age of the patients and family members who will be in the waiting room. Caution must be used if small children are often in the area. For example, a video about preventing sexually transmitted diseases may provide information appropriate for a family practice office, but it would not be appropriate to show the video in the reception area.

CHECKPOINT QUESTION

4. What option should you offer hearing-impaired patients if they wish to watch television?

Guidelines for Pediatric Waiting Rooms

Pediatric offices tend to be very busy practices with a multitude of reasons for patient visits. Generally, visits to the pediatrician can be divided into three types: well child checks, sick child visits, and follow-up visits. Because of the large volume of sick child visits, most pediatric waiting room areas are broken into two sections, one for well children and the other for sick children. Parents may have to be instructed by you as to which side of the waiting room they should sit in. According to the American Academy of Pediatrics (AAP), no studies document the effectiveness of segregated waiting room areas. The recommendation of the AAP is to move children with a communicable disease into an examination room as quickly as possible. Your employer will provide you with instructions and guidelines for dealing with sick children.

A children's play area must be closely watched and monitored. Toys should be kept away from the general seating area. Here are some guidelines for toys:

- Toys should be simple and easy to clean, without sharp edges.
- A policy must be in place for routine cleaning of these toys.
- Toys should be checked daily to ensure that they are not broken. Toys that are broken must be thrown away. Toys should never be glued or taped together.
- Battery-powered toys that make loud noises are not permissible.
- Toys can be a choking hazard. According to the American Heart Association, small children should never to be given toys that can fit inside a standard toilet paper roll. Although older children would like to play with toys like Legos, these toys should not be present. Older children should be expected to sit quietly while waiting for their appointment.

A good selection of books should be present for parents to read to their children. Books must be checked periodically to ensure that they are clean and no pages have been torn out. A small table and chairs will give children a place to read or color.

Americans with Disabilities Act Requirements

The US Department of Justice is responsible for ensuring that all people are treated without discrimination of any kind. Under this department is the Americans with Disabilities Act (ADA). This act prohibits discrimination on the basis of a person's disability. The ADA Title III act requires that all public accommodations be accessible to everyone. This includes access into medical facilities. It is important that you be aware of the basic concept of the ADA rules. Table 5-2 lists some of the basic facility requirements. Additional information is available on the ADA website.

The existing structural dimensions are not something that you have control of, but you need to ensure that there is a clear path to the physician's office at all times. Here are some steps that you can take to ensure this:

- Check that deliveries are left in a safe place. They must not be left in the waiting area or block the door.
- Keep toys clear of entrance pathways.
- Check that chairs are not moved, creating obstacles that might limit wheelchair accessibility.
- Ensure that doors are not blocked or propped opened with objects.
- Limit the amount of stacked papers on counters that may limit the patient's access to you.
- Check the restroom regularly to make sure the entrance is open and not obstructed.

TABLE 5-2	Summary of ADA Requirements for Public Buildings
Area	**Specifics**
Access	Route must be stable, firm, and slip resistant.
	Route must be 36 inches wide.
Ramps	Ramps longer than 6 feet must have two railings.
	Railings must be 34–38 inches high.
	Ramp must be 36 inches wide.
	Ramps and elevators must be available to all public levels.
Entrance and door	Door must be 32 inches wide.
	Door handle must be no higher than 48 inches and must be operable with a closed fist.
	Interior doors must open without excessive force.
Miscellaneous	Carpeting must be no more than 0.5 inch high.
	Emergency egress system must have flashing lights and audible signals.
	Space for wheelchair seating must be available.
	Tables or counters must be 28–34 inches high.
Restrooms	Tactile signs must identify restrooms.
	Doorway must be at least 32 inches wide.
	All doors (including stall doors), soap dispensers, hand dryers, and faucets must be operable with a closed fist.
	Wheelchair stall is required and must be at least 5 feet by 5 feet.

 CHECKPOINT QUESTION

5. What act prohibits discrimination of patients with disabilities?

Infection Control Issues

To prevent the spread of disease, aseptic technique must be used in every aspect of work in the medical office. During the clinical portion of your training, you will learn detailed information about infection control. As a receptionist, however, you need to be aware of a few key points:

- Always follow standard precautions. This means that you must treat all body fluids with precautionary measures.
- Handwashing is the most important practice for preventing the transmission of diseases. You must wash your hands following all direct patient contact (touching the patient) (Fig. 5-3). Since it is not always possible to leave the desk to wash your hands, the CDC has approved the use of alcohol-based antiseptic handwashing solutions for health care providers.
- Patients are often told to bring specimens to the office. Never touch a specimen container without proper gloves and personal protective equipment.

- Patients who arrive coughing and sneezing should be given tissues and instructed to cover their mouth and nose when coughing. Communicate with the clinical staff to have these patients taken directly into examination rooms. Patients who are vomiting, bleeding, or discharging other body fluids must not be left in the waiting room.

Biohazard Waste

All body fluids must be considered infectious and be managed appropriately. All body fluid spills and blood-stained papers must be disposed of in a biohazard container. The spills must be cleaned with an approved germicidal solution. If you have not been trained in handling such waste, do not touch it. Allow the clinical staff to handle the waste. If possible, contain the spill and prevent other patients from touching the area. Here are some examples of biohazard waste that you may encounter:

- Dressing supplies with bloodstains from cuts or wounds
- Tissues from patients with acute nosebleeds
- Urine-saturated diapers left in the restroom
- Vomit
- Saturated tissues with sputum

Figure 5-3 Good handwashing skills are essential to prevent disease transmission.

BOX 5-2

PATIENTS WHO SHOULD NOT BE LEFT IN THE WAITING ROOM

Patients with any of the following diseases or conditions should not be left in the waiting room. These patients should be taken to an examination room as soon as possible:

- Chickenpox
- Conjunctivitis
- Influenza
- Measles and rubella
- Meningitis (or suspected cases)
- Mumps
- Pertussis
- Pneumonia (if patient is coughing)
- Smallpox
- Tuberculosis
- Wounds (if open and draining)

Communicable Diseases

Depending on the type of office you work in, the amount of exposure to communicable diseases will vary. Family practice physicians and pediatricians, for example, treat acute communicable diseases regularly. If you work as a receptionist for a pediatrician, you will need to learn how to look at rashes and determine whether they are contagious.

Good communication between you and the clinical staff is essential to manage patients with communicable diseases. The clinical staff is often aware of patients with such diseases and will communicate it to you. Most infectious diseases cannot be transmitted with routine physical contact (handshaking, talking, touching, sharing pencils, using the telephone). Examples of infectious diseases that cannot be transmitted by routine physical contact include HIV, hepatitis, and the common cold. Some diseases can be easily transmitted, however, and patients with these diseases should not be left in the waiting room. Box 5-2 lists patients who should not be left in the waiting room.

Patients who have an impaired immune system or are taking medications that hinder their immune system (chemotherapy agents) may require immediate place-

ment in an examination room to prevent exposure to otherwise benign organisms. The clinical staff will alert you to these patients.

 CHECKPOINT QUESTION

6. What is the most antiseptic technique for preventing the transmission of diseases?

The End of the Patient Visit

After physicians have completed the examination or other procedures, they generally direct patients to get dressed and wait for their discharge information. In some offices, physicians provide all discharge instructions, while in other office settings, nurses or medical assistants may be assigned to discharge patients. Chapter 4 discusses the information you need to teach your patients. After the medical portion is completed, the patient is escorted to the front desk. It is generally at this time that any fees or copayments are collected by the receptionist. If the doctor has requested a follow-up visit, the appointment should be scheduled. An appointment reminder card is helpful for the patient. You or other administrative personnel may do these tasks. You should bid the patient goodbye in a warm and friendly manner. As patients leave the office, they should feel they have been well cared for by a competent and courteous staff.

TELEPHONE

Importance of the Telephone in the Medical Office

The medical office is filled with expensive scientific equipment used in the diagnosis and treatment of disease, but one of the most important instruments is the telephone. It allows the patient rapid and easy access to medical care. A patient can schedule an appointment, seek medical advice, request prescription refills, obtain test results, question a bill, or report an emergency simply by picking up the telephone. The telephone also links the physician's office to the rest of the medical community, including hospitals, pharmacies, and other doctors.

You must be able to communicate a positive image of the physician and staff over the telephone without the aid of nonverbal cues such as appearance, facial expressions, body language, and gestures. You must be able to use the tone and quality of your voice and speech to project a competent and caring attitude over the telephone.

Basic Guidelines for Telephone Use

Telephone communication is not effective if either party does not fully understand what is being said. Misunderstandings can be embarrassing, frustrating, or even life threatening. To have effective telephone communication, you must be able to overcome various obstacles, such as a noisy environment, a poor telephone connection, a patient's emotional distress, or a patient's hearing or speech impairments

Diction

Diction refers to how words are spoken and enunciated. You should speak clearly and distinctly and use proper grammar. Talk clearly into the mouthpiece; do not prop the handset between your chin and shoulder. Never chew gum or eat while you speak on the telephone. Speak at a moderate pace to avoid slurring your words. Your grammar should be correct.

Pronunciation

Make sure you pronounce words correctly to avoid misunderstandings. Avoid using unfamiliar words, slang, and idiomatic expressions. Most patients do not understand medical terminology, so it is best to use lay terms whenever possible. For example, do not ask the patient, "Are you dyspneic?" Instead ask, "Are you having trouble breathing?"

Expression

Put a smile in your voice by sitting up straight and putting a smile on your lips. Speak with a modulated pitch and volume. Use proper inflection to avoid a droning, monotonous speaking style.

Listening

Be an attentive listener. Focus on the conversation and ignore outside distractions. Guide the conversation to obtain the information you need from the caller. Do not interrupt the speaker. You may have to ask the caller to repeat what was said. Verify your understanding by repeating the message. Some people tend to flood you with information. In order to keep the call concise and to the point, you will need to guide the conversation without being rude. For example, Mrs. Jones calls for an appointment. When you ask her why she needs to see the doctor, she begins a detailed history of her headaches. You have what you need. You could say, "Mrs. Jones, let me interrupt you because I don't want you to have to repeat this to several people. The CMA will record all of this when you see the doctor." Although listening carefully is important, you are handling several telephone lines at the same time.

Courtesy

Always speak politely and courteously. Address the caller by title and last name. Although many telephone calls interrupt your work, do not allow your voice to portray impatience or irritation. Remember that you are there to help the patient (Fig. 5-4).

Figure 5-4 While speaking on the telephone, be courteous and professional.

Never answer the telephone and immediately put the caller on hold. If you need to answer another line or finish a task before you can engage in conversation, ask if the caller would mind holding. Courtesy demands that you wait for an answer before you place the call on hold. Also of great importance, you must determine whether the call is an emergency. If you are unable to take the call after 90 seconds, check back with the caller and ask whether he or she would like to continue holding. Again, wait for an answer before you place the call on hold. If the hold exceeds 3 minutes, you should apologize to the caller for the delay and offer to return the call as soon as you are available.

If you are already engaged in a telephone conversation and have to answer another line, ask the party with whom you are speaking if he or she would mind holding. Again, wait for a reply before answering the second call. Explain to the second caller that you are on the other line and need to complete that call. Do not handle the second call while the first party waits unless the second call is an emergency, a long distance call that cannot be referred to another worker, or a physician calling to speak with your physician.

Quite often you will find that you are juggling the telephones and patients who are in the office. Exercise your best judgment in balancing the tasks. If the call is going to take a long time, ask the caller to wait a moment, address the needs of the patient in the office, and then return to the call. Remember, all information about and conversations with patients are confidential. Use caution when talking on the telephone in front of patients.

CHECKPOINT QUESTION

7. What are the five basic guidelines for telephone use?

Routine Incoming Calls

An incoming call should be given the same courtesy and attention as an arriving visitor. Just as you would not keep a patient waiting without acknowledging his or her presence, so too must you acknowledge an incoming call promptly. Answer the telephone by the second ring if at all possible. Identify both the office and yourself to assure the caller that the correct number has been reached, and offer your assistance. The following are examples of common calls that come into a medical office.

Appointments

New patients call to make appointments, and established patients call to schedule return visits. (See Chapter 6.) Always obtain a new patient's telephone number and

LEGAL TIP

GUIDELINES FOR ENSURING PATIENT PRIVACY AROUND THE RECEPTION AREA

A waiting area and reception desk are places where confidentiality can be breached.

- Close the privacy window when you are not speaking with a patient.
- Never take patient information, demographic or clinical, at the front desk. Have the patient step to a more private area.
- Keep your voice down while discussing patients. Waiting patients may hear what you are saying.
- When making referral calls, use a telephone away from the reception area.
- Keep computer screens, printed appointment lists, appointment books, patient charts, etc. out of the view of patients at the window or around the reception area.
- Do not use a sign-in sheet unless it has a protector over previous names on the sheet.
- Be mindful of patients' right to privacy as you go about your daily duties.

verify an established patient's number in case you need to reach the patient before their appointment.

Billing Inquiries

In some offices, you may be responsible for handling routine inquiries concerning billing, fees, services, and insurance. You may be asked for specific information concerning the cost of services; do not quote exact prices, but tell the patient that costs depend on the type of examination and diagnostic tests performed. Sometimes, third-party callers request information about the patient; remember that no patient information can be given to anyone without a specific release from the patient.

Diagnostic Test Results

Many laboratory and radiology reports are called in to the physician's office before the written copy is sent. Record the information and post it on the front of the chart for the physician to review. If the results are needed at once, bring the information to the physician's attention immediately upon receiving the report. Having at hand a blank laboratory slip or specially designed forms listing the most frequently ordered reports for your office will save time and make it easier to accurately record the results as they are relayed from the laboratory or radiology department. Administrative personnel will place a written copy of test results in the patient's chart.

Routine and Satisfactory Progress Reports

At the end of an office visit, a patient may be told to call in a progress report within a few days. If the patient says he or she is feeling better or getting stronger or the symptoms have resolved, take down the information, record it in the patient's chart, and place it on the physician's desk for review. You may also handle routine progress reports from hospitals, home health agencies, and other allied health professionals. For example, a home care nurse may call and report that a patient's blood pressure is now within normal limits, or a physical therapist may call the office and say that a patient's range of motion is improving. Again, record the information and place it on the physician's desk for review.

Test Results

Patients often call for their test results, and many doctors allow the medical assistant to report favorable test results to patients. Your office will have a specific policy for handling these calls. It is illegal to give information to anyone other than the patient without the patient's specific consent. This consent should be in the form of written permission in the chart, in accordance with HIPAA regulations. Always document the call, as in Figure 5-5.

Unsatisfactory Progress Reports and Test Results

The doctor must speak with patients whose progress or test results are unsatisfactory. The urgency of the patient's condition determines whether the call requires the physician's immediate attention. The physician will discuss serious unsatisfactory test results with the patient. In less serious cases, the physician may ask you to speak with the patient. Never discuss unsatisfactory test results with a patient unless the doctor directs you to do so.

> 11/7/2008   Per Dr. Hedrich, called pt & told her that lab work was normal. She had no questions.
>
> GRM, CMA

Figure 5-5 Charting example.

Prescription Refills

As a medical assistant, you can handle requests for prescription refills if they are indicated on the chart. Most offices have an established protocol for refilling maintenance medications. If there is any doubt, tell the pharmacy or the patient that you will check with the doctor and call back.

Other Calls

Other calls you ordinarily handle include requests for referrals to other physicians, clarifying instructions for patients, and calls concerning routine administrative matters.

Ask the physician which calls he or she prefers to have transferred immediately and which calls can be returned later. Calls from other physicians should be directed to the physician immediately or according to office policy (Box 5-3). Physicians also receive personal calls. Your employer will tell you which calls should be put through immediately. Otherwise, take a message and tell the caller that the doctor will return the call.

BOX 5-3

TELEPHONE ETIQUETTE

- When another physician calls, it is customary to give the call top priority. Many physicians instruct their receptionists to interrupt them. This shows the physician that you respect his time. Always ask the physician if you need to pull a patient chart before you get your doctor. If the call is about a patient, your doctor will need a chart. If it is a personal call or about something other than a patient, the calling doctor will say no. This way you do not have to ask the nature of the call.
- Never put a patient on hold without first asking if they can hold and then waiting for a response.
- Include office extensions in the patient informational brochure so that patients do not have to listen to a long list of options. They can dial an extension to be put through immediately.
- Be respectful of the caller's time.
- Ensure that automated answering systems give the patient instructions to immediately bypass the recorded greetings in case of an emergency. For example, the first thing the caller should hear is "If this is an emergency, please dial `0' now."
- Make an effort to add the human touch to automated systems.

Challenging Incoming Calls

Unidentified Callers

Sometimes, callers who ask to speak with the physician refuse to state their name or the nature of their business. In such instances, you should politely but firmly tell the caller that you cannot interrupt the physician and politely explain that you would be happy to take a message. If the caller persists, ask the caller to call back at a specific time when the physician will be available. Alert the physician that there will be a call for him or her at the specified time. Unidentified callers may be sales representatives.

Irate Patients

When a caller is angry, you must be careful to keep your own temper in check. Try to calm the patient and offer assurance that you want to help. Listen carefully and take notes. If you cannot resolve the situation, let the patient know you must consult with the physician and offer to call back. The physician will probably want to speak with the patient personally. Always tell the physician about complaints regarding fees or care.

 WHAT IF?

An upset patient calls with questions about her bill and demands to speak with the employee who handles accounts receivable, who is at lunch. What should you say?

Patient: "Give me that woman who gets all of my money!"

Medical Assistant (MA): "Mrs. Smith in the Accounts Receivable Department is out of the office for lunch. May I transfer you to her voice mailbox?"

Patient: "Absolutely not! Someone else there must know something about the billing."

MA: "I'll be glad to try and help you, Mrs. McGuire."

If you cannot answer Mrs. McGuire's questions, tell her exactly when she can expect a call from Mrs. Smith. Make sure that happens. By cross-training all employees to understand the billing process, you can give patients better service. Making notes in a memo area of your office computer's system will give every employee an opportunity to look at the patient's account and help patients when they call.

Medical Emergencies

As a medical assistant, you must be able to differentiate between routine calls and emergencies. To do this, first try to calm the caller and ask specific questions concerning the patient's condition. Severe pain, profuse bleeding, respiratory distress, chest pain, loss of consciousness, severe vomiting or diarrhea, and a temperature above 102.0°F are all emergencies, and you should immediately put the call through to the physician or an appropriate health care professional. In some offices, nurses will be assigned to handle these calls.

Determine the patient's name, location, and telephone number as quickly as possible in case you are disconnected or the patient is unable to continue the conversation. This will allow you to direct emergency personnel to the patient's aid. The office should have a policy for handling emergency calls when the doctor is not in the office. Most policies advise you to direct patients to go to the nearest emergency room or walk-in center.

Ask the physician to list instances that might constitute an emergency in his or her specialty and to describe how they should be handled. For example, if you work for a cardiologist, most of your emergency calls will be patients with chest pain and trouble breathing. The cardiologist may instruct you to ask the patient standard questions, have you instruct patients to take certain medications, and then instruct the patient to dial for an ambulance. If you are working for an obstetrician, your emergency calls will be related to patients who have labor concerns or sudden onset of bleeding. Most obstetricians have precise recommendations for when patients in labor should go to the hospital (e.g., contractions lasting more than 1 minute with a frequency of every 5 minutes). Once you have the list of the most common calls and what your response should be, put the list in a prominent place near the telephone.

Triaging Incoming Calls

Usually the office telephone has multiple lines, and frequently, several patients call at the same time. You must be able to **triage** (sort) them into a priority order. For example, any patient with a potentially life-threatening problem, such as chest pain, needs to be taken first. Follow your office policy for emergencies. Patients with serious but non–life-threatening problems should also be handled promptly according to office protocol. Callers who are upset or angry will become increasingly upset the longer they have to wait; handle these calls as quickly as possible. If you need to get back to the caller, do so in a timely manner. Do not leave messages unresolved.

TRIAGE

While answering the telephone, you must handle callers on four different lines:

A. Line 1 is a home care nurse calling the office with a patient status update.

B. Line 2 is a pharmacist questioning a prescription.

C. Line 3 is a mother of a 3-year-old child who has been vomiting for 24 hours.

D. Line 4 is a patient who is having trouble breathing.

How would prioritize these calls? Which one should be handled first? Last?

First, handle the patient on line 4. After gathering information about the patient's complaint and following office protocol, determine the best action. Instruct the patient to come in immediately or to report to the emergency department of a hospital. Next, handle Line 3 using office guidelines as mentioned earlier. Line 2 can be handled next. Even though the patient may be waiting at the pharmacy, the other two calls are more important since they involve the patients' conditions. Lastly, you may record the information on Line 1.

Taking Messages

Taking messages for the physician or other health care professionals will be a large part of your daily responsibilities. Taking messages is easier using notepads designed for this task. Office supply companies have an assortment of pads, or your physician may choose to design his or her own. Carbonless copies give you a record of the messages taken during the day and the action taken.

The minimum information needed for a telephone message includes the name of the caller, date and time of the call, telephone number where the caller can be reached, a short description of the caller's concern, and the person to whom the message is routed.

Before you end the call, tell the patient when to expect a return call. Callback times vary from office to office. Some physicians return calls only at the end of the day, while others return calls randomly. Learn the policy of the office in which you are working.

The patient's chart must document all calls. If you return the call to the patient, document your conversation in the medical record. Some message pads are designed to be added to the progress note on the patient's chart when the call is complete.

 CHECKPOINT QUESTION

8. What is the minimum information needed for taking messages?

Outgoing Calls

General Guidelines for Outgoing Calls

You will make outgoing calls as well as receive incoming calls. You should prepare for your calls carefully; have all information gathered and know what you want to say before you dial the number. If you are calling a patient to reschedule an appointment, be able to explain why the change is necessary and be prepared to offer a new appointment time.

At times, you may have to make long distance calls. You may be required to document calls for the office records. Keep in mind the difference in time zones; if you do not know the time zone of the city you are calling, check the front of the telephone directory. Long distance calls should be dialed directly, without operator assistance. If you dial a wrong number or become disconnected during the call, notify the long distance operator immediately to avoid charges. Never make a long distance call unless you are authorized to do so.

Your employer may ask you to place a conference call, which connects three or more people. Notify all parties of the date and time the call will be made to ensure that everyone will be available to participate. Participants should be given the access phone number and the access code in advance of the scheduled call.

Calling Emergency Medical Services

Some patients will need immediate transport to a hospital. When emergencies occur in the physician's office, the clinical staff will be busy providing life-saving procedures to the patient. As a receptionist, you will be directed to call the local **emergency medical service (EMS)** for transport. In most areas of the United States, the emergency number is 911. Prior to placing the call, obtain the following information:

- Patient's name, age, and sex. (Age is important, especially if the patient is a newborn or child. This will allow the dispatcher to send the most appropriate responders.)
- Nature of the medical problem (chest pain, abdominal pain, bleeding).
- Type of service the physician is requesting. Generally, there are two levels of care: basic and advanced life support. Types of services will vary from community to community.
- Any specific instructions or requests the physician may have. Generally, patients are taken to the nearest

hospital; the physician may have made arrangements for the patient to be admitted at a specific hospital, however, because of a condition or diagnosis. For example, a patient with a high-risk pregnancy may be sent to a hospital with an appropriate newborn nursery instead of the community hospital. It is important that this information be told to the dispatcher so the appropriate team can be sent.

- The location of the office and any specific instructions for access, e.g., 92 Main Street, Medical Office Group, third floor, last door on the left.

After gathering the information, dial the emergency medical service number. Speak in a slow, calm voice to the dispatcher. Give the information. If the dispatcher has additional questions, answer them. Ask the dispatcher the approximate arrival time for the ambulance. Do not end the call until instructed to do so by the dispatcher. (See Figure 5-6.)

After placing the call, alert the staff to the approximate arrival time and any other pertinent information. Ensure that the path for the ambulance personnel is unobstructed and accessible. Reassure other patients in the waiting room. If the patient has any family members present, offer them assistance and reassurance.

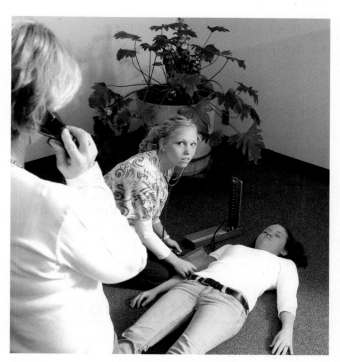

Figure 5-6 No matter what role you play, an office emergency requires all employees to be prepared.

 CHECKPOINT QUESTION

9. What patient information should you know before calling emergency medical services?

Services and Special Features

The telephone system that is used for physician offices should be large enough to serve the needs of the office. For example, if you are working for a single dermatologist, two incoming phone lines may be enough. If you are a receptionist for a large family practice with multiple physicians and other practitioners, however, the number of incoming lines will be greater. Most offices also have unpublished incoming numbers or lines. Staff members, families, and other physicians primarily use these private lines. In addition, most offices have a direct line to the local hospital. A wide variety of communication equipment is available today, and communications consultants can help determine the appropriate services and equipment for your office. At minimum, the phone system should have recall, volume control, intercom, call forwarding, and caller identification. Cordless headsets prevent neck injuries and allow for mobility.

An auto-attendant is the recorded message that answers your phones and instructs callers how to reach the person or department they are looking for. If an office has a high volume of calls, this may be important, or there may be value in having a real person answer every call. You can help callers find the people they need

with dial by name, dial by extension, or dial from directory services.

Phone sets themselves have more standard features, as well. Display phones have a small screen that shows information such as the name and extension of an internal caller, the duration of call, and in some cases, caller ID. Speaker phones are familiar fixtures in many conference rooms but are also now standard on most new handsets. Speaker phones can be half-duplex, which means that only one person on the call can be heard at a time, or full-duplex, which lets both parties talk simultaneously, like a regular phone. Some phones also have a "listen only" mode for speaker phone, which is useful for monitoring a conference call or while on hold. HIPAA guidelines for patient confidentiality must be considered when using speaker phone features. This should only be used in private areas of the office.

Most physicians have a cellular telephone. This number should never be given to anyone, although it should be readily accessible for staff members. Physicians and other health care professionals also have pager systems. Most pager systems allow you to send typed messages to the recipient via the computer. These messages are displayed on the pager, e.g., "Kate Larke's blood sugar was 420," or "Please call Dr. Harrison about Patrick Burke." Typing messages directly into a pager system is good time management. Text messaging or typing on the keypad is also available on most cellular phones. This feature is helpful when it is not necessary to speak with the person or a ringtone would be inappropriate.

CHECKPOINT QUESTION

10. What is text messaging, and when might it be used?

Telecommunication Relay Systems

Patients with hearing or speech impairments often have difficulty communicating with a standard telephone. The ADA requires that telephone companies have telecommunication relay systems (TRS) available 24 hours a day. A relay system allows the caller to type messages into a special telephone that transmits the message across the lines to the other party. The other party reads the message and types a response. The communication continues through written messages. A telephone with an attachment for typing messages is called a **teletypewriter (TTY)**. If the other party does not have the capabilities to read the message, an operator can be used to translate the message. Most physician offices have a TTY phone or access to one. The Federal Communication Commission has set minimum standards for TRS and TTY systems for public buildings. These standards can be found on their website.

español
SPANISH TERMINOLOGY

¡Hola!
Hello!

¿Cómo se llama usted?
What is your name?

¿En qué puedo servirle?
May I help you?

¿Cuál es su dirección?
What is your address?

¿Cuál es el código postal?
What is the zip code?

¿Cuál es su número de teléfono?
What is your phone number?

¿Fecha de nacimiento?
What is your birth date?

¿Cuántos años tiene?
How old are you?

Por favor, siéntese en la sala de espera.
Please have a seat in the waiting room.

Necesito hacerle unas preguntas.
I need to ask you some questions.

Por favor, llene estos papeles.
Please fill out these papers.

 MEDIA MENU

- **Student CD**
  - **Case Study**
    Administrative Interactive Case Study on Maintaining Medical Records and HIPAA; and Managing a Medical Office Emergency
  - **CMA/RMA Certification Exam Review**
- **Premium Online Course**
  http://thePoint.lww.com/Kronenberger3e
- **Internet Resources**

  LiveAdvise Online Tutoring & Competency Training
  http://thePoint.lww.com/LiveAdvise

  American Academy of Pediatrics
  www.aap.org

  American Heart Association
  www.americanheart.org

  CDC
  www.cdc.gov

  Federal Communications Commission
  www.fcc.gov/cib/dro

  Institute for Disabilities Research and Training
  www.idrt.com

  Online Yellow Pages
  www.smartpages.com

  OSHA
  www.osha.gov

  Telecommunications for the Deaf
  www.amrad.org

  US Department of Justice/Americans with Disabilities Act
  www.usdoj.gov/crt/ada

PROCEDURE 5-1: Handling Incoming Calls

Purpose: To receive calls into the practice and route them accordingly or take messages as appropriate
Equipment: Telephone, telephone message pad, writing utensil (pen or pencil), headset (if applicable)

Steps	Purpose
1. Gather the needed equipment	Ensures that all materials are available and ready for use.
2. Answer the phone within two rings.	Demonstrates professionalism and courtesy to the caller.
3. Greet caller with proper identification (your name and the name of the office).	Demonstrates professionalism and courtesy to the caller.
4. Identify the nature or reason for the call in a timely manner.	Allows the call to be appropriately managed.
5. Triage the call appropriately.	Prompt identification of emergency calls is important for good patient care.
6. Communicate in a professional manner and with unhurried speech.	Demonstrates compassion and caring for the patient. An unhurried speech pattern is reassuring to the patient.
7. Clarify information as needed.	Prevents errors in communication.
8. Record the message on a message pad. Include name of caller, date, time, telephone number wherethe caller can be reached, description of the caller'sconcerns, and person to whom the message is routed.	Promotes good communication between you and recipient of the message.

FOR DOCTOR *Stephens*	DATE 4/4/08	URGENT ☐
PATIENT *Tommy Taylor*	TIME 10 am	REFILL ☐
CALLER TEL. 312-462-5515	AGE 42	TEMP N/A
MEDICATION N/A		WT. N/A
MESSAGE *Per your instructions, pt. called to report improvement. He states he feels "a million times better."*		
PHARMACY / TELEPHONE N/A	ALLERGIES NKDA	RECEIVED BY LF, CMA

Step 8. Record the message.

9. Give the caller an approximate time for a return call.	Provides reassurance to the patient that the call will be handled promptly and timely.
10. Ask the caller whether he or she has any additional questions or needs any other help.	Confirms that the patient's needs have been met.
11. Allow the caller to disconnect first.	Ensures that the caller has completed the communication.
12. Put the message in an assigned place.	Having a certain place assigned ensures that the call will be handled correctly and the intended recipient gets the information.
13. Complete the task within 10 minutes.	Ensures that the call is handled promptly and efficiently.

PROCEDURE 5-2: Calling Emergency Medical Services

Purpose: To initiate the 911 emergency system when a patient needs transport to another facility for emergency care

Equipment: Telephone, patient information, writing utensil (pen, pencil)

Steps	Purpose
1. Obtain the following information before dialing: patient's name, age, sex, nature of medical condition, type of service the physician is requesting, any special instructions or requests the physician may have, your location, and any special information for access.	Information is necessary for quick and correct dispatch of EMS personnel. Certain types of patients require special teams for transport.
2. Dial 911 or other EMS number.	The call cannot be placed if the number is not dialed correctly.
3. Calmly provide the dispatcher with the above information.	Allows information to be communicated quickly and professionally
4. Answer the dispatcher's questions calmly and professionally.	Allows dispatcher to obtain any additional information and verify the message.
5. Follow the dispatcher's instructions, if applicable.	Following instructions provides good patient care.
6. End the call as per dispatcher instructions.	Ensures that all communication needs have been met.
7. Complete the task within 10 minutes.	Prompt access to EMS promotes good patient care and is essential for good outcomes.

PROCEDURE 5-3: Explain General Office Policies

Purpose: To instruct a new patient about office policies based on their individual needs and level of comprehension

Equipment: Patient's chart, office brochure

Steps	Purpose
1. Assess the patient's level of understanding.	Patients may have hearing difficulties, mental deficiencies, inability to read, etc.
2. Review important areas and highlight these in the office brochure.	Information about hours of operation, refill request procedures, etc. would be needed more than directions to the office, for example.
3. Ask the patient if he or she understands or has any questions.	Ensures that patient understood the information you provided and gives the patient an opportunity to clarify information or ask any additional questions.
4. Give the patient the brochure to take home.	Patients can read printed materials to refresh the memory.
5. Put in place a procedure for updating information and letting patients know of changes.	A printed announcement of changes in hours, availability, services, etc. will keep patients informed.

- As the receptionist, you are the most visible and accessible representative of the medical practice. Duties and responsibilities of a receptionist vary among office settings.
- The key to being a good receptionist is to demonstrate tact and diplomacy in all interactions with patients. Providing a positive attitude will ease the patient's anxiety and ensure the best and most confident image of the practice is projected.

- Proper telephone etiquette and manners are essential for good patient care and to achieve effective communication among various health care providers. Triaging incoming calls is a skill that you must master if you are to be an effective receptionist.
- Excellent customer service is crucial to a successful medical practice.

Warm Ups for Critical Thinking

1. How would you calm an irate patient on the telephone? Identify some phrases that you might use to calm the caller. What phrases may make the situation worse?

2. Assume you are working in an obstetrician's office. What kinds of educational videos might be appropriate for the waiting room? What if you were working in an orthopedic office or for a surgeon?

3. Describe how you would handle a patient who is vomiting in the waiting room.

4. Assume you are working for a pediatrician. A mother arrives carrying an 18-month-old child with symptoms of a respiratory illness. As per office policy, you direct her to sit in the sick child area. The mother refuses. What do you do?

5. A caller asks to speak to the office manager about a supply order on line 1, a patient is on line 2 complaining of chest pain, and line 3 is another patient needing a stronger pain medication. How would you handle these three callers?

6. A caller asks to speak to the physician directly. How would you respond?

Answers to Checkpoint Questions

1. You can demonstrate a professional image by transmitting a positive attitude, acting as a role model, using courtesy and diplomacy, and making a positive first impression.

2. Messages can be retrieved from answering services, voice mail, electronic mail, and facsimile machines.

3. The purpose of an ergonomic workstation is to prevent injuries to employees and to increase employee satisfaction and work efficiency.

4. Patients who are hearing impaired should be offered closed captioning if they are requesting to watch television.

5. The Americans with Disabilities Act prohibits discrimination against people with disabilities.

6. The most antiseptic technique for preventing the transmission of diseases is handwashing.

7. The five basic guidelines for proper telephone use are good diction, pronunciation, expression, listening, and courtesy.

8. The minimum information needed for a telephone message includes name of the caller, date and time of the call, telephone number where the caller can be reached, a short description of the caller's concern, and the person to whom the message is routed.

9. Before calling emergency medical services, you should know the name, age, and sex of the patient, nature of the medical problem, type of service the physician is requesting, and any special instructions the physician may have.

10. Text messaging is done with the keypad of a cellular phone and sends a readable message to the recipient. It might be used when it is not necessary to speak with the person or a ringtone would be inappropriate.

CHAPTER 6

Managing Appointments

Outline

Appointment Scheduling Systems
Manual Appointment Scheduling
Computerized Appointment Scheduling

Types of Scheduling
Structured Appointments
Flexible Hours
Open Hours

Factors That Affect Scheduling
Patients' Needs
Providers' Preferences and Needs

Physical Facilities

Scheduling Guidelines
New Patients
Established Patients

Preparing a Daily or Weekly Schedule

Patient Reminders
Appointment Cards
Telephone Reminders
Mailed Reminder Cards

Adapting the Schedule
Emergencies
Patients Who Are Acutely Ill
Walk-in Patients

Late Patients
Physician Delays
Missed Appointments

Cancellations
Cancellations by the Office
Cancellations by the Patient

Making Appointments for Patients in Other Facilities
Referrals and Consultations
Diagnostic Testing
Surgery

When the Appointment Schedule Does Not Work

Learning Objectives

Upon successfully completing this chapter, you will be able to:

1. Spell and define the key terms

2. Describe the various systems for scheduling patient office visits, including manual and computerized scheduling

3. Identify the factors that affect appointment scheduling

4. Explain guidelines for scheduling appointments for new patients, return visits, inpatient admissions, and outpatient procedures

5. List three ways to remind patients about appointments

6. Describe how to triage patient emergencies, acutely ill patients, and walk-in patients

7. Describe how to handle late patients

8. Explain what to do if the physician is delayed

9. Describe how to handle patients who miss their appointments

10. Describe how to handle appointment cancellations made by the office or by the patient

Upon successfully completing this chapter, you will be able to:

1. Schedule an appointment for a new patient (Procedure 6-1)

2. Schedule an appointment for a return visit (Procedure 6-2)

3. Schedule an appointment for a referral to an outpatient facility (Procedure 6-3)

4. Arrange for admission to an inpatient facility (Procedure 6-4)

Competencies

CAAHEP

- Schedule and manage appointments
- Schedule inpatient and outpatient admissions and procedures
- Apply third-party guidelines
- Apply managed care policies and procedures

ABHES

- Schedule and monitor appointments
- Schedule inpatient and outpatient admissions

Key Terms

acute	consultation	referral	tickler file
buffer	double booking	STAT	wave scheduling
chronic	matrix	streaming	system
clustering	precertification		
constellation of symptoms	providers		

Responsibility for scheduling and managing the flow of patient care in a medical office or clinic is one of the most important duties assigned to a medical assistant. As appointment manager, you make the first, last, and most durable impression on the patient and **providers**. Depending on your demeanor and actions, that impression can be favorable or unfavorable. A properly used appointment system helps maintain an efficient office. If improperly used, it can mean confusion and chaos; more important, it can waste precious time for the patient, the provider, and the staff.

To use the office facilities and the physician's availability most efficiently, determine which patients will be seen, when they will be seen, and how much time to allot to each of them, depending on their problems. Of course, every practice will have occasional delays and emergencies. Your responsibility is to manage all of this while maintaining a calm, efficient, and polite attitude.

Appointment Scheduling Systems

There are two systems of appointment scheduling for outpatient medical facilities: the manual system, which uses an appointment book, and a computerized scheduling system. The choice of systems will depend on the size of the practice, how many providers' schedules must be managed, and the preferences of the staff responsible for the daily schedule. Whether a medical office uses a manual or computerized system, many of the guidelines for effectively scheduling the workday discussed in this chapter are the same.

Manual Appointment Scheduling

Medical offices may choose to use a manual appointment scheduling system even if the other administrative functions in the office are computerized.

The Appointment Book

If your medical office uses a manual system of scheduled appointments for patient office visits, you will need an appointment book. An appointment book provides space for noting appointments for an entire year. It may have a single sheet for each day and a separate page for each provider or show an entire week on two facing pages. Some offices prefer an appointment book with pages showing only one day at a time; others may want to see a whole week at a glance. A different color page for each day may also be desired.

The more information required for scheduling, the larger the pages should be. Make sure the book has enough space for all pertinent information (e.g., patient's name, telephone number, reason for visit), is divided into time units appropriate for your practice (e.g., 10- or 15-minute intervals), can open flat on the desk where it will be used, and fits easily into its storage place when not in use.

Establishing a Matrix

Before you begin using the appointment book, you will have to set up a **matrix**. A matrix is established by crossing out times that providers are unavailable for patient visits (Fig. 6-1). For example, the physician may have a breakfast meeting and not be in the office until 10:00 AM This is indicated by crossing out the blocks from 8:00 to 10:00 AM. Write in the reason for crossing off the space (e.g., vacation, meeting, hospital rounds). Some practices reserve specific times or even days for certain activities, such as physical examinations and surgery. Also, it is advisable to block off 15 to 30 minutes each morning and afternoon to accommodate emergencies, late arrivals, and other delays. Some physicians want their professional or personal obligations noted on the appointment schedule so that patients are not booked immediately before these times.

Once you have acquired and prepared an appointment book, it is not enough to schedule a time and date for a patient visit and hope everything will run smoothly. Before actually making an appointment, you should review the schedule carefully, evaluating the needs of each patient and considering the physician's preferences and availability of the office facilities. At the beginning of each day, copies of the schedule should be distributed to all staff members. Along with the notations in a patient's chart, the pages of the appointment book provide documentation of a patient's visits and

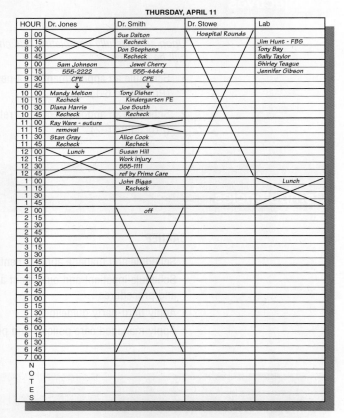

THURSDAY, APRIL 11

HOUR		Dr. Jones	Dr. Smith	Dr. Stowe	Lab
8	00		Sue Dalton	Hospital Rounds	
8	15		Recheck		Jim Hunt - FBS
8	30		Don Stephens		Tony Bay
8	45		Recheck		Sally Taylor
9	00	Sam Johnson	Jewel Cherry		Shirley Teague
9	15	555-2222	555-4444		Jennifer Gibson
9	30	CPE	CPE		
9	45	↓	↓		
10	00	Mandy Melton	Tony Disher		
10	15	Recheck	Kindergarten PE		
10	30	Diana Harris	Joe South		
10	45	Recheck	Recheck		
11	00	Ray Ware - suture			
11	15	removal			
11	30	Stan Gray	Alice Cook		
11	45	Recheck	Recheck		
12	00	Lunch	Susan Hill		
12	15		Work injury		
12	30		555-1111		
12	45		ref by Prime Care		
1	00		John Biggs		Lunch
1	15		Recheck		
1	30				
1	45				
2	00		off		
2	15				
2	30				
2	45				
3	00				
3	15				
3	30				
3	45				
4	00				
4	15				
4	30				
4	45				
5	00				
5	15				
5	30				
5	45				
6	00				
6	15				
6	30				
6	45				
7	00				
N O T E S					

Figure 6-1 Sample page from manual appointment book.

any changes, such as cancellations and rescheduled appointments. This provides further legal documentation to protect the physician and the patient in case of a dispute, as discussed in Chapter 2.

Computerized Appointment Scheduling

Medical management software designed to assist with administrative functions includes systems for appointment scheduling. Computerized scheduling often saves time. Information used to establish a matrix (e.g., hospital rounds 7:30–8:30, lunch 12:30–1:30) has to be entered only once.

Any medical office software will have an appointment toolbar that requires one click to add a patient, add to the waiting list, see a calendar, or search for available times. Many software packages offer an advanced search that defines the resources required for a certain type of appointment.

This quick method allows you to search for available appointment times. Typically, you enter the desired date, and the computer displays the schedule for that day, showing any available time slots. Another feature allows you to search the appointment database for the next available time slot. For example, a patient is instructed to return in 3 months and has a preference for the time of day. You can search for the first available afternoon appointment with that particular provider.

Depending on the specific software, you can also print numerous documents, such as the daily or weekly appointment schedule, appointment reminders, or billing slips. Once the daily schedule is printed, this important document is referred to as the daily activity sheet or the day sheet and is the guide for everyone involved in the flow of patient care. Figure 6-2 shows a computer-generated daily activity sheet.

An important advantage to computerized appointment scheduling is the easy access to billing information. For example, a patient may call for an appointment, and the medical assistant can inform the patient that he needs to pay his balance due of $32 when he comes in to be seen. Credit and collections are discussed in Chapter 12.

CHECKPOINT QUESTION

1. What is the purpose of a matrix?

Figure 6-2 A computer-generated appointment schedule with space for all providers of care. (Courtesy of MICA Information Systems, Winston-Salem, North Carolina.)

Types of Scheduling

Structured Appointments

Most medical offices use a system of structured or scheduled appointments for office visits. Each patient is assigned a time on the schedule and allotted a specific period for examination and treatment. Box 6-1 shows examples of time allotment. The advantages of this system include good time management and optimum use of the office facility. Additionally, a daily schedule may be developed and charts may be prepared in advance of patient arrival.

A disadvantage of this system is that a patient may need more of the physician's time than you have scheduled. Therefore, it is important that you ask the proper questions at the time the appointment is made to anticipate the time needed. Such questions might include "Why do you need to see the doctor?" The patient's reply will tell you how many issues will be addressed. "Do you have a form to be completed for your physical?" The answer to this question will tell you whether this is a school physical or a complete physical.

The practice of adding **buffer** time to the schedule gives extra time to accommodate emergencies, walk-ins, and other demands on the provider's daily time schedule that are not considered direct patient care. Such tasks include returning phone calls, reviewing records, and transcribing reports. For example, you may cross off 30 minutes at the beginning and end of the daily schedule to be used as a buffer.

Methods of scheduling patients include clustering, wave, modified wave, stream, and double booking.

BOX 6-1

HOW MUCH TIME DO I ALLOT?

Every outpatient medical facility has variables that determine the time allotted for each service. Factors like the number of providers, the number of examination rooms, and the size of the office must be considered when establishing the appointment scheduling guidelines. This partial list of typical outpatient services shows an estimate of the time needed for each.

Complete physical examination	1 hour
School physical	30 minutes
Recheck	15 minutes
Dressing change	10 minutes
Blood pressure check	5 minutes
Patient teaching	30 minutes–1 hour

Clustering

Clustering is grouping patients with similar problems or needs. For example, an obstetrics and gynecology practice may see all pregnant patients in the morning and other patients in the afternoon. A pediatrician may schedule vaccinations on certain days of the week. Special tests like sigmoidoscopies may be scheduled one morning a week. Advantages to clustering include maximum use of special equipment, ease in maintaining control of the schedule, the ability to provide many patients with information about their particular situation at the same time, and efficient use of employees' time.

Wave and Modified Wave

Outpatient medical facilities may use the **wave scheduling system** or modify the wave system in ways that work for their particular specialty. With the wave system, several patients are scheduled the first 30 minutes of each hour. They are seen in the order that they arrive at the office. The second half of each hour is left open. This technique works well in large facilities with several departments giving medical care. For example, several patients may arrive for a 9:00 appointment, be seen by the physician, be sent to the laboratory for blood work, and return to the physician 20 minutes later. The physician has the second part of the hour to see these patients after their testing. That second half of each hour is used as a buffer or extra time that can be used for emergencies, walk-ins, returning phone calls, and tasks other than direct patient care. Modifications to this system may include seeing new patients who will have complete physical examinations on the hour with three or four rechecks scheduled on the half hour. For example, a 75-year-old man being seen for a complete physical would be scheduled at 9:00 AM, with a 22-year-old being seen for a follow-up of strep throat and a 6-year-old being seen for recheck of an ear infection scheduled at 9:30 AM.

Fixed Scheduling

Fixed scheduling is the most commonly used method. It divides each hour into increments of 15, 30, 45, or 60 minutes. The reason for each patient's visit will determine the length of time assigned. Patients who are late or do not report for their appointment can cause major problems in the flow of the day. It is helpful to schedule chronically late patients at the end of the day. Another tactic is to tell the patient to arrive 30 minutes prior to the time you schedule.

Streaming

Streaming is a method that helps minimize gaps in time and backups. Appointments are given based on the needs of the individual patient. If a patient is being seen for a complete physical, 1 hour may be allotted. The next patient seen may need a blood pressure recheck, which would be allotted a 15-minute slot. Although this method ensures a smooth work flow, the medical assistant scheduling the appointment must understand the procedures and guidelines for deciding the time that should be allotted. Box 6-1 outlines examples of services and their probable time allotments.

Double Booking

With **double booking**, two patients are scheduled for the same period with the same physician. This works well when patients are being sent for diagnostic testing because it leaves time to see both patients without keeping either one waiting unnecessarily.

Flexible Hours

Offices that operate with flexible hours are open at different times throughout the week. For example, Monday, Wednesday, and Friday office hours might be from 8 AM to 5 PM, and Tuesday and Thursday office hours might be from 8 AM to 8 PM. Some offices may also be open on Saturdays for all or part of the day. Patients still have scheduled appointments, but this greater range of available appointment times better accommodates work and family schedules. Your main challenge with flexible hours is to determine which patients really need to be scheduled for these special times. For example, Saturday appointments may be reserved only for patients whose work schedules do not permit weekday appointments. Flexible hours are most often used by clinics, group practices, and family physicians.

Open Hours

A medical office that operates with open hours for patient visits is open for specified hours during the day or evening. Patients may arrive at any time during those hours to be seen by the physician in the order of their arrival; there are no scheduled appointments. This system is commonly seen in emergency walk-in clinics and eliminates patient complaints such as "I had an appointment at 2 PM but had to wait until 3 PM to be seen." Open-hour scheduling, however, has some clear disadvantages:

- Effective time management is almost impossible.
- The facilities may be overloaded at some times and empty at other times.
- Charts must be pulled and prepared as each patient arrives.

So that patients are seen in the order in which they arrive, some offices use sign-in sheets. Some sign-in sheets require that patients record the reason for their visit. The use of sign-in sheets is discouraged under the Health Insurance Portability and Accountability Act of 1996 regulations, as discussed in Chapter 8. Sign-in sheets are considered a breach of confidentiality, since patients signing the sheet can see the names and medical conditions of other patients.

 CHECKPOINT QUESTION

2. What are the three systems that can be used for scheduling patient office visits?

Factors That Affect Scheduling

Patients' Needs

People express their needs in varied ways. A patient might be feeling uncertainty, embarrassment, shyness, or fear. With a patient in an emotional state, even the slightest real or imagined miscommunication can lead to negative response from the patient. Be courteous and maintain your professionalism.

Before scheduling an appointment, you should determine:

- Why the patient wishes to see the physician
- How long the patient has had the symptoms
- Whether the problem is **acute** (abrupt onset) or **chronic** (longstanding)
- The most convenient time for the patient to come in (e.g., early morning or evenings)
- Any special transportation services the patient requires (community or hospital van services operate only during certain hours)
- Whether the patient needs to see other office staff
- Any third-party payers' constraints
- Receipt of necessary documentation for referrals when the patient is enrolled in a program that requires such documentation (third-party payers are discussed further in Chapter 14)

Control of the appointment schedule is your responsibility. Strive to accommodate a patient's requests whenever possible but not if it will overload the schedule. For example, if a patient requests a 2 PM appointment this Tuesday and you already have patients in that time slot, politely explain that you cannot schedule the appointment then unless you have a cancellation. You might offer a later time on Tuesday or on another day at 2 PM. You can also ask if the patient wishes to be put on a move-up list to be notified if an earlier appointment opens up. In other words, you control the schedule. Do not let it control you. The entire medical office team depends on a well-managed schedule.

E T H I C A L   T I P

Think Before You Speak

As discussed throughout the text, it is illegal and unethical to release patient information without the patient's consent. You may be breaching confidentiality without even realizing it. Consider this: You are a receptionist in a busy OB/GYN practice. A former classmate comes in for a pregnancy test. While you are making her return appointment, she tells you that the test was positive. Later, while having lunch at a nearby restaurant, you see her mother. You congratulate her on her new grandchild and quickly realize that she doesn't know yet. You have just breached the patient's confidentiality.

What if the scenario had been like this: "Hi, Mrs. Roberts. What a conicidence; I just saw Susie this morning." Mrs. Roberts says, "Where did you see her?" You reply, "At work." You have just told Mrs. Roberts that her daughter was at an OB/GYN office. This innocent exchange is a serious violation of the Privacy Rule of HIPAA. Most employers consider this to be reason for immediate dismissal. Be careful.

Providers' Preferences and Needs

The management of the practice depends on the desires and requirements of the providers working in it. Providers in a medical practice may include the physician, nurse practitioner, or physician's assistant. Some providers often run behind schedule; others are extremely punctual. Recognize your providers' habits and communicate any problems to a supervisor. The physician may allow you to adjust the schedule to accommodate his or her habits. If you are employed to assist the physician with clinical duties (e.g., removing sutures, performing electrocardiograms, giving injections), the schedule can be adjusted to accommodate a larger number of patients while still allowing the provider enough time to give each patient personal attention.

As discussed earlier, the physician also needs time to receive and return telephone calls, review laboratory and pathology reports, dictate chart notes or correspondence, and so on. If your physician is on the staff of a teaching hospital, you may also have to block off time for clinic conferences and other teaching duties.

The physician will need time to meet with unscheduled office visitors other than patients. Such visitors might include other physicians and sales representatives from medical supply or pharmaceutical companies. You should determine in advance how the physician wants you to handle these visitors. For example, the physician may want to be notified immediately if another physician comes to the office. With salespersons or pharmaceutical representatives, however, the physician may have another staff member meet with them or may request that an appointment be scheduled for a more convenient time.

Physical Facilities

The physical facilities available in the medical office will affect the management of the appointment schedule. Consider these points: How many providers use the facility? How many examination rooms are there? Is it necessary to resterilize instruments between procedures, or is more than one set of instruments available? You would not want to schedule two sigmoidoscopies at the same time, for example, if the office has only one appropriately equipped examination room. You must thoroughly understand the requirements for procedures to be performed in the office to schedule appointments accurately.

 CHECKPOINT QUESTION

3. What are three factors that can affect appointment scheduling?

Scheduling Guidelines

Whether the patient is making an appointment by telephone or in person, be pleasant and maintain a helpful attitude. Always write the patient's telephone number on the schedule when making appointments. Emergencies and delays are unavoidable, and schedule corrections can be made quickly if the telephone number is handy. Leave some time slots open during each day, perhaps 15 to 20 minutes in the morning and in the afternoon. Invariably, problems will arise (e.g., late patients, emergencies) and disrupt the regular appointment schedule. These open blocks can allow the schedule to catch up. Also, patients calling for appointments will not appreciate being told that no time is available for 2 or 3 weeks. Open slots can be used to schedule brief appointments as needed. Procedure 6-1 describes the steps for scheduling appointments for new patients.

New Patients

Most appointments for new patients are made by telephone. The information you exchange at this encounter is crucial, and entering the patient's data accurately is imperative. The first encounter with a new patient is discussed in Procedure 6-1.

An office brochure can be mailed to the patient in advance of the appointment. Some offices send new-patient forms to be filled out and brought in at the appointment. When scheduling an appointment for a new patient, follow these guidelines:

1. Allow an adequate amount of time for the appointment. To do so, obtain as much information as possible from the patient:
   • Full name and correct spelling
   • Mailing address
   • Day and evening telephone numbers
   • Reason for the visit
   • Name of the referring physician or individual
   • Responsible party and third-party payer (insurance plan)
2. Explain the office's payment policy. Most offices require full or partial payment at the time of an initial visit, and patients must understand this policy. Instruct patients to bring all pertinent insurance information.
3. Be sure patients know your office location; if needed, give them concise directions. You may also want to tell patients how long they can expect to be at the office.
4. Some patients are sensitive about messages left on an answering machine or given to a co-worker. To avoid violating confidentiality, ask the patient if it is permissible to call at home or at work and include this information in the patient's chart.
5. Before ending the call, confirm the time and date of the appointment. You might say, "Thank you for calling Mr. Brown. We look forward to seeing you on Tuesday, December 10, at 2 PM."
6. Always check your appointment system or book to be sure that you have placed the appointment on the correct day in the right time slot.
7. If the patient was referred by another physician, you may need to call that physician's office in advance of the appointment for copies of laboratory work, radiology and pathology reports, and so on. Remember, the patient must give authorization to release medical documents (see Chapter 9). Give these reports to the physician prior to the patient's appointment.

Established Patients

Established patients will be given return appointments when necessary. Most return appointments are made before the patient leaves the office. Procedure 6-2 describes the steps for scheduling a return appointment.

When making a return appointment, follow these guidelines:

1. Carefully check your appointment book or screen before offering an appointment time. If a specific examination, test, or x-ray is to be performed on the return visit, avoid scheduling two patients for the same examination at the same time.

2. Offer the patient a specific time and date. For example, you might say, "Mrs. Hernandez, I have next Tuesday, the 15th, available at 3:30 PM" (Avoid asking the patient when he or she would like to return, as this can elicit indecision.) If the offered appointment is not convenient, offer another specific time and date.

3. Write the patient's name and telephone number in the appointment book, or enter in the information on the appointment screen.

4. Transfer the pertinent information to an appointment card and give it to the patient. Computerized systems print an appointment card. Repeat aloud the appointment day, date, and time to the patient as you hand over the card (Fig. 6-3).

5. Double-check your book or screen to be sure you have not made an error.

6. End your conversation with a pleasant word and a smile.

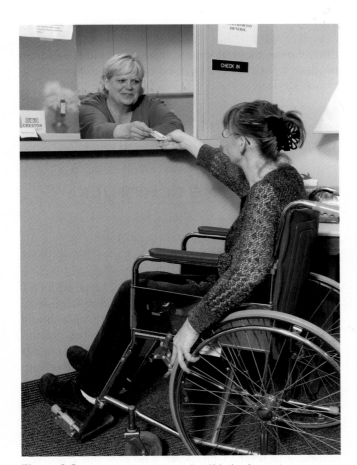

Figure 6-3 An appointment card will help the patient remember his or her appointment and reduce no shows.

Preparing a Daily or Weekly Schedule

In most offices, as medical assistant, you are responsible for preparing a daily and weekly schedule of appointments. Make a copy for the providers and other office staff members. When there are changes in the schedule, ensure that corrections are made on all copies. Place the next day's schedule on the physician's desk before he or she leaves for the day. Give the next week's schedule to the physician before he or she leaves on Friday. Schedules should include not only patients' appointments but also hospital rounds, surgeries, meetings, and any personal engagements on the schedule. Computer systems print a daily or weekly schedule, but you must remember to make changes manually as the day progresses.

Patient Reminders

Offices use various kinds of reminders to tell a patient about an appointment that should be made or to remind them that an appointment has been made on a specific date and time. These reminders are the appointment card, the telephone call, and the mailed card.

Appointment Cards

An appointment card is given to the patient when he or she leaves the office. It should have the following information:

- Patient's name
- Day, date, and time of the return visit
- Physician's name and telephone number

If the patient requires a series of appointments, try to make them on the same day of the week and at the same time of day. This will make it easier for the patient to remember the appointments. Unless your appointment card allows you to list the complete series of appointments, however, give the patient a card for the next appointment only and repeat this procedure after each subsequent visit. When the patient has to save several cards, they can easily be lost or cause confusion. If using a manual system, write on the card with ink so that it cannot be altered. Computer appointment scheduling software provides appointment cards that can be printed on special perforated paper.

Telephone Reminders

All new patients and patients with appointments scheduled in advance should receive a telephone reminder the day before their appointment. Computer systems can place the call to the programmed number and remind the patient of the appointment with a prerecorded message. Remember, do not call a patient at work or leave a message unless you have been given permission to do so. Make the telephone reminder simple. Identify your office and yourself, and state the date and time of the appointment. For example, you might say, "This is Ms. Sprinkle from Dr. Yokley's office. I'm calling to confirm your appointment for tomorrow, Thursday, February 10, at 3:30 PM." Unless the patient has a question, then say, "Thank you and goodbye." This reminder helps jog the patient's memory, and if the patient must cancel or reschedule an appointment, you will have time to fill the slot. Keep a list with the names and phone numbers of patients who have asked to be called or who need to be seen sooner than their next appointment. This list may be called a cancellation list, a waiting list, or a move-up list. Make a notation on the appointment schedule, such as confirmed, left message, or no answer.

Mailed Reminder Cards

Some offices send reminder cards instead of making phone calls. Reminder cards are also used to remind patients who could not be reached by phone that it is time to keep an upcoming scheduled appointment. These should be mailed at least a week before the date of the appointment. In addition, reminder cards are sent after a set period since a patient's last appointment. Reminder cards are often used to alert patients to the need for annual examinations (e.g., Pap smears, mammograms, prostate examinations).

To handle this kind of reminder, keep a supply of preprinted postcards in the office (Fig. 6-4). The cards should have a simple one- or two-sentence message, such as, "According to our records, you are due for your annual physical. If you would kindly call the office, we will be glad to arrange an appointment for you." The physician's name, address, and telephone number should be printed on the card. Place the card in a tickler file (Box 6-2) and mail it at the appropriate

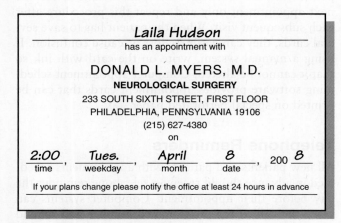

Figure 6-4 Sample reminder postcard.

Laila Hudson
has an appointment with

DONALD L. MYERS, M.D.
NEUROLOGICAL SURGERY
233 SOUTH SIXTH STREET, FIRST FLOOR
PHILADELPHIA, PENNSYLVANIA 19106
(215) 627-4380
on

2:00	*Tues.*	*April*	*8*	200 *8*
time	weekday	month	date	

If your plans change please notify the office at least 24 hours in advance

---

BOX 6-2

A TICKLER FILE CAN TICKLE YOUR MEMORY

A **tickler file** helps remind you to do something by a certain time in the future. It can be something as simple as a card file box (like a recipe box) or an accordion folder with insert guides in chronological order. The guides may be in weekly or monthly divisions. Put patient appointment reminder cards in the appropriate location in the file. Check the file each week or month, depending on the divisions, then mail the reminders.

Medical office computer software often offers help with patient reminders. With a search of the database, a report of every female patient over age 50, for example, could be generated. Some systems even generate patient reminders based on preprogrammed criteria.

time. Some medical management software packages produce a list that can be used to alert patients of necessary services.

CHECKPOINT QUESTION

4. What are the three types of patient reminders?

ADAPTING THE SCHEDULE

Emergencies

When a patient calls with an emergency (Fig. 6-5), your first responsibility is to determine whether the problem can be treated in the office. The office should have a policy for evaluation of the situation. The word **STAT** is used in the medical field to indicate that something should be done immediately (Box 6-3). You also should have a list of appropriate questions to ask the patient, such as "Are you having chest pain? Are you having difficulty breathing? How long have you had the symptoms?" (Box 6-4). When several symptoms occur together, they may indicate a particular problem. This group of complaints is referred to as a **constellation of symptoms**. One group of symptoms found to indicate a certain disorder is severe right lower quadrant pain, nausea, and fever. A physician who sees this constellation of symptoms considers appendicitis.

Figure 6-5 When a patient calls from home with a possible heart attack, you will call 911.

Patients Who Are Acutely Ill

Patients who are acutely ill often have serious, although not life-threatening, conditions. These patients need to be seen as soon as possible but not necessarily on that same day. Obtain as much information about the patient's medical problem as you can so your message to the physician will allow him or her to decide how soon the patient should be seen. Place the chart with a note in the location selected by the physician, and tell the patient you will call back as soon as the physician makes a decision.

BOX 6-3

WHEN DOES THE PATIENT NEED TO BE SEEN NOW?

When the patient calls with any of the following complaints:

- Shortness of breath
- Severe chest pain
- Uncontrollable bleeding
- Large open wounds
- Potential accidental poisoning
- Bleeding in a pregnant patient
- Injury to a pregnant patient
- Shock
- Serious burns
- Severe bleeding
- Any symptoms of internal bleeding (dark, tarry stools; discoloration of the skin)

Note: Remember to check with the physician for proper procedures concerning triage.

BOX 6-4

WHEN A PATIENT COULD BE HAVING A HEART ATTACK

When a patient calls complaining of the following constellation of symptoms, you should assume that this is a potential heart attack:

- Shortness of breath
- Chest pain
- Arm or neck pain
- Nausea and/or vomiting

Just one of these symptoms alone may not indicate a cardiac event, but when there is more than one, you should be alert to the fact that this may be a heart attack. Studies have shown that, in women, early symptoms of a heart attack are different from those in men. These symptoms include jaw, neck, and back pain and severe fatigue. Keep this in mind when questioning the patient. Call 911 and stay on the line with the patient. Do not advise the patient to drive to the hospital. Follow office policies for such an emergency.

Walk-in Patients

Walk-in patients are those who arrive at the office without a scheduled appointment and expect to see the physician that day. Typically, the physician will have a set protocol, or prescribed list of steps, for handling such situations. In general, you must first determine the reason for the walk-in. Patients with medical emergencies need to be seen immediately. Other patients can be asked to have a seat in the waiting room while you inform the physician of the patient's presence. The physician can then make the decision to see the patient or not.

If the patient is to be seen, explain that you will work him or her into the schedule as soon as possible for a brief examination. When the patient leaves the office, you might apologize for the delay and then ask the patient to schedule an appointment for the next visit.

If the physician decides not to see a walk-in patient, you will have to ask the patient to schedule an appointment and to return later.

Late Patients

Patients who are late cause problems in the schedule. You should gently but firmly apologize for any delay but tell the patient, "You were late, and Dr. Wooten is seeing another patient now. The doctor should be able to see you in about 15 minutes." Patients who are routinely late should be politely advised that "According to our office policy, patients who are more than 15 minutes late will have to be rescheduled." Some offices have found that scheduling the habitually late patient at the end of the day is helpful. In addition, ask patients to call the office if they know ahead of time that they are going to be late.

Physician Delays

Of course, sometimes the physician calls in to say he or she has been delayed and will be in the office later. If office hours have not yet begun, call patients with appointments scheduled early, and give them the option of coming in later in the day or rescheduling the appointment for another day. If patients are waiting in the office, inform them immediately if the physician will be delayed. For example, you might say, "Dr. Franklin has been delayed and will probably be 20 to 30 minutes late. Would you like to wait, or would you prefer to reschedule for another time?" Always keep your patients informed; most people will understand if they know you have not ignored or forgotten them. Most patients appreciate the fact that the physician would also be available to them in an emergency. If you reschedule an appointment, note in the patient's chart the reason for the cancellation or rescheduling.

Missed Appointments

A missed appointment, or no-show, occurs when a patient neglects to keep an appointment and does not notify the office. When this happens, call the patient to try to determine why the appointment was missed and to reschedule for another time. If you are unable to reach the patient by telephone, send a card asking the patient to call the office to reschedule. Note in the patient's chart the missed appointment and that you have either rescheduled the appointment or mailed a card to schedule another appointment. Even if the facility does not routinely remind patients of appointments, be sure to call and remind habitually late patients the day before the appointment.

Continued failure to keep appointments should be brought to the attention of the physician, who may want to call the patient personally (particularly if the patient is seriously ill) or send a letter expressing concern for the patient's welfare. In extreme cases, the physician may choose to terminate the physician–patient relationship. See Chapter 2 for the proper procedure for this action. Notations of all actions and copies of any letters sent to the patient should become a permanent part of the individual's medical record. Box 6-5 is an example of a chart note.

LEGAL TIP
DOCUMENT, DOCUMENT, DOCUMENT!

When a patient does not show up for his appointment, you must make an entry in the chart. Because your physician has a legal contract with the patient, he has an obligation to treat him as long and as often as necessary. If the patient does not report for his scheduled appointments, the patient is breaking the contract. This would be an important factor in a court cases involving a physician being sued for abandonment. The chart is the physician's defense. Being diligent with documentation is not optional.

Example:

10/07/07. Mr. Quinn did not report for his appointment at 10 AM today. I called him at 11:00 AM, and he stated that he did not want to reschedule. He says he is doing fine and will call next week to reschedule. LM, RMA

Cancellations
Cancellations by the Office

You may have to cancel a patient's appointment if the physician is ill, has an emergency, or has personal time off. Patients who must be rescheduled need not be told the specific reason for the physician's absence. These cancellations should be noted in the patient's medical record.

When you have advance notice, write a letter to patients with appointments you must cancel, indicating that the physician will be away from the office but will return by a certain date. Patients should be alerted to cancellations a week before their appointments. Ask the patient to call the office to reschedule. If you have to cancel on the day of the appointment, call the patient and explain. For example, you might say, "Dr. Flora has been called out of the office unexpectedly. Would it be convenient to reschedule your appointment for sometime next week?" If the patient arrives at the office before you can contact him or her, apologize and politely explain the situation. Most patients will be understanding. When a physician is unavailable for an extended period, another physician must cover the practice or be on call. Everyone in the office should have a list of names and addresses of on-call physicians, and you should give this information to your patients, according to your office policy. When a locum tenens, or substitute physician, is employed, the office appointments will not be interrupted (see Chapter 2).

BOX 6-5

CHARTING EXAMPLE

05/12/08–1530

Mrs. Parrish was called regarding missing scheduled appointment for today at 9:30 AM Patient said she forgot about the appointment. Appointment was rescheduled for 05/14/08 at 10:00 AM. Patient was advised of the need to have regular prenatal checkups. Patient verbalized understanding. Dr. Wong was notified that appointment was missed and rescheduled.
—Lois Samuels, RMA

Cancellations by the Patient

When a patient cancels an appointment, ask the reason for the cancellation and mark it on your appointment schedule and in the patient's chart. Offer to reschedule at another time. If the patient is being seen for a continuing problem, be sure he or she understands the necessity for the follow-up visit. If the patient wants to call back for an appointment, make a note to yourself to check on the call-back in a few days. If a patient cancels appointments frequently, bring this to the physician's attention.

If a patient cancels an appointment and you have a full schedule, no action is needed. If your schedule is light, however, refer to your move-up list to try to fill the vacancy.

Making Appointments for Patients in Other Facilities

Referrals and Consultations

When the provider requests assistance from another physician in **consultation** or makes a **referral** to another physician for the patient, make certain that the referral meets the requirements of any third-party payers. Managed care companies like HMOs have strict requirements regarding **precertification** and documentation for referrals to specialists and other facilities. If the patient's third-party payer requires a referral form, you will need to complete it with the referral approval number that you must obtain from the insurance company. Figure 6-6 is a sample referral form. (See Chapter 13.) Be sure the physician you are calling is on the preferred provider list for the patient's insurance company. Patients should be given a choice when being referred to a specialist.

When calling another physician's office for an ap-

pointment for your patient (Procedure 6-3), provide the following information:

- Physician's name and telephone number
- Patient's name, address, and telephone number
- Reason for the referral
- Degree of urgency
- Whether the patient is being sent for consultation or referral (see Box 6-6 for an explanation of the terms referral and consultation)

Record in the patient's chart the time and date of the call and the person who received your call. Tell the person you are calling that you wish to be notified if your patient does not keep the appointment. If this occurs, be sure to tell the physician and enter this information in the patient's record.

Write the name, address, and telephone number of the referral doctor on your office stationery and include the date and time of the appointment. Give or mail this information to your patient. The patient may call the referring physician to make his or her own appointment. If this is the situation, ask the patient to call you with the appointment date and document it in the chart.

Figure 6-6 Sample referral form.

BOX 6-6

REFERRAL OR CONSULTATION?

It is important to know the difference between a referral and a consultation. According to the coding guidelines in the *Current Procedural Coding Terminology*, a consultation is a request for the opinion of a colleague. A letter is provided to the referring physician by the consultant and contains the consulting physician's impression and recommendations for the patient, but the patient returns to the referring physician for treatment. For example, an orthopedist may send a patient with rheumatoid arthritis to a rheumatologist for medication management, but the orthopedist will continue the patient's care based on the rheumatologist's recommendations.

A referral usually involves a specialist and requires that the patient's care be transferred to that specialist. For example, a patient may see his family physician for an ingrown toenail. That physician refers the patient to a podiatrist for care. That care will continue simultaneously with any other care by the family physician until the problem is resolved.

Diagnostic Testing

Sometimes, patients are sent for diagnostic testing or treatment at another facility. Such testing includes laboratory tests, radiology, computed tomography, magnetic resonance imaging, and nuclear medicine studies. These appointments are usually made while the patient is still in the office. Before scheduling, determine the exact test or tests the physician requires and how soon the results are needed. (Be sure to indicate to the facility if the results are needed immediately, or STAT.) Also, check with the patient for any time restrictions he or she may have. Give the facility the patient's name, address, telephone number, the exact test or tests required, and any other special instructions from the physician. Give the patient a laboratory or x-ray referral slip with the time and date of the appointment and the name, address, and telephone number of the outside facility.

Some laboratory studies or x-ray tests require advance preparation by the patient. Give your patient a written and verbal explanation of the required preparation, and be sure he or she understands the importance of following the instructions. On the patient's chart, note the name of the outside facility and the date and time of the appointment. Also place a reminder in your tickler file or on your appointment schedule to be sure the test results are received as requested. See Procedure 6-3.

Surgery

You also assist with the scheduling of procedures in a hospital operating room or an outpatient surgical facility. Determine the patient's need for precertification with the insurance carrier. You may have to call the number on the back of the patient's insurance card for a precertification number. Call the participating facility chosen by the patient and specify the time and date the physician has requested. The operating facility will need to know the exact procedure, the amount of time needed, the type of anesthesia required, and any other special instructions your physician may have. The facility will also need the patient's name, age, address, telephone number, insurance information, and the precertification number if required.

If the hospital has supplied your office with preadmission forms, give a copy to the patient and make sure he or she understands the need to complete and return the form in a timely manner. Follow the policies of the surgical facility regarding preadmission testing, which may include laboratory studies, x-rays, or autologous blood donation (donation of a person's own blood in advance). Write down all appointment dates, times, and locations for the patient and be certain he or she understands where to go and when.

Finally, note in the patient's record the name of the operating facility and the date and time the surgery is scheduled. You may also need to arrange for hospital admission by providing the same information to the hospital admitting department (Procedure 6-4).

 CHECKPOINT QUESTION

5. What information should be readily available when calling to schedule a patient for surgery in another facility?

When the Appointment Schedule Does Not Work

No appointment schedule runs smoothly all the time, and an occasional glitch is to be expected. If, however, you find that your schedule is chaotic nearly every day, you should determine the cause. Evaluate the schedule over time, generally 2 to 3 months. For example, make a list of all patients seen, their arrival times, the amount of time they spent with the physician, the time they left, and the amount of time needed to perform each examination or treatment. Since the work flow of the office affects every staff member, involve all employees in your study.

Office meetings are an ideal way to identify scheduling problems. Your evaluation may reveal that many of your patients are arriving late or that you have not allotted enough time for certain procedures. Sometimes, a habitually delayed physician is the problem. You may find that too many staff people are making appointments. If this is the case, you can assign only one staff person to handle all scheduling. Some problems may never be completely solved. If they are identified, however, you can often make adjustments to avoid causing frustration for both patients and office personnel.

MEDIA MENU

- **Student CD**

  - **Case Study**
    Interactive Administrative Case Study 2: Managing a Medical Office Emergency

  - **CMA/RMA Certification Exam Review**

  - **Video Procedures**
    Procedure 6-1 video clip

- **LWW's Medical Assisting Skills DVD**
  Procedures 6-1, 6-2, 6-3, 6-4

- **Premium Online Course**
  http://thePoint.lww.com/Kronenberger3e

- **Internet Resources**

  LiveAdvise Online Tutoring & Competency Training
  http://thePoint.lww.com/LiveAdvise

español
SPANISH TERMINOLOGY

A que se debe su visita?
    Why do you need to see the doctor?
Desde cuando se siente mal?
    How long has this been going on?
Prefiere la cita en la manana o en la tarde?
    Would you prefer morning or afternoon?
Llamo para recordarle su cita.
    I am calling to remind you of your appointment.
Le dare una cita para que vea al Doctor nuevamenta.
    I will give you an appointment to return to see the doctor.
Para su proxima visita, por favor traiga su tarjeta del seguro y todas las medicinas que esta tomando.
    Please bring your insurance card and medicine bottles with you for your next appointment.

Dias de las semana	**Horas del dia**
Days of the week	Times of the day
Domingo	**A la una**
Sunday	One o'clock
Lunes	**El medio pasado uno**
Monday	1:30
Martes	**Dos en punto**
Tuesday	2:00
Miercoles	**Son las dos y media**
Wednesday	2:30
Jueves	**Tres en punto**
Thursday	3:00
Viernes	**Son las tres y media**
Friday	3:30
Sabado	**Siete en punto**
Saturday	7:00
	Son las siete y media
	7:30
	Ocho en punto
	8:00
	Son las ocho y media
	8:30
	Nueve en punto
	9:00
	Son las nueve y media
	9:30

PROCEDURE 6-1: Making an Appointment for a New Patient

Purpose: To secure an allotted time for a patient who is new to your facility to see the provider
Equipment: Patient's demographic information, patient's chief complaint, appointment book or computer with appointment software

Steps	Reasons
1. Obtain as much information as possible from the patient, such as: • Full name and correct spelling • Mailing address (not all offices require this) • Day and evening telephone numbers • Reason for the visit • Name of the referring person	To stay on schedule, you must allow enough time for the appointment. This information will help determine appointment needs and save time at the first visit.
2. Determine the patient's chief complaint or the reason for seeing the physician.	The reason for the visit will determine the time allotment, use of special rooms or equipment, etc.
3. Explain the payment policy of the practice. Most offices require payment at the time of an initial visit. Instruct patients to bring all pertinent insurance information.	Patients must understand this policy if they are to follow it.
4. Be sure patients know your office location; give concise directions if needed. You may also want to give patients an idea of how long they can expect to be at the office.	Helps patients arrive on time and lets them budget their time.
5. To avoid violating confidentiality, ask the patient if it is permissible to call at home or at work.	HIPPA's Privacy Rule prohibits leaving messages on an answering machine or giving any information to another individual who has not been named by the patient.
6. Before ending the call, confirm the time and date of the appointment. Say, "Thank you for calling, Mr. Brown. We look forward to seeing you on Tuesday, December 10, at 2 PM"	Repeating the appointment time will ensure that effective communication has taken place and increase the likelihood that the patient will be there on time.
7. Always check your appointment book to be sure that you have placed the appointment on the correct day in the right time slot.	Failure to record every appointment in the proper location can cause overbooking, frustrated physicians and staff, and irate patients.
8. If the patient was referred by another physician, you may need to call that physician's office before the appointment for copies of laboratory work, radiology, pathology reports, and so on. Give this information to the physician prior to the patient's appointment.	Remember, the patient must give authorization to release medical documents (see Chapter 9).

PROCEDURE 6-2: **Making an Appointment for an Established Patient**

Purpose: To secure an allotted time for a patient who is returning to your office as an established patient
Equipment: Appointment book or computer with appointment software, appointment card

Steps	Reasons
1. Determine what will be done at the return visit. Check your appointment book or computer system before offering an appointment.	If a specific examination, test, or scan is to be performed, you will want to avoid scheduling two patients for the same examination at the same time.
2. Offer the patient a specific time and date. Avoid asking the patient when he or she would like to return, as this can cause indecision.	Give the patient a choice, and if neither time is convenient, offer another specific time and date. Giving a patient a choice is good practice. "Mrs. Chang, we can see you next Tuesday, the 15th, at 3:30 PM or Wednesday, the 16th, at 9:00 AM."
3. Write the patient's name and telephone number in the appointment book or enter it in the computer.	Writing the phone number in the appointment book or making a notation in the computer will give you a quick reference if you need to call the patient to change the appointment.
4. Transfer the pertinent information to an appointment card and give it to the patient. Repeat aloud the appointment day, date, and time to the patient as you hand over the card (see Fig. 6-4).	Repeating the information reinforces the patient's memory and helps ensure that the appointment will be kept.
5. Double-check your book or computer to be sure you have not made an error.	Errors in appointments waste the patient's, staff's, and physician's time.
6. Whether in person or on the phone, end your conversation with a pleasant word and a smile.	A smile always feels good to a patient who may be apprehensive about needing to return to the doctor.

PROCEDURE 6-3: Making an Appointment for a Referral to an Oupatient Facility

Purpose: To secure an allotted time for a patient who needs to be seen in another facility

Equipment: Patient's chart with demographic information; physician's order for services needed by the patient and reason for the services; patient's insurance card with referral information, referral form, and directions to offce

Steps	Reasons
1. Make certain that the requirements of any third-party payers are met.	Some third-party payers require that referrals be precertified. Pre-existing conditions may not be covered for referral. Most companies require that only the patient's primary care physician (PCP) or gatekeeper make referrals. It is important to research each situation. Telephone numbers for pre-certification and questions will be printed on the back of the insurance card.
2. Refer to the preferred provider list for the patient's insurance company. Allow the patient to choose a provider from the list.	Managed care companies have strict requirements for precertification and documentation for referrals (see Chapter 13). If there is more than one provider with the same qualifications, the patient should always be given a choice.
3. Have the following information available when you make the call: • Physician's name and telephone number • Patient's name, address, and telephone number • Reason for the call • Degree of urgency • Whether the patient is being sent for consultation or referral	The referred or consulting physician's office needs to know these things to serve the patient well.
4. Record in the patient's chart the time and date of the call and the name of the person who received your call.	This is necessary for proper documentation of the patient's care.
5. Tell the person you are calling that you wish to be notified if your patient does not keep the appointment. If this occurs, be sure to tell your physician and enter this information in the patient's record.	Anyone in the office who needs this information will have it.
6. Write down the name, address, and telephone number of the doctor you are referring your patient to and include the date and time of the appointment. Give or mail this information to your patient. Be certain that the information is complete, accurate, and easy to read.	It is important that the patient keep their appointment. The physician is responsible for the patient's care and should know if the appointment is not kept.
7. If the patient is to call the referring physician to make the appointment, ask the patient to call you with the appointment date, and then document this in the chart.	Recording the appointment information in the patient's chart completes the transaction and proves that the physician's order was carried out.

PROCEDURE 6-4: Arranging for Admission to an Inpatient Facility

Purpose: To arrange admission to an inpatient facility providing all necessary information and to provide instructions to the patient

Equipment: Physician's order with diagnosis, patient's chart with demographic information, contact information for inpatient facility

Steps	Reasons
1. Determine the place that the patient and/or physician wants the admission arranged.	Physicians may have privileges at one hospital or several hospitals. The patient's insurance carrier may have a preferred facility list as well.
2. Gather information for the other facility, including demographic and insurance information.	Having the patient's demographic and insurance information handy avoids delays.
3. Determine any precertification requirements. If needed, locate contact information on the back of the insurance card and call the insurance carrier to obtain a precertification number.	Most insurance carriers must be notified in advance of an admission to an inpatient facility. You will be given a precertification number that must be given to the hospital admissions department. This number will follow the patient through the claims later filed for that admission.
4. Obtain from the physician the diagnosis and exact needs of the patient for an admission.	The hospital admissions department will need the patient's exact diagnosis. They will also need to know of any special requirements, such as a private room, isolation, etc.
5. Call the admissions department of the inpatient facility and give information from Step 2.	The admissions department handles all preliminary information, insurance information, etc. before assigning the patient a room.
6. Obtain instructions for the patient and call or give the patient instructions and information.	Patients should be given complete information in writing if possible. Patients may be afraid and emotional when they are being admitted to a hospital. Be sure they understand their instructions.
7. Provide the patient with the physician's orders for their hospital stay, including diet, medications, bed rest, etc.	If the patient is not at your office, the physician must call in this information. Most hospitals prefer that patients bring this information.
8. Document time, place, etc. in patient's chart, including any precertification requirements completed.	Any appointments made for the patient must be documented in the patient's chart. This provides the information to anyone in the office who needs it.

- The outpatient medical facility can be chaotic without an efficient appointment system. Moving patients through the facility while treating each person equally and thoroughly is one of the biggest challenges in the medical office.
- It is difficult for a busy practice to run smoothly all of the time. You need structure, but you must be flexible. Available times, equipment and room usage, and personnel coverage must be considered when finding just the right formula for a well-run and efficient office.
- The goals of the outpatient medical facility are to provide quality patient care and maintain financial stability. To reach those goals, an office must have a plan for the efficient scheduling and carrying out of the daily activities.
- Appointment scheduling systems include manual systems using appointment books and computerized systems that render helpful reports and daily activity sheets. The size of a practice, the number of physicians, the types of services, and so on are considered when establishing an appointment scheduling system.
- Sick patients calling to make appointments should be given priority, and there are established guidelines for determining the urgency of a patient's problem. Other functions, such as phone calls, reviewing records, and lunch breaks, are also scheduled into the daily activities of the office.
- An established protocol or list of steps should be in place to handle pharmaceutical representatives and other visitors to the office. As the medical assistant at the front desk, you will be one of the most important factors in the daily operation of the outpatient medical facility.
- As a medical assistant, you will make appointments, document encounters with patients that deal with appointments, and make referrals to other health care facilities. Learning the issues involved in successful appointment scheduling will help you make sure your facility runs smoothly.

Warm Ups for Critical Thinking

1. Assume that you are the office manager in a physician's office. Create a policy and procedure for scheduling patients.

2. Sign-in sheets can cause a breach in patient confidentiality. What other methods could you use that would limit the potential for invasion of patient privacy?

3. You notice that patients typically wait 30 to 45 minutes past their scheduled appointment times because of the physician. How would you approach a physician who chronically runs late?

Answers to Checkpoint Questions

1. A matrix is established to indicate times of each day that are not available for patient appointments.

2. The three systems that can be used for patient office visits include scheduled appointments, flexible hours, and open hours.

3. The three factors that can affect scheduling are patients' needs, physicians' preferences, and the physical facilities.

4. The three types of reminders are appointment cards, telephone reminders, and mailed reminder cards.

5. When scheduling a patient for surgery, the following information is needed: demographic and insurance information; the patient's name, age, address, telephone number, precertification number (if required), and diagnosis; surgery planned; and any special instructions.

Outline

GUIDELINES FOR PRODUCING PROFESSIONAL AND MEDICAL DOCUMENTS
Basic Grammar and
    Punctuation Guidelines
Basic Spelling Guidelines
Accuracy
Capitalization
Abbreviations and Symbols
Plural and Possessive
Numbers
PROFESSIONAL LETTER DEVELOPMENT
Components of a Letter

Letter Formats
Composing a Business Letter
Types of Business Letters
MEMORANDUM DEVELOPMENT
Components of a
    Memorandum
COMPOSING AGENDAS AND MINUTES
Agendas
Minutes

SENDING WRITTEN COMMUNICATION
Facsimile Machines
Electronic Mail
United States Postal Service
Other Delivery Options
RECEIVING AND HANDLING INCOMING MAIL
Types of Incoming Mail
Opening and Sorting Mail
Annotation

Learning Objectives

Upon successfully completing this chapter, you will be able to:

1. Spell and define the key terms

2. Discuss the basic guidelines for grammar, punctuation, and spelling in medical writing

3. Discuss the 11 key components of a business letter

4. Describe the process of writing a memorandum

5. List the items that must be included in an agenda

6. Identify the items that must be included when typing minutes

7. Cite the various services available for sending written information

8. Discuss the various mailing options

9. Identify the types of incoming written communication seen in a physician's office

10. Explain the guidelines for opening and sorting mail

Upon successfully completing this chapter, you will be able to:

1. Compose a business letter (Procedure 7-1)
2. Open and sort mail (Procedure 7-2)

Competencies

CAAHEP

- Respond to and initiate written communications

ABHES

- Fundamental writing skills
- Applications of electronic technology
- Adapt communications to individual's ability to understand
- Respond to and initiate written communications
- Utilize electronic technology to receive, organize, prioritize, and transmit information
- Use correct grammar, spelling, and formatting techniques in written word.

Key Terms

agenda	enclosure	margin	semiblock
annotation	font	memorandum	template
BiCaps	full block	proofread	
block	intercaps	salutation	

Good written communication skills are important for success. In the medical office, written communication is generated in several forms, such as reports (Table 7-1) and letters. Medical assistants commonly compose collection letters, patient reminders, and notifications of test results. You may also have an opportunity to produce memoranda, agendas, and minutes for meetings. Another important form of written communication is the handwritten entry in a patient's medical record. No matter which form it takes, your written communication must be clear, concise, and correct. Poorly written documents reflect negatively on the physician's practice and on you. Written communication may be sent or received through facsimile machines, electronic mail, delivery services, or United States postal service. As discussed throughout this text, HIPAA's Privacy Rule protects the confidentiality of all medical communication. Sending and receiving written communication according to the rules of confidentiality are also discussed. This chapter discusses guidelines for composing letters, writing memoranda, and composing agendas and minutes with proper grammar, spelling, and punctuation.

TABLE 7-1	Medical Reports
Hospital (inpatient) documents and medical office (outpatient) documents are different. You need to become familiar with the reports generated in a hospital because they become a part of the office chart and are needed for patient care, coding insurance claims, etc. Appendix F contains samples of typical reports generated in a hospital or inpatient setting.	

Medical Office Documents	Hospital Documents
The most common documents generated in a medical office are: • history and physical examination (H&P) reports • consultation reports • progress reports • diagnostic test reports (if the practice offers diagnostic tests) Other types of documents in outpatient facilities include: • reports of minor surgical procedures • legal abstracts • general office correspondence	Documents generated in the hospital setting include: • H&Ps • consultation reports • radiology and pathology reports • transfer summaries • discharge and death summaries • autopsy reports

Guidelines for Producing Professional and Medical Documents

Basic Grammar and Punctuation Guidelines

Professional writing requires that you follow the appropriate rules of grammar and punctuation. Box 7-1 provides a helpful list of key rules you will need to know.

Basic Spelling Guidelines

Good spelling skills take time to acquire. Box 7-2 lists basic tips for spelling. Many words sound exactly alike but are spelled differently and have different meanings. Be very careful with these words. Which of the following sentences has a spelling error?

- Wound cultures were taken from the left lower leg site.
- Wound cultures were taken from the left lower leg cite.

The first sentence is correct. Site and cite sound alike, and both are spelled correctly, but in the second sentence, the wrong word was used.

Spell check in word processing programs can be a great asset, but they have limitations. Medical terminology spell check software should be added to your computer and be updated frequently. You can add medical terms into your computer's spell check dictionary, but make sure that any word you add is spelled correctly!

Spell checks can never be 100% stocked with all the needed terms, especially in the medical profession, as new technologies, medications, and treatments arise daily.

Remember, spell check will not recognize words that are spelled correctly but misused. Even if you use spell check, you should proofread your document for other errors.

For example, the following sentence would pass spell check but is incorrect.

- The patient has inflammation of the prostrate.

Prostrate is an adjective that means face down. "The patient was in a prostrate position." The patient has inflammation of the *prostate*, the male sex gland.

- The physician received a plague.
- The physician received a plaque.

There is a big difference between plaque (commemorative item) and plague (bacterial disease)! These types of errors occur as a result of poor word usage and poor spelling. Box 7-3 lists some commonly used medical words that can easily be misspelled or misused.

Accuracy

Many of the medical documents or letters that you will write contain information that requires precision, accuracy, and careful attention to details. Inaccurate information in some letters can lead to injury of a patient and lawsuits and can harm the physician's practice.

BOX 7-1

BASIC GRAMMAR AND PUNCTUATION TIPS

Punctuation

- Period (.)—Used at end of sentences and following some abbreviations.
- Comma (,)—Used to separate words or phrases that are part of a series of three or more. The final comma before the "and" may be omitted. A comma can also be used after a long introductory clause or to separate independent clauses joined by and, but, yet, or, and nor.
- Semicolon (;)—Used to separate a long list of items in a series and to separate independent clauses not joined by a conjunction (e.g., and, but, or).
- Colon (:)—Used to introduce a series of items, to follow formal salutations, and to separate the hours from minutes indicating time.
- Apostrophe (')—Used to denote omissions of letters and to denote the possessive case of nouns.
- Quotation marks (" ")—Used to set off spoken dialogue, some titles (e.g., journal articles, newspaper articles, television and radio program episodes), and words used in a special way (Table 7-2).
- Parentheses [( )]—Used to indicate a part of a sentence that is not part of the main sentence but is essential for the meaning of the sentence. Also used to enclose a number, for confirmation, that is spelled out in a sentence.
- Ellipsis (…)—Used in place of a period to indicate a prolonged continuation of a conversation or list. Also used to display individual items or to connect phrases that are loosely connected.
- Diagonal (/)—Used in abbreviations (c/o), dates (2003/2004), fractions (3/4), and to indicate two or more options (AM/FM).

Sentence Structure

- Avoid long, run-on sentences.
- A verb must always agree with its subject in number and person.
- Ensure that the proper pronoun (he or she) is used.
- Adjectives should be used when they add an important message. Don't overuse adjectives or adverbs. Remember, double negatives used in one sentence make the sentence positive.

Capitalization

- Capitalize the first word in a sentence, proper nouns, the pronoun "I," book titles, and known geographical names.
- Names of persons, holidays, and trademark items should be capitalized.
- Expressions of time (AM and PM) should not be capitalized.

TABLE 7-2	The Use of Other Punctuation With Quotation Marks
Rule	**Example**
Place commas and periods inside quotation marks.	"Your bill," explained the patient, "has not come in the mail."
Place colons and semicolons outside quotation marks.	She said, "The doctor told me to come back on Friday"; however, he has no openings.
Place other punctuation inside quotation marks only if they belong in the quotation.	The student asked, "Is that going to be on the test?"
Place commas and periods outside quotation marks when used with single letters or single words.	Even though she earned an "A", she felt it was not her best work.

BOX 7-2

BASIC SPELLING TIPS

When in doubt about the spelling of a word, always use a dictionary or a spell check. Keep in mind that a computer spell check will check for spelling but will not alert you to inappropriate word usage.

Remember this rhyme: I comes before e, except after c, or when sounded like a as in neighbor and weigh. Examples: achieve, receive. (The exceptions are either, neither, weird, leisure, and conscience.)

- Words ending in -ie drop the e and change the i to y before adding -ing. Examples: die, dying; lie, lying.
- Words ending in -o that are preceded by a vowel are made plural by adding s. Example: studio, studios; trio, trios. Words ending in o that are preceded by a consonant form the plural by adding es. Examples: potato, potatoes; hero, heroes.
- Words ending in -y preceded by a vowel form the plural by adding s. Examples: attorney, attorneys; day, days. For words ending in -y that are preceded by a consonant, change the y to i and add es. Examples: berry, berries; lady, ladies.
- The final consonant of a one-syllable word is doubled before adding a suffix beginning with a vowel. Examples: run, running; pin, pinning. If the final consonant is preceded by another consonant or by two vowels, do not double the consonant. Examples: look, looking; act, acting.
- Words ending in a silent -e generally drop the e before adding a suffix beginning with a vowel. Examples: ice, icing; judge, judging. The exceptions are dye, eye, shoe, and toe. The e is not dropped, however, in suffixes beginning with a consonant unless another vowel precedes the final e. Examples: pale, paleness; argue, argument.
- For all words ending in -c, insert a k before adding a suffix beginning with e, i, or y. Examples: picnic, picnicking; traffic, trafficker.

BOX 7-3

COMMONLY MISUSED OR MISSPELLED MEDICAL TERMS

- anoxia and anorexia
- aphagia and aphasia
- bowl and bowel
- emphysema and empyema
- fundus and fungus
- lactose and lactase
- metatarsals and metacarpals
- mucus and mucous
- parental and parenteral
- postnatal and postnasal
- pubic and pubis
- rubella and rubeola
- serum and sebum
- uvula and vulva

is to be as accurate as possible and to question anything about which you are unsure. Here are some examples of inaccuracy:

- You wrote, "The patient was started on the MVP chemotherapy regimen." The physician, however, had written "MVPP." These are two completely different regimens. MVP is used for treating lung cancer, and MVPP is used for Hodgkin's lymphoma.
- The nurse practitioner dictated, "Patient was told to take Dristan Cold tablets." You rearranged the sentence, however, and typed, "The patient had a cold and was told to take Dristan tablets." Dristan Cold contains an antihistamine medication that plain Dristan does not. Never edit a physician's sentence unless you are sure that it will not affect the meaning.
- The physician said, "There is no reason for him to start radiation therapy at this time." You wrote, "Per Dr. Smith, there is reason for him to start radiation therapy at this time." The simple elimination of the word "no" completely changes the meaning of the sentence and can lead to errors in patient care.
- The physician's assistant dictated, "Hospitalization is needed because the patient continues to be violent." However, you typed, "Hospitalization is needed because the patient continues to be violet." The meaning of the sentence has been changed by the elimination of one "n" in violent.

Some of your letters will be placed in the patient's permanent medical record. Most letters will start with the physician asking you to draft a letter. He may or may not give you some notes to follow. He may dictate the letter. Either way, your responsibility in typing the letter

CHECKPOINT QUESTION

1. What are three consequences that could arise from inaccurate information in a business letter?

Capitalization

It is important to know when to capitalize and when to use lowercase letters. Following standard guidelines for using capital letters applies to most correspondence, but there are some exceptions and additional rules when typing medical documents. Never change how a word is capitalized unless directed to do so. Ask for clarification and mark the proof letter with a question mark for the physician to assist.

Use capital letters:

1. For headings: CHIEF COMPLAINT or Chief Complaint.

2. For eponyms (terms formed using the name of a person, usually the name of the researcher or physician who identified a disorder or the inventor of equipment, instruments, supplies, and so on); the second word in the phrase is not capitalized. *Note:* Recent revisions in punctuation guidelines eliminate the possessive apostrophe.

   Down syndrome
   Foley catheter
   Healy clamp

3. For trade or brand names of drugs and products. Do not capitalize generic names of drugs and products.

   diazepam   Valium
   tissue   Kleenex

4. For the genus of an organism. An example of this classification system of living organisms is *Staphylococcus aureus*. *Staphylococcus* is the genus, and *aureus* is the species. A singular genus is capitalized and italicized. If the genus is plural or used as an adjective, it is lower case and not italicized. Use lowercase letters and italics for the species.

   As noun: *Staphylococcus aureus*
   As adjective: staphylococcal infection

5. For a department name when the name is the proper title of a place, but not for department names within a facility.

   The patient was taken to the emergency room.
   The patient was taken to the Forsyth Medical Center Emergency Room.

6. For proper names of languages, races, and religions. Do not capitalize informal designations such as white or black.

   She is a 23-year-old Hispanic woman.

7. For acronyms (words formed from initials of words in a phrase).

   NKDA (no known drug allergies)
   CABG (coronary artery bypass graft)

8. To draw attention to vital information, such as allergies.

   ALLERGIES: The patient is allergic to PENICILLIN.

9. **Intercaps** or **BiCaps** are abbreviations, words, or phrases with unusual capitalization. Note that the accepted format should be used. For example, m-BACOD is a very different medication regimen from M-BACOD.

   pH, RhoGam, rPA, ReoPro, aVR

Abbreviations and Symbols

Abbreviations and symbols can save time in long handwriting and with typing. When you use abbreviations in medical documents, your reader must be able to recognize or translate the abbreviation. Abbreviations are not used as often as they once were. The possibility of confusion is not worth the time saved by using an abbreviation. When in doubt, spell it out. Abbreviations are also discussed in Chapter 8.

LEGAL TIP

BE CAUTIOUS WHEN USING ABBREVIATIONS

Here are some abbreviations that could be misinterpreted:

- The physician wrote, "The patient had good BS." You assumed that BS meant bowel sounds, so you typed "The patient had good bowel sounds," but the physician meant the abbreviation BS to mean breath sounds.

- Do not change < or > signs to *less than* or *greater than* unless you are sure of what the statement is saying. For example, "The patient will not be admitted to the hospital until her hemoglobin is less than 13." If you made a mistake and typed "greater than 13," confusion could occur.

- The symbols for male (♂) and female (♀) are commonly used in handwritten notes, but you should replace these symbols with words when writing a business or professional letter.

Medical facilities accredited by The Joint Commission are required to "standardize" the abbreviations, acronyms, and symbols used by their employees. Standardization includes having a process to identify accepted abbreviations and then making sure all employees are informed of and have access to a list of these approved abbreviations. The list should be updated regularly. In cases where there may be more than one definition of an established abbreviation, you must identify the definition to be accepted by the facility. The Joint Commission also requires facilities to make and communicate a "do not use" list, which should include abbreviations and symbols that could be ambiguous. (See Chapter 8 and Appendix D for more information.)

Some facilities have local abbreviations that are specific to the facility. Like words in English, many abbreviations have two meanings. Some abbreviations have become accepted because they are used more than the long form. BP has come to be easily recognized as blood pressure when used in the vital sign section of the report. In a hospital setting, the use of abbreviations in some typed reports is forbidden. For example, you are not allowed to abbreviate the diagnosis on an operative report.

Most doctors' offices use standard abbreviations when writing in patient charts, but when you are typing a formal report, it is risky to use abbreviations. If it is the policy of your facility to use abbreviations in letters and formal reports, spell out the words the first time the abbreviation is used, with the abbreviation following in parentheses. For example, "The patient had a coronary artery bypass graft (CABG) in 1987." Become familiar with the abbreviations and symbols that are used where you work. Appendix D lists the most common abbreviations.

Plural and Possessive

Converting words to plural or possessive form can be tricky in English. Most medical terms have a Latin or Greek origin and have their own set of rules for pluralization. Box 7-4 shows the rules for pluralizing most medical terms. You should be accurate because mistakes can cause confusion. For example, "The patient's coming in Monday to be taught to give herself allergy injections. This will require the patient's undivided attention and the CMA's patience."

To show possession, use an apostrophe and add an S to the word: "The patient's appointment is tomorrow." To show possession in a plural word, place the apostrophe after the S: "The medical assistants' credentials are verified before they are hired."

It is common in the medical world to hear possessive units of time: "The patient will return in 2 weeks' time." or "Tuesday's patients will have to be rescheduled."

Numbers

In general, numbers one to ten should be spelled out, except when used with units of measurement (e.g., 5 mg), and numbers over ten may be expressed as a numeral. When several numbers are used in a sentence,

---

BOX 7-4

RULES FOR PLURALIZING MEDICAL TERMS

A add an E	bulla becomes bullae
UM changes to a	ovum becomes ova
US changes to I	bronchus becomes bronchi
ON changes to A	phenomenon becomes phenomena
IS changes to ES or IDES	testis becomes testes, epididymis becomes epididymides
AX or IX: change the X to C and add ES	thorax becomes thoraces
EX changes to ICES	index becomes indices
EN: drop the EN and add INA	lumen becomes lumina
MA changes to MATA	carcinoma becomes carcinomata
NX or YNX change to NGES	phalanx becomes phalanges, larynx becomes larynges

---

this ruled is ignored in order to maintain consistency. All numbers in the sentence should be written in the same form. For example, "There are 21 students in the 2-year medical assisting program."

Here are some important tips you will need to remember about numbers:

- Numbers referring to an obstetrical patient's medical history are not written out: "The patient is a gravida 3, para 2." Do not convert these numbers.
- Watch decimal point placement. There is a huge difference in medication between 12.5 mg and 1.25 mg.
- Double-check that you have not transposed numbers. For example, you typed, "The patient's red blood cell count was 5.1," but it was actually 1.5. A red blood cell count of 1.5 is incompatible with life.
- Roman numerals should never be changed to words. For example, "lead II of the patient's electrocardiogram" should never be changed to "lead two of the patient's electrocardiogram."
- Many health care professionals use military time. Time that is written in military style does not have to

be changed if the recipient of the letter is familiar with it (doctors, nurses). If the letter is going to a patient or other person who may not be able to interpret it, however, either convert the time or express the standard time in parenthesis; for example, "The patient's next appointment is at 1430 hours (2:30 PM)." No colons are used in military time.

- Temperatures must always have the correct symbol for Celsius or Fahrenheit included (98.6°F or 37°C).
- Telephone numbers should include the area code in parentheses or followed by a hyphen, then the number with a hyphen. Add extensions to the number by placing a comma after the last digit of the number, then type Ext. and the number: (800) 555-0000, Ext. 6480. Periods may replace hyphens and parentheses: 800.555.0000.

 CHECKPOINT QUESTION

2. Why should all numbers in a sentence be written in the same way regardless of the rule?

Professional Letter Development

Professional writing is different from writing letters to your friends or family members. The goal of professional writing is to get information communicated in a concise, accurate, and comprehensible manner. Slang or idiomatic terms that are commonly used in writing letters to friends are not appropriate for business letters. For example, "Drop by and say hi" is not suitable for a professional letter, even if you know the recipient personally.

Writing effective business letters is a skill that requires practice and careful attention to detail. To write a professional business letter, you must:

- Understand the components of a letter
- Use the correct letter format
- Ensure that the message is clear, concise, and accurate

These skills are described in the following sections.

Components of a Letter

A typical business letter has 11 components. We will explore each one, beginning at the top of the page. For easy reference, Figure 7-1 displays a sample business letter with these components marked.

1. *Letterhead.* The letterhead consists of the name of the practice or physician, address, telephone number, fax number, and sometimes the company logo. The letterhead is often embossed in color and centered on the top of the page. The letterhead may also be preset into a **template**. (Templates are discussed later in the chapter.)

2. *Date.* The date includes the month, day, and year. It should be positioned two to four spaces below the letterhead. The date must be typed on only one line, and abbreviations should not be used.

3. *Inside address.* The inside address refers to the name and address of the person to whom the letter is being sent. A nine-digit zip code should be used if available. The inside address is placed two spaces down from the date unless the letter is being mailed with a window envelope and it will not be aligned correctly. Never abbreviate city or town names. States can be abbreviated. (See Appendix C for a list of abbreviations approved by the postal service.) Never abbreviate business titles (e.g., President, Chief Executive Officer). Here are some other points to remember:

   - If the letter is going to a business, type the name of the addressee, followed by his or her title, the name of the business on the next line, and then the address.
   - If the letter is being addressed to two or more people at different addresses, type the individual address block one line space under the other or place the addresses side by side.
   - If the letter is going to two people at the same address but with different last names, type the woman's name on the first line, man's name on the second line, then the address. If the sexes are the same, do them in alphabetical order, followed by the address.

4. *Subject line.* The subject line, an optional component, is used to state the intent of a letter or to indicate what the letter is regarding. It is placed on the third line below the inside address and is written as Re: (an abbreviation for regarding) followed by the subject. For example, Re: Blood tests.

5. *Salutation.* The **salutation** is the greeting of the letter. It is placed two spaces down from the inside address or the subject line. Capitalize the first letter of each word in the phrase, and end the phrase with a colon. It is permissible to eliminate the salutation if the letter is informal or if a subject line has been used. When writing to a physician, write out the word doctor. Here are some recommendations when writing salutations:

   - If the letter is going to one person and the gender is known, write "Dear Mr. Rogers."
   - If the letter is going to one person and the gender is *not* known, write "Dear Pat Smith" (use the person's first name).
   - If the letter is going to a woman and a man with different last names, always address the woman first: "Dear Ms. Ray and Mr. Oscar."
   - If the letter is going to several people, place them

Benjamin Matthews, M.D.
999 Oak Road, Suite 313
Middletown, Connecticut 06457
860-344-6000
①

February 2, 2008 ②

Dr. Adam Meza
Medical Director ③
Family Practice Associates
134 N. Tater Drive
West Hartford, Connecticut 06157

Re: Ms. Beatrice Suess ④

Dear Doctor Meza: ⑤

Thank you for asking me to evaluate Ms. Suess. I agree with your diagnosis of rheumatoid arthritis. Her prodromal symptoms include vague articular pain and stiffness, weight loss and general malaise. Ms. Suess states that the joint discomfort is most prominent in the mornings, gradually improving throughout the day.

My physical examination shows a 40-year-old female patient in good health. Heart sounds normal, no murmurs or gallops noted. Lung sounds clear. Enlarged lymph nodes were noted. Abdomen soft, bowel sounds present, and the spleen was not enlarged. Extremities showed subcutaneous nodules and flexion contractures on both hands.

⑥

Laboratory findings were indicative of rheumatoid arthritis. See attached laboratory data. I do not feel x-rays are warranted at this time.

My recommendations are to continue Ms. Suess on salicylate therapy, rest and physical therapy. I suggest that you have Ms. Suess attend physical therapy at the American Rehabilitation Center on Main Street.

Thank you for this interesting consultation.

Yours truly, ⑦

Benjamin Matthews, MD
Benjamin Matthews, MD ⑧

BM/es ⑨

Enc. (2) ⑩

c: Dr. Samuel Adams ⑪

Figure 7-1 Components of a business letter. This letter is done in full block format and contains the following elements: (1) letterhead, (2) date, (3) inside address, (4) subject line, (5) salutation, (6) body, (7) closing, (8) signature and typed name, (9) identification line, (10) enclosure, and (11) copy.

in alphabetical order: "Dear Mr. Andersen, Mr. Cats, Ms. Dart, and Mr. Raymond."

- To Whom It May Concern, Dear Sir, or Dear Madam should not be used.

6. *Body of the letter.* The body of the letter contains the message. It should be single-spaced with double spacing between the paragraphs. Here are some guidelines for writing the body of the letter:

- If the letter is more than one page long, try to avoid dividing a paragraph at the end of a page. If you must, leave at least two sentences at the bottom of the first page. Use the widow and orphan control feature of your word processor program to prevent orphan lines from appearing.
- Tables and graphs should not be broken. They should appear on one page only.
- Web addresses and e-mail addresses should fit on one line and never be continued to another page.
- If the letter is more than one page long, page numbers should be used.
- Use a bulleted format to highlight key points for the reader. For example, "The possible side effects of this medication are:" (then list them vertically with a bullet symbol).
- The letterhead is used only on the first page of the letter. The second page should be the same quality paper as the letterhead. Start the second page with a continuation line (name of person the letter is going to and the date of the letter). Continue the letter two lines down from the continuation line. Your **margins** must be the same as those on page 1. Most templates type the continuation line for you.

7. *Closing.* The closing concludes the letter. Some common closings are: Sincerely, Yours truly, Regards, Respectfully, and Cordially yours. Only the first word is capitalized, and a comma follows the phrase. Closings are placed two spaces down from the end of the letter. Never put the closing alone on a page.

8. *Signature and typed name.* The name of the person sending the document is typed four spaces below the closing, with the person's title typed directly below. The physician will read and sign the letter above the typed name. If you are instructed to sign the letter, sign the physician's name followed by a slash mark and your name, e.g., Susan James, MD/Raymond Smith, RMA.

9. *Identification line.* The identification line, an optional component, indicates who dictated the letter and who wrote it. It consists of abbreviations only. The initials of the person who dictated the letter are capitalized (generally the physician); the initials of

the writer of the letter are in lowercase (generally these will be yours). The identification line can also be called the reference line.

10. *Enclosure.* An **enclosure** is something that is included with a letter. It is abbreviated Enc. and is placed two spaces down from the identification line. The number of documents included is placed in parentheses; if only one document is included, just the abbreviation Enc. is used.

11. *Copy.* The abbreviation c is used to indicate that a duplicate letter has been sent. It is typed two spaces below the enclosure line. Usually, letters are copied to managers, supervisors, or to the physician who requested that the given information be dispersed.

Letter Formats

There are three basic types of letter formats: **full block**, **semiblock**, and **block**. Office policy or the physician preferences will dictate which format you use. Full block is shown in Figure 7-1, which shows the components of a business letter. The elements of the block letter are seen in Figure 7-2, and the semiblock format is seen in Figure 7-3. Semiblock is also referred to as modified block.

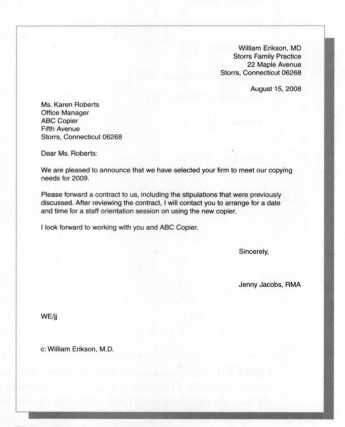

Figure 7-2 Sample block letter.

Elizabeth Jones, M.D.
750 East Street, Suite 205
Hialeah, Florida 33013
305-311-2666

June 12, 2008

Margaret Trent
18 Cambridge Street
Hialeah, Florida 33013

Dear Ms. Trent:

As per our phone conversation, your blood glucose level remains elevated. It is essential that we stabilize your blood sugar level.

In order to achieve normal blood sugar levels, you must follow the enclosed diet. A meeting with a Registered Dietitian can be arranged for you to discuss any dietary concerns you may have.

I am also enclosing patient education instructions for the use of a glucometer. You must test your blood sugar every morning and keep a diary of your results. Glucometers can be purchased from any pharmacy. If you need assistance in using the glucometer, please contact Raymond Smith, CMA, at 555-6423.

Presently, I do not wish to prescribe any medications. If we are unable to get your blood sugar under control, I will prescribe an oral diabetic medication.

Please call my office and schedule an appointment for the week of June 20 for a blood draw and a follow-up visit.

Sincerely,

Elizabeth Jones, M.D.

EJ/rs

enc. (2)

Figure 7-3 Sample semiblock letter.

Composing a Business Letter

To create a professional business letter, follow these three steps: preparation, composition, and editing. Box 7-5 gives you some guidelines for starting to write a letter.

 CHECKPOINT QUESTION

3. Whose address is typed as the inside address? What is the purpose of the salutation? What is the purpose of the identification line?

Composition

The goal of composition is to ensure that your message is transmitted clearly, concisely, and accurately to your reader. As you did during preparation, focus on the message, not on the mechanics.

A clear message ensures that your reader knows precisely what is expected; an unclear message leaves room for doubt.

Unclear: Please contact me.
Clear: Please contact me by Thursday, October 1.

BOX 7-5

HOW TO START WRITING A LETTER

By determining the answers to these four questions, you can better prepare the message of your letter.

1. Who is my reader?

   It is very important that you use proper gender identification. Be especially careful with names that can be used for males or females (e.g., Sam, Kelly, Ronnie, Alex, Tracy). Determine the reader's comprehension level. Letters to physicians will be more technical and will use medical terminology. Letters to patients will be less technical and use medical terminology sparingly.

2. What do I want my reader to do?

   This is your call to action; make it clear and specific. For example, you might write, "Please complete the enclosed insurance form (2 pages). Be sure to include all necessary information and sign your name. Place the form in the enclosed envelope, and return it to our office by June 15, 2003." Avoid using "at your earliest convenience"; include a date for the required action. If possible, include a response mechanism, such as a self-addressed, stamped envelope.

3. What do I want to say?

   Briefly list the necessary information. To help you remember all of the necessary information, ask yourself who, what, where, when, why, and how.

4. How will I organize my message?

   Here are three basic ways that you can organize your message:

   • Chronological: Discuss items in a sequential manner, beginning with the earliest date and proceeding to the most recent date. For example, when discussing the physician's career, list his or her earlier experiences before the most recent career achievements.

   • Problem oriented: Let the reader know about a specific problem and provide instructions for correcting the problem. For example, if a patient's blood work came back with abnormal findings, a letter would be sent identifying the problem (e.g., low hematocrit) and advising the patient on the possible causes, treatments, and follow-up procedures.

   • Comparison: Evaluate the effectiveness of two or more items. For example, as an office manager, you may have to write to the physician comparing two service contracts or two sample computer software packages.

Unclear: You need to make an appointment for blood work.

Clear: Call Temple Hospital laboratories (555-4010) and make an appointment for a blood glucose test on March 13.

A concise message is short and to the point. Wordy phrases with many adjectives should not be used.

Not concise: Please enclose a check in an envelope for exactly $50.

Concise: Please enclose a $50 check.

An accurate message includes the correct date, time, figures, and information. Inaccurate messages cause delays and confusion and can lead to poor public relations.

Editing

After you have composed the letter, edit it for both grammatical errors and factual information. Editing is a key step in making your letter a success. Editing entails two steps: proofreading and corrections.

Proofreading

Whenever possible, have a colleague **proofread** (read text and check for accuracy) your letter and provide constructive criticism. Be sure to maintain confidentiality. If you are using a computer, consider printing out a hard copy of your document for proofreading; some individuals find it difficult to proofread a document on the computer screen. Check for the following items:

- Accuracy of all information
- Clarity and conciseness
- Grammar
- Spelling
- Punctuation
- Paragraphs appropriate in length and limited to one subject
- Capitalization
- Logical organization and flow

Use proofreaders marks (Box 7-6) to speed up the editing process. These are standard marks used to indicate corrections. You should become familiar with the basic marks.

 CHECKPOINT QUESTION

4. What is the purpose of proofreading?

Corrections

After making corrections, print a final copy of the letter. Remember, a computer spell check should be used with caution because it highlights misspelled words but not incorrectly used words.

BOX 7-6

STANDARD PROOFREADER MARKS

Mark	Meaning
♂ or ♄ or ⫮	delete; take it out
◡	close up; print as one word
♂	delete and close up
∧ or > or ⋏	caret; insert here (something
#	insert a space
eq #	space evenly where indicated
stet	let marked text stand as set
tr	transpose; change order the
/	used to separate two or more marks and often as a concluding stroke at the end of an insertion
[	set farther to the left
]	set farther to the right
⌒	set æ or fl as ligatures æ or fl
⹀	straighten alignment
‖	straighten or align
✕	imperfect or broken character
□	indent or insert em quad space
⊓	begin a new paragraph
SP	spell out (set 5 lbs as five pounds)
cap	set in capitals (CAPITALS)
sm cap or s.c.	set in small capitals (SMALL CAPITALS)
lc	set in lowercase (lowercase)
ital	set in italic (*italic*)
rom	set in roman (roman)
bf	set in boldface (**boldface**)
= or -/ or ⌢ or /H/	hyphen
$\frac{1}{N}$ or en or /N/	en dash (1965–72)
$\frac{1}{M}$ or em or /M/	em—or long—dash
∨	superscript or superior (∨² as in πr²)
∧	subscript or inferior (∧₂ as in H₂O)
◇ or ✕	centered (◇ for a centered dot in *p • q*)
⌃	comma
⌄	apostrophe
⊙	period
; or ;/	semicolon
: or ⊙	colon
⌵ ⌵ or ⌵ ⌵	quotation marks
(/)	parentheses
[/]	brackets
OK/?	query to author: has this been set as intended
⌐ or ⌐¹	push down a work-up
ℓ¹	turn over an inverted letter
wf¹	wrong font; a character of the wrong size or esp. style

¹ The last three symbols are unlikely to be needed in making proofs of photocomposed matter.

Types of Business Letters

You will be asked to create and type various letters. Letters that you write will be sent to patients, insurance companies, other health care providers, pharmaceutical companies, and various businesses. Here are some common types of letters that you may write:

- Letters welcoming new patients to the practice
- Letters to patients regarding their test results
- Consultation reports to other health care professionals
- Workers' compensation letters verifying the patient's injury or treatment
- Justification or explanation of treatments to insurance companies
- Cover letters for transferring patients' records to another practice
- Clarification or explanation to patients regarding fees or billing concerns
- Thank you letters to sales representatives
- Physician changes for on-call schedules (generally sent to the hospital and covering physicians)
- Announcements of new services, hours, or office location changes

Memorandum Development

A **memorandum** (often called a memo) is for communication within the office or with another department only; it is never sent to patients. It is less formal than a letter and is generally used for brief announcements.

Components of a Memorandum

A memorandum contains the standard elements in the following list. Use these guidelines to complete each element. Figure 7-4 shows a sample memorandum.

1. *Heading.* The word Memorandum is typed across the top of the page.
2. *Date.* Use the same rules for letters when typing the date for memorandums.
3. *To.* List the names of all recipients in either alphabetic or hierarchic order. If the memorandum is going to a particular group (e.g., all department managers, all employees), it can be addressed to the group.
4. *From.* List the name and title of the person sending the memorandum.
5. *Subject.* Insert a brief phrase describing the purpose of the memorandum.
6. *Body.* Write the message of the memorandum here.
7. *Copy (c).* Use the same rules as for letters when sending duplicate copies of memorandums.

Salutations and closings are not used in memorandums. All lines in a memorandum are justified left, and 1-inch margins are used. Writing a memorandum entails the same steps (preparation, composition, editing) as writing a business letter. The memorandum should be read and initialed by the physician before it is distributed. Your computer software will have a memorandum template.

 CHECKPOINT QUESTION

5. What are memorandums used for?

Composing Agendas and Minutes

Two other forms of written communication are agendas and minutes.

Agendas

The purpose of an **agenda** is to outline briefly the topics to be discussed at a meeting. It allows the meeting participants to prepare any necessary reports before the meeting and to anticipate questions. Agendas usually begin with a call to order, followed by a review of previous meeting minutes, old business updates, and then new business. Adjournment is the last item on the agenda. The format and amount of detail included in an agenda is determined by the type of group that is meeting. Figure 7-5 shows an appropriate format for the meeting of a professional or civic organization. Your physician may take a leadership role in an organization, and you would be asked to prepare an agenda for the meetings.

Minutes

The minutes of a meeting outline the actions of the group. Members may need to refer back to the minutes

---

Franklin Dermatology Center
123 Main Street
Rockfall, Kansas
913-755-2600

Memorandum

To: All Medical Assistants
From: Patty Stricker, Office Manager
Date: 12/03/04
Re: Holiday time

Please notify me by December 10 of any requests you have for taking time off during Christmas or New Year's. Remember that holiday requests will be based on seniority. The office will be closed at noon on December 24. The office will be closed the 25th and reopen on the 26th. The office will also close on December 31st at noon. The office will be closed on January 1, reopening on the 2nd.

If you have any questions, please e-mail me.

Figure 7-4 Sample memorandum.

Forsyth-Stokes-Davie Chapter of Medical Assistants
Winston-Salem NC
Meeting Agenda
September 13, 2008

Welcome
President
Introductions
Members
Introduction of Speaker
Program Committee Chair
Speaker
Roberta Williams, BSN, OSHA Update
Call to Order
President
Reading of the Minutes of October Mtg.
Secretary
Officers' Reports
Committee Reports
Membership Campaign
New Business
Announcements
Newsletter Deadline Dec. 1
Adjournment

Figure 7-5 Sample meeting agenda.

of a previous meeting. In organizations with officers, the secretary takes notes and/or records the meeting. For other meetings such as committee or board meetings, someone is assigned the task of preparing the minutes. You should type the minutes of a meeting as soon as possible. Record only motions, seconds, and the results of a vote. You may include a brief discussion of the motions, but do not include unrelated items, opinions, or individual members' statements. The minutes of a meeting become an important document in the association's history. Include the following information:

- List of members present
- List of members absent
- Date and time the meeting was called to order
- Statement regarding the acceptance of the previous minutes
- Motions made and the name of the person making the motion.
- Brief report of discussion
- Results of voting, whether the motion passed or not
- List of reports that were submitted
- Date and time of the next meeting
- Adjournment time
- Signature of the person who prepared the minutes and the chairperson's signature

ETHICAL TIP

Be Careful What You Record in the Minutes

Remember, you are recording the happenings of a meeting that will stay on record for years. The minutes of a meeting should not include personal opinions or any information that is not relevant to the BUSINESS of the group. The purpose of minutes is to record the ACTIONS that took place at the meeting, not this:

Sherri Hauser made a motion to have a bake sale for the scholarship fund. Joan Merricks seconded the motion. Discussion followed: Sherri told the group not to tell Mindy about the bake sale. Judy reminded the group about Mindy's ginger cookies that broke Tekoa's tooth that time. Everybody got a good laugh. The motion passed.

A more appropriate entry is as follows:

A motion was made by Sherri Hauser to hold a bake sale on November 2 at the community college from 7:00 AM until 3 PM with proceeds going to the scholarship fund. The motion was seconded by Joan Merricks. Discussion followed. The motion passed.

Sending Written Communication

After the document has been written, proofread, and signed, it is ready for you to send it to its receiver. Fold the letter in thirds, and place it in an envelope. Most professional letters are sent through the postal service. Other types of written communications are sent through facsimile machines or by electronic mail. Here are two key steps to remember when sending any type of written communication:

- All attempts must be made to ensure patient confidentiality. The outside of envelopes should be marked confidential when the correspondence contains information about a patient. Send letters only to known or confirmed addresses.
- Return addresses must be used so that mail can be returned if the recipient is no longer at the given address.

Facsimile Machines

Facsimile, or fax, machines allow the medical office to send and receive printed material over a phone line. These machines offer a convenient and cost-effective way to transmit records, orders, prescriptions, test results, and other materials that require quick receipt. Always use a cover sheet (Fig. 7-6) when sending papers

Cardiology Associates
Maria Sefferin, MD
897 Bayou Drive
Philadelphia, PA
215-112-9999

facsimile transmittal

To: _____ Fax: _____

From: _____ Date: _____

Re: _____ Pages: _____

CC: _____

☐ Urgent ☐ For Review ☐ Please Comment ☐ Please Reply ☐ Please Recycle

Comments:

CONFIDENTIAL INFORMATION

The information in the facsimile message and any accompanying documents is confidential. This information is intended only for use by the individual or entity name above. If you are not the intended recipient of this information you are hereby notified that any disclosure, copying or distribution of this information is strictly prohibited. Please notify the sender immediately by telephone.

Figure 7-6 Sample fax cover sheet

through a fax machine. At minimum, a cover sheet should have the following information:

- Name, address, telephone, and fax number of the physician's practice
- Name of the intended receiver of the fax
- Number of pages being sent, counting the cover sheet
- Telephone number of the fax machine of the intended recipient
- Date and time the fax was sent
- Confidentiality statement (e.g., "The information in the facsimile message and any accompanying documents is confidential. This information is intended only for use by the individual or entity name above. If you are not the intended recipient of this information, you are hereby notified that any disclosure, copying, or distribution of this information is strictly prohibited. Please notify the sender immediately by telephone.").

When you receive a fax, forward it to the appropriate person. The fax machine should be checked regularly throughout the day, and all items should be sorted quickly.

Sometimes when you fax a given letter, the fax machine may be busy, or the number dialed may be busy. If the number is busy, it is not acceptable to leave the fax papers in the machine for redial unless you are sure that no one else will have access to that document. Never leave documents unattended.

Electronic Mail

Electronic mail, or e-mail, allows computer-to-computer communication, whether within the same facility or anywhere throughout the world. The communication occurs through a modem. Each computer must be linked to an online service provider. Chapter 9 discusses electronic mail in more detail. Here are a few things you should remember about sending letters via electronic mail:

- Confidentiality cannot be guaranteed.
- Follow the usual steps of preparation, composition, and editing.
- You can attach letters to an e-mail by clicking on the file attachment icon, locating the letter, and inserting it. It is always a good idea to open the attachment to make sure that you are attaching the correct letter or version.

United States Postal Service

Written communication is commonly sent via the United States Postal Service (USPS). Envelopes must be correctly prepared so that the optical character readers (OCR) used by the USPS can sort the mail quickly and efficiently. The OCR reads the envelope, scanning for information. The OCR scans all envelopes using these margins: 1/2 inch on either side and 5/8 inch from the top or bottom of the envelope. Addresses or notations outside of these margins will not be read.

Addressing Envelopes

The standard business envelope is no. 10. USPS regulations state that the minimal size of an envelope is 3 1/2 × 5 inches. It must be rectangular and no less than 0.007 inch thick. The standard no. 10 business envelope is 4 1/8 × 9 1/2 inches.

The requirements for addressing an envelope are necessary because the postal service uses optical character readers (OCR), which quickly and efficiently sort the mail. As the mail travels through the scanning devices, it is sorted electronically.

The return address is placed in the upper left hand corner. It should not exceed five lines. The return address is typed with the same guidelines as for letters and is single spaced. Often, medical offices have the return address preprinted on the envelope.

The recipient's address is typed 12 spaces down from the top and centered on the face of the envelope. All words of the address should be capitalized. Only

PIEDMONT INTERNAL MEDICINE
1050 S MAIN STREET
ASHEBORO NC 26092-1050

SEAMSTER JANITORIAL SERVICE
P O BOX 5030
RALEIGH NC 25532-5030

Figure 7-7 Sample envelope

postal abbreviations for states should be used, and no punctuation is used between the postal abbreviation and the zip code. All addresses must include the five-digit zip code; whenever possible, the four-digit expanded zip code should also be used. The expanded zip code allows the USPS to sort and route the mail faster and more accurately. Envelopes should not be handwritten, as this does not portray a professional image. The entire address should not exceed five lines. Your software may allow you to insert a USPS PostNet bar code. This is generally inserted two to three lines below the address. This bar code accelerates USPS sorting. Always check your software to make sure it is certified by the USPS.

Special notations such as "confidential" or "personal" are placed on the left-hand side of the envelope two lines below the return address. Notations for hand canceling and special delivery are made in the upper right-hand corner of the envelope below the postage. Nothing should be printed in the right lower corner of the envelope because the USPS uses that space for its bar codes. Figure 7-7 displays a properly addressed envelope.

Here are some additional things to remember regarding envelopes:

- Be sure that graphics or logos do not impede the OCR's ability to read the address.
- Do not use fancy **fonts** that may impede the OCR's ability to read the address.
- A minimum of eight-point type is recommended by the USPS.
- USE ALL CAPS.
- Do not use dark envelopes.
- White or tan envelope with black type is preferred.
- Do not use the **#** sign; if it cannot be avoided, leave one space between the **#** sign and the number (this is a USPS recommendation).
- If you are using an envelope with a window frame, there should be an eighth-inch clearance around the address.

 CHECKPOINT QUESTION

6. What does an optical character reader do?

Affixing Postage

Proper postage must be affixed to the envelope by a stamp, permit imprint, or a postage meter machine. Postage meter machines are in-house machines that are regulated by the USPS. They contain a prepaid amount of postage and can imprint the postage stamp either directly on the envelope or onto an adhesive tape that is applied to the envelope. Some machines weigh, stuff, and seal the envelopes. The date on the postage machine must be changed daily, and the ink roller must be kept full.

The physician may opt to use the USPS permit imprint program. In this case, you take the mail, sealed and ready to be sent, to the post office. The postal clerk passes your letters through the USPS machine, and a permit stamp is placed on the envelope. The postal clerk deducts the postage charges from your prepaid account. The advantages to this system are that is saves time and does not require the office to care for the postal meter machine.

USPS Mailing Options

Mail can be sent in a variety of ways based on its urgency and value. The following is a brief description of the services offered by the USPS:

- Express mail, the fastest service, ensures delivery of your package by the next day (by noon in most areas). Express mail is delivered 7 days a week. Express mail is automatically insured for $500. Additional insurance is available.
- Priority mail, the second fastest service, offers 2-day delivery to most destinations. The maximum weight is 70 pounds, and the maximum size is 108 inches combined length and girth. The rate is based on the weight of the package. You can purchase up to $5,000 of insurance for packages.
- First-class mail is the service used for sending standard mail (letters and postcards) weighing up to 13 ounces. Mail weighing more than 13 ounces will be considered priority mail.
- Standard mail (A) is used by companies to mail books and catalogs. Standard mail (B) is used to mail packages weighing more than 1 pound. The maximum weight is 70 pounds, and the maximum measurement is 130 inches combined length and girth.
- Postal rates, fees, and services are subject to change. You must stay abreast of the latest information. Use the USPS website for additional information and updates.

USPS Special Services

A certificate of mailing is used to prove that a document was mailed. No record is kept at the post office. It does

Figure 7-8 Certified mail receipt.

not provide proof that the letter was received by the addressee.

Certified mail provides a mailing receipt and a record of the mailing at the local post office (Fig. 7-8). This service is available only for first-class and priority mail. Return receipts can be purchased in conjunction with this. Return receipts are used to prove that the recipient received the document (Fig. 7-9).

Registered mail provides the most protection for valuables. It is available only for priority and first-class mail. The maximum insurance that can be obtained is $25,000. This service can be combined with return receipts. International rates are available from your local post office. Type the address as discussed earlier, and type the name of the country on the last line without abbreviations (Japan, Korea). All physician offices should have a supply of express and priority mail envelopes along with a current fee schedule.

Other Delivery Options

Many other companies specialize in document and package delivery, particularly with next-day or sec-

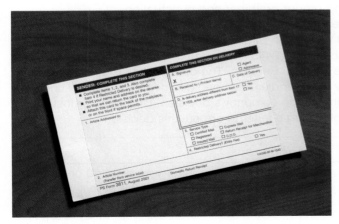

Figure 7-9 Return receipt.

ond-day delivery services. Examples of these companies include Airborne Express, Federal Express, and United Parcel Service (UPS). Use the company with which the physician has an account. Fees vary, so you may have to contact each company for prices and available services. These companies offer services such as tracking, pick-up services, money back guarantees, and proof of delivery. The tracking service can be done through their websites.

Receiving and Handling Incoming Mail

Part of the daily routine for a medical assistant is handling the incoming mail. Sort the mail quickly and promptly to ensure efficient functioning of the office.

Types of Incoming Mail

Many types of mail are received daily in a physician's office:

- Advertisements
- Bills for office services
- Consultation letters
- Hospital communications and newsletters
- Laboratory and radiographic reports
- Office supply magazines
- Patient correspondence
- Payments from insurance companies and patients
- Professional journals
- Literature from professional organizations
- Samples (drugs, laboratory test kits)
- Waiting room magazines

Opening and Sorting Mail

Each physician will have an individual policy on which mail you should open and how you should process it. Any mail marked urgent should be handled first, followed by mail about patient-related issues. Promotional materials should be handled last. Some physicians will have you sort, file, and respond to mail without their review. In some practices, however, all mail is placed in a special file folder and handled only by the physician or office manager. Procedure 7-2 outlines the steps for opening and sorting the mail. Most physicians will open and handle their own e-mail. If the physician is on vacation, he or she will apply an auto reply response to his or her e-mail address.

When the physician is away, personal mail is placed on his or her desk and left for the physician to handle. Mail that pertains to patient care issues should be opened and handled appropriately. Ask your supervisor if you are unsure which pieces of mail you should open.

If the mail requires an urgent response, the covering physician should be contacted unless otherwise directed. Mail should never be allowed to accumulate in outside mailboxes because patient information is confidential.

 CHECKPOINT QUESTION

7. What mail must be opened first?

Annotation

Some physicians request that letters be annotated. **Annotation** involves reading a document and highlighting the key points. If the letter is very detailed, a summary of the key points should be written in the margins. The summary should be factual and not editorialized.

SPANISH TERMINOLOGY

¿Donde está la oficina de correos?
Where is the post office?

Tengo que enviar esta carta.
I need to mail this letter.

¿Cuanto cuesta el franqueo?
How much does the postage cost?

MEDIA MENU

- **Student CD**
  - **Case Studies**
    Administrative Interactive Case Study 1: Maintaining Medical Records and HIPAA
    Administrative Interactive Case Study 2: Managing a Medical Office Emergency
    Clinical Interactive Case Study 1: Triage in an Emergency Situation, Communication and Documentation
    Clinical Interactive Case Study 3: Dealing with a Sick Patient, Infection Control, and Medication Administration
  - **CMA/RMA Certification Exam Review**
- **Premium Online Course**
  http://thePoint.lww.com/Kronenberger3e
- **Internet Resources**
  LiveAdvise Online Tutoring & Competency Training
  http://thePoint.lww.com/LiveAdvise
  Airborne Express
  www.airborne.com
  Federal Express
  www.fedex.com/us/
  Medical dictionary
  www.medical-dictionary.com
  Merriam-Webster's Dictionary
  www.m-w.com
  United Parcel Service
  www.ups.com
  United States Postal Service
  www.usps.com

PROCEDURE 7-1: Composing a Business Letter

Purpose: To construct a clear and concise letter using proper grammar and punctuation
Equipment: Computer with word processing software, 8 ½ × 11 white paper, #10 sized envelope
Scenario: Type a letter from Dr. Tom Chandler (1200 West Main Street, Suite 103, Danberry, VA 24451) to patient James Heffernan (1010 Chestnut Street, Danberry, VA 24451). The letter is in reference to the denial of his insurance claim by Unique Comprehensive Medical Benefits. The denial letter, dated May 28 of the current year, states that the procedure planned by Dr. Chandler has been deemed as medically unnecessary. The letter should inform Mr. Heffernan of his insurance company's decision. Dr. Chandler instructs you to advise the patient that he has every intention of writing a letter to appeal this decision.

Steps	Reasons
1. Move cursor down two lines below the letterhead and enter today's date, flush right.	Use the date that the letter was dictated or constructed by the sender, not the date it was typed.

(continued)

PROCEDURE 7-1:   Composing a Business Letter *(continued)*

Steps	Reasons
2. Flush left, move cursor down two lines and enter the inside address using the name and address of the person to whom you are writing.	Check the incoming correspondence or directory for the exact spelling of the name of the recipient.
3. Double space and type the salutation followed by a colon.	Using a proper salutation and colon denotes professionalism.
4. Enter a reference line.	At a glance, the reader will know what or who the letter is about. Those filing the letter have a quick reference, as well.
5. Double space between paragraphs.	This is block letter style.
6. Double space and flush right, enter the complimentary close.	The close should be professional in a business letter. "Later," would not be an appropriate closing.
7. Move cursor down four spaces and enter the sender's name.	This leaves space for the sender's signature.
8. Double space and enter initials of the sender in all caps.	Reference initials let the sender and recipient know who composed and dictated the letter.
9. Enter a slash and your initials in lowercase letters.	Lowercase initials indicate the person who typed the letter. If necessary, that person can be identified in case of error, omission of enclosures, etc.
10. Enter c: and the names of those who get copies of the letter.	In the days of carbon paper and typewriters, cc: meant carbon copy. Using a single c: is now acceptable to indicate that a copy of this letter was also sent to the person listed.
11. Enter Enc: and the number and description of each enclosed sheet.	If there are enclosures, the reader can see what the sender intended to be included in the envelope with the letter. These enclosures may or may not be mentioned in the body of the letter.
12. Print on letterhead.	Letterhead gives the correspondence a professional look. If no letterhead is available, you may construct it using the name, address, and phone number of the sender.
13. Proofread the letter.	This is the most important step in this procedure. No matter how well written a letter is, errors indicate a lack of professionalism.
14. Attach the letter to the patient's chart.	When the sender of the letter receives the letter for signature, he or she may need to refer back to the information used to compose the letter.
15. Submit to the sender of the letter for review and signature.	The sender should review the letter carefully. It is the sender who is ultimately responsible for the content and condition of the correspondence.
16. Make a copy of the letter for the patient's chart.	Medical documentation guidelines require you to keep copies of every transaction and communication with or on behalf of a patient.
17. Address envelopes using all caps and no punctuation.	In order for the USPS' optical character recognition (OCR) equipment to read an envelope, it should be typed in all capital letters or written in block with no punctuation.

PROCEDURE 7-2:   Opening and Sorting Incoming Mail

Purpose: To efficiently and accurately open and sort mail to be distributed to the appropriate persons in the office

Equipment: Letter opener, paper clips, directional tabs, date stamp

Steps	Reasons
1. Gather the necessary equipment.	An efficient medical assistant has her tools at her fingertips.
2. Open all letters and check for enclosures.	If the letter states that enclosures were sent but they are not in the envelope, contact the sender and request them. Indicate on the letter that the enclosures were missing and the name of the person you contacted.
3. Paper clip enclosures to the letter.	Paper clipping enclosures to a letter reduces the chance of misplacing.
4. Date-stamp each item.	Stamping each piece of correspondence with the date it was opened gives more authenticity to a letter. It also lets the reader know when action should be taken.
5. Sort the mail into categories and deal with it appropriately. Generally, you should handle the following types of mail as noted: *Correspondence regarding a patient:* a. Use a paper clip to attach letters, test results, etc. to the patient's chart. b. Place the chart in a pile for the physician to review. *Payments and other checks:* a. Record promptly all insurance payments and checks and deposit them according to office policy. b. Account for all drug samples and appropriately log them into the sample book.	Using these guidelines helps ensure the proper handling of all incoming mail.
6. Dispose of miscellaneous advertisements unless otherwise directed.	Dispose of items only when instructed to do so by the recipient of the mail. Your idea of junk mail and the recipient's may be different.
7. Distribute the mail to the appropriate staff members. For example, mail might be for the physician, nurse manager, office manager, billing clerk, or other personnel.	Take care that the appropriate person gets each piece of mail. Many times, a letter has the name of someone who is not really the person in the office who should get this type of information. Determine the right person to receive the correspondence.

- As a medical assistant, you need excellent written communication skills.
- Careful attention to detail is essential.
- Medical information is crucial to patient care and must be prepared with proper grammar, punctuation, and spelling.
- You will write letters, memorandums, and other correspondence with patients, physicians, and businesses.

- After preparing your document, you must be able to select the appropriate service for mailing your letters.
- Medical information is confidential and must be handled according to HIPAA guidelines
- Your primary goal with all written communication is to get your message across in a clear, concise, and accurate manner.

Warm Ups for Critical Thinking

1. Create a business letter. Include all the components and use the full block format. Print your unedited copy and, using proofreaders marks, indicate your corrections. Make the corrections and reprint a final copy. Ask your instructor to review both copies.

2. Write 10 sentences using terms from Box 7-3. Use some terms correctly and others incorrectly. Exchange your sentences with another student. Correct your peer's sentences.

3. Collect five pieces of mail that you have received at home. What method of affixing postage did they use? Go to your local USPS office. Obtain either a priority mail or express mail envelope. Correctly address the envelope.

4. Suppose the physician told you to read his e-mails while he was on vacation. In doing so, you come across a personal piece of information that you know he would not want you to see. How would you handle it? Would you tell anyone that you saw it? Would you question the physician about it?

Answers to Checkpoint Questions

1. Inaccurate information in a business letter can lead to injuries to the patient and lawsuits and can harm the physician's practice.

2. This practice ensures consistency, a mark of professional writing.

3. The inside address is the address of the person to whom the letter is going. The salutation is the greeting. The identification line shows the initials of the person who dictated the letters and the initials of the person who typed the letter.

4. Proofreading allows you to check the accuracy and content of the letter.

5. Memorandums are used for communication within the office and with other departments.

6. The USPS uses optical character readers to quickly and efficiently sort the mail electronically.

7. Any mail marked urgent must be opened first.

Outline

**The Health Insurance
    Portability and
    Accountability Act of 1996**
Covered Entities
Administrative Simplification
The HIPAA Officer
**Releasing Medical
    Information**
HIPAA's Privacy Rule
Releasing Records to Patients
Legally Required Disclosures
Standard Medical Records
Contents of the Medical
    Record
Electronic Health Records
Adopting Electronic Health
    Records Technology

Features and Capabilities of
    Electronic Health Records
Billing and Coding Using
    Electronic Health Records
The Medical Assistant's Role
Electronic Health Record Security
Medical Record Organization
Provider Encounters
Documentation Forms
Medical History Forms
Flow Sheets
Progress Notes
Medical Record Entries
Charting Communications With
    Patients
Additions to Medical
    Records

**Workers' Compensation
    Records**
Storing Medical Records
Medical Record Preparation
Filing Procedures
Filing Systems
Alphabetic Filing
Numeric Filing
Other Filing Systems
Storing Health Information
Electronic Data Storage
**Storage of Standard Medical
    Records**
**Classification of Medical
    Records**
Medical Record Retention

Learning Objectives

*Upon successfully completing this chapter, you
will be able to:*

1. Spell and define the key terms

2. Explain the requirements of the Health
   Insurance Portability and Accountability
   Act relating to the sharing and saving of
   personal and protected health information.

3. Describe standard and electronic health
   record systems

4. Explain the process for releasing medical
   records to third-party payers and individual patients

5. List and explain the EHR guidelines established to protect computerized records

6. List the standard information included in
   medical records

7. Identify and describe the types of formats
   used for documenting patient information
   in outpatient settings

8. Explain how to make an entry in a patient's
   medical record, using abbreviations when
   appropriate

9. Explain how to make a correction in a
   standard and electronic health record

10. Compare and contrast the differences be-
    tween alphabetic and numeric filing sys-
    tems and give an example of each

11. Identify the various ways medical records
    can be classified for storage

12. Explain the guidelines of sound policies for
    record retention

Upon successfully completing this chapter, you will be able to:

1. Establish, organize, and maintain a patient's medical record (Procedure 8-1)
2. File a medical record (Procedure 8-2)

Competencies

CAAHEP

- Establish and maintain the medical record
- Organize a patient's medical record
- File medical records
- Identify and respond to issues of confidentiality
- Perform within legal and ethical boundaries

ABHES

- File medical records
- Use appropriate guidelines when releasing records or information

Key Terms

alphabetic filing	electronic health records (EHR)	numeric filing	reverse chronological order
chief complaint	flow sheet	present illness	SOAP
chronological order	medical history forms	problem-oriented medical record (POMR)	subject filing
clearinghouse	microfiche		workers' compensation
covered entity	microfilm	protected health information (PHI)	
cross-reference	narrative		
demographic data			

Medical records have a vital role in ensuring quality patient care. The health care industry is moving slowly but surely toward the electronic management of patient information. Some studies show that physicians are not making the change to electronic health records as readily as they could. The number of physician practices going paperless is expected to grow, however, as the new technology-savvy generation of physicians emerges. Chances are good that, at some point in your career, you will work with a completely computerized and paperless record system. The outpatient medical facility in today's world may be in any phase of computerization depending on geographic location, availability of funds, and personal preferences of the physicians and owners. Whether information is maintained on paper or in electronic form, proper management of the information requires adherence to certain legal, moral, and ethical standards. If these standards are disregarded, a breach of contract between patient and physician may occur, exposing the patient to potential embarrassment or harm and making the physician vulnerable to fines and/or lawsuits (see Chapter 2).

A thorough and accurate medical record furnishes documented evidence of the patient's evaluation, treatment, change in condition, and communication with the physician and staff. Medical records have many other uses as well, including research, quality assurance, and patient education. Information gathered from medical records aids the government in planning for future health care needs and protecting the health of the public. In 1996, HIPAA was enacted to provide consumers with greater access to health care insurance, to protect the privacy of health care data, and to promote more standardization and efficiency in the health care industry.

The Health Insurance Portability and Accountability Act of 1996

Congress addressed the need for reform in the health care industry by passing the Health Insurance Portability and Accountability Act of 1996 (HIPAA). The act includes five "titles." The titles of HIPAA and their subject matter are outlined in Table 8-1.

HIPAA's goals include:

- Simplifying the health insurance claims process and speeding up the process of reimbursement
- Providing greater access to health care insurance when individuals change employers
- Addressing issues dealing with funds set up by employers to pay for health care costs

- Requiring ease of electronic transmissions by establishing a Standard Unique Employer Identifier, which provides complete but coded information about the holder of the code.
- Protection of communication of health information between physicians and insurance companies

In addition to these issues addressed by HIPAA, the rapid advancement of technology in medical information maintenance caused the need for strict regulations to keep electronically transmitted and stored **protected health information (PHI)** safe from unauthorized releases. Confidentiality has always been required in the medical world, but each state had its own laws regarding the exchange of medical information. HIPAA also addresses important new issues that arose after medical facilities became computerized. The use of the internet brought concerns about hackers obtaining personal health information.

Physician offices must also take appropriate steps to ensure that any company they are associated with also follows HIPAA regulations. Physician offices often have

TABLE 8-1	Titles of HIPAA
Title	**Action**
Title I, Health Insurance Access, Portability, and Renewal	Amended the Employee Retirement Income Security Act of 1974 (ERISA) and the Public Health Act. Changed the rules about pre-existing condition exclusions by insurance companies. Prohibited discrimination based on health status by insurance companies.
Title II, Preventing Health Care Fraud and Abuse	Is concerned with how health care providers interact with the insurance network. Includes the Privacy Rule. Prevents fraud and abuse in the delivery of and payment for health care. Improves the Medicare program and others. Establishes standards and requirements for all electronic transmission of certain health information.
Title III, Tax-Related Provisions	Deals with MSAs (Medical Savings Accounts). Consumers deposit money into the account and withdraw it as needed for medical bills only. The money deposited is tax free. Concerned with how employers handle these funds.
Title IV, Group Health Plan Requirements	Amends earlier legislation regarding group insurance. Allows people to carry the same health insurance coverage to a new job. Avoids starting over again with waiting periods for pre-existing conditions. Costs are high without employer's contribution.
Title V, Revenue Offsets	Changes to the Internal Revenue Code of 1986 to generate more revenue to offset the HIPAA-required costs.

a variety of business partnerships that help keep the office flowing professionally and effectively. Some examples of business partnerships are cleaning services, document-shredding companies, laboratory and specimen transport personnel, temporary staffing agencies, and educational facilities. Contracts among physicians and their business partners should reflect that the business adheres to HIPAA regulations. For example, for The Joint Commission to meet HIPAA regulations and ensure security and privacy of patient information during the site visit, health care settings being surveyed must sign a business associate agreement prior to inspection. Students completing externships are also required to sign confidentiality agreements.

Covered Entities

HIPAA uses the language "**covered entity**" to describe those who must adhere to these regulations. A covered entity is defined as health insurance plans, health care **clearinghouses** (entities that receive, review, send, and manage insurance claims for physicians), and health care providers who use electronic billing, funds transfers, and **electronic health records (EHR)**. In some instances, HIPAA identifies covered entities as those meeting the criteria above with more than 25 employees. Civil and criminal penalties are set by the federal act, but each state has enacted regulations governing insurance companies. Covered entities are subject to individual state laws, but if state and federal laws are different, you must follow the strictest laws. In the medical office, you will be concerned with the administrative simplification and privacy rules.

Administrative Simplification

There are four parts to HIPAA's Administrative Simplification section. They include electronic transactions, privacy requirements, security requirements, and national identifier requirements.

The HIPAA Officer

Each health care provider must have certain policies in place to comply with the rulings. In most cases, as long as reasonable care is taken to comply with the intent of the ruling and that effort is documented, providers are considered compliant with HIPAA. HIPAA requires that at least one employee be designated as the HIPAA Officer and one as a Privacy Officer. This requirement varies with the size of the practice or business. The HIPAA Officer coordinates and oversees the various aspects of compliance. Covered entities are subject to inspections by representatives of the Centers for Medicaid and Medicare Services (CMS). Any audits would be coordinated through the HIPAA officer. The Privacy

---

BOX 8-1

RESPONSIBILITIES OF A HIPAA OFFICER

1. Assess, establish, and review policies and procedures to ensure continuous HIPAA compliance.
2. Coordinate mandatory training of employees including specific rules and regulations, reporting any event that might compromise the protection of information, explanation of privacy issues, etc. For example, proper log in and log off procedures.
3. Monitor the access to health information by periodically checking for security threats or gaps when changes occur in equipment or software.
4. Ensure sound practices by the human resources department as employees leave the workforce or move from one department to another. Passwords and access to certain information should be adjusted as employees change responsibilities according to the minimum necessary information needed as stated in the privacy rule. For example, does the appointment secretary need access to the entire chart in order to schedule an appointment?
5. Maintain the integrity of the system by ensuring data and information have not been altered or destroyed in an unauthorized manner by designing and monitoring tracking reports.

Officer keeps track of who has access to protected health information. The responsibilities of these employees are listed in Box 8-1. These duties should be listed on the job descriptions of these appointed employees.

Releasing Medical Records

The protection of personal information is crucial to the privacy of patients. Although the physical medical record legally belongs to the physician, the information belongs to the patient. Any release of records must first be authorized by the patient or the patient's legal guardian. When releasing a medical record, provide a copy only. *Never* release the original medical record except in limited circumstances.

Insurance companies, lawyers, other health care practitioners, and patients themselves may request copies of medical records. All requests should be made in writing, stating the patient's name, address, and social security number, and must contain the patient's *original* signature authorizing the release of records. Never release information over the telephone. You will have no way of verifying that the person with whom you are speaking is actually the person who has authorization.

State laws allow facilities to charge a fee for copying the medical record. The AMA published guidelines for physicians to ensure ethical business practices. They recommend a reasonable fee for reproduction of records to be no more than $1 per page or $100 for the entire record, whichever is less. If the record is less than 10 pages, the office may charge up to $10 to cover postage and miscellaneous costs associated with the retrieval process. Laws may vary from state to state.

WHAT IF?

You work in a family practice office where your physician treats many children. How long should you keep the children's records? The statute of limitations in your state is 3 years from the date of the last treatment.

By law, when a physician treats an adult, the record should be kept until the statute of limitations expires. A minor has the right to bring suit against a health care provider when he becomes of legal age. Therefore, the minor's records should be kept at least 3 years past the 18th birthday.

HIPAA's Privacy Rule

HIPAA provides protection of the sharing of what is referred to as protected health information (PHI). PHI is any information that can be linked to a specific person. A diagnosis alone without a full name is not identifiable, but a first and last name associated with a diagnosis is identifiable; therefore, it is protected health information. For example, the Centers for Disease Control and Prevention (CDC) publishes information to cite statistics about communicable diseases. Since the names of the people who have been diagnosed with the diseases are not published, this information is not protected.

The privacy rule establishes safeguards to protect the confidentiality of medical information. Covered entities must:

- Share health information for health purposes only
- Provide the minimum amount of information necessary
- Adopt written privacy procedures
- Designate a Privacy Officer
- Train employees

ETHICAL TIP

HIPAA Says Patients Have Rights

Through HIPPA, the federal government recognizes that it is ethical to give patients certain rights. HIPAA protects the rights of patients by allowing them to:

- Ask to see and get a copy of their health records
- Have corrections added to their health information
- Receive a notice that tells them how their health information may be used and shared
- Decide if they want to give permission before their health information can be used or shared for certain purposes, such as for marketing
- Get a report on when and why their health information was shared for certain purposes
- If patients believe their rights have been denied or their health information is not being protected, they can file a complaint with the provider or health insurer.
- File a complaint with the U.S. Government

Patients can learn about their rights, including how to file a complaint, from the website at www.hhs.gov/ocr/hipaa/ or by calling 1-866-627-7748.

 CHECKPOINT QUESTION

1. What is the purpose of HIPAA?

Releasing Records to Patients

As discussed previously, releasing medical records is an important part of any medical facility. When patients request copies of their own records, the doctor makes the decision about what to copy. Patients aged 17 years and under cannot get copies of their own medical records without a signed consent from a parent or legal guardian, except for emancipated minors. However, they may obtain certain services independently (check your state's law regarding treatment of minors); in such cases, under the law, you are not permitted to contact the parent or guardian. Some states allow minors to seek treatment for sexually transmitted diseases and birth control without parental knowledge or consent. Sometimes, the parent or guardian may still be billed for these services without the bill being itemized. The billing statement should include only the treatment dates and amount due.

LEGAL TIP

SUBPOENA DUCES TECUM

An original record may be released when it is subpoenaed by a court of law. In such situations, the physician may wish to have the judge sign a document stating that he or she will temporarily take charge of the medical record. This signed document should be filed in the medical office until the record is returned. To further ensure the record's safety, a staff member can transport the original record to court on the day it is requested and then return the record at the end of the court session that day. As soon as it is known that a record will be part of a court case, the record should be kept in a locked cabinet. When the court orders that a record be submitted to the court at a given date and time, the legal order is termed *subpoena duces tecum*.

Proper Authorization

You must follow certain guidelines even with a signed release form (Fig. 8-1). The authorization form must give the patient the opportunity to limit the information to be released. Patients may release only information relating to a specific disorder, or they may specify a time limit. They may not, however, ask that the physician leave out information pertinent to the situation.

References to mental health diagnoses or treatments, drug or alcohol abuse, HIV, AIDS, or any other sexually transmitted disease may not be released without specific mention on the signed authorization form. If it is not specifically requested by the patient, when you are copying the record, place a piece of blank white paper over any such areas of information. Never white-out these areas on the original document or mention what these blank areas included.

Protected health information can be shared with proper authorization by the patient. By signing an appropriate authorization, the patient gives permission for the health care provider to share their personal health information with anyone they designate. The form must include the name of the person to receive the information, the name of the provider releasing the information, and the dates of service and/or certain conditions covered by the authorization. It is recommended that there also be a witness signature. Figure 8-1 is a sample of a proper authorization form.

CHECKPOINT QUESTION

2. What is required for a legal disclosure of a patient's HIV status?

I, _____, give my permission for _____ to release information generated in my medical record between the dates of _____ and _____ to _____ .

Signature _____ Date _____

Witness_____ Date _____

Or

I, _____, give my permission for _____ to release information in my medical record regarding the care and treatment of _____ to _____ .

Signature _____ Date _____

Figure 8-1 A proper authorization for release of information.

Legally Required Disclosures

As previously discussed in Chapter 2, in certain situations, the law requires reporting information to particular authorities. Requirements for reporting vary among states.

As with most laws, there are exceptions to the privacy rule. Certain information is crucial to the patient, needed for the protection of the public, or involves criminal activity and is released without the patient's permission. Such disclosures include:

- Vital statistics
- Child and elder abuse or maltreatment
- Emergency circumstances
- ID of body of deceased person
- Cause of death
- Public health needs, such as communicable diseases
- Research
- Judicial and administrative proceedings
- Law enforcement concerns such as violent criminal activities
- Activities related to national defense and security

PATIENT EDUCATION

PROTECT YOUR PATIENTS BY TEACHING THEM TO READ WHAT THEY ARE SIGNING

Many patients feel inadequate when it comes to understanding the intricacies of the laws that are designed to protect them. Patients are often ready to sign a form handed to them without even reading it. Patients trust and depend on their health care provider to protect their rights to privacy. Whatever form, authorization, or consent the patient is handed should be accompanied by a verbal explanation of what they are signing.

For example, legal experts advise that some forms designed for patients to give their authorization to release their personal information are too general and are not even considered legally binding. Proper authorization should include the elements in Figure 8-1. Patients should understand that it would be improper to sign a form like this:

I, _____, give my permission for the release of my medical records.

Signature: _____

This blanket permission opens the patient up to the possibility of any and all of their information being shared with anyone at anytime. Each time patients need or want their information to be released, they must sign a new authorization outlining the specific information to be released by whom and to whom. Help them understand the importance of knowing what they are signing, and tell them to ask questions if they need any clarification.

 CHECKPOINT QUESTION

3. Why is some information released without a patient's permission?

Standard Medical Records

Even though our expanding technology gives today's medical office the ability to store health information in electronic form, the migration to a paperless environment has been slow. Outpatient medical offices that are not electronic accumulate mounds of paper every day. A medical facility has a variety of options for standard or manual record keeping. The best systems are those that have been tried, revised, and revised again. No matter

how the records are stored, make sure that the information is:

- Easily retrievable
- Kept in an orderly manner
- Complete
- Legible
- Accurate
- Brief

Whether a record is on paper or a computer disk, all medical records have the same contents.

Contents of the Medical Record

A paper medical record in an outpatient facility, often called a chart or a file, contains confidential clinical information about the patient's health and treatment in addition to the billing and insurance information discussed in Chapter 11.

General information, such as name, address, telephone number, date of birth, social security number, credit history, and next of kin, is vital to a complete chart but should never be intermingled with the clinical information. Metal fasteners can be used to keep certain pages on one side of the chart.

The following information is typically found in the clinical section of the medical chart:

- *Chief complaint*—A description of the symptoms that led the patient to seek the physician's care. This information is supplied by the patient during the interview at the beginning of the visit. It is usually stated in the patient's own words in quotation marks. For example, the patient complains of "something stuck in my throat."
- *Present illness*—A more specific account of the chief complaint, including time frames and characteristics. For example: "The patient says it started 2 days ago. She describes the pain as severe and stabbing and reports taking Tylenol with no relief."
- *Family and personal history*—A review of any major illnesses of family members, including grandparents, parents, siblings, aunts, and uncles. Any previous major illnesses and surgeries of the patient are listed under personal history.
- *Review of systems*—A systematic review of the body's 10 systems to detect problems not yet identified. For example, problems with the integumentary system (skin) may be identified if the patient reports a rash, areas of discoloration, or change in a mole.
- *Progress notes*—Documentation of each patient encounter, including information obtained in phone calls and refills of prescriptions.
- *Radiographic reports*—Reports of any x-ray studies performed in the office. If patients are sent to other

facilities for radiographs, a report of that study is placed in the chart.

- *Laboratory results*—A copy of the results of any laboratory work done in the office or a report from an outside facility.
- *Consultation reports*—Any reports from other physicians regarding consultations with the patient.
- *Medication administration*—Some facilities use a separate sheet to log medications given in the office. If an opioid is given, still another form is completed, as discussed in Chapter 2.
- *Diagnosis or medical impression*—The most recent entry on the progress note will contain the provider's opinion of the patient's problems.
- *Physician's and/or medical assistant's identification and signature*—Experts have suggested that you sign your entire name instead of initials, with your credentials written after the name, e.g., Susan Jones, CMA.
- *Documented advance directives, such as living will and power of attorney for medical care*—A copy of any instructions from the patient regarding end-of-life decisions or the appointment of another person who can give consent for treatment for the patient.
- *All correspondence pertaining to the patient*—Any letters or memos generated in the facility and sent out are copied and placed in the chart. Correspondence from other physicians is also included in the chart.

 CHECKPOINT QUESTION

4. What is meant by the heading *chief complaint*?

Electronic Health Records

As the health care community shifts toward greater use of information technology (IT), a primary concern is creating standards for exchanging, integrating, sharing, and retrieving electronic health information. Health Level Seven (HL7) is a not-for-profit organization that was founded to develop such standards. Its website describes HL7 as "an international community of healthcare subject matter experts and information scientists" working to develop health care IT standards that promote high-quality, safe, and economical patient care (www.hl7.org). Many issues addressed by HL7 involve the management and exchange of electronic health information in a hospital setting. However, eventually most physician practices will communicate with other health care facilities, including hospitals, electronically and with ease.

Recent trends show that more physicians are starting to incorporate EHR into their practices. According to the latest data from the CDC's National Center for Health Statistics (www.cdc.gov/nchs), the number of physicians using partial (part paper, part electronic) or full EHR increased from 18.2% in 2001 to 23.9% in 2005—a 31% increase. Full EHR included four basic features: (1) computerized orders for prescriptions; (2) computerized orders for tests; (3) test results; and (4) physician notes. Practices with two or more physicians were more likely to use some form of EHR than solo practitioners, but only one in 10 physicians uses full EHR.

Adopting Electronic Health Records Technology

Changing from a paper-based office environment to one using advanced technology takes time, money, careful decision making, and staff education, among other factors. One of the first steps in the process involves choosing a vendor. Below are some examples of criteria to consider when purchasing electronic health record products:

- The vendor's reputation and history (check references or speak with current customers)
- The vendor's understanding of how your medical office plans to use electronic health records
- The product's use of customizable technology
- Easy access to product support
- Regular product maintenance and updates
- Ability to automate office workflow
- Ease of training and implementation
- Ability to send and receive electronic data to and from other health care entities, such as laboratories or hospitals
- Security of patient information (discussed in greater detail below)

Another factor to assess is whether the product has met the standards established by the Certification Commission for Healthcare Information Technology (CCHIT). CCHIT is an independent, nonprofit organization that certifies ambulatory EHR products, as well as other health care IT products. In developing its product certification criteria, CCHIT took into account HL7's standards for EHR systems. In 2006, CCHIT was named a "Recognized Certification Body" by the US Department of Health and Human Services. Although certification is voluntary, achieving this designation affirms the credibility of the EHR product. (For more information and a list of certified products, visit www.cchit.org.)

Making the Transition

Besides computer workstations, printers, and Internet access, the amount and kind of equipment required for electronic health records depends on the medical office's needs and budget. Other commonly used devices may include laptops, tablet PCs, or hand-held PDAs, which allow greater physician mobility and require less space in exam rooms than desktop PCs. Whatever equipment set up is ultimately chosen, it should not physically impede the physician–patient relationship. For example, avoid set ups where the physician must turn his or her back to patients when inputting information, which might make the physician appear detached or uninterested.

Changeover to electronic health records usually occurs in stages. To avoid problems, the medical office should not eliminate paper charts until the EHR system is consistently working as intended. Integration of paper charts and other records can be accomplished in various ways, depending on office goals and the amount of data to be input. Some facilities keep hybrid records; personnel scan and index medical records into the system and then store paper copies in the office for a few months before destroying them. Other facilities transfer old paper records to microfiche or CD-ROM for storage and then destroy the paper sources. Off-site medical record storage facilities can house the records until time of disposal or indefinitely, whatever the physician wants. Keep in mind that implementing EHR will not eliminate the need to maintain paper documents right away. It can take months or years to fully complete the transition.

To work productively with EHR, medical assistants need training and practice. Graduating from an accredited medical assisting program, which includes training in coding, billing, and computer skills, ensures baseline preparation. Adequate education about the specific EHR system used by the medical office is also required. Medical assistants and other office staff usually undergo 1 to 2 days of initial training; after that, daily practice with EHR in the medical office allows users to get comfortable with the system. Workflow will be set by the facility according to their policies and procedures for EHR. One key point to remember is that, when implementing new technology, everyone must be willing to change. Staff may need to adjust some processes so that EHR can work effectively for the office.

Features and Capabilities of Electronic Health Records

The goal of EHR is to improve patient care while boosting efficiency in the medical office. Some of the key features of electronic health records are discussed in the following list:

- Point-of-care charting—Touch screens make inputting easy, and drop-down menus takes less time than handwriting notes, improving quality and productivity in charting.
- Improved documentation—Problems with illegibility are eliminated, decreasing errors. Physicians can also include drawings to support documentation and use graphing features to transfer numeric data (height, weight, vital signs, etc.) into chart form.

- Data collection from multiple sources—Data from the hospital, pharmacy, laboratory, radiology, and other departments are stored in EHR for quick retrieval.
- Medication management—Computerized prescription order entry helps prevent medication errors by providing warnings about patient allergies, contraindications, or possible interactions. It also avoids problems at the pharmacy due to poor handwriting by the prescriber.
- Assistance with clinical decision making—Alerts, reminders, and patient care recommendations give providers valuable information at their fingertips.
- Improved communication—Easy access to information enhances communication among medical office staff, as well as with patients and other health care entities.
- Support for administrative, financial, and operational functions—Electronic health records assist with storage of patient **demographic data**, appointment scheduling, insurance billing and coding (see next section), accounting procedures, and inventory and supply tracking, among other tasks. EHR may even help increase revenue by (eventually) allowing the practice to eliminate the file room and turn the extra space into exam rooms or office space. EHR also reduces medical transcription costs.

Electronic health records do have some disadvantages, however, including cost, potential software or hardware damage or failure, and the need for in-depth staff training. The task of inputting data from hundreds or thousands of charts into the computer is time consuming but must be done before the system is used. Sometimes, in the beginning stages, implementing EHR can actually reduce physician and staff productivity instead of increasing it. But over time, the benefits should outweigh the drawbacks.

Billing and Coding Using Electronic Health Records

In later chapters, you will learn the world of coding. Selecting the various levels of patient visits to the office is based on many factors. Physicians must choose the level based on the amount of information gathered, the extent of the physical examination performed, and the level of decision making the patient's care required. Many EHR software companies include drop-down lists and preset menus to help providers select the appropriate code based on the information entered for that visit. This is an important feature because every office that accepts Medicare and/or Medicaid is subject to government audits. These audits are designed to verify that the level of office visit charged to the patient is consistent with the criteria outlined by the Centers for

Medicare and Medicaid Services (CMS). If discrepancies are found, the office may be fined. Software that assists with these coding issues can have many benefits, such as avoiding returned claims, preventing insurance fraud, decreasing staff data entry errors, reducing the possibility of an audit, and increasing revenue through streamlined and timely billing processes.

The Medical Assistant's Role

As a medical assistant, you have the same roles and responsibilities related to EHR as with paper records. The difference is that you will perform more of your regular tasks using the computer. Two of your main responsibilities are data collection and patient care. Electronic health records allow you to quickly and accurately record chart notes, look up test results, call in medication orders, and so on. With computers in exam rooms, no time is wasted looking for missing patient data; records are easily stored and retrieved. EHR may also help you gather more complete patient information by prompting you to ask questions that might otherwise be missed before allowing you to move on to the next screen. Tools such as tickler messages can also remind you to provide patient teaching on topics such as vaccines, yearly checkups, BP checks, mammograms, and so on.

Medical assistants can also provide assurance to patients about the safety and security of their health information. In order to comply with HIPAA, electronic health record systems have built-in features to decrease the risk of stolen or misused data. These safeguards include password protections, electronic firewalls that block access by unauthorized users, audit trails that can track who accessed a record and when, data encryption, and more. By explaining the privacy safeguards integrated into EHR, you promote patient confidence in the medical practice. (See Electronic Health Record Security section for more details about EHR security.)

 WHAT IF?

What if the EHR system goes down due to a power outage?

If the lights go out, return to the old paper system, and then input the data when the electricity comes back on again. Use backup reports and schedules that were printed ahead of time. Backup tapes should be done at the end of every workday to save information in case a problem occurs. Always have contingency plans for data backup, disaster recovery, or other emergencies ready to be implemented if needed.

Electronic Health Record Security

The American Medical Association (AMA) and many risk management companies have published guidelines for the EHR. Following are suggestions and guidelines based on HIPAA's requirements for practices using computers to transfer or store patient information. Experts advise physicians and office managers considering software programs to look for the following capabilities:

- User-friendly commands that allow users to move easily within the system.
- Spell check and free text fields for inserting corrections and late entries. The electronic record is corrected by using the same rules as in the standard record. Entries are not deleted but corrected, with an explanation to avoid the appearance of hiding information.
- Security levels to limit entry to all functions. For example, a receptionist does not need access to the physician's personal taxes.
- A system, including encryption, to repel hackers. Evidence shows that persons with access to technology can invade patients' records stored on computer databases. This is a breach of confidentiality and is illegal.

To maintain security, facilities are urged to do the following:

- Keep all computer backup disks in a safe place away from the practice.
- Store disks in a bank safe-deposit box.
- Use passwords with characters other than letters and encrypt the passwords.
- Change log-in codes and passwords every 30 days.
- Prepare a backup plan for use when the computer system is down.
- Turn terminals away from areas where information may be seen by patients.
- Keep the fax machines and printers that receive personal medical information in a private place.
- Ensure that each user is restricted to the information needed to do his or her job.
- Train employees on confidentiality and each person's responsibility to adhere to HIPAA's Privacy Rule.
- Design a written confidentiality policy that employees sign.
- Conduct routine audits that produce a trail of each employee's movement through the EHR system.
- Include disciplinary measures for breaches of confidentiality.

Providers may use a handheld personal data device (PDA), laptop, or personal computer (PC) in central areas or examination rooms. The same security measures apply to these items. Patients should not have access to computer screens in the examination room. The physician should take care in keeping a personal data system, just as he or she protects the prescription pad. The personal data device may contain the entire *Physicians' Desk Reference*, giving the provider information needed for prescribing drugs at the fingertips. Other applications of the PDA include downloading patient education materials and documenting and transferring information about patient encounters when the office is closed. In this era of paperless medical offices, care must be taken to protect the privacy of the patient as carefully as in the world of paper.

Medical Record Organization

Information in the paper medical record is usually organized in a standard chart order and placed in a specially designed folder. The order in which documents are placed in the medical record depends on the physician's preference. As mentioned earlier, the demographic information is kept separate from the clinical information. The clinical portion of the medical record is organized in either a source-oriented or a problem-oriented format. In source-oriented medical records, all similar categories or sources of information are grouped together. The typical groupings:

- Billing and insurance information
- Physician orders
- Progress notes
- Laboratory results
- Radiographic results (magnetic resonance imaging, computed tomography, ultrasound)
- Patient education

All documentation in these categories is placed in **reverse chronological order**; that is, the most recent documents are placed on top of previous sheets.

Provider Encounters

Whether the patient is new or established or seen by a physician assistant, nurse practitioner, or physician, the visit must be documented. It may be handwritten, typed, or entered into a computer, but in any event, it must be recorded. In the paperless office, you will complete the information gathered at the patient's visit by choosing items from a drop-down box that appears when you click on a particular field.

Some offices record new patients' encounters in the history and physical format. Visits of established patients returning for follow-up are documented in a different format. Although some offices use the same format for new and established patients, the most common formats used to document each established patient encounter are narrative, SOAP, and POMR.

Narrative Format

Some providers document visits in the narrative form. **Narrative** is the oldest documentation form and the least structured. It is simply a paragraph indicating the contact with the patient, what was done for the patient, and the outcome of any action. In the sample page shown in Figure 8-2, the chart entries made are in narrative format.

SOAP Format

The **SOAP** (subjective-objective-assessment-plan) format is one of the most common methods for documenting patient visits. The *subjective* component is a statement of what the patient says. Whenever possible, actual quotations by the patient should be used. The *objective* component is what is observed about the patient when the medical assistant begins the assessment and when the provider does the examination. The *assessment* portion is a phrase stating the impression of what is wrong or the patient's diagnosis. If a final diagnosis cannot be made yet, the provider lists possible disorders to be ruled out, called the differential diagnosis. The *plan* is a list of interventions that are to be carried out. In Box 8-2, the second note is written in the SOAP format.

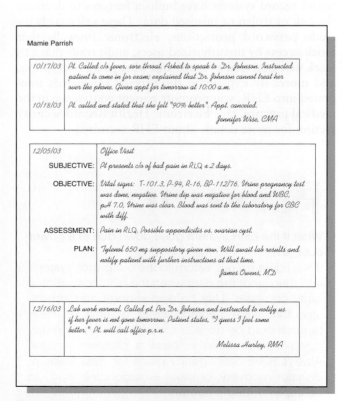

Mamie Parrish

| 10/17/03 | Pt. Called c/o fever, sore throat. Asked to speak to Dr. Johnson. Instructed patient to come in for exam; explained that Dr. Johnson cannot treat her over the phone. Given appt for tomorrow at 10:00 a.m. |
| 10/18/03 | Pt. called and stated that she felt "90% better". Appt. canceled.
Jennifer Wise, CMA |

12/05/03	Office Visit
SUBJECTIVE:	Pt presents c/o of bad pain in RLQ x 2 days.
OBJECTIVE:	Vital signs: T-101.3, P-94, R-16, BP-112/76. Urine pregnancy test was done, negative. Urine dip was negative for blood and WBC, pH 7.0. Urine was clear. Blood was sent to the laboratory for CBC with diff.
ASSESSMENT:	Pain in RLQ. Possible appendicitis vs. ovarian cyst.
PLAN:	Tylenol 650 mg suppository given now. Will await lab results and notify patient with further instructions at that time. James Owens, MD

| 12/16/03 | Lab work normal. Called pt. Per Dr. Johnson and instructed to notify us if her fever is not gone tomorrow. Patient states, "I guess I feel some better." Pt. will call office p.r.n.
Melissa Hurley, RMA |

Figure 8-2 Sample page from patient's chart.

BOX 8-2

SOAP METHOD TO DOCUMENT PATIENT INFORMATION

Jennifer Mosley states that her daughter, Marcia, has been vomiting all night. She also states that Marcia had diarrhea for 2 days before her appointment and has only eaten crackers and bananas since 6:00 PM last night. Dr. Gibson's notes indicate that Marcia has lost 3 pounds since her last visit and that she appears pale, weak, and slightly dehydrated. He suspects a viral infection.

Dr. Gibson ordered a stool culture along with a complete blood count (CBC) with differential. He prescribed the BRAT diet and suggested that Mrs. Mosley give Marcia Imodium A-D for the next 48 hours. He also told Mrs. Mosley to call the office if Marcia's symptoms worsen and to bring her back for a recheck if the symptoms are not cleared up by the end of the week.

S: According to the patient's mother, the patient has been vomiting all night and has had diarrhea for the past 2 days. She has eaten only crackers and bananas since 6:00 PM the night before.

O: Patient appears pale, weak, and slightly dehydrated and has lost 3 pounds since her last visit.

A: Possible viral infection.

P: Stool culture, CBC with differential, BRAT diet, and Imodium for the next 48 hours. Call office if symptoms worsen; return to office if patient not well by the end of the week.

lem develops and is resolved, the problem number will be terminated by a single strikethrough with a date beside it or by adding an X to a heading that indicates resolution of problems. Chronic problems, such as hypertension and hyperglycemia, will be retained by number for as long as the patient remains with the practice. These may be divided by headings of acute and chronic or short-term and long-term for convenience.

POMR documents are divided into four components:

1. *Database.* This contains the following:

   - Chief complaint (Fig. 8-3 shows charting for a chief complaint and history of present illness)
   - Present illness
   - Patient profile
   - Review of systems
   - Physical examination
   - Laboratory reports

2. *Problem list.* This includes every problem the patient has that requires evaluation, including social, demographic, medical, and surgical problems. (Demographic problems relate to statistical characteristics of certain populations.)

3. *Treatment plan.* This includes management, additional workups that may be necessary, and therapy.

4. *Progress notes.* These are structured notes corresponding to each problem.

 CHECKPOINT QUESTION

5. What are three common formats used to document patient–provider encounters?

Documentation Forms

Using printed forms and flow sheets in the medical record saves space and time and allows for easy re-

POMR Format

The **problem-oriented medical record (POMR)** lists each problem of the patient, usually at the beginning of the folder, and references each problem with a number throughout the folder. This method was developed by Dr. Lawrence Weed and is a common method of compiling information because of its logical flow and the ease with which information can be reviewed. In group practices where patients may be seen by more than one physician, the POMR format makes it easier to track the patient's treatment and progress. For instance, if Mr. Jones has hypertension and hyperglycemia, each diagnosis will be assigned a problem number as soon as the diagnosis is made:

2/4/9 #1. Hypertension
2/4/9 #2. Hyperglycemia

At each subsequent visit made by Mr. Jones, these problems will be referenced by these numbers. If a prob-

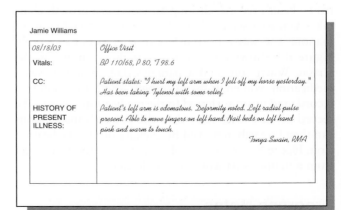

Figure 8-3 Charting a chief complaint and history of present illness.

trieval of information. They are usually customized to meet the needs of the individual practice. Some forms, like vaccination records, are required by federal law. In the paperless office, these forms are completed by the patient and transferred to the patient's electronic record by data entry, and then the completed form is shredded.

Medical History Forms

Medical history forms are commonly used to gather information from the patient before the visit with the physician (see Chapter 18, Fig. 18-1). Some medical offices mail these forms to new patients and have them bring the completed form to their visit. This gives the patient the opportunity to concentrate on the questions, gather information about the family history, and give a more complete history. Whether the patient brings the completed form or fills out the history form in the office, you will review the information with the patient to clarify any questions and add additional information gathered in the interview. Specialty practices use forms designed to gather the type of information they will need to manage the patient's care. For example, an orthopedist's history form might include fields for prior orthopedic injuries, accident information, and physical therapy visits.

Flow Sheets

The **flow sheet** is designed to limit the need for long, handwritten care notes by allowing information to be recorded in either graphic or table form. Generally, flow sheets are designed for a given task. Color-coded sheets for medication administration, vital signs, pediatric growth charts, and so on eliminate the need to read through the pages of a chart to retrieve information. For example, if the physician asks you what the baby weighed 3 months ago, you find the pink growth chart, which saves time and frustration. An advantage of using electronic health records is the capability of converting such information to charts, graphs, and flow sheets. In an electronic health record, clicking an icon for a growth chart takes you to a screen that allows you to enter the information. The software transfers the numbers to a graph. Figure 8-4 shows the growth chart that appears on the screen. When you refill a patient's daily blood pressure medication, you enter the information into the computer record, and it is transferred to the medication record. The record of all entries related to the patient's medications can then be easily retrieved by clicking on the medication icon. Figure 8-5 is an example of a medication flow sheet from a fictitious patient's electronic chart.

Progress Notes

Progress notes are statements about various aspects of patient care. The entries in Figure 8-2 are typical

Figure 8-4 Growth chart from electronic health records.

progress notes. Some facilities use a lined piece of paper with two columns. The left column is used to document the date and time, and the right column is used to write the note. Others use a plain or lined piece of paper without columns. The progress notes will reflect each encounter with the patient chronologically, whether by phone, by e-mail, or in person. In the electronic health record, you will record vital signs, information given by the patient, etc. The results of lab work done in one area of a practice can be entered into the computer. The computer screen in the examination room will then display the results. This immediate availability makes patient care more efficient and convenient for the physician and the patient. No matter what form is used for documenting, you must always include the date, time, your signature, and your credential. The electronic health record has a feature that allows you to assign your signature electronically. A typical user message might say "press enter to sign."

 CHECKPOINT QUESTION

6. List three advantages of using flow sheets in a medical chart.

Medical Record Entries

Proper medical record entries are necessary for efficient communication and for legal considerations. The medical record allows health care practitioners to communicate among themselves and therefore provide the best care possible for the patient. Good communication fosters continuity of patient care.

Ardmore Family Practice, P.A.
2805 Lyndhurst Avenue
Winston-Salem, NC 27103
PHONE: 336-659-0076
FAX: 336-659-0272

Patient: MICHAEL FIELDS   **Date:** 02-12-2003 9:06 AM

MEDICATIONS

Date	Drug Name	Strength/Form	Dispense	Refill	Sig	Last Dose/ Disc Date	Status
1/28/03	SINGULAIR	10 MG TABS	5	0	1 PO BID		NEW
1/28/03	ZITHROMAX	200 MG/5ML SUSR	5	0	1 P.O Q DAY		NEW
1/22/03	ACCUPRIL	10 MG TABS	34	4	1 PO QD	1/28/03	CONTINUE
1/22/03	ADVIL	200 MG TABS	1	1	1/2 Q A.M.	1/25/03	NEW
1/22/03	ALTACE	5 MG CAPS	60	5	ONE TWICE DAILY	1/28/03	CONTINUE
1/22/03	MACROBID	100 MG CAPS	14	0	1 PO BID	1/28/03	CONTINUE
8/26/02	ALTACE	5 MG CAPS	60	5	ONE TWICE DAILY		CONTINUE
8/7/02	PRECOSE	25 MG CAPS	60	0	1/2 B.I.D.	10/5/02	NEW
5/2/01	ACCUPRIL	10 MG TABS	34	4	1 PO QD		NEW
5/2/01	ACCUPRIL	20 MG TABS	30	0	1 PO QD		NEW
5/2/01	ACCUPRIL	40 MG TABS	30	5	1 PO QD		NEW
4/25/01	ACCUPRIL	20 MG TABS	30	0	1 PO QD	4/25/01	NEW
4/25/01	ACCUPRIL	40 MG TABS	30	5	1 PO QD		NEW
4/25/01	MACROBID	100 MG TABS	14	0	1 PO BID	5/1/01	NEW
3/2/01	ACIPHEX 20 MG	TABS	30	6	1 PO QD		NEW
3/2/01	ACTOS 30 MG	TABS	30	2	1 PO QD		NEW
1/23/01	ENTEX PSE	120-600 MG TB12	45	0	1 PO BID		NEW
1/23/01	NASONEX	50 MCG/ACT SUSP	1	3	2 SPRAYS EACH NOSTRIL QD		NEW
8/24/99	ADALAT CC	60 MG TBCR	34	5	1 PO QD	8/24/99	NEW
7/8/99	NITROGLYCERIN	0.4 MG/DOSE AERS	100	1	1 TAB SL Q 5 MIN X 3, IF CHEST PAIN PERS	7/8/99	NEW
6/26/99	CLARITIN	10 MG TABS	30	5	ONE EVERY MORNING		NEW
6/23/99	CELEBREX 100 MG	CAPS	90	3	1 PO Q AM AND 2 PO Q PM		NEW
6/3/99	GLUCOPHAGE	850 MG TABS	90	6	ONE 3 TIMES DAILY	6/3/99	NEW
6/3/99	HYTRIN	5 MG CAPS	30	6	ONE EVERY DAY	6/3/99	NEW

Figure 8-5 Medication administration flow sheet.

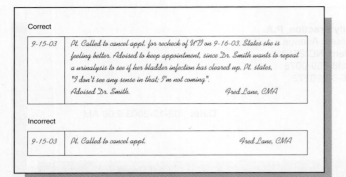

Correct	
9-15-03	Pt. Called to cancel appt. for recheck of UTI on 9-16-03. States she is feeling better. Advised to keep appointment, since Dr. Smith wants to repeat a urinalysis to see if her bladder infection has cleared up. Pt. states, "I don't see any sense in that; I'm not coming". Advised Dr. Smith. Fred Lane, CMA

Incorrect	
9-15-03	Pt. Called to cancel appt. Fred Lane, CMA

Figure 8-6 Charting example showing correct and incorrect entries.

The medical record is a legal document that can be subpoenaed in a malpractice suit. If the documentation is accurate, timely, and legible, it can help win a lawsuit or prevent one altogether. If the documentation is messy, inaccurate, or improperly done, however, it can raise questions that might cause the practice to lose a malpractice suit. Figure 8-6 is a charting example that shows the difference between a well-written chart note and one that leaves what really happened in question. The golden rule in documentation is that if it is not documented, it was not done. Therefore, all patient procedures, assessments, interventions, evaluations, teachings, and communications must be documented. Box 8-3 lists guidelines for documenting in patients' medical records.

LEGAL TIP

ABBREVIATIONS? WHEN IN DOUBT, SPELL IT OUT

The Joint Commission is charged with monitoring and accrediting inpatient and outpatient medical facilities. Recent changes in standards regarding some ambiguous handwritten abbreviations reflect the growing feeling that many commonly used abbreviations are overused, used incorrectly, open to interpretation, or easily confused with another abbreviation. For instance, the abbreviation BS might stand for bowel sounds, breath sounds, or blood sugar. In addition to requiring facilities to keep a list of acceptable abbreviations used in the facility, The Joint Commission issues a "Do Not Use" list that can be found at www.jointcommission.org. Even though some abbreviations can be confusing and should not be used, many continue to be used. Appendix D has a general list of commonly used abbreviations. The Joint Commission is covered in more detail in Chapter 10.

BOX 8-3

DOCUMENTATION GUIDELINES

1. Make sure you know the office policy regarding charting. Find out who is allowed to write in the chart and the procedures for doing so.
2. Make sure you have the correct patient chart. If the patient's name is common, ask for a birth date or social security number as a double check.
3. Document in ink.
4. Sign your complete name and credential.
5. Always record the date of each entry. Some outpatient facilities record the time as well. Using military time will eliminate the need to use AM and PM (Fig. 8-7)
6. Write legibly. Printing is more legible than cursive writing.
7. Check spelling, especially medical terms, before entering them into the chart. Chapter 7 offers help with spelling.
8. Use only abbreviations that are accepted by your facility. Because abbreviations can cause confusion and errors in patient care, the use of certain handwritten abbreviations has been prohibited by The Joint Commission. (See Legal Tip: Abbreviations? When in Doubt, Spell It Out.)
9. When charting the patient's statements, use quotation marks to signify the patient's own words. For example, "My head is killing me."
10. Do not attempt to make a diagnosis. For

Figure 8-7 Military time.

(continued)

BOX 8-3   *(continued)*

example, if the patient says, "My throat is sore," do not write pharyngitis. It is not within the scope of your training to diagnose.

11. Document as soon as possible after completing a task to promote accuracy.
12. Document missed appointments in the patient's chart. Chart your attempts to reach the patient to remind him or her of the appointment.
13. Document any telephone conversations with the patient in the chart.
14. Be honest. If you have given a wrong medication or performed the wrong procedure, as soon as the appropriate supervisor is notified, document it, and then complete an incident report (see Chapter 11). State only the facts; do not draw any conclusions or place blame.
15. Never document for someone else, and never ask someone else to document for you.
16. Never document false information.
17. Never delete, erase, scribble over, or white-out information in the medical record because this can be construed as attempting to cover the truth and tampering with a legal document. If you do make an error, draw a single line through it, initial it, and date it. Then write the word "correction" and document the correct information (Fig. 8-8)

You can click on an icon to make a correction in the electronic chart, but the original information is not deleted. For example, if you discover that you have entered the wrong date of birth after the patient's information has been saved, you can correct it, but most systems allow only certain users to make changes in the saved database.

When correcting a charting error, draw a single line through the error, initial it, date it, and document the correct information.

left 05/15/03 TW

05/15/03 Patient presents today complaining of pain in ~~right~~ eye. Tracy Wiles, CMA

Figure 8-8 Correcting an error in a medical record.

Charting Communications With Patients

As discussed earlier, in addition to documenting patient visits to the facility, other encounters and communications may occur and should become a part of the permanent record. To ensure continuity of care and patient safety, charts should contain a progress sheet or some sort of tool to record each communication with a patient. Actions taken by the physician or employees as directed by the physician on behalf of the patient should be charted. For example, when a prescription is phoned to a pharmacy, the action is recorded. The physician may give instructions to be carried out regarding a patient, such as calling the patient with normal test results. This should be concisely explained in the chart. These entries should appear in **chronological order.** Dates that are out of order and gaps between entries may confuse the reader and give the appearance of poor service. For this reason, entries should be made immediately after communications with the patient.

Telephone or electronic communications with patients are typically recorded in a narrative manner. When a patient calls or e-mails the office, the conversation must be documented in the chart immediately. Phone calls should be documented with the time and date of the call, patient's problem or request, and actions taken by the person making the entry. If special telephone message pads are used, a copy should be placed in the patient's chart. E-mails from patients should be printed and kept in the chart. Replies to a patient's e-mail should be printed out and included with the progress sheet. Remember, care must be taken to adhere to HIPAA's Privacy Rules to ensure protection of the patient's privacy when using electronic means to communicate.

Additions to Medical Records

Any additions to a medical record, such as laboratory results, that are smaller than the standard 8.5 × 11 inches should be transcribed onto a full sheet of paper or shingled and placed in the appropriate area of the chart. Shingling is taping the paper across the top to a regular-size sheet. Each sheet is then added under the current one with a piece of tape across the top. Each sheet can be lifted to view the entire document. Most laboratory reports are computer generated and will come ready to insert into the chart. All additions to the medical record (e.g., laboratory results, radiographic reports, consultation reports) should be read and initialed by the physician before you put them in the chart.

 CHECKPOINT QUESTION

7. What is the golden rule in documentation?

Workers' Compensation Records

From time to time, a patient who is active in your practice may seek treatment for a **workers' compensation** case or an injury or illness related to employment. The government requires employers to provide insurance for care when an injury occurs at work. Workers' compensation is discussed in Chapter 13. When this occurs, do not simply add the information to the patient's medical record. Instead, start a new record. A workers' compensation medical record actually belongs to the employer, so the data in that record can be reviewed by the employer's insurance carrier. Information about the patient's previous health or family history that is not pertinent to the workplace incident should NOT be made available to the insurance carrier.

Workers' compensation cases are kept open for two years after the last date of treatment for any follow-up care that may be required. After that time, care may not be covered under the same case. Even after the care is complete, the separate record is kept with the patient's other record, and information is incorporated into the original record as needed.

LEGAL TIP

VERIFYING WORKERS' COMPENSATION CASES

Before treating a patient for a possible workers' compensation illness or injury, you must first obtain verification from the employer unless the situation is life threatening. Be sure to document the name of the person who authorizes treatment as well as any other information that becomes available during the verification process.

 CHECKPOINT QUESTION

8. Why is it necessary to make a new chart for an established patient who is being seen for an injury sustained at work?

Storing Medical Records

Using electronic health records eliminates the need for filing, but manual records must be prepared and kept in a way that promotes easy retrieval. Since the medical record is the foundation for patient care, much care and attention is given to the process of storing and retrieving medical charts.

Medical Record Preparation

To start filing, you need folders, labels, and any other appropriate supplies. Keep these supplies on hand and follow the same steps every time you put together and

file a medical record. Procedure 8-1 outlines the steps for establishing and maintaining a medical record. Over the course of many years, you may have to replace worn-out folders or peeling labels and stickers. Do so before the folder tears or the labels fall off.

After preparing the folders, you may also want to prepare several out guides, that is, plastic sheets with a tab (projection) and a pocket for index cards. Type "Out guide" on the tabbed edge of the sheet. Then, when you remove a chart, write the date, name of the patient, your initials, and where the chart can be found on an index card. Place the card inside the out guide, and put the out guide in the spot in the file cabinet where the chart was. An out guide indicates that the chart has been removed and where it can be found. Hospitals and larger clinics often use a wand to keep track of charts and radiographs. When a chart arrives in a certain location, a wand is passed over a bar code. When the patient's number is entered into the computer, the screen shows the location of the patient's chart at the moment. If it is in the file cabinet, that is also indicated.

 CHECKPOINT QUESTION

9. What is the purpose of an out guide?

Filing Procedures

Every day in the medical office, information is added to a patient's chart. It is best to keep this information filed on a daily basis. Pieces of paper to be added can be kept in a central location until filed so that employees can retrieve it if needed before the patient's next visit. This holding area should be used only until the daily filing can be done. In a paperless office, these additions to the medical record are scanned into the system, and the original paper is shredded. Procedure 8-2 describes how to file manual records.

To ensure efficient and speedy filing and document retrieval, follow these four steps:

1. *Condition.* Prepare items by removing loose pieces of tape or paper clips. Make sure each sheet of paper includes the patient's name in case a second page gets separated from the first page.
2. *Index.* Separate business records from patient records.
3. *Sort.* Put each group of records in proper order to be filed on shelves, either alphabetic or numeric. This makes actual filing go much faster because you are not moving up and down and back and forth to find the proper letter area; you will just move down in order.
4. *Store.* Place each record in the proper storage area, as described next.

Filing Systems

The two main filing systems are alphabetic and numeric. In some practices you may use both systems, each for different types of files.

Alphabetic Filing

As the name implies, **alphabetic filing** is a system using letters. Begin alphabetic filing by distinguishing the first, second, and third unit as described in Box 8-4. (A unit

---

BOX 8-4

INDEXING RULES FOR ALPHABETIC FILING

When filing records alphabetically, use these indexing rules to help you decide the placement of each record. Indexing rules apply whether you use the title of the record's contents or a person's name.

File by name according to last name, first name, and middle initial, and treat each letter in the name as a separate unit. For example, Jamey L. Crowell should be filed as Crowell, Jamey L. and should come before Crowell, Jamie L.

- Make sure professional initials are placed after a full name. John P. Bonnet, D.O., should be filed as Bonnet, John P., D.O.
- Treat hyphenated names as one unit. Bernadette M. Ryan-Nardone should be filed as Ryan-Nardone, Bernadette M. not as Nardone, Bernadette M. Ryan.
- File abbreviated names as if they were spelled out. Finnigan, Wm. should be filed as Finnigan, William, and St. James should be filed as Saint James.
- File last names beginning with Mac and Mc in regular order or grouped together, depending on your preference, but be consistent with either approach.
- File a married woman's record by using her own first name. Helen Johnston (Mrs. Kevin Johnston) should be filed as Johnston, Helen, not as Johnston, Kevin Mrs.
- Jr. and Sr. should be used in indexing and labeling the record. Many times, a father and son are patients at the same facility.
- When names are identical, use the next unit, such as birth dates or the mother's maiden name. Use Durham, Iran (2-4-94) and Durham, Iran (4-5-45).

- Disregard apostrophes.
- Disregard articles (a, the), conjunctions (and, or), and prepositions (in, of) in filing. File *The Cat in the Hat* under Cat in Hat.
- Treat letters in a company name as separate units. For ASM, Inc., "A" is the first unit, "S" is the second unit, and "M" is the third unit.

---

is each part of a name or title that is used in indexing.) Using the first letter of the first unit, place your records in small groups in order from A to Z. After that, take each small group and gradually work through the second and consecutive letters to put the small groups in order. Using this process allows you to work in a progressive order as you add records to existing files.

If the entire first unit is the same, move onto the second unit. If the second unit is still the same, move onto the third unit. Occasionally, you will have records whose units one, two, and three are identical. In such cases, it does not matter which one is filed first; use extreme caution, however, when retrieving records with identical units to prevent errors. Asking the patient to provide his or her birthday will ensure that you have the right patient and avoid confusion.

With alphabetic filing, color coding may also be used. Letters of the alphabet are color-coded and affixed to each folder, or a color-coded bar is placed next to the label with the patient's name. For example, names beginning with A to F may be blue; G to L, green; M to T, yellow; and U to Z, purple. Using this system, Michele Beals would have a blue strip, Laurie Palmer would have a yellow strip, Lauren Kayser would have a green strip, and Dana Warbeck would have a purple strip. Finding misfiled charts is easier. With one glance at the cabinet, for example, you can spot one purple tab in the middle of the green ones.

Numeric Filing

Numeric filing uses digits, usually six. The digits are typically run together but read as three groups of two digits. For example, the record filed as 324478 is read as 32, 44, 78. Commas are not placed or any separation used when applying the labels to the tabbed edge of the file folder. The records are placed in numeric order without concern for duplication, which may sometimes happen with the alphabetic system. If you use this technique, it is called straight digit filing because you are reading the number straight out from left to right.

Sometimes, the file label will look the same, 324478, but will be read in the reverse order: 78, 44, 32. This technique is called terminal digit filing; that is, the groups of numbers are read in pairs from right to left. Be careful not to mix the two filing systems. If using both techniques within your office, be sure to keep them separate by changing the folder color or some other means to prevent errors. The chart is filed by using the last pairs of digits.

Numeric filing plays an important role in the medical office. With HIPAA's Privacy Rule requirements, the use of numeric filing makes sense. When this technique is used, it is important to keep a **cross-reference** in a secure area, away from patient areas, listing the numeric code and the name of the patient. Such a reference is called a master patient index. This way, a limited number of people know who the patient is, which maintains privacy. Boxes 8-5 and 8-6 describe how to file patient records alphabetically or numerically.

Other Filing Systems

The medical office keeps files other than patient records. An office manager keeps files on employees, insurance policies, accounts payable, and so on. For this type of filing, systems include **subject filing**, in which documents are arranged alphabetically according to subject (e.g., insurance, medications, referrals); geographic filing, in which documents are grouped alphabetically according to locations, such as state, county, or city; and chronological filing, in which documents are grouped in the order of their date.

BOX 8-5

ALPHABETIC FILING EXAMPLES

The following patient records are to be filed alphabetically:

Mary P. Martin
Floyd D. Huey, Sr.
Susan Bailey
Ellen P. Parrish
Karen Hart
Susan Roberts-Hill
Sister Mary Margarita
Cher
Clayton A. Parker, MD
Mrs. John Moser (Donna)

The correct order is:

Susan Bailey
Cher
Karen Hart
Floyd D. Huey, Sr.
Mary P. Martin
Donna Moser
Clayton A. Parker
Ellen P. Parrish
Susan Roberts-Hill
Sister Mary Margarita

BOX 8-6

NUMERIC FILING EXAMPLES

The following patient records are to be filed numerically:

Ramsey, LeRoy	213456
Flora, Curtis	334387
King, Sharon	979779
Moore, Cathy	321138

In straight digit filing, the proper order is:

213456
321138
334387
979779

In terminal digit filing, the proper order is:

321138
213456
979779
334387

With files in which one or two groups of numbers are the same numbers, you refer to the second or third groups of numbers. For example, in straight digit filing (reading from left to right) the number 003491 comes before 004592. The first group of numbers (00) is the same for both files, so you determine the order of filing by the second group of numbers; in this case, 34 comes before 45.

In terminal digit filing (reading from right to left), 456128 would come before 926128. The first two groups of numbers (28 and 61) are the same for both files, so you go to the third group of numbers; in this case, 45 comes before 92.

A well-kept, complete, and accurate medical record and the ability to quickly retrieve information are reflections of the quality and efficiency of the medical facility in which they are generated.

 CHECKPOINT QUESTION

10. What are the two main filing systems? Briefly describe each.

Storing Health Information

Whether a facility uses an electronic form, a manual system, or a combination of both, the records used in the delivery of health care must be stored safely and privately. A goal of a good system includes easy retrieval of the information. Logical organization and policies that ensure that information is safe, secure, and easily accessed make for an efficient medical office.

Electronic Data Storage

The paperless medical office must consider storage of data other than using paper and folders. HIPAA's Administrative Simplification section addresses the issues involved in storing electronically generated transmissions and storage. Backup copies of computerized records must be made daily and stored in a safe, fireproof location. Security experts advise storing backup disks off site. HIPAA mandates that offices establish a disaster plan that includes emergency storage of data and security and safety of that data. Any computer infrastructure should allow for chart availability in a disaster situation. A medical office may choose to outsource the off-site storage of their data. Health information stored off site may be classified as "hot," which means the records are accessible and usable. A storage backup would need activation for use. The speed of computer technology promises changes and new practices. In order to optimize efficiency, you must keep abreast of these new technologies.

Storage of Standard Medical Records

Medical offices use a variety of storage methods for active files that are used on a daily basis. Shelf files are stationary shelves. Shelving units are stacked on each other or placed side by side. These shelves may also be custom-ordered to the width you need. Records are stored horizontally, and labels are read from the side. Figure 8-9 shows an example of shelving units.

Drawer files are a type of filing cabinet. The drawer pulls out for easy access and visibility of all records. This type of filing system allows you easier access to all sides of files, which can help in searches for missing files

that may have been pushed to the back or behind other files. Drawer files also allow easier filing because you can read from above the files, rather than squatting to read the labels from the sides as you work your way down to the lower shelves. A disadvantage is that these files take up a great deal of space.

Rotary circular or lateral files allow records to be stored in units that either spin in a circle or stack one behind the other, enabling you to rotate different units to the front. This system allows for maximum use of office space and is suggested for a medical office with large quantities of records to be stored. With shelf or drawer units, more wall space is needed to spread out each unit, but with rotary files, less wall space is needed.

Classification of Medical Records

For the purpose of storing records, they may be classified in three categories: active, inactive, or closed. Active records are those of patients who have been seen within the past few years. The exact amount of time is designated within each practice; it usually ranges from 1 to 5 years. Keep these records in the most accessible storage spot available because you will be using them regularly.

Inactive records are those of patients who have not been treated in the office for a set time. Most offices consider files inactive after 2 to 3 years. You will still keep inactive records in the office, but they do not have to be as accessible as the active files. Usually, they are placed on bottom shelves to eliminate constant bending when reaching for active files, or they may be stored in another room within the office. They can be stored in the office in an out-of-the-way area, such as a basement or attic. They may even be kept in the physician's home. This practice is permitted because the records belong to the physician, but it is not recommended because, at any time, the office staff may need access to these records. "Inactive" patients have not formally terminated their contact with the physician, but they have either not needed the physician's services or have not informed the office regarding a move, change in physician, or death.

Closed records are those of patients who have terminated their relationship with the physician. Reasons for such termination might include the patient moving, termination of physician–patient relationship by letter, no further treatment necessary, or death of the patient.

Many practices use **microfilm** or **microfiche** to store closed records. Microfilm and microfiche are ways to photograph documents and store them in a reduced form. Microfilm, a popular method for storing large volumes of records, particularly in hospitals and clinics, uses a photographic process that develops medical records in miniature on film. Information is stored on cards holding single film frames or in reels or strips for

Figure 8-9 File cabinets.

projection on compact electric viewers placed at convenient office locations. The cost of the equipment is declining, making this a more practical method for storing and retrieving inactive files.

Microfiche is a miniature photographic system that stores rows of images in reduced size on cards with clear plastic sleeves rather than on film strips. Information can be handled manually, examined on a viewer that enlarges the record, or reproduced as hard copy on a high-speed photocopier. A standard microfiche card holds more than 60 pages of information. The microfiche process allows 3200 papers to be reduced to fit on a single 4- to 6-inch transparency.

Medical Record Retention

As discussed in Chapter 2, the statute of limitations is the legal time limit set for filing suit against an alleged wrongdoer. The time limit varies from state to state. You must observe the statute of limitations in your particular state to know how long medical and business records should be kept in storage.

MEDIA MENU

- **Student CD**
  - **CMA/RMA Certification Exam Review**
- **Premium Online Course**
  http://thePoint.lww.com/Kronenberger3e
- **Internet Resources**

  LiveAdvise Online Tutoring & Competency Training
  http://thePoint.lww.com/LiveAdvise

  US Department of Health and Human Services, CMS, HIPAA — General Information
  http://www.cms.hhs.gov/HIPAAGenInfo/

  US Department of Health and Human Services, CMS, National Provider Identifier Standard
  http://www.cms.hhs.gov/NationalProvIdentStand/

  American Health Information Management Association
  http://www.ahima.org

  Health Level Seven (HL7)
  http://www.hl7.org

  Certification Commission for Healthcare Information Technology (CCHIT)
  http://www.cchit.org

  Office of the National Coordinator for Health Information Technology (ONC)
  http://www.hhs.gov/healthit/hithca.html

It is recommended that medical records be stored permanently because, in some states, malpractice lawsuits can be filed within 2 years of the date of discovery of the alleged malpractice. The statute of limitations for minors is extended until the child reaches legal age in every state; the time given past the legal age varies, however.

When a health care provider's practice ends, either from retirement or death, notice to all patients with records stored in the facility is required. This notice can be in the form of a letter to each patient and/or a newspaper notification advising patients of the closing of the practice and giving them a reasonable length of time in which to pick up their records. Since the facility no longer exists, you may release the original record to the patients. As discussed previously, the record itself belongs to the facility, but the information in the record belongs to the patient. Since the facility no longer exists, it is felt that the record now belongs to the patient. Retiring physicians or the families of deceased physicians may ask a colleague to maintain storage of any patient records that are not claimed. This location should be given to the patients in their written notification. Of course, the statute of limitations for legal action and the need for these records should be taken into consideration. Most risk management experts advise that the records should be kept in some form forever, but this is not always feasible. At the least, every reasonable attempt should be made to notify patients and disseminate the information maintained by the retiring or deceased physician.

CHECKPOINT QUESTION

11. How long should medical records be kept?

español SPANISH TERMINOLOGY

Necesitaremos copias de su historia medical de los archivos de su médico anterior.

We will need copies of your medical records from your previous doctor.

Por firmar aquí, usted nos da permiso de compartir su información medical con su compañía de seguro.

By signing here, you are giving us permission to share your medical information with your insurance company.

PROCEDURE 8-1: Establishing, Organizing, and Maintaining a Medical File

Purpose: To create a file that will organize and save a patient's medical information, including records of transactions and interactions with the office and its staff

Equipment: File folder, metal fasteners, hole punch, five divider sheets with tabs, title, year, and alphabetic or numeric labels

Steps	Reasons
1. Decide the name of the file (a patient's name, company name, or name of the type of information to be stored).	Properly naming a file allows for easy retrieval.
2. Type a label with the title *in unit order* (e.g., Lynn, Laila S., *not* Laila S. Lynn).	Typing the label in unit order helps avoid filing errors.
3. Place the label along the tabbed edge of the folder so that the title extends out beyond the folder itself. (Tabs can be either the length of the folder or tabbed in various positions, such as left, center, and right.)	This ensures easy readability when the folder is in a storage cabinet.

Step 3: Place label along tabbed edge of folder.

Steps	Reasons
4. Place a year label along the top edge of the tab before the label with the title. This will be changed each year the patient has been seen. *Note:* Do not automatically replace these labels at the start of a new year; remove the old year and replace with a new one only when the patient comes in for the first visit of the new year.	Doing this makes removing inactive files more time efficient. At the beginning of each new year, you can easily spot the records that are years beyond your storage time limit in the active file area. Doing this also can help you locate inactive files if patients return years later. (By determining the last year the patient was seen, you can narrow your search to files with a matching year label.)
5. Place the appropriate alphabetic or numeric labels below the title.	This aids in accurate filing and retrieval.

(continued)

PROCEDURE 8-1: Establishing, Organizing, and Maintaining a Medical File *(continued)*

Steps	Reasons
6. Apply any additional labels that your office may decide to use.	Labels noting special information (e.g., insurance, drug allergies, advanced directives) act as quick and easy reminders.
	Step 6: Apply additional labels as needed.
7. Punch holes and insert demographic and financial information using top fasteners across the top.	General information should not be intermingled with clinical information.
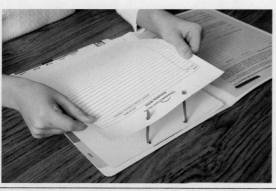	**Step 7:** Punch holes and insert pages in chart.
8. Make tabs for: Ex. H&P, Progress Notes, Medication Log, Correspondence, and Test Results.	This will allow quick and easy retrieval of specific information.
9. Place pages behind appropriate tabs.	Misplacing charts or sheets out of charts creates big problems for everyone.

PROCEDURE 8-2:   Filing Medical Records

Purpose: To place medical information in a designated location that will facilitate easy retrieval and the safety of the record

Equipment: Simulated patient file folder, several single sheets to be filed in the chart, file cabinet with other files

Steps	Purpose
1. Double-check spelling of names on the chart and any single sheets to be placed in the folder.	You can never be too careful with patient identification.
2. Condition any single sheets, etc.	Removing staples, paper clips, and tape will keep paper from getting torn.
3. Place sheets behind proper tab in the chart.	Organizing documents and placing tabs allows for easy retrieval of specific information.
4. Remove out guide.	The out guide will serve as a double-check for the proper placement of the chart.
5. Place the folder between the two appropriate existing folders, taking care to place the folder between the two charts.	It is easy to accidentally place a folder within a folder.
6. Scan color coding to ensure none of the charts in that section are out of order.	Color-coded tabs enable you to spot a misfiled chart easily.

- Medical records are not only a means of communication among health care providers but also are legal documents depicting the quality of patient care.
- HIPAA ensures confidentiality of all medical information. The patient's privacy must be protected at all times.
- You must adhere to strict guidelines when sharing protected health information electronically and releasing any information in patients' medical records.
- You must use sound practices when entering information into a patient's chart.

- To ensure efficient recording and retrieval, you must be familiar with the varied documentation forms as well as the different kinds of filing systems.
- The system of storage of medical information used by a provider must ensure the safety, security, and confidentiality of the patient's protected health information.
- You must follow sound guidelines regarding the retention of records in order to safeguard the patient's rights to their personal medical information.
- The quality, use, and care of the medical record are reflections of the quality of the medical facility itself.

Warm Ups   for Critical Thinking

1. Interview a fellow student with a hypothetical illness. Document the visit with the chief complaint.

2. Compare and contrast alphabetic filing with numeric filling. Which system do you think works better? Explain your response.

3. Role play with a fellow student who is requesting their medical records for a new doctor. Construct a proper authorization for release of information form and have the "patient" complete it.

4. Write an office policy for maintaining confidentiality with electronic modalities, such as fax machines, printers, laptops, and computer screens.

5. You work for an orthopedist who is retiring in 3 months. He asks you to construct a letter to be sent to all of the patients informing them of his retirement and instructing them to come in and pick up their records. List the hours the office will be open and the deadline for picking up the records. Include in the letter the location of the records after that deadline.

Answers   to Checkpoint Questions

1. The Health Insurance Portability and Accountability Act was established in order to provide consumers with greater access to health care insurance, to protect the privacy of health care data, and to promote more standardization and efficiency in the health care industry.

2. Permission to release information about a patient's HIV status must be specifically given on the release form that is signed by the patient.

3. Certain types of information are considered legally required disclosures. These include vital statistics, child and elder abuse or maltreatment,

emergency circumstances, ID of body of deceased person, cause of death, public health needs such as communicable diseases, research, judicial and administrative proceedings, law enforcement concerns such as violent criminal activities, and activities related to national defense and security.

4. The patient's chief complaint is the reason the patient is seeing the physician.

5. Narrative, SOAP, and POMR are three common formats for recording patient–provider encounters.

6. The advantages of using flow sheets in the medical chart are that they limit the need for long hand-

written notes, save time and space, and make it easier to locate information.

7. The golden rule in documenting is that if it is not documented, it was not done.

8. The chart of the patient injured on the job has information that should not be available to the employer, who has access only to the information about the worker's injury.

9. An out guide is used to save the place of a chart in use by someone. The location of the chart is recorded on the out guide so that anyone looking for the chart will know where it is.

10. The two main filing systems are alphabetic (using letters to file records) and numeric (using digits to file records).

11. Medical records should be kept at least as long as the statute of limitations for the state in which they were generated. Experts recommend keeping them forever.

CHAPTER

9

Computer Applications in the Medical Office

Outline

THE COMPUTER
Hardware
Peripherals
Care and Maintenance of the
System and Equipment
INTERNET BASICS
Getting Started and Connected
Security of Electronically
Shared Health Information
Internet Security
Viruses
Downloading Information
Working Offline

ELECTRONIC MAIL
Access
Attachments
Opening Electronic Mail
**MEDICAL APPLICATIONS OF
THE INTERNET**
Search Engines
Professional Medical Sites
Patient Teaching Issues
Regarding the Internet
INTRANET
**MEDICAL SOFTWARE APPLI-
CATIONS**

Clinical Applications
Administrative Applications
HANDHELD COMPUTERS
PURCHASING A COMPUTER
TRAINING OPTIONS
COMPUTER ETHICS

Learning Objectives

Upon successfully completing this chapter, you will be able to:

1. Spell and define the key words

2. Identify the basic computer components

3. Explain the basics of connecting to the Internet

4. Discuss the safety concerns for online searching

5. Describe how to use a search engine

6. List sites that can be used by professionals and sites geared for patients

7. Describe the benefits of an intranet and explain how it differs from the Internet

8. Describe the various types of clinical software that might be used in a physician's office

9. Describe the various types of administrative software that might be used in a physician's office

10. Describe the benefits of a handheld computer

11. Describe the considerations for purchasing a computer

12. Describe various training options

13. Discuss the ethics related to computer access

Upon successfully completing this chapter, you will be able to:

1. Care for and maintain computer hardware (Procedure 9-1)

2. Search a given topic on the Internet (Procedure 9-2)

CAAHEP

- Perform routine maintenance of administrative and clinical equipment
- Perform within legal and ethical boundaries
- Demonstrate knowledge of federal and state health care legislation and regulations

ABHES

- Receive, organize, prioritize, and transmit information expediently
- Application of electronic technology
- Apply computer concepts for office procedures
- Locate resources and information for patients and employees
- Evaluate and recommend equipment and supplies for practice

cookies	Ethernet	literary search	virus
downloading	Internet	search engine	virtual
encryption	intranet	surfing	

Computers play a major role in the physician's office. Computers are used for both clinical and administrative applications. A few examples of administrative applications are appointment scheduling, billing, staff scheduling, and insurance filings. Clinical software programs are used for many areas, such as reading laboratory and radiology reports and helping the physician to prescribe medications. Computers promote communication among health care professionals and provide access to new treatment options. You will need excellent computer skills to work as a medical assistant. This chapter will help you to improve your existing skills. It provides a basic review of computer components. You will learn how the Internet is used in health care settings and some precautions. Various medical software applications will also be discussed. You will learn about training options and how to purchase a computer.

The Computer

A computer system is roughly divided into two areas, hardware and peripherals.

Hardware

Computer hardware consists of seven key elements (Fig. 9-1). Here is a review of their parts:

Figure 9-1 The computer consists of the CPU, keyboard, monitor, hard drive, printer, and secondary storage systems. Additional peripherals include the mouse, battery backup, and modems.

- *Central processing unit.* The central processing unit (CPU), or microprocessor, is the circuitry imprinted on a silicon chip that processes information. The CPU consists of a variety of electronic and magnetic cells. These cells read, analyze, and process data and instruct the computer how to operate a given program. All CPUs function basically the same way, but chips differ dramatically in capabilities and speeds. Your CPU has many ports to connect the printer, mouse, and speakers. At minimum, it has two serial ports, one parallel port, and two universal serial bus (USB) ports. Serial ports are used for items like modems; parallel ports are used for connecting printers and backup drives to the CPU; and USB ports allow the computer to connect with various instruments.
- *Keyboard.* The keyboard is the primary means by which information is entered into the computer. Besides the typical letter and number keys, you will find special function keys that provide increased capabilities. Examples of special function keys are Alt, Ctrl, Insert, and Esc. Each of these keys has a specific function that is determined by the software program. These functions may include searching for and replacing words, moving blocks of text, indenting or centering text, and spell checking.

- *Monitor.* Monitors, also called the visual display terminals, come in various sizes and qualities. The quality of the image is based on the DPIs (dots per inch). The more DPIs there are, the clearer the picture. There are adjustment dials for brightness and contrast. Flat-panel LCD monitors are popular and provide the most protection from unauthorized eyes.
- *Hard drive.* The hard drive provides storage for programs, data, and files. The capacity of a hard drive (i.e., the quantity of program and data it can hold) is measured in megabytes or gigabytes. Originally, hard drives could hold 5 MB (equivalent to about 2000 typed pages), but today they have much more capacity.
- *Printer.* The printer transfers information to paper (hard copy). Printers use various technologies, operate at various speeds, and print in either black or color. The printer allows you to generate bills, print letters, and produce a daily schedule. The most commonly used printer is a laser printer, which focuses a laser beam to form images that are transferred to paper electrostatically.
- *Scanner.* A scanner allows you to take a picture or report and read it into the computer. In offices with no paper charts, you scan laboratory reports, radiology reports, discharge summaries, letters, and any other paper documents into a patient's file. This is also helpful when a new patient arrives with reports from a previous physician. Patient education materials can also be scanned into the computer and then adjusted to meet the needs of your office. Keep in mind that you need to adhere to copyright laws.
- *Secondary storage systems.* All computers have multiple methods for saving data. Examples include floppy diskettes, compact disks, digital video disks, and zip drives. Cartridges are used by hospital for large storage systems. When saving any type of data, remember that good organization skills are essential. Name your files appropriately and place files in properly identified folders. Most computers have preset timing systems that automatically save data. Check your default setting and readjust as needed.

CHECKPOINT QUESTION

1. What do the CPU cells do?

Peripherals

Computers can have many peripheral connections. Three key computer peripherals that you need to know are:

- *Mouse.* The mouse can be used to control the cursor on the display screen. Although you cannot type in characters using the mouse, you can move or delete individual characters, words, or entire blocks of text with it. The track ball is an alternative to a mouse. Your finger rotates the ball to move the pointer. It takes less space than a mouse and is used based on personal preference.

- *Battery backup*. A battery backup allows the computer system to function in the event of a power failure. Batteries come in various sizes depending on the size of your computer and the amount of work to be done during a power failure.
- *Modem*. A modem is a communication device that connects your computer with other computers, including the Internet, online services such as bulletin boards, and electronic mail systems. The faster the modem is, the faster the transmission. Modems may be connected through cable systems or through the telephone. Digital subscriber line (DSL) is the preferred method. To use a cable or DSL connection, your computer must have an **Ethernet** port or an Ethernet interface card. Ethernet is a type of networking technology for local area networks; coaxial cable carries radiofrequency signals between computers at a rate of 10 megabits per second.

Figure 9-2 A messy desk can be a disaster for the hardware components of a computer.

 CHECKPOINT QUESTION

2. What is an Ethernet, and why should your computer have an Ethernet port or Ethernet interface card?

Care and Maintenance of the System and Equipment

As with any piece of equipment in the medical office, it is necessary to maintain your computer on a regular basis. Some maintenance agreements require that a service representative clean and inspect the system on a regular basis. Each employee should take the responsibility of taking care of the equipment in an office. A computer and its accessories will last longer and perform better with care and maintenance. Most equipment in a medical office is very expensive. Its accuracy is crucial. Imagine the inefficiency that would be created if a physician's office could not make copies or receive faxes because of equipment failure. Just as the human body performs better with health maintenance, computer hardware and other equipment and machinery perform better when care and maintenance are carried out. A messy desk (Fig. 9-2) can be disaster for the hardware components of a computer. Procedure 9-1 outlines the general care guidelines for a computer.

Internet Basics

Most physicians' offices can connect to the **Internet**. The Internet is used for both clinical and administrative reasons. The first thing you need to know is how to get your computer connected.

Getting Started and Connected

The Internet is used for access to the World Wide Web (WWW) and for electronic mail (e-mail). To get connected, you will need an Internet connection company and appropriate Internet software.

There are three ways that your computer can connect to the Internet. One is an Internet service provider (ISP). The ISP is a company that connects your computer's modem to the Internet through the phone line. It is often called a dial-up service. This method provides the slowest service but is the cheapest. The second option is your cable television company. This system provides a faster connection. The third option is a digital subscriber line (DSL). This is the fastest connection but is not available in all areas. DSL is the most expensive connection system. If you need to download large files through the Internet, you should use either a DSL or cable connection. If you are having trouble accessing the Internet because of either slow service or connection troubles, speak to the physician or office manager to determine whether a different connection or ISP is needed. Wireless options are emerging, and the technology for accessing the Internet without a land line will continue to grow and improve.

Second, your computer will need a Web browser. A Web browser is software that communicates with your computer and the Internet. Two common examples are Internet Explorer and Netscape Navigator. Most computers are preloaded with a Web browser. Clicking on the Web browser icon makes the actual connection to the Internet. Depending on how your system is set up, you may have to use a password.

 CHECKPOINT QUESTION

3. Which two types of Internet connections are recommended for downloading large files?

Security of Electronically Shared Personal Health Information

As previously discussed, the federal government regulates the sharing and storage of protected health information. The HIPAA legislation mandates that, when a health care provider and health plan transmit and receive PHI (personal health information) electronically, the transmission must comply with certain standards. There are code sets to identify the physician's specialty, training, and payment policies, the status of a claim, why claims have been denied or adjusted, types of health plans, benefits, patient eligibility, provider organization types, and disability types. This simplification of information exchange ultimately results in increased efficiency and available cash flow.

The HIPAA Security Rule requires covered entities to implement policies and procedures designed to prevent, detect, and contain any breaks in security. The HIPAA Officer in a physician's practice is required to monitor the security of their electronic information by conducting a risk analysis. This analysis includes following the path of each type of transmission or movement of data to look for problems. They also periodically check for security threats or gaps by reviewing audit logs and other security tracking measures.

Internet Security

If you choose correct sites and follow some general safety tips, the Internet is a safe way to obtain and transfer patient information. Here are a few key points:

- Never send any patient information over the Internet to a site that does not have a secure sockets layer (SSL). This scrambles your information as it leaves your computer and unscrambles it when it arrives at its designated address.
- Look for a lock icon on the status bar.
- Set limits on your Web browser for **cookies**. A cookie is a tiny file from a website left on your computer's hard drive without your permission. By examining your cookies, a website can learn what sites you have visited, products for which you have been searching, and files that you have downloaded. You may control your computer's cookies by setting limits on your Web browser software. Limit setters can generally be found on your toolbar under Internet options, then under either privacy or security.

Viruses

Virus protection is an important security issue. A virus is a dangerous invader that enters your computer through some source and can destroy your files, software programs, and possibly even the hard drive. A worm is a specific type of virus that affects e-mail. Most

WHAT IF?

Parents ask you how to keep their child safe on the Internet. What should you say?
First and foremost, explain to the parent that direct parental observation is the best method. Encourage parents to have an open and honest discussion with their child regarding the dangers on the Internet. Computers should be kept in living rooms or family rooms. Advise parents not to let children have a computer with Internet access in their bedroom. Parents can require a password to be entered for Internet access. This prevents access when the parent is not present. Most Web browser programs let the parent allow access only to "safe" sites. A few sites can add filters or safety nets to a child's computer. These sites are Net Nanny (www.netnanny.com), Internet Guard Dog (www.mcafee.com), and CyberPatrol (www.cyberpatrol.com).

computers come with virus protection software. This software will identify and stop harmful transmission. However, virus protection is not 100% guaranteed. Some ways that you can protect your computer are:

- Do not open any attachments from unknown or suspicious sites.
- Update your virus protection software regularly. Most virus protection programs offer an updating service. Virus protection updates address new worms, as well.
- Remember, new viruses are detected daily.

Downloading Information

The Internet is filled with great patient teaching resources and other information. You may decide to copy some of this material into your computer. This is **downloading**. Downloading transfers information from an outside location to your computer's hard drive. Download only files that pertain to work. Do not download screen savers, news releases, recipes, or other personal information. Do not assume that you can photocopy any material that you have downloaded and distribute it. Always ask for permission from the author. Some government and professional medical websites state that their material can be freely copied and used. A good example of this is the United States Department of Agriculture (USDA) website, which allows the food pyramids to be copied and used for teaching.

Working Offline

It is possible to access Web pages without connecting your computer to the Internet. To do this, save your commonly accessed sites on your Web browser. (If you are unsure how to do this, search your help topics for working offline). Then, to view the pages offline, click on the connection icon, select work offline, and locate your file. Remember, Web pages are regularly updated, and a page that you have saved to view offline may not be the latest version. Periodically view the online site and resave the site.

Electronic Mail

Electronic mail provides many benefits to the health care system. E-mail promotes good patient care, enhances communication, promotes teamwork, eliminates phone tag, and provides written documentation of messages. Since e-mail messages cannot be guaranteed to provide confidentiality, you must use reasonable measures to ensure compliance with HIPAA's Privacy Rule when handling e-mails from patients. When an e-mail is received from a patient or another sender about a patient, the message should be recorded in the patient record and then deleted from the computer. If you are using a manual or paper chart system, print the e-mail and either enter the information in the record or place the correspondence in the chart. Once the information is recorded in the chart, any paper copies should be shredded. Be sure to document any action taken or reply sent. Issue passwords for those who need access to e-mails from patients.

Here are some general tips for using e-mail:

- Use the office e-mail address only to send work-related messages. Do not send personal messages.
- Do not participate in chain letters.
- Download your e-mail and read it offline unless you are using a DSL or cable connection.
- All e-mail messages should be professional.
- Read your e-mail's **encryption** feature and activate it. Encryption is a process of scrambling messages so that they cannot be read until they reach the recipient.
- Always leave a message on your e-mail system when you will be out of the office for a vacation or other reason. This message is automatically sent to the incoming e-mail senders. This alerts the sender that you will not be reading their message. Include the date when you will be returning to the office and instructions on who they should contact in case of emergencies. This feature is often called the "out-of-office assistant." Following is an example of a good message: "I will be out of the office from 1/20 through 1/28. If this e-mail requires immediate attention, please forward it to Barbara Smith. I will respond to your e-mail when I return."

 CHECKPOINT QUESTION

4. What does the encryption feature do?

Access

Access to your e-mail account is through either the Internet or intranet. The intranet is discussed later in the chapter. To access your e-mail, locate the mail icon, double-click it, and then enter appropriate information. A password is generally required. See the Legal Tip for some guidelines for password use.

 LEGAL TIP

PASSWORD GUIDELINES TO ENSURE SECURITY

- Establish written policies for the assignment and use of passwords to protect personal health information.
- Make unique passwords (combine letters and numbers).
- Do not use your initials, birth date, or phone number.
- System-wide passwords that allow access to the computer should be changed after an employee leaves the practice.
- Do not share your password with your colleagues.
- Do not tape your password on the computer monitor or leave it on your desk.
- Have additional password verifications for certain secure sites (laboratory reports).

Composing Messages

When composing a message, follow the guidelines in Chapter 7 for writing business letters . Here are a few additional tips:

- Check your spelling, grammar, and punctuation before sending any messages.
- Keep messages short, concise, and to the point.
- Flag messages of high importance. This will alert the recipient that the message is important and should be read first. Do not overuse this feature. Flag only messages that warrant immediate response or attention. Never send an e-mail about a patient who is having an emergency. Always call or page the physician instead. The following is an example of an inappropriate e-mail: "Ms. Smith's water broke. Do you want her to go the hospital or come into the office?"

- Use appropriate fonts and an appropriate font size.
- Generic or plain stationery should be used. Do not use stationery that has cute figures or looks busy.
- Always complete the subject line. Keep the subject line short and use only a few key words, for example, *Staff meeting tomorrow.*
- It is a good idea to restrict e-mail messages to only one topic.
- Paragraphs are not indented on e-mail messages. Skip a line between paragraphs.
- You can add a permanent signature to all outgoing e-mails. Your signature should include your name, credentials, and phone number with extension.

Address Books

Your e-mail software will allow you to create address books. An address book is a collection of e-mail addresses. Additional information, such as phone numbers, fax numbers, and street addresses, can be added. A few tips regarding address books are:

- Keep your addresses up to date.
- Organize your addresses in folders or categories. For example, one folder may contain all the cardiologists in the area, and another may contain just insurance-related addresses.

Attachments

An attachment is a file that is sent along with an e-mail. You attach a single file (letter) or several documents at one time. Remember these guidelines:

- When you receive an e-mail with an attachment, open the attached file or letter. File it in an appropriate place on your computer. If appropriate, print the attachment and distribute it as needed.
- If you are sending an e-mail and need to attach a file, compose your message first. Then attach the file by going into the tool bar and locating the menu for file attachments. Click Browse to find the file on your computer, and then click to attach it. It is a good idea before sending the attachment to open it to be sure that you have selected the correct file or version of the document.

Opening Electronic Mail

Some general guidelines regarding opening an e-mail message follow:

- Open only your own e-mail messages unless otherwise instructed.
- After reading the e-mail, either delete it or place it in a folder. Do not allow multiple e-mails to clog your inbox.

- Always open flagged messages first and respond to them immediately.
- If you receive a message that you cannot address or resolve, forward the message to your supervisor and alert the sender that the message has been forwarded.
- If you start receiving bulk mail, either block the sender or ask to be deleted from that mailing list. This can be accomplished by clicking on "unsubscribe," usually at the end of the message.

 CHECKPOINT QUESTION

5. List three steps to take to ensure the privacy of an e-mail from a patient.

Medical Applications of the Internet

Besides e-mail, the Internet offers the World Wide Web, which provides health care professionals with great resources and information. Navigating through the Web quickly and efficiently takes skill and practice. The process of searching the Internet is called **surfing**. Surfing that is unorganized and not focused can be time consuming and unproductive.

Before surfing for information, you need to remember one important rule: Not all of the information on the Web is accurate or truthful. Anyone can post anything or make any claim. Since the information that you obtain from the Web will affect patient care, all steps must be taken to ensure that only accurate information is found and used. First, look for the logo of a verification program such as the HON (Health on the Net) seal. Verification does not guarantee that the information is correct or truthful but does certify it is a good starting point. Keep in mind that many good sites, for example government sites, do not have this seal. The Patient Education Box provides some guidelines for selecting safe sites.

 PATIENT EDUCATION

Guidelines for Selecting Safe Websites

Remember these key points when recommending the internet to a patient:

- Beware of phrases like breakthrough, medical miracle, and secret formula.
- Avoid sites that advertise that they have cured a disease.
- Use caution when you see the phrase "ancient remedy."

(continued)

- Use caution when you find a site that will treat a whole list of diseases with the same treatment.
- Do not believe every testimonial that you read.
- If the site claims that the government is hiding information to cure a disease, use extreme caution.
- Use caution when the treatment can "only be bought here."
- If the site suggests that you not tell your doctor about it, stay away.
- See www.quackwatch.com.
- You can send complaints to the Federal Trade Commission at www.ftc.gov about sites that provide information that is misleading and wrong.
- Do not try to learn lifesaving skills, such as cardiopulmonary resuscitation, on the Internet. No matter how good the information or site is, you need to take a professional class.

Search Engines

A **search engine** allows you to find sites that have the information that you need. There are numerous search engines (Google, Yahoo, Lycos, Excite, Dogpile). These sites are best used for searching out general information. Once you arrive at the search engine page, you must enter some key words. Your key words should be focused to limit the number of responses or "hits" that you will get. For example, if you type in the key word "heart," you will get thousands of sites that pertain to the heart. Some of these sites will be referring to the heart as an organ, and other sites will address how to mend a broken heart. If you had selected your key words to be "heart attack," however, you would narrow your search tremendously. To further narrow your search, use the advanced search feature. Click on advance search, and use the key words "heart and attack and prevention." By doing this, you will obtain the information you want faster and more efficiently. Unless you are using a medical search engine, avoid using medical terms. For example, use the word lung instead of pulmonary. When you need to find medical information, use a medical search or a megamedical site with links. Procedure 9-2 lists the steps necessary to search the Internet. See the listing of websites at the end of this chapter for some good places to start searching for medical information.

✓ CHECKPOINT QUESTION

6. What is a search engine?

Professional Medical Sites

At the end of the chapters in this book you see various Web addresses listed that provide you with more information on that chapter's content. These are good starting points for professional topics. But keep in mind that Web addresses change frequently. If you are unable to access a site, try eliminating the letters and symbols after a slash (/). Use the primary site address. For example, suppose you want to enter this site: www.fda.gov/cder/drug/consumer/buyonline/guide.htm. If you cannot access that site, try www.fda.gov and advance from there. Most sites will link you automatically to a new home page. Also, depending on your Web browser, you may not have to type in www. In this case, you would just type in fda.gov.

The Internet can help you communicate with patients who speak a foreign language. Some websites translate phrases and words. Box 9-1 lists sites that physicians are most likely to use. All medical specialties have their own special site. Hospitals have their own sites also. When you start working as a medical assistant, learn the Web addresses of the specialty of your physician. For example, if you work for a neurologist, you will frequently use www.aan.com (American Academy of Neurology).

These sites will help you translate between English and Spanish:

- AltaVista – www.altavista.com (click on translate)
- Free English to Spanish translations – www.freetranslation.com

---

BOX 9-1

SITES PHYSICIANS USE

Physicians and other health care professionals are likely to use these sites:

Journal of the American Medical Association
   www.jama.com
New England Journal of Medicine
   www.nejm.org
The Lancet
   www.thelancet.com
Annals of Internal Medicine
   www.annals.org
AMA
   www.ama-assn.org
The Joint Commission
   www.jointcommission.org
CDC
   www.cdc.org
Clinical trials
   www.clinicaltrials.gov

The CDC site is also available in Spanish. You can give the following address to patients who want to view the site in Spanish: http://www.cdc.gov/spanish/.

Literary Searches

According to the American Medical Association, approximately 80% of practicing physicians regularly surf the Internet for medical research information. Most research information is found through a **literary search**. A literary search involves finding journal articles that present new facts or data about a given topic. Physicians who specialize in a given area and have conducted a controlled research study write these articles. Various databases can be used to do a literary search:

- OVID will search for articles as far back as 1966. It contains access to more than 4000 professional journals. Its address is http://gateway.ovid.com/.
- PubMed will search for journal articles back to 1966 from the National Library of Medicine.
- CINAHL contains journal articles published since 1982. It has primarily journals for nurses and other allied health care professionals.

Most literary search databases require an annual subscription fee. Once you arrive at the site, you can start to search for the information. First, enter your key words. To narrow the search, you can request journal articles from all countries or limit it to the United States. You can also limit the search by selecting a time line, such as the past 6 months. Once you have done your search, a list of articles will be displayed, and you can highlight the ones you wish to see. You will be asked whether you want to see the whole article or only the abstract. An abstract is a summary of the article. It is always a good idea to print only the abstracts and allow the physician to decide which full articles he or she will want to see. Fees for downloading the complete journal article vary. Abstracts can generally be downloaded free. Your local hospital librarian is often available to assist you with literary searches and may be able to get the article for free. Some libraries will do searches for physicians on staff at no charge. Use this service if it is available.

 CHECKPOINT QUESTION

7. How is a literary search different from a search on an Internet website?

Health-Related Calculators

The Web has numerous calculators that can be used for various health care topics:

- Basal metabolic rate calculator — www.global-fitness.com/BMR_calc.html
- Due date calculator — www.babycenter.com/calculators/duedate
- Ovulation calculator — www.babycenter.com/calculators/ovulation
- Target heart rate — www.webmd.com/heartrate
- Body mass index or BMI — www.cdc.gov

Insurance-Related Sites

The insurance world can seem like an endless maze of papers and regulations. The Internet can help you sort through and clarify some information. Your first stop should be the patient's insurance company. Its Web address is usually listed on the back of the patient's insurance card. Bookmark these sites. Chapter 13 will get into more details on this issue. Following are a few sites that can also help you and your patients:

- For information on buying health insurance online: www.ehealthinsurance.com.
- The Medicare site (www.medicare.gov) discusses the basics of Medicare programs, eligibility, enrollment, drug assistance programs, and many frequently asked questions. This site will link you to various other options. You will also find links to report Medicare fraud and abuse.
- Patients who express concern about their health records being red-flagged because of an illness (HIV, cancer) can check a database that alerts insurance companies to "red-flagged" patients. This site is www.mib.com. There is a fee for using this site.

Patient Teaching Issues Regarding the Internet

Some of your patients will be very skilled at using the Internet. As discussed in Chapter 4, they can find enormous amounts of information regarding their disease, treatment options, and medications. The guidelines discussed in the Patient Education Box pertain to patients who surf the Internet. You cannot stop or limit the information that patients will search and find. Keep in mind that patients often turn to the Internet when they feel confused or hopeless about their disease or anger about the medical profession. If a patient communicates any such feelings, alert the physician.

Teach patients to acquire reliable medical information and advise them of the dangers on the Web. Some physician offices print brochures with recommended Web addresses. This is a very good education tool for patients. Some areas you should be aware of are discussed in the following sections.

Buying Medications Online

As the cost of prescription medications soar, patients look for options. It is possible to buy prescription medications over the Internet. A good Internet pharmacy will provide information on what the medication is used for, possible side effects, dosage recommendation, and safety concerns. If patients want to purchase prescriptions online, advise them to use only sites that are certified by the Verified Internet Pharmacy Practice Site (VIPPS). This certification comes from the National Association of Boards of Pharmacy and indicates that the site has been checked and is monitored for safety and quality care. Advise patients to purchase only medications that have been prescribed by the physician. For consumer safety tips, advise patients to use www.fda.gov/cder/drug/con sumer/buyonline/guide.htm.

 CHECKPOINT QUESTION

8. If you find misleading or erroneous information on a product website, who can you notify?

Financial Assistance for Medications

In 2006, after many years of debate, the federal government provided drug coverage for Medicare beneficiaries. Part D Medicare provides seniors and people with disabilities with a comprehensive prescription drug benefit under the Medicare program. If a patient's coverage does not include a certain prescribed medication and a patient cannot pay for their medications, they can find many financial resources on the Web. First, you should advise patients to search the drug company's homepage, for example, www.Pfizer.com. Patients on Medicare will find assistance on www.medicare.gov/prescription/home.asp. Another good site is www.needymeds.com. Physicians can access www.Rxhope.com to find local financial resources for patients.

Medical Records

Patients may choose to create their own "medical records" and store personal health information on sites. Patients who travel frequently may opt for this. Two sites that offer this are www.personalmd.com and www.mywebmd.com. Patients can store information about their medications, immunizations, laboratory tests, surgeries, and so on. Remind patients that this information is not secure and could be accessed by unauthorized people. A more secure way to keep this information is to download medical record forms, complete the printed copy, and store them safely.

Medical Record Forms

The American Health Information and Management Association provides forms online for patients to record their health histories. These are available at www.ahima.org/consumer/index.html. The American

College of Emergency Physicians has an emergency consent form (www.acep.org) that parents can sign giving permission for another person to consent to their child to be treated in case of an emergency. This is valuable for parents who travel on business and have their child stay with a relative or friend.

Advance directives and legal forms for medical power of attorney are also available online. Patients should be advised to seek legal counsel and speak to the physician before completing these forms. The federal government has cards available online for patients to complete and carry with them regarding their wishes to be an organ and tissue donor at this website: http://www.organdonor.gov/donor/index.htm.

Injury Prevention

Injuries are a leading cause of death for children. The American Academy of Pediatrics (www.aap.org) has reference materials that can help parents with safety tips. The federal government sites (www.cdc.gov and www.nih.gov) also have good information that you can direct parents to search. The National Safe Kids foundation is another excellent resource (www.safekids.org). Questions regarding product recalls can be found at http://www.cpsc.gov/.

Intranet

An **intranet** is a private network of computers that share data. Intranets, sometimes called internal Webs, are used in large multiphysician practices. An intranet is more secure than the Internet. The only people with access to an intranet homepage are people with an affiliation to the practice. Access may be limited to those within the offices or may allow for access from home computer systems. The benefits of an intranet are enhanced communication, quick access to needed information, increased productivity, and enhanced security. Common examples of data found on an intranet are:

- Policy and procedure manuals
- Marketing information
- Minutes from meetings and upcoming agendas
- Staff schedules
- Local hospital announcements or information
- Commonly used forms
- Internal newsletters
- Internal job postings
- Phone lists
- Video conference support
- Links to specialty sites

 CHECKPOINT QUESTION

9. What are the benefits of an intranet?

Medical Software Applications

The types of medical applications and their possibilities are endless. Every day, thousands of new software packages are released into the market. Upgrades and new versions of existing packages are also released daily. Each type of software program will have good benefits and will lack some features. The type of software that you will use will vary among different physician offices. The selection of software is based on the size of the practice, number of physicians, specialty, and the affiliated hospital's software. If the hospital software is compatible, interchanging information is relatively easy. Physician and office manager preferences play a role in the software selection. Other factors include how many users can use software at one time, can the software be used with multiple windows open, how often does the company plan to update it, and is the software HIPAA compliant with regard to security and code sets.

Never buy or install a new software program or update an existing version without permission from either the office manager or the physician.

Learning to use a particular software program and navigate quickly and efficiently through its features takes time. Most programs come with a tutorial program. On-site training is often included in the purchase price of major software applications. Training options will be discussed later in the chapter.

Medical software applications can be divided into two main groups: clinical and administrative. Clinical software packages help the physician or health care professional provide the best possible medical care to patients. Administrative software packages focus on tasks to keep the office flowing efficiently and financially strong. The next sections introduce you to what types of software capabilities are available and most commonly used. Keep in mind that new technologies are emerging every day. Box 9-2 lists some companies that sell medical software.

Clinical Applications

As discussed in Chapter 8, clinical software is designed to help the physician, nurse, medical assistant, or other health care professional provide the most efficient, safest, and most reliable health care available. Here are some examples of the benefits that clinical software programs can bring into the physician's office:

1. Create a **virtual** patient chart. A virtual chart is a paperless chart in which all documentation is stored on the computer. Some offices create dual charts (virtual and paper), and other offices will keep one or the other.

   The advantages to a virtual charting system are that it saves filing space, increases access to patients' charts for all staff members, eliminates hunting for misplaced charts, and keeps the charts better organized and neater. Since the charting is done through keyboarding, the notes are always readable.

BOX 9-2

MEDICAL SOFTWARE COMPANIES

Numerous companies sell medical office software programs. Here are a few sites that you can visit:

Advanced Medical Management
    www.amdsoftware.com
AltaPoint Practice Management
    www.altapoint.com
American Medical software
    www.americanmedical.com
EZ Claim Medical Billing
    www.ezclaim.org
Find Medical Billing Software
    www.findaccountingsoftware.com
Medical Manager
    www.medicalmanager.com
Medical Software products
    www.medsoftware.com
NextGen
    www.nextgen.com
Plexis Health Care
    www.plexisweb.com
SoftAid
    www.soft-aid.com
Web-based appointment scheduling
    www.compassscheduling.com

---

2. Clinical software can maintain an up-to-date list of clinical tasks organized by employee's name. For example, suppose you just discharged a patient and made a note on his chart that you need to check his laboratory tests tomorrow. The task manager would automatically assign this task to your list of duties for tomorrow. Or a physician may discharge a patient and want you to call that patient in the morning for a follow-up. The physician could assign this task to your list. This promotes organization and decreases the potential for tasks to get overlooked or forgotten.

3. The software available for prescription management and drug information is tremendous. A good program that focuses on pharmaceutical information will decrease medication errors, increase patient satisfaction, and provide better patient care, and it can be financially beneficial to the patient and to the practice. At minimum, the software should enable the physician to find the patient's name in a database, virtually write the prescription, and download it directly to the patient's pharmacy. This allows the pharmacist to fill the prescription before the patient arrives. Thus, the patient gets the medication much faster. More important, since most prescription filling errors are due to physicians' poor handwriting, this potentially lethal error is prevented. Most med-

ication software packages red flag the physician if the prescription is contraindicated for the patient. Medications can be contraindicated because of a particular disease (e.g., asthma or diabetes), interaction with other medications the patient is taking, or an allergy. For example, assume the physician has written a prescription for Bactrim, which contains a sulfonamide. The software would find in the patient's medical record that the patient is allergic to sulfonamides. The computer would alert the physician, and the physician would select a different medication. Software also allows the physician to save the patient money. Each insurance company and hospital has a formulary of medications that it reimburses. If the physician orders a medication that is on the patient's insurance formulary, the patient saves money. If the physician selects a medication outside the formulary, the insurance company may refuse to pay some or all of the cost of the medication.

4. Computer programs can insert laboratory reports directly into the patient's records. This is more time efficient than faxing or manually recording the results. It also eliminates transcription errors. Most software will alert the physician when a new laboratory report has been received. Laboratory reports of serious or life-threatening findings will still be telephoned to the office.

5. Perhaps one of the greatest technologies is the importing of the actual imaging study into a patient's chart. Some software allows the physician to see the radiograph or computed tomograph from the office. Without this program, the physician gets a typed written report, such as "chest radiograph shows left lower lobe infiltrate." With this technology, the physician can see the radiograph itself and thus make better clinical decisions.

6. Plastic surgeons use a wide variety of image reconstruction programs in their office. This software allows the physician to insert a picture of the patient and contrast it with the expected outcomes of the surgery. This helps patients both to decide whether the surgery is warranted and to develop realistic expectations of the surgery.

7. Many physicians' offices have a special defibrillator called an automated external defibrillator (AED). Once the AED is used on a patient, the information from the machine must be downloaded to the patient's chart for legal documentation. After use, the AED is attached to a desktop computer, and the AED sends the report into the computer and then into the patient's record. If the patient's chart is not on computer, the data can be printed on paper and placed in a conventional chart.

8. Some programs can help you with telephone triage. Triage is sorting patients. The software allows you to select a caller's topic and displays a list of relevant questions. The software also provides you some in-

structions for the patient. For example, assume you have a caller with abdominal pain. You type the key words "abdominal pain," and a list of questions appears. These programs log the calls with the date, time, and instructions, which provides legal protection for you.

 CHECKPOINT QUESTION

10. What is a virtual chart?

Administrative Applications

There are hundreds of administrative software packages available for physician offices. Most systems have a combination of features. Some examples of benefits administrative software can bring to the physician's office follow:

1. Appointment making and tracking are more efficient with a computer program than with a book format. As discussed in Chapter 6, good appointment software will allow you to enter appointments quickly and make changes more easily. It should allow for an unlimited comment area near the patient's name. The comment area allows you to add special notes, such as "patient is requesting a pregnancy test." Appointment software can keep a waiting list of patients who are looking for appointments or wanting to move their appointment date and time to the first available time. Appointment software can also automatically print notices to remind patients of the need to make appointments. For example, the program can be set to alert patients who have an annual Pap smear to be sent a letter each year reminding them when it is time for the next one. Appointment software can be integrated with other physicians' offices to allow you to have access to their appointment books. This allows you to see when the next available appointment is. For example, assume your physician makes a referral for Mr. Kearns to see a dermatologist. You would be able to view the schedule of the dermatologist and see when he could get an appointment and then later see if he went for his appointment. Software programs allow appointments to be made only when certain equipment is available. For example, the patient needs a biopsy that is done with a particular laser machine. The machine is available only on Tuesdays, so the program would automatically set the appointment for the patient on a Tuesday.

2. Software can allow you or the office manager to track patient flows. This can be helpful to adjust staff scheduling needs, with more help at the busiest hours or days and less staff on slower days. It can alert managers to productivity of staff members. For example, one physician may average 45 minutes per pa-

tient, while another may average 30 minutes. This allows you to schedule appointments at various intervals and thus promotes patient flow. It can track the time patients wait in the waiting room or examination room. Examining such information allows the staff to change the office flow to decrease waiting times or to indicate the need for additional staff. It can also highlight the days when patients are most likely to cancel their appointments. Patient demographics can be obtained, used for marketing, and allow the office to apply for special funding based on these demographics.

3. Software programs are needed to send insurance claims electronically. You will be able to send claims and track their progress. This allows for faster reimbursement to the practice and can identify problems of reimbursement earlier. The programs that you will use should have access to numerous plans and can be updated frequently and easily.

4. Software programs can allow integration with insurance companies and other businesses to allow for automatic quick payment and posting. This saves time and is less complicated to use than traditional accounting books.

5. Physicians' offices should have software that allows for credit card authorization. A variety of card types should be available (Visa, MasterCard, American Express).

6. Insurance software can allow you to check for patient eligibility. Most programs have enough room for the addresses and phone numbers of the primary, secondary, and tertiary providers. Case manager names should be added when available. Software can also allow for preadmission certifications to be completed and electronically submitted. Preadmission or preauthorization allows you and the patient to verify that the insurance company will cover the procedure or admission. Some software programs come with codes (ICD-9, CPT, HCPCS) and anesthesia codes preinstalled.

7. Again, programs must aim to comply with HIPAA's Privacy Rule; these programs allow you to document your adherence to these rules and regulations.

8. Other programs alert you to send collection letters. These programs have a variety of template collection letters. Always double-check the information before sending a collection letter. More information on how to collect past due accounts is discussed in Chapter 13.

9. A variety of financial software programs track accounts receivable and accounts payable. You may need to adjust the billing cycles to meet the needs of the office in which you are working. Software programs can also automate the tickler system.

10. Automated payroll software can automatically calculate tax deductions and other deductions. You will be able to arrange for direct deposit of employee checks through these software programs.

11. You will find transcription systems in most physicians' offices. These programs help you transcribe various medical reports quickly and effectively.

12. A medical office cannot run effectively without a word processing system. These systems help you write letters and other types of documentation.

13. An important part of any administrative software is the section that handles the personnel records. Contracts, disciplinary reports, performance evaluations, and so on can all be stored in a virtual personnel record.

Paging System Software

Some physicians carry a pager. In some offices, other staff members may also be assigned pagers. Always double-check to make sure that the physician you are paging is the one on call. Most paging systems allow you to type alphabetic (alpha) messages versus a numerical code. A numerical message is simply a telephone number. An alpha message is a written message that is displayed on the pager; for example, "Call the office regarding Ms. Home's blood gas results." Here are some guidelines regarding paging:

- Always provide a return phone number unless you are asking the physician to call the office.
- Watch your spelling on alpha pages.
- Keep the message short and concise.
- Keep track of what time the message was sent, and repage if there is no response.
- If it is an emergency page and there is no response, repage or page another physician as per office policy.
- Never give out pager numbers to patients or sales representatives.
- If you are given a pager, do not give the pager number to anyone. Insert fresh batteries when the battery icon is first showing; treat the pager with care and respect. Notify the office manager immediately if it is lost or stolen.

 CHECKPOINT QUESTION

11. What items may be included in a virtual personnel record?

PowerPoint

Physicians are often asked to do formal presentations. These presentations may be made at support group meetings or hospital staff meetings or to other physicians or professional inservices. The most popular program used to write presentations is PowerPoint. Using this software, the physician will create slides. The slides can then be shown on a projection screen by connecting a computer to a projector. Most often a laptop computer is used. PowerPoint can also be used to produce handouts, posters, etc. You may be asked to print slides or handouts for the program or to transfer files. Use the tutorial software for tips on making presentations.

Meeting Maker

Meeting Maker is a common package that promotes internal coordination of meetings and calendars. This system is primarily used in large practices with multiple offices and multiple administrative personnel. This is how the system works. Everyone is listed as a user. Each user enters his or her schedule into a personal calendar. Calendars can be seen daily, weekly, or monthly. For example, you may type in, "Monday, Kernersville office, 8 AM–4 PM; Tuesday, Southside office, 10 AM–5 PM" The system allows you to view other people's calendars. It is possible to allow other people to enter data into your calendar. You can also maintain a list of tasks and print your schedule. If you are asked to arrange a staff meeting, you enter the names of the people who should come, and the computer will select a date and time that is convenient for everyone.

Handheld Computers

Some physicians use a handheld computer, or personal digital assistant (PDA). A handheld device can do almost anything that your desktop computer can do. Companies that make PDA software can be found at the following three Web addresses: www.pdacortex .com, www.skyscape.com, and www.handheldmed .com. At minimum, handheld computers come with software that can do these functions:

* Address book
* Calendar
* Memo pad
* E-mail
* Word processing

Information can be entered into the handheld device either with a stylus (pen) or on a small keyboard. It is possible to attach a regular-size keyboard to a PDA. Information can be sent back and forth between a PDA and a desktop computer in either of two ways. The PDA can be placed in a cradle that is connected via a cable to the desktop ("hot sync"), or information can be sent via e-mail. PDAs can beam information among themselves (business cards, memos) and can attach their modem through a cellular phone for Internet access.

Physicians often add software that allows them to:

* Access patients' charts
* Set up a virtual office
* View financial data
* Use pharmacy and formulary dosing tools
* Access Micromedx (drug information, toxicology, databases)
* View procedures that they may not routinely do, enhancing lifesaving skills

Purchasing a Computer

Purchasing a new office computer system or updating an existing one is a very important business decision. All key members of the staff should be consulted prior to such a purchase and should be actively involved in selecting the hardware and software. Here are some general guidelines to follow when shopping for a computer and software:

* Determine your specific needs. For example, do you need both clinical and administrative applications?
* Visit physicians' offices and clinics to see what other medical office staff are using. Ask questions: How user friendly are the programs? How long did it take to educate the staff? What does the staff like and dislike about the programs?
* Try out many software packages. Most have demonstrator disks that can be used to evaluate the system.
* Interview and compare different computer vendors. Find out:

1. How long they have been in service
2. How many service representatives they have and whether they are available 24 hours a day
3. Specifics of the system
4. Specifics of any service and warranty contracts they provide
5. What training they provide and at what additional cost
6. How to transfer data into the new system
7. How much the system costs
8. Whether the software can be customized and at what cost
9. What is their response time for service or technical support calls
10. Whether their programs are HIPAA compliant

Independent computer consultants can be hired to evaluate your particular office and make specific recommendations. This option is often more expensive initially but can save money in the long run.

Training Options

To achieve the optimal benefit from any computer or software package, you must be trained in its use. There are a number of ways that this can be accomplished:

* The company from which the computer was purchased may provide personnel to train you and other staff members.
* A user manual will come with your system. You can refer to it when you have problems.
* Help screens installed with every software package allow the user to self-teach. The disadvantage of this method is that it is often time consuming.
* Most software packages come with a tutorial. This is an on-screen short course on the use of the software.
* Most computer manufacturers and software programs

will have a service called a help desk, which provides technical support. It is usually accessed by calling a toll-free number and is manned by computer professionals who can answer your questions concerning the system.

A combination of these methods is the best approach to learning about your computer and software.

Computer Ethics

The computer is a must in all physicians' offices. Its capabilities are endless. It can, however, lead to invasion of patients' privacy and unethical behavior. Some key points to keep in mind are:

- Never give out your login password. New employees must be issued their own password.
- Never leave a screen open with patient information and walk away from the computer. Exit the file.
- Only key people need access to sensitive patient information. Some programs, such as those with laboratory results, should have individual passwords.
- Physicians can often access patient data (e.g., radiology and laboratory reports) from the hospital computers. The hospital gives the physician a special code. It is not appropriate for the physician to share this with staff members. Never use another person's password to get patient information unless instructed to do so by a supervisor. You should be given your own code by the administrator of the program.
- Do not use the office Internet access for anything other than work-related tasks. It is inappropriate to surf the Internet for personal reasons while at work.
- E-mails should be read only by the person to whom they were sent. To avoid conflicts, the physician should have his or her own e-mail account, and the practice should have a generic e-mail address. It is never appropriate for you to receive personal e-mail messages on the office's e-mail address. It is also inappropriate to access your personal e-mail while at work.
- Sensitive patient data should not be sent via e-mail from one office to the other unless it is clearly known that the recipient of the e-mail is the only one with access to it. It is a common practice to send patient information to the consulting physician. This information may include cancer diagnosis, HIV testing, and drug abuse reports. Extreme caution must be used.
- If you are allowed access to local laboratories to obtain laboratory results, it is to be used only on patients in your practice. It is unethical and illegal to obtain other people's reports. For example, if your son had a throat culture done at the pediatrician's office and sent to the laboratory you have access to, you should not look up his results.
- Do not take advantage of your position in the medical field. Remember, you have a legal and ethical responsibility to protect patient information.

CHECKPOINT QUESTION

12. What is a tutorial?

SPANISH TERMINOLOGY

Asegurese de buscar los iconos en el sitio de web para asegurarse de su credibilidad.
  Be sure you look for the icons on a website to ensure its credibility.

Tenga cautela al comprar medicamentos en el internet.
  Be careful if you buy medications online.

Nuestro sistema computarizado es securo y privado.
  Our computer system is secure and private.

MEDIA MENU

- **Student CD**
- **Case Study**
  Administrative Interactive Case Study 3: Conduct Patient Teaching
- **CMA/RMA Certification Exam Review**
- **Premium Online Course**
  http://thePoint.lww.com/Kronenberger3e
- **Internet Resources**

LiveAdvise Online Tutoring & Competency Training
http://thePoint.lww.com/LiveAdvise

OSHA Safety and Health Topics: Ergonomics
www.osha-slc.gov/SLTC/ergonomics/index.html

Typing Injuries Frequently Asked Questions
www.tifaq.com

U.S. Department of Health and Human Services
www.healthfinder.gov

Medline Plus
www.medlineplus.gov

HealthCentral
www.healthcentral.com

WebMD
www.mywebmd.com

Mayo Clinic
www.mayoclinic.com

FamilyDoctor
www.familydoctor.org

Rare Disease Search Engine
www.raredisease.org (this site has a database of over 1000 rare diseases and over 900 drugs that can be used to treat rare diseases)

PROCEDURE 9-1: Caring For and Maintaining Computer Hardware

Purpose: To prolong the life of computer hardware by following certain guidelines and performing preventative maintenance

Equipment: Computer CPU, monitor, keyboard, mouse, printer, duster, simulated warranties

Steps	Reasons
1. Place the monitor, keyboard, and printer in a cool dry area out of direct sunlight.	Sunlight can damage casings, and heat and cold are also harmful to hardware.
2. Place the computer desk on an antistatic floor mat or carpet.	Static electricity can cause memory loss, inaccurate data collection, and other adverse reactions.
3. Clean the monitor screen with antistatic wipes.	Glass cleaner is not recommended.
4. Use dust covers for the keyboard and the monitor when they are not in use.	Dust can accumulate and cause the keyboard and mouse to stick and malfunction.
5. When moving the computer, lock the hard drive.	This will protect the CPU and disk drives.
6. Keep keyboard and mouse free of debris and liquids. Dust and/or vacuum the keyboard periodically to eliminate dust particles under the key pads.	Dust and debris can be hazardous to the keyboard and cause the keys to stick, etc. Never eat or drink when using the computer.

Step 6: Keep the keyboard free of dust and debris.

Steps	Reasons
7. Create a file for maintenance and warranty contracts for the computer system.	This will allow quick and easy retrieval of phone numbers, etc. if a representative is needed.
8. Handle data storage disks with special care.	Scratches, fingerprints, etc. can corrupt data

PROCEDURE 9-2: Searching on the Internet

Purpose: To quickly and effectively search the Internet, resulting in good time management
Equipment: Computer with Web browser software, modem, active Internet connection account

Steps	Purpose
1. Connect your computer to the Internet.	An Internet connection is necessary to search the Internet.
2. Locate a search engine.	A search engine is necessary to find information on the Internet.
3. Select two or three key words and type them at the appropriate place on the Web page.	Key words tell the search engine what to look for.
4. View the number of search results. If no sites were found, check spelling and retype or choose new key words.	The search engine was unable to find sites that can provide the information you requested.
5. If the search produced a long list, do an advanced search and refine your key words.	Reading through numerous sites is not time efficient.
6. Select an appropriate site and open its home page.	This allows you to view the information on the website.
7. If you are satisfied with the site's information, either download the material or bookmark the page. If you are unsatisfied with its information, either visit a site listed on the results page or return to the search engine.	Downloading or bookmarking the information gives you access to it in the future.

- Computers are an essential piece of technology in the medical office.
- As a medical assistant, you will use the computer for both clinical and administrative tasks. Computers will help you perform your job more efficiently, timely, and professionally.
- You will take precautions to comply with HIPAA's Administrative Simplification and Privacy Rules.
- Computers promote good patient care.
- You will be able to communicate with various health care professionals by using electronic mail.

- The Internet plays a key role in medicine.
- Patients, physicians, and medical assistants use the Internet to find new medical cures and for seeking current information about various health topics.
- You will need to be able to navigate the Web quickly and safely.
- It is essential that you stay abreast of computer technology, as it changes and improves daily.

Warm Ups for Critical Thinking

1. Log on to the Internet and locate a search engine. Search for a medical topic. It can be administrative or clinical. What are your key words? How many sites are listed? Now, using the same key words, use the advanced search engine. How many sites are listed? What are the benefits of using the advanced search method?

2. Select any five Web addresses listed in this chapter, and view the homepage. What benefits do the sites offer? What information or topics were missing?

3. Review the Patient Education Box about selecting websites safely. Find three websites that use these types of phrases or words. Do you think these sites are misleading? Do you think they pose a danger to patients?

4. Your office manager asks you to serve on a committee to purchase an electronic medical record system. Formulate a list of questions that you can ask a vendor before buying a computer system.

5. List five Web addresses for a patient who has just been diagnosed with type 2 diabetes.

Answers to Checkpoint Questions

1. The CPU cells read, analyze, and process data and instruct the computer how to operate a given program.

2. Ethernet is a type of networking technology for local area networks. Your computer should have an Ethernet port or Ethernet interface card so that it can be connected to a cable or DSL provider.

3. The two types of Internet connections that are recommended for downloading large files are DSL and cable.

4. The encryption feature scrambles messages as they leave your site and unscrambles them when they arrive at the receiver's site.

5. In order to protect the privacy of an e-mail message sent from a patient, you should print or record the information in the e-mail, delete or shred the paper copy, and issue passwords to those who need to see e-mails from patients.

6. A search engine allows you to find the sites that will have the information that you need quickly and efficiently.

7. A literary search is different because it is searching for a professional journal article that addresses a topic versus searching for general information.

8. Questionable websites can be reported to the Federal Trade Commission (FTC) at www.ftc.gov.

9. The benefits of the intranet are enhanced communication, quick access to needed information, increased productivity, and enhanced security.

10. A virtual chart is a paperless chart that holds all necessary documents on the computer.

11. Contracts, disciplinary reports, and performance evaluations can all be stored in a virtual personnel record.

12. A tutorial is an on-screen short course on the use of a certain software.

Outline

OVERVIEW OF MEDICAL OF-FICE MANAGEMENT
Organizational Structure
The Medical Office Manager
RESPONSIBILITIES OF THE MEDICAL OFFICE MAN-AGER
Communication
Staffing Issues
Policy and Procedures Manuals

Developing Promotional Materials
Financial Concerns
Office Maintenance
Management of Inventory and Supplies
Education
RISK MANAGEMENT
Liability Insurance
Incident Reports

QUALITY IMPROVEMENT PRO-GRAMS
Regulatory Agencies
DEVELOPING A QUALITY IM-PROVEMENT PROGRAM
Seven Steps for a Successful Program
PUTTING IT ALL TOGETHER: A CASE REVIEW

Learning Objectives

Upon successfully completing this chapter, you will be able to:

1. Spell and define the key terms

2. Describe what is meant by organizational structure

3. List seven responsibilities of the medical office manager

4. Explain the five staffing issues that a medical office manager will be responsible for handling

5. List the types of policies and procedures that should be included in a medical office's policy and procedures manual

6. List five types of promotional materials that a medical office may distribute

7. Discuss financial concerns that the medical office manager must be capable of addressing

8. Describe the duties regarding office maintenance, inventory, and service contracts.

9. Discuss the need for continuing education

10. Discuss the need for general liability and medical malpractice insurance

11. List three services provided by most medical malpractice companies

12. List six guidelines for completing incident reports

13. List four regulatory agencies that require medical offices to have quality improvement programs

14. Describe the accreditation process of The Joint Commission

15. Describe the steps to developing a quality improvement program

16. Explain how quality improvement programs and risk management work together in a medical office to improve overall patient care and employee needs

Competencies

CAAHEP

- Use methods of quality control
- Demonstrate knowledge of federal and state health care legislation and regulations
- Perform within legal and ethical boundaries

ABHES

- Monitor legislation related to current health care issues and practices
- Perform risk management procedures
- Maintain physical plant
- Maintain liability insurance

Key Terms

budget	incident reports	organizational chart	quality improvement
compliance officer	job description	policy	sentinel event
expected threshold	mission statement	procedure	task force

A successful medical practice needs an effective medical office management process. This process must be a team effort among the physicians, nurse managers, and the office manager. A medical practice must manage risk and engage in ongoing quality improvement procedures. This chapter provides an overview of medical office management, a medical office manager's specific responsibilities, as well as a discussion of risk management and quality improvement.

Overview of Medical Office Management

Each medical office is organized in a slightly different manner, depending on the size and complexity of the setting.

Organizational Structure

The medical office's organizational structure, or chain of command, is depicted in an **organizational chart**, a flow sheet that allows the manager and employees to identify their team members and to see where they fit into the team. Figure 10-1 displays a sample organizational chart for a physician's office in which there is a partnership between two physicians. In this example, it is assumed that the physicians have an equal partnership in the practice.

 CHECKPOINT QUESTION

1. What is the purpose of an organizational chart?

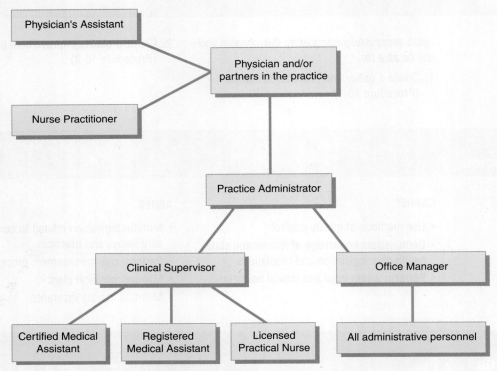

Figure 10-1 Sample organizational chart.

The Medical Office Manager

The medical office manager must be multiskilled, multi-talented, and able to prioritize a variety of issues, juggle responsibilities, and communicate effectively with patients, staff, and physicians. In some settings, the medical office manager may be referred to as the business manager. Managers may be nurses, medical assistants, or administrative support personnel. Although the qualifications and educational requirements for the position vary greatly among health care organizations, a successful medical office manager must be:

- Flexible
- A positive role model for employees
- Honest and fair
- A good communicator
- A resource person for employees
- Supportive of all management decisions
- Well organized
- Able to focus on a given task
- Able to resolve conflicts
- Able to see the big picture
- A continuous learner

A medical office manager's responsibilities include varied tasks:

- Communicating with patients, physicians, and staff
- Handling staffing issues
- Writing and revising policy and procedures manuals
- Developing promotional materials

- Handling financial concerns
- Handling office maintenance
- Managing supplies and inventory
- Ensuring that the staff receives appropriate education
- Maintaining budgets
- Enforcing HIPAA regulations and other accrediting agency regulations

A medical office manager also must keep abreast of important legal issues, such as medical practice acts, employment and safety laws, patient care laws, billing and insurance regulations, and more. See Chapter 2 for more details on these topics.

Responsibilities of the Medical Office Manager

Communication

Perhaps one of the hardest and yet most important aspects of being an effective manager is being able to communicate with fellow employees, colleagues, physicians, and patients. (The techniques for effective communication are discussed in Chapter 3.) You must be a good listener, have good interpersonal skills, and be aware of your own nonverbal language.

Communicating With Patients

Communication with patients on a management level can often be challenging. Patients come to you with a variety of complaints, such as incorrect billing, poor care, or long waits to see physicians. Of course, you must always be diplomatic. Your goal should be to correct the problem in a timely and professional manner and to alleviate any negative feelings the patient may have.

Communicating With Staff

Communication with staff members can be difficult, depending on the number of employees, number and locations of satellite centers, and the variety of shifts that are in place. There are three ways to promote communication with staff members: staff meetings, bulletin boards, and communication notebooks. It is a good idea to ask your staff for input in deciding the best way to communicate with them.

Staff Meetings

Staff meetings should be scheduled at a predictable frequency and time to allow the staff to plan (e.g., they might be held the first Monday of every month at 8 AM). *Meetings should never be canceled except in a true emergency.*

Staff meetings must be well organized and should begin and end on time. Agendas should be created prior to the meeting and posted for staff review. (See Chapter 7 for information on agendas.) The agenda should be followed as closely as possible. Individual staff concerns or complaints should not be handled during a general staff meeting; the meeting should remain focused and constructive and not turn into a battleground for staff disagreements. Minutes should be taken and kept in a notebook for staff to review as needed. (See Chapter 7 for information on minutes.)

Staff meetings should be conducted in a private area out of patients' sight and hearing (Fig. 10-2). All interruptions, except for emergencies, should be avoided.

Have the telephone covered by an answering service or a prerecorded message informing callers of the time

Figure 10-2 Staff meeting being conducted in a private area.

the staff will be unavailable. Lock the door, and place a sign with the time the office will reopen. Of course, you will give clear instructions to callers or visitors who have an emergency. The personnel manual should clearly state the attendance policy for staff meetings. In addition, some offices include attendance as a duty in each employee's **job description** (statement of work-related responsibilities). To improve attendance at staff meetings, consider serving food or including an educational presentation. Involve staff as much as possible when setting the meeting agenda.

Bulletin Boards

Bulletin board postings allow employees to get a quick and easy look at new polices or procedures. To encourage staff members to read the postings, make sure the bulletin boards are attractive, well organized, and updated regularly. It is a good idea to have employees initial all messages on the bulletin board after reading them.

Communication Notebooks

A simple notebook can serve as a two-way communication tool: You can write messages to employees, and they can write back to you. Such a notebook is usually kept in the staff lounge. Again, staff members should initial any important messages after reading them. If the message is directed to you, be sure to respond as soon as possible. One medical office places a note book with pertinent information for employees in staff restrooms and titles it "Potty Training."

Communicating Electronically

E-mail has become popular and is an easy and time-saving way to communicate with staff. Messages can be printed and kept in a binder for easy reference. E-mail messages eliminate the need for memos that must be posted or circulated. Your e-mail system will provide you with an address book that can be customized to include groups such as all employees, all clinical employees, employees and physicians, and so on.

Sometimes, the stress of daily duties prevents managers from communicating with staff members on a personal level. To be an effective manager, you should communicate not only bad news but also positive messages to your employees. You can communicate positive messages through birthday and holiday cards and employee recognition awards. Send thank you notes to the staff to compliment them when they go above and beyond the call of duty.

CHECKPOINT QUESTION

2. What are three ways to promote communication with staff members?

Staffing Issues

Staffing issues will occupy most of your time as an office manager. These concerns include writing job descriptions, hiring new employees, evaluating present employees, taking disciplinary actions, handling terminations, and scheduling. Sometimes an office manager also becomes a coach and a counselor.

Writing Job Descriptions

Each job must have a description. The purpose of a job description is to inform the employee about the essential job duties and expectations for a given position. Job descriptions also help you in interviewing applicants and evaluating existing employees.

Each employee should receive a copy of his or her job description at the time of hiring and after any revisions to the description are made. Some medical offices have a policy requiring the employee to read and sign the job description at the time of hiring and for each annual evaluation.

Formats for writing job descriptions vary among offices. In general, the following elements are included: job title, supervisor, position summary, hours, location, employment requirements, physical requirements, duties, and the evaluation process (Fig. 10-3). The description should also include the date it was written and date of any revisions.

If possible, involve staff members in writing and revising their job descriptions. Employee participation leads to greater cooperation.

LEGAL TIP

MAKE SURE YOUR INTERVIEW QUESTIONS ARE APPROPRIATE

Title VII of the Civil Rights Act prohibits discrimination in the workplace. To ensure that hiring practices are fair and nondiscriminatory, be careful and consistent in the types of questions asked in an interview. You may ask work-related questions like, "Are you proficient in typing?" Avoid questions that might give the appearance of discrimination. You may not ask applicants their age, race, religion, or marital status. You cannot ask about children, day care, or plans for future children.

Hiring and Interviewing Employees

Only after creating or reviewing an existing job description can you begin the process of interviewing and hiring a new employee. You can seek applicants through advertising in local newspaper classified sections, place-

ment personnel at local schools that offer medical assisting programs, networking, and employment agencies.

All applicants should complete an application. State laws vary regarding the types of questions that can be asked on applications. In general, you must avoid any questions pertaining to an applicant's age, sex, race, national origin, religion, and physical or mental disabilities. If your medical facility requires a criminal background check and drug testing, the form should include this information with a place for the applicant to give necessary permission with a signature. Any employee application form should be reviewed by legal counsel prior to its use. It is always a good idea to request that the applicant bring a résumé to the interview.

Before interviewing an applicant, prepare a list of questions. Again, use caution; under law, you are not permitted to ask about some topics. Ask only questions that are job related. Ask questions like, "Tell me about a time when you disagreed with your supervisor. How did you handle it?" This type of "behavioral interviewing" will give the interviewer the most information about the candidate's job knowledge and behavior. During the interview, assess the applicant's ability to do the following:

- Perform technical skills
- Treat patients in a caring manner
- Fit into your organization
- Communicate in a professional yet friendly manner
- Remain flexible

Be consistent and fair when selecting the best candidate.

ETHICAL TIP

Tough Spot

Consider this scenario: A co-worker tells you that a newly hired employee says she is a CMA, but you have a mutual friend who says this person never passed the exam. Should you share this information with anyone? YES. This would constitute fraud. Unfortunately, some people are dishonest and unethical. It would be unethical for you to ignore the information. Tell the office manager who can then verify the employee's stated credentials by calling the appropriate state licensing board or certification registry. You can check any license or certification for currency. A CMA's status can be obtained by calling 1-800-ACT-AAMA. Many state medical assisting societies also have certification registries. Try going to the particular profession's website.

Job Description

Title: Medical Assistant

Supervisor(s): Clinical Supervisor

Office Manager for Administrative Duties

Position summary: This is a 40-hour position that will require the employee to perform various duties including administrative, clinical, and laboratory procedures. Scheduling will be variable to meet the needs of the office.

Hours: Hours will vary to meet the needs of the office. Hours will rotate from 8:00 AM–4:30 PM and 10:00 AM–6:30 PM. You will be expected to work one Saturday per month.

Location: Our main office is located at 129 South Main Street. The satellite office is located at 56 West Road, Suite 102. This position will primarily require you to work at our main office. However, occasional days may be assigned at the satellite office.

Employment Requirements: The employee must have graduated from a medical assisting program. CMA or RMA is preferred. The employee must have a current CPR and First Aid card. One year of experience or completion of an externship is preferred.

• *Language skills:* The employee must be able to read and interpret documents and respond appropriately (verbally and/or in writing). Must be able to document in a professional manner.

• *Mathematical skills:* The employee must be able to add, subtract, multiply, and divide whole numbers and fractions.

Physical requirements: The following are physical requirements for this job: Standing: 6–8 hours/day; Sitting: 6–8 hours/day; Lifting: 50 pounds; Twisting and rotating: 45 degrees; Squatting: As needed to assist patients or to perform office tasks.

Duties: You will be expected to perform the following duties after completing the orientation process. This is a partial list; and other duties can be added as necessary.

Administrative:
Scheduling appointments
Transcribing documents
Filing
Completing insurance forms

Processing mail
Operating the telephone
Providing patient education

Clinical/Laboratory:
Operating centrifuge
Performing phlebotomy
Performing HCT/HGB/CBC
Performing pregnancy and monospot tests
Obtaining visual acuities

Obtaining vital signs
Administering vaccines and other medications
  as ordered
Providing patient education
Assisting the physician as directed

Evaluation process: Three evaluations will be conducted in the first year. Thirty days from start date, ninety days from start date, and then at the one-year anniversary date. Following the first year of employment, annual evaluations will be done.

I have read my job description, and I understand what is expected of me. I am able to physically perform all the required duties.

Signature of employee: _____ Date: _____

Signature of supervisor: _____ Date: _____

Signature of supervisor: _____ Date: _____

Figure 10-3 Sample job description

WHAT IF?

You receive a call requesting a reference for an employee who was fired. What should you say?

Be careful! This situation can turn into a legal and ethical nightmare if not handled appropriately. If you give a wonderful report to the potential employer and say, "She was great; never had any problems," you and the office may be sued by the former employee for wrongful discharge. In court, you would be asked, "If she was so wonderful, why did you fire her?" On the other hand, if you say, "She was a terrible employee, and we fired her," you can be sued for defamation of character. Because of the legal concerns in providing employment references, most organizations have a policy stating that the only information to be released is verification of employment dates and job titles. When in doubt, give no information. Ask for the caller's name and phone number; discuss the issue with the physician in charge, and then return the phone call.

Evaluating Employees

All employees must be evaluated annually. The evaluation should be a positive experience for the employee. Employee evaluations must be fair, accurate, and objective. Some type of written evaluation should be given to the employee to read, sign, and comment on. Most forms ask employees to list their objectives and goals for the coming year. Figure 10-4 displays a sample evaluation form. Some organizations call evaluations performance appraisals.

New employees should be evaluated 1 month after their start date, again in 90 days, and then at their 1-year anniversary date. This process helps new employees gain confidence and improve weaknesses. Coaching and counseling should occur throughout the year. The employee should know what will be said during the feedback because the manager has communicated with them throughout the year. An employee should never be surprised by the feedback.

Taking Disciplinary Action

Most offices have policies regarding documentation of disciplinary action. Disciplinary actions can be verbal or written. Verbal warnings are generally done for a first-time minor occurrence (e.g., not showing up for work and not calling in). A note should go into the employee's file stating that a verbal warning was given, the date, any actions that were taken, and any comments that the employee made.

Written notices are used for more serious problems (e.g., breaching patient confidentiality, substance abuse) or recurrent minor ones. Employees should sign any written warning notices. These documents can be used as evidence in the event that the person is fired and brings a lawsuit for wrongful discharge. Figure 10-5 shows a sample written disciplinary action form. Determine whether the employee's credentialing agency should be notified of serious infractions.

Terminating Employees

Having to terminate (fire) an employee is never an easy or pleasant task. It is essential that policies regarding termination be followed precisely. All disciplinary actions must be clearly and objectively stated. Terminating employees for unlawful reasons or failing to follow the organization's termination policy can result in lawsuits against you and the office. When disciplining an employee, make sure to ask yourself if other employees have committed the same policy violations. Have they all been treated the same? Some reasons for termination include:

- Excessive tardiness or absenteeism
- Inappropriate dress or behavior
- Alcohol or drug use
- Endangering patients
- Lying or stealing
- Falsifying medical records or time sheets
- Breaching patient confidentiality

Scheduling

The primary goal of scheduling is to meet the needs of the office. The secondary goal is to meet the requests of your employees. You must be fair in scheduling and always follow your organization's policies for weekend and holiday or personal day requests. If possible, employees should be given time off with pay when attending seminars and meetings of their professional organization. This practice will keep morale high and encourage employees to stay current with their skills. Depending on the number of employees that you have to schedule and the complexity of the hours or shifts, you can either schedule by hand or use a computer program. If your organization is small and cohesive, you may want to assign a senior staff member to do the scheduling, or you might allow the employees to self-schedule. No matter what scheduling format is used, you are ultimately responsible for ensuring that the appropriate number and type of employees needed are scheduled.

Requests for time off should be put in writing. Depending on the size of the organization, such requests may have to be received by a given date or time. For ex-

Employee Evaluation Form

Employee: *Jackie England*
Evaluation Date: *5/2/08*
Job Title: *CMA*
Ratings:

Traits	Score
Appearance	5
Communication Skills	3
Attendance	4
Quality of work	5
Reliability	4
Initiative	4
Other: *Willingness to work as a team*	5
Total Score:	30

Rating scale:
5—excellent
4—above average
3—meets job expectations
2—below job expectations
1—does not meet job expectations

Supervisor comments:
Is an excellent CMA. She is shy with patients + co-workers, but improving

Employee goals for the next year (to be completed by employee):
I will continue to attain CEU's for recertifiction. I plan to take class on being assertive.

Employee Comments:
I love working here and appreciate having good + fair bosses.

Supervisor signature: *Diane Hall*   Date: *5/2/08*
Employee signature: *Jackie England*   Date: *5/2/08*

Figure 10-4 Sample employee evaluation form.

ample, the policy may read, "A request for a day off in May should be submitted by April 15. Any requests for time off filed after the cutoff date will be approved whenever possible." This eliminates repeated adjustment of the staffing schedule.

 CHECKPOINT QUESTION

3. What is the medical office manager's primary goal in scheduling?

Policy and Procedures Manuals

Every business needs written rules and regulations to ensure that its practices are within legal and ethical boundaries. Employees need written procedures to ensure consistency in the practices of the business. In the outpatient medical facility, these written policies and procedures are *required* by regulatory and accrediting agencies.

It is the office manager's responsibility to coordinate the orientation and training of any new employee. A

Discipline Record

Employee Name: _Billie Elliott_ #: _26_ Date of Warning: _5/28/08_

Warning

Date of Violation: _5/28/08_ Time: _9:15 AM_ Place: _Exam Room 1_

Description of Violation:

Billie was assisting Dr. Bay c̄ minor surgery. She took no action when the sterile field was compromised. The possibly contaminated field was not reset. She told no one. It was questioned by the patient.

_____ Verbal Warning
_____ Written Warning
__✔__ Probation ___30___ Days
_____ Suspension _____ Days
_____ Termination
Dana Hudson, CMA
Supervisor's Signature

Action To Be Taken:
Billie is placed on probation for 30 days. Another occurrence will mean possible dismissal.

_____
Date

Employee's Remarks

Do you agree with the details above: Yes: __✔__ No: _____

Comments: _I understand the seriousness of my error. It will never happen again._

Employee's Signature: _Billie Elliott_ Date: _5/28/08_

Figure 10-5 Sample disciplinary action form.

personnel manual that includes the organization's policies and outlines step-by-step procedures for each task performed in the facility becomes the new employee's information source. Even veteran employees may have to refer to the proper procedure for a task. As new procedures become available or existing procedures are changed, this is added to the procedures manual. Tips regarding policy and procedures manual are detailed in Box 10-1.

Most organizations create a policy and procedures manual that is written, maintained, and regarded as one document. A **policy** is a statement regarding the organization's rules on a given topic. A **procedure** is a series of steps required to perform a given task. Policies and procedures must be written in a clear, concise, and understandable format. Each policy or procedure is signed by the employees, indicating they have read, understand, and will adhere to the policy or procedure. Policies regarding medical office management are signed by the physician and supervisory staff.

Types of Policies and Procedures

There are many types of policies and procedures. In general, the following areas are included in a policy and procedures manual:

1. Mission statement
2. Organizational structure
3. Human resources or personnel
4. Quality improvement and risk management
5. Clinical procedures
6. Administrative procedures
7. Infection control

Section 1: Mission Statement.

A mission statement describes the goals of the practice and whom it serves. Often a mission statement provides a philosophical look at an organization. It is generally one to two paragraphs long (Fig. 10-6).

The mission statement should not only be included in the policy and procedures manual; it should also be

BOX 10-1

TIPS REGARDING PERSONNEL MANUALS

- Form a personnel committee. If staff members help develop the policies and procedures, they are more likely to follow them.

- Determine the rules and regulations of the office with the physician and managers.

- Contact local organizations, medical offices, or ambulatory care centers and ask for copies of their personnel manuals including policies and procedures.

- Research state and federal laws that regulate the medical office.

- Ensure compliance by appointing a **compliance officer.**

- Keep personnel manuals in a central location so they are available to each employee for review.

- Review all policies and procedures annually to make sure they are up to date and accurate.

BOX 10-2

TYPES OF HUMAN RESOURCES POLICIES

Absentee policies
Cafeteria plans
Confidentiality policy
Continuing education requirements
Disciplinary action procedures
Emergency procedures
Employee benefits (health and dental insurance)
Evaluation and performance appraisals
Grievance procedures
Grooming, uniforms, appearance
Holiday coverage and compensation for holidays
Jury duty
Office hours
Orientation
Overtime reports
Parking
Payroll
Personal phone calls
Resignations
Sexual harassment
Sick leave and family leave
Staff meetings
Tardiness
Termination process
Time recording
Vacation days

available to patients. Often it is framed and placed in the waiting room or printed in the practice brochure.

Section 2: Organizational Structure

The organizational chart is included in this section along with policies regarding the following:

- Chain of command
- How and when to contact various members of the team
- Coverage for managers
- Physician on-call policies

Section 3: Human Resources or Personnel

This section consists of policies relating to staff responsibilities, benefits, and rules and regulations for employ-

North Shore Family Practice is a group practice dedicated to providing quality care through compassion, innovation, performance and education. It is our goal to provide medical care to the community of Rochester, New York. The physicians, nurse practitioners, and all staff members are committed to working together as a team to provide the patient with the best care possible.

Figure 10-6 Sample mission statement

ees. Box 10-2 lists the kinds of policies found in this section of the manual. A sample human resources policy is displayed in Figure 10-7.

Section 4: Quality Improvement and Risk Management

This section includes policies outlining who is in charge of **quality improvement,** the steps for developing a quality improvement plan, and explanations of incident reporting, discussed later.

Section 5: Clinical Procedures

Any task that requires intervention with a patient should be listed in this section. (Some offices separate laboratory procedures into a different section for convenience.) In addition, clinical procedures should include specific infection control guidelines for the particular procedure, patient education guidelines, and instructions for documentation. Sample documentation forms should be included in this section. It is a good idea to complete the sample form correctly so that it can serve as a model. In the medical office, these procedures

Benjamin William, MD
2295 Matthews Drive
Boca Raton, Florida 33432
POLICY AND PROCEDURE MANUAL

Policy title: Human Resources, Absences
Purpose: The purpose of this policy is to advise all employees of the policy for absences and to prewarn employees regarding the disciplinary steps that will be taken as a result of not complying with this policy.
Equipment/Forms necessary: No equipment or forms are required.
Explanation:

• If you are going to call in sick, you must call in two hours prior to your assigned time. Messages should be left with the answering service if the office is not open.
• If you have personal days accrued, you can use them for compensation.
• If you are going to be out sick for more than three consecutive working days, you will need to obtain a physician's note to document the illness.
• Employees are allowed six (6) absences per year without disciplinary action. Seven (7) absences will result in a verbal warning regarding attendance. Eight (8) absences will result in a written warning. Nine (9) absences will result in termination. Exceptions to disciplinary action will be reviewed on an individual basis and are at the joint discretion of the office manager and physician.

_____   _____
Susan Rogers, RMA   Benjamin William, MD
Office Manager

date: original policy - 06/96, revised 07/08
HR: 14

Figure 10-7 Sample human resources policy.

may vary slightly to meet the needs of the office, physicians' requests, or manufacturers' guidelines.

Section 6: Administrative Procedures

This section includes procedures on all tasks that the administrative office staff must perform. Sample forms should also be included and updated as necessary. Examples of administrative tasks are as follows:

• Accounting and bookkeeping
• Appointment scheduling
• Collections
• Computer care and operations
• Insurance filings
• Medical records management
• Mail and postal machine operations

Section 7: Infection Control

Depending on the length of this section, some offices opt for a separate manual dedicated to infection control and prevention. Examples of these policies are as follows:

• Types of personal protection equipment available
• Biohazardous waste disposal
• Handling of various disease identities

• Handling of employee exposures and needlesticks
• Documentation required by the Occupational Safety and Health Administration (OSHA)
• Employee education for infection control

 CHECKPOINT QUESTION

4. Which seven elements must be included when writing a policy or procedure?

Developing Promotional Materials

The medical office manager is often responsible for developing and distributing promotional literature for the practice. Depending on the budget, promotional materials can be created and produced at commercial printing shops or done in the office with desktop publishing programs. Examples of promotional materials follow:

• Education pamphlets and booklets for patients. Be sure to use educational information that has been accredited or approved by an appropriate authority (Fig. 10-8).
• Practice brochures (Box 10-3)
• Newsletters

Figure 10-8 Sample patient brochure.

- Holiday cards
- Birthday cards (usually used by pediatricians)
- Newspaper articles
- Yellow pages
- Direct mail
- Business cards

    Follow these guidelines when creating promotional materials:

- Double-check all spelling and grammar.
- Ensure accuracy.
- Use clear and specific language.
- Avoid abbreviations and complex medical terms.
- Use brightly colored materials.
- If you are using a commercial printer, be sure to review the proofs carefully before the final printing.

Financial Concerns
Budgets

A **budget** is a financial planning tool that helps an organization estimate its anticipated expenditures and revenues. Budgeting has many purposes for an organization:

- Forcing the manager and physician to plan
- Causing managers and staff to become cost conscious
- Promoting communication among staff and managers
- Helping the organization achieve a financial goal

BOX 10-3

INFORMATION TO BE INCLUDED IN AN OFFICE BROCHURE

A well-written, attractive informational brochure will help the office run efficiently and reduce patient questions and confusion. Having this important information in one handy place will not only help patients, but will also provide confidence that you are giving all patients complete and consistent information.

    A patient information brochure should include the following information:

- Name and address of practice with directions
- Office hours
- Provider's names, credentials, and specialties
- Physician's assistants, nurse practitioners, counselors, etc., and their credentials
- Services provided
- Payment policies, insurance claim filing information, major third-party payers accepted
- Phone numbers and extensions for all departments, including emergency numbers
- Procedures for reaching providers after hours
- A statement about how the office handles phone calls, medication refills, triage, etc.
- Be sure to update information as changes occur
- If space allows, you may include all employee names and positions, short biographies of the physicians, etc.

    The medical office generally has both an operating and a capital budget. Operating budgets consist of all costs to run the office. These include but are not limited to payroll, office and medical supplies, education, promotional materials, electricity, telephone services, etc. Capital budgets consist of large outlays of money. These include large purchases (usually over $500), building maintenance, property management, and equipment.

    Developing and writing a budget takes practice and instructions from the financial officer or physician. In general, the previous year's expense report is reviewed, revenues are projected for the following year, and figures are assigned to ensure that income balances with the outgoing expenses.

 CHECKPOINT QUESTION

5. What is the definition of a budget?

Payroll

Another financial concern for the manager is payroll. All employees expect to receive the correct amount of pay on time, and those expectations must be met. Payroll is a complex task that must satisfy state and federal laws regarding deductions for Social Security and other taxes. Because of this and because payroll is so time consuming, some offices outsource this service.

Office Maintenance

One of the medical office manager's key responsibilities is to keep the office neat, clean, safe, efficient, and well organized. Most offices have outside agencies to clean and maintain the lobby, examination rooms, and offices, to do laundry and landscaping, to manage heating and air conditioning, etc. OSHA requires that you use a licensed vender for biohazardous waste disposal. Office manager duties include managing and scheduling these service vendors. These services would be considered accounts payable, which is covered in Chapter 12.

A well-lit, attractive entrance and waiting area reflect quality throughout the facility. Staff should be encouraged to check the lobby periodically for neatness and to assist in routine cleaning and straightening. Remember, special attention to waiting room toys is necessary because they can pose a safety threat to children (see Chapter 5).

Management of Inventory and Supplies

There should be a policy outlining who is responsible for ordering supplies and the procedure for ordering. There also must be some process to check that deliveries of supplies are complete and accurate. Most medical software has a feature for keeping up with supplies. In a manual system, a tickler file can be used. Ordering and receiving supplies is an important part of the office manager's job. In addition to clinical and office equipment, extensive supplies are needed for a medical office. As a medical office manager, you must develop a logical system to keep track of supplies. A tickler system can be used to organize vendor information, supply lists, reorder information, etc. Many computer systems have inventory control and accounts payable capabilities. A spreadsheet can easily be constructed to save information about vendors, dates supplies were ordered, etc. Ordering supplies and accounts payable are covered more thoroughly in Chapter 12.

Office staff members who receive the supplies must check the packing slip against the actual contents to ensure that all supplies are in the shipment. The person should initial the packing slip, which shows that all goods were received. When it is time to issue checks for payables, the assistant can then pay the invoice or bill. These receipts or packing slips should be placed in a bills pending file for payment.

Service Contracts

The medical office manager is responsible for keeping track of all service contracts. A service contract is an agreement between the medical organization and a service company in which the company agrees to perform regular inspections of and care for a specific piece of equipment. Service contracts are usually obtained for copiers, computers, fax machines, and other large and expensive pieces of equipment.

Education
Staff Education

The medical office manager must keep the staff up to date on medical procedures, drugs and vaccines, insurance coding and billing regulations, and any other topics that promote good patient care. In addition to these topics, annual education is usually conducted on cardiopulmonary resuscitation (CPR), infection control, and fire and electrical safety. Most allied health professionals are required to accumulate continuing education units (CEUs). CMAs must receive 60 CEUs every 5 years to retain the CMA credential. The office manager may choose to keep a file for each employee with the necessary documentation. This will assist the staff in the recertification process.

As the medical office manager, you should select an educational topic for each month. In some offices, the educational topic is covered during the monthly staff meetings, whereas other offices have separate educational programs. After choosing the monthly topic, select an appropriate presenter. Suggestions for presenters include colleagues, physicians, sales representatives, local hospital staff development coordinators, and specialists. Presenters for CPR classes must be CPR instructors who are approved by a national organization. To promote attendance, create informative flyers and distribute them to all staff members. Keep attendance records for all classes given.

In addition to formal educational programs, there are other ways to keep your staff up to date. For instance, educational videos and DVDs can be rented or purchased for staff viewing; consider developing a posttest to assess for comprehension. Also, many professional magazines have continuing education articles on various topics, usually accompanied by a posttest. Finally, staff members should be sent to one or two seminars a year. Outside seminars help increase employee productivity, self-esteem, and retention.

Patient Education

All members of the health care team must constantly contribute to educating patients. As a manager, you may not provide patient education directly, but you are responsible for assisting the staff in performing this task. You can help the staff with patient education by creating booklets, developing posters, and by teaching your staff how, when, and what to teach patients and families.

Patient education brochures should be colorful and easy to read. Close attention to spelling, grammar, punctuation, and accuracy is essential. All brochures should be reviewed by a physician. Depending on your office's clientele, the brochures should be printed in various languages. Refer to Chapter 4 for more details on creating patient education brochures.

Manager Education

Managers should attend workshops and conferences and read appropriate printed materials to enhance their knowledge and skills in managing a medical office. All new managers can benefit from courses on time management, stress management, solving personnel conflicts, and budget preparation. Memberships in professional organizations can also assist the new office manager. Two such organizations are:

Medical Office Management Association
1355 South Colorado Boulevard, Suite 900
Denver, CO 80222-3331

Professional Association of Health Care Office
   Management
2929 Langley Avenue, Suite 102
Pensacola, FL 32504-7355

Risk Management

Risk management is an internal process geared to identifying potential problems before they cause injury to patients or employees. Potential problems are related to risk factors. A risk factor is any situation or condition that poses a safety or liability concern for a given practice. Examples of risk factors are poor lighting, clutter, unlocked medication cabinets, failure to dispose of needles properly, and faulty patient identification procedures. Such factors may lead to patient falls, medication errors, employee needlesticks, and mistakes in therapeutic intervention. Risk factors for a particular health care organization are identified through a study of patterns.

Liability Insurance

Doctors today face challenges that those of a generation ago never imagined. As discussed in Chapter 2, physi-cians are at risk for malpractice suits and must use sound practices to decrease this risk. New medical procedures, treatments, and drugs require regular review to ensure each practice meets high standards of safety and care. Physicians need malpractice insurance to protect them from financial loss in the event of a successful lawsuit or settlement. Nurses also carry malpractice insurance, and many allied health professionals are now opting for coverage.

Many malpractice insurance companies offer services such as teaching employees to take preventative measures and to identify problems before they become threats. They also conduct risk inspections, supply self-auditing tools, and provide bulletins. Malpractice insurance websites have many helpful tools for office managers.

A medical office is not just subject to liability regarding patients; since it is a public place, any visitor to the office could slip and fall on a wet floor or be hurt by a picture falling from a wall. As office manager, you should assess the coverage needs of your employees and investigate the possibility of a policy that would cover any employees who need it. Insurance is a large expense but one that a medical practice must incur.

CHECKPOINT QUESTION

6. Why do physicians need malpractice insurance?

Incident Reports

Incident reports, sometimes referred to as occurrence reports, are written accounts of untoward (negative) patient, visitor, or staff events. Such events may be minor or life or limb threatening. The insurance company that provides the institution's liability insurance often requires incident reports.

An incident report is written or completed by the staff member involved in or at the scene of the incident. The report is reviewed by a supervisor for completion and accuracy and is then sent to a central location. In a hospital, incident reports are sent to the risk manager. In a medical office, incident reports are usually given to the office manager or the physician. Depending on the type of event and organizational policy, a physician may or may not document the event on the incident report. If an unusual event happens to a patient, however, the physician should assess the patient and document the findings on the incident report. Figure 10-9 is a sample incident report.

When to Complete an Incident Report

Even in the safest settings, undesirable things can happen to patients. These events sometimes result from human

Workplace Requirements Program for Safety and Health

SUPERVISOR'S ACCIDENT REPORT FORM

This form is to be completed by the supervisor and forwarded to the Payroll Coordinator along with a copy of the North Carolina Industrial Commission Form 19 (Workers Compensation Form) within five days of the accident. All accidents involving serious bodily injury or death must be reported to the safety and health officer immediately.

ACCIDENT DATA

1. NAME OF EMPLOYEE:
   or Patient

2. ADDRESS AND PHONE NO:

| 3. WORK DEPT. OR DIVISION: | 4. SEX: ☐ MALE ☐ FEMALE | 5. DATE AND TIME OF INJURY: |

| 6. NATURE OF INJURY: | 7. PART OF BODY INJURED: |

| 8. CAUSE OF INJURY: | 9. LOCATION OF ACCIDENT: |

| 10. OCCUPATION AND ACTIVITY OF PERSON AT TIME OF ACCIDENT: | 11. STATUS OF JOB OR ACTIVITY: (CHOOSE ONE) Halted |

12. NAME AND PHONE NO. OF ACCIDENT WITNESS:

13. LIST UNSAFE ACT, IF ANY:

14. LIST UNSAFE PHYSICAL OR MECHANICAL CONDITION, IF ANY:

15. UNSAFE PERSONAL FACTOR:

16. LIST HAZARD CONTROLS IN EFFECT AT TIME OF INJURY DESIGNED TO PREVENT INJURY:

17. PERSONAL PROTECTIVE EQUIPMENT BEING USED AT TIME OF ACCIDENT:
    GLOVES, SAFETY GLASSES, GOGGLES, FACE SHIELD, OTHER

18. BRIEF DESCRIPTION OF ACCIDENT:

19. CORRECTIVE ACTION TAKEN OR RECOMMENDED TO DEPARTMENT SAFETY COMMITTEE:

TREATMENT DATA

20. WAS INJURED TAKEN TO (CHOOSE ONE): Hospital
21. DIAGNOSIS AND TREATMENT, IF KNOWN:

| 22. ESTIMATED LOST WORKDAYS: (EXCLUDING DAY OF ACCIDENT) | 23. DATE OF REPORT: Month Day Year |

24. REPORT PREPARED BY:

25. SIGNATURE OF SUPERVISOR:

26. SIGNATURE OF AGENCY SAFETY AND HEALTH OFFICER:

Figure 10-9 Sample incident report.

error (e.g., giving the wrong medication), or they may be idiopathic. Idiopathic means that something occurred for unknown reasons and was unavoidable (e.g., an allergic reaction). Incident reports must be completed even if no injury resulted from an event. A few examples of situations requiring an incident report are:

- All medication errors
- All patient, visitor, and employee falls
- Drawing blood from a wrong patient
- Mislabeling of blood tubes or specimens
- Incorrect surgical instrument counts following surgery
- Employee needlesticks
- Workers' compensation injuries

The rule of thumb is, when in doubt, always complete an incident report

Information Included in an Incident Report

Although every agency has its own form, the following data are always included in an incident report:

- Name, address, and phone number of the injured party
- Date of birth and sex of the injured party
- Date, time, and location of the incident
- Brief description of the incident and what was done to correct it
- Any diagnostic procedures or treatments that were needed
- Patient examination findings, if applicable
- Names and addresses of witnesses, if applicable
- Signature and title of person completing form
- Physician's and supervisor's signatures as per policy

Guidelines for Completing an Incident Report

When completing an incident report, follow these guidelines:

1. State only the facts. Do not draw conclusions or summarize the event. For example, if you walk into the reception room and find a patient on the floor, do not write, "Patient tripped and fell in reception area," because that draws a conclusion. Instead, document the incident as follows: "Patient found on the floor in the reception area. Patient states that he fell."
2. Write legibly and sign your name legibly. Be sure to include your title.
3. Complete the form in a timely fashion. In general, incident reports should be completed within 24 hours of the event.
4. Do not leave any blank spaces on the form. If a particular section of the report does not apply, write n/a (not applicable).
5. Never photocopy an incident report for your own personal record.
6. Never place the incident report in the patient's chart. Never document in the patient's chart that an incident report was completed. Only document the event in the patient's chart. (By writing in the medical record that an incident report was completed, it opens the potential for lawyers to subpoena the incident report, should there be a lawsuit.)

Trending Incident Reports

After incident reports are completed, they are reviewed and tracked to highlight specific patterns. The resulting statistical data can be used to identify problem areas, which can be corrected through quality improvement (QI) programs. Examples of statistical data that can be found in incident reports include:

- Particular days of the week when most negative events happen (if most events occur on Friday afternoons, perhaps staffing on Friday afternoons should be re-evaluated)

- Most common area for patient falls (if most falls happen in the lobby, a QI program may need to be established to assess why falls occur there)
- Medications that are routinely given incorrectly (educating staff and using colored labels to highlight similar drug names may correct this)
- The age group most likely to have problems (if most of your incident reports reflect problems in the geriatric population, a QI program focusing on geriatric care may be needed)

Incident reports should be kept in a special file in the manager's office (some managers file these reports according to dates, whereas others file them according to the problem).

WHAT IF?

You give the wrong medication, and the patient has a bad reaction to it. Would you be better off not documenting the medication error?

NO! By not documenting the incident, you place yourself at risk. These risks can include allegations of falsifying medical records, tampering with medical records, and failing to follow reporting policies and procedures. On the incident report, do not say, "I gave the wrong medication"; just state the facts: "X medication was ordered. I gave Y medication." Then document who you told and when, what you were advised to do, and any other pertinent information. Your supervisor or the risk manager may call the medical office's insurance company to alert them to the incident. If the incident results in a malpractice lawsuit, an accurately completed incident report can prove helpful to your organization's attorney.

Quality Improvement Programs

Regulatory Agencies

One of the most challenging problems for risk managers is to prevent noncompliance with regulatory agencies. As discussed earlier, numerous agencies regulate health care settings, and these rules and regulations change frequently. You can stay up to date with new changes by reading newsletters from these organizations, attending your state and local professional meetings, and frequently visiting various professional websites. Most states publish a monthly bulletin that reports new legislation. Every state has a website that will link you to legislative action. Read these regularly. Each office should have legal counsel who can assist in interpreting

legal issues. It is important for a new manager to meet with the medical office's attorney to discuss legal concerns for the practice. These regulatory agencies monitor medical practices to ensure quality of care, protection of employees, and sound practices.

Occupational Safety and Health Administration (OSHA)

OSHA is a federal agency that regulates health and safety concerns in the workplace. OSHA requires that QI programs be in place to protect the health and welfare of patients and employees. OSHA's mission is to save lives, prevent injuries, and protect the health of America's workers. Many rules under OSHA affect your job. Examples are rules for blood-borne pathogen protection, use of personal protective equipment (PPE), tuberculosis prevention, management of biohazardous waste, ergonomics, and laser protection. Laser protection is needed if you are working with a physician who is operating a laser in the office. These rules and other guidelines can be found on the OSHA website. Unlike The Joint Commission, compliance with OSHA regulations is not voluntary. Noncompliance with OSHA regulations can result in fines and closure of the health care organization.

CHECKPOINT QUESTION

7. What is the mission of OSHA?

The Joint Commission

The Joint Commission is a private agency that sets health care standards and evaluates an organization's implementation of these standards for health care settings. Prior to the mid 1990s, the primary focus of The Joint Commission was on evaluating hospitals and inpatient care institutions such as nursing homes. In 1996, The Joint Commission expanded its jurisdiction to outpatient and ambulatory care settings. This change was, in part, due to the shift of patient care from inpatient to outpatient services. As mentioned in Chapter 8, The Joint Commission sets standards and evaluates the care in the various health care settings. Box 10-4 lists various types of freestanding facilities for which The Joint Commission sets standards and provides accreditation.

The Joint Commission surveys these centers and then assigns them an accreditation title. A survey is an on-site evaluation of the organization's facility and policies. Participation in The Joint Commission is voluntary for health care organizations; without accreditation, however, the health care organization may not be eligible to participate in particular federal- and state-funded programs, such as Medicare and Medicaid. In

---

BOX 10-4

TYPES OF FACILITIES

The Joint Commission accredits a variety of health care settings. These are some types of centers that can be accredited:

- Ambulatory care centers
- Birthing centers
- Chiropractic clinics
- Community health organizations
- Corporate health services
- County jail infirmaries
- Dental clinics
- Dialysis centers
- Endoscopy centers
- Group practices
- Imaging centers
- Independent practitioner practices
- Lithotripsy centers
- Magnetic resonance imaging centers
- Oncology centers
- Ophthalmology surgery centers
- Pain management centers
- Podiatry centers
- Physician offices
- Rehabilitative centers
- Research centers
- Sleep centers
- Student health centers
- Women's health centers

---

addition, accreditation indicates to the community that an organization has met basic practice standards, which is important for marketing its services.

The Joint Commission Accreditation Process

The process of obtaining and maintaining accreditation by The Joint Commission occurs in various stages:

1. The health care organization files a survey application and a business associate agreement with The Joint Commission. The business associate agreement is a new requirement that is part of the Health Insurance Portability and Accountability Act regulations. These regulations are discussed later in the chapter. The application, which is sent from The Joint Commission headquarters, consists of inquiries regarding the following:

   - Ownership of the organization
   - Demographics (e.g., address and phone number)
   - Types of services provided
   - Volume of patients served per year

2. The health care organization prepares for the survey by reviewing each The Joint Commission standard and assessing its own compliance. The Joint Commission standards can be found in its publications or on its website. In addition, the organization to be inspected reviews and updates all policy and procedure manuals. Personnel records are checked for accuracy and completion. Staff members are taught about the survey process and are provided with sample questions that they may be asked during the survey.

3. The Joint Commission informs the health care organization of the date, time, and duration of the survey. The length of the survey depends on the size and complexity of the setting. A first-time survey visit usually lasts 2 to 4 days. The Joint Commission surveyors who specialize in health care standards conduct the survey.

4. The Joint Commission conducts the survey, which consists of reviewing patient records, interviewing patients and family members, and touring the facility. Employees are interviewed to determine whether they know where the policy and procedure manuals are kept, what is in the manuals, and safety rules. An exit conference in which preliminary findings are discussed is held between the surveyors and the administration (leadership) of the health care organization.

5. The Joint Commission mails the accreditation decision to the health care organization within 60 days after the survey. An organization can appeal to The Joint Commission for re-evaluation of its assigned title. The organization receives a certificate indicating the level of accreditation that it has achieved. The certificate is posted at the facility.

6. If the initial site review identified some unsatisfactory areas, a second survey, called a focus survey, may be required to prove that corrections have been made. This type of survey generally lasts 1 to 2 days.

7. After 3 years (the period for which accreditation by The Joint Commission is valid), the health care organization submits a renewal application, resuming the cycle.

Approximately 50% of The Joint Commission standards are directly related to patient safety issues. As of January 2003, all site surveys are based on a new set of national goals aimed at improving the overall safety of patient care in hospitals and in other health care settings. All settings must show that they have reached these six goals:

- Improved accuracy of patient identification. (Always use two methods to identify patients.)
- Improved effectiveness of communication among caregivers.
- Improved safety of using high-alert medications. (These medications are given only in hospitals by registered nurses. Examples of high-alert medications are chemotherapy agents and potassium injections.)

- Eliminate wrong-site, wrong-patient, and wrong-procedure surgeries. (All steps must be taken to prevent procedures on a wrong patient. Wrong procedures can be simple errors, such as drawing blood from a wrong patient, or serious life-changing mistakes.)
- Improved safety of infusion pumps. (Examples of infusion pumps are pain management devices and insulin administration devices.)
- Improved effectiveness of clinical alarm systems. (All alarms must be checked on a regular basis and must be audible to everyone.)

In addition, The Joint Commission requires accredited health care organizations to have a **sentinel event** policy and alert forms. A sentinel event is an unexpected death or serious physical or psychological injury to a patient. Any time a sentinel event occurs, the organization must determine the cause, implement improvements to prevent a repeat occurrence, and monitor the effectiveness of its plan. The Joint Commission publishes a newsletter, *The Sentinel Event Alert*, discussing reported events to alert other facilities to potential problems, and copies can be viewed on its website. The sentinel event alert has raised awareness in the health care community and in the federal government about the occurrences of adverse events and ways these events can be prevented.

Physicians who perform office-based surgery need to follow the standards set forth by The Joint Commission in the *Standards Manual for Office-Based Surgery*. The manual addresses certain standards, such as customer service, quality of care, qualified and competent staff levels, patient safety, leadership, and improving care and health. The manual provides the standards, the in-

tent or purpose of the standards, and some tips for compliance. Table 10-1 displays a sample standard. If office-based surgeries are performed where you work, you should be familiar with these standards. Questions on how to implement these standards can be answered via the The Joint Commission website or through its hotline.

 CHECKPOINT QUESTION

8. What are the benefits of being accredited by The Joint Commission?

Centers for Medicare and Medicaid Services (CMS)

The Centers for Medicare and Medicaid Services (CMS) [formerly the Health Care Financing Administration (HCFA)], a division of the United States Department of Health and Human Services, regulates and runs various departments and programs, including Medicare and Medicaid. This federal agency is assigned to monitor and follow two key regulations that will affect your job as a medical assistant. These two laws are the Clinical Laboratory Improvement Amendments Act (CLIA) and the Health Insurance Portability and Accountability Act (HIPAA). See Chapter 8 for information on HIPAA.

State Health Departments

Each state has a specific agency to license and monitor health care organizations and monitor public health. Each state has specific guidelines for required QI programs. As in participation with OSHA regulations, par-

TABLE 10-1	Sample Standard	
The practice demonstrates respect for the following needs of patients:		
Standard	**Intent**	**Tips for Compliance**
RI.1.5 Privacy	Confidentiality of information gathered during treatment Privacy during care Security of self and property	Private examination rooms and treatment areas Staff members who demonstrate concern for patients' privacy Gowns provided when clothing must be changed
RI.1.6 Communication	Effective communication that considers hearing, speech, and visual impairments	Interpreters available when needed Staff age-specific training Patient information packets, educational materials, and consent forms available in the patients' languages
RI 1.7 Resolution of complaints	The right to complain about care and to have complaints reviewed and resolved	Documentation on investigation of patients' complaints or issues regarding care

ticipation with state regulations is not optional. The rules and regulations vary among states. It is important that you be aware of the regulations in your state. For example, in some states, medical assistants cannot administer medications, while in other states, they can. Using your Internet search engine, type in the key words "public health department" and look for your state's health department website.

Developing a Quality Improvement Program

The size and complexity of an organization's QI program depends on the organization's particular needs. In large facilities, numerous committees may be assigned to monitor and implement QI plans. Examples of QI plans are fall prevention, needlestick surveillance, and laboratory contamination rates. The committees will consist of staff members, including physicians. Most facilities have a specific person assigned to oversee all of these committees.

In the medical office and ambulatory care settings, QI programs tend to be more informal. Usually the office manager or senior physician is responsible for monitoring and implementing QI plans. As more outpatient centers become accredited by The Joint Commission, however, QI programs have become more structured. A few examples of quality issues that can be monitored in the physician offices are:

- Patient waiting times
- Unplanned returned patient visits for the same ailment or illness
- Misdiagnosed illnesses that are detected by another partner in the practice
- Patient or family complaints
- Timely follow-up telephone calls to patients
- Patient falls in physician's office or office building
- Mislabeled specimens sent to the laboratory
- Blood specimens that are coagulated or contaminated

Seven Steps for a Successful Program

The following seven steps are essential for creating an effective QI program:

1. *Identify the problem or potential problem.* All organizations can improve their delivery of patient care. Suggestions for improving care can come from many resources, including the following:

   - Office managers
   - Physicians (recommendations and complaints)
   - Other employees (e.g., nurses and medical assistants)
   - Patients (interviews)
   - Incident report trending (discussed earlier)

The person responsible for QI in the medical office reviews all QI problems or potential problems and selects the one to be addressed first. Problems given top priority are those that are high risk (most likely to occur) and those that are most likely to cause injury to patients, family members, or employees.

2. *Form a task force.* A **task force** is a group of employees with different roles within the organization brought together to solve a given problem. In a medical office, the task force usually consists of a physician, nurse, medical assistant, and office manager. In large hospitals, various department managers are generally involved.

3. *Assign an expected threshold.* The task force establishes an **expected threshold** (numerical goal) for a given problem. Thresholds must be realistic and achievable. For example, if the problem is needlestick injuries, the expected threshold is a realistic number of employee needlestick injuries that the task force considers acceptable in a given period. For instance, the threshold may be one employee stick per month. It is not realistic to set the goal at zero; this may be optimal but is not achievable.

4. *Explore the problem and propose solutions.* The task force investigates the problem thoroughly to determine all potential causes and possible solutions. After various solutions are discussed, the task force decides what solution or solutions are to be implemented.

5. *Implement the solution.* The key to successful implementation of the solution is staff education. All staff members must be taught about the problem and the plan to decrease the problem. The type of implementation will be based on the problem. For example, if the problem is patients falling at the entrance to the building, fixing the problem is likely to be complex and expensive. It may involve reengineering and construction of new walkways. If the problem is mislabeling or misspelling patients' names on laboratory specimens, the implementation will be simpler, possibly printing labels from the computer database.

6. *Establish a QI monitoring plan.* After implementation, the solution must be evaluated to determine whether it worked and, if so, how well. QI monitoring plans have three elements:

   - Source of monitoring, that is, where the numerical data will be obtained (e.g., medical record review, incident reports, laboratory reports, office logs)
   - Frequency of monitoring, that is, how often the data will be monitored and tallied (e.g., once a week, once a month)
   - Person responsible for monitoring, that is, who collects the data and presents the results in graphic form, allowing for easy comparison of data from before and after implementation of the solution

7. *Obtain feedback*. The members of the task force must review the graphs in relation to their expected threshold. Did they meet the threshold? If yes, the problem has been resolved. If the threshold was not met, the task force must determine whether the expected threshold was unrealistic or the solutions were inadequate. In either case, the problem has not been resolved; therefore, the task force must review each of the steps and make appropriate changes.

 CHECKPOINT QUESTION

9. What are the three elements of a QI monitoring plan?

Putting It All Together: A Case Review

Following is a case study in which the elements of successful QI and risk management programs are put into action.

You are working in a busy family practice. The average number of patients seen daily is 92. The physicians, nurses, and medical assistants are responsible for labeling specimen containers before they go to the laboratory. On the average, 15 specimens are collected daily. The hospital laboratory that analyzes the specimens reports that an average of seven specimens are mislabeled monthly.

The office manager brings to a staff meeting a graph (Fig. 10-10) depicting the number of mislabeled specimens that occurred over a 4-month period. She notes that most mislabelings occurred on Monday and Friday afternoons. It is decided that this is a significant patient care issue and that a QI program to address and resolve the problem is needed.

A task force is formed. It includes a physician, a nurse, and a medical assistant. The task force identifies the problem as a high-risk issue and assigns the expected threshold to be fewer than two mislabeled specimens per month. The task force identifies the factors re-

lated to the problem, which includes lack of sufficient labels in patient rooms, high patient volumes on Monday and Friday afternoons, and overall need for educating all staff members about the importance of labeling specimens correctly.

Solutions to these three problems are created:
Problem: Insufficient labels in the rooms.
Solution: Additional specimen labels are placed in every room. Also, specimen labels will be already printed and waiting for patients who arrive for an anticipated specimen collection (stool, urine, skin biopsy).
Problem: Large volume on Monday and Friday afternoons.
Solution: The medical assistant's hours will change to 10:00 AM to 6:30 PM on Monday and Fridays instead of 8:00 AM to 4:30 PM. This creates more staff coverage during peak hours.
Problem: Lack of knowledge.
Solution: A representative for the hospital laboratory will conduct an in-service review for all staff members. He or she will explain the implication of mislabeled specimens and how they can impair patient care. Let's say that both Mrs. Brown and Mrs. Eubanks came into the office for skin biopsies. The specimens were taken and placed in bottles. The bottles were put next to each other on the shelf. The name labels were reversed on the specimens. One specimen showed a malignancy. Which patient would get treated? The wrong patient would be treated, causing unnecessary expense and distress and probably even a lawsuit. The patient with the malignancy would not be treated and might get sicker.

After these steps were taken, a new graph was developed showing the improvement (Fig. 10-11). Because the threshold has been met, the task force does not think any more changes are needed, and the QI mislabeling program is ended.

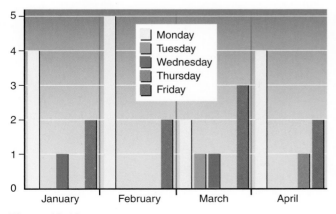

Figure 10-10 Frequency of mislabeled specimens by day of the week and by month.

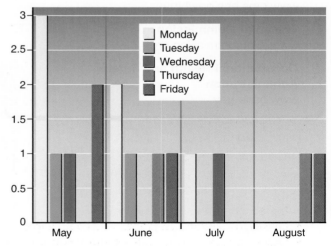

Figure 10-11 Frequency of mislabeled specimens by day of the week and by month after a QI plan was carried out. Note the change in the numerical system on the graph.

MEDIA MENU

- **Student CD**
  - **CMA/RMA Certification Exam Review**
- **Premium Online Course**
  http://thePoint.lww.com/Kronenberger3e
- **Internet Resources**

  LiveAdvise Online Tutoring & Competency Training
  http://thePoint.lww.com/LiveAdvise

  Medical Group Management Association
  www.mgma.org

  Physicians Practice Group
  www.physicianspractice.com

  Family Leave Act/Department of Labor
  www.dol.gov

  Americans with Disabilities Act/US Department of Justice
  www.ada.gov
  www.usdoj.gov

  Centers for Medicare and Medicaid Services
  www.cms.gov

  Clinical Laboratory Improvement Amendments Act
  www.cms.hhs.gov/clia/

  Health Care Report Cards
  www.healthgrades.com

  Health Insurance Portability and Accountability Act
  www.cms.hhs.gov/hipaa

  The Joint Commission
  www.jointcommission.org

  Occupational Health and Safety Administration
  www.osha.gov

español
SPANISH TERMINOLOGY

Busco un trabajo.
I am looking for a job.

¿Tiene usted cualquier abîerto?
Do you have any openings?

¿Dónde estan las aplicaciones?
Where are the applications?

Soy el director.
I am the manager.

¿Vio usted lo que pasó?
Did you see what happened?

¿Cayo usted?
Did you fall?

¿Está lastimado usted?
Are you hurt?

¿Quiere usted ver un doctor?
Do you want to see a doctor?

Usted necesita obtener una radiografía.
You need an x-ray.

PROCEDURE 10-1: Create a Procedures Manual

Purpose: To communicate the proper policies and procedures to be used by all employees in a practice in order to ensure consistent, accurate, and efficient patient interaction and care

Equipment: Word processor, three-ring binder, paper, choose any procedure approved by your instructor

Steps	Reasons
1. Check the latest information from key governmental agencies, local and state health departments, and health care organizations, such as OSHA, CDC, JCAHO, etc., to make sure that the policies and procedures being written comply with federal and state legislation and regulations.	Serious consequences can occur if you are not conscientious about keeping abreast of changes in the medical and legal worlds. This information can be found on the Internet and in published reports.
2. Gather product information; consult government agencies, as needed. If the procedure is for using new equipment, ask the sales representative for training pamphlets.	This ensures that you are using products and equipment according to the manufacturer's suggestions and that you are practicing within legal and ethical boundaries.
3. Title the procedure, e.g., Infection Control Procedure for Handwashing.	A logical, easily identifiable format will allow easy retrieval.
4. Number the procedure, e.g., "HR 14" means human resource section, policy 14.	All policies and procedures should be numbered to allow for easy access and identification.
5. Define the overall purpose of the procedure. This should be a sentence or two at most explaining the intent of the procedure.	Provides the staff with a rationale for the procedure.
6. List any necessary equipment or forms. Include everything needed to complete the task. Also indicate if no special equipment or forms are necessary.	The employee will be prepared before beginning the procedure if he or she has everything needed at hand.
7. List each step with its rationale. The steps must be complete and in order. Never assume the reader knows how or when to perform a given step, such as handwashing. The employee will be able to follow specific steps, ensuring patient safety.	Listing the steps in order promotes compliance and accuracy for procedure completion.
8. Provide spaces for signatures. Administrative procedures are signed by the physician and office manager. Clinical procedures usually are signed by the clinical manager and a physician. Employees must have a space to sign.	The employee's signature will verify that he or she has read and understands the procedure.
9. Record the date the procedure was written. If changes are needed, the procedure is rewritten, signed, and dated again. The previous dates also are generally listed.	By recording the date, you ensure that you are reading the most current revision. It will also help you know when a new revision should be considered.

PROCEDURE 10-2: Create a Quality Improvement Program

Purpose: To implement practices that will help ensure high-quality patient care and service

Equipment: Paper, pen, or word processing equipment; scenario

Steps	Reasons
1. Identify the problem or potential problem.	Pinpointing the problem is the first step in solving it.
2. Form a task force of employees from different departments or areas. Select a group of other students to work with.	People working together can accomplish more. Using people from the specific area in question along with employees from other areas gives the discussion an objective and fresh approach.
3. Assign an expected threshold using measurable, realistic goals.	Assigning a number to the desired outcome allows a more concrete way to measure success.
4. Explore the problem and propose solutions.	Brainstorming is a great tool for gathering ideas. Using different viewpoints and perspectives adds to the success of the group.
5. Implement the solution. Write a memorandum to the employees with instructions for the implementation.	Making sure all employees are informed will help with morale and ensure that everyone is "on the same page."
6. Establish a QI monitoring plan. Make a list of the source, frequency, and person responsible for collecting data.	The only way to know if the expected threshold is reached is to monitor data, actions, and results.
7. Obtain feedback. Review data collected in the monitoring process.	Without proper follow-up, the success of the improvement process cannot be properly evaluated.
8. Document the entire process.	Documentation protects the information for future use. You may need to readdress the situation at a later date.

Chapter Summary

- Effective management of the medical office is essential for a health care organization to succeed in the competitive marketplace.
- A good manager must be able to perform a variety of tasks in an organized and efficient manner.
- An office manager will be communicating with patients and staff, handling staffing issues, developing policy and procedures manuals, creating promotional materials, preparing budgets, and overseeing educational programs.
- The medical office manager must keep current on legal requirements related to office operations.
- Quality improvement programs have many benefits

to health care organizations. They can identify potential problems for patients and employees.
- After identifying the problem, a task force can create solutions to resolve them.
- QI programs are also required by various agencies. Four important agencies are The Joint Commission, OSHA, CMS, and your state health department. You must stay alert to new regulations from these agencies. Patients place trust in all health care workers and health care settings. We must all work hard to provide good quality care to all patients every time they are treated.

1. Review the list of qualities that a manager should have. Which ones do you have? How would you acquire the others? Should any other qualities be listed?
2. Review the types of sections that are often included in policy and procedures manuals. Now assume that you are to help a physician set up a practice. How would you organize your policy and procedures manual? Create one sample sheet for each section of your manual. Be sure to include all necessary elements when you write your policies and procedures.
3. Create a list of potential patient or employee problems that could be solved with a QI program. Be sure to include some administrative, clinical, and laboratory examples. Then select three problems and develop a list of solutions for each problem.
4. Search The Joint Commission website. What information can you find regarding sentinel events? What steps can be taken to prevent them?

Answers to Checkpoint Questions

1. An organizational chart is a flow sheet that allows the manager and employees to identify their team members and to see where they fit into the team.
2. Three ways to communicate with staff members are through bulletin boards, staff meetings, and communication notebooks.
3. The primary goal of scheduling is to ensure that the needs of the office are met.
4. The elements that must be in a policy or procedure are document name, purpose, equipment or forms needed, steps or explanations, signatures, numbering system, and dates.
5. A budget is a financial planning tool that helps an organization estimate its anticipated expenditures and revenues.
6. Physicians need malpractice insurance to protect them from financial loss in the event of a successful lawsuit. Insurance companies offer services such as teaching employees to take preventative measures, helping to identify problems, conducting risk inspections, supplying self-auditing tools, and providing bulletins.
7. OSHA's mission is to save lives, prevent injuries, and protect the health of America's workers.
8. The benefits of being accredited by The Joint Commission are that the health care organization is eligible for state and federal funding programs and that accreditation proves to the community that the facility has met basic standards of care.
9. The three elements of a QI monitoring program are the source of monitoring, the frequency of monitoring, and the person responsible for monitoring,

UNIT TWO

Power Critical Thinking Exercises

FUNDAMENTALS OF ADMINISTRATIVE MEDICAL ASSISTING (CHAPTERS 5-10)

1. The physician has ordered diagnostic testing for your patient, Jake Moore. Mr. Moore has been experiencing severe indigestion, nausea, and diarrhea off and on for about 3 months. The doctor asks you to schedule an abdominal CT and a colonoscopy. He wants to see Mr. Moore again after his tests.

    A. What type of facility will offer these services? (knowledge)

    B. What is the reason for the testing? (comprehension)

    C. What information will the facility need? (application)

    D. How would you sequence the tests? (analysis)

    E. How would your actions change if Mr. Moore did not have his own transportation? (synthesis)

    F. What are the goals you want to accomplish when making multiple appointments for patients? (evaluation)

2. Your office has just implemented a new electronic medical records system. Although the transition was a challenge, you know the effort will be worth it. Your physician wants to make use of every feature. He asks the employees to brainstorm and come up with ways the computer can be used.

   A. What feature might be used for sending out patient notifications? (knowledge)
   B. How would you ensure having the desired features available in your new system? (comprehension)
   C. How would you handle documents after they are scanned into a computerized patient record? (application)
   D. List some advantages and disadvantages of the EMR as it relates to a patient's privacy. (analysis)
   E. Which features of electronic medical records would save the most time? (synthesis)
   F. How do you see the future of medical records as technology progresses? (evaluation)

3. It is your first day on the job as office manager for a new podiatrist. He will open his practice in 3 months. You are responsible for hiring the employees and preparing the office for business.

   A. What characteristics will you look for in your applicants? (knowledge)
   B. What manuals will you need to design? (comprehension)
   C. How would you prioritize your duties? (application)
   D. Based on the specialty of the practice, what procedures will need to be included in a manual? (analysis)
   E. How will you determine how many employees to hire? (synthesis)
   F. What goals will the practice want to achieve? (evaluation)

Managing the Finances in the Practice

Good management of finances is essential for a medical practice to succeed. This unit introduces you to various aspects of medical office finances, beginning with a chapter on credit and collections, in which you learn the process of collecting fees. Next, you will learn bookkeeping and banking skills as well as other accounting responsibilities. Most of the income for the physician's practice is through insurance reimbursements. To be able to collect fees from insurance companies, you must understand coding. This information is covered in the last three chapters. A financially strong practice is good for the patients, the community, and you.

CHAPTER

11 Credit and Collections

Outline

Fees
Fee Schedules
Discussing Fees in Advance
Forms of Payment
Payment by Insurance
   Companies
Adjusting Fees

Credit
Extending Credit
Legal Considerations
Collections
Legal Considerations
Collecting a Debt
Collection Alternatives

Learning Objectives

Upon successfully completing this chapter, you will be able to:

1. Spell and define the key terms

2. Explain the physician fee schedule

3. Discuss forms of payment

4. Explain the legal considerations in extending credit

5. Discuss the legal implications of credit collection

6. Describe three methods of debt collection

Upon successfully completing this chapter, you will be able to:

1. Evaluate and manage a patient account (Procedure 11-1)
2. Write a collection letter (Procedure 11-2)

CAAHEP

- Perform accounts receivable procedures
- Perform billing and collection procedures

ABHES

- Perform billing and collection procedures
- Use physician fee schedule

adjustment

aging schedule

collections

credit

installment

participating providers

patient co-payment

professional courtesy

write-off

The medical practice must operate in a financially sound manner to continue to serve the patient's needs. The office depends on the fees generated by patient visits, laboratory work, and in-office procedures. Without these fees, the medical office would be unable to pay for staff, office space, and supplies. Therefore, collecting fees, whether paid by the patient, an insurer, or a third party, is essential for the medical practice to succeed. Box 11-1 shows how to determine whether your office is collecting fees satisfactorily.

Fees

Fee Schedules

Generally, the physician sets the fees for office visits, laboratory work, and in-office procedures based on the UCR concept: (1) U (usual) fair value of the service; (2) C (customary) competitive rates charged by other physicians; and (3) R (reasonable), that which meets the other two cri-

teria. Fee setting also considers the resource-based relative value scale (RBRVS), by which fees are based on the relative value of a particular service and adjusted for geographical differences. (See Chapter 13 for more information about UCR fees and Chapter 15 for more information about RBRVS.) A physician's fee schedule also takes into consideration the costs of operating the office, such as rent, utilities, malpractice insurance, salaries, and so on. A list of the services and procedures offered in an office along with descriptions, procedure codes, and prices must be available to patients. Federal regulations require that a sign to this effect be posted in the office.

There may be several fee schedules based on the reimbursement schedules of different insurance companies. **Participating providers** are doctors who agree to participate with managed care contracts and other third-party payers in exchange for building a solid patient base. Patients covered under participating plans will have a different fee schedule from patients who are private payers (paying with no money from insurance). Each managed

BOX 11-1

DETERMINING A PRACTICE'S COLLECTION PERCENTAGE

Medical practices should evaluate their method of collections periodically to determine the effectiveness of their practices. A collection analysis lets you identify the strengths and weaknesses of the system.

To do a collection analysis, determine the monthly production from the first day of each month to the last day. This will be the total charges posted to all patients' accounts. Next, determine the revenues the practice received. Computer systems will automatically total payments received during a specified time. Divide revenue by production to determine the collection percentage. Analysis of the collection percentage should reveal the percentage of the collection of all outstanding debts to the practice.

Collection percentage = monthly production ÷ monthly revenue received

Most medical practices average 8% to 20% loss yearly. Experts consider a collection percentage above 80% to be reasonable. Performing a 2-year collection percentage comparison analysis will help you evaluate past collection effectiveness.

Code	Key	Mod	Par Fee	Non Par Fee	Limiting Charge
50010			$690.30	$655.79	$754.16
50010			$690.30	$655.79	$754.16
50020			$1,112.72	$1,057.08	$1,215.64
50021			$522.30	$496.19	$570.62
50040			$1,009.84	$959.35	$1,103.25
50045			$921.52	$875.44	$1,006.76
50060			$1,116.74	$1,060.90	$1,220.04
50065			$1,128.28	$1,071.87	$1,232.65
50070			$1,172.52	$1,113.89	$1,280.97
50075			$1,451.88	$1,379.29	$1,586.18
50080			$976.28	$927.47	$1,066.59
50081			$1,336.92	$1,270.07	$1,460.58
50100			$1,033.66	$981.98	$1,129.28
50120			$945.54	$898.26	$1,033.00
50125			$980.30	$931.29	$1,070.98
50130			$1,010.09	$959.59	$1,103.53
50135			$1,110.42	$1,054.90	$1,213.14
50200			$138.72	$131.78	$151.55
50205			$696.55	$661.72	$760.98
50220			$1,015.02	$964.27	$1,108.91
50225			$1,168.36	$1,109.94	$1,276.43

Figure 11-1 Sample Medicare fee schedule.

care plan, workers' compensation company, Medicaid carrier, and Medicare plan has a different fee schedule. See Chapter 15 for further discussion of third-party payers.

A Medicare fee schedule has three columns. A participating fee is the amount paid to physicians who participate or agree to accept a certain fee. A nonparticipating fee is the amount paid to physicians who do not have agreements with Medicare. A limiting charge is the amount a physician can charge a Medicare patient. Figure 11-1 is a sample Medicare fee schedule.

 CHECKPOINT QUESTION

1. What is meant by "participating provider?"

Discussing Fees in Advance

It is always a good policy to discuss fees with patients in advance. This ensures that patients are aware of the charges. Patients will need to know in advance whether the medical office is a participating provider with their insurance carrier. Managed care companies usually require that the patient pay a certain share of the bill, known as the **patient co-payment,** or co-pay. A good and easy way

to initiate a discussion of fees is by providing an office brochure that lists not only the office's address, telephone number, and hours but also office policies regarding fees and collections, third-party payments, and how they are handled. Patients should understand that co-pays are to be paid at the time of service. Such information should be included in the office brochure. Many offices post a sign in the waiting area stating this.

Ideally, you should collect the entire amount due from a new patient on the first visit. Obviously, the less credit you extend, the lower your accounts receivable and the better the cash flow. As discussed in Chapter 5, many problems associated with collection (acquiring funds that are due) come from patients who move and leave no forwarding address or those who go from one practice to another. Be sure you get complete information including the names, numbers, and relationships of contacts able to give you information about a patient's new location. You should also get a picture identification, such as a driver's license, on a patient's first visit. (See Chapter 5, The First Contact: Telephone and Reception.)

Forms of Payment

Depending on the medical office's policies, patients can usually pay for services in several ways: cash, personal check, debit card, or credit card (e.g., Visa, MasterCard, Discover). If a new patient is paying by check, get two forms of identification.

By agreeing to accept a credit card payment, the medical office also agrees to pay the credit card company a percentage (usually 1.8%) of the total charge. Although this may seem costly, it is sometimes more cost effective to receive payment by credit card than to receive it in installments—or not at all—from the patient.

CHECKPOINT QUESTION

2. List four forms of payments accepted by most physician offices.

Payment by Insurance Companies

By far, the largest proportions of fees are paid by insurance companies. Therefore, it is imperative that patients' insurance information be kept current. Most medical practices require that a patient submit a medical insurance card for each visit; this way, changes in insurance can quickly and easily be noted. Remember, always make a copy of both sides of the patient's insurance card and place it in the appropriate section of the chart for billing reference. Most insurance companies offer online services such as checking coverage, eligibility for procedures, co-pays, etc.

Adjusting Fees

Sometimes, **adjustments** (changes in a posted account) must be made to a standard fee, as when the medical office accepts a set insurance rate for a service that is lower than the practice's rate. You must charge the patient the regular fee for the service; when the insurance carrier sends payment, however, the explanation of benefits (EOB) will show how much you may collect for the service. The difference between the physician's normal fee and the insurance carrier's allowed fee will be adjusted in the credit adjustment column on the patient's account.

Other fee adjustments include **professional courtesy** fees, in which other health care professionals are charged a reduced rate. The physician may choose not to charge a fee at all; this too is considered a professional courtesy and should not be confused with writing off a fee. (A **write-off** is cancellation of an unpaid debt; these generally can be claimed as deductions on the practice's federal taxes.) Again, you charge the regular fee and then adjust the designated amount in the adjustment column with "professional courtesy" in the description column. Some practices offer discounts for paying in full. You would handle this as earlier described for adjustments (charge the full amount and adjust off the discount).

CHECKPOINT QUESTION

3. What is the difference between a fee adjustment and a write-off?

Credit

Extending Credit

It is not always possible for patients to pay the entire bill when costs are incurred. Depending on the medical office's policy, **credit** may be extended to patients on an installment plan. Collection experts have estimated that billing one patient costs the practice about $8 per month. This total includes the time it takes to prepare the statements, the supplies needed, and so on. Extension of credit to a patient is a decision that is sometimes made solely by the physician. The practice will make the decision to extend credit in house or to arrange financing through a bank or other lending facility. If the credit is extended by the practice without the use of a third party, credit to a patient should be extended only after checking the patient's credit history (Box 11-2). Many offices outsource their credit and billing functions. There are medical billing companies that manage the practice's accounts receivable, prepare the insurance claims, offer training to the employees, and provide other related services.

Legal Considerations

When a medical practice extends credit to a patient, it may charge interest on the patient's unpaid balance. If this is the case, the medical office is legally required to disclose this information to the patient, along with any other fees or charges incurred by the patient's acceptance of credit. This legal documentation, called a truth-in-lending statement, must be filed in the patient's medical chart.

Different states have different laws concerning the extension of credit. Generally, credit cannot be denied based on age, gender, race, marital status, religion, national origin, or source of income (e.g., if a patient receives public assistance). If your facility has given credit to one patient, you typically may not refuse the same arrangement to another patient. Some states have laws

---

BOX 11-2

WHAT IS A CREDIT SCORE?

There are three major credit reporting firms—Experian, Transunion, and Equifax. Credit reports can help you make better-informed decisions about granting credit. A credit rating or score is assigned to consumers who have credit. It is a number between 300 and 850 that evaluates your risk as a lender. This score will determine whether you extend credit and also determines interest rates if you charge interest. The website addresses for these companies are listed at the end of the chapter.

ETHICAL TIP

Paying the Doctor With Eggs?

There was a time when patients paid for their medical care with eggs from their farm. Those days are long gone. In today's complicated financial world, it is necessary for a physician practice to behave as any other "business." Although it is legal to charge patients reasonable interest rates, finance charges, and late payment fees, risk managers suggest avoiding them. Even the American Medical Association, which advises physicians on matters such as ethical principles and finances, warns that patients may be put off by their doctor charging these fees. Doctors are in the business of taking care of people, but they must pay their bills. These charges may create bad will or be seen as a conflict from a caring and helpful physician.

bills to its patients who have unpaid balances. Larger offices set up a billing cycle and divide the alphabet, sending statements once a week to each selected group. For example, patients with names beginning with the letters A to G might be billed on the 1st of the month, H to N on the 8th, O to S on the 15th, and T to Z on the 22nd. If your facility changes a billing cycle, you are legally required to notify patients of the change three months before the change takes effect.

The uncomputerized office normally just copies the ledger cards of the patients who owe balances. It is important to make each entry on the ledger card with consistency and provide a key for office codes or abbreviations. The patient should be able to understand each entry. When a practice is computerized, the staff can easily send statements. Medical office software usually gives the option of printing a separate message at the bottom. For instance, you may add "Happy Holidays" to every patient's December statement or "Time for your flu shot" in the September statements.

limiting the amount of interest that can be charged. The practice's accountant should be able to provide the information required by the state and municipality.

CHECKPOINT QUESTION

4. On what grounds is it illegal to deny credit?

Collections

When a patient has an unpaid bill or has not paid an installment per a credit agreement, those funds must be collected. Collecting an unpaid debt is costly to any business. Collecting fees can also be time consuming, and collecting practices are regulated by a variety of consumer protection laws. Many medical practices outsource their billing to companies specializing in billing and debt collection.

Legal Considerations

Certain procedures should be followed in attempts to collect a debt. A debt collector—in this case, the medical assistant or billing clerk—must exercise reasonable restraint when contacting a patient about a bill. Attempting to collect a debt from a patient's estate requires particular diplomacy.

Collecting a Debt
Monthly Billings

The easiest way to collect a debt or an installment is by monthly billing. Once a month, the medical office sends

LEGAL TIP

STAY WITHIN THE LAW WITH COLLECTION ATTEMPTS BY PHONE

When attempting to collect a debt by telephone, a debt collector **should never:**

- Contact the patient before 8:00 a.m. or after 9:00 p.m.
- Contact the patient at his or her place of employment if the employer objects
- Contact the patient at all if the patient's account has been turned over to a collection agency or the patient has filed for bankruptcy
- Harass or intimidate the patient; that is, use abusive language, provide false or misleading information, or pose as someone other than a debt collector
- Make threats of actions on the account without taking the action. For example, you tell the patient that you are going to turn the account over to a collection agency if payment is not received by a certain date. Payment is not received, but you do not turn the account over.
- Tell anyone other than the patient or responsible party about a debt without court authorization

Remember that, even though the patient owes you money, you must treat him or her with courtesy and respect.

WHAT IF?

What should you do if you need to collect a debt from a patient's estate?

Collecting debts from an estate requires professionalism and tact. When a patient dies, give the family time to grieve. Never contact the family regarding a debt immediately after a patient's death. Most offices have a policy stating that family members of deceased patients will not be contacted until at least a week after the funeral. At the appropriate time, call the next of kin listed in the patient's chart. Offer your sympathy and ask for the name of the patient's executor, the individual responsible for handling the patient's affairs after death. The executor may be an attorney, spouse, friend, or other relative. Call the executor and introduce yourself. Obtain the executor's address and send a final bill. It is important that all claims on a patient's estate be made promptly. If the estate does not have enough funds to meet all of its debts, the probate court will decide the priority list and percentages for debt collection. If your bill is not in the list of debts, it will not be paid.

If the account is on an **installmentt** plan, the patient receives a bill that lists the amount due for that month, any third-party payments or adjustments applied to the account, the total amount due, and the amount the patient owes. This way, the patient has the option of paying more than is due for that particular month (and thereby reducing the amount of any interest charged) and is aware of the current balance.

Aging Accounts

Unpaid accounts must be monitored to determine how far overdue they are. You will base your actions on the age of the account. Aging of an account is determining the amount of time between the date of the first bill sent to the patient and the date of the last payment. Note that it is calculated from the first date of billing, not by the procedure or service date. For example, a patient has an office visit on April 5 and the first statement is sent on May 1. The account will be 30 days old on June 1.

In a computerized accounting system, an **aging schedule** lists the patient's name, balance, any payments, and comments, such as reminders or second notices sent. In a manual system, such a schedule can be kept on a large sheet of paper. Figure 11-2 is a sample of a manual report. Figure 11-3 shows a screen that au-

---

Aging of Accounts Receivable Report: April 30, 2008

Patient Name	Account Number	Due Date	Amount
Accounts 30 Days Past Due:			
Doe, John C.	000-00-0000	3/6/08	625.00
Graham, Paula R.	000-00-0000	3/29/08	450.00
O'Toole, William Q.	000-00-0000	3/13/08	25.00
Parker, Mary W.	000-00-0000	3/25/08	299.00
Reeves, Chris A.	000-00-0000	3/11/08	58.00
South, Cheryl C.	000-00-0000	3/8/08	385.00
Yarkony, Ralph M.	000-00-0000	3/11/08	108.00
Accounts 60 Days Past Due:			
Forest, Patricia L.	000-00-0000	2/19/08	476.00
Heany, Beverly O.	000-00-0000	2/13/08	57.00
Thomas, Walter T.	000-00-0000	2/27/08	185.00
Accounts 90 Days Past Due:			
Glick, Rhonda K	000-00-0000	1/4/08	28.00
Payne, Robert A.	000-00-0000	1/25/08	456.00
Accounts 120 Days or More Past Due:			
Baird, Jane C.	000-00-0000	10/3/07	45.00
Wallace, Michael S.	000-00-0000	12/15/07	349.00
Total Overdue Accounts Receivable			**$3,546.00**

Figure 11-2 Manual aging schedule.

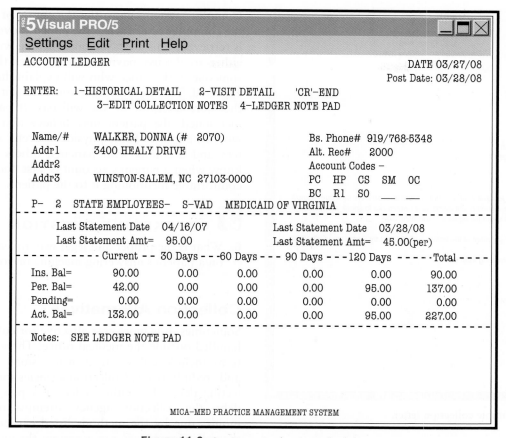

Figure 11-3 Computerized aging schedule.

tomatically places the amounts charged under the proper heading based on the age of the account. This account shows that $132 of the charges are current charges, or less than 30 days old. The $95 represents charges that were incurred and posted at least 120 days ago.

Aging of accounts is a measure of the practice's ability to collect its fees. Nearly all fees (80%) should be collected within 30 days. If the aging shows a high percentage (50%) of fees being collected 30 days or more after billing, the practice's billing and collection procedures should be reviewed. Procedure 11-1 outlines the steps in aging accounts.

 CHECKPOINT QUESTION

5. What is meant by aging of accounts?

Collecting Overdue Accounts

The three most common ways of collecting an overdue account are sending an overdue notice to the patient, telephoning the patient to let him or her know the account is overdue, and informing the patient at their next office visit.

Overdue Notices

With a manual system, overdue notices are fairly simple to prepare. Often, they consist of a copy of the patient's monthly billing with the words "overdue" or "second notice" stamped in red. Alternatively, a form letter with spaces for the patient's particulars may be sent. Figure 11-4 is a sample collection letter. If a computer billing program is used, the computer often can automatically generate overdue notices. Procedure 11-2 describes how to compose a collection letter.

Telephoning the Patient

If written notices bring no response, you may have to telephone the patient to inquire about an overdue account. Always ask when payment may be forthcoming and document the reply on the patient's account. If payment is not received as promised, contact the patient again. (See Legal Tip.)

In-Office Reminders

A patient can be reminded of an overdue balance when he or she comes to the office to see the physician. To handle this situation discreetly, simply give the patient a copy of the most recent overdue notice. Once again, ask when payment may be forthcoming and follow through.

Elkin Neurologic Center
1222 Brook Blvd
Edenton South Carolina 22617
331-561-8821

June 20, 2008

Christine Stultz
149 Fourth Street
Reedtown, SC 22617

Dear Mrs. Stultz,

This is to inform you that your account is more than 90 days past due. I know that you value your good credit rating, and I would like to speak with you as soon as possible about taking care of this oblication.

I will expect your payment of the balance of $250.00 by Friday, June 30, 2008.

I look forward to hearing from you.

Sincerely,

Tiffany Stone, CMA
Credit Manager

Figure 11-4 Sample collection letter.

Computer systems may offer the option of a message on the computer screen when the patient's overdue account is retrieved. This alerts anyone working with the patient either to discuss payment or to refer the patient to someone in the office who will explain that payment is expected. The more contact you have with the patient, the more likely he or she will pay. If payment is not mentioned, the patient may believe that you are not worried about it. Some physicians prefer not to discuss fees and accounts with patients; others will want to know when a patient's account is past due and will feel comfortable mentioning it to the patient.

 CHECKPOINT QUESTION

6. What is the proper and legal way to leave a message on a patient's answering machine or voice mail?

Collection Alternatives

Sometimes, it is more cost effective for **collections** to be handled outside the medical office. Three common options include collection agencies, small claims court, and credit bureaus. Collection agencies specialize in collecting debts. For either a fee or a percentage of the debt, the collection agency attempts to collect the monies due by the methods listed earlier. In addition, the collection agency can represent the medical practice in small claims court and can have the bad debt listed with credit-reporting agencies.

The medical practice can, of course, sue patients in small claims court or list patients with credit bureaus, but it is often more time and cost effective to hire an outside agency.

 CHECKPOINT QUESTION

7. What are three ways of collecting overdue accounts?

 LEGAL TIP

BE CAREFUL WHEN LEAVING MESSAGES ON ANSWERING MACHINES

Many people work during the day, and you will leave a message for the patient to call you back. Because you cannot be sure who will retrieve the message, you must protect the patient's rights. HIPAA's Privacy Rule prohibits disclosing information that would link the patient to a particular physician or medical treatment. Your message must not include any such information. For example, it would be improper to leave a message asking for payment on a past due account. It would be within the law, however, to ask the person to call you back. You should only give your first name and telephone number. Do not state the nature of the call.

español
SPANISH TERMINOLOGY

Necesito recoger el total en su cuenta.
I need to collect the balance on your account.

¿Puede pagar usted algunos de su deuda?
Can you pay some of your balance?

Esto es una carta de la colección.
This is a collection letter.

Usted debe este dinero a esta oficina.
You owe this office money.

MEDIA MENU

- **Student CD**
  - **CMA/RMA Certification Exam Review**
- **Premium Online Course**
  http://thePoint.lww.com/Kronenberger3e
- **Internet Resources**

  LiveAdvise Online Tutoring & Competency Training
  http://thePoint.lww.com/LiveAdvise

  Credit and Collections World
  www.collectionsworld.com

  Fair Debt Collection Practice/Federal Trade Commission Statutes
  www.ftc.gov

National Credit Systems
www.nationalcredit.com

Experian
www.experian.com

Transunion
www.transunion.com

Equifax
www.equifax.com

PROCEDURE 11-1:   Evaluate and Manage a Patient's Account

Purpose: To monitor the activity on a patient's credit account in order to keep the collection ratio at a maximum rate

Equipment: Simulation including scenario; sample patient ledger card with transactions; yellow, blue, and red stickers:

Yellow for accounts 30 days past due
Blue for accounts 60 days past due
Red for accounts 90 days past due

Scenario: Stephen Hill was seen first on March 3, 2008. His total bill that day was $250.00 for a level 2 consultation. He paid $50.00 as he was leaving. He returned to the office on April 9, 2008, for a revisit. His limited office visit was $50.00. He paid nothing that day. He has no insurance. It is now May 4, 2008. Post the charges and payment on a ledger card. Make a copy of the ledger card and place the appropriate sticker.

Steps	Purpose
1. Review the patient's account history to determine the "age" of the account. If payment has not been made between 30 and 59 days from today's date, the account is 40 days past due, and so on.	Aging accounts lets you know what action to take.
2. Flag the account for appropriate action. Place a yellow flag (sticker) on accounts that are 30 days old. Place a blue flag on accounts that are 60 days old. Place a red flag on accounts that are 90 days old.	Color coding the ledger cards lets everyone know the status of the account. In a computerized accounting system, the status of the account is determined automatically.

(continued)

PROCEDURE 11-1: Evaluate and Manage a Patient's Account (continued)

3. Set aside accounts that have had no payment in 91 days or longer.	You will write collection letters to these patients (see Procedure 11-2).
4. Make copies of the ledger cards.	These copies will serve as the patient's monthly statement.
5. Sort the copies by category: 30, 60, or 90 days.	Keeping each type together will make the next step quicker and easier.
6. Write or stamp the copies with the appropriate message, for example, "30 days past due" or "Your account is 30 days past due, please remit."	The messages you placed on the accounts will hopefully generate payment. The messages will be designed to become stronger as the account ages. In these cases, the patient may need more than a gentle nudge.
7. "Mail" the statements to the patients.	
8. Follow through with the collection process by continually reviewing past due accounts.	Following up on collection attempts and promises is the most important part of the process. Patients need to know that there will be continuous and consistent attempts to receive payment. They will be more apt to pay

PROCEDURE 11-2: Composing a Collection Letter

Purpose: To obtain payment from a patient whose account is more than 90 days old
Equipment: Ledger cards generated in Procedure 11-1, word processor, stationery with letterhead

Steps	Purpose
1. Review the patients' accounts and sort the accounts by age.	Sorting the accounts will make the task quicker and easier.
2. Design a rough draft of a form letter that can be used for collections.	A rough draft gives you the opportunity to review and edit your letter.
3. In the first paragraph, tell the patient why you are writing.	Let the patient know that you are attempting to collect a debt.
4. Inform the patient of the action you expect. For example: "To avoid further action, please pay $50.00 on this account by Friday, May 1, 2008."	Being specific will let the patient know exactly what you expect and enable you to follow up more efficiently.
5. Proofread the rough draft for errors, clarity, and accuracy, and then retype.	Errors in a letter may translate to the patient as inattention to detail and, therefore, to your collection follow through.
6. Take the collection letter to a supervisor or physician for approval.	Since you are serving as an agent of the facility, you should be sure the contents of the letter are appropriate.
7. Fill in the appropriate amounts and dates on each letter. Ask for at least half of the account balance within a 2-week period.	Each letter will have a different amount based on the account activity.
8. Print, sign, and mail the letter.	

Chapter Summary

- The financial status of a medical office is based on the ability of the staff to collect the physician's fees.
- Fee collection must be done in a professional manner and in accordance with state and federal laws. Technology affords the medical office the ability to streamline procedures, and collection practices are more efficient with computer systems.
- Aging accounts and communicating with patients in a fair and professional manner ensures a constant cash flow and success in managing the finances of the outpatient medical practice.
- Keeping the delicate balance between taking care of people and running a business can be a challenge.

Warm Ups for Critical Thinking

1. Write a script for leaving a message on a patient's answering machine asking them to return your call.

2. A patient has an overdue account balance. She is coming in for a visit today. What would you say to her?

3. A patient tells you that he does not believe he owes the amount on his statement. He says his insurance will pay. You have received a statement from his insurance indicating that he owes the balance on the account. What do you say to him?

4. Create a collection letter that you would send to a patient's executor or patient's estate.

5. A patient promises to come by and bring you $100.00 on Friday. The payment is now 5 days late. What will you say when you call the patient?

Answers to Checkpoint Questions

1. Participating providers are doctors who agree to participate with managed care contracts and other third-party payers in exchange for building a solid patient base.

2. Four forms of payment accepted by most physician offices include cash, check, debit card, and credit card.

3. A fee adjustment is a reduced rate; a write-off is cancellation of an unpaid debt.

4. Credit cannot be denied based on age, gender, race, marital status, religion, national origin, or source of income.

5. Aging of an account is determining the amount of time between the date of the first bill sent to the patient and the date of the last payment.

6. Do not leave a message on an answering machine disclosing information that would link the patient to a particular physician or medical treatment. Ask that the patient return your call, but only give your first name and phone number. Do not state the nature of the call.

7. Overdue accounts can be collected by sending notices, telephoning patients, and informing patients at the next office visit.

Outline

**Accounts Receivable and
Daily Bookkeeping**
Manual Accounting
Pegboard Bookkeeping System
Posting a Charge
Posting a Payment
Processing a Credit Balance
Processing Refunds
Posting a Credit Adjustment
Posting a Debit Adjustment
Posting to Cash-Paid-Out
Section of Day Sheet
Computerized Accounting

Posting to Computer Accounts
Computer Accounting Reports
Banks and Their Services
Types of Accounts
Bank Fees
Types of Checks
Banking Responsibilities
Writing Checks for Accounts
Payable
Receiving Checks and Making
Deposits
Reconciling Bank Statements
Petty Cash

Overview of Accounting
Accounting Cycle
Record-Keeping Components
Accounts Payable
Ordering Goods and Services
Receiving Supplies
Paying Invoices
Preparation of Reports
Assisting with Audits

Learning Objectives

*Upon successfully completing this chapter, you
will be able to:*

1. Spell and define the key terms

2. Explain the concept of the pegboard bookkeeping system

3. Describe the components of the pegboard
system

4. Identify and discuss the special features of
the pegboard daysheet

5. Describe the functions of a computer accounting system

6. List the uses and components of computer
accounting reports

7. Explain banking services, including types
of accounts and fees

8. Describe the accounting cycle

9. Describe the components of a record-
keeping system

10. Explain the process of ordering supplies
and paying invoices

Upon successfully completing this chapter, you will be able to:

1. Post charges on a daysheet (Procedure 12-1)
2. Post payments on a daysheet (Procedure 12-2)
3. Process a credit balance (Procedure 12-3)
4. Process refunds (Procedure 12-4)
5. Post adjustments (Procedure 12-5)
6. Post collection agency payments (Procedure 12-6)
7. Post NSF checks (Procedure 12-7)
8. Balance a daysheet (Procedure 12-8)
9. Complete a bank deposit slip and make a deposit (Procedure 12-9)
10. Reconcile a bank statement (Procedure 12-10)
11. Maintain a petty cash account (Procedure 12-11)
12. Order supplies (Procedure 12-12)
13. Write a check (Procedure 12-13)

CAAHEP

- Prepare a bank deposit
- Post entries on a daysheet
- Post adjustments
- Process credit balance
- Process refunds
- Post NSF checks
- Post collection agency payments
- Perform an inventory of supplies and equipment

ABHES

- Prepare a bank statement and deposit records
- Reconcile a bank statement
- Post entries on a daysheet
- Prepare a check
- Establish and maintain a petty cash fund
- Post adjustments
- Process credit balance
- Process refunds
- Post NSF funds
- Post collection agency payments
- Use physician fee schedule
- Inventory equipment and supplies

accounting cycle	charge slip	Internal Revenue Service (IRS)	posting
accounts payable	check register		profit-and-loss statement
accounts receivable	check stub	invoice	
adjustment	credit	ledger card	purchase order
audit	daysheet	liabilities	returned check fee
balance	debit	packing slip	service charge
bookkeeping	encounter form	payroll	summation report

Bookkeeping and banking are important facets of medical office management. In most medical practices, bookkeeping and banking involve maintaining both patient and office account records, including petty cash, **accounts receivable** (money owed to the practice), and **accounts payable** (money owed by the practice). Most medical practices use computer accounting systems, although some smaller practices and satellite offices still use manual systems. When a computerized system is down, the pegboard serves as a backup. Although daily bookkeeping practices are handled in the office, the office also employs an accountant who receives reports of the daily financial functions.

Accounts Receivable and Daily Bookkeeping

Bookkeeping is defined as an organized and accurate record-keeping system of financial transactions for a business. The daily financial transactions of a medical office include patient payments that arrive through the mail, patient payments from patients seen in the office, and patient charges that are added to the accounts receivable. Most medical practices use the single-entry bookkeeping system.

The foundation of accounting is this equation:

$$\text{Assets} = \text{liabilities} + \text{equity}$$

Assets are all things of value owned by or relating to the practice. Liabilities are monies owed. Equity refers to the amount of capital the physician has invested in the practice. Because the two sides of the accounting equation must always **balance** (be equal), each transaction requires a **debit** (charge) on one side of the equation and a **credit** (payment) on the other side of the equation; the amount of the debit and credit must be equal. Double-entry systems are usually used by accounting firms and corporations.

Most medical facilities use the *cash basis* type of accounting, which means that income is considered as income only when money is collected and that payables (money owed) are considered expenses only when money is paid.

The most popular formats for daily bookkeeping are the manual pegboard system and computer systems.

Manual Accounting

Pegboard Bookkeeping System

The pegboard, or write-it-once, bookkeeping system uses a board with pegs running down the left side. The pegs hold a **daysheet,** or daily journal, in place on the board. All transactions for the day are recorded on this daysheet. Each patient has a **ledger card** (record of the patient's financial activities). When a patient transaction occurs, the bookkeeper places the ledger card over

the daysheet and the **charge slip** (preprinted patient bill) over the ledger card on the next available entry line and makes the appropriate entry on the ledger card. Figure 12-1 is a sample daysheet.

Daysheets come with a sheet of carbon paper; thus, the entry recorded on the ledger card, even when a charge slip is not used, is also recorded on the daysheet. When a payment received in the mail is posted, for example, no charge slip is needed. As the day progresses, each patient's ledger card is placed on the next available line on the daysheet, so that the day's entries appear consecutively. At the end of the day, all of the transactions are added.

The various components used in a pegboard system and the specific steps for recording patient transactions are discussed in greater detail next.

 CHECKPOINT QUESTION

1. What is an asset?

Daysheet

The daysheet keeps track of daily patient transactions, such as charges for services to patients, payments received from patients and insurance carriers, and adjustments to patient accounts. A daysheet should be kept for each day that the physician sees patients; on busy days or for practices with more than one physician, more than one daysheet may be required.

The daysheet has several sections: a deposit slip, distribution columns, a section for payments, a section for adjustments, and a section for **posting** proofs (listing financial transactions in a ledger).

The deposit slip is a detachable portion of the daysheet. All payments received are noted on the deposit slip, and at the end of the day, it is separated from the daysheet and deposited with that day's payments.

The distribution columns are used to assign charges for various services. How these columns are used de-

Figure 12-1 Sample daysheet with ledger card and charge slip (to fill in before sending). (Courtesy of Control-o-fax, Waterloo, IA.)

pends on the needs of the individual practice. In a group practice, each practitioner has his or her own column. Some practices may assign columns to the various insurance plans they accept. Finally, these columns can be used to provide information on quality improvement issues. The distribution columns, regardless of how they are assigned, provide the physician with important information about how the practice earns its income.

An **adjustment** is an entry to change an account. The adjustments section allows for reductions in office fees, as with professional courtesy discounts and insurance disallowances. The adjustments section also allows for crediting an account for uncollectible monies without using the payment column. It can also be used to return charges to an account if the patient's payment has been returned by the bank for insufficient funds.

The posting proofs section is where the day's totals are entered and the daysheet is balanced, much as one would balance a checkbook. Once the daysheet is complete, each column or section is totaled individually. It is best to total each column twice to make sure that no errors have been made. After all the columns have been totaled, the posting proofs section is filled out.

If the posting proofs do not balance, an error has been made on the daysheet. To locate the error, go over each transaction one by one. Add the previous balance to the fee or subtract the payment from the previous balance to check whether the new balance listed is correct. If the posted charges are correct, total each column again. Do not erase or white-out errors; draw a line through the erroneous entry and enter the transaction on a new line. When you re-enter a transaction on the daysheet, use the ledger card again.

The daysheet is important because it keeps track of accounts receivable. The accounts receivable total changes every time a charge, payment, or adjustment is made to an account. You should perform a trial balance at the end of each month. Add the totals of each ledger card with an outstanding balance. The total should match the running total kept on the daysheet. This practice ensures the accuracy of your financial records.

Completed daysheets are filed chronologically in a ledger (a book of accounts) with the most recent daysheet on top. Completed daysheets are important legal documents and must be kept for at least 7 years for tax purposes. They should be stored in a safe, dark area to avoid loss or fading.

 CHECKPOINT QUESTION

2. What are five sections of a pegboard daysheet?

Ledger Cards

The **ledger card** is a financial record for each patient. Most ledger cards include areas for the responsible per-

son's name, address, telephone number, and insurance information. Figure 12-2 is a sample ledger card. Patient information appears on the top of the ledger card; the bottom portion is used to record the patient's financial activities.

A photocopy of an individual's ledger card is sent as a bill. If you use a copy of the ledger card for billing, make sure that no information other than the billing name and address is visible through the window of the envelope. Allowing other information to be visible is a breach of privacy.

The ledger card is a legal document and should be kept for the same length of time as the patient's medical record. Ledger cards are filed alphabetically in a ledger tray. A medical practice may require more than one ledger tray. Ledger cards with outstanding balances are kept separate from paid ledger cards; this makes it easier to photocopy the monthly bills or find a ledger card when a patient calls about an outstanding bill. If the office uses only one ledger tray, the ledger cards with outstanding balances are filed alphabetically in the front of the ledger tray, with the paid ledger cards filed alphabetically in the back.

Encounter Forms and Charge Slips

The **encounter form** and the charge slip are preprinted patient statements that list codes for basic office charges and have sections for the patient's current balance and next appointment. Most encounter forms and charge slips have three-part copies:

1. The first copy is kept by the facility for auditing purposes (all are numbered).

DATE	DESCRIPTION	CHARGES	CREDITS PYMNTS.	ADJ.	BALANCE	
		BALANCE FORWARD ➔			20	00
5/2	OV	50 00			70	00
5/10	BC/BS ck (5/2)		60 00	10 00	-0-	
5/25	OV, Lab	120 00			120	00

FORM MR 10   PLEASE PAY LAST AMOUNT IN BALANCE COLUMN ➔

Figure 12-2 Sample ledger card.

2. The second copy is given to the patient for insurance filing (if the patient files the insurance claims).
3. The third copy, which has a carbon line at the top to match your ledgers and daysheets, is given to the patient as a receipt of services.

Charge slips are smaller versions of an encounter form and are designed to be used in conjunction with ledger cards. They often have different-colored no-carbon-required (NCR) copies. Figure 12-3 shows a computer-generated encounter form and a charge slip used in a manual system.

 CHECKPOINT QUESTION

3. What is an encounter form?

Posting a Charge

The charge column of the daysheet is for original charges incurred for services received by the patient from the physician or staff on a specific date. Examples include office visits, electrocardiograms, blood work, hospital visits, consultations, and fees for returned checks. As discussed previously, charges in a medical office are based on a fee schedule or list of charges determined by the usual, customary, and reasonable charges of similar providers in similar localities who practice under similar circumstances. Procedure 12-1 outlines the steps for posting a charge.

Posting a Payment

Payments received by the practice may include insurance checks received in the mail, money orders, credit card payments, or cash received from patients. Procedure 12-2 outlines the steps for posting payments and adjustments.

Processing a Credit Balance

Sometimes an account is overpaid, either by the patient or the insurance company. Such an overpayment is termed a credit (money owed to the patient or insurance carrier). This will show on the patient's ledger card as the last balance, with brackets (e.g., [25]) indicating a credit (Procedure 12-3). Brackets indicate the opposite of the column's usual meaning. For example, the balance column normally shows patients' debits, or amounts patients owe to the doctor. Brackets around an amount indicate the opposite, namely, that the doctor owes the patient money.

Processing Refunds

Credits are handled in one of two ways: (1) the credit stays on the account and is subtracted from the charges on the patient's next visit, or (2) the patient is mailed a refund for the amount of the overpayment. How an overpayment is handled depends on office policy and the amount of the overpayment. Generally, overpayments under $5 are left on account as a credit, whereas overpayments over $5 are refunded. Procedure 12-4 indicates how to process refunds.

Posting a Credit Adjustment

The adjustments section is used to indicate nonstandard office fees and to credit an account for uncollectible monies. Below are three specific situations that require a credit adjustment.

Example 1. The physician wishes to give a registered nurse a 25% professional discount on charges incurred for an office visit. You enter the fee from the fee schedule in the charge column, show in the description column an office visit with a professional discount of 25%, and put the 25% in the adjustment column. Assume an office visit is $40. You put $40 in the charge column and $10 (25% of $40) in the adjustment column. The patient owes your facility $30 for this visit.

Example 2. Most medical offices participate with certain insurance groups, which means the physician has signed an agreement with the insurance carrier to accept the fee for services set by that carrier instead of the physician's normal fee. Again, you must charge the same fee for the procedure. When payment is received, however, the explanation of benefits from that carrier will show the agreed-on amount for that procedure. You will post the payment in the normal way, but you must write off the difference between the physician's standard fee for this procedure and the agreed-on amount. Assume the doctor charged $40 for an office visit and the insurance carrier's agreed-on amount was $35. You would post $40 in the payment column and $5 in the adjustment column to arrive at the agreed-on amount.

Example 3. Most facilities require that you write off the balance of an account when you turn it over to a collection agency to keep better control of the accounts receivable. Therefore, if the patient's balance is $1200, you would show "collection agency" in the description column of the ledger and put the $1200 in the adjustment column, which would bring the balance to 0. Procedures 12-5 and 12-6 list the steps for posting an adjustment and collection agency payment.

Patient Name: _____   Encounter #: _____

Patient ID #: _____ DOB: _____ Sex: _____   Service Provider: _____

PCP: _____   Appt. Status: ☐ Scheduled ☐ Same Day ☐ Walk-in

SSN: _____ Financial Class: _____   Check-in Time: _____ Check-out Time: _____

Escorted to Exam Room: _____ Time Patient Seen: _____

Phone: _____ (home) _____ (work)   Appointment Time: _____

Medical Record #: _____ Date of Service: _____   Is Patient Being Seen in Relation to:
☐ Motor Vehicle Accident ☐ Workman's Compensation

Benefit Pkg: _____ Copay $ _____   Appointment Failure Reason:
☐ Patient Cancel ☐ No Show ☐ Walk Out ☐ PHA Cancel

TYPE OF VISIT

✓	CODE	DESCRIPTION	FEE	✓	CODE	DESCRIPTION	FEE	✓	CODE	DESCRIPTION	FEE	✓	CODE	DESCRIPTION	FEE
		OFFICE VISITS-EST.				**OFFICE VISITS-NEW CONT.**				**PREVENTATIVE, NEW**				**COUNSELING**	
	99211	Minimal			99204	Compreh.			99385	E&M 18-39			99401	15 Min.	
	99212	Focused			99205	Comp. & Complex			99386	E&M 40-64			99402	30 Min.	
	99213	Expanded				**NURSE VISIT**			99387	E&M 65 & over			99403	45 Min.	
	99214	Detailed			99211	Minimal				**CONSULTATION**			99404	60 Min.	
	99215	Compreh.				**PREVENTATIVE, EST.**			99241	Focused					
		OFFICE VISITS-NEW			99395	E&M 18-39			99242	Pre-Op Consult					
	99201	Focused			99396	E&M 40-64			99244	2nd Opinion					
	99202	Expanded			99397	E&M 65 & over									
	99203	Detailed													

PROCEDURES

✓	CODE	DESCRIPTION	FEE	✓	CODE	DESCRIPTION	FEE	✓	CODE	DESCRIPTION	FEE	✓	CODE	DESCRIPTION	FEE
	88170	Aspiration - Cyst			11200	Skin Tag Removal				**IMMUNIZATIONS/INJECTIONS**				**IMMUNIZATIONS/INJECTIONS CONT.**	
	20600	Aspiration - Joint (Small)			20550	Trigger point/Tendon Inj.			G0009	Administration Fee - Pneumovax			J2203	Triamcinolone Inj.	
	20605	Aspiration - Joint (Interm.)							G0010	Administration Fee - Hepatitis B			J3420	Vitamin B₁₂	
	20610	Aspiration - Joint (Large)				**SPECIALTY SERVICES**			95115	Allergy Injection Single				**IN-HOUSE LABORATORY**	
	16020	Burn Dressing			99070	Ace Bandage			95117	Allergy Injection Multiple			89050	Cell Count, except blood	
	69210	Ear Irrigation			E0110	Crutches			90788	Antibiotic IM			89060	Crystalanalysis	
	10120	Foreign Body Removal, Skin			29130	Finger Splint			J2910	Aurothioglucose			82948	Glucose	
	10060	I&D Abscess, simple			29125	Wrist Splint			G0008	Flu Vaccine			85013	HCT	
	90780	IV Infusion Therapy			99080	Form Completion			J1600	Gold Injection			85018	Hemoglobin Screen	
	12001	Laceration Repair, Simple				**TESTING/SCREENING**			90731	Hepatitis B			81025	Pregnancy	
	13160	Laceration Repair, Extens.			95004	Allergy - Skin Test			90741	Immune Globulin			81002	Urinalysis, Dipstick	
	64450	Medial Nerve Infiltration			92557	Audiometry			90724	Influenza			81000	Urinalysis, Full	
	17110	Molluscum/Wart Rmvl			93000	EKG			J9217	Lupron 3.75 mg			G0001	Venipuncture	
	94640	Nebulizer			92506	Hearing Screen			J9217	Lupron 7.5 mg				**OTHER PROCEDURES**	
	82270	Stool for Blood (Hemocult)			86580	PPD			J9250	Methotrexate 2-5 mg					
	12001	Suturing, Superficial			94010	Pulmonary Function			90732	Pneumovax					
	13100	Suturing, Complex			94760	Pulse Oximetry, Single			90718	Td					
	11050	Skin Les./Wart Cautery			45330	Sigmoidoscopy, Flexible			90782	Therapeutic SQ or IM					

P = PRIMARY   S = SECONDARY   S1-S9 = NUMBERED SECONDARY

DIAGNOSIS

✓	CODE	DESCRIPTION	✓	CODE	DESCRIPTION	✓	CODE	DESCRIPTION
	789.0	Abdominal Pain		780.6	Fever		462	Pharyngitis (sore throat)
	879.8	Abrasion/Laceration		704.8	Folliculitis		486	Pneumonia
	995.3	Allergic Reaction		535.5	Gastritis		V70.3	Pre-Marital Testing
	477.9	Allergic Rhinitis		558.9	Gastroenteritis		V72.81	Pre-op Cardiac Exam
	285.9	Anemia		274.9	Gout		V72.83	Pre-op Exam, Other
	413.9	Angina		V72.3	Gyn Exam		601.0	Prostatitis
	300.00	Anxiety		784.0	Headache		600	Prostatism
	716.90	Arthritis		389.9	Hearing Loss		782.1	Rash
	427.9	Arrhythmia		536.8	Heartburn/Indigestion		569.3	Rectal Bleeding
	493.90	Asthma		573.3	Hepatitis		530.81	Reflux
	611.72	Breast Lump		455.6	Hemorrhoids		V81.2	Screening for Cardiac Condition
	490	Bronchitis		553.9	Hernia		780.3	Seizure Disorder
	727.3	Bursitis		401.9	Hypertension (NOS)		473.9	Sinusitis
	354.0	Carpal Tunnel Syndrome		272.4	Hyperlipidemia		848.9	Strain/Sprain
	682.9	Cellulitis		242.00	Hyperthyroidism		438	Stroke
	786.50	Chest Pain		251.2	Hypoglycemia		305.90	Substance Abuse
	575.1	Cholecystitis		380.4	Impacted Cerumen		099.9	STD
	372.3	Conjunctivitis		780.52	Insomnia		727.00	Tenosynovitis, Tendonitis
	496	COPD		564.1	Irritable Bowel Syndrome		451.9	Thrombophlebitis
	414.9	Coronary Artery Disease		719.40	Joint Pain		246.9	Thyroid Disease
	290.9	Dementia		592.0	Kidney Stones		435.9	TIA
	311	Depression		464.0	Laryngitis		463	Tonsillitis
	692.9	Dermatitis		724.2	Low Back Pain		011.90	Tuberculosis
	250.01	Diabetes, IDDM		710.0	Lupus		465.9	Upper Respiratory Infection
	250.00	Diabetes, NIDDM		V70.0	Medical Exam/Physical		599.0	Urinary Tract Infection
	558.9	Diarrhea		346.9	Migraine		V04.8	Vaccination, Flu
	562.10	Diverticular Disease		278.0	Obesity		V03.9	Vaccination, Pneumovax
	780.4	Dizziness		382.9	Otitis Media		616.10	Vaginitis
	995.2	Drug Reaction		614.9	Pelvic Inflammatory Disease		424.9	Valvular Heart Disease
	782.3	Edema		533.9	Peptic Ulcer Disease		079.9	Viral Syndrome
	780.7	Fatigue/Tiredness/Malaise		443.9	Perpheral Vascular Disease			

Comments: _____

PREVIOUS BALANCE	$
TODAY'S CHARGES	$
PAYMENT	$
BALANCE	$

RETURN APPOINTMENT: ____ Days ____ Weeks ____ Months
APPT. LENGTH: _____ PROVIDER: _____

APPT. REASON: _____

PROVIDER SIGNATURE: _____

Adult

Philadelphia Health Associates
Tax ID #23-2350500
PHA Group # PH75923

☐ 3550 Market Street Philadelphia, PA 19104 (215) 823-8660
☐ The Bourse Building 111 S. Independence Mall East • 7th Floor Philadelphia, PA 19106 (215) 625-9100

PHA-019 (6/95)

OTHER DIAGNOSIS

✓	CODE	DESCRIPTION	✓	CODE	DESCRIPTION

Figure 12-3 Sample encounter form and charge slip.

Posting a Debit Adjustment

Generally, a credit adjustment reduces the patient's account balance, whereas a debit adjustment adds to the patient's account balance. Below are three specific situations that require a debit adjustment.

Example 1. You receive a nonsufficient funds (NSF) check from the bank today. The check was given to you by a payment made earlier in the month and posted as such to his account. (See What If? box.) The previous payment is no longer valid. Therefore, you must eliminate that payment because the patient now owes it again. Because this is not an original charge, you may not use the charge column for this entry. To post this debit adjustment to the patient's account, you will show NSF in the description column and the amount of the NSF check in the adjustment column with brackets. Procedure 12-7 describes the steps for processing NSF checks.

Example 2. Assume that you have turned over an account to a collection agency and the patient comes in later to pay the amount owed. You must first put the money back on the account, or you will create a credit balance. Place the ledger card on the daysheet, and in the description column, write "reverse collection." Again, this is not an original or new charge, so you do not use the charge column. Show the amount in the adjustment column in brackets because you are adding the amount to the patient's balance. You may now show the payment in the payment column.

Example 3. Your office requires that you refund all money over $5 to the patient or insurance carrier. You must also post this to eliminate the credit balance on the account. Place the ledger card on the daysheet, and in the description column, write "refund to patient" (or insurance carrier). To eliminate a credit balance, you must debit the account. You put the amount of the refund in the adjustment column in brackets, indicating that it is a debit, not a credit adjustment. Procedure 12-4 describes the steps in processing refunds.

 CHECKPOINT QUESTION

4. How does a credit adjustment differ from a debit adjustment?

Posting to Cash-Paid-Out Section of Daysheet

Some insurance carriers adjust for money overpaid to your facility by holding that amount out of money they are paying your facility for other patients. Although you are posting the correct amounts in the payment c0olumn for each patient, the check amount from the insurance carrier is short the refund or kept-out money.

 PATIENT EDUCATION

Physician Charges: What Happens to the Difference?

The concept of writing off the difference in the amount the physician charges and the amount a third-party payer pays is often misunderstood by patients. Many patients think that this means the physician has overcharged them. You can help clear up confusion by saying something like this: "The doctor charges $50.00 for a level 1 exam. When we file a claim with your insurance company, they only `allow' $40.00 for that particular exam. The doctor has made an agreement with your insurance company to accept less in exchange for being your choice of physician."

Let's say a patient's coverage requires her to pay 20% of the bill. Insurance will pay their portion of what they allowed, which would be 80% of $40.00 or $32.00. The patient pays $8.00. This would leave a balance of $10.00, which is the difference in what was charged and what was allowed. This $10.00 is adjusted off of the account. This amount is written off only when the doctor is a participating provider with the insurance company. If you break it down, most patients will understand and appreciate the lesson.

You write this in the cash-paid-out section of the daysheet, explaining, "insurance refund on account of [patient's name]." It is also a good idea to make a copy of the explanation of benefits and staple it to the back of your daysheet for future reference. Procedure 12-8 describes how to balance a daysheet.

Computerized Accounting

Most medical office accounting software available today is easy to use and requires a minimum of computer skills. Computer programs fulfill many of the same functions as a pegboard system but do so much faster. Instead of recording entries on a daysheet, you key entries into a computer. You can print out invoices and receipts for patients and insurance companies. Since most practices have computer stations in several locations, the patient's account can be quickly and easily retrieved in all areas of the office, enabling everyone involved in the patient's care to access information about third-party coverage, co-payments required, and so on.

Computer bookkeeping programs have a variety of advantages over pegboard bookkeeping. Computer programs work as expanded calculators and perform the arithmetic functions, such as balancing individual accounts and the day's totals. Many bookkeeping programs also can write checks. Some programs manage electronic banking between the office and bank. The office may have computerized many functions, including bookkeeping, making appointments, and generating other office reports, such as forms for insurance reimbursement. It is essential that data stored on computer be backed up in a reliable way in case the computer crashes.

Posting to Computer Accounts

If you understand the fundamentals of accounting and how to post entries manually, you will be able to use a computer system with ease. To post payments, first retrieve the patient's account. The software will take you through the process. You enter the source and amount of the payment, the allowed amount for the service, and any necessary adjustments. As in a manual system, this information is provided on the insurance carrier's explanation of benefits (EOB). Calculations are automatic and error free.

When you post charges into the computer database, in most systems, you use a local or access code to indicate a certain procedure or service. For example, you may enter 211 to post a level 2 office visit for a new patient. When the information prints on the claim form, the CPT (Current Procedural Terminology) code 99212 will appear (see Chapter 15).

Computer Accounting Reports

Depending on the software package, you can easily generate daily, monthly, and yearly reports on transactions of an individual physician in a group practice. Daily and weekly reports provide the same information found on the bottom of a daysheet in a manual accounting system. At any given time, you can request a report that displays the practice's period-to-date and year-to-date financial status.

Computer systems record the daily activities described earlier for the manual system, and bookkeeping software enables you to create a closing report that prints a list of the day's financial activities. You may run a trial daily report or a final daily report. In a trial report, the information keyed in that day is printed for review. You correct any errors before running a final report. As on the daysheet, you categorize receipts as cash, check, and so on. A check register report can print the amount of the daily deposit and a list of checks for the day.

 CHECKPOINT QUESTION

5. What is a local or access code?

Banks and Their Services

Types of Accounts

Besides physical location, several factors are important when choosing a bank for the office business account. These factors include the monthly service fees, overdraft protection programs (protection against bouncing checks), interest-bearing accounts, and returned check fees.

Checking Accounts

A checking account allows you to write checks for funds that are deposited in the account. Each day, you will deposit to a checking account the money collected in the office. At the time a new checking account is opened, checks are ordered with a check order form. The administrative medical assistant must maintain the checkbook and ensure that checks are reordered as needed.

Banks offer a variety of options for checking accounts. Variables include monthly service charges, maximum amounts of checks written, minimum balance requirements, and so on. Interest-bearing checking accounts pay interest if the balance is kept above a certain amount. Most banks set the minimum checking account balance at $500 to $2500. The bank pays this interest in exchange for the use of your money for loans and other transactions. If you drop below the minimum balance, however, you will not earn interest. Most banks also charge a monthly service fee and a fee for each check written for the period the balance was below the limit. Some banks waive the monthly service fee if the office agrees to maintain a minimum balance in another account, such as a savings account.

Savings Accounts

The medical practice may use a savings account for money that is put aside for long-term plans or money that is not needed for writing checks. A savings account pays interest at a higher percentage rate than a checking account, allowing the money to grow. Funds can be transferred to the checking account as needed.

Money Market Accounts

Money market accounts are a combination of a savings account and an interest-bearing checking account. The minimum balance is usually much higher than that of a checking account (as much as $2500), but the interest rate also is much higher. These accounts offer limited check-writing privileges, including an initial deposit of $2000 and minimum balance of $500 per check.

Bank Fees

Banks charge fees for services. In an effort to get new business, banks offer special services and plans for small business, including the medical office.

Monthly Service Fees

Bank policies concerning monthly fees or service charges vary widely. A **service charge** is a fee charged monthly for using an account. The charge can be a fixed amount or may be an individual charge for each check written on the account. As discussed, some banks do not levy a service charge if a specific minimum balance is maintained for the account.

Overdraft Protection

Overdraft protection guarantees that checks written against the account will be paid even when there is not enough money in the account at the time. Usually, the bank pays the checks and retrieves the money owed to it when the account balance is restored. Many banks offer overdraft protection only up to a certain dollar amount.

Returned Check Fee

Some banks charge a **returned check fee**, which is a fee charged for any check that is deposited into the checking account but that is later returned to the bank because the account it was issued from had insufficient funds with which to pay the check. Such a check is often

W H A T   I F ?

What if a patient's check is returned for nonsufficient funds?

As a courtesy, you may call the patient and explain that the check has been returned for nonsufficient funds. Many times, the patient will instruct you to send the check back through the bank. You will need to make a separate deposit slip from the daily deposit of money taken in that day.

If this is not an option, then the patient should come into the office and pay the amount of the check plus any fees your office charges for a returned check. The returned check would then be given back to the patient since he or she has now paid cash for the amount. It is a good practice to flag the patient's account and even to demand cash only for future payments. Some businesses use a check service that electronically approves a check. There is a fee for this service.

referred to as a bounced check. Most facilities charge this amount to the patient. Because this is an original charge, the bad check fee is listed in the charge column of the patient ledger and daysheet, with the amount of the check being recorded as a debit adjustment.

Types of Checks

Most medical offices use the standard business check, but when certain circumstances require, there are other types available:

- Certified checks are stamped and signed by the bank to verify that the amount of the check is being held in the account for payment. The check is written from the customer's account.
- Cashier's checks are sold to a customer for cash or a personal check. The check is written by the bank, giving the recipient the added guarantee that the check is good.
- Traveler's checks are a convenient and safe way to carry cash when traveling. They are available in denominations of $10, $20, and $50, and if lost, they can be replaced. Traveler's checks are signed when bought and are countersigned (signed again) in the presence of the payee.
- Money orders, although not checks, can be purchased with cash from a bank or the US Postal Service. Money orders, which guarantee payment to the recipient, are often used for mailing payments since it is not safe to mail cash.

Box 12-1 highlights other terms used in the language of banking.

Banking Responsibilities

Writing Checks for Accounts Payable

Another financial responsibility of the medical assistant may be to handle accounts payable, or pay the bills. The accounts payable in a medical office usually include rent, utilities, taxes, salaries, vendors of supplies and services, patient refunds, and petty cash reimbursement. The accounts are usually paid by check. Banks require signature cards for each person authorized to sign checks. In most cases, this is limited to the physician or physicians. Some medical offices require two signatures, especially if the check is over a certain amount. Computer systems allow you to enter information in the proper field and print checks. Software systems also keep track of every transaction using a check. When using a manual system, type or write legibly. Use the current date and write the amount of the payment in both figures and words and the name of the payee. Complete the memo line for reference. Record the date, check number, amount of the check, and payee on the check registry. Post this transaction to the appro-

BOX 12-1

COMMON BANKING LANGUAGE

ABA number: A number originated by the American Bankers Association to identify the bank on which the check is written. It is written in the form of a fraction and is usually found above or below the check number. The top number of the fraction indicates the geographic location, and the bottom number identifies the bank.

ATM: Automated teller machines (ATM) have made 24-hour banking possible. With the use of a card you insert into a slot and a personal identification number (PIN), you can make deposits, withdrawals, and transfers at an ATM. If your bank owns the ATM, this convenience is usually free. If you use any other ATM, a service fee of up to $3.50 is charged. The ATM screen gives you the opportunity to cancel the transaction if you are not willing to pay the service fee.

Debit card: A card with a magnetic strip that is presented for payment directly from your checking account. When a transaction occurs, you record it in your check registry.

Online banking: Electronic or online banking gives you the opportunity to view your account at any time. Withdrawals and deposits are listed and can be printed, and transfers can be made.

Stale check: A check that has not been cashed within a certain time, usually 6 months. Some checks must be cashed within a shorter time, but that requirement must be printed on the check.

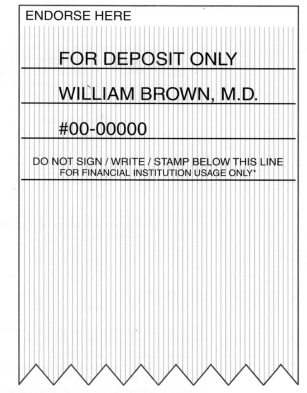

Figure 12-4 An endorsed check.

priate account in the general ledger or apply it to the proper category in a computer system by entering the type of payment on the proper screen. Recording transactions in the proper account or category is important when preparing the office taxes. Subtract each amount from the check register balance.

Receiving Checks and Making Deposits

When checks are received in the office, they are first endorsed. To endorse a check requires writing (or rubber stamping) on the back of the check the name and number of the account into which it will be deposited (Fig. 12-4). This way, if the payments are lost or stolen, no one else can cash them. It also ensures that the bank deposits the payments to the correct account. An endorsement stamp can be purchased from your bank or an office supply store.

After all payments are posted, total all of the checks and all cash received that day. This total should match the totals of the payments column on your daysheet. Detach the deposit sheet from the daysheet and stamp the back with the endorsement check stamp. If a computer program is used, print out a deposit slip. Wrap the deposit slip around the checks and complete a bank deposit slip for the account to which the deposit is made. The deposit can be hand delivered or mailed to the bank.

A hand-delivered deposit may be taken to a teller, who will issue a deposit receipt, or dropped in a depository. If the deposit is mailed, make sure sufficient postage has been affixed to the envelope. Never include cash payments in a deposit that is mailed or placed in a depository. Cash deposits should always be hand delivered, and a teller's receipt should always be obtained. Procedure 12-9 describes how to make a bank deposit.

Reconciling Bank Statements

All banks mail monthly statements to account holders on which are listed all transactions since the last closing date. This bank statement must be reconciled, or compared for accuracy, with your records each month.

The statement consists of a list of all checks written and their amounts, all deposits made and their amounts,

1. Subtract any fees or charges that appear on this statement from your checkbook balance.
2. Add any interest paid on your checking account to your checkbook balance.
3. List the checks you have written that have not been paid (these checks did not yet appear on your bank statement). You can also include in this list any withdrawals you have made since the ending date of the banking statement that do not appear on the statement.

Check Number	Amount
6217	32.94
6218	50.00
6219	119.24
Total	202.18

4. If you have entered deposits or other additions to your checkbook that do not appear on the statement, list them here:

Date	Amount
12-8-08	592.00
Total	592.00

5. Enter the ending balance from your statement here: 9542.91
    Add the total deposits from Step 4: + 595.00
    Subtract the total from Step 3: − 202.18
    Total (this should equal your checkbook balance): 9932.73

If these balances do not equal your checkbook balance:
*   Check the addition and subtraction in your checkbook
*   Check the amount of each transaction in your checkbook with the amount shown on your statement
*   Check to see that all transactions from your previous statement have been accounted for
*   Call your bank manager for assistance

Figure 12-5 Completed reconciling worksheet.

any electronic transactions, and any service charges. Verify that all checks and deposits are listed correctly. Make a check mark on the checkbook stub of each check that has been paid by the bank. On the back of the statement is a worksheet that explains how to balance the account (Fig. 12-5). Following the steps listed on the worksheet makes balancing the account fairly easy. The steps for reconciling a bank statement are listed in Procedure 12-10.

 CHECKPOINT QUESTION

6. What information is found on a bank statement?

Petty Cash

A petty cash account is a cash fund kept in the office specifically for small purchases, such as buying postage stamps or office supplies. The value of the petty cash account should always remain the same. A petty cash fund is always a designated sum of money. When money is

ETHICAL TIP

Honesty IS the Best Policy

A physician-employer puts his trust in his employees every day. In the clinical area, he trusts that his assistants will be conscientious and careful. In the administrative area, he trusts that employees will be completely honest and trustworthy. Borrowing $5.00 out of petty cash for lunch is not acceptable. When handling money for the facility, follow established procedures to the letter. Cross every "t" and dot every "i" so there will be no reason to doubt you. Fortunately, most physicians and their medical assistants enjoy a mutual respect and loyalty. By following the rules, you will prove to your employer that you are worthy of his trust.

PETTY CASH RECEIPT

_____ 12/1 20 _08_

Supplies:		
	14.	32
Postage:		
	1.	17
Travel Expenses:		
	—0—	
Other:		
fish food	4.	00
Approved 12/1/08		
L. Davis, CMA	TOTAL	19.49

Received Above Amount

19.49   HP, CMA

Figure 12-6 Completed petty cash receipt.

taken from the fund, a voucher (Fig. 12-6) or receipt is placed in the fund to verify the purchase. The remaining cash and the sum of the vouchers should always equal the designated sum; for example, a petty cash fund of $40 with $13 in actual cash should have receipts that amount to $27.

Petty cash funds should be kept separate from patient cash payments. All cash should be kept in a securely locked area. One person should be designated to maintain the petty cash fund and issue vouchers. A voucher with an attached receipt should always be placed in the petty cash box, both to provide proof of the purchase and to keep the account balanced. The petty cash fund normally is replenished once a month. To replenish the fund, cash a check in the amount of the total of the vouchers. The money is placed in the fund, and the vouchers are removed and filed (Procedure 12-11).

Some offices keep a petty cash expense record. This record is similar to a checkbook that keeps track of the account balance as checks are written, such as personal checkbook. This expense record also categorizes purchases so that they can be included with the monthly office expenses. Purchases such as stamps and office and medical supplies can be deducted as office expenses and added to the accounts payable expense record.

 CHECKPOINT QUESTION

7. List six guidelines for managing petty cash.

Overview of Accounting

Accounting is the compilation of a business's financial records. It is necessary for assessment of the practice's financial history and current financial stakes, which serves as the basis for sound financial management. The medical office, like other businesses, requires strict adherence to sound record-keeping practices. Records must be maintained in an orderly fashion so you can retrieve financial information at any time and to present an organized picture of the business's finances. A system of checks and balances is an integral part of record management. Generally, the check-and-balance status of accounts is examined monthly by comparing the total of all accounts with outstanding balances against the running total taken from the daily logs of all financial transactions. The practice's accountant will also closely scrutinize these records at scheduled intervals for tax-reporting purposes.

Although manual accounting systems are still used, computer accounting is available as part of most medical software packages, and the many advantages include efficient tracking and analysis of critical information, improved productivity, and smarter business decisions. General ledger, payables, receivables, inventory, purchasing, cash flow, bank reconciliation, collections, fixed assets, and many other applications integrate with each other so you can manage the office's core processes efficiently and effectively.

 LEGAL TIP

CORRECT IT CORRECTLY

It is illegal to falsify any financial documents. Accurate record keeping is essential. The IRS will examine the practice's financial records. You may be held liable for errors or omissions to these documents. White out is a great product, but should not be used in a medical office. There are documented cases of suspected fraud when financial records were corrected with white out. Corrections to ledger cards, daysheets, petty cash records, etc. are made just as they are in the medical record. Draw a single line through the wrong number, and place the correct one above or below. You should be able to see the item being corrected. If the space is too small for this, cross out the entire transaction and start a new one. Initial the correction.

Accounting Cycle

The finances of medical practices operate in one of two 12-month intervals or durations. The office **accounting cycle** follows either a fiscal year (a consecutive 12-month period starting with a specified date) or a calendar year (January through December). The yearly interval used depends on the way the practice's accountant has structured the business. For example, the medical practice can exist as a sole proprietorship or as a professional corporation.

The federal **Internal Revenue Service (IRS)** examines a business's income statements for the amount of profit and owed tax four times a year by quarterly estimated tax returns. The practice's annual tax return is a summary of the quarterly returns and reports the final year-end profit or loss (income minus expenses equals profit or loss) for the fiscal or calendar reporting period. If financial records are scrupulously maintained all year, preparation of the annual income tax return should merely be a summation of existing accounting facts. Well-maintained office records not only facilitate IRS returns but also provide data that define the practice's business picture.

There are many reasons for a physician along with an accountant to review financial data on a regular basis. Financial records reflect growing expenditures and growth in the business. Conclusions drawn from financial data can affect future financial decisions. For example, analysis of the practice's accounts receivable can predict the amount of salary increases. Tax records must be available in case of an IRS inquiry or **audit** (review of accounts). Records such as receipts should be retained for 7 years, but records such as bank statements, canceled checks, and IRS tax returns should be kept for the duration of the business.

Record-Keeping Components

The practice's financial records should include a running record of income, accounts receivable, and total expenditures, including **payroll** (employee salaries), cash on hand, and **liabilities** (amounts the practice owes). Expenditures can be broken down into categories (Box 12-2). This is important because it enables the record keeper to track the practice's expenses and provide the physician and accountant with a cohesive picture of the practice's expenses at tax time.

Categories can be accommodated by several types of bookkeeping systems; a simple business checkbook does not allow this. Pegboard systems allow the bookkeeper to write the check once over the **check register** (a place to record checks) or the ledger sheet and then have multiple pages with columns to distribute an expense into categories, including a back sheet for payroll. These columns are totaled and balanced at the completion of each check register sheet and can be subtotaled

---

BOX 12-2

CATEGORIES OF EXPENDITURES

- Office supplies: items used by the facility's employees, such as paper, pencils, daysheets, and ledger cards
- Medical supplies: items used for patients, such as examination gowns, electrocardiograph paper, syringes, and tongue depressors
- Drugs: drug purchases, such as injectables; some facilities keep a separate column for these purchases, and others put this amount in the medical supplies category
- Payroll: gross amount paid to employees
- Taxes: taxes paid, such as FICA, Medicare, federal withholding, state withholding, listed separately
- Rent: amount paid to rent the facility
- Utilities: gas, electric, telephone
- Maintenance: routine care of the facility, such as cleaning personnel
- Travel: physician's car lease payment, gas mileage if paid to employees, and so on
- Personal: any money used personally by the physician

---

monthly, quarterly, and annually (discussed later in the chapter). Keeping a monthly accounts payable disbursement sheet lets the administrative medical assistant easily compare past years' expenses for the same part of the year.

Software packages offer the most sophisticated way to maintain financial records, not just for the categorization of expenses but also for the rapid formation of financial reports. Automating accounts payable does, however, require a personal computer (PC), software, and the training to use it.

There are advantages and disadvantages to both computer systems and paper records. Each practice should make this decision based on its particular volume and needs. Either system (pegboard or computer) can provide the practice and its accountant with the ability to pay and track expenses and to furnish the financial data necessary to create reports.

Multiple **summation reports**, such as the payroll report, itemized category report, account balances, and the **profit-and-loss statement**, must be prepared for the practice's accountant. If financial data are entered diligently into the bookkeeping system, preparing monthly, quarterly, or yearly reports should not be a daunting task. Income tax accounting cycles are divided into quarters: January through March, April through June, July through September, and October through December. Payroll reports show the amount of taxes being withheld and made monthly, quarterly, or annually. Normally, the practice's accountant will send you necessary reports and have you mail the checks.

Accounts Payable

Ordering Goods and Services

There are many economical ways to purchase office supplies or equipment. For instance, purchasing cooperatives (co-ops) offer bulk rate discounts by allowing physicians to order in a pool with other purchasers. Vendors may offer discounts for buying in volume or for paying promptly. Large warehouse-type merchandisers and companies with discount catalogs also offer competitive prices. Researching and cost-comparing office products and medical supplies can be time consuming, but it is worth the effort, especially for items used frequently. Compare past invoices with prices in new catalogs.

Besides cost, other considerations come to bear when purchasing office supplies. For example, office supply companies often provide free delivery, but office warehouse chains may charge a fee or require a minimum order for free delivery. Quality also plays a role. Supplies should be of standard quality as well as economical. It is common to use several office supply vendors according to quality or pricing of specific goods.

Office supplies or equipment can be ordered in a number of ways. Once an account is set up, offices can place orders by telephone, fax, mail, or e-mail. These orders can be paid monthly by check or by credit card. It is preferable to pay for supplies by check or credit card rather than by cash, but when cash purchases are necessary, retain a detailed receipt for tax purposes. Credit card purchases can be made online, over the telephone, or by mail, but for security reasons credit card account numbers should not be faxed.

When placing orders for supplies, give the office's account number to the vendor or write it on the order form. It is a good idea to use a **purchase order** that lists the supplies ordered and their order numbers, so that order numbers for frequently ordered items can be pulled from the previous purchase order; this saves time with subsequent orders. Be sure to record the charges for your order and verify them against the bill later. It is also handy to keep a list of all vendors, telephone numbers, and account numbers. Procedure 12-12 lists the steps for ordering supplies.

CHECKPOINT QUESTION

8. When purchasing office supplies, what factors besides price should you consider?

Receiving Supplies

When goods are delivered to the office, a receipt or **packing slip** listing the enclosed items should always accom-

WHAT IF?

What if all of the supplies ordered from a particular vendor are not in the shipment?
Check the packing slip to see that the item was actually sent (Fig. 12-7). The form should indicate whether the item or items are being shipped separately, out of stock, or discontinued. If the item is listed on the form as having been shipped, you will need to call the supplier. The supplier will need an order number from the packing slip. The missing item may have just been left out. Be sure to document the date, findings of the call, and name of the person you spoke with. Place a reminder on your calendar to follow up if the item is not there when promised. Don't pay for something you don't get.

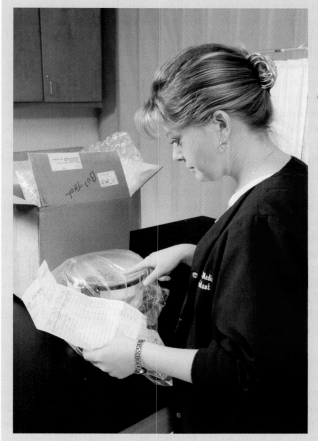

Figure 12-7 The medical assistant should be sure supplies are received and checked carefully.

pany the order. The office staff member who receives the supplies must check the packing slip against the actual contents to ensure that all supplies are in the shipment. The person should initial the packing slip, which shows that all goods were received. When it is time to issue checks for payables, the assistant can then pay the **invoice** or bill. These receipts or packing slips should be placed in a bills pending file, so that they may be compared to the bill when it arrives. If the bill has already been paid by check or credit card, the invoice should be placed in the appropriate accounts paid file; there should be such a file for each fiscal or calendar year.

Paying Invoices

Invoices for supplies and other types of bills payable by the practice should be kept together in a bills pending file to avoid loss or misplacement of a bill. Bills can be paid daily, weekly, biweekly, or monthly.

Manual Payment

Manual payment of bills requires a checkbook and checks (Procedure 12-13). The practice's accountant may recommend use of a log or record book into which is entered information about each check, such as payroll taxes or the breakdown of expenses for a monthly credit card bill. The large checks and checkbooks available from banks and business printers offer more space for writing memos or itemizing a check. Each check, once written, is detached from a **check stub**, which remains in the checkbook. If you make a mistake while writing a check, void the check and stub and staple the voided check to the stub. Never make corrections on the facility's checks. Check stubs should be filed with other fiscal or calendar year records and kept for the life of the practice.

The information recorded on the check stub includes the check number, the date the check was issued, the payee (the party to whom the check was written), and the full amount of the check. Notes should be written on both the memo section of the check and on the check stub. For example, when entering the purchase of a new beeper, the note might read, "payee: Office Communications" or "new beeper for Dr. Smith." The check is then attached to the bill or invoice and signed by an authorized individual.

Memos or notations on check stubs can be referenced later if a question arises concerning payment by a particular check. A log or record book enables the bookkeeper to make entries for each expense, categorize expenses, and maintain detailed payroll records. Unlike one-write (pegboard) or computer systems, multiple entries must be made by hand to track office bill paying. This can seem laborious when compared to other bookkeeping systems, but it may be ideal for smaller practices.

Pegboard Payment

The same pegboard system that is used for accounts receivable may be used for bill paying; it has several advantages over the ordinary manual method of paying bills. Instead of using a daysheet, a **check register** page is used to record the checks that have been written. The check is then aligned on the pegboard over the register page and is filled out as with any other check (Fig. 12-8). Pegboard checks have a carbon or transfer strip, and on this strip is written the date, the payee, the check number, and the amount. The information written on the strip is recorded automatically on the check register. These check-writing systems are referred to as one-write systems for this reason. The check can be addressed directly beneath the payee line and mailed in a window envelope, which saves the time it would take to address an envelope.

The pegboard check register has approximately 20 columns that can be used to categorize expenses, such as rent, insurance, office supplies, utilities, service contracts, postage, and any other applicable categories. All entries on the check register are totaled when the register is completed; these totals are carried forward to the new register page. Each fiscal or calendar year begins with a new first page (page 1), and the last check register page will have totals for the entire year. The check register provides a system of checks and balances even before the bank statement arrives because the check register must be balanced, as with a bank statement.

The check register also allows entries for bank deposits, and the back page of the register is used for payroll record keeping. As with pegboard accounts receivable, completed pegboard check registers are filed in a separate binder in chronological order, with the most recent register on top.

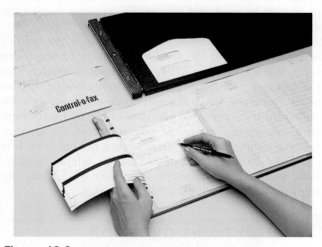

Figure 12-8 Sample pegboard check and check register. (Courtesy of Control-o-fax, Waterloo, IA.)

Computer Payment

A computer accounts payable system has all the advantages that a pegboard system offers: access at a glance to check registers, itemized categories and their totals, payroll records, and entries for bank deposits. To use such a system, you must have a PC, accounts payable program software, printer, and bank checks that are compatible with the software and printer. The initial expense with a computer system is much higher than that of manual or pegboard systems. Office personnel will need computer training to use the program. Also, since it runs on electricity, a computer may not work during power failures. A good computer accounting program will, however, provide functions for both accounts receivable and accounts payable. Financial data should be recorded in three forms: on the computer's hard drive, on a magnetic tape or CD, and in printout form (hard copy).

Although entering data in the computer may be time consuming at first, this becomes less of a concern with practice. Furthermore, financial reports can be compiled and printed in a fraction of the time required with manual or pegboard systems. The computer program can also perform the record-keeping arithmetic; as a result, mathematical errors are practically nonexistent.

Paying bills by computer requires using the software to open the check-writing file. Checks are presented on the computer screen in the same way that a paper check would normally appear, and the information that is required to appear on the check is entered on the computer keyboard. The information is stored, and the check is printed out; the computer program automatically subtracts the amount of the check from the account's balance. The bookkeeper can print one check at a time or a batch of checks together.

The computer can "memorize" checks so that the information on them can be recalled and reprinted without re-entering it; this is especially helpful with payroll checks. A good accounting program also allows for bill and backup reminders. Of course, it is essential to back up financial data in case of computer problems.

 CHECKPOINT QUESTION

9. Whether using a manual, pegboard, or computer accounts payable system, two steps must always occur when ordering and receiving supplies. What are they?

Preparation of Reports

The bookkeeper must also prepare reports for the practice's accountant or the IRS based on financial data stored in the office's bookkeeping system. For this reason, care should always be taken when recording financial data.

The manual system, when assisted by the use of a log or record book, should be able to provide monthly, quarterly, and annual summaries for income, expenditures, and payroll. It is advisable to have subtotals and totals for these periods for tax payment purposes.

The pegboard system is also practical for providing summaries of income, expenses, and payroll and can be totaled monthly, quarterly, and yearly. Each daysheet, check register, and payroll journal is individually totaled, with all balances forwarded to the next page. These records are stored in binders and kept for future reference.

A computer system of accounting offers all of the previously mentioned reports along with other more complicated reports that generally require more advanced accounting skills. The great advantage with a report generated by a computer is that the computer will perform all of the mathematical calculations for the time frame requested.

Assisting With Audits

An **audit** may be informal (in-house) and used to assist the practice's accountant with tax preparation, or it may be a formal audit by the IRS. If meticulous attention to record keeping has been paid throughout the year, the preparation time needed for such an audit should be minimal. It is important to save all bank statements, copies of annual and quarterly tax returns, and receipts for expenditures. Canceled checks and payroll records should be readily available.

Manual and pegboard systems can provide spending category and payroll summaries in addition to examination of the actual entries for the period being audited. A computer accounting system can provide all of this plus reports such as profit-and-loss statements, which normally would be compiled by an accountant.

español
SPANISH TERMINOLOGY

Los impuestos deben ser sacados de su cheque.
Taxes must be taken out of your paycheck.

Usted necesita completar estas formas.
You need to complete these forms.

Gracias para su pago.
Thank you for your payment.

Gracias para su cheque.
Thank you for your check.

Esto es su recibo.
This is your receipt.

Esto es su total.
This is your balance.

Esto es su crédito.
This is your credit.

No pague esta cuenta.
Do not pay this bill.

Su cheque se volvió para fondos de insuficiente.
Your check was returned for insufficient funds.

Su cuenta ha sido mandada a una agencia de la colección.
Your account has been sent to a collection agency.

MEDIA MENU

- **Student CD**
- **Case Study**
  Interactive Case Study 4: Accounting and Billing in the Medical Office
- **CMA/RMA Certification Exam Review**
- **Premium Online Course**
  http://thePoint.lww.com/Kronenberger3e
- **Internet Resources**

LiveAdvise Online Tutoring & Competency Training
http://thePoint.lww.com/LiveAdvise

Superbill Forms and Creations
www.physicianshelp.com

Comptroller of Currency Administrator of National Banks
www.occ.treas.gov

The Accounting Library (TAL)
www.accountinglibrary.com

Quickbooks Online
www.quickbooks.com

Microsoft Business Solutions
www.microsoft.com/businesssolutions

Internal Revenue Services
www.irs.gov

Payroll Taxes
www.payroll.com

PROCEDURE 12-1:   Post Charges on a Daysheet

Purpose: To keep a daily and running account of all charges to patients in the medical practice

Equipment: Pen, pegboard, calculator, daysheet, encounter forms, ledger cards, previous day's balance, list of patients and charges, fee schedule

Computer and medical office software: Follow the software requirements for posting credits to patient accounts

Steps	Purpose
1. Place a new daysheet on the pegboard and record the totals from the previous daysheet.	A new sheet should be used each day. Transferring the totals from the day before enables you to keep a running total.
2. Align the patient's ledger card with the first available line on the daysheet.	Each line should be used. It is easy to accidentally overlap entries.
3. Place receipt to align with the appropriate line on the ledger card.	Proper alignment makes neat and legible entries.

(continued)

PROCEDURE 12-1: Post Charges on a Daysheet *(continued)*

Steps	Purpose
4. Record the number of the receipt in the appropriate column.	This enables you to cross reference and provides two forms of tracking.
5. Write the patient's name on the receipt.	This is the section that will appear in the name section.
6. Record any existing balance the patient owes in the previous balance column of the daysheet.	This total must be added to any charges because this amount is already owed.
7. Record a brief description of the charge in the description line.	This will tell you and the patient what the charges were for.

Statement						
DATE	DESCRIPTION	CHARGES	CREDITS		BALANCE	
			PYMNTS.	ADJ.		
	BALANCE FORWARD ➞					
	OV, Lab					

Step 7. Write description in proper line of daysheet.

Steps	Purpose
8. Record the total charges in the charge column. Press hard so that marks go through to the ledger card and the daysheet.	Totaling the charges for a visit saves room on the ledger cards and the daysheets.
9. Add the total charges to the previous balance and record this number in the current balance column.	The current balance is what is already owed plus the new charges.
10. Return the ledger card to appropriate storage	Cards should be returned promptly for quick and easy retrieval.

PROCEDURE 12-2: Post Payments on a Daysheet

Purpose: To keep a daily and running account of all payments made to accounts in the medical practice
Equipment: Pen, pegboard, calculator, daysheet, encounter forms, ledger cards, previous day's balance, list of patients and charges, fee schedule
Computer and medical office software: Follow the software requirements for posting credits to patient accounts

Steps	Purpose
1. Place a new daysheet on the pegboard and recorded the totals from the previous daysheet.	A new sheet should be used each day. Transferring the totals from the day before enables you to keep a running total.
2. Align the patient's ledger card with the first available line on the daysheet.	Proper alignment makes neat and legible entries.
3. Place receipt to align with the appropriate line on the ledger card.	Each line should be used. It is easy to accidentally overlap entries.
4. Record the number of the receipt in the appropriate column.	This enables you to cross reference and provides two forms of tracking.
5. Write the patient's name on the receipt.	This is the section that will appear in the name section.

(continued)

PROCEDURE 12-2: Post Payments on a Daysheet *(continued)*

Steps	Purpose
6. Record any existing balance the patient owes in the previous balance column of the daysheet.	This total must be added to any charges because this amount is already owed.
7. Record the date of service being paid for, source, and type of the payment in the description line.	Such information makes tracking the payment easier and gives vital information that can be easily retrieved.
8. Record appropriate adjustments in adjustment column.	In many cases, it is illegal not to write off certain adjustments.
9. Record the total payment in the payment column. Press hard so that marks go through to the ledger card and the daysheet.	Because you are using a write-it-once system, your marks must go through three thicknesses.
10. Subtract the payment and adjustments from the outstanding/previous balance, and record the current balance.	Subtracting these amounts will give you the current amount owed.
11. Return the ledger card to appropriate storage.	Cards should be returned promptly for quick and easy retrieval.

PROCEDURE 12-3: Process a Credit Balance

Purpose: To determine and record monies that have been paid on an account beyond what is owed
Equipment: Pen, pegboard, calculator, daysheet, ledger card
Computer and medical office software: Follow the software requirements for processing a credit balance in patient accounts

Steps	Purpose
1. Determine the reason for the credit balance and be sure it is recorded in the explanation column of the ledger card.	An explanation will help you discuss the account with the patient.
2. Place brackets around the balance indicating that it is a negative number.	Brackets indicate the opposite of the usual action of a certain column. For example, when totaling the daysheet, a number in brackets would be subtracted instead of added.

	Statement				
			CREDITS		
DATE	DESCRIPTION	CHARGES	PYMNTS.	ADJ.	BALANCE
	BALANCE FORWARD ──────→				
			‹47│00›		

Step 2. Place brackets around number.

Steps	Purpose
3. Write a refund check by following the steps in Procedure 12-4.	A credit indicates that a patient's account has been overpaid.

PROCEDURE 12-4: Process Refunds

Purpose: To return money to the proper person or company when more money has been paid on an account than is owed

Equipment: Pen, pegboard, calculator, daysheet, ledger card, checkbook, check register, word processor letterhead, envelope, postage, copy machine, patient's chart, refund file

Steps	Reasons
1. Determine who gets the refund—the patient or the insurance company.	The explanation of benefits will list the patient's responsibility.
2. Pull patient's ledger card and place on current daysheet aligned with the first available line.	Proper alignment makes neat and legible entries.
3. Post the amount of the refund in the adjustment column in brackets, indicating it is a debit, not a credit, adjustment.	The brackets will instruct you to perform the opposite action of the column.
4. Write "Refund to Patient" or "Refund to _____" (name of insurance company) in the description column.	This information will be needed to discuss the account with the patient.
5. Write a check for the credit amount made out to the appropriate party. (See Procedure 12-13.)	Refunds should be made in a timely fashion. It is unethical to keep money that does not belong to the practice.
6. Record the amount and name of payee in the check register.	This follows proper procedure for writing a check.
7. Mail check with letter of explanation to patient or insurance company.	Place any identifying numbers in the letter to help match the refund to the proper person. Again, this should be done as soon as possible after writing the check.
8. Place copy of check and copy of letter in the patient's record or in refund file.	You must keep complete and accurate records of all transactions.
9. Return the patient's ledger card to its storage area.	Cards should be returned promptly for quick and easy retrieval.

PROCEDURE 12-5: Post Adjustments to a Daysheet

Purpose: To keep a daily and running account of all adjustments made to patients' accounts in the medical practice

Equipment: Pen, pegboard, calculator, daysheet, encounter forms, ledger cards, previous day's balance, list of patients and charges, fee schedule

Computer and medical offie software: Follow the software requirements for posting credits to patient accounts

Steps	Reasons
1. Pull the patient's ledger card and place on current daysheet aligned with the first available line.	Proper alignment makes neat and legible entries.
2. Post the amount to be written off in the adjustment column. Press hard so that marks go through to the ledger card and the daysheet.	Because you are using a write-it-once system, your marks must go through three thicknesses.

(continued)

PROCEDURE 12-5:   Post Adjustments to a Daysheet *(continued)*

Steps	Reasons
3. Subtract the adjustment from the outstanding/ previous balance, and record in the current balance column.	Subtracting these amounts will give you the current amount owed.
4. Return the ledger card to appropriate storage.	Cards should be returned promptly for quick and easy retrieval.

PROCEDURE 12-6:   Post Collection Agency Payments

Purpose: To apply payments made to collection agencies to patient's accounts, adjusting any amount paid to the collection agency.

Equipment: Pen, pegboard, calculator, daysheet, patient's ledger card

Steps	Reasons
1. Review check stub or report from the collection agency explaining the amounts to be applied to the accounts.	There may be more than one patient's account paid in a single check. You must determine the amount for each individual account.
2. Pull the patients' ledger cards.	Pulling all cards that are needed will minimize interruptions.
3. Post the amount to be applied in the payment column for each patient.	This amount should be subtracted from the outstanding amount for a particular date of service.
4. Write "payment from collection agency" in the explanation column.	This makes tracking the amount owed easier.
5. Adjust off the amount representing the percentage of the payment charged by the collection agency.	Subtracting the amount paid to the collection agency clears out the outstanding balance.

PROCEDURE 12-7: Process NSF Checks

Purpose: To document, record, notify patients, charge back amount "paid," assess fees and retrieve funds when the medical practice has a check returned due to nonsufficient funds (NSF)

Equipment: Pen, pegboard, calculator, daysheet, patient's ledger card

Steps	Purpose
1. Pull patient's ledger card and place on current daysheet aligned with the first available line.	Proper alignment makes neat and legible entries.
2. Write the amount of the check in the payment column in brackets indicating it is a debit, not a credit, adjustment.	Brackets tell you to do the opposite action of that expected in a particular column. Normally, the adjustment column is subtracted from the outstanding balance. Brackets instruct you to add the amount instead.
3. Write "Check Returned for Nonsufficient Funds" in the description column.	An explanation will make it easier to track transactions and determine specific reasons.
4. Post a returned check charge with an appropriate explanation in the charge column.	If the office charges a returned check fee, it should be posted here. This amount is designed to discourage returned checks and to cover administrative costs.
5. Write "Bank Fee for Returned Check" in the description column.	If the bank charges the practice with a fee, then you will pass this charge along to the patient.
6. Call the patient to advise him or her of the returned check and the fee.	The patient should be notified immediately in order to rectify the situation.
7. Construct a proper letter of explanation and a copy of the ledger card and mail to patient.	Even though the patient is notified by phone, details should also be recorded in writing.
8. Place a copy of the letter and the check in the patient's file.	A copy of the letter placed in the patient's chart proves the communication with the patient actually happened.
9. Make arrangements for the patient to pay cash to cover the check and fees.	Requiring cash will eliminate the possibility of another returned check.
10. Flag the patient's account as a credit risk for future transactions.	It is helpful to know of possible future problems with payment of an account.
11. Return the patient's ledger card to its storage area.	Cards should be returned promptly for quick and easy retrieval.

PROCEDURE 12-8: Balance a Daysheet

Purpose: To ensure an accurate daily total of charges, payments, and adjustments to patients' accounts in the medical practice
Equipment: Daysheet with totals brought forward, calculator, pen

Steps	Purpose
1. Be sure the totals from the previous daysheet are recorded in the column for previous totals.	You must have these previous totals in order to keep a running balance of the accounts receivable.
2. Total the charge column and place that number in the proper blank.	
3. Total the payment column and place that number in the proper blank.	
4. Total the adjustment column and place that number in the proper blank.	
5. Total the current balance column and place that number in the proper blank.	
6. Total the previous balance column and place that number in the proper blank.	
7. Take the grand total of the previous balances, add the grand total of the charges, and subtract the grand totals of the payments and adjustments. This number must equal the grand total of the current balance.	This will prove that the daysheet is balanced and there are no errors.
8. If the numbers do not match, calculate your totals again, and continue looking for errors until the numbers match.	The daysheet must be accurate before moving onto a new daysheet.
9. Record the totals of the columns in the proper space on the next daysheet.	You will be prepared for balancing the new daysheet.

PROCEDURE 12-9: Complete a Bank Deposit Slip and Make a Deposit

Purpose: To place money collected in the medical practice into a safe and secure bank account
Equipment: Calculator with tape, currency, coins, checks for deposit, deposit slip, endorsement stamp, deposit envelope

Steps	Reasons
1. Separate the cash from the checks.	These will be recorded separately on the deposit slip.
2. Arrange bills face up and sorted with the largest denomination on top.	Most bill counters in banks are loaded in this manner. Sorting the bills is also a courtesy to the bank.
3. Record the total in the cash block on the deposit slip.	

(continued)

PROCEDURE 12-9: **Complete a Bank Deposit Slip and Make a Deposit** *(continued)*

Steps	Reasons
4. Endorse the back of each check with "For Deposit Only."	This is one safety practice to reduce the possibility of fraud and/or forgery.
5. Record the amount of each check beside an identifying number on the deposit slip.	This helps ensure the identity and accuracy of each check
6. Total and record the amounts of checks in the line on the deposit slip labeled "total of checks."	This amount will be added to the amount of cash.
7. Subtotal and record the amount of cash and checks.	Add the amount of cash and the amount of checks for the total deposit.
8. Record the total amount of the deposit in the office checkbook register.	This step will keep the checkbook balance accurate and current.
9. Make a copy of both sides of the deposit slip for office records.	Keeping records helps you prove any errors or future discrepancies.
10. Place the cash, checks, and completed deposit slip in an envelope or bank bag for transporting to the bank for deposit.	Deposits should be made as soon as possible to prevent loss or theft. If using a night deposit box, pay close attention to your surroundings and stay safe.

PROCEDURE 12-10: **Reconcile a Bank Statement**

Purpose: To ensure the accuracy and sound financial practices of the bank accounts of the medical practice
Equipment: Bank statement, reconciliation worksheet, calculator, pen

Steps	Purpose
1. Compare the opening balance on the new statement with the closing balance on the previous statement.	You must know where your last bank statement ends and where the current one begins.
2. List the bank balance in the appropriate space on the reconciliation worksheet	Since there is no standard format for a reconciliation statement, be sure you are using the proper blank.
3. Compare the check entries on the statement with the entries in the check register. Place a check mark beside each check listed as paid on the statement.	This will help you identify the outstanding checks.

Withdrawals / Debits

DATE	AMOUNT	DESCRIPTION	REFERENCE #
02-12	38.90	Food Lion	436674796
02-12	500.00	Melton Custodial Servic	426580282
02-13	1200.00	Lewis Realty	446480157
02-13	22.00	John Little	456974902
02-14	150.00	HS Brown, Florist	466748392

Step 3. Place check marks next to checks listed as paid.

Steps	Purpose
4. List the amounts of the checks without checkmarks (outstanding checks).	These have not cleared the bank.

(continued)

PROCEDURE 12-10:   Reconcile a Bank Statement *(continued)*

Steps	Purpose
5. Total outstanding checks.	
6. Subtract from the checkbook balance items such as withdrawals, automatic payments, or service charges that appear on the statement but not in the checkbook.	These transactions are reflected in the bank statement but not in the checkbook.
7. Add to the bank statement balance any deposits not shown on the bank statement.	This gives you the proper current balance in the account.
8. Make sure that the balance in the checkbook and the bank statement agree.	This will ensure the accuracy of the current balance in the account.

PROCEDURE 12-11:   Maintain a Petty Cash Account

Purpose: To keep a small amount of cash on hand to cover expenses such as postage due, reimbursement for emergency supplies, etc.

Equipment: Daysheet and an exercise from the workbook about establishing and maintaining a petty cash fund

Steps	Reasons
1. Count the money remaining in the box.	This amount will remain in the box.

Step 1. Count the cash from the box.

Steps	Reasons
2. Total the amounts of all vouchers in the petty cash box to determine the amount of expenditures.	This total will represent the amount of money used.
3. Subtract the amount of receipts from the original amount in petty cash.	This should equal the amount of cash remaining in the box.
4. When the cash has been balanced against the receipts, write a check only for the amount that was used.	You will keep the same amount of petty cash unless instructed otherwise.

(continued)

PROCEDURE 12-11: Maintain a Petty Cash Account *(continued)*

Steps	Reasons
5. Record totals on the memo line of the check stub.	This is proper procedure for writing a check.
6. Sort and record all vouchers to the appropriate accounts.	The next step in the accounting practice is to post the amounts to the individual accounts of the practice.
7. File the list of vouchers and receipts attached.	Records of all business transactions must be kept.
8. Place cash in petty cash fund.	Added to the amount already in the box, this will replenish the petty cash box.

PROCEDURE 12-12: Order Supplies

Purpose: To maintain the materials and supplies needed to operate a medical practice efficiently
Equipment: 5 × 7 index cards, file box with divider cards, computer with internet (optional), medical supply catalogues

Steps	Purpose
1. Create a list of supplies to be ordered.	Employees will report supply needs as they occur. Knowing what supplies you are ordering will help you know what catalogues will be needed. Making a list of all the needed items will help you organize the ordering process.
2. Create an index card for each supply on the list by placing the name of the supply in the top left corner and including name and contact information of vendor(s) and product identification number.	This establishes a record of the supplies used in the facility.
3. File the index cards in the file box with divider cards alphabetically or by product type.	This allows for quick access and makes reordering easier.
4. Record the current price of the item and how the item is supplied. Make a note of any price breaks on larger quantities, etc.	The price should be written in pencil because this allows you to change the price as needed. You will save money by taking advantage of special discounts for larger quantities.
5. Record the reorder point. This is the point where you reorder an item.	When supplies on hand reach half of the amount you need, you will know to reorder.

PROCEDURE 12-13: Write a check

Purpose: To disperse money to individuals or companies from the medical practice by preparing checks from a checking account

Equipment: Simulated page of checks from checkbook, scenario giving amount of check, check register

Steps	Purpose
1. Fill out the check register with the following information: a. check number b. date c. payee information d. amount e. previous balance f. new balance	This is all crucial information and must be recorded accurately.
2. Enter the date on the check.	Dates are also crucial to a bookkeeping system.
3. Enter the payee on the check.	Without a payee, the check is nonnegotiable
4. Enter the amount of the check using numerals	This is the amount paid by the bank. It will be compared to the written amount below, ensuring that the amount has not been tampered with.
5. Write out the amount of the check beginning as far left as possible and making a straight line to fill in space between dollars and cents.	This practice creates a double check system that helps to verify the authenticity of the check.
6. Record cents as a fraction with 100 as the denominator.	According to banking guidelines, this is the customary way to write a check
7. Obtain appropriate signature(s).	Many offices require more than one signature to help reduce the possibility of employee theft.

Step 7. A properly completed check.

8. Proofread for accuracy.	Accuracy is important in everything a medical assistant does.

- Accounting is a complex process involving many legal issues. As a medical assistant, you must keep neat and well-organized accounting records.
- Whether a medical practice uses a manual bookkeeping system, such as the pegboard system, or a computer system, you may be responsible for keeping records of accounts payable, accounts receivable, and petty cash.
- You may also be responsible for banking functions, such as receiving checks, making deposits, and reconciling monthly bank statements. To carry out these responsibilities effectively, you must record all transactions accurately and promptly.
- Computers have made the daily bookkeeping practices much easier, but you must understand the principles of accounting applied in the manual system if you are to use the computer system.
- Using the appropriate banking services will allow the day-to-day financial operations to be efficient, accurate, and secure.
- Managing the supplies and equipment in a practice, ordering goods and services efficiently and economically, and paying invoices are important duties of a medical assistant.
- With the computer being used for many administrative medical office functions, it is imperative that you keep abreast of changes and new opportunities to make this process more efficient and up-to-date.

Warm Ups for Critical Thinking

1. Your daysheet deposit slip and your posting proofs do not agree. How do you find the error?

2. Your office is considering going from a pegboard system to a computer bookkeeping system. What features should you look for in the software?

3. Explain the advantages of using computerized accounting systems.

4. When might a manual bookkeeping system using a pegboard be used?

5. A vendor continually mixes up your orders, and the physician asks you to look for a new vendor. How do you decide which one to recommend? What factors influence your choice of one office supply vendor over another?

6. The physician asks you, the office manager, how much money is owed to him. How do you gather the information needed to answer his question?

Answers to Checkpoint Questions

1. An asset is a thing of value owned by or relating to a business.

2. Five sections of a pegboard daysheet include the distribution columns, adjustment column, deposit slip, payments section, and posting proofs section.

3. Ledger cards include the name, address, phone number, and insurance information of the patient.

4. Generally, a credit adjustment reduces the patient's account balance, whereas a debit adjustment increases the patient's account balance.

5. A local or access code is one that indicates a certain procedure or service for one particular system.

6. The statement consists of one or more pages that lists all checks written and their amounts, all deposits made and their amounts, any electronic transactions, and any service charges.

7. These are the six guidelines for managing petty cash:
   - Keep petty cash separate from patient cash payments.
   - Keep in a secure, locked area.
   - Designate one person to maintain the petty cash fund and issue vouchers.
   - Place a voucher with an attached receipt in the petty cash fund.
   - Replenish the petty cash fund once a month.
   - Remove and file all vouchers.

8. Besides price, you should consider delivery charges and product quality when purchasing office supplies.

9. The bookkeeper must write out a purchase order and compare the packing slip and final invoice to the purchase order.

CHAPTER

13

Health Insurance

Outline

Health Benefits Plans
Group Health Benefits
Health Care Savings Accounts
Individual Health Benefits
Government-Sponsored
(Public) Health Benefits

Managed Care
Health Maintenance
Organizations
Preferred Provider
Organizations
Physician Hospital Organizations
Other Managed Care Programs

Workers' Compensation
Filing Claims
Electronic Claims Submission
Explanation of Benefits
Policies in the Practice

Learning Objectives

Upon successfully completing this chapter, you will be able to:

1. Spell and define the key terms

2. Describe group, individual, and government-sponsored (public) health benefits and explain the differences between them

3. Explain the differences between Medicare and Medicaid

4. Explain how managed care programs work

5. Explain the differences between health maintenance organizations, preferred provider organizations, and physician hospital organizations

6. List the information required on a medical claim form and explain why each piece of information is needed

7. Name two legal issues affecting claims submissions

Performance Objectives

Upon successfully completing this chapter, you will be able to:

1. Complete a CMS-1500 claim form (Procedure 13-1)

CAAHEP

- Complete insurance claim forms
- Apply managed care policies and procedures
- Apply third-party guidelines

ABHES

- Apply managed care policies and procedures
- Apply third-party guidelines

Key Terms

Assignment of bene-
   fits
balance billing
birthday rule
capitation
carrier
claims
claims administrator
coinsurance
coordination of bene-
   fits
co-payments

crossover claim
deductible
dependent
eligibility
employee
explanation of bene-
   fits (EOB)
fee-for-service
fee schedule
group member
Healthcare Savings

Account
health maintenance
   organization (HMO)
health insurance
independent practice
   association (IPA)
insured
managed care
Medicare
peer review organiza-
   tion
physician hospital or-

ganization
plan maximum
pre-existing condi-
   tion
preferred provider
   organization (PPO)
third-party administ-
   trator
usual, customary,
   and reasonable
   (UCR)
utilization review

In the United States, **health insurance** is funded by a combination of employer and employee contributions and tax-funded coverage. In addition to the numerous Blue Cross and Blue Shield plans, health benefits also are provided by other insurance companies, self-funded group plans, and government plans such as Medicare and Medicaid. The benefits vary with each plan and from state to state. Approximately 80% of Americans are enrolled in health benefits plans of one sort or another. Consequently, most of the patients you will encounter in the physician's office have some type of health insurance. With so many different companies and plans, it would be impossible for you to know each patient's insurance plan requirements, but as a medical assistant, you will need to know where and how to obtain such information so that you can complete and file claim forms appropriately. You must keep abreast of changes as you are notified. You will also need to learn the special terminology associated with health insurance claims. In addition, you may need to instruct patients about insurance matters.

Health Benefits Plans

Group Health Benefits

Group health benefits are sponsored by an organization, such as an employer, a union, or an association. A person covered by group health benefits is either an **employee** or a **group member,** who by virtue of employment or membership in an organization may participate in and receive benefits from a health plan. Coverage in health plans differs greatly, so you need to know the **eligibility** of the patient for services being provided by your office. For example, birth control is frequently not covered unless there is medical necessity.

Benefits may be either **insured** or self-funded. Commonly, health benefits are referred to as insurance. It is, however, important to distinguish between the actual benefits and the vehicle used to fund and provide them.

With insured benefits, the employer, employee, or both pay a monthly premium to an insurance company. The insurance company, in turn, is obligated to pay for any eligible health benefits. Self-funded benefits on the surface appear the same as insured benefits. They are paid for in the same manner as group health benefits, but instead of the employer paying the insurance company to invest the money to cover payments, they invest it themselves. They pay an insurance company or other agency to process **claims** and make payments on their behalf. Any payment for medical services that are not paid by the patient or physician is said to be paid by a *third-party payer*. In this case, the payer is an agent for the self-funded plan and is, therefore, known as a **third-party administrator** (TPA). Many employers now choose to self-fund their group benefit plans rather than insure them.

You will need to be aware of these funding differences as they relate to state and federal regulations. For instance, insured benefit plans are subject to state regulations. Many states mandate that certain types of benefits be included in any insurance plan. These mandated benefits vary from state to state but often include such medical services as childhood immunizations, routine diagnostic care, and treatment for substance abuse.

For a group benefit plan to cover (pay for) eligible expenses, the patient must meet several criteria, called eligibility requirements. These are defined in the policy or plan document and may include a minimum number of hours worked per week and a waiting period from the date of employment before benefits become effective.

The eligibility of a **dependent** (spouse, children) is based on the employee's eligibility. Certain eligibility limitations apply to dependent children. For example, children are usually eligible until they are 18 or 21 years old. The age limitation is usually extended if the child is disabled or a full-time student. Eligibility usually requires that children be the unmarried natural or adopted children of the employee, unmarried stepchildren, or children for whom the employee has legal guardianship.

To confirm a patient's eligibility, check the back of the patient's identification (ID) card (Fig. 13-1) for a web address or phone number to contact the **claims administrator** for the health benefits plan.

Group and individual health benefits describe contractual agreements and how the policies are paid. Both groups and individuals can choose from many different types of plans, such as traditional, HMO, and PPO. These types are further discussed later in this chapter.

Health Care Savings Accounts

Health Care Savings Accounts (HSAs) are often offered as an employee benefit. Employees save money through payroll deduction to accounts that can only be used for medical care. Money is put into a health savings account before it is taxed and can be withdrawn instantly for qualified medical expenses as needed; any dollars remaining can be carried over to be spent in future years or invested to accumulate savings for health needs after retirement. HSAs are not designed to replace a regular health insurance policy but work in conjunction with a high-deductible health insurance policy, which costs less. In effect, an employee would pay for medical care, using his tax-free HSA dollars, until he spends up to the deductible. Once he meets the deductible, the health insurance pays for most or all of his medical expenses for the rest of the year. Employees choose their own doctor

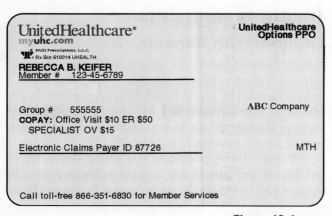

Figure 13-1 Patient identification card.

and level of care. HSAs are gaining popularity, and experts say they are here to stay.

 CHECKPOINT QUESTION

1. Under what circumstances is a dependent eligible for coverage by a parent's insurance policy?

Individual Health Benefits

Individual health benefits policies are purchased by an individual from an insurance company. The individual pays premiums directly to the insurance company, and the insurance company pays either the doctor or the hospital directly if they are a participating provider or reimburses the individual for eligible medical expenses.

For patients with individual health benefits, the criteria for completing and filing claims are the same as for patients with group health benefits. Individual health policies commonly have less generous coverage, however, than group health plans have. An individual policy may also have a rider that limits or eliminates benefits for certain illnesses or injuries based on the determination of the underwriter at the time the policy was issued. The Health Insurance Portability and Accountability Act of 1996 (HIPAA) includes a provision to protect employees changing jobs from being denied benefits for pre-existing conditions (see Appendix A). There can, however, be a waiting period for coverage of pre-existing conditions.

With the cost of health care skyrocketing and more insurance companies limiting what they will cover, many people have more than one health care insurance policy. It is extremely important that you know which insurance you bill first (primary) and which to bill the remainder of the charges (secondary).

Government-Sponsored (Public) Health Benefits

Government-sponsored benefit programs are funded and regulated by the federal government or individual states. Government programs have been developed over the years to assist persons who do not otherwise have health benefits, such as the elderly, the indigent, and others unable to obtain benefits. Government programs include Medicare, Medicaid, TRICARE/CHAMPVA, and workers' compensation.

Medicare

In 1965, the Social Security Act established **Medicare** to provide health insurance for the elderly. Elderly persons were defined as Social Security recipients age 65 or older. In 1972, amendments to the Social Security Act expanded Medicare coverage to two additional high-risk groups: disabled persons who have been receiving Social Security benefits for 24 months and persons suffering from end-stage renal disease.

Medicare Part A covers hospital expenses and is provided at no additional charge to persons eligible for Social Security benefits. Medicare Part B pays for physician fees, both inpatient and outpatient, diagnostic testing, certain immunizations (influenza and pneumonia), and specific screening tests (PSA, mammograms, Pap smears, bone density testing, colorectal screening). Part B Medicare is optional, and the participant is charged a monthly fee. The fee is deducted from the monthly Social Security benefits.

Persons signing up for or receiving Social Security benefits are automatically enrolled in both Part A and Part B Medicare when they reach 65. If they do not wish to participate in Part B, they must decline it. Both Part A and Part B of Medicare have deductibles and co-payments, and as with most health insurance policies, these generally increase yearly.

A patient with Medicare coverage who is actively employed and covered by the employer's plan will have secondary Medicare benefits. A retired person age 65 or over who has health insurance in addition to Medicare will have primary Medicare benefits. Physicians are required to submit claims to Medicare on behalf of Medicare patients. These claims must be filed within 1 year of the time the service is incurred. (See section on filing claims for more information.)

After the **deductible** has been met, Medicare Part B reimburses the physician 80% of the Medicare-approved charges. The patient is responsible for the remaining 20% of the Medicare-approved fee. Under certain circumstances, if paying the 20% causes undue financial hardship, the physician may not charge the remaining 20%. The Centers for Medicare and Medicaid Services (CMS) can provide forms with the requirements, and the forms should always be used. In addition to Medicare, the Social Security Act of 1965 established Medicaid, a program of health care coverage for the poor. If patients are financially unable to pay the 20%, they may be eligible for Medicaid. This is referred to as a **crossover claim** because the patient is eligible under both Medicare and Medicaid, and the claim crosses over automatically from one coverage to the other. In this situation, Medicare is primary, and Medicaid is secondary. Medicare will accept original claims (no copies) filed on CMS-1500 universal claim forms only.

The CMS, which was known as the Health Care Financing Administration (HCFA) prior to July 1, 2001, is a government agency that oversees the financial aspects of health care in the United States (Box 13-1). The CMS has adopted a revised Current Procedural Terminology (CPT) coding system that must be used for Medicare claims. Medicare B claims use the standard

BOX 13-1

WHAT IS THE CMS?

The CMS is the federal agency that administers Medicare, Medicaid, and the State Children's Health Insurance Program (SCHIP). About 100 million people—1 in 3—now have government coverage through Medicaid, Medicare, or military or federal employee health plans. More than 10 million others are eligible for Medicaid but have not signed up. The CMS also performs quality-focused activities, including regulation of laboratory testing, development of coverage policies, and quality-of-care improvement. The CMS maintains oversight of the survey and certification of nursing homes and continuing care providers, including home health agencies and intermediate-care facilities for the mentally retarded. It makes available to beneficiaries, providers, researchers, and state surveyors information about these activities and nursing home quality.

To ensure public and expert involvement in running their programs, the CMS maintains a number of chartered advisory committees. These committees, whose meetings are open to the public, provide advice or make recommendations on a variety of issues relating to CMS's responsibilities and activities.

CPT codes. For equipment, supplies, and services not listed in the CPT code, the CMS has established the Healthcare Common Procedure Coding System (HCPCS) codes (see Chapter 15).

It is important to ask the patient about supplemental or secondary coverage. This policy, which patients may purchase on their own, usually covers the deductible and charges not covered by Medicare. In this case, filing a second claim is necessary.

 CHECKPOINT QUESTION

2. What is the difference between parts A and B of Medicare coverage?

Medicaid

Medicaid provides health benefits to low-income or indigent persons of all ages. Often, eligibility for Medicaid is based on a patient's eligibility for other state programs, such as welfare assistance. Medicaid is governed by both federal and state statutes and rules and then implemented on a state and local level. Although the federal government stipulates the minimum health care coverage, states can provide cover-

age beyond the minimum. Therefore, Medicaid eligibility and benefits vary from state to state. At a minimum, Medicaid provides 100% coverage for the following:

- Inpatient hospital care
- Outpatient treatment and services
- Diagnostic services
- Family planning
- Skilled nursing facilities
- Diagnostic screenings for children

Many states use a managed care type of Medicaid coverage in which recipients make a co-payment based on their income and are assigned a primary care physician as a "gatekeeper."

Since circumstances that make recipients eligible for coverage change from month to month (i.e., employment), Medicaid patients receive a new ID card each month. Make a photocopy of the card for the patient's file on the first visit of each month. Most states have online eligibility and authorization verification capabilities. Because reimbursement is considerably less than other insurances, not all physicians accept Medicaid patients, nor are they required to do so. If Medicaid patients are accepted, you need to be familiar with Medicaid as administered in your state.

 CHECKPOINT QUESTION

3. List six types of medical expenses that are covered at 100% by Medicaid.

TRICARE/CHAMPVA

TRICARE is administered by the US Department of Defense and provides medical coverage for dependents of active service personnel, dependents of service personnel who died during active duty, and retired service personnel. When Congress realized that CHAMPUS costs could be controlled with managed care, they mandated that HMOs and PPOs (discussed later in this chapter) be added to the coverage. This three-part system is now called TRICARE. This system requires that participants be assigned a primary care manager (PCM). The PCM is named on the beneficiary's card.

If a patient lives within 40 miles of a uniformed services hospital and that facility is unable to handle the needs of patients covered by TRICARE, a statement of unavailability is required for treatment by a physician's office or civilian hospital. Patients who live more than 40 miles from a uniformed services hospital do not need this statement to be treated in a physician's office or civilian hospital and for the physician or hospital to be reimbursed.

The Civilian Health and Medical Program of the Veterans Administration (CHAMPVA) covers dependents of veterans who have total and permanent service-connected disabilities. CHAMPVA is administered by the area Veterans Administration hospital. Once admitted to the CHAMPVA program, patients select their own physician; this allows them the same benefits as private insurance.

Managed Care

Health care costs in the United States have grown at about twice the general rate of inflation. As a result, the United States now spends more for health care services than any other industrialized nation, both as a percentage of gross national product and per person. In the United States, most people obtain health coverage through their employer. The exceptions are Medicare for the elderly, TRICARE for retired military personnel and their dependents, Medicaid for low-income Americans, and those who buy their own health insurance.

The rapid rate of health care inflation encouraged employers to begin offering **managed care** programs, which are typically less costly than traditional insurance coverage systems. Managed care programs vary greatly, but all involve a different relationship between the insurer, health care provider, and covered individual from that of traditional insurance programs. To understand this difference, we first discuss the traditional insurance system.

In traditional insurance systems, the covered patient may seek care from any provider. Normally, the patient and physician decide what care is needed. Then, services are rendered, and the insurer pays a portion of the provider's bills (after deductibles and coinsurance). The insurer has no relationship with the provider.

In managed care systems, however, the insurer has a contractual relationship with the provider. The contract usually establishes what prices will be charged for each service and the conditions under which a service would be covered. Most managed care programs contain the following elements:

- *Precertification of hospital admissions* (often also called utilization management [UM] or **utilization review** [UR]). A patient can be admitted to a hospital for certain conditions only if that admission has been certified (approved) by the insurer. The goal of this requirement is to ensure that a patient's care is provided in the most cost-effective setting. For example, many surgical procedures that used to require an inpatient hospital stay can now be performed in an outpatient setting if proper education and support are available to the patient. Conflict between a UR guideline and the physician's requirements for the patient can be appealed to an impartial **peer review organiza-**

tion composed of physicians and specialists who will review the case and make the final recommendation.
- *Approved referrals.* As discussed in Chapter 6, Managing Appointments, in many managed care plans, a specialty physician can provide services to a managed care patient only on referral from the patient's primary care physician. The purpose is to ensure that the services provided by the specialist are medically necessary and, again, provided in the most cost-effective setting. Payment of a claim depends on the completion of the appropriate form.
- *Network.* A network consists of providers (physicians, hospitals, pharmacies, and other providers and suppliers) who have signed contracts with the insurer or **health maintenance organization** (**HMO**) to provide services to covered persons in individual, group, or public health plans. A patient is normally required to use network providers to receive full coverage. The financial penalties (lost coverage) are often very high if a patient does not use these providers.
- *Assignment of benefits.* By contract, the network provider cannot bill the patient for any amounts not paid by the insurer (no **balance billing**) except for copayments, coinsurance, and deductibles. If payment for a service provided by a network physician or hospital is denied by the insurer because it was not properly authorized, the provider cannot bill the patient for these services unless the contract does not contain a hold-harmless clause for the patient. This puts teeth in the control features of the managed care program.

Most physicians have contracts with more than one managed care program, and each of these programs has its own requirements and reimbursement schedules. So that the physician can provide the patient with needed health care services, while ensuring that the physician is paid for his or her services, it is necessary to consider the requirements of each patient's program. UM or precertification requirements are extremely important. Check the patient's ID card for details (Fig. 13-1). UM requirements may apply to inpatient services or to a variety of outpatient and doctor office services.

Until you are very familiar with the requirements of each of your patient's managed care programs, you should call the number on the ID card before a patient is admitted to a hospital (on a nonemergency basis), referred to another physician, or scheduled for specific laboratory, radiologic, or other tests or evaluations. For inpatient admissions, the UM firm may ask for the diagnosis, the procedure or procedures to be performed, and other related information before approving the admission. Once the procedure is approved, the UM firm may only approve a specified length of stay in the hospital. Failure to comply with the precertification requirements results in a financial penalty for the patient and possibly also for the physician and the hospital.

It is important to be familiar with physicians within the network. The physician, hospital, laboratory, or other provider you normally refer a patient to may not be in the patient's managed care network. By calling the UM number to check, you can avoid penalties and improve the satisfaction of the patient with your services. Many times, these requirements can be met electronically as companies improve their technology.

 CHECKPOINT QUESTION

4. What are the four key elements of a managed care program?

Health Maintenance Organizations

It is easiest to understand how an HMO functions if we contrast it with a traditional health insurance program. In the traditional insurance system, the relationship between the covered individual and the insurer or self-insurer is purely financial. In return for receiving a paid monthly premium, the insurer promises to reimburse (indemnify) the individual if he or she incurs certain types of covered medical expense. There are often limits to coverage (exclusions and limitations), and normally, the coverage has a **deductible** (amount below which services are not reimbursable) and **coinsurance** (the patient pays a percentage of the medical expense after the deductible is satisfied). For example, the patient pays the first $200 (deductible) in physician charges each year starting January 1; then insurance pays 80% of covered charges, and the patient must pay the other 20%.

The covered individual seeks medical services and thereby incurs an expense. The individual, not the insurer, must pay for this expense. If the medical treatment is covered as defined in the insurance policy, the insurer will reimburse the patient a portion of the amount incurred after deductibles and coinsurance.

In contrast to traditional insurance companies, an HMO promises to provide covered services rather than pay for them. In this respect, the HMO acts as both an insurer and a provider of service. HMO policies are written differently from insurance policies. The HMO policy lists the medical services that the member is entitled to receive and the physicians and hospitals that will provide these services. The HMO has a contract with both the patient and provider. It must provide covered services to the member either directly from its own physician staff and hospitals or indirectly from physicians and hospitals contracted to provide the services promised to the member. The HMO, rather than the patient, is responsible for the costs of medical services, and providers bill the HMO rather than the patient when a reimbursable service is rendered to an HMO member.

This is one reason HMOs do not normally use deductibles and coinsurance, which are standard features of health insurance programs. A patient does not receive a provider's bill, so deductibles and coinsurance cannot apply. Instead, HMOs use predetermined **co-payments** (e.g., $10 per physician office visit) to reduce premium prices.

HMOs come in many forms. An HMO contracts with employers to cover their employees. The medical group and hospitals contract with the health plan to provide the services required in the health plan's contract with employers. Rather than paying for these services on a **fee-for-service** basis, a company pays the physicians per employee. Consistent with its history, the health plan does not pay the medical group a fee for each service provided. Instead, it pays each party based on the number of members enrolled in the health plan. This is often called **capitation** because there is one payment per member. Capitation payments are also used by other types of HMOs.

As group model HMOs developed (they were called prepaid group practices until 1973 federal legislation changed their names), nongroup physicians organized into an entity called an **independent practice association (IPA)**. The early IPA HMOs were often sponsored by a local medical society and were developed to allow independent physicians to compete with prepaid group practices.

IPA HMOs contract with employers in the same manner as group model HMOs, and their members receive covered services from IPA physicians. The HMO's contracts with physicians are different, however, because these physicians are not organized into a single multispecialty group practice. IPA physicians are paid in a number of ways. Some are paid on a capitation basis, and some may be paid on a fee-for-service basis using a **fee schedule** established by the HMO. Often, a portion of any reimbursement is withheld by the HMO and paid only if the HMO's total medical expense is within budget; this encourages the physician to be cost conscious in caring for patients.

In some of these HMOs, the IPA is a separate corporation, often owned by physicians. With this structure (still called an IPA HMO), the IPA contracts with physicians, and the HMO contracts with the IPA instead of directly with each physician.

Over the years, HMOs have continued to evolve, and many are now a mixture of these discussed models. As a medical assistant, you must know what type of relationship the practice has with an HMO before you can determine how the practice is reimbursed. Most HMOs require claims to be submitted even if payment is capitation rather than fee-for-service. Many HMOs also require the collection and transmission of other patient information, which is not required in the traditional insurance industry. Of course, this information is provided with the patient's permission.

CHECKPOINT QUESTION

5. How does an HMO differ from a traditional health insurance program?

 PATIENT EDUCATION

Help Patients Understand Their Obligation

As discussed in Chapter 2, the contract between a physician and his patient implies that the *patient* will pay the physician for his services, not the patient's insurance company. When a physician participates with an insurance company, he may be required to file a patient's claims, but this is not the case with all third-party payers. Although patients have the ultimate responsibility of paying the physician, they tend to think that a physician should wait for their insurance to pay. A physician who does not choose to participate with a particular third-party payer is not obligated to extend credit to a patient. Of course, most practices choose to offer filing the patient's claim as a courtesy. Because of the nature of a physician's work, most physicians are willing to make reasonable credit arrangements, but patients should understand that their physician is not legally obligated to file their claims or extend credit.

Understanding the claims filing process will give patients the opportunity to take a more active role in their physician's reimbursement. Direct patients to their insurance company's website, keep abreast of changes, and be willing to discuss these matters openly. Help patients understand their obligations to the physician and their insurance company's obligations to them. This approach will not only benefit the patients, but will also improve your collection ratio.

Preferred Provider Organizations

Whereas HMOs promise to provide services and have a financial risk in their relationships with subscribers, a **preferred provider organization (PPO)** is a type of health benefit program whose purpose is simply to contract with providers and then lease this network of contracted providers to health care plans. The PPO network is not risk bearing; it does not have any financial involvement in the health plan. PPOs are typically developed by hospitals and physicians as a vehicle to attract patients, although some are developed and managed by insurance **carriers**.

PPOs contract with participating providers, including hospitals and physicians. These contracts allow the PPO to contract with insurers and other purchasers of health care services on behalf of the participating providers, who typically accept less than their normal charges and agree to follow the UM and other administrative protocols as specified by the PPO.

Typically, a health plan with a PPO offers benefits at two levels, commonly referred to as in network and out of network. Unlike in an HMO, patients may visit any provider they wish for services. If the provider is in network (a participating provider), the levels of benefit for the patient are greater than if the patient receives services from an out-of-network (nonparticipating) provider.

A typical health plan with a PPO may look like the breakdown shown in Figure 13-2.

As you can see from the example, each time the patient sees an in-network provider, he or she receives significantly better benefits. A primary difference between an HMO and PPO, therefore, is that patients can see any physician of their choice and receive benefits; they simply have an incentive in the form of higher benefits when they see an in-network provider.

As part of your responsibilities, you should identify the PPOs with which the physician has contracted and determine the administrative requirements set forth by each PPO in the contract. To understand the necessary administrative procedures agreed to by the physician, review all managed care contracts carefully. Also be aware that most PPOs have a provider relations representative who works with the contracted providers (physicians) to answer questions and clarify procedures. The PPO is typically operated by a group of hospitals or physicians or by an insurance company or independent organization. Physicians agree to participate in PPOs to serve their existing patients who now have PPO plans and sometimes to gain additional patients who seek the services of a PPO physician.

Participating physicians have agreed to perform certain administrative services for PPO patients. Commonly, the physician's office must accept assignment of benefits and provide claims filing services for the patient. The physician agrees to accept the reimbursement by the claims administrator as payment in full and agrees not to

Example of a Health Plan With a PPO		
Benefit	In-network	Out-of-network
Deductible	$100	$300
Coinsurance	90%	70%
Routine care	$200 per calendar year	-0-
Mental health	80%	50%
Office visit	$10 co-pay; no deductible	70%

Figure 13-2 A health plan with a PPO.

bill the patient for any difference between the physician's usual charge and the PPO-negotiated charge for the service. The participating physician is responsible for collecting any co-pay amount at the time of service. The physician also agrees to comply with any precertification requirements stipulated by the plan.

 CHECKPOINT QUESTION

6. What is the primary difference between an HMO and a PPO?

Physician Hospital Organizations

Physicians and hospitals have become more active in developing managed care alternatives. A **physician hospital organization** (PHO) is a coalition of physicians and a hospital contracting with large employers, insurance carriers, and other benefits groups to provide discounted health services. There are numerous variations of PHOs. A PHO may look much like a PPO with no risk-bearing elements, in which case the network of providers constituting the PHO are under no financial obligation to subscribers. Alternatively, a PHO may be more like an HMO, wherein the participating providers in the PHO do have a risk-bearing contract and assume responsibility for the overall medical budget of subscribing units. Physician organizations (POs) are such groups consisting of physicians only. As with any managed care program, it is important to know and understand the particulars of each managed care contract and the requirements of the provider and obligations to patients and the managed care entity.

Other Managed Care Programs

Although HMOs, PPOs, and increasingly PHOs are the most common managed care programs, many others cover patients today, and still more are being developed.

Although requirements vary, a gatekeeper provision is common. A gatekeeper is a primary care physician. Participants are required to see a primary care physician for all nonemergency services. That physician will either treat the patient or, if necessary, refer the patient to a specialist. The physician must complete and submit a referral form or call the claims administrator for approval of the referral. (See Box 13-2.)

The gatekeeper provision seeks to reduce the plan cost of specialists. For example, without such a provision, a patient might see a specialist first at a more costly fee, even though the condition may have been adequately treated by a less costly primary care physician. The gatekeeper approach also encourages patients to establish a relationship with a primary care physician, who is then in a position to manage the patient's care.

ETHICAL TIP

When a Provider Is Unethical

The following scenario may occur in a medical office. While you are filing an insurance claim, the physician tells you to "readjust" the laceration length from 4 cm to 9 cm. (The physician can bill more for a 9-cm laceration.) When you question him about this, he says, "Don't worry. The patient isn't paying the difference, the insurance company is, and they have plenty of money." How should you handle this situation?

Ethically and legally, you cannot change the length of a laceration on the medical record or the bill. This is fraud. You must explain to the physician that you are uncomfortable with this request and that you are ethically and legally bound to truthful billing. Any requests to alter or misrepresent the medical records or claims of a patient must be firmly denied.

A physician who operates in an unethical manner should be reported. If he or she is a partner in a practice, alert the other physicians about the suspect actions. You can also contact your state medical association, the American Medical Association, or the institutional review board at the hospital where your physician is affiliated.

BOX 13-2

REFERRALS ARE MORE THAN JUST PHONE CALLS

As discussed in Chapter 6, when a patient has third-party coverage that requires precertification for a referral to a specialist, you must follow the steps and complete the proper forms in order for the patient to be covered for the specialist's services. You will know the patient's requirements by looking at the card or going to a website listed on the card. For example, your physician employer is Mr. Smith's primary care physician (PCP) or gatekeeper. Mr. Smith's policy requires precertification for referrals. Mr. Smith is complaining of frequent and severe headaches. Your doctor wants him to see a neurologist to rule out migraine headaches. Before calling to make an appointment with the neurologist, you must contact the third-party payer for approval. They will want to know the patient's situation, the physician's plans for him, the rationale for the referral, etc. If the referral is approved, they will give you a referral approval number that will be placed on the referral form. You must give this completed form to the patient, who must take it to the neurologist.

Workers' Compensation

Workers' compensation benefits were developed to cover the expenses resulting from a work-related illness or injury. In the event of a work-related illness or injury, claims submitted to the group or individual health benefits plan will be returned with instructions to file with the workers' compensation administrator, who determines the validity of the claim and reimburses accordingly. Because your practice will likely be taking care of the patient for both routine medical care and work-related illness or injury, it is important to determine at the time services are rendered whether the illness or injury is work related and, if so, to account and file for those services separately.

You are responsible for knowing your state's workers' compensation regulations and procedures. Consult your state's office for workers' compensation or your state's designated claims administrator of the workers' compensation program for specific information.

Filing Claims

If the provider requires patients to make full payment at the time of the visit, the physician may still submit a claim on the patient's behalf; however, the patient may need to submit claims to the claims administrator for reimbursement. Most providers accept assignment of benefits, however. To do this, the patient must give written authorization for the claims administrator to reimburse the physician for billed charges. As a medical assistant, you may be responsible for obtaining all necessary claims information from the provider and the patient and then submitting a claim for payment to the claims administrator.

As discussed in Chapter 5, the patient's ID card is a source of information necessary for complete and accurate claims submission. Keep a copy of this card in the patient's file and be sure to update it at least yearly and preferably at each visit, since the patient's employment and eligibility may change.

In addition, a patient may be covered by more than one group plan. For example, a patient may be covered both on an employer's group plan and as a dependent on his or her spouse's group plan. The primary plan—the one that pays first—is the plan provided by the patient's employer. Any unpaid amount is then considered for payment by the spouse's group plan, which is considered secondary. This is called **coordination of benefits**.

Dependent children may be covered under one or two parents' plans. Unless the plans state otherwise, the plan of the parent whose birthday occurs first each calendar year (not necessarily the oldest parent) is the primary plan. This is known as the **birthday rule**. This rule is commonly used by benefit plans and claims administrators to coordinate the benefits of dependent children covered by two plans. If the parents are legally separated or divorced, however, the primary plan is the plan of the parent who has custody or, in some instances, is subject to a court order or divorce decree.

After establishing the primary plan and the claims submission destination, you prepare the claim for filing. The CMS-1500 was developed by the American Medical Association to standardize an acceptable claim form for different plans and different claims administrators. It is the most widely used method of filing a health claim (Fig. 13-3). The CMS-1500 is accepted by most claims administrators, including Blue Cross and Blue Shield, Medicare, Medicaid, and TRICARE/CHAMPVA. Procedure 13-1 explains how to complete a CMS-1500 claim form.

Most plans include a clause that excludes coverage for a stated period (usually 12 months) for a condition that existed before the plan's effective date; this is known as a **pre-existing condition**. For example, a patient with a diagnosis of depression before the effective date of his or her plan would be covered for all other conditions from the effective date forward but would not be covered for services related to the diagnosis or treatment of depression for the pre-existing exclusion period (in this example, 12 months).

Many pieces of information are needed for timely and efficient claims processing. The insurance company or managed care plan cannot process claims with incomplete or inaccurate information and will return them to the provider for completion, correction, and resubmission. This lengthens the time the provider must wait for reimbursement, making accurate claims submission a critical aspect of your responsibilities. Table 13-1 describes the most frequent causes for denial of a claim and the corrective actions that you can take.

WHAT IF?

What if a patient comes in to see the physician but does not have her Medicaid card?

Most states offer Medicaid providers the ability to verify eligibility on any given date of service online. By searching for the Department of Human Services on the web in almost any city, you can be directed to this feature. This is especially helpful since Medicaid eligibility is managed on a monthly basis, and sometimes patients will not receive their card before the first day of a new month. Before this capability existed, many times patients were sent away if they did not have their cards with them. As long as you have an ID number or Social Security number, you can verify eligibility instantly.

PLEASE
DO NOT
STAPLE
IN THIS
AREA

CARRIER →

HEALTH INSURANCE CLAIM FORM

| | | | | | PICA | | | | | PICA | |

| 1. | MEDICARE | MEDICAID | CHAMPUS | CHAMPVA | GROUP HEALTH PLAN | FECA BLK LUNG | OTHER | 1a. INSURED'S I.D. NUMBER | (FOR PROGRAM IN ITEM 1) |
| | (Medicare #) | (Medicaid #) | (Sponsor's SSN) | (VA File #) | (SSN or ID) | (SSN) | (ID) | | |

| 2. PATIENT'S NAME (Last Name, First Name, Middle Initial) | 3. PATIENT'S BIRTH DATE MM DD YY | SEX M F | 4. INSURED'S NAME (Last Name, First Name, Middle Initial) |

| 5. PATIENT'S ADDRESS (No., Street) | 6. PATIENT RELATIONSHIP TO INSURED Self Spouse Child Other | 7. INSURED'S ADDRESS (No., Street) |

| CITY | STATE | 8. PATIENT STATUS Single Married Other | CITY | STATE |

| ZIP CODE | TELEPHONE (Include Area Code) ( ) | Employed Full-Time Student Part-Time Student | ZIP CODE | TELEPHONE (INCLUDE AREA CODE) ( ) |

| 9. OTHER INSURED'S NAME (Last Name, First Name, Middle Initial) | 10. IS PATIENT'S CONDITION RELATED TO: | 11. INSURED'S POLICY GROUP OR FECA NUMBER |

| a. OTHER INSURED'S POLICY OR GROUP NUMBER | a. EMPLOYMENT? (CURRENT OR PREVIOUS) YES NO | a. INSURED'S DATE OF BIRTH MM DD YY SEX M F |

| b. OTHER INSURED'S DATE OF BIRTH MM DD YY SEX M F | b. AUTO ACCIDENT? PLACE (State) YES NO | b. EMPLOYER'S NAME OR SCHOOL NAME |

| c. EMPLOYER'S NAME OR SCHOOL NAME | c. OTHER ACCIDENT? YES NO | c. INSURANCE PLAN NAME OR PROGRAM NAME |

| d. INSURANCE PLAN NAME OR PROGRAM NAME | 10d. RESERVED FOR LOCAL USE | d. IS THERE ANOTHER HEALTH BENEFIT PLAN? YES NO If yes, return to and complete item 9 a-d. |

READ BACK OF FORM BEFORE COMPLETING & SIGNING THIS FORM.

12. PATIENT'S OR AUTHORIZED PERSON'S SIGNATURE I authorize the release of any medical or other information necessary to process this claim. I also request payment of government benefits either to myself or to the party who accepts assignment below.

SIGNED _____ DATE _____

13. INSURED'S OR AUTHORIZED PERSON'S SIGNATURE I authorize payment of medical benefits to the undersigned physician or supplier for services described below.

SIGNED _____

| 14. DATE OF CURRENT: MM DD YY | ILLNESS (First symptom) OR INJURY (Accident) OR PREGNANCY(LMP) | 15. IF PATIENT HAS HAD SAME OR SIMILAR ILLNESS. GIVE FIRST DATE MM DD YY | 16. DATES PATIENT UNABLE TO WORK IN CURRENT OCCUPATION MM DD YY MM DD YY FROM TO |

| 17. NAME OF REFERRING PHYSICIAN OR OTHER SOURCE | 17a. I.D. NUMBER OF REFERRING PHYSICIAN | 18. HOSPITALIZATION DATES RELATED TO CURRENT SERVICES MM DD YY MM DD YY FROM TO |

| 19. RESERVED FOR LOCAL USE | 20. OUTSIDE LAB? $ CHARGES YES NO |

| 21. DIAGNOSIS OR NATURE OF ILLNESS OR INJURY. (RELATE ITEMS 1,2,3 OR 4 TO ITEM 24E BY LINE) 1. 3. 2. 4. | 22. MEDICAID RESUBMISSION CODE ORIGINAL REF. NO. 23. PRIOR AUTHORIZATION NUMBER |

24. A DATE(S) OF SERVICE From MM DD YY To MM DD YY	B Place of Service	C Type of Service	D PROCEDURES, SERVICES, OR SUPPLIES (Explain Unusual Circumstances) CPT/HCPCS MODIFIER	E DIAGNOSIS CODE	F $ CHARGES	G DAYS OR UNITS	H EPSDT Family Plan	I EMG	J COB	K RESERVED FOR LOCAL USE
1										
2										
3										
4										
5										
6										

| 25. FEDERAL TAX I.D. NUMBER SSN EIN | 26. PATIENT'S ACCOUNT NO. | 27. ACCEPT ASSIGNMENT? (For govt. claims, see back) YES NO | 28. TOTAL CHARGE $ | 29. AMOUNT PAID $ | 30. BALANCE DUE $ |

| 31. SIGNATURE OF PHYSICIAN OR SUPPLIER INCLUDING DEGREES OR CREDENTIALS (I certify that the statements on the reverse apply to this bill and are made a part thereof.) SIGNED _____ DATE _____ | 32. NAME AND ADDRESS OF FACILITY WHERE SERVICES WERE RENDERED (If other than home or office) | 33. PHYSICIAN'S, SUPPLIER'S BILLING NAME, ADDRESS, ZIP CODE & PHONE # PIN# GRP# |

PATIENT AND INSURED INFORMATION →
PHYSICIAN OR SUPPLIER INFORMATION →

(APPROVED BY AMA COUNCIL ON MEDICAL SERVICE 8/88) **PLEASE PRINT OR TYPE**

APPROVED OMB-0938-0008 FORM CMS-1500 (12-90), FORM RRB-1500,
APPROVED OMB-1215-0055 FORM OWCP-1500, APPROVED OMB-0720-0001 (CHAMPUS)

Figure 13-3 CMS-1500 claim form. This is known as the universal claim form. On the facing page you will find a detailed list explaining how to complete each line of the form.

TABLE **13-1**	Frequent Causes for Claim Denial and Corrective Actions
Causes for Claim Denial	**Corrective Actions**
The patient cannot be identified as a covered person.	Confirm that coverage information on file is current, including insurance company and group number, and that the Social Security number is accurate.
Coding is deemed inappropriate for services provided.	Review provided services and recode as necessary.
The patient is no longer covered by the plan.	Bill the patient for the charges. The patient may provide confirmation of new coverage.
The data are incomplete.	Complete the required data and resubmit the claim. Flag it as a resubmission.
Services are not covered by the plan.	Bill the patient for the charges unless there is a basis for an appeal.

Electronic Claims Submission

Although some practices continue to submit claims on paper through the mail and most claims administrators continue to accept this practice, most practices submit at least their Medicare and Medicaid claims electronically. Remember, HIPAA requires covered entities to submit electronic information safely and confidentially. The CMS requires that all government-sponsored insurance claims be submitted electronically. The physician's office computer software includes the CMS-1500 format for convenient and automated claims filing. With a computer and a modem, health claims can be filed immediately, reducing the time for the reimbursement cycle. You will need to work closely with your practice's software vendor to ensure compatibility with the insurance companies' computer systems.

Several regional and national clearinghouses receive health benefits claims and electronically direct them to the appropriate claims administrators. This system allows you to file all electronic claims through one clearinghouse rather than filing separately with each claims administrator.

The system requires that all fields on the electronic claim form be completed and in the required format. If the claim is incomplete or inaccurate, the system will not transmit the form. You can complete or correct the form online, allowing the form to be transmitted. Claims submitted electronically that do not meet the plan's criteria will be rejected by the clearinghouse and must be submitted by mail. In addition, claims that are particularly complicated or cumbersome, have attachments, or are otherwise unsuitable for electronic submission should be filed on paper with the claims administrator.

Explanation of Benefits

When the claims administrator settles a claim, that is, makes a payment, an **explanation of benefits** (EOB) is issued to both the provider and the patient (Fig. 13-4). The EOB tells how the payment was made, including deductible and coinsurance information. Some EOBs include information for several claims on several patients

LEGAL TIP

SIGNATURE ON FILE

Keeping patient information confidential is a primary concern in all medical practices. To adhere to HIPAA's regulation, you should not release any information about the patient to any party, including the claims administrator, without the written authorization of the patient or the patient's guardian. Obtain a written authorization to release information to the patient's insurance company from each patient on his or her first visit to the practice. Keep this signature in the patient's file. Any claims submitted by the physician's office should have "signature on file" on the claim form. A new authorization should be signed at the beginning of each year. This written authorization for the release of information only pertains to the insurance company specified. Only such information as is pertinent to the claim and necessary for the processing of that claim should be released. Releasing any patient information without written consent is a breach of confidentiality and a HIPAA violation.

that may have been processed during a particular period. You must check the EOB to be sure that all payments made to the physician are for the appropriate procedures and in the correct amounts. Claims that are denied should be corrected and resubmitted if possible.

Policies in the Practice

Managed care contracts and negotiated services affect many practice policies. You must be knowledgeable and precise in administering practice policies, especially with regard to assignment of benefits and balance billing.

Assignment of benefits is a service the practice may provide. If assignment of benefits is accepted, the patient's signature must be on file, authorizing the claims administrator to reimburse the physician. Managed care plans require physicians to accept assignment, although many physicians do not accept assignment for non–managed care patients. If assignment is not accepted, the patient is responsible for paying all charges and filing a claim with the claims administrator for reimbursement directly to the patient.

Balance billing is prohibited by most managed care contracts. The physician cannot charge the patient the difference between the physician's usual charge and the allowable charge specified by the contract. For other types of plans, however, balance billing is not restricted, and the practice may bill the patient for any difference between the physician's charged fee and the amount allowable by the plan according to **usual, customary, and reasonable (UCR)** tables.

A few national firms provide UCR data to claims administrators who use that information to determine the maximum amount payable for any given service (the **plan maximum**). UCR data are calculated from surveys of the amount physicians charge for each service or procedure.

MEDIA MENU

- **Student CD**
  - **Case Studies**
    Administrative Interactive Case Study 1:
      Maintaining Medical Records and HIPAA
    Administrative Interactive Case Study 4:
      Accounting and Billing in the Medical Office
  - **CMA/RMA Certification Exam Review**
- **Premium Online Course**
  http://thePoint.lww.com/Kronenberger3e
- **Internet Resources**

  LiveAdvise Online Tutoring & Competency Training
  http://thePoint.lww.com/LiveAdvise

  Centers for Medicare and Medicaid Services
  www.cms.gov

  Medicare for recipients
  www.Medicare.gov

  BlueCross BlueShield Association
  www.bluecares.com

  Local medical review policies
  www.LMRP.net

  American Medical Association
  www.AMA-assn.org

  All government agencies, federal and state
  http://www.usa.gov/

That amount is calculated on a geographic basis to reflect regional variations in health care costs. Non–managed care plan physician reimbursements are based on a maximum allowable charge as specified in the UCR data. The physician may choose to bill the patient for the difference between the amount charged and the UCR amount.

español
SPANISH TERMINOLOGY

¿Tiene usted seguro médico?
   Do you have medical insurance?
¿Qué es el nombre del seguro?
   What is the name of the insurance?
¿Qué es el número de su póliza?
   What is the number of your policy?
¿Va a pagar el hospital?
   Will it pay for the hospital?
¿Tiene Medicare?
   Do you have Medicare?
¿Tiene su tarjeta de Medicare?
   Do you have your Medicare card?

Explanation of Benefits

Employee Name: Joe Doe
SSN: 555-55-5555 **1**
Group No. 55555
Patient Name: Joe Doe

Date of Service: 6-15-2008
Provider: Dr. Jones
Provider TIN: 35-5555555

Date of Service **2**	Comment Code **3**	Amount of Charge **4**	Amount Allowed **5**	At **6**	Amount Paid **7**
6-15-2004	57	87.00	82.00	80%	65.60
			Total **8**		65.60
			Less Deductible **9**		25.00
			Amount Paid **10**		40.60

Payable to: Dr. Jones
                 Address

Comment Code:
57 - The amount charged exceeds Usual and Customary

Reading the EOB (Explanation of Benefits)

After the claim has been processed, an EOB will be issued. Although each payer has his or her own EOB format, this sample EOB illustrates the key points included in an EOB. The terms used may differ, and the formats differ widely.

1 The top section typically includes the name of the employee and the Social Security number (SSN) or other identifying number, as well as the name of the patient, the group number, the date of service and provider name, and employer identification number (EIN) (Federal identification number assigned to the physician).

2 The date of service is included and is shown as the date the service is actually rendered, not the date that was posted or billed.

3 The Comment Code is a tool used on many EOBs to indicate a coded comment that is on the bottom as exceeding" Usual and Customary." In this situation, the claim will be processed on the Usual and Customary amount. The difference between the amount charged ($87.00) and the amount allowed ($82.00) is $5.00. Unless the physician is contractually bound by an agreement with a managed care plan that forbids the practice of balance billing, that difference of $5.00 may be billed to the patient.

4 Amount of Charge shows the amount that the physician's office billed for the service.

5 Amount Allowed shows the amount of charge upon which the claim processing will be based (in this example, it is the amount of Usual and Customary).

6 This indicates the percentage of co-insurance payable by the plan.

7 Amount Paid shows the amount payable by the plan after co-insurance has been applied, but is not necessarily the amount that is actually paid (see #10).

8 The Total shows the total submitted and payable after the claim has been processed.

9 After all processing on the claim has been completed, any deductible is applied. In this example, Joe still had $25.00 to be applied to his annual deductible. Therefore, $25.00 is deducted from the amount paid and the actual reimbursement to the physician is $40.60. The amount applied to the deductible should be billed to the patient.

10 The amount actually reimbursed.

Figure 13-4 Explanation of benefits.

PROCEDURE 13-1:   Completing a CMS-1500 Claim Form

Purpose: To ensure competency in completing a CMS-1500 claim form accurately and completely using managed care policies and procedures and third-party guidelines

Equipment: Case scenario, completed encounter form, blank CMS-1500 claim form, pen

Scenario: Naomi A. Dishman is an established leukemia patient who was seen in your office on June 20, 2008, 30 minutes after falling down the steps of her home. She is complaining of pain and swelling in her right ankle. Her charges and codes for the visit are: Established Patient Office Visit Level III (99213) and x-ray, right ankle, two views (73600). Her diagnosis is listed as ankle sprain.

Steps	Purpose
1. Using the information provided in Figure 14-5, complete the demographic information in lines 1 through 11d.	This section includes vital information to identify the policyholder and start the process of paying the claim.
2. Insert "SOF" (signature on file) on lines 12 and 13. Check to be sure there is a current signature on file in the chart and that it is specifically for the third-party payer being filed.	It is fraudulent to say there is a signature on file if there is not one in the chart. Patients should sign a separate authorization for each recipient of their information. If there is no SOF, you must call the patient to come in and sign one or mail them a form to be signed and sent back.
3. If the services being filed are for a hospital stay, insert information in lines 16, 18, and 32.	These fields are used for hospital services only.
4. If the services are related to an injury, insert the date of the accident in line 14.	If the date of accident field is not completed and an ICD-9 code for an injury is used, the payer's computer system will reject the claim.
5. Insert dates of service.	You must be accurate with the dates of service. Each line may be a different date of service.
6. Using the encounter form, place the CPT code listed for each service and procedure checked off in column D of lines 21–24 on the form.	The codes on the encounter form are current and accurate because the form has been reviewed before using any revised or new codes every January.
7. List the reason for the encounter on line 21.1 and any other diagnoses listed on the encounter form that relate to or affect the services or procedures.	All diagnoses or concurrent conditions that will affect the current treatment should be communicated to the third-party payer. For example, diabetes should be listed for a podiatric service.
8. Reference the codes placed in lines 21 (1–4) to each line listing a different CPT code by placing the corresponding one digit in line 24, column E.	Each line that lists a CPT code must also list a reason for that particular service or procedure. This reason will justify the medical necessity of the service or procedure.

- Most patients in the physician's office have some type of health care plan.
- Types of plans include group, individual, and government-sponsored health benefits, such as Medicare or Medicaid.
- Many physicians have contracts with managed care plans, such as HMOs and PPOs.
- Each type of plan has certain requirements regarding eligibility and claims submission, and you must be knowledgeable about those requirements.
- In particular, one of your primary duties is to file claims in a timely and accurate manner to ensure appropriate reimbursement for the physician.
- When filing claims, you must be careful to maintain patient confidentiality and to avoid fraud.

Warm Ups   for Critical Thinking

1. Jane and Joe are married, and both are employed and cover themselves and their two children on their health plans. Jane's birthday is July 23 and Joe's birthday is August 9. Joe is 2 years older than Jane. When claims are submitted for their two children, which spouse's plan is primary? Show which plan is primary and secondary for each family member.

	Primary	Secondary
Jane		
Joe		
Child 1		
Child 2		

2. The requirements for Medicaid vary from state to state. How do you determine the Medicaid requirements for your particular state? Locate the name, address, and telephone number of your state's resource.

3. As discussed in Chapter 8, HIPAA requires certain procedures and practices when transmitting insurance claims electronically. Search the HIPAA law for these guidelines and create a procedure for ensuring compliance regarding electronic claims filing. You can find this information by going to http://www.hhs.gov/news/press/2002pres/hipaa.html. See also Appendix A for excerpts from HIPAA's Administrative Simplification section.

Answers   to Checkpoint Questions

1. A dependent is usually eligible for coverage until the age of 18 or 21. This coverage may be extended if the adult child is disabled or a full-time student.

2. Persons enrolled in Social Security are automatically enrolled in Medicare Part A, which covers hospital services and expenses only, and Medicare Part B, which covers the physician's charges for inpatient or outpatient care as well as diagnostic services. Part B does not cover routine examinations, well care, routine immunizations, or cosmetic surgery. Part A is provided at no charge to Social Security recipients, and Part B carries a monthly fee. If Part B is not wanted, it must be declined.

3. Inpatient hospital care, outpatient treatment and services, diagnostic services, family planning, skilled nursing facilities, and diagnostic screenings for children are covered at 100% by Medicaid.

4. The four elements of managed care programs are precertification of hospital admissions (often also called utilization management or utilization review—UM or UR), approved referrals, network, and assignment of benefits.

5. In a traditional insurance system, the individual, not the insurer, seeks medical services and thereby incurs the expense. An HMO promises to provide covered services rather than pay for them.

6. A primary difference between an HMO and a PPO is that patients with PPO coverage can see any physician of their choice and receive benefits; they simply have an incentive in the form of higher benefits when they see an in-network provider.

Outline

Diagnostic Coding
Inpatient Versus Outpatient
Coding
ICD-9-CM: The Code Book
Volume 1: Tabular List of
Diseases
Volume 2: Alphabetic Index to
Diseases
Volume 3: Inpatient Coding

Locating the Appropriate Code
Using the ICD-9-CM
Conventions
Main Term
Fourth and Fifth Digits
Primary Codes
When More Than One Code Is
Used
Coding Suspected Conditions

Documentation Requirements
**The Future of Diagnostic
Coding: International
Classification of Diseases,
Tenth Revision**

Learning Objectives

*Upon successfully completing this chapter, you
will be able to:*

1. Spell and define the key terms

2. Describe the relationship between coding
   and reimbursement.

3. Name and describe the coding system used
   to describe diseases, injuries, and other reasons for encounters with a medical provider

4. Explain the format of the ICD-9-CM

5. Give four examples of ways E codes are
   used

6. List the steps in locating a proper code

7. Explain common diagnostic coding guidelines

Performance Objectives

*Upon successfully completing this chapter, you
will be able to:*

1. Locate an appropriate ICD-9-CM code
   (Procedure 14-1)

Key Terms

advance beneficiary notice

audit

conventions

cross-reference

E-codes

eponym

etiology

inpatient

International Classification of Diseases, Ninth

Revision, Clinical Modification

late effects

main terms

medical necessity

outpatient

primary diagnosis

service

specificity

V-codes

Coding, at its simplest, is the assignment of a number to a verbal statement or description. Medical coding is anything but simple. The **International Classification of Diseases, Ninth Revision, Clinical Modification** (ICD-9-CM) is a system for transforming verbal descriptions of disease, injuries, conditions, and procedures into numeric codes. It is essential that the physician and medical assistant work together to achieve accurate documentation, code assignment, and reporting of diagnoses and procedures. Use of standardized codes makes it easier for third-party payers to understand the reason for the patient's encounter with the health care provider and increases the likelihood of timely processing of claims and prompt payment when appropriate.

Coding is a way to standardize medical information for purposes such as collecting health care statistics, performing a medical care review, and indexing medical records. It is also used for health insurance claims processing (see Chapter 13). Because coding is the basis for reimbursement, it is imperative that you code patient visits accurately and precisely. Incorrect, insufficient, or incomplete coding on claims forms can lead to nonpayment for the physician as well as incorrect information in the insurance companies' databases, which may affect the patients' insurability. For example, if a patient complaining of chest pain is coded as having "acute myocardial infarction" instead of "chest pain," that pa-

tient may be incorrectly labeled as having heart disease. The Current Procedural Terminology (CPT) codes, which are used to report services and procedures performed by health care providers, determine the amount paid (see Chapter 15), but the code assigned to the diagnosis or reason for the service or procedure proves the medical necessity for the services or procedures so that claims are paid. The third-party payer needs to know why the service was performed to assess **medical necessity**. Medical necessity means the procedure or service would have been performed by any reasonable physician under the same or similar circumstances. The ICD-9 diagnostic codes convey this information. Is a chest radiograph medically necessary for a patient who has gout? No, but it may be necessary for a patient with acute bronchitis. The diagnosis justifies the procedure.

Since Medicare considers certain procedures medically necessary only at certain intervals, having the patient sign an **advance beneficiary notice** (ABN) will ensure payment of treatments and procedures that will likely be denied by Medicare. An example is a Pap smear for a low-risk woman, which will be paid for once every 2 years. If the physician considers it *not* to be medically necessary, but the patient wants a Pap test, the patient will be responsible for payment and must sign an ABN.

CHECKPOINT QUESTION

1. What is meant by medical necessity?

Diagnostic Coding

The ICD-9-CM is a statistical classification system based on the International Classification of Diseases, Ninth Revision (ICD-9), developed by the World Health Organization (WHO). The CM, which stands for clinical modification, addresses the intent of these codes to describe the clinical picture of the patient. These codes are much more precise than those needed for statistical grouping and trend analysis found in the ICD-9 and used in hospital coding.

The ICD-9-CM, which is now mandated by the Health Insurance Portability and Accountability Act of 1996 (HIPAA), is the most comprehensive statistical classification of its kind. Containing more than 10,000 diagnostic codes and 1000 procedure codes, it consists of three volumes:

- Volume 1: Tabular List of Diseases
- Volume 2: Alphabetic Index of Diseases
- Volume 3: Tabular List and Alphabetic Index of Procedures

The ICD-9-CM code books are available from several publishers, and although the presentation of the material may be different, the content must be the same. Depending on the publisher, these three volumes may be included within one book. In the physician's office, only Volumes 1 and 2 are used. Volume 3 is used by hospitals.

The diagnostic classification systems in Volumes 1 and 2 are maintained by a federal government agency, the National Center for Health Statistics (NCHS); the procedure classification (Volume 3) is maintained by the Centers for Medicare and Medicaid Services (CMS), the federal agency that regulates health care financing. All three volumes are updated regularly, with codes being added, revised, and sometimes deleted. Changes in the ICD-9-CM are published by NCHS and CMS with the approval of WHO. Both the American Health Information Management Association (AHIMA) and the American Hospital Association (AHA) advise and assist in keeping the classification system current.

CHECKPOINT QUESTIONS

2. What organization must approve any changes in the disease classification system?

LEGAL TIP

DOES EVERYONE NEED TO KNOW?

Remember that the ICD-9 codes placed on the CMS-1500 are confidential and should be protected as much as any other medical information. Forms left lying in common areas in the office may be seen by other patients. Keep printers and copies of these forms in a private place, and share the diagnosis codes only with those who need the information to carry out their duties. Patients have the right to keep their diagnoses private.

Inpatient Versus Outpatient Coding

There is a big difference between coding medical claims in a hospital or other inpatient facility and coding for the physician in an outpatient medical practice. The systems and references used to assign codes to third-party claims is only one difference in the coding requirements and practices of the physician and the inpatient medical facility. Volumes 1 and 2 of the ICD-9-CM are used to report the diagnostic code that justifies physician services whether those services are provided in the office or in the hospital. Hospital coders use Volume 3 to report inpatient procedures, services, and supplies, as well as the reasons for the services.

The UB-92 (uniform bill) is used by institutions to report inpatient admissions and outpatient and emergency department services and procedures. These charges are for nursing services, building maintenance, and all costs associated with running the institution. These charges do not include physician services. The CMS-1500 (universal claim form) is used to report physician services, whether the physician sees the patient in the office, emergency department, hospital, or nursing home, because even though the physician may have been in the hospital, it is his **service** for which we are billing in the medical office.

The term **outpatient** is used to describe patients treated in the following places:

- Health care provider's office
- Hospital clinic
- Emergency department
- Hospital same-day surgery unit or ambulatory surgical center that releases the patient within 23 hours
- Observation status in a hospital (the patient is admitted for a short time for observation only, and the physician bills for his or her service during the stay)

The term **inpatient** refers to a patient who is admitted to the hospital for treatment with the expectation that the patient will remain in the hospital for 24 hours or more.

Hospital coders code only services provided by the hospital and hospital employees. Coders who are employed by the physician practice are concerned with the services provided by the physician no matter where the services are provided. For example, the hospital room, meals, and laboratory testing that a patient receives are billed and coded by the hospital billing department. The daily visits the physician makes to the patient are billed and coded by the physician's office.

Since the focus of this textbook is medical assisting, we concentrate on outpatient coding.

 CHECKPOINT QUESTION

3. Name and give uses for the three volumes of the ICD-9-CM.

ICD-9-CM: The Code Book

Coding books are available from several publishers, such as Ingenix and Medicode. The AMA (American Medical Association) Press also publishes coding books and training materials. The classification system is also available as part of a medical software package; one of these packages is CodeManager from the AMA. Although each publisher offers special features and helpful aids, the format remains the same. Some coders become comfortable with certain special features (i.e., AMA publications are spiral bound) and, since the content is the same, can choose among the various publications based on organization, illustrations, tabs, bullets, and color coding.

To become an expert medical coder, you need general knowledge of human anatomy and medical terminology. In addition to using a code book, you will need reference materials such as a medical dictionary and/or medical dictionary software.

To ensure accurate coding, update your ICD-9-CM coding books and software as needed. (Updates and addenda can be purchased from the publisher of your coding book.) You must update codes on superbills (preprinted bills listing a variety of procedures) or any other forms you use. Experts have estimated that millions of dollars in reimbursement have been lost because an incorrect code was taken from a standardized form that had not been updated. New codes are published each October, and third-party payers require their use after January 1.

 CHECKPOINT QUESTION

4. How often is the ICD-9-CM updated? When is the use of the new codes required?

Volume 1: Tabular List of Diseases

Volume 1 contains the classification of diseases (conditions) and injuries by code numbers. Figure 14-1 shows the table of contents from this volume. These 17 chapters cover groupings of diseases and injuries by **etiology** or cause (e.g., infectious diseases) and by anatomic system (e.g., digestive, respiratory). Figure 14-2 is a sample page from the tabular list showing each level of classification. Note that each chapter has a heading or title [e.g., 16, Symptoms, Signs, and Ill-Defined Conditions (780–799)]. Following the title in parentheses is the range of three-digit categories included in that chapter. In each chapter, you will find subtitles in large type followed by a range of three-digit categories in parentheses [e.g., 16, Symptoms (780–789)]. These sections describe general disease. Three-digit codes followed by a title, the category codes, describe specific diseases (e.g., 780, general symptoms). The fourth digit further breaks down the category (e.g., 780.0, alteration of consciousness), and the fifth digit is the highest level of definition (e.g., 780.01, coma).

You must always code a diagnosis to its highest definition. Volume 1 tells you how many digits are required to code a diagnosis correctly and to a level that most third-party payers will accept. Volume 1 also includes five appendices, which are outlined in Table 14-1.

Supplementary Classifications

Supplementary classifications in Volume 1 include V- and E-codes.

V-Codes

V-codes, which range from V01 to V82, provide a means of indexing the reason for hospital or physician office care for other than current or genuine illness, such as a history of illness, immunizations, or live-born infants according to type of birth. An example of a V-code is V10.04, which is used for a person with a personal history of a malignant neoplasm of the stomach. Because of this history, it would be important for this patient to have regular checkups. You would not want to code the visit 230.2, neoplasm of the stomach, because that would imply the patient has the malignant neoplasm at this visit. V-codes may be used alone if no disease diagnosis is appropriate or as the second or third code to help better explain the reason for the visit.

E-Codes

E-codes, which range from E800 to E999, are used to classify external causes of injuries and poisoning. Specificity is limited to the fourth-digit level. E-codes are used in conjunction with codes in Chapters 1 to 17. They help to provide information of interest to industrial medicine, insurance underwriters, national safety programs, public health agencies, and others concerned

TABLE OF CONTENTS

Preface .... *iii*
Acknowledgments .... *v*
Introduction .... *xiii*
Conventions Used in the Tabular List .... *xxi*
Guidance in the Use of ICD-9-CM .... *xxiii*

Classification of Diseases and Injuries
1. Infectious and Parasitic Diseases 1
2. Neoplasms 81
3. Endocrine, Nutritional, and Metabolic Diseases and
      Immunity Disorders 154
4. Diseases of the Blood and Blood-Forming Organs ... 188
5. Mental Disorders 204
6. Diseases of the Nervous System and Sense Organs 251
7. Diseases of the Circulatory System 358
8. Diseases of the Respiratory System 404
9. Diseases of the Digestive System 432
10. Diseases of the Genitourinary System 481
11. Complications of Pregnancy, Childbirth, and the
      Puerperium 527
12. Diseases of the Skin and Subcutaneous Tissue 569
13. Diseases of the Musculoskeletal System and
      Connective Tissue 593
14. Congenital Anomalies 639
15. Certain Conditions Originating in the Perinatal Period ... 683
16. Symptoms, Signs, and Ill-Defined Conditions 707
17. Injury and Poisoning 735

Supplementary Classification
    Classification of Factors Influencing Health Status and
      Contact with Health Service 880
    Classification of External Causes of Injury and Poisoning 930

Appendices
A. Morphology of Neoplasms 1055
B. Glossary of Mental Disorders 1077
C. Classification of Drugs by American Hospital
      Formulary Service List Number and Their *ICD-9-CM*
      Equivalents 1127
D. Classification of Industrial Accidents According to
      Agency 1137
E. List of Three-Digit Categories 1143

Figure 14-1 Table of contents from ICD-9-CM, Volume 1.

with causes of injuries (e.g., auto accidents, accidents caused by heavy industrial machinery). These codes do not affect reimbursement.

Volume 2, Section 3, has a separate index to access E-codes, the Alphabetic Index to External Causes of Injury and Poisoning.

 CHECKPOINT QUESTION

5. List four reasons for using E-codes.

Volume 2: Alphabetic Index to Diseases

Volume 2, the Alphabetic Index to Diseases, contains many diagnostic terms that do not appear in Volume 1. For example, itch, barbers, beard, and scalp are all listed under *Itch* in Volume 2. In Volume 1, they are all listed under code 110.0. The index is arranged by condition. Always check all indentations in the index under the condition to ensure that you have the one most appropriate to the diagnosis you intend to code.

✓5th **780.5** **Sleep disturbances**
> **EXCLUDES** *that of nonorganic origin (307.40-307.49)*

780.50 Sleep disturbance, unspecified

780.51 Insomnia with sleep apnea
DEF: Transient cessation of breathing disturbing sleep.

780.52 Other insomnia
Insomnia NOS
DEF: Inability to maintain adequate sleep cycle.

780.53 Hypersomnia with sleep apnea
DEF: Autonomic response inhibited during sleep; causes insufficient oxygen intake, acidosis and pulmonary hypertension.

780.54 Other hypersomnia
Hypersomnia NOS
DEF: Prolonged sleep cycle.

780.55 Disruptions of 24-hour sleep-wake cycle
Inversion of sleep rhythm
Irregular sleep-wake rhythm NOS
Non-24-hour sleep-wake rhythm

780.56 Dysfunctions associated with sleep stages or arousal from sleep

780.57 Other and unspecified sleep apnea

780.59 Other

✓4th **780 General symptoms**

✓5th **780.0** **Alteration of consciousness**
> **EXCLUDES** *coma:*
> *diabetic (250.2-250.3)*
> *hepatic (572.2)*
> *originating in the perinatal period (779.2)*

780.01 Coma
DEF: State of unconsciousness from which the patient cannot be awakened.

780.02 Transient alteration of awareness
DEF: Temporary, recurring spells of reduced consciousness.

780.03 Persistent vegetative state
DEF: Persistent wakefulness without consciousness due to nonfunctioning cerebral cortex.

780.09 Other
Drowsiness	Stupor
Semicoma	Unconsciousness
Somnolence	

780.1 **Hallucinations**
Hallucinations:	Hallucinations:
NOS	olfactory
auditory	tactile
gustatory	

> **EXCLUDES** *those associated with mental disorders, as functional*
> *psychoses (295.0-298.9)*
> *organic brain syndromes (290.0-294.9, 310.0-310.9)*
> *visual hallucinations (368.16)*

DEF: Perception of external stimulus in absence of stimulus; inability to distinguish between real and imagined.

✓5th **779.8** **Other specified conditions originating in the perinatal period**

779.81 Neonatal bradycardia
> **EXCLUDES** *abnormality in fetal heart rate or rhythm*
> *complicating labor and delivery*
> *(763.81-763.83)*
> *bradycardia due to birth asphyxia (768.5-768.9)*

779.82 Neonatal tachycardia
> **EXCLUDES** *abnormality in fetal heart rate or rhythm*
> *complicating labor and delivery*
> *(763.81-763.83)*

779.89 Other specified conditions originating in the perinatal period

Figure 14-2 Sample page from ICD-9-CM, Volume 1, showing categories, subheadings, and so on.

TABLE **14-1** ICD-9-CM Appendices	
The following five appendices are found in Volume I.	
Title	**Description**
Appendix A: Morphology of Neoplasms	This appendix is used in conjunction with Chapter 2 in ICD-9-CM when coding neoplasms. It lists the five-digit alphanumeric codes used to identify the morphology of a neoplasm. For example, in the morphology code M8070/3, the 8070 indicates that the morphology is squamous cell carcinoma. The /3 indicates that it is the primary site.
Appendix B: Glossary of Mental Disorders	Alphabetic list of mental disorders, including detailed descriptions of each disease.
Appendix C: Classification of Drugs by American Hospital Formulary Service (AHFS) List Number and the ICD-9-CM Equivalents	This appendix lists the AHFS list number (e.g., 24:04 for cardiac drugs) and the ICD9-CM code number for each one (e.g., 24.04 cardiac drugs would be equivalent to category 972.9, the ICD9-CM category of "other and unspecified agents primarily affecting the cardiovascular system").
Appendix D: Classification of Industrial Accidents by Agency	This includes codes that can be used as a supplement to describe types of equipment or materials that may be responsible for an industrial accident or illness.
Appendix E: List of Three-Digit Categories	This is a list of all three-digit categories in ICD-9-CM.

Note: Appendices A through D are not recognized by most government programs, such as Medicare and Medicaid. As previously mentioned, ICD-9-CM has other uses, however, and you may find that you need the appendices to track such things as disorders treated.

LEGAL TIP

DON'T GIVE PATIENTS A DISEASE THEY DON'T HAVE!

It is important that you use the code that explains the patient's situation accurately. Coding AIDS before that diagnosis is made could be construed as defamation of character and even libel. Some patients just want to be tested for HIV, but there are no signs or symptoms.

The ICD-9-CM offers a variety of codes for HIV testing. For a patient who has the test simply because he or she wants to know, you will use V72.6, which is simply "laboratory examination." The code used for a patient who has known exposure is V01.79, which is "contact with or exposure to communicable diseases, other viral diseases." For patients who want to be tested because they are worried about exposure, V69.2 is used. This code is "high-risk sexual behavior." In this case, two codes would be used: V69.2 and V01.79. This approach will ensure that a patient is not assigned a diagnosis code for a problem he or she does not have.

The alphabetic index is organized into three sections:

- Section 1, Alphabetic Index to Diseases and Injuries, is organized by **main terms** printed in boldface type. Section 1 is used for reporting the reason for patient encounters for most insurance claims. Following the main term is a code number, which refers you to the tabular listing (Volume 1). You must not accept this number as the correct code without a **cross-reference** or check of the tabular list. Never code directly from the alphabetic index. This could result in an incomplete or incorrect coding assignment. For example, if you have a patient with fluid overload and you look under fluid, it may seem logical to code the first code under fluid, which is abdomen, 789.5, but your patient is generally retaining fluid. If you use the alphabetic index only, you do not know that the correct code is 276.6, fluid overload, which excludes ascites, 789.5, and localized edema, 782.3. Box 14-1 outlines several exceptions to the main term rule.

- Section 2, Table of Drugs and Chemicals, includes an extensive listing of drugs, chemical substances, and toxic agents. It also shows E-codes and American Hospital Formulary Service (AHFS) list numbers, which are in the table under the main term *drug*.

BOX 14-1

EXCEPTIONS TO THE MAIN TERM RULE

Sometimes, you have to think outside the box. Most of the time, locating the condition instead of the location works well, but sometimes a diagnosis will stump you.

1. Obstetric conditions may be found under the main terms *delivery, pregnancy,* and *puerperal.*
2. Complications of medical or surgical procedures or primary diagnoses can be found under complications. For example, complications of pneumonia would be found under *complications*—not *pneumonia.*
3. Conditions arising from an earlier problem or procedure are called late effects and can be found under the words *late effects, due to, as a result of, residual,* etc.
4. Lacerations can be found under *wounds.*
5. V-Codes are codes used for patients who are not sick. They may be found by looking for terms such as *admission, examination, history of…, observation, problem with, status, vaccination, encounter for, follow-up,* etc.

• Section 3, Alphabetic Index to External Cases of Injuries and Poisonings, leads you to codes that describe circumstances of injuries, accidents, and violence. These codes are not used for medical diagnoses. Main entries in this section usually are a type of accident or violence (e.g., assault, fall, collision). These codes can supplement the diagnostic code, but they should never be used alone or as principal diagnosis codes. E-codes are frequently used with these codes. For example, a person who fractured a tibia in a fall off a sidewalk curb would be given a code from Chapter 17, Volume 1, in the ICD-9-CM for the injury (e.g., fracture of tibia, closed, is 823.80), and an additional code, E880.0, indicates that the accident was a fall off a sidewalk curb.

 CHECKPOINT QUESTION

6. What are V-codes used for?

Volume 3: Inpatient Coding

Volume 3, the Tabular List and Alphabetic Index of Procedures, is used in inpatient facilities and is based on anatomy, not surgical specialty. There are no alphabetic characters in these procedure codes. The codes are two-digit categories with a maximum of two decimal digits where necessary. Most refer to surgical procedures, and the rest cover miscellaneous diagnostic and therapeutic procedures. An example of a procedure code is 31.61, larynx laceration suture. Volume 3 is used for inpatient coding only.

Locating the Appropriate Code

Box 14-2 outlines CMS guidelines for diagnostic coding. These are explained next.

Using the ICD-9-CM Conventions

Figure 14-3 lists the conventions used in the ICD-9-CM indexes. **Conventions** are rules that apply to the assignment of the ICD-9 codes. They are found throughout both the Index to Diseases and the Tabular List and include general notes using specific terms, cross-references, abbreviations, punctuation marks, symbols, typeface, and format. They direct and guide the coder to the appropriate code and should be strictly adhered to. Each publisher uses these same conventions, and many add more to assist coders in providing the most complete and accurate reason for the encounter. For example, when you locate the word itch, you will find "see pruritus," the medical term for severe itching. This is a helpful tool for coders who are unfamiliar with medical terminology.

Main Term

When trying to locate a diagnosis with more than one word, look first under the main term or condition. Often, a diagnosis may be an **eponym** (e.g., Ménière's disease or syndrome). These terms can be found under the main term *disease* or *syndrome.* In the diagnosis of breast cyst, the main term is *cyst.* Find the condition, not the location. Imagine how large the ICD-9-CM code book would have to be to list every condition possible for the leg, the arm, or any other location. Instead, the condition is listed, and the arm or leg would be found under that term. For example, the diagnosis code for fracture of the left tibia would be found by looking up the main term fracture, not tibia.

Fourth and Fifth Digits

In many instances, a fourth digit has been added to a category to provide more detail, or **specificity.** These are subcategory codes. Some codes also have a fifth digit because of the need to code to a higher specificity. For example, diabetes mellitus is category 250. It is

BOX 14-2

CMS DIAGNOSTIC CODING GUIDELINES

CMS defines specific guidelines that provide the basic knowledge necessary to apply the correct ICD-9 codes. Although these guidelines were developed for use in submitting government claims, most insurance companies have also adopted them. Many variations exist among the private insurance companies; therefore, care must be taken in recognizing the different requirements for each third-party payer. Most coders operate on the assumption that the government regulations are the strictest, and following those guidelines will satisfy most third-party payers.

1. Identify each service and procedure, or supply with an ICD-9 code from 001.0 through V82.9 to describe the diagnosis, symptom, complaint, condition, or problem.
2. Identify services or visits for circumstances other than disease or injury, such as follow-up care after chemotherapy, with V-codes provided for this purpose.
3. Code the reason for the visit first and code any coexisting conditions that affect the treatment of the patient for that visit or procedure as supplementary information. Do not code a diagnosis that is no longer applicable.
4. Code to the highest degree of specificity. Carry the numeric code to the fourth or fifth digit when necessary.
5. Code a chronic diagnosis as often as it is applicable to the patient's treatment.
6. When only ancillary services are provided, list the appropriate V-code first and the problem second. For example, if a patient is receiving only physical therapy, list the V-code first, followed by the code for the condition on line 24E on the CMS-1500 form.
7. For ambulatory or outpatient surgical procedures, code the diagnosis applicable to the procedure. If the postoperative diagnosis is different from the preoperative diagnosis, use the postoperative diagnosis.

necessary to use one of the fourth-digit subcategories to indicate the specific complications that may accompany the diabetes and then add a fifth digit to indicate whether the diabetes is insulin dependent or noninsulin dependent. Those codes requiring a fifth digit are iden-

tified in both Volumes 1 and 2. Incomplete coding here affects reimbursement and causes data errors. Figure 14-4 shows samples of fifth-digit classifications from the ICD-9-CM, Volumes 1 and 2. The code 807.1 tells the third-party payer that the patient was seen for an open fracture of a rib. The fifth digit is added to describe how many ribs. A patient who fractured two ribs would be assigned the code 807.12. This gives a more thorough picture of the patient's problem and enables the payer to determine whether the treatment is medically necessary.

Primary Codes

In outpatient coding, the **primary diagnosis** is simply the patient's chief complaint or the reason the patient sought medical attention today. It may be a routine follow-up visit, or there may be a new problem. The primary code is listed first on the CMS-1500.

When More Than One Code Is Used

In many cases, more than one code is used for a single patient visit. When patients have more than one diagnosis, it is necessary to convey an accurate picture of the patient's total condition. For example, an elderly patient may have the following diagnoses listed each time she visits the doctor: degenerative arthritis, type 2 diabetes mellitus, macular degeneration, hypertension, and pernicious anemia. If any of these conditions is related to or affects her treatment, they should be listed as supplementary information. If she visits the doctor because she has influenza and her other diagnoses are not addressed at the visit, it is not necessary to list all the diagnoses given. The primary diagnosis is her reason for coming to the office (symptoms of influenza). But the fact that she is diabetic will affect her treatment and makes her visit medically necessary. Multiple codes should be sequenced with the proper service or procedure code on the proper line of the CMS-1500. Figure 14-5 shows the proper sequencing for another patient's CMS-1500. On Line 1 of Section 24 on the CMS-1500, you place the code and charge for the visit. In Block 24E, the diagnosis code for the ankle injury appears first because that is what brought the patient to the office today. On Line 2 of 24A, the laboratory work is listed but is also referenced to the diagnosis on Line 21, Item 2, which is the proper code for the patient's diabetes; this is referenced to Item 2 on Line 24. If the patient did not have diabetes, the laboratory work would not be considered reasonable for a patient with an ankle injury. If this procedure were not followed, the laboratory work would be seen as medically unnecessary, and the physician would not be reimbursed.

Conventions

Braces { }   These are used in the Tabular List to connect a series of terms to a common stem. Each term on the left of the brace is incomplete without one of the terms to the right of the bracket.

Brackets [ ]   Brackets enclose synonyms, alternate wording, or explanatory phrases.

Colon :   A colon is used after an incomplete term that needs one or more of the modifiers that follow to make it assignable to a given category.

Parentheses ( )   Parentheses enclose supplementary words that may be present or absent in the statement of a disease or procedure, without affecting the code number to which it is assigned.

NEC (not elsewhere classifiable)   Alerts the coder that the specified form of the condition is classified differently. Codes following NEC should be used only when the coder lacks the information necessary to code the term in a more specific category.

NOS (not otherwise specified)   The coder should continue to look for a more specific code.

Note   Used to define terms and give coding instructions. Found most often with list of fifth digits.

"Includes"   Indicates separate terms as adjectives that further modify sites and conditions or to further define or give examples of the content of a certain category.

"Excludes"   A box with "excludes" in italics draws the reader's attention to instructions that direct the coder to the proper code. This convention is found in the Tabular List.

"See," "See Also," and "See Category"   Direct the coder to other terms or sections that should be considered. ALWAYS follow these instructions.

"Use additional code"   This directs the coder to add another code to further explain and give the third-party payer a better understanding of a diagnosis.

"Code First Underlying Disease"   This direction is used in the tabular list when a reason for an encounter results from another disorder. The coder is instructed to indicate the underlying disease that caused the current problem or symptom that brought the patient to the office.

Index to Disease Example

478.1   Other diseases of nasal cavity and sinuses

Abscess
Necrosis } Of nose (septum)
Ulcer

422.92   Septic myocarditis
Myocarditis, acute or subacute:
  Pneumococcal
  Staphylococcal
Use additional code to identify infectious organism [e.g., Staphylococcus 041.1]

See above example 478.1 (septum) may or may not be present in the diagnosis given.

Infection
  Streptococcal NEC 041.00
    Group
      A 041.01
      B 041.002

As soon as the bacterium is identified, code for specific infection.

At the time of the service, it has not been established whether a neoplasm is benign or secondary, for example. Remember, you are coding for a date of service with the information documented for that date of service.

	Allergic rhinitis (nonseasonal)
INCLUDES	477 Allergic rhinitis (seasonal)
	Hay fever
EXCLUDES	Allergic rhinitis with asthma (bronchial) (493.0)

Itch (see also Pruritus) 698.9

See 422.92 examples above.

362.72   Retinal dystrophy in other systemic disorders and syndromes
  Code first underlying disease, as:
    Bassen-Kornzweig syndrome (272.5)
    Refsum's disease (356.3)

Figure 14-3 Conventions used in ICD-9.

WHAT IF?

You need to code a condition described as acute, chronic, or both. What code should you use?
When a particular condition is described as both acute and chronic, code it according to the subentries in the alphabetic index (Volume 2) for the condition. If there are separate entries listed for acute, subacute, and chronic, use both codes. The first code listed should be for the acute condition, the reason the patient came to the office today. Respiratory and orthopedic conditions tend to be acute and chronic. That is, a patient with emphysema will always have underlying symptoms of progressive disease, but during the spring, pollen may aggravate the condition and cause acute breathing problems.

A   INJURY AND POISONING   807–808.49

☑4th **807 Fracture of rib(s), sternum, larynx, and trachea**

The following fifth-digit subclassification is for use with codes 807.0-807.1:

  0 rib(s), unspecified
  1 one rib
  2 two ribs
  3 three ribs
  4 four ribs
  5 five ribs
  6 six ribs
  7 seven ribs
  8 eight or more ribs
  9 multiple ribs, unspecified

☑5th **807.0 Rib(s), closed**   MSP
☑5th **807.1 Rib(s), open**   MSP
807.2 Sternum, closed   MSP
    DEF: Break in flat bone (breast bone) in anterior thorax.

807.3 Sternum, open   MSP
    DEF: Break, with open wound, in flat bone in mid anterior thorax.

807.4 Flail chest   MSP
807.5 Larynx and trachea, closed   MSP
    Hyoid bone   Trachea
    Thyroid cartilage

807.6 Larynx and trachea, open   MSP

B   Fracture — *continued*
                                       multiple — *continued*
                                        skull, specified or unspecified bones, or
                                          face bone(s) with any other bone(s) —
                                            continued

┌───┐
│ Note — *Use the following fifth-digit*   │
│ *subclassification with categories 800, 801,* │
│ *803, and 804:*   │
│   │
│ 0   *unspecified state of consciousness*   │
│ 1   *with no loss of consciousness*   │
│ 2   *with brief [less than one hour] loss*   │
│   *of consciousness*   │
│ 3   *with moderate [1-24 hours] loss of*   │
│   *consciousness*   │
│ 4   *with prolonged [more than 24 hours]*   │
│   *loss of consciousness and return to*   │
│   *pre-existing conscious level*   │
│ 5   *with prolonged [more than 24 hours]*   │
│   *loss of consciousness, without*   │
│   *return to pre-existing conscious level* │
│ *Use fifth-digit 5 to designate when a*   │
│   *patient is unconscious and dies*   │
│   *before regaining consciousness,*   │
│   *regardless of the duration of the*   │
│   *loss of consciousness*   │
│ 6   *with loss of consciousness of*   │
│   *unspecified duration*   │
│ 9   *with concussion, unspecified*   │
└───┘

                                       with
                                        contusion, cerebral 804.1 ☑5th
                                        epidural hemorrhage 804.2 ☑5th
                                        extradural hemorrhage 804.2 ☑5th
                                        hemorrhage (intracranial) NEC
                                          804.8 ☑5th
                                        intracranial injury NEC 804.4 ☑5th
                                        laceration, cerebral 804.1 ☑5th
                                        subarachnoid hemorrhage 804.2 ☑5th
                                        subdural hemorrhage 804.2 ☑5th

Figure 14-4 Samples of fifth-digit classifications from ICD-9-CM. (**A**) Volume 1. (**B**) Volume 2.

PLEASE
DO NOT
STAPLE
IN THIS
AREA

↑ CARRIER

| | PICA | | | | | | | **HEALTH INSURANCE CLAIM FORM** | | PICA | | |

1. MEDICARE MEDICAID CHAMPUS CHAMPVA GROUP HEALTH PLAN FECA BLK LUNG OTHER **1a.** INSURED'S I.D. NUMBER (FOR PROGRAM IN ITEM 1)

[X] (Medicare #) [ ] (Medicaid #) [ ] (Sponsor's SSN) [ ] (VA File #) [ ] (SSN or ID) [ ] (SSN) [ ] (ID)   000-00-0000A

2. PATIENT'S NAME (Last Name, First Name, Middle Initial)
Naomi A Dishman

3. PATIENT'S BIRTH DATE MM 04 DD 14 YY 24 SEX M [ ] F [X]

4. INSURED'S NAME (Last Name, First Name, Middle Initial)
Same

5. PATIENT'S ADDRESS (No., Street)
405 Carolina Ave

6. PATIENT RELATIONSHIP TO INSURED
Self [ ] Spouse [ ] Child [ ] Other [ ]

7. INSURED'S ADDRESS (No., Street)

CITY
Danville   STATE VA

8. PATIENT STATUS
Single [ ] Married [X] Other [ ]

CITY   STATE

ZIP CODE 24540   TELEPHONE (Include Area Code) (434) 555-5555

Employed [ ] Full-Time Student [ ] Part-Time Student [ ]

ZIP CODE   TELEPHONE (INCLUDE AREA CODE) ( )

9. OTHER INSURED'S NAME (Last Name, First Name, Middle Initial)
NONE

10. IS PATIENT'S CONDITION RELATED TO:

11. INSURED'S POLICY GROUP OR FECA NUMBER

a. OTHER INSURED'S POLICY OR GROUP NUMBER

a. EMPLOYMENT? (CURRENT OR PREVIOUS)
YES [ ] NO [X]

a. INSURED'S DATE OF BIRTH MM DD YY SEX M [ ] F [ ]

b. OTHER INSURED'S DATE OF BIRTH MM DD YY SEX M [ ] F [ ]

b. AUTO ACCIDENT?
YES [ ] NO [X]   PLACE (State)

b. EMPLOYER'S NAME OR SCHOOL NAME

c. EMPLOYER'S NAME OR SCHOOL NAME

c. OTHER ACCIDENT?
YES [X] NO [ ]

c. INSURANCE PLAN NAME OR PROGRAM NAME

d. INSURANCE PLAN NAME OR PROGRAM NAME

10d. RESERVED FOR LOCAL USE

d. IS THERE ANOTHER HEALTH BENEFIT PLAN?
YES [ ] NO [ ]   *If yes,* return to and complete item 9 a-d.

READ BACK OF FORM BEFORE COMPLETING & SIGNING THIS FORM.
12. PATIENT'S OR AUTHORIZED PERSON'S SIGNATURE I authorize the release of any medical or other information necessary to process this claim. I also request payment of government benefits either to myself or to the party who accepts assignment below.

SIGNED Signature on File   DATE 052808

13. INSURED'S OR AUTHORIZED PERSON'S SIGNATURE I authorize payment of medical benefits to the undersigned physician or supplier for services described below.

SIGNED

14. DATE OF CURRENT: MM 05 DD 28 YY 08   ◄ ILLNESS (First symptom) OR INJURY (Accident) OR PREGNANCY(LMP)

15. IF PATIENT HAS HAD SAME OR SIMILAR ILLNESS. GIVE FIRST DATE MM DD YY

16. DATES PATIENT UNABLE TO WORK IN CURRENT OCCUPATION FROM MM DD YY TO MM DD YY

17. NAME OF REFERRING PHYSICIAN OR OTHER SOURCE

17a. I.D. NUMBER OF REFERRING PHYSICIAN

18. HOSPITALIZATION DATES RELATED TO CURRENT SERVICES FROM MM DD YY TO MM DD YY

19. RESERVED FOR LOCAL USE

20. OUTSIDE LAB? YES [ ] NO [ ] $ CHARGES

21. DIAGNOSIS OR NATURE OF ILLNESS OR INJURY. (RELATE ITEMS 1,2,3 OR 4 TO ITEM 24E BY LINE)

1. 845.03
2. 250.00
3. ___.___
4. ___.___

22. MEDICAID RESUBMISSION CODE   ORIGINAL REF. NO.

23. PRIOR AUTHORIZATION NUMBER

24. A DATE(S) OF SERVICE						B Place of Service	C Type of Service	D PROCEDURES, SERVICES, OR SUPPLIES (Explain Unusual Circumstances) CPT/HCPCS MODIFIER	E DIAGNOSIS CODE	F $ CHARGES	G DAYS OR UNITS	H EPSDT Family Plan	I EMG	J COB	K RESERVED FOR LOCAL USE
From MM	DD	YY	To MM	DD	YY										
05	28	08	05	28	08	11		99213	1	100 00	1				
05	28	08	05	28	08	11		82947	2	25 00	1				

25. FEDERAL TAX I.D. NUMBER SSN [ ] EIN [ ]
54-0000000

26. PATIENT'S ACCOUNT NO.
1234

27. ACCEPT ASSIGNMENT? (For govt. claims, see back)
[X] YES [ ] NO

28. TOTAL CHARGE
$ 125 00

29. AMOUNT PAID
$

30. BALANCE DUE
$ 125 00

31. SIGNATURE OF PHYSICIAN OR SUPPLIER INCLUDING DEGREES OR CREDENTIALS (I certify that the statements on the reverse apply to this bill and are made a part thereof.)

SIGNED   DATE

32. NAME AND ADDRESS OF FACILITY WHERE SERVICES WERE RENDERED (If other than home or office)

33. PHYSICIAN'S, SUPPLIER'S BILLING NAME, ADDRESS, ZIP CODE & PHONE #
JOSEPH G NORTH, MD
1111 GRAYSON STREET
DANVILLE VA
PIN#   GRP#

(APPROVED BY AMA COUNCIL ON MEDICAL SERVICE 8/88)   *PLEASE PRINT OR TYPE*   APPROVED OMB-0938-0008 FORM CMS-1500 (12-90), FORM RRB-1500, APPROVED OMB-1215-0055 FORM OWCP-1500, APPROVED OMB-0720-0001 (CHAMPUS)

PATIENT AND INSURED INFORMATION → PHYSICIAN OR SUPPLIER INFORMATION

Figure 14-5 Sample CMS-1500 claim form indicating proper sequencing.

Late Effects

Late effects are symptoms or conditions arising from an acute illness. The effects are present after treatment for the acute illness or injury has ended. Proper coding sequence requires that you list the code number identifying the residual or current condition first, with the code number identifying the cause or original illness or injury listed second. Key words used in the patient's medical records defining late effects include late, due to an old injury, due to a previous illness/injury, due to an illness or injury occurring a year or more ago, sequela of . . . ,

as a result of . . . , resulting from . . . , and so on. Patients who are status post cerebrovascular accident (CVA) may have residual effects from their original stroke, for example, and may have a diagnosis of left hemiparesis as a result of CVA 3 years ago. Figure 14-6 is a sample listing of a late effect from the ICD-9-CM.

Coding Suspected Conditions

In the inpatient setting, coders list conditions after the patient's testing is complete. In other words, they are coding

---

A **LATE EFFECTS OF INJURIES, POISONINGS, TOXIC EFFECTS, AND OTHER EXTERNAL CAUSES (905-909)**

Note: These categories are to be used to indicate conditions classifiable to 800-999 as the cause of late effects, which are themselves classified elsewhere. The "late effects" include those specified as such, or as sequelae, which may occur at any time after the acute injury.

☑4ᵗʰ **905 Late effects of musculoskeletal and connective tissue injuries**

905.0 **Late effect of fracture of skull and face bones**
Late effect of injury classifiable to 800-804

905.1 **Late effect of fracture of spine and trunk without mention of spinal cord lesion**
Late effect of injury classifiable to 805, 807-809

905.2 **Late effect of fracture of upper extremities**
Late effect of injury classifiable to 810-819

905.3 **Late effect of fracture of neck of femur**
Late effect of injury classifiable to 820

905.4 **Late effect of fracture of lower extremities**
Late effect of injury classifiable to 821-827

905.5 **Late effect of fracture of multiple and unspecified bones**
Late effect of injury classifiable to 828-829

905.6 **Late effect of dislocation**
Late effect of injury classifiable to 830-839

905.7 **Late effect of sprain and strain without mention of tendon injury**
Late effect of injury classifiable to 840-848, except tendon injury

905.8 **Late effect of tendon injury**
Late effect of tendon injury due to:
open wound [injury classifiable to 880-884 with .2, 890-894 with .2]
sprain and strain [injury classifiable to 840-848]

905.9 **Late effect of traumatic amputation**
Late effect of injury classifiable to 885-887, 895-897
EXCLUDES *late amputation stump complication (997.60-997.69)*

B

Late

Late — *continued*
  effect(s) (of) — continued
    tuberculosis — *continued*
      genitourinary (conditions classifiable to 016) 137.2
      pulmonary (conditions classifiable to 010-012) 137.0
      specified organs NEC (conditions classifiable to 014, 017-018) 137.4
      viral encephalitis (conditions classifiable to 049.8, 049.9, 062-064) 139.0
    wound, open
      extremity (injury classifiable to 880-884 and 890-894, except .2) 906.1
      tendon (injury classifiable to 880-884 with .2 and 890-894 with.2) 905.8
      head, neck, and trunk (injury classifiable to 870-879) 906.0

Figure 14-6 Sample section of late effects in ICD-9-CM. (**A**) Volume 1. (**B**) Volume 2.

with complete information. In outpatient settings, however, the coder reports the reason for the patient visit as it occurs. When filing claims, the coder is limited by the information and documentation on hand at the time of the patient visit. If at the end of the visit the diagnosis is not confirmed, the physician may indicate "rule out," "suspected," or "probable." For example, a patient who comes in complaining of headache may be sent for magnetic resonance imaging (MRI) of the head because the physician suspects a serious disorder. On the patient's encounter form, the physician may list the diagnosis as "rule out brain tumor." It is not accurate to code the visit as brain tumor before it is confirmed by MRI. On this first visit to the physician's office, the reason for being seen is headache. The patient's symptom (headache) is the only confirmed reason for the encounter at this point. On the second visit to the doctor, the MRI has confirmed a glioma in the frontal lobe. For the second and all subsequent visits, glioma is coded as the reason for the encounter. Figure 14-2 shows a page from the ICD-9-CM that includes many of the symptom codes.

ETHICAL TIP

Don't Break the Rules

Imagine an unethical patient asking a physician to break the rules. Unfortunately, it happens. Some insurance companies still offer limited coverage when the patient is not sick. Routine exams and tests may be covered at a reduced rate or not at all. For this reason, some patients may think that if the doctor codes the claim with a diagnosis, then that makes the service medically necessary, and their insurance will pay. Coding based on anything other than the documentation proves is wrong. It is not only unethical, it is illegal. If a patient asks you to be dishonest, explain that this would be unethical. Tell the patient that random audits are often carried out by the CMS to ensure that the medical chart indicates that the services and procedures on claims were actually performed and the reasons were legitimate.

 CHECKPOINT QUESTION

7. When coding a visit on a date before a definitive diagnosis is made, what is coded?

Documentation Requirements

As discussed throughout this chapter, you should choose the code assigned to any given claim for a service or procedure based on the documentation available in the pa-

tient's record at the time of the service. An **audit** is conducted by the government, a managed care company, and a health care organization to determine compliance and to detect fraud. Remember, if it's not in the chart, it did not happen. Auditors verify the codes used based on information recorded in the chart on the date of service.

The Future of Diagnostic Coding: International Classification of Diseases, Tenth Revision

A new edition of the ICD, the International Classifica-tion of Diseases, Tenth Revision (ICD-10), is scheduled to be implemented at some point in the future. The WHO is responsible for revising the ICD to improve the quality of data input into clinical databases. The ICD-10-CM includes more codes and will be used by every type of health care provider for all encounters, including hospice and home health care. ICD-10 codes are alphanumeric, but the format of the index is similar to the ICD-9-CM. Two new chapters relating to disorders of the eye and the ear have been added to the ICD-10. Computer software will be revised, and the ICD-9-CM code books will be obsolete.

 CHECKPOINT QUESTION

8. List two reasons for a chart audit.

 MEDIA MENU

- **Student CD**
  - **CMA/RMA Certification Exam Review**
- **Premium Online Course**
  http://thePoint.lww.com/Kronenberger3e
- **Internet Resources**

  LiveAdvise Online Tutoring & Competency Training
  http://thePoint.lww.com/LiveAdvise

  World Health Organization
  www.who.int

  US Department of Health and Human Services
  www.hhs.gov

  Centers for Medicare and Medicaid Services
  www.cms.gov

  American Health Information Management Association
  www.ahima.org

español

SPANISH TERMINOLOGY

¿Qué son todo estos números?
   What are all these numbers? Is that my bill?
No, estos números se utilizan para su seguro.
   No, these numbers are used for your insurance.
Estos se llaman los números de codificación.
   These are called coding numbers.

PROCEDURE 14-1: Locating a Diagnostic Code

Purpose: To quickly and accurately locate a code based on reasonableness for the medical service or procedure performed
Equipment: Diagnosis, ICD-9-CM Volumes I and II Code Book, medical dictionary

Steps	Purpose
1. Using the diagnosis "chronic rheumatoid arthritis," choose the main term within the diagnostic statement. If necessary, look up the word(s) in your dictionary. *(main term is "arthritis")*	In a diagnosis that has more than one word, choosing the condition, not the location, helps find the code quickly. If you don't know what the word(s) means, you cannot make the most accurate choice.
2. Locate the main term in Volume 2. **Step 2.** Locate the main term.	The alphabetic list is in Volume 2
3. Refer to all notes and conventions under the main term.	These notes and conventions are there for a reason. In order to find the correct code, you should pay close attention to them.
4. Find the appropriate indented subordinate term. *(appropriate indented subordinate term is "rheumatoid")*	The indented terms go with the terms above them.
5. Follow any relevant instructions, such as "see also."	If the book wants you to see another code, you should go there to determine if the code you have chosen is the correct code.
6. Confirm the selected code by cross-referencing to Volume 1. Make sure you have added any necessary fourth or fifth digits.	Volume 1 will tell you if there is a fourth or fifth digit to further specify a diagnosis. Remember, if there is a fifth digit, it must be used.
7. Assign the code.	Without an appropriate code to explain the medical necessity of a service, insurance will not pay!

- Medical outpatient diagnostic coding involves the use of numbers to describe diseases, injuries, and other reasons for seeking medical care. ICD-9-CM provides an index to report and track diseases. Diagnostic coding is linked to reimbursement because it assures that the physician's service or procedure was medically necessary.

- As a medical assistant, you must understand the format and guidelines for assigning a code or reason for each encounter, treatment, and/or service.

Warm Ups for Critical Thinking

1. Tom Barksdale has been seen by the physician for controlled non–insulin-dependent type 2 diabetes mellitus for about 10 years. While being seen for a routine check of his blood sugar, he complains of numbness and tingling in his left lower leg and foot. An x-ray of both legs is performed because poor circulation in the extremities can be a complication of diabetes. The x-ray confirms the diagnosis of peripheral neuropathy. Which ICD-9 code should be listed with the office visit? Which code indicates the reason for the x-ray? Which code should be placed on the CMA-1500 first as the primary diagnosis or reason for the visit?

2. Determine the main term for the following multiple word diagnoses: gestational diabetes; amyotrophic lateral sclerosis; benign, localized hyperplasia of prostate; and nursemaid's elbow.

3. A patient calls complaining of pain and swelling in the right hand since awakening this morning. The patient comes in, sees the doctor, and returns to the front desk with an encounter form that states his diagnosis is "gout." In order to make this diagnosis, the physician would need to know the patient's uric acid level. You know that the patient just had blood drawn for the test. It is a test that must be sent to an outside lab. Do you still code today's visit as "gout"? What would you do?

Answers to Checkpoint Questions

1. Medical necessity means a particular service or procedure is reasonable.

2. The World Health Organization must approve any changes in the ICD-9-CM system.

3. Volumes 1 and 2 of the ICD-9-CM are used to report the diagnostic code that justifies physician services whether those services are provided in the office or in the hospital. Hospital coders use Volume 3 to report inpatient procedures, services, and supplies, as well as the reasons for the services.

4. ICD-9-CM is updated annually in October. You must start using the new book on January 1.

5. E-codes are used to provide information to (1) industry, (2) insurance underwriters, (3) national safety programs, and (4) public health agencies and others concerned with injuries and poisonings.

6. V-codes are used to report reasons for receiving services other than illness.

7. Before a definitive diagnosis is assigned to a patient, services must be coded with the patient's symptoms at the time he or she was seen.

8. Chart audits are conducted to assess compliance and to detect fraud.

Outpatient Procedural Coding

Outline

**Healthcare Common
Procedure Coding System**
**Physician's Current Procedural
Terminology (CPT)**
Performing Procedural Coding
The Layout of CPT-4
The Alphabetic Index
Reading Descriptors
Place of Service
Section Guidelines

Unlisted Procedures and Special
Reports
**Evaluation and Management
Codes**
Key Components
**Other Categories of Evaluation
and Management Codes**
Anesthesia Section
Surgery Section
Radiology Section

Pathology and Laboratory
Section
Medicine Section
CPT-4 Modifiers
Reimbursement
Diagnostic Related Groups
Resource-Based Relative Value
Scale
Fraud and Coding

Learning Objectives

*Upon successfully completing this chapter, you
will be able to:*

1. Spell and define the key terms

2. Explain the Healthcare Common Procedure
   Coding System (HCPCS), levels I and II

3. Explain the format of level I, Current
   Procedural Terminology (CPT-4) and its use

4. Explain what diagnostic related groups
   (DRGs) are and how they are used to determine Medicare payments

5. Discuss the goals of the resource-based relative value system (RBRVS)

6. Describe the relationship between coding
   and reimbursement

Performance Objectives

*Upon successfully completing this chapter, you
will be able to:*

1. Perform procedural coding (Procedure
   15-1)

Key Terms

Current Procedural
Terminology
descriptor
diagnostic related
group

Healthcare Common
Procedure Coding
System
key component

modifiers
outlier
procedure

resource-based rela-
tive value scale
upcoding

As discussed in Chapter 14, coding is a way to standardize medical information for purposes such as collecting health care statistics, performing a medical care review, and indexing medical records. It is also used for health insurance claims processing (see Chapter 13 for more information). Because coding is linked to reimbursement, you must code accurately and precisely. Incorrect, insufficient, or incomplete coding on claims forms can lead to improper reimbursement for the physician as well as recording and possibly passing along inaccurate patient information. Because learning to code is an ongoing process, continuing education is vital. This can be accomplished by attending workshops in your geographic area or by joining a local association of coders, which may also sponsor coding clinics. Two organizations are the American Academy of Professional Coders (AAPC) and the American Health Information Management Association (AHIMA). Other sources are local medical societies and your school.

Healthcare Common Procedure Coding System

The **Healthcare Common Procedure Coding System** (HCPCS) is divided into two principal subsystems, referred to as level I and level II. Level I of the HCPCS is comprised of Current Procedural Terminology (CPT), a numeric coding system maintained by the American Medical Association (AMA). Level II of the

BOX 15-1

HCPCS LEVEL II CODES

Because Medicare and other insurers cover a variety of services, supplies, and equipment that are not identified by CPT codes, the level II HCPCS codes were established for submitting claims for these items. The development and use of level II of the HCPCS began in the 1980s. Level II codes are also referred to as alpha-numeric codes because they consist of a single alphabetical letter followed by four numeric digits, whereas CPT codes are identified using five numeric digits. The HCPCS level II code listing comes out once a year in the National Coding Manual, which can be ordered from the American Hospital Association, American Medical Association, or other publishers of the CPT coding book. It includes the following sections:

- Chemotherapeutic drugs
- Dental services
- Durable medical equipment
- Injections
- Ophthalmology services
- Orthotics
- Some pathology and laboratory and rehabilitation supplies
- Vision care

HCPCS is a standardized coding system that is used primarily to identify products, supplies, and services not included in the CPT codes, such as ambulance services and durable medical equipment, prosthetics, orthotics, and supplies when used outside a physician's office. Box 15-1 describes level II codes. Level III codes, also referred to as local codes, were established when an insurer preferred that suppliers use a local code to identify a service, for which there was no level I or level II code. In the interest of standardizing code sets, The Health Insurance Portability and Accountability Act of 1996 (HIPAA) required the elimination of level III local codes, which took effect on December 31, 2003.

 CHECKPOINT QUESTION

1. What are level II codes? List their sections.

Physician's Current Procedural Terminology (CPT)

HCPCS level I codes, or the Physician's **Current Procedural Terminology (CPT)**, is a comprehensive listing of medical terms and codes for the uniform coding of procedures and services provided by physicians. The fourth edition, CPT-4, contains more than 7000 new codes. CPT-4 is updated annually, with the newest version available each October. Providers are required to use the updated codes by January of each year. The CPT-4 allows insurance companies to:

• Communicate easily with one another
• Compare reimbursable amounts for procedures
• Speed claims processing

Performing Procedural Coding

Every code means something unique and is used only to describe a specific **procedure**, service, or medical supply provided by physicians to their patients. This is true for inpatients and outpatients. Codes and descriptions are updated, revised, or changed yearly. If your physician's office uses an encounter form or preprinted routing slip that lists the procedures performed, you must update this form yearly and work with your software vendor to update your computer software. The CPT-4 code selected will be placed on the CMS-1500 universal claim form in Section 24, Box D, along with any modifiers used. Procedure 15-1 outlines the steps in performing procedural coding. Figure 15-1 is a sample universal claim form showing the proper placement of codes for consultation and chest radiography. The general layout and features of the CPT-4 book published by the American Medical Association are user-friendly. There are definitions, diagrams, simple explanations, examples, and instructions.

The Layout of CPT-4

CPT-4 is divided into six major sections: Evaluation and Management, Anesthesia, Surgery, Radiology, Pathology and Laboratory, and Medicine. These sections are followed by explanations and listings of the Category I and Category II codes, which are explained in Box 15-2.

Next are the appendices. The appendices most widely used in the outpatient arena are Appendices A through C. Appendix A is a listing of the modifiers available to help further explain a code. Appendix B is a summary of the additions, deletions, and revisions made since the last edition of the CPT-4. Appendix C includes clinical examples designed to assist providers in the selection of Evaluation and Management levels. Appendices D through I are seldom used in the medical office. You may refer to the CPT-4 code book to see their content.

The Alphabetic Index

The CPT alphabetic index is located in the back of the book and is organized by main terms like the ICD-9-CM book (Fig. 15-2). Unlike the ICD-9 index, you can locate codes by finding the procedure, the location, or the condition. For example, the code for removal of a colon polyp could be found under *removal*, *colon*, or *polyp*. When you find the service or procedure, you will see either one code or a range of codes. Cross-reference by finding this section in the tabular section to be sure you have the correct code.

Reading Descriptors

When reading a code's **descriptor**, or description, you will read up to the semicolon and then look down for any indentations using the same words before the semicolon. Refer to Figure 15-2, and locate the code for incision and drainage of an infected bursa. The proper code is 27604. It is indented under the code 27603. Read up to the semicolon in the code above. The descriptor for 27603 reads, "Incision and drainage, leg or ankle; deep abscess or hematoma." If the incision and drainage was done in an infected bursa of the leg or ankle, then the code is 27604. This descriptor is "Incision and drainage, leg or ankle; infected bursa." You would use 27603 for an incision and drainage of a leg or ankle for a deep abscess or a hematoma. Use of the indentation and the semicolon organizes the codes in a way that also saves space and keeps the CPT books

Figure 15-1 Sample CMS claim form for consultation and chest radiography.

from becoming too large. Although the manual coding process is still widely used, CPT software is available and is growing in popularity.

✔ **CHECKPOINT QUESTION**

2. What is the significance of the semicolon in a CPT descriptor?

Place of Service

The CPT-4 book begins with "Place of Service Codes for Professional Claims." Most payers require that place of service codes be placed on each line of Section 24, Column B of the CMS-1500 claim form. Since the CMS maintains these place of service codes, you should make sure that a certain payer recognizes the codes listed in CPT-4. For example, if a procedure is performed in the physician's office, the place of service

BOX 15-2

CPT-4 CATEGORIES

CPT-4 includes three categories of codes. Category I codes include all current US Food and Drug Administration–approved physicians' procedures and services. The AMA developed it in collaboration with various other health organizations.

Category I CPT codes describe a procedure or service identified with a five-digit CPT code and descriptor nomenclature. The inclusion of a descriptor and its associated specific five-digit identifying code number in this category of CPT codes is generally based upon the procedure being consistent with contemporary medical practice and being performed by many physicians in clinical practice in multiple locations.

Category II CPT codes are intended to facilitate data collection by coding certain services and/or test results that are agreed upon as contributing to positive health outcomes and quality patient care. This category of CPT codes is a set of optional tracking codes for performance measurement. These codes may be services that are typically included in an Evaluation and Management (E/M) service or other component part of a service and are not appropriate for Category I CPT codes. The use of tracking codes for performance measures will decrease the need for record abstraction and chart review, thus minimizing administrative burdens on physicians and survey costs for health plans.

Once approved by the Editorial Panel, the newly added Category III CPT codes will be made available on a semiannual (twice a year) basis via electronic distribution on the AMA/CPT website. The full set of Category III codes will be included in the next published edition for that CPT cycle.

Source: http://www.ama-assn.org/ama/pub/category/12886.html.

code recognized by Medicare and Medicaid is 11. The most commonly used place of service codes are found in Table 15-1.

Section Guidelines

Each section begins with its own specific guidelines and a listing of specific procedures and services applicable in that field. The guidelines contain definitions, explanatory notes, a listing of the previously unlisted procedures found in that particular section, directions on how to file a special report, modifiers for use in that particular section, and definitions to assist the coder.

Unlisted Procedures and Special Reports

CPT provides unlisted codes at the beginning of each section for use when an unusual, variable, or new procedure is done. When an unlisted code is used, however, you must submit a copy of the procedure report with the claim. Each section's guidelines list the information to be included in a special report. This information includes:

1. Definition or description of the nature, extent, and need for the procedure
2. Time, effort, and equipment necessary to provide the service
3. Complexity of symptoms
4. Final diagnosis
5. Pertinent physical findings
6. Diagnostic and therapeutic procedures
7. Concurrent problems
8. Follow-up care

Evaluation and Management Codes

Evaluation and Management (E/M) codes are five-digit numbers that begin with the number 9. These are the most frequently used codes. E/M codes describe various patient histories, examinations, and decisions physicians must make in evaluating and treating patients in various settings (e.g., office, outpatient, hospital). In essence, the E/M codes address what the physician does when interacting with the patient. For this reason, the physician's documentation must meet standards so the physician and coder (medical assistant) can decide which level or type of code to use for a specific patient–physician encounter.

Key Components

To code the services described in the E/M section, you must be sure that the patient's medical record indicates that certain **key components** are present. Two of three key components are required for established patients, and three of three are required for new patients. These components are the elements that make up the visit. All E/M codes contain the following components:

• History
• Physical examination
• Medical decision making
• Counseling

Leg (Tibia) and Fibula) and Ankle Joint

Incision

27600   Decompression fasciotomy, leg; anterior and/or lateral compartments only

27601   posterior compartment(s) only

27601   anterior and/or lateral, and posterior compartment(s)

     (For incision and drainage procedures, superficial, see 10040-10160)

     (For decompression fasciotomy with debridement, see 27892-27894)

27603   Incision and drainage, leg or ankle; deep abscess or hematoma

27604   infected bursa

27605   Tenotomy, percutaneous, Achilles tendon (separate procedure); local anesthesia

27606   general anesthesia

27607   Incision (eg, osteomyelitis or bone abscess), leg or ankle

27610   Arthrotomy, ankle, including exploration, drainage, or removal of foreign body
     CPT Assistant Nov 98:9

27612   Arthrotomy, posterior capsular release, ankle, with or without Achilles tendon lengthening
     CPT Assistant Nov 98:8

     (See also 27685)

Excision

27613   Biopsy, soft tissue of leg or ankle area; superficial

27614   deep (subfascial or intramuscular)
     CPT Assistant Nov 98:8

     (For needle biopsy of soft tissue, use 20206)

27615   Radical resection of tumor (eg, malignant neoplasm), soft tissue of leg or ankle area

27618   Excision, tumor, leg or ankle area; subcutaneous tissue

27619   deep (subfascial or intramuscular)

27620   Arthrotomy, ankle, with joint exploration, with or without biopsy, with or without removal of loose or foreign body

27625   Arthrotomy, with synovectomy, ankle;
     CPT Assistant Nov 98:8

27626   including tenosynovectomy

27630   Excision of lesion of tendon sheath or capsule (eg, cyst or ganglion), leg and/or ankle

27635   Excision or curettage of bone cyst or benign tumor; tibia or fibula;

27637   with autograft (includes obtaining graft)

27638   with allograft

27640   Partial excision (craterization, saucerization, or diaphysectomy) bone (eg, osteomyelitis or exostosis); tibia

27641   fibula

27645   Radical resection of tumor, bone; tibia

27646   fibula

27647   talus or calcaneus

Introduction or Removal

27648   Injection procedure for ankle arthrography

     (For radiological supervision and interpretation, use 73615. Do not report 76003 in addition to 73615)

     (For ankle arthroscopy, see 29894-29898)

Repair, Revision, and/or Reconstruction

27650   Repair, primary, open or percutaneous, ruptured Achilles tendon;

27652   with graft (includes obtaining graft)

27654   Repair, secondary, Achilles tendon, with or without graft

27656   Repair, fascial defect of leg

27658   Repair, flexor tendon, leg; primary, without graft, each tendon
     CPT Assistant Nov 98:8

27659   secondary, with or without graft, each tendon

27664   Repair, extensor tendon, leg; primary, without graft, each tendon
     CPT Assistant Nov 98:8

27665   secondary, with or without graft, each tendon
     CPT Assistant Nov 98:8

27675   Repair, dislocating peroneal tendons; without fibular osteotomy

27676   with fibular osteotomy

27680   Tenolysis, flexor or extensor tendon, leg and/or ankle; single, each tendon
     CPT Assistant Nov 98:8

27681   multiple tendons (through separate incision(s))
     CPT Assistant Nov 98:8

27685   Lengthening or shortening of tendon, leg or ankle; single tendon (separate procedure)
     CPT Assistant Nov 98:8

27686   multiple tendons (through same incision), each
     CPT Assistant Nov 98:8

= Revised code   = New code   = Contains new or revised text   = References: see p xv for details

Figure 15-2 Sample page of 2007 CPT book.

TABLE 15-1	Place of Service Codes Used in Physician Coding
Place of Service	**Code**
Physician's office	11
Patient's home	12
Assisted living facility	13
Urgent care facility	20
Inpatient hospital	21
Outpatient hospital	22
Emergency room–hospital	23
Ambulatory surgical center	24
Skilled nursing facility	31
Hospice	34

These two-digit codes are placed on each line of Section 24, Column B.
Source: Current Procedural Terminology, CPT 2006 Professional Edition; American Medical Association.

- Coordination of care
- Nature of presenting problem
- Time

History, physical examination, and medical decision making are three key components for a visit.

> Mr. Fowler was seen today for follow up of his bacterial pneumonia. He has finished his course of antibiotics and reports feeling much better. His sputum culture on the day of his discharge shows no growth. On exam, his chest is clear, there is no wheezing, and he is breathing well. I explained to the patient that his pneumonia was probably contracted when he was exposed to a co-worker with the same illness. He was reminded of the importance of frequent handwashing. He will return in 3 months.

Key: Red = history; green = physical exam; yellow = medical decision making

Charting example showing history, physical exam, and medical decision making.

History

The amount of history documented in a patient's record determines which of the four classifications or levels is assigned. The classifications of the type of history taken from the patient are:

- Problem focused
- Expanded problem focused
- Detailed
- Comprehensive

Table 15-2 lists the classifications and gives a general description and examples of each. The provider must select one of these based on the documentation in the patient's record. Note that the times listed in the table are not regulated; they are used only for describing a typical level.

Examination

The examination levels are the same as for the history taken. A review of systems is a systematic way to assess the body when doing a physical exam. The level of an examination depends on how many body systems were examined. CPT recognizes the following body systems: eyes; ears, nose, mouth, and throat; cardiovascular; respiratory; gastrointestinal; genitourinary; musculoskeletal; skin; neurologic; psychiatric; and hematologic/immunologic (laboratory tests). Analyze the following chart note to assign the proper level of exam.

> Patient presents with complaints of runny nose and sore throat x 3 days. Patient states the urinary tract infection we treated two weeks ago is better. On examination her eyes are red, nose is boggy, throat is red and swollen. Patient reports no more urinary problems since finishing the Bactrim DS. Urinalysis is clear.

Charting example showing examination level.

At this visit, the patient had an expanded problem-focused examination. The doctor examined her eyes, nose, and throat (her problem area) and also did a urinalysis to confirm that an earlier treatment took care of her previous urinary tract infection. Note that, even if the doctor examined the patient's skin, arm strength, etc., if it is not in the chart note, it cannot be considered in the selection of the level of her examination.

Medical Decision Making

The third key component, medical decision making, is defined in CPT-4 as:

- Straightforward
- Low complexity
- Moderate complexity or
- High complexity

Medical decision making refers to the kinds of things the physician must do to establish a diagnosis for the patient. A provider must consider and determine the number of diagnoses and/or management options avail-

TABLE **15-2**	**History and Physical Examinations**	

The physician or provider must select which history and physical examination code to use. You, however, should have a basic understanding of each category. It is important to note that there are separate codes for each category and separate codes for both new and established patients.

Type of History and Physical Examination	Patient Problems and Physician Time Required	Examples
Problem focused	Patient problems are self-limited and minor. Physician time: usually 10 minutes	9-month-old patient with diaper rash 40-year-old patient with sunburn 18-year-old patient with poison ivy 60-year-old patient with a routine blood pressure check
Expanded problem focused	Patient problems are mild to moderate. Physician time: 15–20 minutes	55-year-old patient with recurrent urinary tract infection 16-year-old patient with chronic asthma presenting with a cold 76-year-old patient with osteoarthritis 56-year-old patient with a stomach ulcer
Detailed	Patient problems are moderate to severe. Physician time: usually 30 minutes	18-year-old patient with first Pap smear and contraceptive education 67-year-old patient with the new onset of dysuria 18-month-old patient with delayed motor skill development 34-year-old patient with diabetes requiring insulin dose changes
Comprehensive	Patient problems are moderate to severe. Physician time: usually 45 minutes	36-year-old patient with infertility 8-year-old patient with new onset of diabetes 65-year-old patient with history of left-sided weakness and confusion

able, the amount and complexity of any data to be reviewed, and the risk of complications or other problems the patient has. To use a particular decision-making level, the physician must document the information to justify his level selection. For example, a doctor may write a chart note like this:

> *Mr. Jones presents today for follow up of his severe back pain. He is no better. I offered him several options, including physical therapy, anti-inflammatories, and surgery. I reviewed 35 pages of records from his surgery in Baltimore, MD, five years ago. He has cardiac problems that may make another surgery too risky.*

Charting example showing medical decision making.

This visit would qualify for a level of moderate complexity. The documentation states the number of management options and the amount of data reviewed and lists the patient's other problems.

Time

Time is not considered a key component unless more than half of the visit is spent counseling the patient. Time spent with a patient (e.g., counseling or coordinating care) is sometimes the key component in determining E/M codes. When time spent with the patient is more than 50% of the typical time for the visit, time becomes the deciding factor in choosing an E/M code. For example, if a physician spends an additional 15 minutes counseling a patient in what would normally be only a 10-minute expanded problem-focused history and physical examination, the counseling was more than 50% of the typical 25-minute face-to-face time. The appropriate E/M code is one with a 25-minute time frame (10 minutes and an extra 15 minutes for counseling).

CHECKPOINT QUESTION

3. List three things a physician must consider when assigning a level of medical decision making.

WHAT IF?

What if a patient's visit turns out to be mostly counseling?

A 42-year-old established patient with a family history of alcoholism sees her family doctor for an annual exam. She tells the doctor that she is doing fine, but her exam reveals some tenderness over her liver, and there is a faint odor of vodka on her breath. After a few minutes, the patient admits to the doctor that she is having marital problems and has been drinking excessively lately. The rest of the visit is spent explaining the dangers of drinking and the effects of alcohol on the liver. The doctor spends time giving her information about Alcoholics Anonymous and other resources. The chart notation reads: "Visit began at 9:15 AM Patient states she is doing well. On palpation of the liver, there is guarding and tenderness. There is a faint odor of ETOH. I spent 30 minutes of a 45-minute appointment counseling the patient and arranging a referral to Southside Drug and Alcohol Rehabilitation Center. Her husband was given several brochures, information about Al-Anon (an arm of Alcoholics Anonymous for family members of alcoholics), and hints about finding online resources. She left in the care of her husband who was instructed to take the patient to the rehab center now. Time 10:00 AM"

Time is the only factor when selecting the level for this office visit. Remember, the documentation must clearly state that more than half of the visit was spent counseling a patient face to face. According to CPT, the time counted can be with the patient and/or family members or caretaker. Using the times listed in the descriptors in CPT, locate the proper category (office visit for established patient), and find the level that describes the amount of time the physician spent with the patient. The chart states the entire visit was 45 minutes; therefore, the correct code would be 99215.

Other Categories of Evaluation and Management Codes

As a medical assistant, you will be responsible for billing for your provider-employer. Although many of these services are performed in the medical office, physicians also visit and care for patients in other places. You will assist the physician in assigning codes for these visits and procedures. Other categories in the E/M section include observation codes and hospital inpatient services including initial care and subsequent care. There is a section for consultations ordered by other physicians. (Box 15-3 outlines the difference between a consultation and a referral.)

Emergency department service codes are used only when the service is rendered in a 24-hour hospital-based facility that specializes in providing treatment of unscheduled events. Nursing homes, rest homes, and home visits are listed. Critical care, preventive medicine, and newborn care are other sections used by physicians for their direct care of patients. For a complete list of the subsections and categories, refer to the CPT code book.

CHECKPOINT QUESTION

4. To code for a service in the E/M section, what three key elements are considered?

Anesthesia Section

Anesthesia codes are five-digit codes that begin with 0. Anesthesia codes are divided by anatomic site and by specific type of procedure. For example, head, neck, and thorax are anatomic sites, and the codes in each section represent the specific procedure, such as plastic repair of cleft lip. Medical assistants in an anesthesiology practice code anesthesia procedures provided in the hospital setting, even though the office is an outpatient facility.

Two types of **modifiers** (letters or numbers added to a code to add detail to the code) are used in the anesthesia section. One type is the standard modifier that is found in all sections of CPT. The other type is the physical status modifier, a two-digit code beginning with the letter P and ending in a number from 1 to 6. These physical status modifiers indicate the patient's condition at the time of anesthesia and the corresponding complexity of services (e.g., P1 indicates a normal, healthy patient, and P5 indicates a patient who is not expected to survive without the procedure).

Surgery Section

The surgery section is organized by body systems. Surgery codes begin with numbers 1 through 6. The CPT-4 codes in this section include surgery packages.

BOX 15-3

IS IT A REFERRAL, A CONFIRMATORY CONSULTATION, OR JUST A CONSULTATION?

There are four subcategories of consultations: office, initial inpatient, follow-up inpatient, and confirmatory (in any setting). Each subcategory has specific reporting instructions.

When a physician asks another provider to offer an opinion or advice regarding evaluation and management of a specific problem, the second provider becomes a consultant for the patient. The initial encounter is coded as a consultation, and the documentation must support the encounter. A letter should accompany the patient seeing a consulting physician, and the advising physician should send a letter back to the patient's primary physician outlining the findings. If the consulting physician takes over part or all of the patient's care, follow-up or subsequent visits are coded as regular subsequent visits. A confirmatory consultation is considered a second opinion, and the physician should offer only an opinion or advice to the patient.

A confirmatory consultant does not take over the treatment of the patient. A referral is defined as passing on a patient to another physician. Referrals are coded as new patients, not consultations. Consider the following scenario. A 17-year-old girl sees her family physician for recurrent sore throats. When the family physician realizes that the girl probably needs a tonsillectomy, the patient is *referred* to an otorhinolaryngologist for evaluation and possible surgery. The patient has been referred to the surgeon, who will take over that part of her care. When she has recovered from the procedure, she is discharged from the care of the surgeon and returns to her family physician for continued care.

In another example, a patient may be seen by an orthopedic surgeon for arthritis. When it is determined that the patient's problem may be rheumatoid arthritis, he may be sent to a rheumatologist for consultation. The rheumatologist advises the orthopedic surgeon on a treatment plan, but the orthopedic surgeon continues to see the patient and carries out that plan. Written communications between the two physicians are kept in the chart. The significant difference between a consultation and a referral is whether or not the patient's treatment is transferred to another physician for that problem.

When an operation is performed, CPT requires that the doctor's fee includes the following: the surgical procedure; normal, uncomplicated follow-up care; and local infiltration, metacarpal, metatarsal, or digital block or topical anesthesia. General anesthesia must be given by an anesthesiologist.

You cannot bill separately for preoperative and postoperative visits unless you use a modifier to explain the circumstances. For example, a patient has a cholecystectomy (gallbladder removal). The fee charged for the surgery covers three office visits after the surgery. Between the first and second visit, the patient develops symptoms associated with appendicitis. The doctor can charge for this office visit because it is not related to the cholecystectomy. The surgery package does not apply.

The Centers for Medicare and Medicaid Services (CMS) has defined the surgical package for Medicare recipients somewhat differently. According to CPT-4, no complications or problems related to the surgery are included in the surgical package. If additional procedures are performed to correct or alleviate these problems, they should be coded separately. According to CMS, however, complications that do not require a revisit to the operating room are included in the price of surgery.

Third-party payers have different rules about what constitutes a surgery package, so the coder must check with the relevant third-party payers. Some insurance carriers have a set number of follow-up days that is consistent for all surgical services. Check with the carrier to learn what these are so you can bill for the additional office, outpatient, or hospital visits. The fees for fracture care and deliveries also include the care given before and after the service.

 CHECKPOINT QUESTION

5. What items are included in a surgical package?

Content of the Surgery Section

The subheadings in the surgery section are as follows: integumentary system, musculoskeletal system, respiratory system, cardiovascular system, hemic and lymphatic system, urinary system, digestive system, male genital system, intersex surgery, female genital system, maternity care and delivery, endocrine system, nervous system, eye and ocular adnexa, and auditory system. Each subheading contains subsections that organize the procedures by location and type. For example, in the musculoskeletal system section, the subcategories begin with the head and move down the body. The first heading is "Head." Under this heading are the following procedures that are done to the head: incision; excision; introduction or removal; repair, revision, and/or reconstruction; skull, facial, and nasal fractures and/or dislo-

TABLE 15-3	Medical Terminology Refresher		
Words that end in the following suffixes are related to surgical procedures.			
CPT Subcategory		**Suffix**	**Meaning**
Incision		-tomy	Incision into
Excision		-ectomy	Surgical removal
Repair, revision, or reconstruction		-pexy	Surgical fixation
		-plasty	Surgical repair
		-rrhaphy	Suture

cations, etc. The next heading is "Neck (Soft Tissues) and Thorax," which begins with incision, excision, and so on.

It is helpful to be familiar with the suffixes and definitions related to surgical procedures. Table 15-3 provides a refresher on these words and word parts.

Radiology Section

The radiology section of CPT-4 is divided into the following four subsections:

- Diagnostic radiology/diagnostic imaging
- Diagnostic ultrasound
- Radiation oncology
- Nuclear medicine

All radiology codes are five-digit numbers that begin with 7. They are generally arranged by anatomic site, from the top of the body to the bottom. Many radiology codes indicate the number of views for a particular study. Obviously, the facility must be reimbursed for film, developer, and the radiology technologist's time and service.

Some radiologic tests require the administration of a contrast medium that enhances the image. The descriptors for such tests specify "with contrast" or "without contrast." "With contrast" refers to contrast medium that is given intravascularly. If the contrast medium is given orally or rectally, you use the code "without contrast."

If a physician performs the procedure and supervises and interprets a procedure (e.g., injects contrast medium and then supervises and interprets), two codes should be used. A written report in the patient's medical record is necessary for billing these codes. The code for the procedure can be found in the surgery, medicine, or radiology section, and the code for supervision and interpretation is found in the radiology section. If two physicians are participating (e.g., a surgeon and radiologist), the radiology portion is billed by the radiologist.

Pathology and Laboratory Section

All codes in pathology and laboratory work are five-digit numbers that begin with 8. These codes are divided into sections for panels of tests, drug testing, consultations with pathologists, urinalysis, chemistry testing, antibody testing, cytopathology, and so on. The last part of the pathology and laboratory section includes services and procedures provided by a pathologist, including gross (can be seen by the naked eye) and microscopic examination of tissue removed in surgery. Each tissue specimen is submitted under a different identifying code for diagnosis by the pathologist. The codes represent the level of the physician's work. Postmortem examination or autopsy is performed by a pathologist, and CPT-4 provides codes to report such examinations.

A subsection, automated multichannel tests, deserves a special note. When coding, check that the tests performed are included in the lists under this subsection. For example, the physician may perform the following three tests for a patient: bilirubin, direct; cholesterol; and blood urea nitrogen (BUN). To code this, you assign the code 80003, three clinical chemistry tests, because all of these tests are listed under the automated multichannel test subsection. If the tests performed were bilirubin, direct; cholesterol; and blood acetaldehyde, however, you would code 80002, two clinical chemistry tests, and 82000, blood acetaldehyde. That is because blood acetaldehyde was not on the list of clinical chemistry tests in the automated multichannel test subsections.

Also of note are the terms *qualitative* and *quantitative* used in the drug screening section. Patients who are on certain medications, such as digoxin for the heart or Dilantin for seizures, have regular drug levels tested to be sure the amount of drug in the blood is at the proper therapeutic level. These tests are quantitative because the doctor is looking for the amount of drug in the blood. When testing for illegal drugs, however, the amount does not matter. The mere presence of the drug makes the test positive and provides the information wanted. This is qualitative information.

Medicine Section

Like the E/M codes, medicine codes are five-digit numbers that begin with 9. Like the other five sections of the CPT-4, this section includes guidelines for appropriate coding.

The first subsection in the medicine section is for immunization injections and includes codes from 90701 to 90749. Typically, immunization injections are given when the patient comes to the physician's office for either a routine physical examination or for a minor problem, such as a sore throat. When the injection is given at the time of such a visit, use two codes—one for the service (usually an E/M code) and one for the immunization injection. For example, an established patient may come into the physician's office for a brief examination for a minor problem (e.g., controlled hypertension blood pressure check). The patient may be examined briefly by a nurse or medical assistant while the physician is in the office and may also be given an immunization for poliomyelitis. The codes for this are:

1. 99211, office and other outpatient visit for the evaluation and management of an established patient, which may not require the presence of a physician. Usually, the presenting problems are minimal. Typically, 5 minutes are spent performing or supervising services. (This code is generally used for examination by employees of the practice while a physician is in the office but not performing the examination.)
2. 90713, poliomyelitis vaccine.

Next, CPT lists codes for therapeutic or diagnostic injections (codes 90782–90799). Consider the code 90782, therapeutic injection of medication (specify); subcutaneous or intramuscular. This code is the same for most injectable therapeutic substances. In order to be reimbursed for the medication itself, an additional, more specific code is necessary. Injection codes begin with a J and can be found in the HCPCS level II codes. Other injections in this section include infusions and chemotherapy. (See Box 15-1.) Using the most specific codes for injectable substances and supplies while keeping invoices to document actual cost helps verify charges submitted for these services.

The medicine section also includes codes used by psychiatrists and codes for biofeedback; dialysis; esophageal procedures; eye surgery and other ophthalmologic services; speech and hearing services including cochlear implants; cardiac diagnostic testing, such as electrocardiography and echocardiography; CPR; vascular studies like cardiac catheterization; allergy testing; electroencephalography; sleep studies; and other miscellaneous services and procedures.

 CHECKPOINT QUESTION

6. Why is it necessary to use two codes for an injection?

CPT-4 Modifiers

CPT-4 provides a way to give additional information about a procedure through the use of additional two-digit numbers called modifiers.

There are two ways to write modifiers. You can write the five-digit code with a hyphen followed by the two-digit modifier (e.g., 28702-22). Any modifier can be added to 999 and placed on a separate line on the CMS-1500. If multiple modifiers are used, write the five-digit code with the first modifier as -99 (multiple modifiers), followed by the additional modifiers (e.g., 28702-99922). Of course, the modifier can never appear on the claim form by itself because it refers to the procedure and must be directly below it on the claim form.

Box 15-4 provides a few examples of modifiers. The modifiers used for certain sections are listed in the section guidelines. A separate listing of available modifiers can be found in Appendix A of CPT-4. Check Appendix A first; then go to the guidelines of the appropriate section to verify that the modifier may be used with the specific CPT code. Failure to use an appropriate modifier causes database and reimbursement errors.

BOX 15-4

EXAMPLES OF CPT-4 MODIFIERS

Here are just a few examples of CPT-4 modifiers. A complete list can be found in Appendix A of CPT-4.

- *20 microsurgery or 99920:* This modifier signifies that the surgeon used an operating microscope to perform a procedure.
- *23 unusual anesthesia or 99923:* This modifier signifies that anesthesia was used in a procedure that normally would not require it.
- *26 professional component or 99926:* This modifier signifies that there are two components to the procedure, a professional one and a technical one; for example, a physician who does not perform a particular test, but interprets the test and dictates a report.

CHECKPOINT QUESTION

7. What are modifiers?

ETHICAL TIP

Be Diligent About Accuracy

Even if you pay attention to detail and strive for accuracy, there are times when mistakes are still made. In some cases, you will learn to code by trial and error. It is important, however, not to make the same error twice. Examine every explanation of benefits for problems. Develop a system to remember and track rejected claims. Do what it takes to correct any coding problems in order to get reimbursement. When a claim is pending, patients usually receive a letter from their insurance company telling them that they have asked for additional information from their doctor. Often, patients receive this letter before you receive the request for information. Be as prompt as possible in answering these requests. Patients will depend on you to assist them with their claims. It is your ethical responsibility to take care in getting the proper reimbursement.

Reimbursement

Diagnostic Related Groups

Diagnostic related groups (DRGs) are categories into which inpatients are placed according to the similarity of their diagnoses, treatment, and length of hospital stay. Initially, these categories were developed by researchers at Yale University in the mid 1970s to aid the process of utilization review. Some 13,000 codes were run through a computer and grouped according to their clinical similarities (including similarities in resources used). Today, DRGs are used to determine reimbursement for Medicare patients' inpatient services. The fee attached to each DRG is based on the national average of all Medicare charges and is adjusted for regional differences in hospital wages and updates. Hospitals are paid a set amount for each DRG regardless of actual costs for treating the patient. For example, if a hospital uses fewer resources to care for a patient and discharges that patient in less time, it may keep the difference between its actual cost and the DRG payment. Conversely, if the patient stays longer than usual and requires more services, the hospital absorbs the loss. A patient who has an unusually long stay or a complicated case is considered an **outlier**, and the hospital may be paid more than the standard DRG rate if the added expenses can be justified. The hospital coder uses ICD-9-CM codes to pick the appropriate DRG. The more information the hospital has prior to admission, the more accurate the coding; for example, for a patient admitted with chest pain, the hospital coder needs to know that the patient also has hypertension and diabetes.

You may be asked to schedule a patient for admission to the hospital. Assigning the correct ICD-9-CM code from the outpatient practice will influence the DRG to which the patient will be assigned. The hospital coder selects the proper DRG based on these factors:

- Principal diagnosis
- Surgeries
- Complications and comorbid conditions

Physicians can help with coding in the following ways:

- Record the appropriate documentation to identify each patient's problems, complaints, or other reasons for the encounter or visit.
- Work with the medical records or the office coding and billing staffs to determine the proper diagnosis to code, using terminology that includes specific diagnoses, symptoms, problems, or reasons for the encounter (ICD-9-CM codes describe all of these).

Resource-Based Relative Value Scale

As part of the 1989 Omnibus Budget Reconciliation Act (OBRA), the US Congress stipulated that reimbursement to physicians for Medicare services is based on a fee schedule. This fee schedule sets a maximal fee for each service based on the **resource-based relative value scale** (RBRVS). The goal of RBRVS is to reduce Medicare Part B costs and to establish national standards for payment based on CPT-4 codes. (Remember, Part B of Medicare covers physicians' services; Part A covers hospital expenses.)

Fee calculations are based on the following factors:

- Intensity of the service
- Time required
- Skills needed
- Overhead expenses
- Malpractice premiums

The particular fee is adjusted by a geographical practice cost index (GPCI), which reflects the difference in health care costs in different parts of the country. This determines the relative value unit (RVU). Finally, a national conversion factor is assigned yearly. The formula looks like this: CPT code 99205 has an RVU of 4.58, and the national conversion factor is 36.7856. The Medicare allowed charge would be $168.48. RVU x national conversion factor = Medicare allowed amount.

CHECKPOINT QUESTION

8. Why are DRGs used?

Fraud and Coding

Billing for services not performed, using another patient's coverage to receive reimbursement, and falsifying records are examples of blatant fraud. Millions of dollars have been budgeted to investigate fraud and abuse. The attorney general of the United States has jurisdiction over such cases, and in most states, the Office of the Inspector General investigates reports of possible fraud. In cases of suspected fraud, peer review organizations have been authorized by CMS to obtain medical records of Medicare beneficiaries for review.

Less severe and nondeliberate fraudulent practices also cause misuse of health care dollars, and CMS remains vigilant by conducting audits. Fiscal intermediaries (organizations under contract with the US government to handle Medicare claims) randomly review and compare the documentation in the record with the information and codes received and report their findings on the particular providers.

Even though the physician may already have been paid for a claim, the medical office may still be audited. As a federal program, Medicare has the same authority as the Internal Revenue Service to audit claims and may do so retroactively. This means that an audit can occur even a couple of years after payment has been received for

claims. If the medical practice is found to be in error, the physician may be required to repay an amount owed plus interest. Even worse, such errors can jeopardize the physician's ability to participate in Medicare-funded programs.

When submitting Medicare or other insurance claims, do not bill for services the physician has not performed, and do not bill more than the proper fee for a service (**upcoding**). Many citations have been handed down for upcoding.

LEGAL TIP

BE CAREFUL

To avoid costly errors, be certain that you can justify your coding:

- Keep adequate, accurate, and complete documentation in medical and billing records.
- Use the proper tools to code. Code books are updated yearly. Always use the most recent book.
- Follow the coding rules.
- Stay abreast of new rules, and keep up-to-date on any changes to existing ones. Medicare has regional updates, usually at no charge, and provides one of the best sources of information.
- Work closely with the provider, and never code anything about which you are not sure.

MEDIA MENU

- **Student CD**
  - **Case Studies**
    Administrative Interactive Case Study 2: Managing a Medical Office Emergency
    Administrative Interactive Case Study 4: Accounting and Billing in the Medical Office
  - **CMA/RMA Certification Exam Review**
- **Premium Online Course**
  http://thePoint.lww.com/Kronenberger3e

- **Internet Resources**

  LiveAdvise Online Tutoring & Competency Training
  http://thePoint.lww.com/LiveAdvise

  Medical Billing Association
  www.e-medbill.com

  American Health Information Management Association (AHIMA)
  www.ahima.org

  American Medical Association
  www.ama-assn.org

PROCEDURE 15-1: Locating a CPT Code

Purpose: To assign the most accurate code for services and procedures rendered by a physician or other provider in order to communicate with a third-party payer

Equipment: CPT-4 code book, patient chart

Steps	Purpose
1. Identify the exact procedure performed. *(muscle biopsy, deep)*	This will ensure accuracy.
2. Obtain the documentation of the procedure in the patient's chart.	The documentation must match the code assigned.
3. Choose the proper code book.	CPT level I and II codes are listed separately.
4. Using the alphabetic index, locate the procedure.	The alphabetic index is a quick reference.
5. Locate the code or range of codes given in the tabular section.	The index lists ranges of codes in many cases. You must select the correct code by cross-referencing to the codes themselves.
6. Read the descriptors to find the one that most closely describes the procedure.	Reading the descriptors carefully ensures accuracy.
7. Check the section guidelines for any special circumstances.	These guidelines are helpful in staying within the coding rules for each section.
8. Review the documentation to be sure it justifies the code.	In the event of a chart audit, the documentation must match the code.
9. Determine if any modifiers are needed.	If there are any unusual circumstances, the modifier will explain.
10. Select the code and place it in the appropriate field of the CMS-1500 form. *(accurate code is 20205)*	Accurate completion of the CMS-1500 form produces clean claims.

Chapter Summary

- Medical coding involves the use of numbers to describe diseases, injuries, and procedures.
- The purposes of coding include indexing medical records, performing medical care reviews, deriving health statistics, and reimbursing physicians and hospitals for services.
- As a medical assistant, you are responsible for knowing the format and usage of CPT-4, the system used to report services and procedures by the physician.
- Accurate and thorough coding is essential to ensure appropriate reimbursement.

- You must assist the physician in making sure the proper documentation is available to substantiate the codes used on a claim.
- As in all other aspects of patient contact and care, coding of patients' records is covered by the Health Insurance Portability and Accountability Act of 1996 (HIPAA). Only those with a need to know should have access to patient records.

1. How would you handle a physician who you think overbills for procedures? To whom would you report this? How might you collect documentation of fraud?

2. Using a CPT-4 code book, find as many different main terms as you can for "removal of ear wax" (69210). Remember, the medical term for ear wax is cerumen. HINT: When thinking of the ear, think auditory canal.

3. By attempting to locate the code for the procedure in the scenario that follows, make a list of any further information needed to select the correct code. A 12-year-old girl presents for headaches. She reports that when she has a headache, she cannot see well. The physician orders an electroencephalogram.

Answers to Checkpoint Questions

1. CPT level II codes are used for services, supplies, and equipment that are not identified by CPT level I. They cover chemotherapeutic drugs, dental services, durable medical equipment, injections, ophthalmology services, orthotics, some pathology and laboratory and rehabilitation supplies, and vision care.

2. When reading a descriptor, you will read up to the semicolon and then look down for any indentations using the same words before the semicolon.

3. The elements that determine the level of medical decision making in Evaluation and Management coding are (1) the number of management options available, (2) the amount and complexity of the data to be reviewed, and (3) the risk of complications or other problems.

4. The three key elements are history, physical examination, and medical decision making.

5. The surgical package consists of local infiltration; metacarpal, metatarsal, or digital blocks; topical anesthesia; the operation; and normal uncomplicated follow-up care.

6. Two codes are needed for injections because one covers the administration of the drug and the other covers the medication itself.

7. Modifiers are two-digit numbers that give the payer additional information about a procedure or service.

8. DRGs are used to determine the reimbursement for Medicare patients' inpatient services.

UNIT THREE

Power Critical Thinking Exercises

MANAGING THE FINANCES IN THE PRACTICE (CHAPTERS 11–15)

1. William Moyer calls the office after receiving his Medicare Explanation of Benefits from his last office visit. The charge was $120.00, but Medicare only allowed $82.00. Mr. Moyer is upset and wants to know why his doctor "overcharged him."

   A. What government entity oversees medical finances in this country? (knowledge)

   B. What is meant by "accepting assignment"? (comprehension)

   C. How is the difference in the amount charged and the amount allowed handled on a daysheet? (application)

   D. Why would accounting practices require you to handle the difference in this way? (analysis)

   E. What would be a possible result of a health care system with no government regulation? (synthesis)

F. What would a health care system without government regulation be like? (evaluation)

2. Tom Barksdale has been seen by the physician for controlled non–insulin-dependent type 2 diabetes mellitus for about 10 years. While being seen for a routine check of his blood sugar, he tells you that he has been having numbness and tingling in his left lower leg and foot. Since poor circulation in the extremities can be a complication of diabetes, the doctor orders a Doppler ultrasound study of both lower legs. The ultrasound confirms the diagnosis of peripheral neuropathy.

   A. What is the patient's reason for his visit? (knowledge)

   B. Why was the Doppler study ordered? (comprehension)

   C. What is the appropriate ICD-9 code for the office visit? (application)

   D. Which code should be placed on the CMA-1500 first as the primary diagnosis or reason for the visit? (analysis)

   E. Which ICD-9 code should be referenced to the office visit charge? (synthesis)

F. Why is it important to use the most accurate code? (evaluation)

3. A patient calls complaining of pain and swelling in the right hand since awakening this morning. The patient comes in, sees the doctor, and returns to the front desk with an encounter form that states his diagnosis is "gout." In order to make this diagnosis, the physician would need to know the patient's uric acid level. You know that the patient just had blood drawn for the test. It is a test that must be sent to an outside lab.

   A. What is the reason for the visit? (knowledge)

   B. What is the main term in the patient's complaint? (comprehension)

   C. What is the appropriate code for the patient's chief complaint? (application)

   D. Do you code today's visit as "gout"? Why or why not? (analysis)

   E. On the patient's next visit, will you be able to code the claim differently? Why or why not? (synthesis)

   F. Identify a possible consequence of mishandling this situation. (evaluation)

PART

III

The Clinical Medical Assistant

UNIT FOUR

Fundamentals of Clinical Medical Assisting

CHAPTER 16

Nutrition and Wellness

Outline

Essentials Of Nutrition
 Nutrients
 Cholesterol
 Fiber
Digestion
Metabolism
Nutritional Guidelines
 MyPyramid
 Understanding Food Labels
Therapeutic Nutrition

Physical Fitness
 Components of Physical
 Fitness
Weight Management
 Physiologic Issues
 Body Mass Index
 Sociologic and Psychological
 Issues
Staying Well
 Stress

Pollution
Seat Belt Use and Airbags
Dental Health
Positive Mental Outlook
Genetics
Infectious Disease Prevention
Substance Abuse
 Alcohol
 Drugs
 Smoking Cessation

Learning Objectives

Upon successfully completing this chapter, you will be able to:

1. Spell and define the key terms

2. Name all of the essential nutrients

3. Describe the body's digestion and metabolism of these nutrients

4. Discuss the body's basal metabolic rate and its importance in weight

5. Understand how to use the food guide pyramid, MyPyramid

6. Read and explain the information on food labels

7. Describe special therapeutic diets and the patients who need them

8. Describe the components of physical fitness

9. Discuss weight management and the elements involved in changing weight

10. List suggestions for a healthy lifestyle

11. Explain the importance of disease prevention

12. Recognize the dangers of substance abuse

13. List and describe the effects of the substances most commonly abused

Upon successfully completing this chapter, you will be able to:

1. Teach a patient how to read food labels (Procedure 16-1)

CAAHEP

• Provide instruction for health maintenance and disease prevention

• Instruct individuals according to their needs

ABHES

• Instruct patients with special needs

• Teach patients methods of health promotion and disease prevention

anabolism
basal metabolic rate
body mass index
calories

catabolize
dental cavities
endorphins
essential amino acids

euphoria
guided imagery
homeostasis

metabolism
minerals
predisposed

The human body requires certain things to maintain its efficiency. Regular exercise and eating properly offer important benefits. For example, with proper nutrition and sufficient amounts of physical activity, children have an increased likelihood of developing at a normal rate. People of all ages can improve their health and well-being by adhering to healthy diet and exercise guidelines. When the general public is in good health, there is a lesser risk for the development of chronic diseases.

Psychological wellness is also crucial to a balanced, healthy life. Avoiding harmful substances and unhealthy practices is as important as doing all the right things. As a medical assistant, you will be a role model for your patients. You will have opportunities to teach patients the essentials of good health, and, in the process, you will learn how to stay healthy, happy, and productive.

Essentials of Nutrition

Making healthy food choices gives you the best chance at being well and maintaining **homeostasis** in the body. When the body is working efficiently and in balance, it is considered to be homeostatic.

Nutrients

Nutrients are essential elements found in the food we eat. These essential nutrients include vitamins, minerals, carbohydrates, proteins, fiber, and certain fats. Micronutrients are elements that are needed in trace amounts.

Carbohydrates

Carbohydrates are chemical substances that provide the body with energy. Carbohydrates are found in foods made from grain products, fruits, vegetables, legumes, and sugars. They are made up of carbon, hydrogen, and oxygen atoms. Complex carbohydrates are starches that are found in grains, legumes, and potatoes. These types of carbohydrates have the most nutrients. Simple carbohydrates are unrefined sugars found in fruits and plants. Refined sugars have a high caloric value but no nutritious value and should be kept to a minimum.

Proteins

Proteins contain amino acids, provide energy, help to build and repair tissue, and assist with antibody production. There are approximately 80 amino acids found in nature, but the human body only needs 20 of them. The body produces 11 of these on its own; the other nine are known as **essential amino acids** and come from your diet. Some animal proteins provide all the necessary amino acids and are called complete proteins. Milk, cheese, eggs, and meat all provide complete proteins. Other proteins do not contain all of the nine essential amino acids. For this reason, they are called incomplete proteins. Plants, such as beans, legumes, nuts, and seeds, are natural sources of incomplete proteins. A combination of both types of proteins will ensure a proper amount of protein in the diet.

Fats

Fats, also known as lipids, serve as a concentrated source of heat production and energy, and they provide essential fatty acids. Many tissues, including heart and skeletal muscle, derive energy from fatty acids. Fats are composed of carbon, hydrogen, and oxygen but in different proportions than those found in carbohydrates. Food must supply essential fatty acids that are necessary for nutritional well-being. If the body has inadequate supplies of glucose to break down for energy, it will **catabolize**, or break down, fats. Fats have important functions within the body. They cushion and protect body organs, sustain normal body temperature, and help cells function properly. While food labels list information about fats, these labels can be confusing. Table 16-1 lists the types, characteristics, and sources of fats.

Vitamins

Vitamins are organic substances that enhance the breakdown of proteins, carbohydrates, and fats. Some vitamins are used in the formation of blood cells and hormones as well as in the production of neurochemical substances necessary for life. Vitamins are categorized as either fat soluble or water soluble.

Vitamins A, D, E, and K are all examples of fat-soluble vitamins. These vitamins are usually absorbed with foods that contain fat and are stored in the liver, kidneys, and body fat. Bile, which is formed in the liver, breaks down fat-soluble vitamins. Too much of these vitamins should be avoided because the body stores these vitamins, and an excess can result in serious illness.

TABLE 16-1	The Good and Bad Fats	
Type of Fat	**What Does It Do?**	**Where Is It Found?**
Monounsaturated (MUFA) fat	Does not raise "bad" cholesterol levels	Olive oil and canola oil
Omega-3 fatty acid	May protect against heart disease	Salmon, albacore tuna, mackerel, sardines, herring, and trout
Polyunsaturated (PUFA) fat	Contains some essential fatty acids; does not raise "bad" cholesterol levels	Natural oils found in certain fish and nuts; vegetable oils such as corn oil, soybean oil, and sunflower oil
Saturated fat	Raises "bad" cholesterol levels, increases risk of heart disease	Meat, poultry, dairy products, processed and fast foods
Trans fat or hydrogenated fat[a]	Raises "bad" cholesterol levels, increases risk of heart disease	Cookies, cakes, margarine, crackers, and some fried foods
Triglycerides	Excess amounts increase risk of heart disease when coupled with other risk factors	Main form of fat in foods, produced by the body and stored as fat from excess calories

[a] Trans fats are created by adding hydrogen to vegetable oil. This process, called hydrogenation, increases the shelf life of certain products. Hydrogenation turns liquid vegetable oils into solid fats.

Sources: http://www.mypyramid.gov, http://www.fda.gov/fdac/features/2003/503_fats.html, and http://www.americanheart.org/presenter .jhtml?identifier=4778.

Vitamin C and the B-complex vitamins thiamin (B1), riboflavin (B2), niacin (B3), and folic acid are examples of water-soluble vitamins. The body does not store these vitamins; an excess amount is excreted. Water-soluble vitamins should be consumed daily.

PATIENT EDUCATION
WOMEN AND FOLIC ACID

Folate, one of the B vitamins, has been found to reduce the risk of neural tube defects in developing fetuses. These types of defects, like spina bifida and anencephaly, affect the fetus' brain and spine during early pregnancy. Neural tube defects can cause paralysis and, in extreme cases, death. In 1998, the March of Dimes, in its dedication to wiping out birth defects, began a national campaign to get the word about folate out to women of childbearing age who may become pregnant. The March of Dimes joined forces with other agencies to provide education, training, and vitamin distribution to women across the nation. Since that time, women have become more aware of the importance of folic acid, and physicians provide more information and assistance to patients.

A daily intake of 400 µg/day of synthetic folate or folic acid from fortified foods or supplements is recommended for women of childbearing age who may become pregnant. Women are encouraged to eat foods naturally rich in folate including liver, avocado, orange juice, boiled asparagus, cooked spinach, and green leafy vegetables. Vegetables should be eaten raw or lightly steamed as cooking may destroy the vitamins. Many breakfast cereals and breads are fortified with folic acid. Women of childbearing age are also encouraged to read labels to see if the amount of folic acid in products meets their daily requirement. The March of Dimes campaign has played a significant role in the incidence of neural tube defects decreasing by 19% over the past 5 years.

Other recommendations for women in this group include eating foods that are high in iron, as well as eating vitamin C-rich foods that enhance the absorption of the iron. Pregnant women should limit their mercury intake by having no more than one can of tuna per week. The March of Dimes has been instrumental in providing research funds and educating the public about birth defects, and it has been through their work that the recommendations have been established. This organization is meeting their ethical responsibility to the babies they work so hard to protect.

CHECKPOINT QUESTION

1. Why is it important to follow the recommended dosage of a fat-soluble vitamin?

Minerals

Minerals are inorganic substances used in the formation of hard and soft body tissue. Minerals are necessary for muscle contraction, nerve conduction, and blood clotting. You get minerals from the foods you eat. The body uses minerals in differing amounts. The minerals sodium, potassium, calcium, phosphorus, magnesium, iron, and iodine are considered major minerals. You also need trace amounts of fluorine, zinc, copper, cobalt, and chromium. These are referred to as the trace minerals.

Cholesterol

Foods such as meat, poultry, seafood, eggs, and dairy products are considered animal products. Cholesterol is found only in animal products; vegetables and vegetable products do not contain cholesterol. Egg yolks and organ meats, such as liver, are particularly high in cholesterol.

The body needs cholesterol to function properly; however, it already manufactures sufficient amounts of cholesterol. A high-cholesterol diet can raise blood cholesterol to unhealthy levels. According to the National Cholesterol Education Program (NCEP), it is recommended that adults consume fewer than 300 mg of dietary cholesterol each day.

Lipoproteins

Lipoproteins are substances composed of lipids and proteins that transport cholesterol between the liver and arterial walls. Food sources do not contain lipoproteins; they are found only in the body. The amounts and types of lipoproteins found in the blood are a good indicator of the risk of heart disease. There are two types of lipoproteins: low-density lipoprotein and high-density lipoprotein.

Low-density lipoprotein (LDL) transports cholesterol from the liver to the walls of large- and medium-sized arteries. Excess LDL in the blood can cause plaques to form, which reduce the flow of blood within the affected artery. Circulation becomes impaired, and as LDL levels rise above the normal range, the risk of heart disease increases. Due to these risks, LDL is occasionally labeled "bad" cholesterol. Factors that contribute to an unhealthy increase in LDL levels include excess body fat and a diet high in saturated fat. An LDL level above 160 mg/dL indicates an increased risk for heart disease.

High-density lipoprotein (HDL) is responsible for carrying cholesterol away from arterial walls back to the liver, which then removes cholesterol from the body. High levels of HDL have been linked to a reduction in the risk of heart disease. For this reason, HDL is sometimes called "good" cholesterol. Regular exercise helps increase HDL levels. An HDL level above 35 mg/dL indicates a lower risk for heart disease.

 CHECKPOINT QUESTION

2. What are complete proteins, and where are they found?

Fiber

Fiber is needed in the diet to help the body with elimination of waste. All vegetables, raw and cooked fruits, and whole-grain foods, including breads, grains, and cereals, contain fiber. Patients with chronic colitis, ileitis, or diverticulitis may be instructed to follow a low-fiber diet, which includes avoiding fresh fruits and vegetables and consuming only broiled, boiled, or baked meats, fish, and poultry; pastas; dairy products; well-cooked vegetables; fruit and vegetable juices; and canned fruit. A high-fiber diet may be recommended for patients with constipation or to regulate bowel movements. These patients would be told to avoid fatty foods and eat lots of whole grains. There are many brands of fiber supplements that can be added to a liquid for daily regularity.

After discussing healthy foods, give patients information about healthy food preparation (Box 16-1).

BOX 16-1

HEALTHY FOOD PREPARATION TIPS

Here are a few guidelines on how to prepare healthy foods that you can teach your patients:

- Broil, boil, bake, roast, or grill meat, poultry, and fish.
- Trim the fat from beef.
- Use a cooking rack so that fat drips away from the meat.
- Remove the skin from chicken. Use caution with raw chicken. Wash hands and cutting surfaces immediately.
- Cook homemade soups or gravies and then chill them. Skim the fat off and then reheat.
- Use unsaturated oils (canola, corn, safflower). Use nonstick spray when possible. Avoid saturated oils (butter, lard).

Digestion

Digestion consists of both the physical and chemical breakdown of complex food into simpler substances that the body can use. When you swallow, food travels down the esophagus and into the stomach. Your saliva contains enzymes that start to break the food down in the mouth as you chew. As the food passes through the digestive tract, enzymes continue to break down food. When the food is small enough, the small intestines absorb the nutrients into the bloodstream, where they are taken to the liver to be further broken down and filtered. The nutrients then make their way to every cell in the body. Any nutrients not needed are eliminated from the body.

Metabolism

There are two phases in the process of **metabolism,** or the change that food undergoes after it is absorbed into the bloodstream. **Anabolism** is considered the constructive phase because smaller molecules are converted to larger molecules. For example, amino acids are converted to proteins. Catabolism is the destructive phase of metabolism in which larger molecules are converted into smaller molecules. For example, glycogen is converted to pyruvic acid. This process releases energy and is measured in **calories.** This energy is needed for cell growth and heat production. The speed of this process is particular to each individual, which is why some people seem to be able to eat more and maintain a healthy weight, while others consume the same amount of food and gain weight.

Nutritional Guidelines

The United States Department of Health and Human Services (DHHS), the United States Department of Agriculture (USDA), the National Academy of Sciences, and the Food and Nutrition Board are all involved in establishing the guidelines recommended for a healthy diet.

MyPyramid

The USDA has developed a food guidance system, MyPyramid, to help people maintain healthy diets and sufficient exercise levels (Fig. 16-1). This system, developed in 2005, is based on the *Dietary Guidelines for Americans, 2005*, published by the DHHS and the USDA. MyPyramid includes five basic food groups, as well as one additional category, oils. The five main food groups are:

1. Grains
2. Vegetables
3. Fruits

Anatomy of MyPyramid

One size doesn't fit all

USDA's new MyPyramid symbolizes a personalized approach to healthy eating and physical activity. The symbol has been designed to be simple. It has been developed to remind consumers to make healthy food choices and to be active every day. The different parts of the symbol are described below.

Activity

Activity is represented by the steps and the person climbing them, as a reminder of the importance of daily physical activity.

Moderation

Moderation is represented by the narrowing of each food group from bottom to top. The wider base stands for foods with little or no solid fats or added sugars. These should be selected more often. The narrower top area stands for foods containing more added sugars and solid fats. The more active you are, the more of these foods can fit into your diet.

Personalization

Personalization is shown by the person on the steps, the slogan, and the URL. Find the kinds and amounts of food to eat each day at MyPyramid.gov.

Proportionality

Proportionality is shown by the different widths of the food group bands. The widths suggest how much food a person should choose from each group. The widths are just a general guide, not exact proportions. Check the Web site for how much is right for you.

Variety

Variety is symbolized by the 6 color bands representing the 5 food groups of the Pyramid and oils. This illustrates that foods from all groups are needed each day for good health.

Gradual Improvement

Gradual improvement is encouraged by the slogan. It suggests that individuals can benefit from taking small steps to improve their diet and lifestyle each day.

MyPyramid.gov
STEPS TO A HEALTHIER YOU

USDA
U.S. Department of Agriculture
Center for Nutrition Policy
and Promotion
April 2005 CNPP-16

USDA is an equal opportunity provider and employer.

GRAINS   VEGETABLES   FRUITS   OILS   MILK   MEAT & BEANS

Figure 16-1 Anatomy of MyPyramid. (Source: http://www.mypyramid.gov/downloads/MyPyramid_Anatomy.pdf)

4. Milk
5. Meat and beans

A person's age, gender, and level of physical activity are all considered in determining the appropriate number of daily servings from each food group. MyPyramid is designed for individuals over 2 years of age in the general public. Those suffering from chronic health conditions should discuss their diet with a qualified health care provider who will be able to develop an eating plan to suit their specific nutritional needs.

Figure 16-2 is a sample food pyramid based on a 2000-calorie diet. The USDA has also developed educational materials for children ages 6 to 11. There is a pyramid designed specifically for children (Fig. 16-3), which is based on a diet of 1800 calories. This pyramid is visually appealing to children and provides parents with examples of the recommended number of daily servings for each food group. When you are teaching nutritional guidelines, provide the patient with a copy of his or her personalized MyPyramid plan. The USDA's website (www.mypyramid.gov) allows users to create

their own personalized food pyramids by entering their age, gender, and level of daily physical activity. Additional resources and materials for children can be found on the website as well. By following these dietary guidelines, you and your patients will have the best chance of fighting disease and staying healthy.

Grains

This food group includes grain products such as bread, cereal, oatmeal, crackers, rice, and pasta. The USDA recommends choosing whole grains (as opposed to refined grains) for at least half of your daily servings. Whole grains are made with the entire grain kernel and contain nutrients such as fiber, certain vitamins, carbohydrates, proteins, and antioxidants. Refined grains, on the other hand, only include part of the grain kernel. These types of grains lack fiber, iron, and some vitamins. Here are some tips to follow when selecting foods from this group:

• Look at the product's ingredient list. Foods with ingredients such as "whole wheat," "bulgur," "whole-

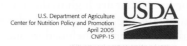

Figure 16-2 MyPyramid guide based on a 2000-calorie diet. (Source: http://www.mypyramid.gov/downloads/MiniPoster.pdf)

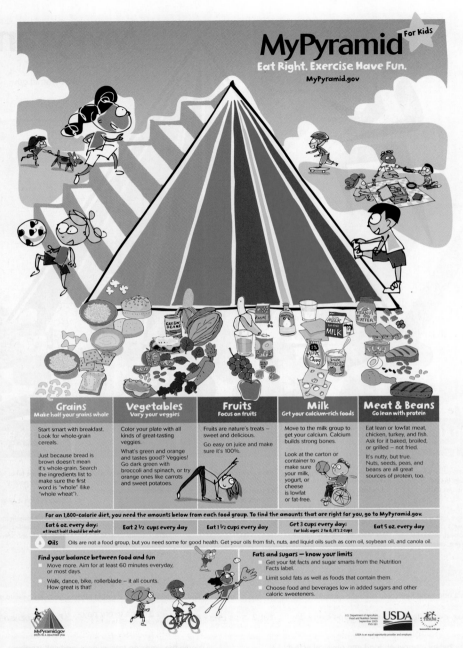

Figure 16-3 MyPyramid guide for children based on a diet of 1800 calories. (Source: http://teamnutrition.usda.gov/Resources/mpk_poster2.pdf)

grain corn," "oatmeal," "whole oats," or "wild rice" at the beginning of the list indicate whole grains.

• Look for foods that are high in dietary fiber. Nutrition labels indicate the percentage of the recommended daily value (DV) that is included in one serving.

• Substitute brown rice or whole-wheat pasta for white rice or pasta made from refined grains. Likewise, substitute whole-wheat bread for white bread.

• When making pancakes or muffins, use recipes that call for whole wheat or oat flour. Use whole-grain flour or oatmeal when baking cakes and cookies.

• Choose whole-grain snacks, such as baked tortilla chips or air-popped popcorn (without added salt or butter), instead of potato chips.

• Eat whole-grain cereals, such as muesli or toasted oat cereal.

Vegetables

The vegetables group is subdivided into five categories: dark green vegetables, orange vegetables, dry beans and peas, starchy vegetables, and other vegetables. The key to choosing foods within this group is to select a variety of vegetables from different categories. Other tips include:

- Eat fresh seasonal vegetables. Fresh vegetables have more flavor and generally cost less than processed vegetables (e.g., canned or frozen vegetables). Processed vegetables may also contain sauces or seasonings that add sodium and fat.
- When buying canned vegetables, look for foods without added salt. Choose vegetables labeled "no salt added," or check the sodium content on the nutrition label.
- Choose foods with high levels of potassium, such as sweet potatoes, tomato paste, beet greens, white potatoes, white beans, soybeans, lima beans, and spinach.
- Eat a green salad with lunch or dinner each day. Add only a small amount of salad dressing.
- Prepare vegetable main dish meals, such as soups, stews, and stir-fries. Include potatoes in soups and stews for added texture and nutrients.

Fruits

The fruits food group includes 100% fruit juice as well as fresh, frozen, dried, and canned fruit. Here are some tips for selecting foods from this group:

- Get most of your daily servings from whole fruit instead of juice. Whole or cut-up fruit contains dietary fiber, while most juices do not.
- When buying packaged fruit, look for items that do not contain added sugar. For example, select canned fruit stored in 100% juice or water instead of syrup.
- Eat a wide variety of fruits to obtain the greatest nutritional benefit. Prune juice, bananas, and dried apricots supply potassium. Pears, raspberries, and blackberries provide dietary fiber. Guava, kiwi, and oranges are good sources of vitamin C.
- Add fresh berries, peaches, or bananas to your cereal at breakfast and drink a glass of 100% orange or grapefruit juice.
- Snack on cut-up or dried fruit. Cut-up fruit is often sold in convenient single-serving packages, and dried fruit can be stored in a bag or desk drawer. One-fourth cup of dried fruit is equal to one-half cup of other fruit.
- When baking cakes, substitute applesauce for some of the oil in the recipe.

Milk

Also referred to as the "milk, yogurt, and cheese group," this food group includes all milk and milk products that retain their calcium content. Found in this food group are liquid milk (including lactose-free milk), milk-based desserts (such as pudding and ice cream), hard and soft cheeses, and yogurt. Not included in this group are milk products such as butter and cream cheese, which do not provide calcium. In choosing foods from this group, it's important to select low-fat or nonfat items. Other tips are:

- Drink a glass of low-fat or fat-free milk with meals.
- Have pudding made from low-fat or fat-free milk for dessert.
- When making hot cereals or oatmeal, use low-fat or fat-free milk instead of water. Also substitute milk for water when preparing condensed cream soups.
- Snack on low-fat or fat-free yogurt topped with fresh fruit.
- Add low-fat cheese to soups, stews, and casseroles. Top vegetables with melted low-fat cheese, or add low-fat or fat-free yogurt to baked potatoes.
- For those who are lactose intolerant, choose lactose-free or lower lactose milk products. Although soy milk, orange juice, and other products may be calcium fortified, these foods do not provide all the essential nutrients supplied by foods within the milk group.

Meat and Beans

The meat and beans group includes all foods made from meat, poultry, eggs, dry beans, peas, nuts, and seeds. The high fat and cholesterol content of some foods in this group (such as beef or egg yolks) makes varying your food choices important. It is also crucial to select a variety of foods to obtain the greatest nutritional benefit. For example, sunflower seeds and almonds are high in vitamin E; salmon and trout contain omega-3 fatty acids; clams and oysters provide iron; beef, lamb, pork, poultry, fish, shellfish, and eggs are good sources of protein.

Here are some guidelines to use when choosing foods from the meat and beans group:

- For vegetarians, alternate protein sources include eggs, beans, nuts, peas, and foods made from soybeans, such as tofu.
- Select lean cuts of beef (round steaks, roasts, top loin, top sirloin) and pork (pork loin, tenderloin, ham). When buying ground beef, look for packages labeled "90% lean," "93% lean," or "95% lean."
- Choose boneless skinless chicken breasts and turkey cutlets, or remove the skin from poultry before cooking.
- Prepare meat, poultry, and fish without adding fat. First, trim off any visible fat and then broil, grill, roast, or boil foods, being careful to drain off excess fat during cooking. Add little or no breading, and avoid using gravies or sauces that are high in fat.
- Prepare meatless main dishes containing dry beans or peas. For example, use kidney or pinto beans to make chili, cook split pea soup or minestrone, add chick-

peas or garbanzo beans to a salad, or prepare tofu or veggie burgers.

- Eat fish more often than you eat meat or poultry. Salmon, trout, and herring are excellent sources of omega-3 fatty acids.
- Substitute nuts in dishes containing meat or poultry. Add pine nuts instead of chicken to pesto sauce, substitute peanuts or cashews for meat in vegetable stir-fries, and add walnuts, almonds, or pecans to green salads instead of meat or chicken.

Oils

One additional category appearing in the food pyramid is oils. Included in this category are fats that are in liquid form at room temperature, such as vegetable oils, and oils that come from other natural plant and fish sources. Fats that are solid at room temperature, such as butter, shortening, and beef or chicken fat, are not considered oils. The recommended daily servings for this category are relatively small (usually several teaspoons, depending on a person's age, gender, and level of physical activity). Therefore, the most important guideline to use when choosing foods in this category is to avoid exceeding recommended amounts. Most people consume enough oils in the foods they eat (e.g., olives, avocadoes, nuts, fish, cooking oils, and salad dressing).

 WHAT IF?

You are assisting your physician-employer in the exam room one afternoon when the two of you see a patient who has gained 30 pounds in a year. She appears depressed and complains of leg pain and increased difficulty getting around. The physician explains that she needs to make some changes and asks you to assist the patient in getting started. Where should you begin?

You should refer to the *Dietary Guidelines for Americans, 2005* from the USDA and the DHHS. Provide the patient with the "Key Recommendations" listing, and go over each item, giving examples and answering any questions.

- *Monitor calories and nutrients.* Eat foods with more nutrients per calorie, and limit saturated and trans fats, added sugars, cholesterol, sodium, and alcohol.
- *Manage your weight.* To prevent weight gain, slightly decrease calories consumed and increase daily physical activity. To maintain a healthy weight, find a balance between the number of calories consumed each day and an appropriate amount of exercise.
- *Exercise regularly.* To prevent unhealthy weight gain, exercise for 60 minutes (moderate to vigorous activity) most days of the week. Include cardiovascular training, flexibility exercises, and weight training to receive the full benefits of physical fitness.
- *Make healthy food choices.* Eat a variety of fruits and vegetables every day, being sure to consume the recommended amount of servings based on energy needs. When selecting foods from the grains food group, choose whole-grain products. Be sure to include the recommended daily servings of milk or milk products in your diet as well.
- *Limit fats.* Try to consume no more than 20% to 35% of calories from fat each day. Most fats in your diet should come from natural sources, such as nuts, vegetable oils, and fish. Limit other fats by selecting foods that are designated as low-fat, nonfat, or lean, and avoid trans fats.
- *Choose healthy sources of carbohydrates.* Select carbohydrate sources that are also high in fiber, such as fruits, vegetables, and whole-grain products. Avoid foods and beverages that contain added sugars or sweeteners.
- *Monitor sodium and potassium intake.* Limit sodium to less than 2300 mg per day. Select foods that are high in potassium, such as fruits and vegetables.
- *Limit alcohol consumption.* Consume alcohol in moderation; women should not exceed one drink per day, and men should not exceed two drinks per day. Those who should avoid alcohol include: pregnant or lactating women, women who may become pregnant, children, adolescents, individuals taking medication that should not be mixed with alcohol, and people who have certain medical conditions.
- *Prevent food-borne illness.* Wash hands, food preparation surfaces, and fruits and vegetables. Cook foods long enough and at high enough temperatures to kill dangerous microorganisms. Properly store perishable items and avoid unpasteurized milk products, raw eggs, undercooked meat or poultry, and raw sprouts.

Remember to document the instructions. Place a copy of the information you gave the patient and/or make a note in the chart. For example: *Gave patient the guidelines for healthy eating from the DHHS. Explained each item. The patient had no questions and stated she would start eating healthier tomorrow. LSD, CMA*

CHECKPOINT QUESTION

3. Who publishes the MyPyramid food guidance system and why?

Understanding Food Labels

The Nutritional Labeling and Education Act (NLEA) was passed in 1990 to help consumers identify nutritional content in food products. Most food manufacturers (except meat and poultry) are required to list the nutritional information prominently on the package. The Food and Drug Administration (FDA) regulates this information. Mandatory food labeling was designed to help consumers make informed food choices. Even fast food restaurants are including labeling as consumers become more health conscious.

The label includes measurements of calories, fat content, cholesterol, sodium, carbohydrates, dietary fiber, protein, vitamins, calcium, and any other nutrients contained in the product. Labels for foods that only have a few of certain nutrients are not required to list them. The food label gives the amount of a particular nutrient in one serving size. The percentage of the total daily intake is listed on the right side of the label. The information on the food label helps you choose the daily allowances of the good nutrients like fiber, protein, vitamins, and minerals and a minimal amount of the things that are harmful like fats, cholesterol, sodium, and sugar. A daily value (DV) of 0% is listed for those things that should be kept to a minimum. The calories listed measure how much energy is received from one serving and how many of those calories are from fat. Calories will be discussed later.

To get the full benefit of food labels, patients must understand how to read them. Figure 16-4 is a sample food label with an explanation of each component. Procedure 16-1 outlines the steps in instructing a patient to read food labels.

 PATIENT EDUCATION

VEGETARIAN DIETS

Patients may ask you about vegetarian diets. There are three types of vegetarian diets. A lacto-ovo-vegetarian diet means that the diet of vegetables is supplemented with milk, eggs, and cheese. A lacto-vegetarian diet means the diet is supplemented only with milk and cheese. A pure vegetarian diet is only vegetables and excludes all foods of animal origin. It is possible to eat healthy and obtain necessary nutrients with all three vegetarian diets. The USDA provides guidelines educating vegetarians about appropriate foods that provide essential nutrients.

 CHECKPOINT QUESTION

4. What information is listed on the right side of a food label?

Therapeutic Nutrition

Each part of the lifespan brings different nutritional needs. These needs are outlined in Figure 16-5.

Sometimes a patient's medical condition or situation will require diet restrictions and special foods. When the physician orders such a diet for a patient, you will teach him or her how to follow the guidelines. Some chronic conditions like diabetes and heart disease require special diets. Patients who are confined to bed, whether due to a chronic condition or a fracture, need to eat certain foods. The purposes of these therapeutic diets are to facilitate the healing process, promote healthy weight, assist with chewing and swallowing, and/or influence the components found in blood, such as cholesterol.

Figure 16-4 Sample food label.

Figure 16-5 You can get exercise while doing something as enjoyable as spending time with the kids.

Table 16-2 shows an example of a special diet, the Dietary Approaches to Stop Hypertension (DASH) eating plan.

 CHECKPOINT QUESTION

5. List four possible reasons for a patient's need for a special therapeutic diet.

Physical Fitness

Physical fitness is characterized by endurance, flexibility, and strength. Along with a healthy and balanced diet, regular exercise is necessary for maintaining physi-

cal fitness. Physical movement helps maintain a healthy musculoskeletal system, a normal weight, and a positive mental attitude. Studies have shown that exercising regularly improves the immune system as well. Physical movement causes the production of **endorphins**, the body's "natural painkillers" that tend to produce **euphoria**, or "good feeling."

Components of Physical Fitness

There are several components of physical fitness:

- *Cardiovascular health and endurance.* Regular exercise, particularly aerobic activities, can improve cardiovascular system functioning and endurance. Benefits of a healthy heart include lowered blood pressure, lower cholesterol levels, and a reduced risk for developing conditions such as type 2 diabetes or heart disease.
- *Flexibility.* Stretching exercises give muscles increased flexibility, or a greater range of motion. Calisthenics, yoga, and other stretching activities improve flexibility. Greater flexibility makes everyday physical tasks easier to accomplish; it also helps decrease the risk of muscle injury.
- *Bone and muscle strength.* Exercise can help build strong bones, while weight lifting and resistance training increase muscle strength and endurance.

 CHECKPOINT QUESTION

6. What types of physical activities promote cardiovascular health and endurance?

TABLE 16-2	Example of a Therapeutic Diet: The DASH Eating Plan	
What Does This Diet Accomplish?	**Who May Follow This Diet?**	**Basic Dietary Guidelines**
• Lowers blood pressure • Reduces the risk of developing hypertension • Lowers "bad" cholesterol levels	• Adults with blood pressure above normal levels	• Consume more servings of grains, vegetables, and fruit. • Limit foods and beverages containing added sugars. • Limit sodium intake to 1500–2300 mg per day. • Increase potassium intake from natural sources, such as potatoes, spinach, bananas, apricots, soybeans, and low-fat or nonfat milk.

Source: http://www.nhlbi.nih.gov/health/public/heart/hbp/dash/introduction.html.

PATIENT EDUCATION

CALCULATING TARGET HEART RATE

Patients who are starting an exercise program may need to learn how to calculate their target heart rate. Aerobic activities, such as running, bike riding, rowing, and swimming, are most effective when target heart rate is maintained. Target heart rate should be anywhere between 60% and 90% of a patient's maximum heart rate. To find a patient's target heart rate, follow these steps:

1. Subtract the patient's age (in years) from 220 (beats/minute) to calculate the maximum heart rate. For example, a 35-year-old patient would have a maximum heart rate of 185.

$$220 - 35 = 185$$

2. Multiply the maximum heart rate by the desired intensity level (60% to 90% of the maximum heart rate) to obtain the target heart rate. A patient with a maximum heart rate of 185 who would like to exercise at 70% intensity would need to maintain a target heart rate of 129.5.

$$185 \times 0.70 = 129.5$$

Weight Management

The rate of obesity in the United States has doubled in the past two decades. Nearly one-third of the adult population is obese, and an estimated 16% of children and adolescents are overweight. During this period of time, the obesity rate has doubled among children and tripled among adolescents. Excess body fat can result in a higher risk of certain health conditions, such as hypertension, heart disease, type 2 diabetes, gallbladder disease, respiratory disorders, and certain kinds of cancers.

When helping overweight children and adolescents, it is important to find ways to slow the unhealthy rate of weight gain. However, it is also necessary that these patients maintain normal growth and development. Children who maintain a healthy weight during their childhood may have a reduced risk of becoming overweight during their adult years. Simple methods for managing body weight include eating more nutritious, lower calorie foods and increasing physical activity. Even losing a small amount of weight (e.g., 10 pounds) can benefit a person's health and help prevent future weight gain.

WHAT IF?

A patient who is a young mother of three says that she would like to stay fit, but she has no time for a fitness plan. What are some ways she can incorporate exercise into her busy schedule?

Remind her that exercise does not have to consist of a 30-minute walk or an hour in the gym. Give her some suggestions for creative ways to be physically active every day. For example, take the stairs instead of the elevator. Take two steps at a time for leg and buttock strengthening. On weekends, take a long walk or run around with the children at the park. Doing yard work is another way to be physically active; mowing the lawn with a push mower and raking leaves are ways to stay active while accomplishing necessary chores. While watching television in the evening, jog in place or do jumping jacks. Do calf raises while waiting in line at the grocery store. While talking on the phone, walk up and down stairs or do leg lifts. A simple trip to the grocery store provides exercise by walking and lifting. While driving in the car, tense up various muscle groups for a few seconds and then release. Do leg lifts with your child sitting across your feet (Fig. 16-5). Even a hearty laugh works the abdominal muscles.

The benefits of regular physical activity go beyond maintaining a healthy level of physical fitness. Being active also helps relieve stress. By taking small steps to be more active every day, you will eventually progress to a point where you will want to engage in more physical activity. Then you can hire a babysitter and go take a kickboxing class. Meanwhile, move more.

Physiologic Issues

Reducing and maintaining a healthy weight for you depends on a familiar formula—moving more + eating less = reduction in body weight. The energy that the body expends burns the calories you consume. You can calculate the amount of calories you should take in to know how to lose or maintain weight. To do this, you must understand the three basic ways the body expends energy. These include:

- Basal metabolic rate (or how many calories the body uses to perform basic functions, such as respiration and heartbeat, while in a resting state)
- Energy expended during physical activity

LEGAL TIP

US GOVERNMENT IS CONCERNED ABOUT AMERICANS' EATING HABITS

The US government is dedicated to improving America's nutritional needs, and this is evident when you consider the many bills passed and programs provided by the agencies of the federal government. Based on data concerning dietary intake and evidence of public health problems, experts say that Americans have formed some poor eating habits. Studies have shown that Americans consume too many calories per day, as well as unhealthy amounts of saturated and trans fat, cholesterol, added sugars, and sodium. In addition, most people do not meet the recommended daily intakes for a number of nutrients. The federal government says most manufacturers must list the nutrients and their amounts in food packaging. The FDA mandates the information included on a food label. A recent new mandate requires manufacturers to list the amount of trans fats in their products.

In the 1960s, the federal government instituted the Presidential Physical Fitness Award, which outlined specific physical programs for school physical fitness programs. The USDA regulates the public school lunch programs and requires lunches to satisfy the recommended daily dietary requirements. Head Start is a federal preschool program that has an excellent food program, ensuring that disadvantaged children get at least one nutritious meal a day. Their food programs, along with agricultural extensions across the nation, train parents in proper nutrition and food preparation through regular workshops and training.

- The thermic effect of food (or how much energy the body expends while processing different foods)

The body's daily caloric needs are most accurately determined by taking into account all three of these components.

Basal Metabolic Rate

As mentioned earlier, metabolism is the process of changing things in the body. An individual's **basal metabolic rate** (BMR) refers to the amount of energy used in a unit of time to maintain vital functions by a fasting, resting subject. Approximately 60% to 70% of the body's energy is expended this way. BMR includes basic activities such as respiration, heartbeat, and maintaining body temperature.

Level of Physical Activity

The second component is your level of physical activity, which makes up 20% to 30% of the body's total energy expenditure. You have already learned the positive effects of physical activity, one of which is to burn calories and maintain a healthy weight. Box 16-2 shows an appropriate workout schedule.

Calories

The third component is the thermic effect of food, which is the increase in energy required to digest food. The amount of energy used by the body can be measured in calories. Four different sources can contribute calories to a person's diet. These sources include carbohydrates, fats, proteins, and alcohol. Together, your BMR, your

BOX 16-2

SAMPLE WORKOUT SCHEDULE

The following is a sample workout schedule that the average healthy patient can follow to maintain physical fitness.

- *Warming up.* Take 5 to 10 minutes to warm up your muscles. Walk or jog at a slow pace to prepare your body for the workout.
- *Stretching exercises.* It's important to stretch your muscles when they are warm; this prevents muscle injury. Spend 10 to 12 minutes on stretching exercises, being careful to move slowly and avoid bouncing. Stretching each day also improves flexibility.
- *Strength training.* To increase muscle strength, lift weights at least twice a week for 20 minutes at a time. Also incorporate resistance exercises such as pull-ups, push-ups, and sit-ups into your workout. These exercises should be done at least three times a week for 30 minutes and should include all major muscle groups.
- *Cardiovascular endurance exercises.* Aerobic activities, including running, bike riding, jumping rope, swimming, and hiking, increase your cardiovascular endurance. Devote 30 minutes or more to aerobic activity at least three times a week.
- *Cooling down.* After each workout, take 5 to 10 minutes to cool down. Several minutes of walking or other low-intensity movement will allow your heart rate to return to normal. It is also important to stretch the muscles that have just been used.

Source: www.fitness.gov/fitness.htm.

level of physical activity, and the thermic effect of food indicate how many calories your body needs each day. If you take in fewer calories than you need, you lose weight.

The combination of these three components can be calculated as follows:

- For those who are not physically active: weight (lbs) × 14 = estimated calories/day
- For those who are moderately active: weight (lbs) × 17 = estimated calories/day
- For active individuals: weight (lbs) × 20 = estimated calories/day

Body Mass Index

Body mass index (BMI) measures an individual's ratio of fat to lean body mass. It can be calculated by using the following formula: [weight (pounds) ÷ height (inches)^2] × 703. With the increased incidence of obesity, physicians are turning to BMI for assessing patients' risk for obesity. For adults who are 20 years of age or older, the condition of being overweight or obese is based on their BMI level only (i.e., regardless of age or gender). For children and adolescents, however, weight status is determined by taking into account not only BMI level, but also age and gender.

Because BMI takes into account both weight and height, it is a more accurate way to measure body fat than by measuring weight alone. It is important to note, however, that BMI is not the sole method used to determine obesity. It does have limitations; BMI can overestimate body fat in someone who is very muscular or underestimate body fat in an individual with decreased muscle mass. Other factors, including age, gender, and ethnicity, also cause variations in the relationship between BMI and body fat. Slightly reducing caloric intake for children who are overweight will decrease their body fat, which will improve their BMI over the course of time.

A BMI over 30 is considered obese. The Centers for Disease Control and Prevention offer a body mass calculator on their website. By going to *www.cdc.gov*, you can search for the BMI calculator, enter the patient's requested information, and print a graph and information about the patient. There are also growth charts available to track BMI (Fig. 16-6).

 CHECKPOINT QUESTION

7. What is meant by BMR?

Sociologic and Psychological Issues

Many people are what researchers have called "emotional eaters." Instead of facing the stresses of everyday life, emotional eaters use food to cope. Others eat when

Figure 16-6 Growth charts track the body mass index.

they are happy as a form of celebration or as a reward for an accomplishment.

Almost every social event you attend involves food. Eating has become entertainment for many people. Food is a part of many of our traditions, e.g., birthday cake, homemade ice cream for summer outings, and sweets and cakes around holidays, etc. You may remember the cookies and milk your mother gave you after school or the lollipop she offered when you scraped your knee.

Food is everywhere; it is necessary for life. Experts warn that we must make some major lifestyle changes, make better food choices, and become more active to stop the growing epidemic of obesity. This starts with changing your bad habits.

 CHECKPOINT QUESTION

8. What are the ill effects of excess body fat?

Staying Well

Maintaining the proper body weight and consuming the right nutrients in the right amounts are necessary for good health, but in our busy world, it is difficult to follow a rigid diet or a confining exercise regimen. With some planning and determination, though, you can make even subtle changes to improve your health and quality of life. Eating more slowly, sleeping more, and taking the stairs instead of an elevator are just a few of the things that you can do every day to make you feel better. A healthy body has a better immune system.

Stress

Although a certain amount of good stress is needed to function and thrive in everyday life, too much stress can be harmful. High stress levels are known to cause a long list of health problems. Everything from headaches to leg cramps can be indicators of too much stress. Keep lists of suggestions in a central patient education area or waiting area of the office. During waiting times in the examination room, talk to patients about their stress levels. To lessen stress, try using some of the following techniques:

- Think positively. Look for the good in each situation instead of focusing on the bad.
- Devote at least 30 minutes of each day to an activity you truly enjoy, such as spending time with friends, reading, or pursuing a favorite hobby.
- Take a moment to calm your thoughts when faced with a situation that causes you to become angry or agitated.
- Know your limits and don't take on too many obligations.
- Get a good night's sleep.

Even leisure activity reduces stress by providing a temporary break from the everyday pressures and obligations that can make life stressful. Not only will you be better equipped to handle life's daily challenges, but you will reduce your physical symptoms of stress as well. High levels of stress and its effects on the body can contribute to heart disease, ulcers, and other conditions in individuals who are **predisposed**, or genetically programmed, for such problems. Stress can also exacerbate chronic conditions, like diabetes, and have a negative impact on a person's emotional health and interpersonal relationships.

Relaxation exercises can calm you down in times of high stress. Sitting or lying comfortably with your eyes closed while imagining a quiet, peaceful place is a self-relaxation technique called **guided imagery**. Meditation is a relaxation technique that calms the mind and the body, relieving physical and emotional stress.

Pollution

Air pollution can negatively affect health. Those who live in areas with high levels of pollution might suffer from respiratory problems and general discomfort due to burning eyes or irritated throats. A number of chemicals detected in polluted air have been linked to birth defects, certain cancers, respiratory disorders, and brain damage. Accidental releases of some chemicals have been known to cause serious injury or even death.

Air pollution also harms the environment by destroying trees and plants, polluting bodies of water, and killing fish and animals. Air pollutants have caused the protective ozone layer above our planet to thin. Environmental changes may result from damage to the ozone layer. Increased instances of skin cancer and eye damage are also likely.

The Clean Air Act of 1990 is a federal law that limits the amounts of certain pollutants that may be released into the air in the United States. The act is designed to provide the same basic health and environmental protection to all Americans. It is up to the states to regulate these levels. States may set up stricter laws concerning pollution, but they may not adopt weaker pollution controls than the federal law mandates. A federal agency, the Environmental Protection Agency (EPA), is in place to help the states meet federal regulations. The EPA conducts research and provides funding to support state programs designed to reduce air pollution.

To minimize the harmful effects of pollution, experts suggest that you avoid secondhand smoke, areas with heavy traffic, and inhaling highway fumes. When exercising outdoors, try to avoid busy roads or high-pollution areas when smog levels are high. Monitor air quality levels. Shrubbery in your yard is recommended because it protects you from breathing in pollution and dirt from the street.

Seat Belt Use and Airbags

It is estimated that 40,000 people die each year in motor vehicle accidents. Thankfully, proper seat belt use can prevent up to half of these deaths. In an automobile accident, when the front of a vehicle hits an unmoving object, the car stops abruptly, but the driver and passengers do not. Momentum keeps moving their bodies forward at the same speed the vehicle was traveling until they are stopped by unmoving objects inside the vehicle (such as the dashboard, steering wheel, or windshield). The impact can cause serious, and sometimes fatal, injuries. However, properly worn seat belts prevent that second crash. Seat belts should fit snugly so the hips and shoulders suffer the greatest impact. These areas of the body can best withstand the impact of a crash. Both the lap belt and shoulder restraint are necessary for the greatest protection. The lap belt keeps the body from moving forward, and the shoulder restraint protects the head and face from coming into contact with the vehicle's dashboard or windshield.

A large percentage of motor vehicle deaths result from frontal impact crashes. Air bags are engineered to protect passengers and drivers involved in these types of accidents. Although air bags can reduce injuries to the head and chest, they are not intended to replace seat belts. In fact, air bags make seat belts even more effective. When air bags are used in addition to lap belts and shoulder restraints, the risk of injury to the head is greatly reduced. The National Highway Traffic Safety Administration estimates an 81% reduction of injuries when both seat belts and air bags are used, whereas the estimated reduction when seat belts alone are used is 60%.

 CHECKPOINT QUESTION

9. What effects are thought to be caused by the loss of the earth's ozone?

Dental Health

Dental health is an important part of a person's overall health (Fig. 16-7). Flossing removes plaque between and around the individual teeth reducing **dental cavities** (holes in the teeth) and promoting healthy gums. Unattended cavities have a profound effect on the gums, as well as on the sinuses and the throat. There are many affordable dental products that make dental health simple for patients, including battery-powered toothbrushes, plastic floss holders, and tongue cleaners. Keeping teeth in good repair with regular dental checkups promotes better general health.

Positive Mental Outlook

Having a positive mental outlook can benefit your health and well-being. Experts say that genetics may play a part in mental attitude, but you also have control over your feelings and emotions. Maybe you cannot control certain events, but you can control your reactions to them or how you let the events affect you. Looking at the bright side of things reduces stress and, ultimately, can even prolong life. There have been many instances of terminally ill patients who fared better than

expected because they maintained a positive outlook. In almost every situation, you can identify positive and negative aspects. If you pay attention to the positive and downplay the negative, you can train your brain to have a positive attitude.

Genetics

It is undeniable that genetics determine a great deal in regard to your health. However, even if your parents suffered from ill health, there are ways of reducing your own health risks. Studies have shown that genetics play a large role in what diseases a person contracts, but patients should not use this as an excuse to ignore risk factors. Even if there has been no lung cancer in a family, tobacco use would still increase the risk. In other words, good genes can be negated by bad health habits.

Infectious Disease Prevention

Fortunately, the body is equipped with a remarkable immune system. The body protects a healthy person from most germs or pathogens. You can control how many of these germs enter the body by taking a few precautions. Proper handwashing is known to be the best defense against illness. Because germs must enter the body to make you sick, the hands are usually the mode of transportation. Wearing personal protective equipment when handling body fluids will protect you in the workplace. As a health care worker, you are trained to stay safe from blood-borne pathogens. These same actions should be taken at home. Using safe practices in the kitchen and bathroom will also reduce the spread of disease. Preventing the spread of infection takes care and attention. Box 16-3 gives some tips for avoiding colds and other contagious illnesses.

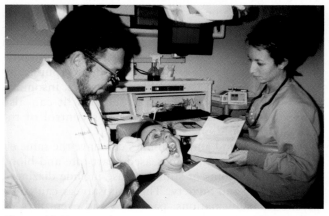

Figure 16-7 Healthy teeth promote general good health.

BOX 16-3

THINGS TO DO TO PREVENT INFECTIOUS DISEASES

- Keep immunizations up to date. Follow recommended immunizations for children and adults. Immunize your pets as well.
- Wash your hands often, especially during cold and flu season. Be sure to wash hands:
  After using the bathroom
  Before preparing or eating food
  After changing a diaper
  After blowing your nose or sneezing or coughing
  After caring for a sick person
  After playing with a pet

(continued)

BOX 16-3 *(continued)*

- Be aware of what you eat, and be careful how your prepare it:

  Keep hot foods hot and cold foods cold until eaten or cooked

  Be sure temperature controls in refrigerators and freezers are working properly

  Wash counters, cutting boards, and utensils frequently with soap and hot water, especially after preparing poultry and other meats

  Wash fresh fruits and vegetables before eating

  Cook ground beef until you can no longer see any pink

- Use antibiotics exactly as prescribed. Take them for the full course prescribed by your doctor, but do not take them for colds or other nonbacterial illnesses. Never self-medicate with antibiotics or share them with family or friends.

- Report to your doctor any quickly worsening infection or any infection that does not get better after you finish a prescribed antibiotic.

- After any animal bite, clean the skin with soap and water, and seek medical care immediately.

- Avoid areas of insect infestation. Use insect repellents on skin and clothing when in areas where ticks or mosquitoes are common. If you have visited wooded or wilderness areas and are now sick, your doctor needs all the details to diagnose both rare and common illnesses quickly.

- If you're sick, don't fly. It would be easy to infect others in a confined area, and you won't enjoy your trip if you're sick. Stay alert to disease threats when you travel or visit undeveloped areas. Get all recommended immunizations, and use protective medications for travel, especially to areas with malaria. Don't drink untreated water while hiking or camping. If you become ill when you return home, tell your doctor where you've been.

- When sick, allow yourself time to heal and recover. Be courteous to others: wash your hands frequently, and cover your mouth when you sneeze or cough.

Source: Rhode Island Department of Health, 3 Capitol Hill, Providence RI 02908; http://www.health.ri.gov/contact.php.

Substance Abuse

Substance abuse is excessive use of and dependency on drugs. Some abused substances are legal (e.g., alcohol, nicotine), whereas others are illegal (e.g., marijuana, cocaine). Patients with substance abuse problems can seek help from trained specialists or counselors. Because substance abuse can be highly detrimental to your patients'

health, it is important that you have information available about substance abuse if they should ask. You can find this information from various national organizations. Your office should also have information available for patients on any local chapters or organizations that may help these patients.

Alcohol

Alcohol is one of the most commonly abused legal substances. While there have been studies done that link a daily glass of red wine to a potential reduced risk for heart disease, overconsumption of alcohol can contribute to certain health problems. These problems include high blood pressure, cardiomyopathy, fetal alcohol syndrome, and, in some cases of long-term alcohol abuse, possible liver damage.

Some people can drink in moderation. Others are prone to addiction, which is an illness and should be treated as such. Because alcohol contains ethanol, it is considered a mind-altering substance. Ethanol works as a depressant within the central nervous system. The effects of alcohol intoxication include a lack of coordination, slurred speech, blurred vision, and impaired brain function. Large quantities of alcohol can have a negative effect on such basic functions as breathing and heart rate. The long-term effects of excessive alcohol use can include cirrhosis of the liver, certain cancers, an increased risk of stroke, and nutritional deficiencies.

Drugs

Marijuana and hashish impair short-term memory and comprehension. They alter the user's sense of time and reduce the ability to perform tasks requiring concentration and coordination. They also increase the heart rate and appetite. Long-term users may develop psychological dependence. Because these drugs are inhaled as unfiltered smoke, users take in more cancer-causing agents and do more damage to the respiratory system than with regular filtered tobacco smoke.

Cocaine and crack cocaine are extremely addictive. These illegal drugs stimulate the central nervous system. Crack cocaine is particularly dangerous because this pure form of cocaine is usually smoked and absorbed rapidly in the bloodstream. It can cause sudden death. Use of cocaine can cause psychological and physical dependency. Side effects include dilated pupils, increased pulse rate, elevated blood pressure, insomnia, loss of appetite, paranoia, and seizures. It can also cause death by disrupting the brain's control of the heart and respiration.

Stimulants and amphetamines can have the same effect as cocaine, causing increased heart rate and blood pressure. Symptoms of stimulant use include dizziness, sleeplessness, and anxiety. These substances can cause psychosis, hallucinations, paranoia, and even physical collapse. The long-term effects of these substances include hypertension, heart disease, stroke, and renal and liver failure.

Depressants and barbiturates can cause physical and psychological dependence. Abuse of these drugs can lead to respiratory depression, coma, and death, especially when they are taken with alcohol. Withdrawal can lead to restlessness, insomnia, convulsions, and death.

Hallucinogens, such as lysergic acid diethylamide (LSD), phencyclidine ("angel dust" or PCP), mescaline, and peyote, all interrupt brain messages that control the intellect and keep instincts in check. Large doses can produce seizures, coma, and heart and lung failure. Chronic users complain of persistent memory problems and speech difficulties for up to a year after discontinuing use. Because hallucinogens stop the brain's pain sensors, drug experiences may result in severe self-inflicted injuries.

Narcotics, such as heroin, codeine, morphine, and opium, are addictive drugs. These drugs can produce euphoria, drowsiness, and blood pressure and pulse fluctuations. An overdose can lead to seizures, coma, cardiac arrest, and death.

It is important to teach all pregnant women the damage substance abuse may do to their unborn child and to refer pregnant patients to support services. The most important role of the medical assistant in educating patients about any type of substance abuse is to be supportive. Provide positive reinforcements as appropriate and offer services to patients for cessation programs.

Smoking Cessation

The health risks associated with smoking have been well documented for many years. Nicotine is highly addictive whether ingested by inhaling or chewing. This drug reaches the brain in 6 seconds, damages the blood vessels, decreases heart strength, and is associated with many can-

cers. The withdrawal symptoms include anxiety, progressive restlessness, irritability, and sleep disturbances. There are numerous methods to try to stop smoking. The methods vary greatly. Some programs have the patient gradually stop, while other programs seek a total, abrupt stoppage. There are research data to support both methods.

PATIENT EDUCATION

SMOKING CESSATION
REQUIRES HELP

Here are some suggestions to help patients stop smoking:

- Find local smoking cessation support groups. Provide phone numbers and contact names of these groups to your patients.
- If there are no local support groups, the American Heart Association, American Lung Association, or American Cancer Society may help.
- Discuss with the physician the options of prescribing various patches, gums, or other interventions for the patient. Some products have side effects, and the physician may opt not to order them based on the patient's age or other medical illnesses.

MEDIA MENU

- **Student CD**
  - **Case Study**
    Administrative Interactive Case Study 3: Conduct Patient Teaching
  - **CMA/RMA Certification Exam Review**
- **Premium Online Course**
  http://thePoint.lww.com/Kronenberger3e
- **Internet Resources**

LiveAdvise Online Tutoring & Competency Training
http://thePoint.lww.com/LiveAdvise

Ten Essential Health Tips
www.health-fitness-tips.com

To download body mass index and other charts
www.cdc.gov/growthcharts

For dietary guidelines
www.health.gov/dietaryguidelines/

US Department of Agriculture's MyPyramid site
www.mypyramid.gov

American Running and Fitness Association
www.americanrunning.org/

The President's Council on Physical Fitness and Sports
www.fitness.gov

American Alliance for Health, Physical Education, Recreation, and Dance
www.aahperd.org

March of Dimes
www.marchofdimes.com

American Heart Association
www.americanheart.org/

American Lung Association
www.lungusa.org

For information on alcoholism
www.cdc.gov/alcohol/faqs.htm

español SPANISH TERMINOLOGY

Debes tener una dieta balanceada. Utiliza la pirámide de alimentos como guía para ayudarte a escojer los alimentos apropiados.

> You should have a balanced diet. Using the food guide pyramid helps you to choose the right foods.

Utilizando estas fotos, yo circularé o marcare los alimentos que debes comer.

> Using these pictures, I'll circle the foods you can have.

Estos son los alimentos que debes evitar.

> These are the foods you should avoid.

Debes hacer ejercicios por lo menos tres veces a la semana.

> You should exercise at least three times a week.

Asegurate de cuidar tus dientes.

> Be sure and take care of your teeth.

PROCEDURE 16-1: Instruct a Patient to Read Food Labels

Purpose: To instruct a patient in how to read a food label so that he or she may make better food choices
Equipment: Two boxes of the same item, one low calorie or "lite," the other regular; measuring cup; two bowls; refer to Figure 16-4 for reference

Steps	Purpose
1. Identify the patient.	
2. Introduce yourself and explain the procedure.	
3. Have the patient look at the labels, briefly comparing the two.	Taking an overall look at the label will show the patient the types of items listed.
4. Ask the patient to pour out a normal serving into a bowl.	The patient's perception of a normal serving may be wrong.
5. Measure the exact serving size printed on the label. Compare the two. Discuss the difference, if any.	Using a measuring cup will show the patient the accuracy of the serving size.

Step 5. Measure the exact serving size.

(continued)

PROCEDURE 16-1: Instruct a Patient to Read Food Labels
(continued)

6. Explain to the patient each section of the label (see Fig. 16-4):
  a. Serving size and servings per package
  b. Column for amount in serving
  c. Column for % daily value (formerly called recommended daily allowance [RDA])
	The patient may be surprised that his or her servings are more or less than on the label, which changes the weights and daily values.

7. Explain calories and calories from fat. Have the patient calculate the percentage of fat calories by multiplying the grams of fat by 9 and dividing that number by the total calories per serving as listed on the label. Multiply the answer by 100. This number is the percentage of calories from fat.	Although manufacturers are required to list this information, patients should know how this number is calculated.
8. Read down the label and discuss each nutrient, pointing out the amounts and percentages.	Seeing the labels will help the patient understand.
9. Have the patient compare the two labels and tell you how many total carbohydrates, sugars, protein, etc. are in each label.	This will ensure that the patient understands how to determine the types and amounts of ingredients.
10. Ask the patient if he or she has any questions.	Having the patient answer your questions and giving him or her an opportunity to ask you questions will ensure the patient's comprehension of the information.
11. Chart the instruction.	The physician and other workers in the office may need to know what the patient has been taught. Remember, if it's not in the chart, it did not happen.

Charting Example:

9/25/08, Taught patient how to read a food label using sample labels. Patient understood and expressed excitement in her plan to be more careful in her food choices. She had no questions. She was instructed to call if she has any questions as she uses her new skill.

—Cindy Parent, CMA

- Good nutrition and a healthy lifestyle are important to everyone. Knowing the guidelines for a healthy and safe life is important, but practicing those guidelines is key.
- There is a growing trend in the United States toward obesity, especially among young people. The federal government is working to reverse this trend.
- Following the helpful information and suggestions that you give your patients also gives you a better chance at good health and longevity.
- There are ways to stay as safe and healthy as possible even during daily activities like driving a car. Medical assistants should be prepared to teach these safe and healthy living habits.

- The same safe practices for reducing the spread of disease in the health care workplace, such as handwashing, can be used at home to keep you and your family safe from pathogens.
- To increase chances of good health, patients should be encouraged to limit or avoid harmful substances such as nicotine, alcohol, and drugs.
- Understanding good nutrition, knowing the benefits of physical fitness, and using suggestions for staying safe and healthy will give patients a good foundation for making the right choices in life-to be as healthy and happy as possible.

Warm Ups for Critical Thinking

1. The physician asks you to assist a 65-year-old patient with a low-cholesterol diet. Write a plan for the instruction. Help her plan several sample meals to help get her started. What would you say to her?

2. A 12-year-old boy presents for his routine yearly physical. His current weight is 150 pounds, and his growth chart indicates a steady increase in body weight. Explain the dangers of obesity to the patient's mother. Go to *www.cdc.gov*, search for body mass index, and click on the BMI calculator. Enter the information to complete a BMI chart for the patient with the following measurements: 5 feet, 5 inches tall, 150 pounds, date of birth 5/28/1994.

3. Keep track of all of the food that you consume over a 24-hour period. Calculate your total fat and total carbohydrate intake. Do your meals follow your MyPyramid guidelines? If not, what do you need to do to improve your nutritional status? Using pictures from magazines, create well-balanced breakfast, lunch, and dinner plates. Hint: your plate should be colorful.

Answers to Checkpoint Questions

1. Fat-soluble vitamins are not absorbed with fatty foods and are stored in the body.

2. A complete protein is one that contains all nine essential amino acids. Complete proteins are found in milk, cheese, eggs, and meats.

3. The USDA publishes the MyPyramid food guidance system to help people maintain healthy diets and sufficient exercise levels.

4. The right side of the food label gives the percentage of the total daily intake recommended that is contained in one serving.

5. The purposes of therapeutic diets are to facilitate the healing process, promote healthy weight, assist with chewing and swallowing, and/or influence the components found in blood, such as cholesterol.

6. Aerobic activities, such as running, bike riding, rowing, and swimming, can improve cardiovascular system functioning and endurance.

7. The BMR is the basal metabolic rate and refers to the rate at which the body performs the basic functions such as heart beat, respiration, and maintaining body temperature.

8. Excess body fat can result in a higher risk of certain health conditions, such as hypertension, heart disease, type 2 diabetes, gallbladder disease, respiratory disorders, and certain kinds of cancers.

9. The loss of our ozone is predicted to cause changes in the environment and increase skin cancer and eye damage.

Outline

Microorganisms, Pathogens, and Normal Flora
Conditions That Favor the Growth of Pathogens
The Infection Cycle
Modes of Transmission
Direct Transmission
Indirect Transmission
Sources of Transmission

Principles of Infection Control
Medical Asepsis
Levels of Infection Control
Occupational Safety and Health Administration Guidelines for the Medical Office
Exposure Risk Factors and the Exposure Control Plan

Standard Precautions
Personal Protective Equipment
Handling Environmental Contamination
Disposing of Infectious Waste
Hepatitis B and Human Immunodeficiency Viruses

Learning Objectives

Upon successfully completing this chapter, you will be able to:

1. Spell and define key terms

2. Describe conditions that promote the growth of microorganisms

3. Explain the components of the infectious process cycle

4. List the various ways microbes are transmitted

5. Explain concepts of medical asepsis and infection control

6. Compare the effectiveness in reducing or destroying microorganisms using the various levels of infection control

7. Define sanitation

8. Distinguish between the need for disinfection and sterilization

9. Discuss risk management procedures relative to the Occupational Safety and Health Administration guidelines for the medical office

10. List the required components of an exposure control plan

11. Explain the importance of following standard precautions in the medical office

12. Identify various personal protective equipment (PPE) items

13. Describe circumstances when PPE items would be appropriately worn by the medical assistant

14. Describe the procedures for cleaning, handling, and disposing of biohazardous waste in the medical office

15. Explain the facts pertaining to the transmission and prevention of the hepatitis B virus and the human immunodeficiency virus in the medical office

16. Describe how to avoid becoming infected with the hepatitis B and human immunodeficiency viruses

1. Perform a medical aseptic handwashing procedure (Procedure 17-1)

2. Remove contaminated gloves (Procedure 17-2)

3. Clean and decontaminate biohazardous spills (Procedure 17-3)

Competencies

CAAHEP

- Perform handwashing
- Dispose of biohazardous materials
- Practice standard precautions

ABHES

- Apply principles of aseptic techniques and infection control
- Dispose of biohazardous materials

Key Terms

aerobe	exposure risk factors	Administration (OSHA)	sanitization
anaerobe	germicide	pathogens	spores
asymptomatic	immunization	personal protective equipment (PPE)	standard precautions
bactericidal	infection		sterilization
biohazardous	medical asepsis	postexposure testing	transient flora
carriers	microorganisms	resident flora	vector
disease	normal flora	resistance	viable
disinfection	Occupational Safety and Health	sanitation	virulent
exposure control plan			

Many patients are seen daily in the medical office for a variety of reasons, including physical examinations for employment, reassurance about a current health problem, and follow-up care for a chronic condition or surgical procedure. In addition, many patients request appointments because of illness. It is important for you to protect patients from each other with regard to contagious diseases and for you to protect yourself from acquiring the many microorganisms with which you will come into contact every day.

To prevent the spread of **disease** in the medical office, medical assistants must meet two goals. First, you must understand and practice **medical asepsis** at all times, using specific practices and procedures to prevent disease transmission. These practices and procedures also allow you to work with ill patients while reducing the chances that you will spread disease to other patients or become infected yourself. Second, you must teach the patients and their families about techniques to use at home to prevent the transmission of disease. Handwashing, the cornerstone of infection control, is discussed in this chapter and is emphasized in all subsequent chapters wherever contact with infectious material might be expected. In addition, this chapter describes how disease is transmitted and, most important, how to prevent the spread of disease.

Microorganisms, Pathogens, and Normal Flora

Microorganisms, living organisms that can be seen only with a microscope, are part of our normal environment.

In addition to our physical environment, many microorganisms can be found on your skin and throughout your gastrointestinal, genitourinary, and respiratory systems, and some of these are required for good health. These microorganisms are normal and are referred to as **normal flora** or **resident flora**. Some microorganisms, however, are not part of the normal flora and may cause disease or **infection**. Disease-producing microorganisms are referred to as pathogens and are classified as bacteria, viruses, fungi, or protozoa. (See Chapter 44 for a more detailed discussion of microorganisms.)

When normal flora become too many in number or are transmitted to an area of the body in which they are not normally found, they are referred to as **transient flora**, which can become pathogens under the right conditions. For example, *Staphylococcus aureus*, a microorganism commonly found on the skin, may get into underlying tissue if the skin is broken. In this situation, the normal flora of the skin has become transient flora and may cause disease. Decreased **resistance** in the host is one condition that may allow transient flora to become pathogenic. Individuals who are elderly, receiving certain drugs to treat cancer, or under unusual stress may have a lowered resistance and be particularly susceptible to infections.

Although the body is protected by many nonspecific defenses against disease, infection or illness may occur if the natural barriers are overpowered or breached. The following are some of the body's natural defenses that may prevent the invasion of pathogens into various body organs:

- Skin. As long as the skin is kept clean and remains intact or unbroken, staphylococcal (Staph) bacteria are not considered dangerous. Washing the skin frequently will flush away many of these bacteria along with any other microorganisms.
- Eyes. The eyelashes act as a barrier by trapping dust that may carry microorganisms before they have an opportunity to enter the eye. If any microorganisms do enter the eye, the enzyme lysozyme normally found in tears will destroy some microorganisms, including bacteria.
- Mouth. The greatest variety of microorganisms in the body is in the mouth. Saliva is slightly **bactericidal**, and good oral hygiene will remove or prevent the growth of many of the pathogens in the mouth.
- Gastrointestinal tract. Hydrochloric acid normally found in the stomach destroys most of the disease-producing pathogens that enter the gastrointestinal system. One bacterium, *Escherichia coli* (*E. coli*), is resident flora found in the large intestine and is necessary for digestion. It does not usually cause disease as long it remains within the gastrointestinal tract. *Helicobacter pylori* also reside in the digestive tracts of some individuals and may cause gastric ulcers.

- Respiratory tract. Hairs and cilia on the membrane lining of the nostrils are early defenses against airborne microorganisms. If these physical barriers do not stop an invasion, mucus from the membranes lining the respiratory tract should trap the microorganisms and facilitate their removal from the respiratory system as the person swallows, coughs, or sneezes.
- Genitourinary tract. The reproductive and urinary systems provide a less hospitable environment for microorganisms. The slightly acidic environment of these body systems reduces the ability of many microorganisms to survive. In addition, frequent urination flushes the urinary tract and removes many transient microorganisms.

Although these systems have protective mechanisms to prevent infection, any of them may be overpowered by a particularly **virulent** organism. Transient flora is not usually pathogenic unless the person's defenses are compromised by a decrease in resistance.

 CHECKPOINT QUESTION

1. What are pathogenic microorganisms? How does the body prevent an invasion and subsequent infection naturally?

Conditions That Favor the Growth of Pathogens

All microorganisms require certain conditions to grow and reproduce. To reduce the number of microorganisms and potential pathogens in a clinical setting, you must eliminate as many of their life requirements as possible. These requirements include the following:

- Moisture. Few microorganisms can survive with little water or moisture. However, some microorganisms form **spores** and remain dormant until moisture is available.
- Nutrients. Microorganisms depend on their environment for nourishment. Surfaces (tables, counters, equipment, etc.) that are contaminated with organic matter (food products, body fluids, or tissue) promote the growth of microorganisms.
- Temperature. Although some microorganisms can survive even in freezing or boiling temperatures, those that thrive at a normal body temperature of 98.6°F are most likely to be pathogenic to humans. Many microorganisms that leave an infected person can survive for awhile at room temperature; therefore, surfaces that are contaminated with dried organic material should be considered possibly pathogenic.
- Darkness. Many pathogenic bacteria are destroyed by bright light, including sunlight.

- Neutral pH. The pH of a solution refers to the measurement of its acid-base balance on a scale of 1 to 14, with 7 being neutral. Many microorganisms are destroyed in an environment that is not neutral. The pH of blood (7.35–7.45) is preferred by microorganisms that thrive in the human body.
- Oxygen. Microorganisms that need oxygen to survive are called **aerobes**. A few, however, do not require oxygen; these are called **anaerobes**. Although most pathogens are aerobic, the microbes that cause tetanus and botulism are anaerobic.

If any one of these conditions is altered in any way, the growth and reproduction of the pathogen will be affected. Your role as a professional medical assistant in a medical office includes using this knowledge of microbial growth to inhibit the growth and reproduction of microorganisms in the office.

 CHECKPOINT QUESTION

2. Given the six conditions that favor the growth of pathogens, explain how you can alter the growth and reproduction of microorganisms by changing these factors.

The Infection Cycle

The infection cycle is often thought of as a series of specific links of a chain involving a causative agent or invading microorganism (Fig. 17-1). The first link in the chain is the reservoir host; this is the person who is infected with the microorganism. While this person may or may not show signs of infection, his or her body is serving as a source of nutrients and an incubator in which the pathogen can grow and reproduce. These persons are also called **carriers**, or reservoirs, of disease.

The reservoir host may transmit disease only when the pathogen has a means of exit. The second link in the chain is the manner in which the pathogen leaves the reservoir host. Means of exit include the mucous membranes of the nose and mouth, the openings of the gastrointestinal system (mouth or rectum), and an open wound.

In addition to the means of exit, the microbe must have a vehicle in which to leave the host. This next link in the chain, the means of transmission, involves the vehicle that is used by the pathogen when it leaves the reservoir host and spreads through the environment. Vehicles include mucus or air droplets from the oral or nasal cavities and direct contact between an unclean hand and another person or object. Sneezing and coughing without covering the nose and mouth are excellent methods of transmitting microorganisms into the environment and potential hosts.

The fourth link in the chain of the infectious process cycle is the portal of entry. This is the route by which the pathogen enters the next host. With inhalation of contaminated air droplets, the respiratory system is the portal of entry. Another portal of entry is the gastrointesti-

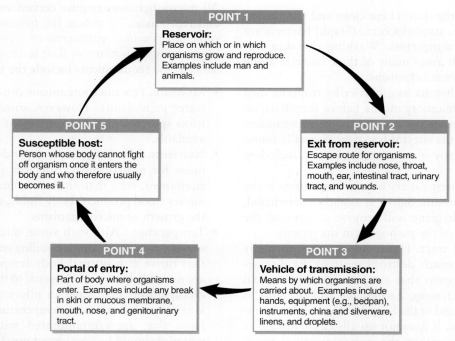

Figure 17-1 The infectious process cycle. Infections and infectious diseases are spread by starting from the reservoir (point 1) and moving in a circle to the susceptible host (point 5). Microorganisms can be controlled by interfering at any point in the cycle.

nal system: the pathogen enters the body in contaminated food or drink. Any break in the skin or mucous membranes can be a portal of entry for pathogenic microorganisms.

The final link in the infectious process cycle is the susceptible host (Box 17-1). This host is one to whom the pathogen is transmitted after leaving the reservoir host. If the conditions in the susceptible host are conducive to reproduction of the pathogen, the susceptible host becomes a reservoir host and the cycle repeats.

 CHECKPOINT QUESTION

3. How are the first and fifth links of the infection cycle related?

Modes of Transmission

In the third link of the infectious process cycle, the vehicle that spreads the microorganism is often called the mode of transmission. It is important for you to understand the mode of transmission used by various pathogens so that you can break this link in the infectious cycle and prevent the spread of disease.

Direct Transmission

Direct contact between the infected reservoir host and the susceptible host produces direct transmission. Direct transmission may occur when one touches contaminated blood or body fluids, shakes hands with someone who has contaminated hands, inhales infected air droplets, or has intimate contact, such as kissing or sexual intercourse, with someone who is contaminated.

Indirect Transmission

Indirect transmission may occur through contact with a vehicle known as a vector. Vectors include contaminated food or water, disease-carrying insects, and inanimate objects such as soil, drinking glasses, wound drainage, and infected or improperly disinfected medical instruments. While visible blood and body fluids are obvious sources of infection, many infectious organisms remain **viable** for long periods on inanimate surfaces that are not visibly contaminated.

Sources of Transmission

Most reservoir hosts are humans, animals, and insects. Human hosts include people who are ill with an infectious disease, people who are carriers of an infectious disease, and people who are incubating an infectious disease but are not exhibiting symptoms. This last group can transmit disease even though they are ambulatory and **asymptomatic** (have no symptoms). Animal sources, which are less common, include infected dogs, cats, birds, cattle, rodents, and animals that live in the wild. Diseases that may be transmitted to humans from infected animals include anthrax and rabies.

In addition to flies and roaches, which carry many diseases, other insect sources feed on the blood of an infected reservoir host and then pass the disease to another victim or susceptible host. Ticks and mosquitoes may transmit diseases, including Lyme disease (ticks) and malaria (mosquitoes). Table 17-1 lists some common diseases and their methods of transmission.

 CHECKPOINT QUESTION

4. The medical office where you work has a policy about not opening windows that do not have screens in examination rooms and the reception area. Why do you think this policy is or is not important?

Principles of Infection Control

Most transmission of infectious disease in the medical office can be prevented by strict adherence to guidelines issued by the Occupational Safety and Health Administration (OSHA) and the Centers for Disease Control and Prevention (CDC). While most medical assistants take extraordinary precautions when dealing

---

BOX 17-1

THE SUSCEPTIBLE HOST

The susceptible host is unable to resist the invading pathogens for a variety of reasons:

- *Age.* As the body ages, defense mechanisms begin to lose their effectiveness. The immune system is no longer as active or as efficient as in youth. The immune system may also not be fully functional in the very young.
- *Existing disease.* The stress of an existing illness may deplete the immune system and allow microorganisms to cause illness in someone who might otherwise be able to fight it naturally.
- *Poor nutrition.* A diet deficient in nutrients such as proteins, carbohydrates, fats, vitamins, or minerals will not allow cells of the body to repair or reproduce as they are weakened by disease.
- *Poor hygiene.* Although multitudes of microbes exist on our skin, keeping the numbers down by practicing good hygiene will reduce the numbers of pathogens.

TABLE 17-1	Common Communicable Diseases
Disease	**Method of Transmission**
AIDS	Contact, or contact with contaminated sharps
Chicken pox (varicella)	Direct contact or droplets
Cholera	Ingestion of contaminated food or water
Diphtheria	Airborne droplets, infected carriers
Hepatitis B	Direct contact with infectious body fluid
Influenza	Airborne droplets, infected carriers or direct contact with contaminated articles such as used tissues
Measles (rubeola)	Airborne droplets, infected carriers
Meningitis	Airborne droplets
Mononucleosis	Airborne droplets or contact with infected saliva
Mumps	Airborne droplets, infected carriers, or direct contact with materials contaminated with infected saliva
Pneumonia	Airborne droplets or direct contact with infected mucus
Rabies	Direct contact with saliva of infected animal such as an animal bite
Rubella (German measles)	Airborne droplets, infected carriers
Tetanus	Direct contact with spores or contaminated animal feces
Tuberculosis	Airborne droplets, infected carriers

PATIENT EDUCATION

BASIC ASEPTIC TECHNIQUE

While performing procedures, take the opportunity to instruct your patients in basic aseptic techniques they can use at home to reduce the spread of disease.

- *Handwashing.* This routine aseptic technique is particularly important for patients and families in preventing the spread of disease. Instruct patients to wash their hands before and after eating meals; after sneezing, coughing, or blowing the nose; after using the bathroom; before and after changing a dressing; and after changing diapers.
- *Use tissue.* Explain to patients with respiratory symptoms that using a disposable tissue to cover the mouth and nose when coughing and sneezing decreases the potential to transmit the illness throughout the household. In addition, immediate and proper disposal of the used tissue is essential to prevent the spread of infection.
- *Changing bandages.* Patients and family members who change dressings on wounds should be instructed in the proper procedure for using sterile dressings and clean bandages. Always demonstrate the procedure for the patient and have the patient or family member return the demonstration to ensure their understanding.
- *Sanitation.* Explain the proper techniques for disposing of waste from members of the household with communicable diseases. If in doubt, consult the local public health department for guidelines.

with patients who are known carriers of infectious microorganisms, you may also treat an estimated five unknown carriers for each patient known to be infectious. Therefore, knowledge and use of effective infection control in relation to all patients is essential.

Medical Asepsis

Medical asepsis does not mean that an object or area is free from all microorganisms. It refers to practices that render an object or area free from pathogenic microorganisms. Commonly known as clean technique, medical asepsis prevents the transmission of microorganisms from one person or area to any other within the medical office (Box 17-2).

Handwashing is the most important medical aseptic technique to prevent the transmission of pathogens. The proper procedure for washing your hands is detailed in Procedure 17-1. Always wash your hands:

BOX 17-2

GUIDELINES FOR MAINTAINING MEDICAL ASEPSIS

- Avoid touching your clothing with soiled linen, table paper, supplies, or instruments. Roll used table paper or linens inward with the clean surface outward.
- Always consider the floor to be contaminated. Any item dropped onto the floor must be considered dirty and be discarded or cleaned to its former level of asepsis before being used.
- Clean tables, counters, and other surfaces frequently and immediately after contamination. Clean areas are less likely than dirty ones to harbor microorganisms or encourage their growth.
- Always presume that blood and body fluids from any source are contaminated. Follow the guidelines published by OSHA and the CDC to protect yourself and to prevent the transmission of disease.

- Before and after every patient contact
- After coming into contact with any blood or body fluids
- After coming into contact with contaminated material
- After handling specimens
- After coughing, sneezing, or blowing your nose
- After using the restroom
- Before and after going to lunch, taking breaks, and leaving for the day

Because you should always assume that blood and body fluids are contaminated with pathogens, you should wear gloves when handling any specimens or when contact with contaminated material is anticipated. However, wearing gloves does not replace handwashing! In fact, your hands should be washed BEFORE you apply gloves and AFTER you remove them in all situations to prevent disease transmission.

Other medical aseptic techniques include general cleaning of the office, including the examination and treatment rooms, waiting or reception area, and clinical work areas. Floors are always considered contaminated, and dust and dirt are vehicles for transmission of microorganisms and should be regularly cleaned from all surfaces, including the floor. In addition, you should teach patients and their caregivers proper medical aseptic techniques for use in the home to prevent the spread of disease.

CHECKPOINT QUESTION

5. Explain why wearing examination gloves does not replace handwashing.

Levels of Infection Control

Sterilization, the highest level of infection control, destroys all forms of microorganisms, including spores, on an inanimate surfaces. Sterilization methods include exposing the articles to various conditions, including steam under pressure in an autoclave; specific gases, such as ethylene oxide; dry heat ovens; and immersion in an approved chemical sterilizing agent (see Chapter 21 for a more complete discussion of sterilization techniques). Instruments or devices that penetrate the skin or come into contact with areas of the body considered sterile, such as the urinary bladder, must be sterilized using one of these methods. To save time, many medical offices use disposable sterile supplies and equipment to eliminate the need for manual sterilization (Fig. 17-2).

The next highest level of infection control is **disinfection.** Disinfectants or germicides inactivate virtually all recognized pathogenic microorganisms except spores on inanimate objects. There are three levels of disinfection—high, intermediate, and low. Each is described in more detail in the following section.

The lowest level of infection control is **sanitization,** which is cleaning any visible contaminants from the item using soap or detergent, water, and manual friction.

Sanitation

Most instruments, equipment, and supplies used in medical offices must be sanitized regularly according to the recommendations of the manufacturer. Sanitation is the maintenance of a healthful, disease-free, and hazard-free environment. **Sanitation** often involves sanitization procedures that reduce the number of microorganisms on an inanimate object to a safe or relatively safe level. This is accomplished by thoroughly cleaning items such as instruments and equipment with warm, soapy water with mechanical action to remove organic matter and other residue. Cleaning or sanitizing must precede disinfection and sterilization.

Disinfection

Disinfectants, or germicides, inactivate virtually all recognized pathogenic microorganisms but not necessarily all microbial forms, including spores, on inanimate objects. The following factors may affect disinfection:

- Prior cleaning of the object. Equipment and supplies that have been sanitized first are more effectively disinfected.

Figure 17-2 Equipment that must be sterile includes items that will penetrate the skin or come into contact with surgical incisions, such as surgical instruments. These items are disposable and meant for one-time use only.

- The amount of organic material on the object. The more organic matter, such as blood or body tissues, on the item, the more disinfectant agent you must use.
- The type of microbial contamination. All blood and body fluids should be considered contaminated with blood-borne pathogens such as hepatitis B and HIV.
- The concentration of the **germicide** or chemical disinfectant that kills pathogens. Disinfectants diluted with water are relatively ineffective at killing microbes.
- The length of exposure to the germicide. The longer the disinfectant comes into contact with the contaminated object, the more thorough disinfection is likely to be.
- The shape or complexity of the object being disinfected. Objects that have rough edges, corners, or otherwise difficult-to-clean areas may require special techniques to disinfect all surfaces.
- The temperature of the process. Most disinfectants work adequately at room temperature.

Disinfection is categorized into three levels—high, intermediate, and low. High-level disinfection destroys most forms of microbial life except certain bacterial spores. This level of infection control, which is slightly less effective than sterilization, is commonly used to clean reusable instruments that come into contact with mucous membrane–lined body cavities that are not considered sterile, such as the vagina and the rectum. Methods of high-level disinfection include immersion in boiling water for 30 minutes (rarely used in the medical office) and immersion in an approved disinfecting chemical, such as glutaraldehyde or isopropyl alcohol for 45 minutes or according to the guidelines in the disinfectant label.

Intermediate-level disinfection destroys many viruses, fungi, and some bacteria, including *Mycobac-terium tuberculosis* (*M. tuberculosis*), the bacterium that causes tuberculosis. However, intermediate disinfection does not kill bacterial spores. Intermediate disinfection is used for surfaces and instruments that come into contact with unbroken skin surfaces, including stethoscopes, blood pressure cuffs, and splints. Commercial chemical germicides that kill *M. tuberculosis* and solutions containing a 1:10 dilution of household bleach (2 oz of chlorine bleach per quart of tap water) are effective intermediate disinfectants.

Low-level disinfection destroys many bacteria and some viruses, but not *M. tuberculosis* or bacterial spores. This type of disinfection is adequate in the medical office for routine cleaning and removing surface debris when no visible blood or body fluids are on the items being disinfected. Disinfectants without tuberculocidal properties are used for low-level disinfection (Fig. 17-3). Table 17-2 describes disinfection methods, uses, and precautions of various chemicals.

✓ CHECKPOINT QUESTION

6. What level of disinfection would you use to clean a reusable instrument that comes into contact with the vaginal mucosa, such as a vaginal speculum? Why?

Occupational Safety and Health Administration Guidelines for the Medical Office

The Occupational Safety and Health Administration (OSHA) is the federal agency responsible for ensuring the safety of all workers, including those in health care.

Figure 17-3 These products destroy many pathogenic microorganisms if used correctly.

TABLE **17-2**	Disinfection Methods
Method	**Uses and Precautions**
Alcohol (70% isopropyl)	Used for noncritical items (countertops, glass thermometers, stethoscopes) Flammable; damages some rubber, plastic, and lenses
Chlorine (sodium hypochlorite or bleach)	Dilute 1:10 (1 part bleach to 10 parts water) Used for a broad spectrum of microbes Inexpensive and fast acting Corrosive, inactivated by organic matter, relatively unstable
Formaldehyde	Disinfectant and sterilant Regulated by OSHA Warnings must be marked on all containers and storage areas
Glutaraldehyde	Alkaline or acid Effective against bacteria, viruses, fungi, and some spores OSHA regulated; requires adequate ventilation, covered pans, gloves, masks; must display biohazard or chemical label
Hydrogen peroxide	Stable and effective when used on inanimate objects Attacks membrane lipids, DNA, and other essential cell components Can damage plastic, rubber, and some metals
Iodine or iodophors	Bacteriostatic agent Not to be used on instruments May cause staining
Phenols (tuberculocidal)	Used for environmental items and equipment Requires gloves and eye protection Can cause skin irritation and burns

DNA, deoxyribonucleic acid; OSHA, Occupational Safety and Health Administration.

OSHA promulgates and enforces federal regulations that must be followed by all medical offices. The practices of individual offices regarding employees' health and safety must be either put into a policy and procedure manual or compiled separately as an infection control manual. Regardless of where the office policies are kept, however, they must be readily available to both employees of the medical office and OSHA representatives.

LEGAL TIP

BLOOD-BORNE PATHOGEN STANDARD TRAINING

According to OSHA, health care facilities, including physician offices, must provide training to newly hired employees who will be exposed to blood or other possibly infectious material while caring for patients. This training must be repeated yearly and include any new issues or policies recommended by OSHA, the CDC, the Department of Health and Human Services, or the US Public Health Service. The following items must be included in the training:

- A description of blood-borne diseases, including the transmission and symptoms
- Personal protective equipment (PPE) available to the employee and the location of the PPE in the medical office
- Information about the risks of contracting hepatitis B and about the HBV vaccine
- The exposure control plan and postexposure procedures, including follow-up care, in the event of an exposure

Exposure Risk Factors and the Exposure Control Plan

Medical offices must provide clear instructions in the policy or infection control manual for preventing employee exposure and reducing the danger of exposure to biohazardous materials. The **exposure risk factor** for each worker by job description must be included in the written policy. It is based on the employee's risk of exposure to communicable disease. Administrative medical assistants have a low exposure risk and require only minimal protection to perform the duties associated with that position. However, clinical medical assistants have a higher exposure risk and require access to a variety of **personal protective equipment (PPE)**, such as gloves, goggles, and/or face shields, depending on the task at hand, and **immunization** against hepatitis B at no charge to the employee. The medical office must provide the appropriate equipment and supplies as outlined in this office policy according to OSHA.

Another written policy required by OSHA for offices with 10 or more employees is the **exposure control plan**. The medical office must have a written plan of action for all employees and visitors who may be exposed to **biohazardous** material despite all precautions. In the event of an exposure, you must first apply the principles of first aid and notify your immediate supervisor, office manager, or the office physician. The physician or supervisor should provide guidance regarding **postexposure testing** and follow-up procedures. Next, you should complete and file an incident report (or exposure report) form explaining the circumstances surrounding the exposure. This report form not only documents the incident, but also allows management to establish a policy to prevent this type of exposure in the future. In addition, the employer must record the exposure on an OSHA 300 log (Fig. 17-4) and report the exposure to OSHA if one or more of the following criteria are present:

- The work-related exposure resulted in loss of consciousness or necessitated a transfer to another job.
- The exposure resulted in a recommendation for medical treatment, such as vaccination or medication to prevent complications.
- The exposure resulted in the conversion of a negative blood test for a contagious disease into a positive blood test in the employee who was exposed.

Box 17-3 describes biohazard and safety equipment commonly used in medical offices.

 CHECKPOINT QUESTION

7. Explain the difference between exposure risk factors and the exposure control plan.

Standard Precautions

Standard precautions are a set of procedures recognized by the CDC to reduce the chance of transmitting infectious microorganisms in any health care setting, including medical offices. By presuming that all blood and body fluids, except perspiration, are contaminated and by following these precautions, you can protect yourself and prevent the spread of disease. Specifically, these precautions pertain to contact with blood, all body fluids except sweat, damaged skin, and mucous membranes and require that you:

- Wash your hands with soap and water after touching blood, body fluids, secretions, and other contaminated items, whether you have worn gloves or not.
- Use an alcohol-based hand rub (foam, lotion, or gel) to decontaminate the hands if the hands are not visibly dirty or contaminated.
- Wear clean nonsterile examination gloves when contact with blood, body fluids, secretions, mucous

membranes, damaged skin, and contaminated items is anticipated.
- Change gloves between procedures on the same patient after exposure to potentially infective material.
- Wear equipment to protect your eyes, nose, and mouth and avoid soiling your clothes by wearing a disposable gown or apron when performing procedures that may splash or spray blood, body fluids, or secretions.
- Dispose of single-use items appropriately; do not disinfect, sterilize, and reuse.
- Take precautions to avoid injuries before, during, and after procedures in which needles, scalpels, or other sharp instruments have been used on a patient.
- Do not recap used needles or otherwise manipulate them by bending or breaking. If recapping is necessary to carry a used needle to a sharps container, use a one-handed scoop technique or a device for holding the needle sheath (see Chapter 24).
- Place used disposable syringes and needles and other sharps in a puncture-resistant container (sharps) as close as possible to the area of use.
- Use barrier devices (e.g., mouthpieces, resuscitation bags) as alternatives to mouth-to-mouth resuscitation (see Chapter 26).
- Do not eat, drink, or put candy, gum, or mints into your mouth while working in the clinical area.

 CHECKPOINT QUESTION

8. How will following standard precautions help to protect you against contracting an infection or communicable disease?

Personal Protective Equipment

In any area of the medical office where exposure to biohazardous materials might occur, PPE must be made available and used by all health care workers, including medical assistants. For instance:

- Gloves must be available and accessible throughout the office. If you or a patient is sensitive to the latex found in regular examination gloves, proper alternatives such as vinyl gloves must be available (Box 17-4).
- Disposable gowns, goggles, and face shields must be available in areas where splattering or splashing of airborne particles may occur (Fig. 17-5)
- You must wear gloves when performing any procedure that carries any risk of exposure, such as surgical procedures or drawing blood specimens, disposing of biohazardous waste, or touching or handling surfaces that have been contaminated with biohazardous materials, or if there is any chance at all, no matter how remote, that you may come into contact with blood or body fluids.

OSHA's Form 300

Log of Work-Related Injuries and Illnesses

Year 20____

U.S. Department of Labor
Occupational Safety and Health Administration

Form approved OMB no. 1218-0176

Attention: This form contains information relating to employee health and must be used in a manner that protects the confidentiality of employees to the extent possible while the information is being used for occupational safety and health purposes.

You must record information about every work-related death and about every work-related injury or illness that involves loss of consciousness, restricted work activity or job transfer, days away from work, or medical treatment beyond first aid. You must also record significant work-related injuries and illnesses that are diagnosed by a physician or licensed health care professional. You must also record work-related injuries and illnesses that meet any of the specific recording criteria listed in 29 CFR Part 1904.8 through 1904.12. Feel free to use two lines for a single case if you need to. You must complete an Injury and Illness Incident Report (OSHA Form 301) or equivalent form for each injury or illness recorded on this form. If you're not sure whether a case is recordable, call your local OSHA office for help.

Establishment name _____

City _____ State _____

Identify the person

(A) Case no.	(B) Employee's name	(C) Job title (e.g., Welder)

Describe the case

(D) Date of injury or onset of illness	(E) Where the event occurred (e.g., Loading dock north end)	(F) Describe injury or illness, parts of body affected, and object/substance that directly injured or made person ill (e.g., Second degree burns on right forearm from acetylene torch)
month/day		

Classify the case

Using these four categories, check ONLY the most serious result for each case:

Death (G)	Days away from work (H)	Remained at work — Job transfer or restriction (I)	Remained at work — Other recordable cases (J)

Enter the number of days the injured or ill worker was:

On job transfer or restriction (K)	Away from work (L)
____ days	____ days

Check the "Injury" column or choose one type of illness:

(M)				
Injury (1)	Skin disorder (2)	Respiratory condition (3)	Poisoning (4)	All other illnesses (5)

Page totals ►

Be sure to transfer these totals to the Summary page (Form 300A) before you post it.

Page ____ of ____

Public reporting burden for this collection of information is estimated to average 14 minutes per response, including time to review the instructions, search and gather the data needed, and complete and review the collection of information. Persons are not required to respond to the collection of information unless it displays a currently valid OMB control number. If you have any comments about these estimates or any other aspects of this data collection, contact: US Department of Labor, OSHA Office of Statistics, Room N-3644, 200 Constitution Avenue, NW, Washington, DC 20210. Do not send the completed forms to this office.

Figure 17-4 The OSHA 300 Log. (Courtesy of the US Department of Labor.)

BOX 17-3

BIOHAZARD AND SAFETY EQUIPMENT IN THE MEDICAL OFFICE

- *MSDS binder.* Material safety data sheets (MSDS) are forms prepared by the manufacturers of all chemical substances used in the medical office. The binder should contain sheets for all chemicals used in the office. Each sheet describes how to handle and dispose of the chemical and, most important, the health hazards of the chemical and safety equipment needed when using it.

- *Biohazard waste containers.* Only waste contaminated with blood or body fluids or other potentially infectious material (OPIM) should be placed in biohazard waste containers. Sharps containers are used for disposal of items that have the potential to puncture or cut the skin.

- *Personal protective equipment.* Employers are required to provide PPE appropriate to the risk of exposure. For example, employees who may come into contact with blood, such as the clinical medical assistant giving an injection, need be protected only by wearing gloves. However, situations that may cause a splash or splatter of blood require full coverage of the skin, eyes, and clothing.

- *Eyewash basin.* Pressing the lever on the basin and turning on the faucets produces a stream of water that forces open the caps of the eyewash basin. To remove contaminants or chemicals from the eyes, lower your face into the stream and continue to wash the area until the eyes are clear or for the amount of time recommended on the MSDS.

- *Immunization.* Employers are required by OSHA to provide immunization against blood-borne pathogens if vaccines are available.

BOX 17-4

LATEX ALLERGY AND PREVENTION

The incidence among health care workers of allergic reactions to proteins in latex has increased in recent years. The proteins in latex, a product of the rubber tree that is used to make many products including examination gloves, may cause allergic reactions, especially with repeated exposure. The reactions can be mild (skin redness or rash, itching, or hives) or severe (difficulty breathing, coughing, or wheezing). Respiratory reactions often result when the powder in the gloves becomes airborne and is inhaled as the gloves are removed after use. To protect yourself from exposure and allergy to latex, the following guidelines may be useful:

- Use gloves that are not latex for tasks that do not involve contact or potential contact with blood or body fluids.
- When contact with blood or body fluids is possible, wear powder-free latex gloves. Powder-free gloves contain less protein than the powdered ones, reducing the risk of allergy.
- Avoid wearing oil-based lotions or hand creams before applying latex gloves. The oil in these products can break down the latex, releasing the proteins that cause the allergic reactions.
- Wash your hands thoroughly after removing latex gloves.
- Recognize the symptoms of latex allergy in yourself, your co-workers, and your patients.

✓ CHECKPOINT QUESTION

9. What PPE should you wear when assisting the physician with a wound irrigation?

WHAT IF?

What if your patient is offended that you are wearing gloves when drawing a blood specimen?

Sometimes patients become defensive and make statements to the effect that they are "disease free." If this happens to you, reassure the patient by saying that wearing gloves is a standard practice and is used for the protection of the patient also. Use this occasion to teach the patient about standard precautions and the importance of following these guidelines.

Employers who do not make this equipment available are not in compliance with OSHA regulations and may face significant fines. However, employees are responsible for using the PPE correctly and appropriately and washing their hands frequently throughout the day. Remember, pathogens may be carried home to family members and to other persons who come into contact with you or the patient. When removing PPE after a procedure, remove all protective barriers before removing your gloves. Once you have removed all PPE, including your contaminated gloves (Procedure 17-2), always wash your hands (see Procedure 17-1).

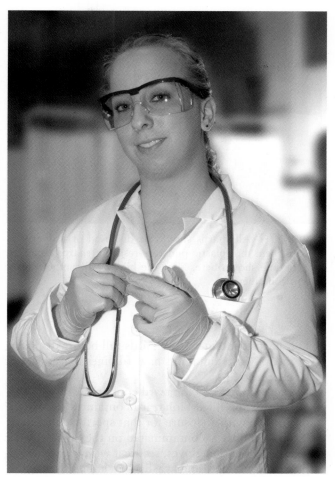

Figure 17-5 Personal protective equipment that must be provided for employees who may come into contact with contaminated materials includes gloves, goggles, face shields, and gowns or aprons to protect clothing.

Handling Environmental Contamination

Although not all equipment or surfaces in the medical office must be sterile (free from all microorganisms), all equipment and areas must be clean. Sanitization is cleaning or washing equipment or surfaces by removing all visible soil. Any detergent or low-level disinfectant can be used to clean and disinfect areas such as floors, examination tables, cabinets, and countertops. Because you may be expected to perform cleaning tasks routinely or when these surfaces become soiled with visible blood or body fluids, you should understand how these procedures are correctly performed.

Any surface contaminated with biohazardous materials should be promptly cleaned using an approved germicide or a dilute bleach solution. OSHA requires that spill kits or appropriate supplies be available, and commercial kits make cleaning contaminated surfaces relatively safe and easy. Commercial kits include clean

gloves, eye protection if there is a risk of splashing, a gel to absorb the biohazardous material, a scoop, towels, and a biohazard waste container to discard all used items (Fig. 17-6). If your office does not purchase commercial kits, you should gather and store the following items together in the event that a biohazardous spill occurs:

- Eye protection, such as goggles
- Clean examination gloves
- Absorbent powder, crystals, or gel
- Paper towels
- A disposable scoop
- At least one biohazard waste bag
- A chemical disinfectant

In some cases, you may need a sharps container (Fig. 17-7) and spill control barriers. If there is a large amount of contamination on the floor, you should put on disposable shoe coverings to avoid transmitting microorganisms on your shoes. All gloves, paper towels, eye protection, and shoe coverings should be discarded in the biohazardous waste bags, which must be disposed of properly. Procedure 17-3 outlines the procedure for an area contaminated with blood or body fluids.

Although most medical offices use disposable patient gowns and drapes, some offices continue to use cloth. Hygienic storage of clean linens is recommended, and proper handling of soiled linens, disposable or not, is required. After applying clean examination gloves, handle soiled linen, including examination table paper, as little as possible by folding it carefully so that the most contaminated surface is turned inward to prevent contamination of the air. Contaminated linen should be placed in a biohazard bag in the examination room where the contamination occurred rather than carried through the hallways of the medical office. Some offices using cloth linens and contract with an outside company for the laundering. If linen materials are laundered at the office, use normal laundry cycles following the recommendations of the washer, detergent, and fabric.

 CHECKPOINT QUESTION

10. How would you respond to an employee in the medical office who is unsure about how to clean up a spilled urine specimen? Is this biohazardous?

Disposing of Infectious Waste

Federal regulations from the Environmental Protection Agency (EPA) and OSHA set the policies and guidelines for disposing of hazardous materials, but individual states determine policies based on these guidelines. As a result, policies vary widely, and you should review your state and local regulations before making waste disposal decisions. Most medical offices are considered small

Figure 17-6 A commercially prepared biohazard spill kit contains gloves, absorbent material, eye protection, and a biohazard bag for proper disposal. (Courtesy of Caltech Industries, Midland, MI.)

Figure 17-7 All sharps should be disposed of properly by placing them in a plastic puncture-resistant sharps container like the one shown here. Note the biohazard symbol on the sharps container.

generators of waste because they produce less than 50 pounds of waste each month. Facilities such as hospitals and large clinics that generate more than 50 pounds are considered large generators and must obtain a certificate of registration from the EPA and maintain a record of the quantity of waste and disposal procedures.

To remain compliant with any state and federal laws, facilities that are considered large generators of infectious waste and some smaller medical offices use an infectious waste service to dispose of biohazardous waste appropriately and safely. These services supply the office with appropriate waste containers and pick up filled containers regularly (Box 17-5). Once the filled containers are picked up by the waste service, the infectious waste is disposed of according to EPA and OSHA guidelines. The service maintains a tracking record listing the type of waste, its weight in pounds, and the disposal destination. When the waste has been destroyed, a tracking form documenting the disposal is sent to the medical office and should be retained in the office records for 3 years. This documentation must be provided to the EPA should an audit be performed to assess compliance. States impose stiff penalties, including fines and/or imprisonment, for violations of regulations involving biohazardous waste.

Because the fee charged by an infectious waste service is based on the type and amount of waste generated, you should follow these guidelines to help keep the cost down while maintaining safety:

• Use separate containers for each type of waste. Don't put bandages in sharps containers (puncture-resistant containers for needles or other sharp items) or paper towels used for routine handwashing in a biohazard bag.

• Fill sharps containers two-thirds full before disposing of them. Most containers have fill lines that must not be exceeded.
• Use only approved biohazard containers.
• When moving filled biohazard containers, secure the bag or top with a closure for that specific container.
• If the container is contaminated on the outside, wear clean examination gloves, secure it within another approved container, and wash your hands thoroughly afterward.
• Place biohazard waste for pick up by the service in a secure, designated area.

 CHECKPOINT QUESTION

11. After drawing a blood specimen from a patient, you notice that the tube of blood is leaking onto the examination table where you put it while finishing the procedure. How do you clean up the blood spill?

Hepatitis B and Human Immunodeficiency Viruses

One of the most persistent health care concerns in the medical office is the transmission of hepatitis B virus (HBV) and human immunodeficiency virus (HIV). Although HIV is the most visible public concern, HBV has been an occupational hazard for health care professionals for many years. HBV is more viable than HIV and may survive in a dried state on clinical equipment and counter surfaces at room temperature for more than a week. In this dried state, HBV may be passed through the medical setting by way of contact with contaminated hands, gloves, or other means of di-

BOX 17-5

BIOHAZARD WASTE DISPOSAL

A regular waste container should be used only for disposal of waste that is not biohazardous, such as paper, plastic, disposable tray wrappers, packaging material, unused gauze, and examination table paper. To prevent leakage and mess, nonbiohazardous liquids should be discarded in a sink or other washbasin, not in the plastic bag inside the waste can. Biohazard liquid spills (any waste containing blood or other body fluids) should be cleaned according to the office policy using the guidelines noted in Procedure 17-3. Never discard sharps of any kind in plastic bags; these are not puncture resistant, and injury may result even with careful handling. Regardless of the type of waste container used (biohazard or nonbiohazard), bags should not be filled to capacity. When the plastic bag is about two-thirds full, it should be removed from the waste can, with the top edges brought together and secured by tying or with a twist tie. Remove the bag from the area and follow the office policy and procedures for disposal. Put a fresh plastic bag into the waste can.

◆ TRIAGE

The following three situations occur at the same time in the office where you are employed:

A. You have just finished changing the dressing on a wound that is draining a moderate amount of blood. You still have your gloves on, but you need to document the procedure in the patient's medical record and instruct the patient regarding wound care.

B. As you are cleaning up the materials used to irrigate the wound, you spill the basin used to collect the irrigating solution and blood obtained from the procedure.

C. Another staff member knocks on the door of the examination room and informs you that you have a phone call.

How do you sort these tasks? What do you do first? Second? Third?

Tell the staff member in situation C that you cannot take a phone call now and ask him or her to take a message or refer the call to another medical assistant. The spill in situation B is a biohazardous spill and should be cleaned up and the area decontaminated immediately. You should be familiar with the policy and procedures of the medical office and clean the spill accordingly. Once the spill is cleaned and decontaminated, remove your gloves and wash your hands. Document the wound irrigation, dressing change, and patient education in situation A only after removing your gloves and washing your hands. To prevent the spread of microorganisms to the medical record, you should never handle the medical record while wearing contaminated gloves.

---

rect transmission. Fortunately, HBV can be contained by the proper use of standard precautions, and it can be killed easily by cleaning with a dilute bleach solution.

HBV and HIV are both transmitted through exposure to contaminated blood and body fluids. Accidental punctures with sharp objects contaminated with blood are one way to become infected, but the viruses may also enter the body through broken skin. Disorders of the skin, including dry cracked skin, dermatitis, eczema, and psoriasis, also allow entrance into the body if contact with contaminated surfaces or equipment occurs.

While there is no vaccine to prevent infection with HIV, employers whose workers, including clinical medical assistants, are at risk for HBV exposure are mandated by OSHA to provide the vaccine to prevent HBV at no cost to the employee. This vaccine is given in a series of three injections that normally produce immunity to the disease. It is recommended that a blood sample be drawn 6 months after the third injection of HBV vaccine to determine whether the person has developed immunity. The blood test can detect the presence, or titer, of antibodies against hepatitis B. The series is repeated if HBV immunity is not found, but the vaccine has been found to be very effective. The immunity may last as long as 10 years. Employees who choose not to receive the vaccine must sign a waiver or release form stating that they are aware of the risks associated with HBV. Individuals who contract hepatitis B may develop cirrhosis (destruction of the cells of the liver) and are at increased risk for developing liver cancer.

In the event of exposure to blood or body fluids infected with HBV, the postexposure plan should include an immediate blood test of the employee. Repeat blood titers should be obtained at specific intervals, usually 6 weeks, 3 months, 6 months, 9 months, and 1 year, as a comparison. If you have been immunized against HBV, usually no further treatment is required. However, if you waive the HBV series, hepatitis B immunoglobulin can be given by injection for immediate short-term protection, and the general series of three immunizations should be started.

The same schedule of evaluation is required after HIV exposure. Again, there is no vaccine to prevent HIV, but other HIV treatments for preventing transmission are being tested.

 CHECKPOINT QUESTION

12. Which virus is more of a threat to the clinical medical assistant: HIV or HBV? Why?

 MEDIA MENU

- **Student CD**
  - **Case Study**
    Clinical Interactive Case Study 3: Dealing with a Sick Patient, Infection Control, and Medication Administration
  - **Video Procedure**
    Procedure 17-1 video clip
  - **CMA/RMA Certification Exam Review**
- **Premium Online Course**
  http://thePoint.lww.com/Kronenberger3e
- **LWW's Medical Assisting Skills DVD**
  - **Procedures 17-1, 17-2**
- **Internet Resources**

LiveAdvise Online Tutoring & Competency Training
http://thePoint.lww.com/LiveAdvise

Occupational Safety and Health Administration (OSHA)
http://www.osha.gov

Latex Allergy Prevention
http://www.cdc.gov/niosh/

Infection Control
http://www.cdc.gov/ncidod/dhqp/index.html

Food and Drug Administration
http://www.fda.gov

PROCEDURE 17-1: **Handwashing for Medical Asepsis**

Purpose: To prevent the growth and spread of pathogens
Equipment: Liquid soap, disposable paper towels, an orangewood manicure stick, a waste can
Standard: This task should take 2–3 minutes.

Steps	Purpose
1. Remove all rings and your wristwatch if it cannot be pushed up onto the forearm.	Rings and watches may harbor pathogens that may not be easily washed away. Ideally, rings should not be worn when working with material that may be infectious.
2. Stand close to the sink without touching it.	The sink is considered contaminated, and standing too close may contaminate your clothing.
3. Turn on the faucet and adjust the temperature of the water to warm.	Water that is too hot or too cold will crack or chap the skin on the hands, which will break the natural protective barrier that prevents infection.
4. Wet your hands and wrists under the warm running water, apply liquid soap, and work the soap into a lather by rubbing your palms together and rubbing the soap between your fingers at least 10 times.	This motion dislodges microorganisms from between the fingers and removes transient and some resident organisms.

Step 4. Wet hands and wrists.

Steps	Purpose
5. Scrub the palm of one hand with the fingertips of the other hand to work the soap under the nails of that hand; then reverse the procedure and scrub the other hand. Also scrub each wrist.	Friction helps remove microorganisms.

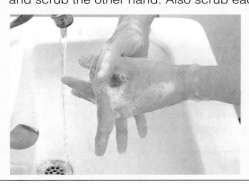

Step 5. Wash hands and wrists with firm rubbing and circular motions.

(continued)

PROCEDURE 17-1: **Handwashing for Medical Asepsis** *(continued)*

Steps	Purpose
6. Rinse hands and wrists thoroughly under running warm water, holding hands lower than elbows; do not touch the inside of the sink. **Step 6.** Rinse hands thoroughly.	Holding the hands lower than the elbows and wrists allows microorganisms to flow off the hands and fingers rather than back up the arms.
7. Using the orangewood stick, clean under each nail on both hands.	Nails may harbor microorganisms. Metal files and pointed instruments may break the skin and make an opening for microorganisms. This may be done at the beginning of the day, before leaving for the day, or after coming into contact with potentially infectious material.
8. Reapply liquid soap and rewash hands and wrists.	Rewashing the hands after using the orangewood stick washes away any microorganisms that may have been removed with the orangewood stick.
9. Rinse hands thoroughly again while holding hands lower than wrists and elbows.	
10. Gently dry hands with a paper towel. Discard the paper towel and the used orangewood stick when finished. **Step 10.** Dry hands gently with a paper towel.	Hands must be dried thoroughly and completely to prevent drying and cracking.
11. Use a dry paper towel to turn off the faucets and discard the paper towel.	Your hands are clean and should not touch the contaminated faucet handles.

PROCEDURE 17-2:   Removing Contaminated Gloves

Purpose: To remove contaminated gloves to prevent the spread of pathogenic microorganisms
Equipment: Clean examination gloves; biohazard waste container
Standard: This task should take 1–2 minutes.

Steps	Purpose
1. Choose the appropriate size gloves for your hands and put them on.	Gloves should fit comfortably, not too loose and not too tight.
2. To remove gloves, grasp the glove of your nondominant hand at the palm and pull the glove away.	To avoid transferring contaminants to the wrist, be sure not to grasp the glove at the wrist. **Step 2.** Grasp the palm of the glove on your nondominant gloved hand.
3. Slide your hand out of the glove, rolling the glove into the palm of the gloved dominant hand.	You should avoid touching either glove with your ungloved hand. **Step 3A.** Carefully remove the glove and avoid contaminating your bare skin. **Step 3B.** Grasp the soiled glove with your gloved dominant hand.

(continued)

PROCEDURE 17-2:   **Removing Contaminated Gloves** *(continued)*

Steps	Purpose
4. Holding the soiled glove in the palm of your gloved hand, slip your ungloved fingers under the cuff of the glove you are still wearing, being careful not to touch the outside of the glove.	Skin should touch skin but never the soiled part of the glove.

Step 4. Slip your free hand under the cuff of the remaining glove.

Steps	Purpose
5. Stretch the glove of the dominant hand up and away from your hand while turning it inside out, with the already removed glove balled up inside.	Turning it inside out ensures that the soiled surfaces of the gloves are enclosed.

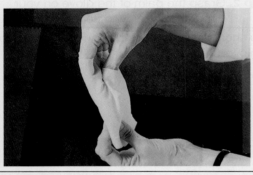

Step 5. Remove the glove by turning it inside out over the previously removed glove.

6. Both gloves should now be removed, with the first glove inside the second glove and the second glove inside out.

7. Discard both gloves as one unit into a biohazard waste receptacle.

8. Wash your hands.   Wearing gloves is NOT a substitute for washing your hands!

PROCEDURE 17-3:   Cleaning Biohazardous Spills

Purpose: To clean contaminated surfaces
Equipment: Commercially prepared germicide OR 1:10 bleach solution, gloves, disposable towels, chemical absorbent, biohazardous waste bag, protective eye wear (goggles or mask and face shield), disposable shoe coverings, disposable gown or apron made of plastic or other material that is impervious to soaking up contaminated fluids
Standard: This task should take 3–5 minutes.

Steps	Purpose
1. Put on gloves. Wear protective eyewear, gown or apron, and shoe coverings if you anticipate any splashing.	A plastic gown or apron will protect your clothing from contaminants.
2. Apply chemical absorbent material to the spill as indicated by office policy. Clean up the spill with disposable paper towels, being careful not to splash.	
	Step 2. Wearing PPE, carefully clean up biohazardous spills immediately after they occur.
3. Dispose of paper towels and absorbent material in a biohazard waste bag.	The bag will alert anyone handling the waste that it contains biohazardous material.
4. Spray the area with commercial germicide or bleach solution and wipe with disposable paper towels. Discard towels in a biohazard bag.	
	Step 4. Place contaminated materials into a biohazard bag.

(continued)

PROCEDURE 17-3:	Cleaning Biohazardous Spills *(continued)*

Steps	Purpose
5. With your gloves on, remove the protective eyewear and discard or disinfect per office policy. Remove the gown or apron and shoe coverings and put in the biohazard bag if disposable or the biohazard laundry bag for reusable linens.	
6. Place the biohazard bag in an appropriate waste receptacle for removal according to your facility's policy.	
7. Remove your gloves and wash your hands thoroughly.	Wearing gloves does not replace proper handwashing.

Chapter Summary

- Following the principles of medical asepsis and infection control helps ensure a safe environment for patients and health care providers in the medical office. If you fail to follow these principles consistently, you will place yourself and others at risk for infection that may impair patients' recovery and affect health care workers' performance.
- Although avoiding contact with microorganisms in the environment is impossible, sanitation and disinfection will reduce the numbers of microorganisms and potential pathogens, making the environment clean and as disease free as possible.

- OSHA and the CDC issue regulations and standards for health care workers who work with blood and body fluids, and you must always follow them, including wearing PPE. In case of exposure, your office must have an exposure control plan and a postexposure plan to assist you in receiving appropriate medical attention and follow-up care.
- *Remember*: Handwashing is the single most effective measure to prevent the spread of infection.

Warm Ups   for Critical Thinking

1. Review Table 17-1 on common communicable diseases. Create a patient education brochure that focuses on the spread of these diseases.

2. A patient who comes into your office has a leg wound that must be cared for at home. When asked about caring for the wound, he tells you that he knows how to do it, but you think he may be confused about the importance of using medical asepsis. How do you handle this situation?

3. On a busy morning in the medical office, you accidentally spill a small amount of urine from a speci-

men container onto the counter. Your co-worker needs you to assist with a pediatric injection in the examination room down the hall. Would it be acceptable to clean up the urine spill after you help your co-worker? Why or why not?

4. Develop a written policy for new employees regarding disinfecting individual examination rooms in the medical office. Be specific and include issues related to safety.

1. Pathogenic microorganisms are microscopic organisms that cause disease. Natural ways that the body stops an invasion or destroys pathogens include tears (wash microbes away from the eyes and contain lysozyme, an effective disinfectant); hydrochloric acid in the stomach (produces a pH that kills many microbes that may get into the stomach); unbroken or intact skin (provides a barrier to invading microorganism); and mucous membranes and cilia lining the respiratory tract (trap microorganisms that may be inhaled).

2. The conditions that favor the growth of microorganisms include moisture, nutrients, a warm temperature, darkness, a neutral or slightly alkaline pH, and oxygen. To prevent the growth of microbes, remove any moisture or sources of nutrition, use heat higher than 98.6°F, expose the area to light, or clean with acidic or alkaline chemicals.

3. The first link in the infection cycle (the reservoir host) provides nutrients and an incubation site for the pathogen. The fifth link (the susceptible host) allows the pathogen to enter and begin growing, thus becoming the new reservoir host, repeating the cycle.

4. Opening screenless windows allows insects to come into the office. Insects may be reservoir hosts to certain diseases and contaminate items in the medical office.

5. Gloves are a barrier to prevent the skin from coming into contact with contaminated materials. However, once they are removed, standard precautions require that the hands be washed as an additional precaution.

6. Items or instruments that come into contact with unbroken mucous membranes in areas of the body that are not considered sterile (like the vagina) may be safely disinfected using a high-level disinfectant for the specified period.

7. Exposure risk factors are associated with specific jobs in terms of exposure to biohazardous or contaminated materials. The exposure control plan is a written document outlining the procedure that an employee or visitor should take to prevent contact with biohazardous material.

8. Following the standard precautions will help to protect you against contracting an infection or disease by preventing entrance of the pathogenic microorganisms into your body.

9. A wound irrigation requires wearing gloves and covering the eyes, nose, and mouth. This procedure has the potential to splash microorganisms into the environment.

10. Urine may be biohazardous and should be cleaned up by applying clean examination gloves, using paper towels or absorbent powder to absorb the urine, and placing all items used for cleaning up the spill into a biohazardous waste container. Once the urine is absorbed and discarded appropriately, the area or floor should be disinfected.

11. Again, all blood should be considered contaminated and should be cleaned up using the commercially prepared spill kit or with items assembled from the office. The broken blood tube should be placed in a sharps container, and once the blood has been wiped up, the table should be disinfected.

12. The virus that is actually more of a threat to the medical assistant is HBV. HBV may live in dried body secretions on an inanimate surface for up to 2 weeks. In the "right" circumstances, contact with these dried secretions may cause infection in the exposed individual. Hepatitis B is a serious disease and may cause scarring and destruction of the liver tissue (leading to liver failure), an increased risk for developing liver cancer, and death.

Medical History and Patient Assessment

Outline

The Medical History
Methods of Collecting
Information
Elements of the Medical
History

Conducting the Patient Interview
Preparing for the Interview
Introducing Yourself
Barriers to Communication

Assessing the Patient
Signs and Symptoms
Chief Complaint and Present
Illness

Learning Objectives

Upon successfully completing this chapter, you will be able to:

1. Spell and define key terms

2. Give examples of the type of information included in each section of the patient history

3. Identify guidelines for conducting a patient interview using principles of verbal and nonverbal communication

4. Explain the difference between a sign and a symptom and give examples of each

5. Discuss open-ended and closed-ended questions and explain when to use each type during the patient interview

Performance Objectives

Upon successfully completing this chapter, you will be able to:

1. Obtain and record a patient history using appropriate communication techniques (Procedure 18-1)

2. Accurately document a chief complaint and present illness (Procedure 18-2)

CAAHEP

- Obtain and record patient history
- Recognize and respond to verbal communications
- Recognize and respond to nonverbal communications
- Document appropriately

ABHES

- Be impartial and show empathy when dealing with patients
- Interview effectively
- Recognize and respond to verbal and nonverbal communication
- Interview and take patient history

Key Terms

assessment	familial	homeopathic	signs
chief complaint	hereditary	medical history	symptoms
demographic	HIPAA	over-the-counter	

To diagnose a patient's present illness, the physician needs the patient's past and current health information. As a professional medical assistant, you are often responsible for obtaining this information as part of the **medical history** and **assessment**. The medical history is a record containing information about a patient's past and present health status, the health status of related family members, and relevant information about a patient's social habits. Assessment begins with gathering information to determine the patient's problem or reason for seeking medical care. Typically, you ask standard questions and document the patient's responses during the assessment on preprinted forms or in a manner decided by the physician and outlined in the medical office policy and procedure manual.

The Medical History

Methods of Collecting Information

To complete the patient's medical history, you and the physician work cooperatively with the patient. In some medical practices, medical assistants gather initial patient information by interviewing the patient using a printed list of questions. Other medical offices ask the patient to fill out a standard form before or during the first appointment. Patients who receive the form in the mail are instructed to bring the completed document to the office at the initial visit. In either case, you must check the form for completeness because the physician uses this information as the basis for more extensive questioning during the examination.

In other practices, the physician may prefer to complete the medical history form during the initial patient interview and examination. In this situation, you should be familiar with the form and ready to assist the physician if needed or asked to do so.

Elements of the Medical History

The medical history forms used by the office may vary with the practice specialty, but most forms are composed of these common elements: identifying data (database), past history (PH), review of systems (ROS), family history (FH), and social history. Figure 18-1 shows a medical history form. This information is confidential and protected by the Health Insurance Portability and Accountability Act, or **HIPAA**, a federal law that protects the privacy of health information. No one except those directly involved in the patient's care may have access to it without the patient's permission.

The following are the main elements of the medical history:

- Identifying data (database). The **demographic** information in this section, required for administrative purposes, always includes the patient's name, address, and phone number. It also includes the name,

Professional Medical Associates – History Form

NAME: _____ DATE OF BIRTH: _____

What is the main reason for your visit to the doctor? _____

_____

Were you referred? _____ if so, by whom? _____

PAST MEDICAL HISTORY:

Are you allergic to any medication? _____

If so, list medications: _____

List current medications, dosage, and how many times a day you take them:

Medication   **Dose**   **Times A Day**

_____

_____

Alcohol Consumption: What type? _____ Amount _____ How Often? _____

                   History of Alcoholism? _____

When was your last TB or Tine test? _____

Have you ever had a positive test for tuberculosis? _____

When was your last Tetanus shot? _____

List all surgeries you have had in the past:

Date   **Type of Surgery**

_____

_____

List all past hospitalizations (not involving surgeries above):

Date   **Reason For Hospital Stay**

_____

List all past problems with trauma (broken bones, lacerations, etc.):

_____

REVIEW OF SYSTEMS, PAST MEDICAL PROBLEMS:
If you have been told you have any of the problems listed below, or are having any of the problems listed below,
please CIRCLE:

1. <u>GENERAL:</u> Weight loss, weight gain, fever, chills, night sweats, hot flashes, tire easily, problems with sleep, crying spells, history of cancer.

2. <u>SKIN:</u> Rash, sores that won't heal, moles that are new or changing, history of skin problems.

3. <u>HEENT:</u> Headache, eye problems, hearing problems, sinus problems, hay fever, dizziness, hoarseness, sores in your mouth that won't heal, dental problems.

    Do you chew tobacco or dip snuff? _____

4. <u>METABOLIC/ENDOCRINE:</u> Thyroid problems, diabetes or sugar problems, high cholesterol.

Figure 18-1 A sample medical history form, front and back.

5. RESPIRATORY: Cough, wheezing, breathing problems, history of asthma, history of lung problems.

   Do you smoke cigarettes or pipe? _____

   How much? _____ For how long? _____

6. BREAST (WOMEN): Breast lumps, changes in nipples, nipple discharge, breast problems, family history of breast cancer. When was your last mammogram? _____

7. CARDIOVASCULAR: Heart murmur, rheumatic fever, high blood pressure, angina, heart problems, heart attack, abnormal heart rhythm, chest pain, palpitations, leg swelling, history of phlebitis or blood clots.

8. GI: Problems with appetite, swallowing, heartburn, nausea, vomiting, pain in the abdomen, constipation, diarrhea, blood in stool, history of ulcers, liver problems, hepatitis, jaundice, pancreas problems, gallbladder problems, or colon problems.

9. REPRODUCTIVE (WOMEN): Problems with irregular menstrual cycles, abnormal vaginal bleeding or discharge, history of sexually transmitted diseases, sexual problems.

   AGE OF FIRST MENSES (PERIOD) _____ AGE OF MENOPAUSE _____

   LAST PAP SMEAR _____ METHOD OF CONTRACEPTION _____

   Obstetric History (Women)

   NUMBER OF PREGNANCIES _____ PLEASE LIST AS FOLLOWS:

   Delivery Date   Pregnancy Complications   Type Delivery   Baby's Weight

   _____

   _____

   MEN: Problems with genital discharge, history of venereal diseases, sexual problems, prostate problems.

   METHOD OF CONTRACEPTION _____

10. UROLOGIC: Problems with painful urination, urinary frequency, blood in urine, weak urinary stream, history of bladder or kidney infections, or kidney stones.

11. MUSCULOSKELETAL: Arthritis, back pain, cramps in legs.

12. NEUROLOGIC: Seizures, stroke, arm or leg weakness or numbness, black-out spells, memory or thinking problems, depression, anxiety, psychiatric problems.

13. HEMATOLOGIC: Anemia, bleeding problems, enlarged lymph nodes.

HAVE YOU EVER HAD A BLOOD TRANSFUSION? _____ DATE _____

FAMILY HISTORY:

List any medical problems that run in your family and which family members have these problems.

_____

_____

SOCIAL HISTORY:

MARITAL STATUS: _____

OCCUPATION: _____

EDUCATION: _____

HOBBIES: _____

WHAT DO YOU DO FOR ENJOYMENT? _____

Figure 18-1 *(continued)*

TRIAGE

While working in the medical office, you begin the day by placing the following three patients into examination rooms:

A. Patient A, a new patient, arrives on time and was given the two-page medical history form to complete.

B. Patient B is an established patient who is scheduled to have his blood pressure checked today because he started a new antihypertensive medication last month.

C. Patient C is a 1-year-old baby who is scheduled to be seen today for a well-child checkup and immunizations.

How would you sort these patients? Who should be seen first? Second? Third?

Patient B should be called back first, since he will probably take the least amount of time. Unless this patient's blood pressure is not responding to the antihypertensive medication or he has unanticipated problems, this type of visit is typically conducted in a timely manner as a convenience to the patient. Patient C should be seen next, since infant checkups usually require additional procedures that may require more time from the medical assistant and physician. Patient A should be given an adequate amount of time to complete the medical history forms, since this information will be necessary for the physician to understand the patient's current and future health problems. The patient should not be rushed to complete this paperwork. If necessary, you may call the patient back and assist with completion of the form, especially if the patient is having difficulty due to a physical disability, such as visual impairment, deformity, or trouble holding a pen or pencil because of arthritis.

address, and phone number of the patient's employer and insurance carrier and the patient's health insurance policy number, social security number, marital status, gender, and race.

- Past history (PH). This section addresses the patient's prior health status and helps the physician plan appropriate care for any present illness. Information in this section typically includes allergies, immunizations, childhood diseases, current and past medications, and previous illnesses, surgeries, and hospitalizations.
- Review of systems (ROS). A thorough review of each body system may elicit information that the patient forgot to mention earlier or thought was irrelevant. Specific questions, such as symptoms or known diseases, related to each system of the body are included in this section.
- Family history (FH). This section contains the health status of the patient's parents, siblings, and grandparents. This information is important because certain diseases or disorders have **familial** or **hereditary** tendencies. Familial diseases tend to occur often in a particular family, whereas hereditary diseases are transmitted from parent to offspring. If any immediate family member is deceased, the cause of death should be documented.
- Social history. The social history covers the patient's lifestyle, such as marital status, occupation, education, and hobbies. It may also include information about the patient's diet, use of alcohol or tobacco, and sexual history. This information may help the physician understand how present illness, including any treatment, may affect the lifestyle or how the lifestyle may affect the illness. The social history may also provide a guide for patient education, since some behaviors, such as tobacco use or a diet high in fat, may not yet be causing illness but can cause illness in the future.

 CHECKPOINT QUESTION

1. What is the difference between the past history and the family history?

Conducting the Patient Interview

Preparing for the Interview

As a medical assistant, your primary goal during a patient interview is to obtain accurate and pertinent information. To do this, you need to understand the basic components of communication and to use active listening skills. You should also use a variety of interviewing techniques, including reflecting, paraphrasing, asking for examples, asking questions, summarizing, and allowing silence (see Chapter 3, Communication Skills). Communication also includes observation. Specifically, any objective or observable information concerning the patient's physical or mental status should be noted and documented in the patient's record as appropriate. Examples of observations about a patient's physical status include the general appearance (bruising or injury, pale or flushed skin). The mental or emotional condition of the patient includes observations such as lethargy, crying, tearfulness, and confusion. Judgments made about these observations should not be documented in the patient's record because the terminology used (depressed, abused) may be diagnostic, which is out of the scope of training for the medical assistant. In the case of suspected abuse, you should document the observable information in the medical record and alert the physician regarding your suspicions. Procedure 18-1 outlines the process for conducting a successful patient interview.

PATIENT EDUCATION
GENETIC DISEASES

The patient's family history can provide you with many teaching opportunities. If a patient indicates that previous members of his or her family had certain diseases, then there may be a genetic link. A genetic disease is noted by a mark on the DNA (genetic material) for a specific illness or disease. The patient receives this mark from either or both parents. Some common examples include some forms of high blood pressure, diabetes, heart disease, obesity, and certain cancers. Examples of less common genetic disorders are Tay-Sachs disease, Marfan syndrome, and Huntington disease. Great strides have been made in genetic testing. This allows the patient to have the DNA examined for potential markers of diseases. For example, color blindness is a genetic disorder that can easily be seen on a DNA chain. Patients can have genetic testing done to see whether they carry a particular disease marker. Genetic counseling may also be appropriate depending on the type of genetic disorder. Some insurance plans will pay for genetic testing and counseling. Advise the patient to contact his or her insurance company directly for specific coverage guidelines.

Before you start interviewing the patient, make sure you are familiar with the medical history form and any previous medical history provided by the patient. Shuffling papers while the patient is talking or asking questions out of order may distract the patient and disrupt the flow of the interview. If the patient is new to the medical practice, review the new patient questionnaire before beginning. Review the chart of any established patient, and update information as indicated.

To safeguard confidential patient information and allow for open communication, conduct the interview in a private and comfortable place. Avoid public areas, such as the reception area, where distractions are likely and where others may hear the patient's answers. Interview the patient alone unless he or she wishes to have family members or significant others present (Fig. 18-2).

LEGAL TIP
SAFEGUARDING PATIENT INFORMATION

You are responsible for ensuring that information in the patient's medical history is kept confidential. Legally and ethically, the patient has a right to privacy concerning his or her medical records, which includes storage in a secure place. Only health care providers directly involved in the patient's care should be allowed access to the records.

Introducing Yourself

Always begin the interview with new or established patients by identifying yourself, your title, and the purpose of the interview. For example, you might say, "Good morning, Mr. Frank. My name is Angela, and I'm Dr. Martin's medical assistant. I would like to ask you a few questions that will help the doctor diagnose and treat you appropriately. Please be assured that your responses will be kept in strict confidence." Under no circumstance should you identify yourself as a nurse because it is unethical and illegal to give the patient a false impression of your credentials.

The initial impression you make will be a lasting one, so be sure that your demeanor and words communicate genuine respect and concern. By developing professional rapport, you will gain the patient's confidence and trust in you, the physician, and the office staff. Some patients may be reluctant to share private information with you until a sense of trust has been established. This makes the professional role of the medical assistant as a caring and empathic health care worker even more important.

Barriers to Communication

As you begin speaking with the patient, you must assess any barriers to communication, such as unfamiliarity with English, hearing impairment, or cognitive impairment. Note the patient's verbal and nonverbal behavior during the interview and adjust your questioning if necessary. Avoid using highly technical or medical terminology when conversing with most patients. If the patient has impaired hearing or vision or difficulty understanding or speaking English, adjust your interviewing techniques to fit the patient's needs; however, remember that raising your voice is not necessary and will not improve communication or understanding with these patients. Instead, it is best to face the patient and maintain eye contact when speaking and use physical cues as appropriate. (See Chapter 3 for more details about overcoming communication barriers.)

Figure 18-2 Conduct the patient interview in a private office or exam room.

 CHECKPOINT QUESTIONS

2. Why is it important for the medical assistant to review the medical history form before beginning the interview?
3. Why should you let the patient know that any information shared during the interview will be kept confidential?

Assessing the Patient

Signs and Symptoms

During the interview, listen carefully as the patient describes current medical problems to identify **signs** and **symptoms.** Signs are objective information that can be observed or perceived by someone other than the patient. Signs include such things as rash, bleeding, coughing, and vital sign measurements. Signs may also be found during the physician's examination.

Symptoms, or subjective information, are indications of disease or changes in the body as sensed by the patient. Usually, symptoms are not discernible by anyone other than the patient. They include complaints such as leg pain, headache, nausea, and dizziness. Observable signs that may indicate that a patient is having these symptoms include facial expressions, such as wincing during pain, holding onto rails or furniture for balance when walking, and gagging.

Chief Complaint and Present Illness

After recording the patient's medical history and reviewing the information for accuracy and clarity, you must find out exactly why the patient has come to see the physician for this appointment (Procedure 18-2). Ask an open-ended question to encourage the patient to describe the chain of events leading to this visit. Open-

 PATIENT EDUCATION

GENERAL TOPICS

While assessing a patient, you can also teach. Your teaching may include information about a specific disease or general care. For example, a diabetic patient may need instruction on glucose testing or diet control. General topics for all patients can include the following:

- Blood pressure management
- Stress management
- Diet or weight control tips
- The importance of exercise
- The effects of alcohol and tobacco
- Instructions for conducting breast or testicular self-examinations
- The importance of proper immunizations
- Cancer warning signs and prevention tips

ended questions allow the patient to answer with more than one or two words. For example, you might ask, "What is the reason for your appointment today?" or "Can you describe what has been going on?" Such questions require the patient to explain the visit by giving additional information. In contrast, answers to closed-ended questions usually necessitate only one or two words. Examples of closed-ended questions are "Do you have pain?" and "Are you able to sleep?" These questions can be answered with a simple yes or no and are not going to elicit responses that will be useful to the physician attempting to make a diagnosis.

When open-ended questions are used to determine the reason for the visit, the patient's answer will reveal the **chief complaint** (CC). The CC, which is one statement describing the signs and symptoms that led the patient to seek medical care, is documented in the patient's medical record at each visit. Examples of a CC might include "I've had a headache for the past 3 days" or "Yesterday I lifted a heavy crate and hurt my back." You should document the CC on the progress report form in the patient's record, using the patient's own words in quotation marks whenever possible. The entry should include the date (day, month, and year) and the time of day.

Once you have obtained the CC, continue to probe for more details to further define the patient's present illness (PI). The PI includes a chronologic order of events, including dates of onset and any home remedies or other self-care activities, including **over-the-counter** and **homeopathic** medications. Over-the-counter medications are those that are available without prescriptions. They include natural drugs, such as herbs, vitamins, and some homeopathic agents. Homeopathic medications include small doses of agents that cause similar symptoms in healthy individuals and are given to a person who is ill to help cure the disease causing the symptoms. The following questions could be used to obtain the PI:

- Chronology. How did this first begin?
- Location. Can you explain or show me exactly where the pain is?
- Severity. Can you describe the pain? Is the pain constant?
- Self-treatment. What medications have you taken for the pain? Do they help?
- Quality. Does anything that you do make the symptoms better or worse?
- Duration. Have you had these symptoms before?

Avoid suggesting answers with questions such as "Is the pain sharp?" or "Is the pain worse when you walk?" Many patients will agree or answer positively because they think this must be the expected answer. In addition, do not coax patients by making suggestions of

symptoms you might expect them to have based on the chief complaint. Some patients may agree to have the symptoms you describe if they feel that you are suggesting those that "should" be present.

After asking several open-ended questions, it may be appropriate to ask closed-ended questions to obtain specific data. For example, you might ask the patient, "How long have you had this pain?" This kind of question requires only a short answer, not a lengthy description.

Of course, not all patients visit the doctor because they are ill. Some appointments are for routine examinations or tests. In this case, the CC will include a statement about the reason for the visit (e.g., annual physical examination, employment examination); however, you should obtain any additional PI information as appropriate.

 CHECKPOINT QUESTION

4. Explain the difference between a sign and a symptom, and give one example of each.

 WHAT IF?

What if the patient appears highly anxious or intimidated about procedures that seem routine?

You can help put patients at ease by following these steps:

- Treat each patient as an individual with unique needs. Help elderly or disabled patients onto the examination table. If they are unsteady, keep them seated in a regular chair.
- When weighing patients, do not announce their weight aloud, since they may be embarrassed. Instead, ask them in the privacy of the examination room if they want to know their weight.
- Always offer a sheet or blanket to a patient who must change into an examination gown.
- When preparing a patient for a gynecologic examination, have her sit on the examination table until the physician is ready.
- If the physician is delayed, let the patient know. Explain generally the reason for the delay (e.g., an emergency), and let the patient know the approximate length of the delay.

 PATIENT EDUCATION

PREVENTATIVE MEDICINE

While interviewing the patient about their chief complaint, you may have an opportunity to teach the patient about various topics. Emphasize to the patient that illnesses can often be treated easier and quicker if prompt medical attention is received. This is a very important point to stress to older patients with chronic medical problems such as diabetes. For example, a diabetic patient who presents with a small foot ulcer in its early stages may be able to be treated with medicated dressings. However, if the ulcer goes untreated and gets bigger, the patient may need surgery to clean the wound and may even require hospitalization for antibiotics. While interviewing the patient about their chief complaint, take the opportunity to stress the importance of preventative medicine

MEDIA MENU

- **Student CD**
  - **Case Studies**
    Administrative Interactive Case Study 2:
      Managing a Medical Office Emergency
    Clinical Interactive Case Study 3: Dealing
      With a Sick Patient, Infection Control,
      and Medication Administration
    Clinical Interactive Case Study 4: Patient
      Interviewing, Education and
      Confidentiality, and Specimen Handling
  - **CMA/RMA Certification Exam Review**

- **Premium Online Course**
  http://thePoint.lww.com/Kronenberger3e

- **Internet Resources**

  LiveAdvise Online Tutoring & Competency Training
  http://thePoint.lww.com/LiveAdvise

  The Health Insurance Portability and Accountability Act (HIPAA)
  www.cms.hhs.gov/hipaa

  American Autoimmune Related Diseases Association
  www.aarda.org

  March of Dimes
  www.marchofdimes.com

  Genetic Alliance
  www.geneticalliance.org

PROCEDURE 18-1: Interviewing the Patient to Obtain a Medical History

Purpose: Complete the various sections of a medical history form while interviewing a patient
Equipment: Medical history form or questionnaire, black or blue pen
Standard: This task should take 10 minutes.

Steps	Reasons
1. Gather the supplies.	You have everything you need before you begin.
2. Review the medical history form.	Be familiar with the order of the questions and the type of information required to allow for smooth communication with the patient.
3. Take the patient to a private and comfortable area of the office.	A private place prevents distractions and ensures confidentiality.
4. Sit across from the patient at eye level and maintain frequent eye contact.	Standing above the patient may be perceived as threatening and may result in poor communication
5. Introduce yourself and explain the purpose of the interview.	This helps to establish a professional rapport with the patient.
6. Using language the patient can understand, ask the appropriate questions, and document the patient's responses. Be sure to determine the patient's CC and PI.	You must obtain accurate and complete data for the physician.
7. Listen actively by looking at the patient from time to time while he or she is speaking.	Patients can sense when the interviewer is not listening, so be sure that you show interest in what the patient is saying.
8. Regardless of the confidences shared by the patient, avoid projecting a judgmental attitude with words or actions.	Maintain professionalism, and ensure the patient's trust.
9. If appropriate, explain to the patient what to expect during examinations or procedures at that visit.	Keeping the patient informed about his or her care may decrease anxiety.
10. Thank the patient for cooperating during the interview, and offer to answer any questions.	Courtesy encourages the patient to have a positive attitude about the physician's office.

Charting Example:

> 10/14/2008 11:00 AM CC: New pt. checkup. Medical hx form complete, pt. indicates no physical or health problems at this time. Family history of colon cancer and hypertension noted.
>
> —E. Parker, CMA

PROCEDURE 18-2: Document a Chief Complaint (CC) and Present Illness (PI)

Purpose: Accurately record a CC and PI using open-ended and closed-ended questions while interviewing the patient
Equipment: A cumulative problem list or progress notes form, black or blue ink pen
Standard: This procedure should take 10 minutes or less.

Steps	Reasons
1. Gather the supplies, including the medical record containing the cumulative problem list or progress note form.	You have everything you need before you start.
2. Review new or established patient's medical history form.	Be as familiar as possible with the patient to help you obtain a complete CC and PI.

Professional Medical Associates – History Form

NAME: _Fred Smart_   DATE OF BIRTH: _09-15-1945_

What is the main reason for your visit to the doctor? _Physical Exam_

Were you referred? _No_   if so, by whom?

PAST MEDICAL HISTORY:

Are you allergic to any medication? _Yes_

If so, list medications: _Penicillin_

List current medications, dosage, and how many times a day you take them:

Medication	Dose	Times A Day
Multivitamin	1 tablet	every day

Alcohol Consumption: What type? _Beer_   Amount _2-3_   How Often? _Every week_
                        History of Alcoholism? _No_

When was your last TB or Tine test? _I can't remember_

Have you ever had a positive test for tuberculosis? _No_

When was your last Tetanus shot? _Last year, I cut my finger when fishing._

List all surgeries you have had in the past:

Date	Type of Surgery
1952-childhood?	Tonsillectomy

List all past hospitalizations (not involving surgeries above):

Date	Reason For Hospital Stay
Spring, 1999	Pneumonia

List all past problems with trauma (broken bones, lacerations, etc.):
Cut my finger while fishing last year. I had a broken leg from a car accident in 1984.

REVIEW OF SYSTEMS, PAST MEDICAL PROBLEMS:
If you have been told you have any of the problems listed below, or are having any of the problems listed below, please CIRCLE:

1. GENERAL: Weight loss, weight gain, fever, chills, night sweats, hot flashes, tire easily, problems with sleep, crying spells, history of cancer.

2. SKIN: Rash, sores that won't heal, moles that are new or changing, history of skin problems.

3. HEENT: Headache, eye problems, hearing problems, sinus problems, hay fever, dizziness, hoarseness, sores in your mouth that won't heal, dental problems.
   Do you chew tobacco or dip snuff? _No_

4. METABOLIC/ENDOCRINE: Thyroid problems, diabetes or sugar problems, high cholesterol.

Step 2A.
Completed
Medical History
Form—Front

(continued)

PROCEDURE 18-2: Document a Chief Complaint (CC) and Present Illness (PI) *(continued)*

Steps	Reasons

5. <u>RESPIRATORY:</u> (Cough,) wheezing, breathing problems, history of asthma, history of lung problems.

   Do you smoke cigarettes or pipe? *Cigarettes*

   How much? *1 pack a day*   For how long? *20 years*

6. <u>BREAST (WOMEN):</u> Breast lumps, changes in nipples, nipple discharge, breast problems, family history of breast cancer. When was your last mammogram? _____

7. <u>CARDIOVASCULAR:</u> Heart murmur, rheumatic fever, high blood pressure, angina, heart problems, heart attack, abnormal heart rhythm, chest pain, palpitations, leg swelling, history of phlebitis or blood clots.

8. <u>GI:</u> Problems with appetite, swallowing, heartburn, nausea, vomiting, pain in the abdomen, constipation, diarrhea, blood in stool, history of ulcers, liver problems, hepatitis, jaundice, pancreas problems, gallbladder problems, or colon problems.

9. <u>REPRODUCTIVE (WOMEN):</u> Problems with irregular menstrual cycles, abnormal vaginal bleeding or discharge, history of sexually transmitted diseases, sexual problems.

   AGE OF FIRST MENSES (PERIOD) _____ AGE OF MENOPAUSE _____

   LAST PAP SMEAR _____ METHOD OF CONTRACEPTION _____

   Obstetric History (Women)

   NUMBER OF PREGNANCIES _____ PLEASE LIST AS FOLLOWS:

   Delivery Date   Pregnancy Complications   Type Delivery   Baby's Weight

   _____

   _____

   <u>MEN:</u> Problems with genital discharge, history of venereal diseases, sexual problems, prostate problems.

   METHOD OF CONTRACEPTION _____

10. <u>UROLOGIC:</u> Problems with painful urination, urinary frequency, blood in urine, weak urinary stream, history of bladder or kidney infections, or kidney stones.

11. <u>MUSCULOSKELETAL:</u> Arthritis, back pain, cramps in legs.

12. <u>NEUROLOGIC:</u> Seizures, stroke, arm or leg weakness or numbness, black-out spells, memory or thinking problems, depression, anxiety, psychiatric problems.

13. <u>HEMATOLOGIC:</u> Anemia, bleeding problems, enlarged lymph nodes.

   HAVE YOU EVER HAD A BLOOD TRANSFUSION? _____ DATE _____

FAMILY HISTORY:

List any medical problems that run in your family and which family members have these problems.

Grandmother had colon cancer; Father has high blood pressure

_____

SOCIAL HISTORY:

MARITAL STATUS: *Married for 30 years*

OCCUPATION: *Mail Carrier*

EDUCATION: *Graduated high school 1963*

HOBBIES: *Fishing, camping*

WHAT DO YOU DO FOR ENJOYMENT? _____

Step 2B.
Completed
Medical History
Form—Back

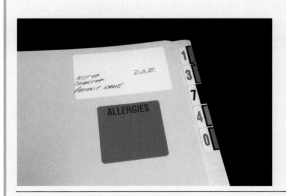

Step 2C.

(continued)

PROCEDURE 18-2:   **Document a Chief Complaint (CC) and Present Illness (PI)** *(continued)*

Steps	Reasons
3. Greet and identify the patient while escorting him or her to the examination room.	Greeting the patient by name helps develop a professional rapport and eases patient's anxiety. Correctly identifying the patient may help to prevent errors.

Step 3.

Steps	Reasons
4. Using open-ended questions, find out why the patient is seeking medical care; maintain eye contact.	Maintaining eye contact demonstrates that you are actively listening.
5. Determine the PI using open-ended and closed-ended questions,	Use closed-ended questions to obtain specific data only after the patient has responded to open-ended questions.
6. Document the CC and PI correctly on the cumulative problem list or progress report form.	Documentation should include the date, time, CC, PI, and your signature (first initial, last name, and title). Use only correct medical terminology and approved abbreviations.

(continued)

PROCEDURE 18-2: Document a Chief Complaint (CC) and Present Illness (PI) *(continued)*

Steps	Reasons

```
09/15/2008

9:45 a.m. CC: Pt. c/o headache ad nausea x3
days. Has taken ibuprofen for the pain with
"some relief." The pain is a "dull ache" in the
frontal area of the head and face. Denies
emesis. Face flushed, skin warm and dry.
T 98.9°F, P88, R24, BP 190/110 (L) sitting.

                              S. Vincer, CMA
```

Step 6.

7. Thank the patient for cooperating, and explain that the physician will soon be in to examine the patient.	Courtesy encourages a positive attitude about the physician's office. If you indicate a time frame in reference to the physician coming into the examination room, be honest.

Charting Example:

> 09/15/2008 9:45 AM CC: Pt. c/o headache and nausea ×3 days Has taken ibuprofen for the pain with "some relief." The pain is a "dull ache" in the frontal area of the head and face. Denies emesis. Face flushed, skin warm and dry. T 98.8°F, P 88, R 24, BP 190/110 (L) sitting.
>
> —S. Vincer, CMA

Chapter Summary

- In every medical practice, a history is taken from each patient.
- As a professional medical assistant, you need to know the components of a standard medical history form. You may be required to obtain and document the information on the history form and to interview the patient to elicit the chief complaint and present illness.

- The physician relies on the information that you gather and document for diagnosing and treating patients, so it is essential that you question the patient carefully and document accurately.

1. Mrs. Smythe has always been impeccably groomed, articulate, and punctual for her monthly blood pressure checks. Today, she was 15 minutes late, her hair was not combed, she wore no makeup, and her clothes did not match. Are any of these observations worth noting on her chart?

2. After reviewing the following items, determine in which section of the medical history the information should be included and explain why. Identify any items that are irrelevant.

   - Sister died of breast cancer.
   - Son had chickenpox last year.
   - Patient has many allergies.
   - Father died of heart disease.
   - Mother is alive and well.
   - Brother works in real estate.
   - Patient smokes three packs of cigarettes a day.
   - Patient works in a cotton mill.
   - Patient is a runner and teaches aerobics.
   - Patient has recently lost 60 pounds.
   - Patient had an angioplasty last year.

3. Determine which of the following are signs and which are symptoms.

   - Nausea
   - Vomiting
   - Itching
   - Rash
   - Dizziness
   - Abdominal pain
   - Pallor
   - Tingling fingers and toes
   - Ringing in the ears
   - Fever
   - Edema

4. Provide open-ended questions for obtaining additional information from patients with the following complaints:

   - "I am tired; I don't sleep well at night."
   - "I have pain in the bottom of my foot when I walk."
   - "My stomach hurts, and I threw up yesterday."
   - "I have indigestion every day."

5. An elderly patient, Mr. Barnes, comes into the office and is given the medical history form, a pen, and a clipboard. He is unable to hold the pen due to arthritic deformities of his hands. Would it be appropriate to sit with Mr. Barnes in the waiting room and complete the form for him? Why or why not?

1. The past history summarizes the patient's prior health status, whereas the family history summarizes the health status of the patient's parents, siblings, and grandparents.

2. You should be familiar with the medical history form before beginning the patient interview to promote smooth communication during the interview.

3. Yes, it is important to let the patient know that any information shared during the interview will be kept confidential. Understanding this enables patients to trust in the medical staff and encourages them to share important information that allows the physician to provide better care for the patient.

4. A sign is an objective (observable or measurable) indication of disease. An example of a sign is a patient's blood pressure, temperature reading, or noting a laceration or rash on the patient's skin. A symptom is a subjective indication of disease that is felt or noticed by the patient but not directly observable or measurable by the medical assistant or physician. Examples of symptoms include headache, nausea, and pain.

Anthropometric Measurements and Vital Signs

Outline

Anthropometric Measurements
Weight
Height

Vital Signs
Temperature
Pulse

Respiration
Blood Pressure

Learning Objectives

Upon successfully completing this chapter, you will be able to:

1. Spell and define key terms
2. Explain the procedures for measuring a patient's height and weight
3. Identify and describe the types of thermometers
4. Compare the procedures for measuring a patient's temperature using the oral, rectal, axillary, and tympanic methods
5. List the fever process, including the stages of fever

6. Describe the procedure for measuring a patient's pulse and respiratory rates
7. Identify the various sites on the body used for palpating a pulse
8. Define Korotkoff sounds and the five phases of blood pressure
9. Identify factors that may influence the blood pressure
10. Explain the factors to consider when choosing the correct blood pressure cuff size

Performance Objectives

Upon successfully completing this chapter, you will be able to:

1. Measure and record a patient's weight (Procedure 19-1)
2. Measure and record a patient's height (Procedure 19-2)
3. Measure and record a patient's oral temperature using a glass mercury thermometer (Procedure 19-3)
4. Measure and record a patient's rectal temperature (Procedure 19-4)

5. Measure and record a patient's axillary temperature (Procedure 19-5)
6. Measure and record a patient's temperature using an electronic thermometer (Procedure 19-6)
7. Measure and record a patient's temperature using a tympanic thermometer (Procedure 19-7)
8. Measure and record a patient's temperature using a temporal artery thermometer (Procedure 19-8)

9. Measure and record a patient's radial pulse (Procedure 19-9)

10. Measure and record a patient's respirations (Procedure 19-10)

11. Measure and record a patient's blood pressure (Procedure 19-11)

Competencies

CAAHEP

- Obtain vital signs
- Document appropriately

ABHES

- Take vital signs

Key Terms

afebrile	cardinal signs	hypertension	pyrexia
anthropometric	diaphoresis	hyperventilation	relapsing fever
apnea	diastole	hypopnea	remittent
baseline	dyspnea	intermittent	sphygmomanometer
calibrated	febrile	orthopnea	sustained fever
cardiac cycle	hyperpnea	palpation	systole
cardiac output	hyperpyrexia	postural hypotension	tympanic

Vital signs, also known as **cardinal signs**, are measurements of bodily functions essential to maintaining life processes. Vital signs frequently measured and recorded by the medical assistant include the temperature (T), pulse rate (P), respiratory rate (R), and blood pressure (BP). In addition, medical assistants take **anthropometric** measurements, or the height and weight, of patients and document them in the medical record. This information is essential for the physician to diagnose, treat, and prevent many disorders.

Measurements taken at the first visit are recorded as **baseline** data and are used as reference points for comparison during subsequent visits. After the first office visit, the height is usually not taken; however, the vital signs and weight are taken and recorded for each adult patient at each visit to the medical office.

Anthropometric Measurements

Weight

An accurate weight is always required for pregnant patients, infants, children, and the elderly. In addition, weight monitoring may be required if the patient has been prescribed medications that must be carefully calculated according to body weight or for a patient who is attempting to gain or lose weight.

Since most medical practices have only one scale, placement of the scale is important. Many patients are uncomfortable if they are weighed in a place that is not private. Types of scales used to measure weight include balance beam scales, digital scales, and dial scales (Fig. 19-1). Weight may be measured in pounds or kilograms, depending upon the preference of the physician and the

Figure 19-1 The three types of scales used in medical offices include the digital, dial, and balance scale.

type of scale in the medical office. Procedure 19-1 describes how to measure and record a patient's weight.

Height

Height can be measured using the movable ruler on the back of most balance beam scales. Some offices use a graph ruler mounted on a wall (Fig. 19-2), but more accurate measures can be made with a parallel bar moved down against the top of the patient's head. Height is measured in inches or centimeters, depending upon the physician's preference. Procedure 19-2 describes how to measure an adult patient's height. Refer to Chapter 37 for the procedure for measuring the height and weight of infants and children.

CHECKPOINT QUESTION

1. Why is it important to accurately measure vital signs at every patient visit?

Vital Signs

Temperature

Body temperature reflects a balance between heat produced and heat lost by the body (Fig. 19-3). Heat is pro-

duced during normal internal physical and chemical processes called metabolism and through muscle movement. Heat is normally lost through several processes, including respiration, elimination, and conduction through the skin (Table 19-1). Normally, the body maintains a constant internal temperature of around 98.6° Fahrenheit (F) or 37.0° Celsius (C) (centigrade). A patient whose temperature is within normal limits is said to be **afebrile**, while a patient with a temperature above normal is considered **febrile** (has a fever).

Thermometers are used to measure body temperature using either the Fahrenheit or Celsius scale. Box 19-1 compares temperatures taken a variety of ways in Celsius and in Fahrenheit. Since glass or electronic thermometers used in the medical office may be in either scale, you should be able to convert from one scale to another (see Appendix G). The patient's temperature can be measured using the oral, rectal, axillary, or **tympanic** method. The oral method is most commonly used, but use of the tympanic thermometer is also becoming more prevalent, especially in pediatric offices. A newer type of thermometer that you may see is the temporal artery thermometer (Fig. 19-4). This device measures the temperature of the blood within the temporal artery through the skin. If used accurately, both the tympanic thermometer and the temporal artery thermometer give readings that are comparable to the oral temperature.

Figure 19-2 A wall-mounted device to measure height and the sliding bar on the balance scale.

A reading of 98.6°F orally is considered a normal average for body temperature, with the normal range being 97°F to 99°F. Rectal and axillary readings will vary slightly. Generally, rectal temperatures are 1°F higher than the oral temperatures because of the vascularity and tightly closed environment of the rectum. Axillary temperatures are usually 1°F lower because of lower vascularity and difficulty in keeping the axilla tightly closed. When recording the body temperature, you must indicate the temperature reading and the method used to obtain it, such as oral, rectal, axillary, tympanic, or temporal artery. A rectal temperature reading of 101°F is equivalent to 100°F orally, and an axillary reading of 101°F is equivalent to 102°F orally.

Figure 19-3 Factors affecting the balance between heat loss and heat production.

 CHECKPOINT QUESTION

2. How does an oral temperature measurement differ from a rectal measurement? Why?

Fever Processes

Although a patient's temperature is influenced by heat lost or produced by the body, it is regulated by the hypothalamus in the brain. When the hypothalamus senses that the body is too warm, it initiates peripheral vasodilation to carry core heat to the body surface via the blood and increases perspiration to cool the body by evaporation. If the temperature registers too low, vasoconstriction to conserve heat and shivering to generate more heat will usually maintain a fairly normal core temperature. Temperature elevations and variations are often a *sign* of disease but are not diseases in themselves. The following factors may cause the temperature to vary:

- *Age.* Children usually have a higher metabolism and therefore a higher body temperature than adults. The elderly, who have slower metabolisms, usually have lower readings than younger adults. Temperatures of both the very young and the elderly are easily affected by the environment.
- *Gender.* Women usually have a slightly higher temperature than men, especially at the time of ovulation and during pregnancy.
- *Exercise.* Activity causes the body to burn more calories for energy, which raises the body temperature.
- *Time of day.* The body temperature is usually lowest in the early morning before physical activity has begun.
- *Emotions.* Temperature tends to rise during times of stress and fall with depression.
- *Illness.* High or low body temperatures may result from a disease process.

Stages of Fever

An elevated temperature, or fever, usually results from a disease process, such as a bacterial or viral infection. Body temperature may also rise during intense exercise, anxiety, or dehydration unrelated to a disease process, but these elevations are not considered fevers. **Pyrexia** refers to a fever of 102°F or higher rectally or 101°F or higher orally. An extremely high temperature, 105° to 106°F, is **hyperpyrexia** and is considered dangerous because the intense internal body heat may damage or destroy cells of the brain and other vital organs. The fever process has several clearly defined stages:

1. The *onset* may be abrupt or gradual.

TABLE **19-1**	Mechanisms of Heat Transfer	
Mechanism	**Definition**	**Example**
Radiation	Diffusion or dissemination of heat by electromagnetic waves.	The body gives off waves of heat from uncovered surfaces.
Convection	Dissemination of heat by motion between areas of unequal density.	An oscillating fan blows cool air across the surface of a warm body.
Evaporation	Conversion of liquid to vapor.	Body fluid (perspiration and insensible loss) evaporates from the skin.
Conduction	Transfer of heat during direct contact between two objects. The body gives off waves of heat from uncovered surfaces.	The body transfers heat to an ice pack, melting the ice.

Radiation

Convection

Evaporation

Conduction

2. The *course* may range from a day or so to several weeks. Fever may be **sustained** (constant), **remittent** (fluctuating), **intermittent** (occurring at intervals), or **relapsing** (returning after an extended period of normal readings). Table 19-2 describes and illustrates these courses of fever.

3. The *resolution*, or return to normal, may occur as either a *crisis* (abrupt return to normal) or *lysis* (gradual return to normal).

CHECKPOINT QUESTION

3. Explain why the body temperature of a young child may be different from that of an adult.

Types of Thermometers

Glass Mercury Thermometers

Oral, rectal, and axillary temperatures have traditionally been measured using the mercury glass thermometer. This thermometer consists of a glass tube divided into two major parts. The bulb end is filled with mercury and may have a round or a slender tip. Glass thermometers have different shapes for oral and rectal use. Rectal thermometers have a rounded, or stubbed, end and are usually color-coded red on the opposite flat end of the thermometer. Thermometers with a long, slender bulb are used for axillary or oral temperatures and are color-coded blue (Fig. 19-5). When the glass thermometer is placed in position for a specified period, body heat

BOX 19-1

TEMPERATURE COMPARISONS

	Fahrenheit	Centigrade
Oral	98.6°	37.0°
Rectal	99.6°	37.6°
Axillary	97.6°	36.4°
Tympanic	98.6°	37.0°

expands the mercury, which rises up the glass column and remains there until it is physically shaken back into the bulb.

The long stem of the Fahrenheit thermometer is **calibrated** with lines designating temperature in even degrees: 94°, 96°, 98°, 100°, and so on. Uneven numbers are marked only with a longer line. Between these longer lines, four smaller lines designate temperature in 0.2° increments. The thermometer is read by noting the level of the mercury in the glass column. For example, if the level of the mercury falls on the second smaller line past the large line marked 100, the reading is 100.4°F. Celsius thermometers are marked for each degree (35°, 36°, 37°, and so on), with 10 markings between the whole numbers (Fig. 19-6). If the mercury falls on the third small line past the line marked 37, the temperature reading is recorded as 37.3°C.

Before using a glass thermometer, place it in a disposable clear plastic sheath. When you take the thermometer from the patient, remove the sheath by pulling the thermometer out, which turns the sheath inside out and traps the saliva inside it. Dispose of the sheath in a biohazard container, and sanitize and disinfect the thermometer according to the office policy. Usually, washing the thermometers with warm—not hot—soapy water and soaking in a solution of 70% isopropyl alcohol is sufficient for disinfection. In the event that a glass mercury thermometer breaks, you should have a mercury spill kit available and use it to clean the area as indicated in your office policy and procedure manual. Never allow anyone to touch or manipulate the mercury from a broken thermometer.

Figure 19-4 A temporal artery scanning thermometer.

TABLE 19-2 Variations in Fever Patterns: Temperature Comparisons

	Fahrenheit	Celsius
Oral	98.6	37.0
Rectal	99.6	37.6
Axillary	97.6	36.4
Tympanic	98.6	37.0

Sustained
Normal

Remittent
Normal

Intermittent
Normal

Relapsing
Normal

The procedure for measuring an oral temperature using a glass mercury thermometer is described in Procedure 19-3. The procedures for measuring a rectal or axillary temperature using either the glass mercury thermometer or the electronic thermometer are described in Procedures 19-4 and 19-5.

Electronic Thermometers

Electronic thermometers are portable battery-operated units with interchangeable probes (Fig. 19-7). The base unit of the thermometer is battery operated, and the interchangeable probes are color-coded blue for oral or axillary and red for rectal. When the probe is properly positioned, the temperature is sensed, and a digital readout shows in the window of the hand-held base. Electronic thermometers are usually kept in a charging unit between uses to ensure that the batteries are operative at all times. The procedure for taking and recording an oral temperature using an electronic thermometer is described in Procedure 19-6.

Figure 19-5 Glass mercury thermometers. **Front:** Slender bulb, oral. **Center:** Rounded bulb, red tip, rectal. **Back:** Blue tip, oral.

Tympanic Thermometers

Another type of thermometer used in medical offices today is the tympanic, or aural, thermometer. This device is usually battery powered. The end is fitted with a disposable cover that is inserted into the ear much like an otoscope (Fig. 19-8). With the end of the thermometer in place, a button is pressed, and infrared light bounces off the tympanic membrane, or eardrum. When correctly positioned, the sensor in the thermometer determines the temperature of the blood in the tympanic membrane. The temperature reading is displayed on the unit's digital screen within 2 seconds. This device is considered highly reliable for temperature measurement. Procedure 19-7 describes the complete process for obtaining a body temperature with a tympanic thermometer.

Temporal Artery Thermometer

The temporal artery thermometer measures actual blood temperature by placing the unit on the front of

the forehead, depressing the "on/off" button, and sliding the probe scanner over the forehead and down to the temporal artery area of the forehead. Upon releasing the "on/off" button, the temperature is immediately recorded in the digital display box located on the front of the thermometer. Depending on the brand and type of temporal artery thermometer purchased, you should read the manufacturer's instructions carefully for proper use and care of the unit. Procedure 19-8 describes the steps for taking a temperature for taking a temperature using the temporal artery thermometer.

Disposable Thermometers

Single-use disposable thermometers are fairly accurate but are not considered as reliable as electronic, tympanic, or glass thermometers. These thermometers register quickly by indicating color changes on a strip. They are not reliable for definitive measurement, but they are acceptable for screening in settings such as day care centers and schools (Fig. 19-9). Other disposable thermometers are available for pediatric use in the form of sucking devices, or pacifiers, but these are not used in the medical office setting.

 CHECKPOINT QUESTION

4. How is the reading displayed on an electronic, tympanic, and temporal artery thermometer?

Centigrade

Rectal

Oral

Fahrenheit

Rectal

Oral

Figure 19-6 The two glass thermometers on the top are calibrated in the Celsius (centigrade) scale, and the two on the bottom use the Fahrenheit scale. Note the blunt bulb on the rectal thermometers and the long thin bulb on the oral thermometers.

 PATIENT EDUCATION
Fever

When instructing patients about fever, explain that temperature elevations are usually a natural response to disease and that efforts to bring the temperature back to normal may be counterproductive. However, if the patient is uncomfortable or the temperature is abnormally high, it should be brought down to about 101°F; the body's natural defenses may still be able to destroy the pathogen without extreme discomfort to the patient.

(continued)

After consulting with the physician, instruct all patients regarding the following comfort measures:

- Consume clear fluids by mouth as tolerated to rehydrate the tissues if nausea and vomiting are not present.
- Keep clothing and bedding clean and dry, especially after **diaphoresis** (sweating).
- Avoid chilling. Chills cause shivering, which raises the body temperature.
- Rest and eat a light diet as tolerated.
- Use antipyretics to keep comfortable, but *do not* give aspirin products to children under 18 years of age. Aspirin has been associated with Reye's syndrome, a potentially fatal disorder, following cases of viral illnesses and varicella zoster (chicken pox).

Pulse

As the heart beats, blood is forced through the arteries, expanding them. With relaxation of the heart, the arteries relax also. This expansion and relaxation of the arteries can be felt at various points on the body where you can press an artery against a bone or other underlying firm surface. These areas are known as pulse points. With **palpation**, each expansion of the artery can be felt and is counted as one heartbeat. A pulse in specific arteries supplying blood to the extremities also indicates that oxygenated blood is flowing to that extremity.

The heartbeat can be palpated (felt) or auscultated (heard) at several pulse points. The arteries most commonly used are the carotid, apical, brachial, radial, femoral, popliteal, posterior tibial, and dorsalis pedis (Fig. 19-10). Palpation of the pulse is performed by placing the index and middle fingers, the middle and ring fingers, or all three fingers over a pulse point (Fig. 19-11). The thumb is not used to palpate a pulse. The

Figure 19-8 The tympanic thermometer in use.

apical pulse is auscultated using a stethoscope with the bell placed over the apex of the heart (Fig. 19-12). A Doppler unit may be used to amplify the sound of peripheral pulses that are difficult to palpate (Fig. 19-13). This unit is a small battery-powered or electric device that consists of a main box with control switches, a probe, and an earpiece unit that plugs into the main box and resembles the earpieces to a stethoscope. The earpiece may be detached so the sounds can be heard by everyone in the room if desired. Follow the following steps to use a Doppler device:

1. Apply a coupling or transmission gel on the pulse point before placing the end of the probe, or transducer, on the area. This gel creates an airtight seal between the probe and the skin and facilitates transmission of the sound.
2. With the machine on, hold the probe at a 90-degree angle with light pressure to ensure contact. Move the probe as necessary in small circles in the gel until you hear the pulse. When contact with the artery is made, the Doppler will emit a loud pumping sound with each heartbeat. Adjust the volume control on the Doppler unit as necessary.
3. After assessing the rate and rhythm of the pulse, clean the patient's skin and the probe with a tissue or soft cloth. Do not clean the probe with water or alcohol, as this may damage the transducer.

Figure 19-7 Two types of electronic thermometers and probes.

Figure 19-9 Disposable paper thermometer. The dots change color to indicate the body temperature.

A Carotid

B Brachial

C Radial

D Femoral

E Popliteal

F Dorsalis pedis

G Posterior tibial

Figure 19-10 Sites for palpation of peripheral pulses.

Figure 19-11 Measuring a radial pulse.

Pulse Characteristics

While palpating the pulse, you also assess the rate, rhythm, and volume as the artery wall expands with each heartbeat. The *rate* is the number of heartbeats in 1 minute. This number can be determined by palpating the pulse and counting each heartbeat while watching the second hand of your watch either for 30 seconds and then multiplying that number by 2 or for 1 minute. In healthy adults, the average pulse rate is 60 to 100 beats per minute. At other ages, there is a large variance of pulse rates, as shown in Table 19-3.

The *rhythm* is the interval between each heartbeat or the pattern of beats. Normally, this pattern is regular, with each heartbeat occurring at a regular, consistent rate. An irregular rhythm should be counted for 1 full minute to determine the rate, and the irregular rhythm should be documented with the pulse rate.

Volume, the strength or force of the heartbeat, can be described as soft, bounding, weak, thready, strong,

Figure 19-12 Measuring an apical pulse.

Figure 19-13 The dorsalis pedis pulse being auscultated using a Doppler device.

or full. Usually the volume of the pulse is recorded only if it is weak, thready, or bounding.

Factors Affecting Pulse Rates

Many factors affect the force, speed, and rhythm of the heart. Young children and infants have a much faster heart rate than adults. A conditioned athlete may have a normal heart rate below 60 beats per minute. Older adults may have a faster heart rate, as the myocardium compensates for decreased efficiency. Other factors that affect pulse rates are listed in Table 19-4.

The radial artery is most often used to determine pulse rate because it is convenient for both the medical assistant and the patient (Procedure 19-9). If the radial pulse is irregular or hard to palpate, then the apical pulse is the site of choice (Fig. 19-14). To assess the flow of blood into the extremities, you may be asked to palpate peripheral pulses such as the dorsalis pedis. Peripheral pulses that are difficult to palpate may be auscultated with a Doppler unit to check for the presence of blood flow.

 CHECKPOINT QUESTION

5. What characteristics of a patient's pulse should be assessed, and how should they be recorded in the medical record?

TABLE **19-3**	Variations in Pulse Rate by Age
Age	**Beats per Minute**
Birth to 1 year	110–170
1–10 years	90–110
10–16 years	80–95
16 years to midlife	70–80
Elderly adult	55–70

Table 19-4	Factors Affecting Pulse Rates
Factor	**Effect**
Time of day	The pulse is usually lower early in the morning than later in the day.
Gender	Women have a slightly higher pulse rate than men.
Body type and size	Tall, thin people usually have a lower pulse rate than shorter, stockier people.
Exercise	The heart rate increases with the need for increased **cardiac output** (the amount of blood ejected from either ventricle in 1 minute).
Stress or emotions	Anger, fear, excitement, and stress will raise the pulse; depression will lower it.
Fever	The increased need for cell metabolism in the presence of fever raises the **cardiac output** to supply oxygen and nutrients; the pulse may rise as much as 10 beats/minute per degree of fever.
Medications	Many medications raise or lower the pulse as a desired effect or as an undesirable side effect.
Blood volume	Loss of blood volume to hemorrhage or dehydration will increase the need for cellular metabolism and will increase the **cardiac output** to supply the need.

Respiration

Respiration is the exchange of gases between the atmosphere and the blood in the body. With respiration, the body expels carbon dioxide (CO_2) and takes in oxygen (O_2). External respiration is inhalation and exhalation, during which air travels through the respiratory tract to the alveoli so that oxygen can be absorbed into the bloodstream. Internal respiration is the exchange of gases between the blood and the tissue cells. Respiration is controlled by the respiratory center in the brainstem and by feedback from chemosensors in the carotid arteries that monitor the CO_2 content in the blood.

As the patient breathes in (inspiration), oxygen flows into the lungs, and the diaphragm contracts and flattens out, lifting and expanding the rib cage. During expiration, air in the lungs flows out of the chest cavity as the diaphragm relaxes, moves upward into a dome-like shape, and allows the rib cage to contract. Each respiration is counted as one full inspiration and one full expiration.

Observing the rise and fall of the chest to count respirations is usually performed as a part of the pulse measurement. Generally, you should not make the patient aware that you are counting respirations because patients often change the voluntary action of breathing if they are aware that they are being watched. Respirations can be counted for a full minute or for 30 seconds with the number multiplied by 2. When appropriate, a stethoscope may be used to auscultate respirations.

Respiration Characteristics

The characteristics of respirations include rate, rhythm, and depth. *Rate* is the number of respirations occurring in 1 minute. *Rhythm* is the time, or spacing, between each respiration. This pattern is equal and regular in patients with normal respirations. Any abnormal rhythm is described as irregular and recorded as such in the patient's record after the rate.

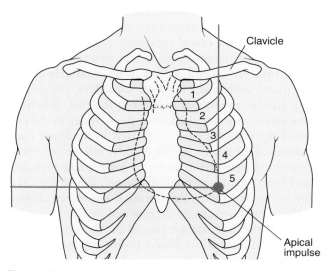

Figure 19-14 The apical pulse is found at the 5th intercostal space at the midclavicular line.

Depth is the volume of air being inhaled and exhaled. When a person is at rest, the depth should be regular and consistent. There are normally no noticeable sounds other than the regular exchange of air. Respirations that are abnormally deep or shallow are documented in addition to the rate. Abnormal sounds during inspiration or expiration are usually a sign of a disease process. These abnormal sounds are usually recorded as crackles (wet or dry sounds) or wheezes (high-pitched sounds) heard during inspiration or expiration.

Factors Affecting Respiration

In healthy adults, the average respiratory rate is 14 to 20 breaths per minute. Table 19-5 shows the normal variations in respiratory rates according to age. Patients with an elevated body temperature usually also have increased pulse and respiratory rates. A respiratory rate that is much faster than average is called tachypnea, and a respiratory rate that is slower than usual is referred to as bradypnea. Further descriptions of abnormal or unusual respirations include the following:

- **Dyspnea:** difficult or labored breathing
- **Apnea:** no respiration
- **Hyperpnea:** abnormally deep, gasping breaths
- **Hyperventilation:** a respiratory rate that greatly exceeds the body's oxygen demand
- **Hypopnea:** shallow respirations
- **Orthopnea:** inability to breathe lying down; the patient usually has to sit upright to breathe

Procedure 19-10 lists the steps for counting and recording respirations.

 CHECKPOINT QUESTION

6. What happens within the chest cavity when the diaphragm contracts?

Blood Pressure

Blood pressure is a measurement of the pressure of the blood in an artery as it is forced against the arterial walls. Pressure is measured in the contraction and relaxation phases of the cardiac cycle, or heartbeat. When the heart contracts, it forces blood from the atria and ventricles in the phase known as **systole**. This highest pressure level during contraction is recorded as the systolic pressure and is heard as the first sound in taking blood pressure.

As the heart pauses briefly to rest and refill, the arterial pressure drops. This phase is known as **diastole**, and the pressure is recorded as the diastolic pressure. Systolic and diastolic pressure result from the two parts of the **cardiac cycle**, the period from the beginning of one heartbeat to the beginning of the next. When measured using a stethoscope and **sphygmomanometer**, or blood pressure cuff, these two pressures constitute the blood pressure and are written as a fraction, with the systolic pressure over the diastolic pressure. Table 19-6 describes the classification of blood pressure readings for adults with normal, prehypertenion, and hypertension blood pressures. A lower pressure may be normal for athletes with exceptionally well-conditioned cardiovascular systems. Blood pressure that drops suddenly when the patient stands from a sitting or lying position is **postural hypotension**, or orthostatic hypotension; it may cause symptoms including vertigo. Some patients with postural hypotension may faint. Extra precautions should be taken when assessing patients going from lying down to sitting or standing.

Two basic types of sphygmomanometers are used to measure blood pressure: the aneroid, which has a circular dial for the readings, and the mercury, which has a mercury-filled glass tube for the readings (Fig. 19-15). Although only one type actually contains mercury, both types are calibrated and measure blood pressure in millimeters of mercury (mm Hg). A blood pressure of 120/80 indicates the force needed to raise a column of mercury to the 120 calibration mark on the glass tube during diastole and to 80 during diastole. The elasticity of the person's arterial walls, the strength of the heart muscle, and the quantity and viscosity (thickness) of the blood all affect the blood pressure.

The sphygmomanometer is attached to a cuff by a rubber tube. A second rubber tube is attached to a hand pump with a screw valve. This device is used to pump air into the rubber bladder in the cuff. When the screw valve is turned clockwise, the bladder in the cuff around the patient's arm is inflated by multiple compressions of the pump. As the bladder inflates, the pressure created against the artery at some point prohibits blood from passing through the vessel. When the screw valve is slowly opened by turning it counterclockwise, the blood pressure can be determined by listening carefully with the stethoscope placed on the artery to the sounds produced as the blood begins to flow through the vessel. Procedure 19-11 describes the steps for correctly obtaining a patient's blood pressure using the radial artery.

TABLE **19-5**	Variations in Respiration Ranges by Age
Age	**Respirations per Minute**
Infant	20+
Child	18–20
Adult	12–20

Table 19-6	Blood Pressure Readings		
	Systolic BP		**Diastolic BP**
Normal	<120 mm Hg	and	<80 mm Hg
Prehypertension	120–139 mm Hg	or	80–89 mm Hg
Hypertension, stage I	140–159 mm Hg	or	90–99 mm Hg
Hypertension stage II	≥160 mm Hg	or	≥100 mm Hg

Source: US Department of Health and Human Services, National Institutes of Health, National Heart, Lung, and Blood Institute

PATIENT EDUCATION

HYPERTENSION

After taking a patient's blood pressure, you should tell the patient what you obtained for the blood pressure reading. Patients with hypertension, or high blood pressure, should be encouraged to keep a personal log of their readings and bring this to each physician office appointment. Because the freestanding blood pressure machines found in pharmacies and supermarkets are not always reliable, you should teach patients with hypertension how to take their blood pressure at home.

CHECKPOINT QUESTION

7. What is happening to the heart during systole? During diastole?

Korotkoff Sounds

Korotkoff sounds can be classified into five phases of sounds heard while auscultating the blood pressure as described by the Russian neurologist Nicolai Korotkoff. Only the sounds heard during phase I (represented by the first sound heard) and phase V (represented by the last sound heard) are recorded as blood pressure. You may hear other Korotkoff sounds during the procedure, but it is not necessary to record them. Table 19-7 describes the five phases of Korotkoff sounds that may be heard when auscultating blood pressure.

Pulse Pressure

The difference between the systolic and diastolic readings is known as the pulse pressure. For example, with the average adult blood pressure of 120/80, the difference between the numbers 120 and 80 is 40. The average normal range for pulse pressure is 30 to 50 mm Hg. Generally, the pulse pressure should be no more than one-third of the systolic reading. If the pulse pressure is more or less than these parameters, the physician should be notified.

Auscultatory Gap

Patients with a history of **hypertension**, or elevated blood pressure, may have an auscultatory gap heard during phase II of the Korotkoff sounds. An auscultatory gap is the loss of any sounds for a drop of up to 30

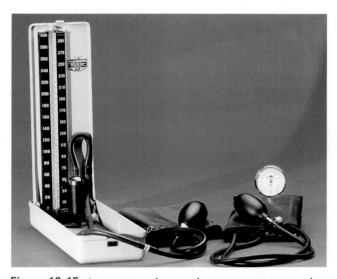

Figure 19-15 A mercury column sphygmomanometer and an aneroid sphygmomanometer.

TABLE 19-7	Five Phases of Blood Pressure
Phase	**Sounds**
I	Faint tapping heard as the cuff deflates (systolic blood pressure)
II	Soft swishing
III	Rhythmic, sharp, distinct tapping
IV	Soft tapping that becomes faint
V	Last sound (diastolic blood pressure)

mm Hg (sometimes more) during the release of air from the blood pressure cuff after the first sound is heard. If the last sound heard at the beginning of the gap is recorded as the diastolic blood pressure, the documented blood pressure is inaccurate and may result in misdiagnosis and treatment of a condition that the patient does not have. As a result, it is important for you to listen and watch carefully as the dial or column of mercury falls until you are certain that you have heard the last sound, or diastolic pressure.

Factors Influencing Blood Pressure

Atherosclerosis and arteriosclerosis are two disease processes that greatly influence blood pressure. These diseases affect the size and elasticity of the artery lumen. The general health of the patient is also a major factor and includes dietary habits, alcohol and tobacco use, the amount and type of exercise, previous heart conditions such as myocardial infarctions, and family history for cardiac disease. Other factors that may affect blood pressure include:

- *Age.* As the body ages, vessels begin to lose elasticity and will require more force to expand the arterial wall. The buildup of atherosclerotic patches inside the artery will also increase the force needed for blood flow.
- *Activity.* Exercise raises the blood pressure temporarily, while inactivity or rest will usually lower the pressure.
- *Stress.* The sympathetic nervous system stimulates the release of the hormone epinephrine, which raises the pressure in response to the fight or flight syndrome.
- *Body Position.* Blood pressure will normally be lower in the supine position.
- *Medications.* Some medications will lower the pressure, while others may cause an elevation.

Figure 19-16 Choosing the right blood pressure cuff.

Figure 19-17 Three sizes of blood pressure cuffs (from left): a large cuff for obese adults, a normal adult cuff, and a pediatric cuff.

Blood Pressure Cuff Size

Before beginning to take a patient's blood pressure, assess the size of the patient's arm, and choose the correct size accordingly. The width of the cuff should be 40% to 50% of the circumference of the arm. To determine the correct size, hold the narrow edge of the cuff at the midpoint of the upper arm. Wrap the width, not the length, around the arm. The cuff width should reach not quite halfway around the arm (Fig. 19-16). Varying widths of cuffs are available, from about 1 inch for infants to 8 inches for obese adults (Fig. 19-17). The blood pressure measurement may be inaccurate by as much as 30 mm Hg if the cuff size is incorrect. Box 19-2 lists causes of errors in blood pressure readings.

 CHECKPOINT QUESTION

8. How are the pulse pressure and the auscultatory gap different?

BOX 19-2

CAUSES OF ERRORS IN BLOOD PRESSURE READINGS

- Wrapping the cuff improperly
- Failing to keep the patient's arm at the level of the heart while taking the blood pressure
- Failing to support the patient's arm on a stable surface while taking the blood pressure
- Recording the auscultatory gap for the diastolic pressure
- Failing to maintain the gauge at eye level
- Applying the cuff around the patient's clothing and attempting to listen through the clothing
- Allowing the cuff to deflate too rapidly or too slowly
- Failing to wait 1–2 minutes before rechecking using the same arm

T R I A G E

While working in a medical office, you have just taken the following three patients' vital signs:

A. A 52-year-old woman complaining of dyspnea. Her respiratory rate is 38, her pulse is 112 and irregular, and her blood pressure is 150/86.

B. A 43-year-old man with a pulse of 54 and blood pressure of 98/52. He denies any shortness of breath, chest pain, or dizziness.

C. A 65-year-old man who had open-heart surgery 2 weeks ago. He states that yellow drainage is coming from the surgical wound on his chest. His temperature is 101.8°F orally, his blood pressure is 188/62, and his pulse is 118 and regular.

How do you sort these patients? Who should be seen first? Second? Third?

Patient A should be seen first. The physician should immediately see any patient complaining of trouble breathing. Her respiratory and pulse rates are faster than normal for an adult. Patient C should be seen second because of his temperature and pulse rate. Patient B should be seen last. A pulse rate of 52 and blood pressure of 98/52 are low, but the patient is not complaining of any symptoms. If he is physically fit, his vital signs may normally be lower than average. If he were complaining of dizziness or feeling faint, he would need to be seen sooner.

 W H A T I F ?

What if a patient has a dialysis shunt (a surgically made venous access port that allows a patient with little or no kidney function to be connected to a dialysis machine) in his left arm? Should you use that arm to take his blood pressure?

NO! By taking a blood pressure in that arm, you could cause the shunt to be permanently damaged, and the patient would not be able to receive dialysis until another shunt was prepared by a surgeon. The patient's chart should be clearly marked indicating that a shunt is in place and which arm it is located in. Most dialysis patients are keenly aware of the importance of this shunt and will alert you to the location of their shunt. Also, you should not draw blood from this arm

español
SPANISH TERMINOLOGY

Voy a tomar su pulso radial.
  I am going to take your radial pulse.
Voy a tomar su presion de sangre.
  I am going to take your blood pressure.
Voy a tomar la temperature.
  I am going to take your temperature.
Fiebre?
  Fever?

 M E D I A M E N U

- **Student CD**
  - **Case Study**
    Interactive Case Study on Vital Signs, Patient Education, and Refusal of Treatment
  - **Video Procedures**
    Procedure 19-9 and 19-10 video clip
  - **Animations**
    Breathing Sounds; Cardiac Cycle; Hypertension
  - **CMA/RMA Certification Exam Review**
- **LWWs Medical Assisting Skills DVD**
  - **Procedures 19-1 and 19-2; 19-6, 19-7, and 19-8; 19-9 and 19-10; 19-11**
- **Premium Online Course**
  http://thePoint.lww.com/Kronenberger3e
- **Internet Resources**

  LiveAdvise Online Tutoring & Competency Training
  http://thePoint.lww.com/LiveAdvise

  National Reye's Syndrome Foundation
  www.reyessyndrome.org

  American Society of Hypertension
  www.ash-us.org

  American Lung Association
  www.lungusa.org

  National Heart Lung and Blood Institute
  www.nhlbi.nih.gov

  American Heart Association
  www.americanheart.org

Procedure 19-1: Measuring Weight

Purpose: Accurately measure and record a patient's weight
Equipment: Calibrated balance beam scale, digital scale, or dial scale; paper towel
Standard: This procedure should take 5 minutes.

Steps	Reasons
1. Wash your hands.	Handwashing before contact with patients aids in infection control.
2. Ensure that the scale is properly balanced at zero. **Step 2.** A balanced scale with the weights at zero.	This helps prevent an error in measurement.
3. Greet and identify the patient. Explain the procedure.	Identifying the patient prevents errors; explaining the procedure promotes cooperation.
4. Escort the patient to the scale, and place a paper towel on the scale.	Since the patient will be standing in bare feet or stockings, the paper towel minimizes microorganism transmission.
5. Have the patient remove shoes and heavy outerwear and put down purse.	Unnecessary items must be removed to get an accurate reading.
6. Assist patient onto the scale facing forward and standing on paper towel without touching or holding on to anything if possible, while watching for difficulties with balance. **Step 6.** The patient should stand erect on the scale.	Some patients may feel unsteady as the plate of the scale settles.
7. Weigh the patient: A. Balance beam scale: Slide counterweights on bottom and top bars (start with heavier bars) from zero to approximate weight. Each counterweight should rest securely in the notch with indicator mark at proper calibration. To obtain	

(continued)

Procedure 19-1:   Measuring Weight *(continued)*

Steps	Reasons
measurement, balance bar must hang freely at exact midpoint. To calculate weight, add top reading to bottom one. (Example: If bottom counterweight reads 100 and lighter one reads 16 plus three small lines, record weight as 116 ¾ lb).	
B. Digital scale: Read and record weight displayed on digital screen.	
C. Dial scale: Indicator arrow rests at patient's weight. Read this number directly above the dial.	Reading at an angle will result in an incorrect measurement.

Step 7. The weight of this patient using the balance beam scale is 175 pounds.

Steps	Reasons
8. Return the bars on the top and bottom to zero.	A balance beam scale should be returned to zero after each use.
9. Assist the patient from the scale if necessary, and discard the paper towel.	Patients may lose balance and fall when stepping down from the scale; they should be observed and assisted as necessary. The paper towel may be left in place on the balance beam scale if the height is going to be obtained using this scale.
10. Record the weight.	If the weight and height are measured at the same time, they will be recorded together (see example in Procedure 19-2).

Procedure 19-2: Measuring Height

Purpose: Accurately measure and record a patient's height
Equipment: A scale with a ruler
Standard: This procedure should take less than 5 minutes.

Steps	Reasons
1. Wash your hands if this procedure is not done at the same time as the weight.	Typically, height is obtained with weight; your hands are already washed.
2. Have the patient remove shoes and stand straight and erect on the scale, with heels together and eyes straight ahead. (Patient may face the ruler, but a better measurement is made with the patient's back to the ruler).	The posture of the patient must be erect for an accurate measurement.
3. With the measuring bar perpendicular to the ruler, slowly lower it until it firmly touches the patient's head. Press lightly if the hair is full or high.	Hair that is full should not be included in the height measurement.

Step 3. Measure where the bar slides out of the scale (or point of movement). This measure reads 63 inches, or 5 feet 3 inches.

4. Read the measurement at the point of movement on the ruler. If measurements are in inches, convert to feet and inches (e.g., if the bar reads 65 plus two smaller lines, read it at 65 ½. Remember that 12 inches equals 1 foot; therefore, the patient is 5 feet, 5 ½ inches tall).	
5. Assist the patient from the scale if necessary; watch for signs of difficulty with balance.	
6. Record the weight and height measurements in the medical record.	

Charting Example:

10/14/2008 9:15 AM Ht. 5 ft, 5 ½ inches, Wt. 136 ¼ lb
—*Y. Torres, CMA*

Procedure 19-3: Measuring Oral Temperature Using a Glass Mercury Thermometer

Purpose: Accurately measure and record a patient's oral temperature using a glass mercury thermometer

Equipment: Glass mercury oral thermometer; tissues or cotton balls; disposable plastic sheaths; biohazard waste container; cool, soapy water; disinfectant solution

Standard: This task should take 10 minutes.

Steps	Reasons
1. Wash your hands and assemble all the necessary supplies.	Handwashing aids infection control.
2. Dry the thermometer if it has been stored in a disinfectant solution by wiping it from the bulb and going up the stem with a tissue or cotton ball. **Step 2.** Dry the glass thermometer beginning at the bulb and moving up the stem.	Removing the wet disinfectant will allow the thermometer to slip easily into the sheath.
3. Carefully check the thermometer for chips or cracks.	A chipped or cracked thermometer could injure the patient.
4. Check the reading by holding the stem horizontally at eye level and turning is slowly	It is easiest to see the mercury in the column in this position.
5. If the reading is above 94°F, shake down the thermometer by securely grasping it at the end of the stem with your thumb and forefinger and snapping your wrist several times. Avoid hitting the thermometer against anything while snapping your wrist.	The reading must be below 94°F to provide an accurate temperature reading. The reading will never decrease in the thermometer unless the mercury is physically forced into the bulb.
6. Insert the thermometer into the plastic sheath. **Step 6.** Place the thermometer into a disposable sheath before using.	Follow the package instructions for placing the thermometer correctly into the sheath.

(continued)

Procedure 19-3: Measuring Oral Temperature Using a Glass Mercury Thermometer *(continued)*

Steps	Reasons
7. Greet and identify the patient. Explain the procedure and ask about any eating, drinking of hot or cold fluids, gum chewing, or smoking within the past 15 minutes.	Eating, drinking, gum chewing, or smoking may alter the oral reading. If the patient has done any of these within 15 minutes, wait 15 minutes or select another route.
8. Place the thermometer under the patient's tongue to either side of the frenulum.	This is the area of highest vascularity and will give the most accurate reading.

Step 8. Place the thermometer to one side of the frenulum.

Steps	Reasons
9. Tell the patient to keep the mouth and lips closed without biting down on the thermometer.	Keeping the mouth and lips closed prevents air from entering the mouth and causing an inaccurate reading. Biting down on the thermometer may break it.
10. Leave the thermometer in place for 3–5 minutes. Note: The pulse, respirations, and blood pressure may be taken during this time (see Procedures 19-9 to 19-11).	The thermometer may be left in place for 3 minutes if there is no evidence of fever and the patient is compliant. It should be left in place for 5 minutes if the patient is febrile or noncompliant (talks or opens mouth frequently).
11. At the appropriate time, remove the thermometer from the patient's mouth while wearing gloves. Remove the sheath by holding the very edge of the sheath with your thumb and forefinger and pulling down from the open edge over the length of the thermometer to the bulb. Discard the sheath into a biohazard container.	

Step 11. Remove the sheath by grasping the end nearest the tip and inverting the plastic toward the bulb. The soiled area should now be inside the sheath.

(continued)

Procedure 19-3: Measuring Oral Temperature Using a Glass Mercury Thermometer *(continued)*

Steps	Reasons
12. Hold the thermometer horizontal at eye level and note the level of mercury that has risen into the column.	
13. Sanitize and disinfect the thermometer according to the office policy and wash your hands. 	Wash the thermometer with cool or tepid soapy water, rinse with cool water, and dry well. Place the thermometer in a disinfectant solution, such as 70% isopropyl alcohol, according to office policy **Step 13.** Store clean thermometers in a covered instrument tray padded with gauze to prevent chipping or cracking the glass.
14. Record the patient's temperature in the medical record.	Procedures are considered not done if they are not recorded. The vital signs (temperature, pulse, respirations, and blood pressure) are usually recorded together.

Charting Example:

09/10/08 8:50 AM T 100.6°F (O)

—L. Ervin, CMA

Procedure 19-4:   **Measuring a Rectal Temperature**

Purpose: Accurately measure and record a rectal temperature using either a glass rectal thermometer or electronic thermometer with a rectal probe attached

Equipment: Glass mercury rectal thermometer or electronic thermometer with rectal probe; tissues or cotton balls; disposable plastic sheaths; surgical lubricant; biohazard waste container; cool, soapy water; disinfectant solution; gloves

Standard: This procedure should take 5 minutes.

Steps	Reasons
1. Wash your hands and assemble the necessary supplies.	Handwashing aids infection control.
2. Insert the thermometer into a plastic sheath. **Step 2.** Rectal thermometers are noted by the red tip.	Follow the package instructions for placing the sheath correctly onto the thermometer. If a glass mercury rectal thermometer is used, follow Steps 2 through 5 in Procedure 19-3 to prepare the thermometer. If an electronic thermometer is used, attach the rectal probe if necessary.
3. Spread lubricant onto a tissue and then from the tissue onto the sheath of the thermometer. **Step 3.** Place lubricant onto a tissue first.	When using a tube of lubricant, avoid cross-contamination by not applying lubricant directly to the thermometer. A lubricant should always be used for rectal insertion to prevent patient discomfort.
4. Greet and identify the patient and explain the procedure.	

(continued)

Procedure 19-4: Measuring a Rectal Temperature *(continued)*

5. Ensure the patient's privacy by placing the patient in a side-lying position facing the examination room door and draping appropriately.

| If the examination room door is opened, a patient facing the door is less likely to be exposed. The side-lying position facilitates exposure of the anus. |

Step 5. The patient is in a side-lying position and draped appropriately.

6. Apply gloves and visualize the anus by lifting the top buttock with your nondominant hand.	Never insert the thermometer without first having a clear view of the anus.
7. Gently insert the thermometer past the sphincter muscle about 1½ inches for an adult, 1 inch for a child, and ½ inch for an infant.	Inserting the thermometer at these depths helps prevent perforating the anal canal.
8. Release the upper buttock and hold the thermometer in place with your dominant hand for 3 minutes. Replace the drape without moving the dominant hand.	The thermometer will not stay in place if it is not held. Replacing the drape will ensure the patient's privacy.
9. After 3 minutes, remove the glass thermometer and the sheath. The electronic thermometer will signal when the reading is obtained. Discard the sheath into an appropriate waste container and note the reading.	The lubricant or sheath may obscure the mercury column in a glass thermometer and should be removed before you read the thermometer. The electronic thermometer will have a digital display of the reading (see Procedure 19-6).
10. Sanitize and disinfect the glass mercury thermometer according to the office policy. Replace the electronic thermometer into the charger as necessary.	
11. Remove your gloves and wash your hands.	This prevents the spread of microorganisms.
12. Record the procedure and mark the letter R next to the reading, indicating that the temperature was taken rectally.	Temperature readings are presumed to have been taken orally unless otherwise noted in the medical record. The vital signs (temperature, pulse, respirations, and blood pressure) are usually recorded together.

Note: Infants and very small children may be held in the lap or over the knees for this procedure. Hold the thermometer and the buttocks with the dominant hand while securing the child with the nondominant hand. If the child moves, the thermometer and the hand will move together, avoiding injury to the anal canal.

Charting Example:

09/11/2008 8:30 AM T 100.2°F (R)

—J. Barth, CMA

Procedure 19-5: Measuring an Axillary Temperature

Purpose: Accurately measure and record an axillary temperature using a glass mercury thermometer or an electronic thermometer

Equipment: Glass mercury thermometer or electronic thermometer (oral or rectal); tissues or cotton balls; disposable plastic sheaths; biohazard waste container; cool, soapy water; disinfectant solution

Standard: This procedure should take 15 minutes.

Steps	Reasons
1. Wash your hands and assemble the necessary supplies.	Handwashing aids infection control.
2. Insert the thermometer into a plastic sheath.	Follow the package instructions for placing the sheath correctly onto the thermometer. If a glass mercury thermometer is used, follow Steps 2 through 5 in Procedure 19-3 to prepare the thermometer.
3. Expose the patient's axilla without exposing more of the chest or upper body than is necessary.	The patient's privacy must be protected at all times.
4. Place the tip of the thermometer deep in the axilla and bring the patient's arm down, crossing the forearm over the chest. Drape the patient as appropriate for privacy.	This position offers the best skin contact with the thermometer and maintains a closed environment.
	Step 4. With the thermometer in the axilla, the arm should be down, and the forearm should be crossed across the chest.
5. After 10 minutes, remove the glass thermometer and the sheath. The electronic thermometer will signal when the reading is obtained. Discard the sheath into an appropriate waste container and note the reading.	Axillary temperatures using a glass thermometer take longer than oral or rectal ones. The sheath may obscure the mercury column in a glass thermometer and should be removed before you read the thermometer. The electronic thermometer will have a digital display of the reading (see Procedure 19-6).
6. Sanitize and disinfect the glass mercury thermometer according to the office policy. Replace the electronic thermometer into the charger as necessary.	
7. Wash your hands.	This prevents the spread of microorganisms.
8. Record the procedure and mark a letter A next to the reading, indicating that the reading is axillary.	Temperature readings are presumed to have been taken orally unless otherwise noted in the medical record. The vital signs (temperature, pulse, respirations, and blood pressure) are usually recorded together.

Charting Example:

02/01/2008 3:45 PM T 97.8°F (A)

—B. DeMarcus, CMA

Procedure 19-6: Measuring Temperature Using an Electronic Thermometer

Purpose: Accurately measure and record a patient's temperature using an electronic thermometer
Equipment: Electronic thermometer with oral or rectal probe, disposable probe covers, biohazard waste container, gloves for taking a rectal temperature
Standard: This task should take 5 minutes.

Steps	Reasons
1. Wash your hands and assemble the necessary supplies.	Handwashing aids infection control.
2. Greet and identify the patient and explain the procedure.	Identifying the patient prevents errors.
3. Choose the most appropriate method (oral, axillary, or rectal) and attach the appropriate probe to the battery-powered unit.	
4. Insert the probe into a probe cover. Covers are usually carried with the unit in a specially fitted box attached to the back or top of the unit.	All probes fit into one size probe cover. If using the last probe cover, be sure to attach a new box of covers onto the unit to be ready for the next patient.
5. Position the thermometer appropriately for the method.	If measuring the temperature rectally, be sure to wear gloves, apply lubricant to the probe cover, and hold the probe in place.
6. Wait for the electronic thermometer unit to "beep" when it senses no signs of the temperature rising further. This usually occurs within 20–30 seconds.	
7. After the beep, remove the probe and note the reading on the digital display screen on the unit before replacing the probe into the unit.	Most units automatically shut off when the probe is reinserted into the unit.
8. Discard the probe cover by depressing a button, usually on the end of the probe, while holding the probe over a biohazard container. After noting the temperature, replace the probe into the unit.	
9. Remove your gloves, if used, wash your hands, and record the procedure.	Be sure to indicate whether the temperature was taken rectally or axillary by placing an R or an A next to the reading in the documentation. The vital signs (temperature, pulse, respirations, and blood pressure) are usually recorded together.
10. Return the unit and probe to the charging base.	Although the unit is battery powered, it should be kept in the charging base so that the battery is adequately charged.

Charting Example:

11/28/2008 10:15 AM T 101°F (O)

—D. Shaper, CMA

Procedure 19-7: Measuring Temperature Using a Tympanic Thermometer

Purpose: Accurately measure and record a patient's temperature using a tympanic thermometer
Equipment: Tympanic thermometer, disposable probe covers, biohazard waste container
Standard: This task should take 5 minutes.

Steps	Reasons
1. Wash your hands and assemble the necessary supplies.	Handwashing aids infection control.
2. Greet and identify the patient and explain the procedure.	Identifying the patient prevents errors.
3. Insert the ear probe into a probe cover.	Always put a clean probe cover on the ear probe before inserting it.
4. Place the end of the ear probe into the patient's ear canal with your dominant hand while straightening out the ear canal with your nondominant hand.	Straighten the ear canal of most patients by pulling the top, posterior part of the outer ear up and back. For children under 3 years of age, pull the outer ear down and back.

Step 4. Place the probe into the ear canal while straightening the ear canal.

Steps	Reasons
5. With the ear probe properly placed in the ear canal, press the button on the thermometer. The reading is displayed on the digital display screen in about 2 seconds.	
6. Remove the probe and note the reading. Discard the probe cover into an appropriate waste container.	The probe covers are for one patient use only.
7. Wash your hands and record the procedure.	Be sure to indicate that the tympanic temperature was taken. The vital signs (temperature, pulse, respirations, and blood pressure) are usually recorded together.
8. Return the unit to the charging base.	The unit should be kept in the charging base so that the battery is always adequately charged.

Charting Example:

04/13/2008 2:00 PM T 99.4°F tympanic

—M. Smythe, CMA

Procedure 19-8:   Measuring Temperature Using a Temporal Artery Thermometer

Purpose: Accurately measure and record a patient's temperature using a temporal artery thermometer
Equipment: Temporal artery thermometer, alcohol wipe
Standard: This task should take less than 5 minutes.

Steps	Reasons
1. Wash your hands and assemble the necessary supplies.	Handwashing aids infection control.
2. Greet and identify the patient and explain the procedure.	Identifying the patient prevents errors.
3. Place the probe end of the hand-held unit on the forehead of the patient. Make sure the patient's skin is dry.	If the patient is diaphoretic, dry the skin with a towel first or take the temperature using another method.

Step 3. The temporal artery thermometer is placed flat against the forehead.

Steps	Reasons
4. With the thermometer against the forehead, depress the on/off button, move the thermometer across and down the forehead, and release the on/off button with the unit over the temporal artery.	Some units may indicate that you should lift the thermometer from the temporal artery and place it behind the ear before releasing the on/off button.

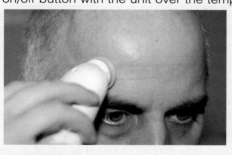

Step 4A. Slide the unit across the forehead.

Step 4B. Stop over the temporal artery before releasing the on/off button.

Steps	Reasons
5. The reading is displayed on the digital display screen in 1–2 seconds.	

(continued)

Procedure 19-8: Measuring Temperature Using a Temporal Artery Thermometer (continued)

Steps	Reasons
6. Properly disinfect the end of the thermometer according to manufacturer instructions.	
7. Wash your hands and record the procedure.	Be sure to indicate that a temporal artery temperature was taken. The vital signs (temperature, pulse, respirations, and blood pressure) are usually recorded together.
8. Return the unit to the charging base.	The unit should be kept in the charging base so that the battery is always adequately charged.

Charting Example:

09/22/2008 9:30 AM T 98.6°F temporal artery
—N. Hoffman, CMA

Procedure 19-9: Measuring the Radial Pulse

Purpose: Accurately measure and record a patient's radial pulse
Equipment: A watch with a sweeping second hand
Standard: This procedure should take 3–5 minutes.

Steps	Reasons
1. Wash your hands.	Handwashing is an infection control technique and should be performed before and after any patient contact.
2. Greet and identify the patient and explain the procedure.	In most cases, the pulse is taken at the same time as the other vital signs.
3. Position the patient with the arm relaxed and supported either on the lap of the patient or on a table.	If the arm is not supported or the patient is uncomfortable, the pulse may be difficult to find and the count may be affected.
4. With the index, middle, and ring fingers of your dominant hand, press with your fingertips firmly enough to feel the pulse but gently enough not to obliterate it (see Fig. 19-11).	Do not use your thumb; it has a pulse of its own that may be confused as the patient's. You may place your thumb on the opposite side of the patient's wrist to steady your hand.
5. If the pulse is regular, count it for 30 seconds, watching the second hand of your watch. Multiply the number of pulsations by 2 since the pulse is always recorded as beats per minute. If the pulse is irregular, count it for a full 60 seconds.	Counting an irregular pulse for less than 60 seconds will give an inaccurate measurement.
6. Record the rate in the medical record with the other vital signs. Also note the rhythm if irregular and the volume if thready or bounding.	Procedures are considered not to have been done if they are not recorded. The vital signs (temperature, pulse, respirations, and blood pressure) are usually recorded together.

Charting Example:

06/12/2008 11:30 AM Pulse 78 and irregular
—E. Kramer, CMA

Procedure 19-10: Measuring Respirations

Purpose: Accurately measure and record a patient's respirations
Equipment: A watch with a sweeping second hand
Standard: This procedure should take 3–5 minutes.

Steps	Reasons
1. Wash your hands.	Handwashing aids in infection control.
2. Greet and identify the patient and explain the procedure.	In most cases, the respirations are counted at the same time as the pulse.
3. After counting the radial pulse and still watching your second hand, count a complete rise and fall of the chest as one respiration. Note: Some patients have abdominal movement rather than chest movement during respirations. Observe carefully for the easiest area to assess for the most accurate reading. **Step 3.** Continue holding the wrist after taking the pulse and begin counting the respirations.	A patient who is aware that you are observing respirations may alter the breathing pattern. It is best to begin counting respirations immediately after counting the pulse without informing the patient.
4. If the breathing pattern is regular, count the respiratory rate for 30 seconds and multiply by 2. If the pattern is irregular, count for a full 60 seconds.	Counting an irregular respiratory pattern for less than 60 seconds may give an inaccurate measurement.
5. Record the respiratory rate in the medical record with the other vital signs. Also, note whether the rhythm is irregular, along with any unusual or abnormal sounds such as wheezing.	Procedures are considered not to have been done if they are not recorded. The vital signs (temperature, pulse, respirations, and blood pressure) are usually recorded together.

Charting Example:

09/15/2008 8:45 AM Resp 16

—J. Thompson, CMA

Procedure 19-11: Measuring Blood Pressure

Purpose: Accurately measure and record a patient's blood pressure
Equipment: Sphygmomanometer, stethoscope
Standard: This procedure should take 5 minutes.

Steps	Reasons
1. Wash your hands and assemble your equipment.	Handwashing aids infection control.
2. Greet and identify the patient and explain the procedure.	Identifying the patient prevents errors and explaining the procedure eases anxiety.
3. Position the patient with the arm to be used supported with the forearm on the lap or a table and slightly flexed, with the palm upward. The upper arm should be level with the patient's heart.	Positioning the arm with the palm upward facilitates finding and palpating the brachial artery. If the upper arm is higher or lower than the heart, an inaccurate reading may result.

Step 3. Support the arm on the patient's lap, slightly flexed with the palm upward.

Steps	Reasons
4. Expose the patient's arm.	Any clothing over the area may obscure the sounds. If the sleeve is pulled up, it may become tight and act as a tourniquet, decreasing the flow of blood and causing an inaccurate blood pressure reading.
5. Palpate the brachial pulse in the antecubital area and center the deflated cuff directly over the brachial artery. The lower edge of the cuff should be 1–2 inches above the antecubital area.	If the cuff is placed too low, it may interfere with the placement of the stethoscope and cause noises that obscure the Korotkoff sounds.

Steps 5 and 6. Center the cuff over the brachial artery.

Steps	Reasons
6. Wrap the cuff smoothly and snugly around the arm and secure it with the Velcro edges.	

(continued)

Procedure 19-11: Measuring Blood Pressure *(continued)*

Steps	Reasons
7. With the air pump in your dominant hand and the valve between your thumb and the forefinger, turn the screw clockwise to tighten. Do not tighten it to the point that it will be difficult to release.	The cuff will not inflate with the valve open. If the valve is too tightly closed, it will be difficult to loosen with one hand after the cuff is inflated. **Step 7.** Holding the bulb and the screw valve properly allows you to inflate and deflate the cuff easily.
8. While palpating the brachial pulse with your nondominant hand, inflate the cuff and note the point or number on the dial or mercury column at which you no longer feel the brachial pulse.	The dial or mercury column should be at eye level. Noting this number gives you a reference point for reinflating the cuff when taking the blood pressure. **Step 8.** Palpate the brachial pulse and place the stethoscope diaphragm bell over this artery.
9. Deflate the cuff by turning the valve counterclockwise. Wait at least 30 seconds before reinflating the cuff.	Always wait at least 30 seconds after deflating the cuff to allow circulation to return to the extremity.
10. Place the stethoscope earpieces in your ears with the openings pointed slightly forward. Stand about 3 feet from the manometer with the gauge at eye level. Your stethoscope tubing should hang freely without touching or rubbing against any part of the cuff.	With the earpieces pointing forward in the ear canals, the openings follow the natural opening of the ear canal. The manometer should be at eye level to decrease any chance of error when it is read. If the stethoscope rubs against other objects, environmental sounds may obscure the Korotkoff sounds.
11. Place the diaphragm of the stethoscope against the brachial artery and hold it in place with the nondominant hand without pressing too hard.	If not pressed firmly enough, you may not hear the sounds. Pressing too firmly may obliterate the pulse. **Step 11.** Hold the stethoscope diaphragm firmly against the brachial artery while taking the blood pressure and listening carefully.

(continued)

Procedure 19-11: Measuring Blood Pressure (continued)

Steps	Reasons
12. With your dominant hand, turn the screw on the valve just enough to close the valve; inflate the cuff. Pump the valve bulb to about 30 mm Hg above the number felt during Step 8.	Inflating more than 30 mm Hg above baseline is uncomfortable for the patient and unnecessary; inflating less may produce an inaccurate systolic reading.
13. Once the cuff is appropriately inflated, turn the valve counterclockwise to release air at about 2–4 mm Hg per second.	Releasing the air too fast will cause missed beats, and releasing it too slowly will interfere with circulation.
14. Listening carefully, note the point on the gauge at which you hear the first clear tapping sound. This is the systolic sound, or Korotkoff I.	Aneroid and mercury measurements are always made as even numbers because of the way the manometer is calibrated.

Step 14A. The meniscus on the mercury column in this example reads 120 mm Hg.

Step 14B. The gauge on the aneroid manometer reads 80 mm Hg.

Steps	Reasons
15. Maintaining control of the valve screw, continue to listen and deflate the cuff. When you hear the last sound, note the reading and quickly deflate the cuff. Note: Never immediately reinflate the cuff if you are unsure of the reading. Totally deflate the cuff and wait 1–2 minutes before repeating the procedure.	The last sound heard is Korotkoff V and is recorded as the bottom number or diastolic blood pressure.
16. Remove the cuff and press the air from the bladder of the cuff.	

(continued)

PROCEDURE 19-11: Measuring Blood Pressure *(continued)*

Steps	Reasons
17. If this is the first recording or a new patient, the physician may also want a reading in the other arm or in another position.	Blood pressure varies in some patients between the arms or in different positions such as lying or standing.
18. Put the equipment away and wash your hands.	
19. Record the reading with the systolic over the diastolic pressure, noting which arm was used (120/80 LA). Also, record the patient's position if other than sitting.	Procedures are considered not done if they are not recorded. The vital signs (temperature, pulse, respirations, and blood pressure) are usually recorded together.

Charting Example:

11/08/2008 3:30 PM T 98.6°F O, P 78, R 16, BP 130/90 LA sitting, 110/78 LA standing

Y. Torres, CMA

- Anthropometric measurements include height and weight. Vital signs include:
  - temperature (T)
  - pulse (P)
  - respirations (R)
  - blood pressure (BP)

- When a patient first visits the medical office, these measurements are recorded as a baseline and used as a comparison for data collected at subsequent visits. These measurements, which provide important data for the physician to use in diagnosing and treating illnesses, are very frequently performed by medical assistants.

Warm Ups for Critical Thinking

1. You are asked to teach a patient, Mr. Stone, how to take his blood pressure at home once in the morning and once at night and record these readings for 1 month. Create a patient education brochure that explains the procedure in understandable terms and design a sheet that Mr. Stone can easily use to record these readings.

2. Ms. Black arrived at the office late for her appointment; she was frantic and explained that she had experienced car trouble on the way to the office, could not find a parking place, and just locked her keys inside her car. How would you expect these events to affect her vital signs? Explain why.

3. What size of cuff would you choose for Mrs. Cooper, an elderly female patient who is 5 feet 3 inches tall and weighs approximately 90 pounds? Why?

4. How would you respond to a patient who asks you to give advice on what type of thermometer to buy for use at home? Would the age of the patient be relevant with regard to the type of thermometer you might suggest?

5. An elderly male patient tells you that he is considering stopping the blood pressure medication the physician ordered at the previous visit. He further explains that he has "read all about this drug on the internet," and he informs you that "it has side effects," although he denies experiencing any at this time. Describe how you would handle this situation.

Answers to Checkpoint Questions

1. Accurately measuring vital signs assists the physician in diagnosing and treating various disorders.

2. Rectal temperature measurements are usually 1° higher than oral measurements because of the vascularity and tightly closed environment of the rectum.

3. A child's body temperature may be slightly higher than an adult's because of the faster metabolism in a child.

4. The electronic, tympanic, and temporal artery thermometers have digital display screens that show the obtained temperature.

5. Measuring a patient's pulse entails assessing and recording the rate (number of heartbeats in 1 minute), rhythm (regular or irregular), and volume (thready, bounding).

6. Contraction of the diaphragm causes negative pressure in the lungs, which respond by filling with inhaled air.

7. During systole, the heart contracts and forces blood out and through the arteries. In diastole, the heart relaxes and fills with blood.

8. The pulse pressure is the difference between the systolic and diastolic blood pressures, and the auscultatory gap is an abrupt, but temporary, end to the tapping sound heard when auscultating the blood pressure.

Outline

**Basic Instruments and
  Supplies**
  Percussion Hammer
  Tuning Fork
  Nasal Speculum
  Otoscope and Audioscope
  Ophthalmoscope
  Examination Light and
    Gooseneck Lamp
  Stethoscope
  Penlight or Flashlight
**Instruments and Supplies
  Used in Specialized
  Examinations**
  Head Light or Mirror

Laryngeal Mirror and
  Laryngoscope
Vaginal Speculum
Lubricant
Anoscope, Proctoscope, and
  Sigmoidoscope
Examination Techniques
  Inspection
  Palpation
  Percussion
  Auscultation
**Responsibilities of the Medical
  Assistant**
  Room Preparation
  Patient Preparation

Assisting the Physician
Postexamination Duties
Physical Examination Format
  Head and Neck
  Eyes and Ears
  Nose and Sinuses
  Mouth and Throat
  Chest, Breasts, and Abdomen
  Genitalia and Rectum
  Legs
  Reflexes
  Posture, Gait, Coordination,
    Balance, and Strength
**General Health Guidelines and
  Checkups**

Learning Objectives

*Upon successfully completing this chapter, you
will be able to:*

1. Spell and define the key terms

2. Identify and state the use of the basic and
   specialized instruments and supplies used
   in the physical examination

3. Describe the four methods used to examine
   the patient

4. State your responsibilities before, during,
   and after the physical examination

5. List the basic sequence of the physical examination

Performance Objectives

*Upon successfully completing this chapter, you
will be able to:*

1. Assist the physician with a patient's physical
   examination (Procedure 20-1)

CAAHEP

- Prepare and maintain examination and treatment areas
- Prepare for and assist with routine and specialty examinations

ABHES

- Prepare patients for procedures
- Prepare and maintain examination and treatment areas
- Assist physician with examinations and treatments

Key Terms

applicator
asymmetry
auscultation
Babinski reflex
baseline
bimanual
bruit
cerumen
clinical diagnosis

diagnosis
differential diagnosis
extraocular
gait
hernia
inguinal
inspection
lubricant
manipulation

nasal septum
occult
palpation
Papanicolaou (Pap) test or smear
percussion
peripheral
PERRLA

range of motion (ROM)
rectovaginal
sclera
speculum
symmetry
transillumination
tympanic membrane

The purpose of the complete physical examination is to assess the patient's general state of health and detect signs and symptoms of disease. New patients usually receive a complete physical examination, which gives the physician **baseline** information about the patient. This baseline information is valuable for future comparison and can aid the physician in **diagnosis** (identifying a disease or condition). Routine examinations are performed thereafter at regular intervals to help maintain the patient's health and prevent disease.

When a patient comes into the office, the physician can make a **clinical diagnosis** based only on the patient's symptoms. At other times, symptoms are vague and could be caused by one of several diseases. In this situation, a **differential diagnosis** is made by comparing symptoms of several diseases. To make any diagnosis, the physician will rely on three basic components: the medical history, the physical examination, and any laboratory and diagnostic tests. Once the data from these three components are collected and evaluated, the physician will make a judgment about the patient's condition and devise a plan of care including appropriate treatment. As a medical assistant, you are responsible for as-

sisting with taking the medical history, preparing the patient for the examination, and assisting the physician during the examination so that a clinical or differential diagnosis can be made as accurately as possible. In addition, you may collect specimens for diagnostic testing. During the examination, you must anticipate the needs of the physician and patient and be prepared to assist as necessary.

Basic Instruments and Supplies

Instruments used during the physical examination enable the examiner to see, hear, or feel areas of the body being assessed. In most cases, it is the physician who uses these instruments, but you must be familiar with instruments and supplies. These instruments should be kept in a special tray or drawer in a convenient location in each examination room. The exact equipment used varies among medical offices according to physicians' preferences and the specialty. Supplies that should be available in the examination room include a tape measure, gloves, tongue depressors, and cotton-tipped **applicators** (Fig. 20-1). The purpose of the most common in-

Figure 20-1 Common supplies used in the adult physical examination: tape measure, gloves, tongue depressor, and cotton-tipped applicator.

struments used in the physical examination is described in the following sections.

 CHECKPOINT QUESTION

1. Why is there variation in the types of instruments and supplies used in each medical office?

Percussion Hammer

The percussion hammer is used to test neurologic reflexes. Also called a reflex hammer, this instrument has a stainless steel handle and a hard rubber head (Fig. 20-2). The head is used to test reflexes by striking the tendons of the ankle, knee, wrist, and elbow. The tip of the handle may be used to stroke the sole of the foot to assess the **Babinski reflex** (a reflex noted by extension of the great

Figure 20-2 A reflex hammer.

Figure 20-3 A tuning fork.

toe and abduction of the other toes). Some hammers have a brush and needle in the handle specifically used to test sensory perception.

Tuning Fork

The tuning fork is used to test hearing. It is a stainless steel instrument with a handle at one end and two prongs at the other end (Fig. 20-3). The examiner strikes the prongs against his or her hand, which causes them to vibrate and produce a humming sound. While vibrating, the handle is placed against a bony area of the skull near one of the ears, and the patient is asked to describe what, if anything, is heard in that ear. Depending on the results of this hearing test, the physician may order additional auditory tests.

Nasal Speculum

The nasal **speculum** is a stainless steel instrument that is inserted into the nostril to assist in the visual inspection of the lining of the nose, nasal membranes, and septum. The tip of the instrument is inserted into the nose, and the handles are squeezed, opening the end and allowing for visualization (Fig. 20-4). Nasal specula are also available in a disposable form.

Otoscope and Audioscope

The otoscope permits visualization of the ear canal and tympanic membrane. The **tympanic membrane**, or

Figure 20-4 A nasal speculum.

eardrum, is a thin, oval membrane between the outer and middle ear that transmits sound vibrations to the inner ear. The otoscope has a stainless steel handle at one end and a head with a light, a magnifying lens, and a cone-shaped hollow speculum at the other end. A portable otoscope has batteries in the handle to operate the light in the head; other otoscopes are part of a unit attached to the wall and plugged into an electrical outlet (Fig. 20-5). In both types, the hollow speculum is covered with a disposable speculum cover before it is placed in the ear canal. An otoscope with a specialized nasal speculum tip may be used to examine the nose.

The audioscope is used to screen patients for hearing loss. Although it looks like an otoscope, the audioscope's handle has a variety of indicators and selection buttons that can be used to adjust its tones. The examiner places the tip of the audioscope in the patient's ear and asks the patient to respond to each of the tones that is produced. The results are recorded in the patient's medical record.

Figure 20-6 A portable ophthalmoscope.

Ophthalmoscope

The ophthalmoscope is used to examine the interior structures of the eyes. Like the otoscope, it may have a stainless steel handle that contains batteries or may be mounted on the wall (Fig. 20-6). The head of the ophthalmoscope also has a light source, magnifying lens, and opening through which to view the eye. Portable units may have a common base handle with various otoscope or ophthalmoscope tips that can be attached for different examinations.

Examination Light and Gooseneck Lamp

Some offices are equipped with an adjustable overhead examination light for better visualization during the examination. The gooseneck lamp is a floor lamp with a movable stand that bends at the neck for use when the overhead lighting is not adequate (Fig. 20-7). You have

Figure 20-5 (A) A portable otoscope. (B) Wall-mounted examination instruments. From left: sphygmomanometer with cuff, ophthalmoscope, otoscope, and dispenser for disposable otoscope speculum covers.

Figure 20-7 An examination light.

Figure 20-8 A stethoscope.

the responsibility to make sure all examination lights are in proper working order and to direct the light toward the area of the body as indicated by the physician.

Stethoscope

The stethoscope is used for listening to body sounds. The bell or diaphragm is at one end and is placed on the patient's body. This end is connected to two earpieces by flexible rubber or vinyl tubing (Fig. 20-8). The two earpieces have plastic or rubber tips that must be adjusted and directed outward before being placed in the examiner's ears. The stethoscope is used to listen to the sounds of the heart, lungs, and intestines. It is also used for taking blood pressure.

Penlight or Flashlight

A penlight or flashlight provides additional light to a specific area during the examination. The penlight is the shape and size of a ballpoint pen and is easily carried in the examiner's pocket (Fig. 20-9). A common flashlight may be used if a penlight is not available. The penlight is often used to examine the eyes, nose, and throat.

Figure 20-9 A penlight.

 CHECKPOINT QUESTION

2. Which instruments are used to test the ears and hearing?

Instruments and Supplies Used in Specialized Examinations

In addition to the basic instruments described previously, specialized equipment may be used during the physical examination. This chapter introduces the specialized examinations and equipment. A more detailed description of specialty examinations is provided in Unit Five.

Head Light or Mirror

An ear, nose, and throat specialist (otorhinolaryngologist) may wear a headlight or head mirror during the examination of these structures. This instrument consists of a light or mirror attached to a headband that fits over the examiner's head (Fig. 20-10). A head light provides direct light on the area being examined; the mirror reflects light from the examination light into the area.

Laryngeal Mirror and Laryngoscope

The laryngeal mirror is a stainless steel instrument with a long, slender handle and a small, round mirror. It is used to examine areas of the patient's throat and larynx that may not be directly visible.

The laryngoscope handle is similar to the battery handle of a portable otoscope or ophthalmoscope, but

Figure 20-10 A head light.

Figure 20-11 A laryngoscope handle and blades (straight and curved).

the head allows attachment of curved or straight laryngoscope stainless steel blades and a small light source (Fig. 20-11). The examiner places the blade in the patient's throat to visualize the larynx or vocal cords, which cannot be seen by simply looking down the patient's throat.

Vaginal Speculum

The general physical examination of female patients may include a pelvic examination and **Papanicolaou (Pap) smear**. This is a simple test in which cells obtained from the cervix or vagina are examined microscopically for abnormalities including cancer. To obtain the cells for a Pap smear, or to visually examine internal female reproductive structures, the vaginal speculum is inserted into the vagina to expand the opening (Fig. 20-12). This instrument is made of stainless steel or disposable plastic.

To obtain vaginal or cervical cells, the physician may use the Ayre spatula or cervical scraper (Fig. 20-13). This

Figure 20-12 Vaginal specula.

Figure 20-13 Cotton-tipped applicator (left), Ayre spatula (center), and histobrush (right). Cotton-tipped applicators of this size are frequently used to remove excess vaginal secretions or to apply medications during the gynecologic examination.

scraper is about 6 inches long and made of plastic or wood. One tip has an irregular shape that is placed in the cervical opening and rotated to collect the specimen; the other end is rounded and may be used to collect cells from the vaginal cul-de-sac. A histobrush may also be used to obtain cells for a Pap smear; it is made of nylon or plastic with soft bristles at one end. The collected cells are transferred to either a glass slide or a liquid preservative and sent to a laboratory for analysis. Chapter 35 has additional information about the gynecologic examination and the role of the medical assistant.

Lubricant

Lubricant is a water-soluble gel used to reduce friction and provide easy insertion of an instrument in the physical examination. After cells are obtained for a Pap smear, lubricant may also be used for a **bimanual** examination. This examination allows the examiner to palpate internal structures of the pelvic cavity with one hand on the abdomen and with two fingers of the other gloved hand inserted into the vagina. Lubricant may also be used for rectal examinations.

Anoscope, Proctoscope, and Sigmoidoscope

The instruments used for examination of the rectum and colon vary in length as appropriate for the structure to be examined. The anoscope is a short stainless steel or plastic speculum that is inserted into the rectum to inspect the anal canal. An obturator with a rounded tip extends beyond the anoscope to allow the instrument to be easily inserted into the rectum (Fig. 20-14). After the

Figure 20-14 The anoscope with the obturator.

anoscope is inserted, the obturator is removed for visualization of the internal lining of the rectum.

The proctoscope is another type of speculum that is used to visualize the rectum and the anus. It is longer than the anoscope and allows the examiner to inspect more areas of the rectum. While it also consists of an obturator that is removed after the instrument is inserted, a fiberoptic light handle and magnifying lens are attached. The tubular part of the scope is marked in centimeters so that the depth of abnormalities in the anal canal can be noted.

A longer instrument used to visualize the rectum and the sigmoid colon is the sigmoidoscope. This instrument consists of a tube with an obturator, fiberoptic light handle, and magnifying lens (Fig. 20-15). It may be rigid and made of stainless steel, or it may be flexible. The advantages of the flexible sigmoidoscope include a smaller diameter, greater depth during the examination, better visualization of the intestinal mucosa, and less discomfort for the patient.

During all rectal examinations, you need a suction machine, cotton-tipped applicators, glass microscope slides, specimen containers, and laboratory request slips available. Tissue or stool specimens obtained during any rectal procedure must be properly preserved and protected for transport to the laboratory for analysis. More information regarding examinations of the colon is found in Chapter 32.

Figure 20-15 A flexible sigmoidoscope.

 CHECKPOINT QUESTION

3. What are the uses of the anoscope, proctoscope, and sigmoidoscope? What is the function of an obturator?

Examination Techniques

While performing the physical examination, the physician uses four basic techniques to gather information. These include **inspection**, **palpation**, **percussion**, and **auscultation**. Each technique is described in more detail in the following sections.

Inspection

Inspection is looking at areas of the body to observe physical features. The examiner inspects the patient's general appearance, including movements, skin and membrane color, contour, and **symmetry** or **asymmetry**, which is equality or inequality in size and shape. Inspection is done both with the naked eye and with instruments, using either room lighting or a special light source. In some cases, inspection includes use of the sense of smell to note any unusual odors of the breath (such as a fruity smell in a diabetic patient) or foul odors from infected wounds or lesions.

Palpation

Palpation is touching or moving body areas with the fingers or hands. The examiner palpates the body to determine pulse characteristics and the presence of growths, swelling, tenderness, or pain. Organs can be palpated to assess their size, shape, and location. Skin temperature, moisture, texture, and elasticity may also be assessed by palpation. Palpation performed with both hands is called bimanual palpation; if the fingers are used, it is called a digital examination. **Manipulation** is the passive movement of the joints to determine the extent of movement or **range of motion (ROM)**.

Percussion

Percussion is tapping or striking the body with the hand or an instrument to produce sounds. Direct percussion is performed by striking the body with a finger. Indirect percussion is done by placing a finger on the area and then striking this finger with a finger of the other hand while listening to the sounds and feeling the vibrations. This allows the examiner to determine the position, size, and density of air or fluid within a body cavity or organ.

Auscultation

Auscultation is listening to the sounds of the body. This examination method uses a stethoscope or the ear placed directly on the patient's body. Areas of the body that can be auscultated include the heart, lungs, abdomen, and blood vessels. In the abdominal examination, auscultation is performed before palpation and percussion, which can affect normal bowel sounds.

 CHECKPOINT QUESTION

4. Which of the examination techniques requires the use of the hands and fingers to feel organs or structures?

Responsibilities of the Medical Assistant

Room Preparation

Medical assistants are usually responsible for preparing the examination rooms, equipment, and supplies in the clinical area. The examination room should be clean, well lighted, well ventilated, and at a comfortable temperature for the patient. The examination table is decontaminated with an appropriate disinfectant between patients, and the paper on the table is removed and replaced with clean paper. At the beginning of each day, you are responsible for checking each examination room for adequate supplies and equipment, including the working condition of equipment. Batteries in otoscopes, ophthalmoscopes, and laryngoscopes are to be checked daily and replaced as needed.

Patient Preparation

Once the examination room is ready, you will call the patient back by name from the waiting room and escort him or her to the treatment room. It is important that you develop rapport with your patients and practice good interpersonal skills. This helps put your patients at ease and increases their confidence in you and the physician. Your goal is to create a positive, supportive, caring, and friendly atmosphere. Treat each patient as an individual, and speak clearly with a confident tone of voice as you explain any procedures.

Before the physician sees the patient, it may be your responsibility to obtain and record the patient's history, chief complaint, and vital signs. If a urine specimen is needed, explain how to obtain the specimen, direct the patient to the bathroom, and explain what to do with the specimen.

Once in the examination room, give the patient instructions for disrobing and putting on the examination gown. Depending on the type of examination to be performed, the patient may wear the gown with the opening in the front or in the back. Leave the room while the patient undresses unless the patient needs help. Then ask the patient to sit on the examination table, helping if needed, and cover the legs with a drape. Place the chart outside the examining room door and notify the physician that the patient is ready.

 CHECKPOINT QUESTION

5. What would be the advantage of checking the working condition of equipment at the beginning of each work day?

 PATIENT EDUCATION

VITAMINS, HERBS, AND NATURAL REMEDIES

When obtaining the patient's history, it is important to ask about medications and treatments that the patient may be using on a regular basis but may not mention. Many times, patients think that vitamins, herbs, and other over-the-counter products are not medications; however, these should be noted in the medical record since they may interact with prescription drugs that the physician has ordered. Although patients may have specific questions about their medications, advise them that the physician will answer specific questions about drug interactions and complications.

Assisting the Physician

During the physical examination, you may assist the physician by handing him or her instruments or supplies and directing the light appropriately. Procedure 20-1 describes the steps for assisting the physician with the physical examination.

Depending on the examination and the physical condition of the patient, you may also assist the patient into an appropriate position and adjust the drape to expose only the body area being examined (Fig. 20-16). Be supportive and offer reassurance to the patient during the examination. Always assess the patient's facial expression and level of anxiety by noting verbal and nonverbal behavior during the examination. Table 20-1 lists standard examination positions, the body parts usually examined in these positions, and the instruments needed by the physician for these examinations.

Figure 20-16 Patient examination positions. **(A)** The erect or standing position. The patient stands erect facing forward with the arms at the sides. **(B)** The sitting position. The patient sits erect at the end of the examination table with the feet supported on a footrest or stool. **(C)** The supine position. The patient lies on the back with arms at the sides. A pillow may be placed under the head for comfort. **(D)** The dorsal recumbent position. The patient is supine with the legs separated, knees bent, and feet flat on the table. **(E)** The lithotomy position is similar to the dorsal recumbent position but with the patient's feet in stirrups rather than flat on the table. The stirrups should be level with each other and about 1 foot out from the edge of the table. The patient's feet are moved into or out of the stirrups at the same time to prevent back strain. **(F)** The Sims position. The patient lies on the left side with the left arm and shoulder behind the body, right leg and arm sharply flexed on the table, and left knee slightly flexed. **(G)** The prone position. The patient lies on the abdomen with the head supported and turned to one side. The arms may be under the head or by the sides, whichever is more comfortable. **(H)** Knee-chest position. The patient kneels on the table with the arms and chest on the table, hips in the air, and back straight. **(I)** Fowler's position. The patient is half-sitting with the head of the examination table elevated 80–90 degrees. **(J)** Semi-Fowler position. The patient is in a half-sitting position with the head of the table elevated 30–45 degrees and the knees slightly bent. **(K)** Trendelenburg position. The patient lies on the back with arms straight at either side, and the head of the bed is lowered with the head lower than the hips; the legs are elevated at approximately 45 degrees.

WHAT IF?

What if you are assisting the physician during a genital and pelvic examination on a disabled female patient who cannot be placed into the lithotomy position?

Both genital and rectal examinations may be performed with the patient in the dorsal recumbent or Sims position for patients who cannot comfortably assume the usual positions, including the lithotomy position.

Postexamination Duties

After the physical examination, you should perform any follow-up treatments and procedures as necessary or as ordered by the physician. Always offer the patient help returning to a sitting position after the examination. Ask the patient to dress, and leave the room unless the patient needs your assistance. Tell the patient what to do after getting dressed. In many offices, the patient gets dressed and remains in the examining room until the medical assistant gives further instructions; in other offices, patients are told to go to the front desk to schedule future appointments or receive further instructions or prescriptions. In either situation, you are responsible

TABLE 20-1 Examination Positions and Their Uses		
Position	**Body Parts**	**Instruments Needed**
Sitting	General Appearance	
	Head, neck	Stethoscope
	Eyes	Ophthalmoscope, penlight
	Ears	Otoscope, tuning fork
	Nose	Nasal speculum, penlight, substances to smell
	Sinuses	Penlight
	Mouth	Glove, tongue blade, penlight
	Throat	Glove, tongue blade, penlight, laryngeal mirror, laryngoscope
	Axilla, arms	
	Chest	Stethoscope
	Breasts	
	Upper back	Stethoscope
	Reflexes	Percussion hammer
Supine	Chest	Stethoscope
	Abdomen	Stethoscope
	Breasts	
Lithotomy, dorsal recumbent, Sims	Female genitalia and internal organs	Gloves, vaginal speculum, Ayre spatula, histobrush, lubricant
Standing, dorsal recumbent, Sims	Male genitalia and hernia	Gloves
	Male rectum	Gloves, lubricant, fecal occult blood test
	Prostate	Gloves, lubricant
	Legs	Percussion hammer
	Spine, posture, gait, coordination, balance, strength, flexibility	
Prone	Back, spine, legs	
Knee-chest	Rectum	Glove, lubricant, anoscope, proctoscope, or sigmoidoscope, fecal occult blood test
	Female genitalia	Glove, lubricant, vaginal speculum, Ayre spatula, histobrush
	Prostate	Glove, lubricant
Fowler's	Head, neck, chest	Stethoscope

LEGAL TIP

During the physical examination, it is recommended that you remain in the examination room if the physician is examining a patient of the opposite gender. For example, if a male physician is performing a gynecologic examination, the medical assistant should remain in the room to protect the physician from being accused of inappropriate behavior. A female physician should also ask the medical assistant to remain present during the examination of a male patient for similar reasons. Although physicians perform these examinations routinely and medical assistants are often busy performing many tasks at once, taking the time to be present during these examinations will provide legal protection for the physician should an accusation of impropriety arise at a later date.

for reinforcing any instructions given by the physician and providing appropriate patient education. Unless the patient was advised to wait in the examination room for instructions after dressing, escort the patient to the front desk for scheduling future appointments and addressing billing issues while maintaining confidentiality. Check the medical record to be sure that all data have been accurately documented before releasing the record to the billing department.

Clean all reusable equipment, and properly dispose of any disposable supplies or equipment used during the examination. Cover the examination table with clean paper, and prepare the room for the next patient.

 CHECKPOINT QUESTION

6. What are your four basic responsibilities in the performance of the physical examination?

Physical Examination Format

The physical examination of the patient begins with the patient seated on the examining table with a drape sheet over the lap and covering the legs. The physician usually progresses through the examination in an orderly, methodical sequence. The patient's general appearance, behavior, speech, posture, nutritional status, hair distribution, and skin are observed throughout the examination. The next sections describe the areas of the body examined, including normal and abnormal findings.

Head and Neck

The patient's skull, scalp, hair, and face are inspected and palpated for size, shape, and symmetry. The examiner looks for nodules, masses, and local trauma. The patient may be asked to roll the head in all directions to assess range of motion and to check for any limitations of movement. The trachea and lymph nodes on the anterior neck are palpated for size and symmetry.

The thyroid gland, also on the anterior neck, is palpated for size and symmetry. The patient may be asked to swallow to facilitate palpating this gland. The carotid arteries are palpated and auscultated on both sides of the neck to check for any **bruit** (abnormal sound) caused by abnormal blockage.

Eyes and Ears

Usually you perform the visual acuity test before the physician's examination (see Chapter 29). The physician also inspects the **sclera**, or fibrous tissue covering the eye, for normal color. The pupils are inspected with a light to see if they are equal in size, round, and nor-

mally reactive to light and accommodation (adjustment). Normal pupil reaction is recorded as **PERRLA**, which means the *p*upils are *e*qual, *r*ound, and *r*eactive to *l*ight and *a*ccommodation. Eye movement is assessed by asking the patient to follow the examiner's fingers. Normal movement may be documented as "EOM intact," which means **extraocular** (outside the eye) movement intact. **Peripheral** vision, or side vision while looking straight ahead, may also be assessed. Using the ophthalmoscope, the physician visualizes the interior of the eye and evaluates the condition of the retina and any pathology of the interlobular blood vessels.

The ears are inspected and palpated for size, symmetry, lesions, and nodules. The otoscope is used to examine the interior of the ear canal, including any **cerumen**, or ear wax. The tympanic membrane is checked for color and intact or broken condition. Normally the tympanic membrane is pearly gray and concave (Fig. 20-17). However, infection may cause discoloration, and fluids behind the eardrum may cause the membrane to bulge outward. Auditory acuity is tested with the tuning fork or the audioscope (see Chapter 29).

Nose and Sinuses

The external nose is palpated for abnormalities and inspected using a nasal speculum and light. The position of the **nasal septum** is noted for any deviation to the right or left. Each nostril is inspected for color of the mucosa, discharge, lesions, obstructions, polyps, swelling, or tenderness. The sense of smell may be assessed by having the patient close the eyes and identify a common substance such as alcohol, lemon, strawberry, or peppermint.

Figure 20-17 A normal tympanic membrane. Reprinted with permission from Moore KL, Agur AM. Essential Clinical Anatomy, 3rd ed. Baltimore: Lippincott Williams & Wilkins, 2007.

The paranasal sinuses are also inspected and palpated. With the technique of **transillumination** to visualize the sinuses, the room is darkened and a penlight or flashlight is placed against the upper cheek or periorbital ridge.

PATIENT EDUCATION

THE SENSE OF TASTE AND SMELL

When obtaining the medical history, ask the patient whether he or she has had any problems with tasting or smelling. A sudden loss in the ability to taste or smell can be the result of medication, sinus infection, and certain types of tumor. Lack of taste sensation can be the result of normal aging. Normally, the tongue is covered with small bumps called papillae. Each papilla holds about 100 taste buds that allow sweet, salty, sour, and bitter tastes to be identified. The average adult has about 10,000 taste buds. The cells that make up the taste buds are replaced about every 2 weeks. Scientists estimate that, by 80 years of age, most people have lost 60% to 80% of their taste buds, and unfortunately, the remaining taste buds are less sensitive than earlier in life. Sweet and salty taste buds tend to be the most affected.

Mouth and Throat

The physician inspects the mucous membranes of the mouth, gums, teeth, tongue, tonsils, and throat using clean gloves, a light source, and a tongue blade. A laryngeal mirror may also be used. The examiner assesses general dental hygiene and salivary gland function and looks for any abnormalities in the oral cavity, including color, ulcerations, and nodules.

CHECKPOINT QUESTION

7. What is the tympanic membrane, and how does infection affect its appearance?

Chest, Breasts, and Abdomen

The anterior chest is examined with the gown removed to the waist. The physician observes the general appearance and symmetry of the chest and breast area, the respiratory rate and pattern, and any obvious masses or swelling. Palpation includes the axillary lymph nodes and the area over the heart. Underlying structures may also be percussed. Using a stethoscope, the examiner auscultates the lungs for abnormal sounds, at which

time the patient may be asked to take deep breaths. The heart sounds and apical pulse are also assessed.

Inspection and palpation of the posterior chest include the muscles of the back and spine. This is followed by percussion of the back to assess lung fields. With a stethoscope, the examiner listens to posterior lung sounds, again with the patient asked to take deep breaths.

The breasts may be palpated in both male and female patients. The supine position is preferred for palpation of the breasts because the breast tissue flattens out, making any abnormalities easier to feel. The tissue subject to breast examination includes not only the breast and nipple, but the tissue extending up to the clavicle, under the axilla, and down to the bottom of the rib cage.

After the breasts are examined, the drape is lowered to expose the abdomen to the pubic area. The patient's chest is draped or gowned to just below the breasts. The abdomen is inspected for contour, symmetry, and pulsations from the aorta, a large artery that extends from the heart down the center of the thoracic and abdominal cavities. The examiner uses the stethoscope to auscultate the bowel sounds. Percussion may be used to determine the outlines of the abdominal organs, and palpation is used to assess any organ enlargement, masses, pain, or tenderness.

The lower abdomen and groin are palpated to assess enlargement of **inguinal** lymph nodes and detect any **hernia.** A hernia is protrusion of an organ, such as the intestines, through a weakened muscle wall. The femoral arteries, which pass through each groin, may also be palpated and auscultated.

CHECKPOINT QUESTION

8. Why is the patient supine for palpation of the breasts?

Genitalia and Rectum

The physician puts on clean gloves to examine the external male genitalia and then the rectum. The male genitalia are inspected to note symmetry, lesions, swelling, masses, and hair distribution. The scrotal contents may be visualized using transillumination in a darkened room. In addition, the scrotum is palpated for testicular size, contour, and consistency. The male patient is then asked to stand and bear down as if having a bowel movement while the examiner places a gloved index finger upward along the side of the scrotum in the inguinal ring to assess for a hernia.

The physician asks the patient either to bend over the examination table or to assume the Sims position to inspect the anus for lesions and hemorrhoids. The examiner inserts a gloved and lubricated finger into the rectum to palpate the rectal sphincter muscle and prostate gland for size, consistency, and any masses. An **occult** blood (hidden blood) stool test may be obtained on any stool obtained from the gloved finger. (Chapter 32 describes the procedure for processing the occult blood stool specimen.)

The female genitalia and rectum are usually examined with the patient in the lithotomy position and with one corner of the drape extending over the genitalia and the other corner covering the patient's chest. A gooseneck lamp is adjusted to direct light on the vaginal area, and the external genitalia are inspected for lesions, edema, cysts, discharge, and hair distribution. With clean gloves, the examiner inserts the vaginal speculum and inspects the condition of the vaginal mucosa and cervix. A Pap smear sample from the cervix is obtained, and the speculum is removed. At this time, the examiner performs a bimanual examination to palpate the internal reproductive organs for size, contour, consistency, and any masses. Two fingers of the gloved dominant hand are inserted into the vagina while the gloved nondominant hand is placed on the lower abdomen to compress the internal organs. (See Chapter 35 for a complete description of the procedure for assisting with a gynecologic examination.)

Sometimes a **rectovaginal** examination is necessary to palpate the posterior uterus and vaginal wall. The examiner places a gloved index finger in the vagina and the middle finger of the same hand in the rectum at the same time. The rectum is usually inspected and palpated for lesions, hemorrhoids, and sphincter tone. A stool specimen may be obtained from the gloved finger to test for occult blood.

Legs

The legs are inspected and the peripheral pulse sites palpated with the patient supine. The patient stands, with assistance if needed, and the peripheral pulse sites may be palpated again and the legs observed for varicose veins.

Reflexes

The examiner uses the percussion hammer to test the patient's reflexes by striking the biceps, triceps, patellar, Achilles, and plantar tendons. The patient is usually sitting when these reflexes are checked but may move to supine for checking the plantar reflexes.

Posture, Gait, Coordination, Balance, and Strength

The general posture of the patient and the spine may be inspected with the patient standing. The patient may be asked to walk and perform other movements so that **gait** and coordination can be observed. A balance test may be done by having the patient stand with the feet together and eyes closed. Range of motion and strength of arms and legs are assessed.

CHECKPOINT QUESTION

9. What is the function of the rectovaginal and bimanual pelvic examinations?

General Health Guidelines and Checkups

Physicians vary as to how often they recommend a complete physical examination. For patients aged 20 to 40 years, physical examinations are scheduled about every 1 to 3 years. Annual examinations are typically performed on patients over age 40 unless a medical condition requires more frequent visits.

For women, the American Cancer Society recommends the first Pap smear when sexual activity occurs, but no later than 21 years of age. This test should be done annually for conventional testing or every 2 years if the practitioner uses a liquid-based Pap test. A breast examination by a physician is recommended every 3 years for women aged 20 to 40 to detect lumps and thickenings that could be malignancies, but breast self-examinations (BSE) should be performed monthly to allow the patient to detect and report any abnormalities in breast tissue between visits to the physician (see Chapter 35). As with most cancers, early detection of breast cancer is the key to survival. A baseline mammogram is recommended for those aged 35 and yearly after 40. If the patient is at risk for developing breast cancer, the physician may recommend mammograms earlier and more often.

The American Cancer Society also recommends that male patients have the prostate-specific antigen (PSA) blood test and digital rectal examination (DRE) yearly beginning at age 50 to detect early signs of prostate cancer. Men who are high risk for developing prostate cancer should have these tests starting at age 45. Risk factors include African-American men and those with close family members (father, brothers, or sons) who were diagnosed with prostate cancer before the age of 65. Again, early detection is important for early treatment, which saves lives.

All patients should have a baseline electrocardiogram (ECG) at age 40 and follow-up ECGs as necessary. In addition, a rectal examination and fecal occult blood test are recommended annually beginning at age 40. At age 50, a proctoscopic examination (colonoscopy) is recommended, and if the results are negative, this exam should be performed every 3 to 5 years thereafter.

The Centers for Disease Control and Prevention recommends the following immunizations for all adults:

- Tetanus booster every 10 years, or sooner if the patient has an open wound.
- Measles, mumps, rubella (MMR) one or two doses between the ages of 19 and 49 years for patients who do not have documentation of having the vaccine or for those who have never had the disease.
- The varicella vaccine (chickenpox) should be given in two doses between the ages of 19 and 49 years for patients who do not have documentation of having the vaccine or for those who have never had the disease.
- One injection of pneumococcal vaccine should be given at age 65 years.
- After age 50, an annual influenza vaccine should be given.
- Some doctors also recommend a series of three hepatitis B injections for any adult patient who has not received this immunization.

You should take every opportunity to educate patients regarding the signs and symptoms that may signal health problems and when to call the physician.

 CHECKPOINT QUESTION

10. Why are monthly breast self-examinations important for women aged 20 to 40 years?

 PATIENT EDUCATION

THE BODY'S WARNING SIGNALS

Teach patient's the CAUTION acronym to recognize these early warning signs of cancer:

C Change in bowel or bladder habits
A A sore that does not heal
U Unusual bleeding or discharge
T Thickening, lumps, or changes in the shape of the breasts or testicles
I Indigestion or difficulty swallowing
O Obvious change in a wart or mole
N Nagging cough or hoarseness of the voice

Frequent, severe headaches and persistent abdominal pain are other signals that should not be ignored. Instruct patients not to overlook the following signs in their children:

- Continual crying for no obvious reason
- Unexplained nausea and vomiting
- General failure to thrive
- Spontaneous bleeding or bleeding that does not stop in the normal amount of time
- Bumps, lumps, masses, or swelling anywhere on the body

 TRIAGE

While working in a family practice office, you have to complete the following three tasks:

A. A patient was just discharged, and the examination room has to be cleaned and restocked.

B. The physician states that she is ready to perform a gynecologic examination and needs your assistance.

C. A suture tray has to be set up for a 3-year-old child with a facial laceration.

How do you sort these tasks? What do you do first? Second? Third?

First, assist the physician with the examination. When possible, limit the waiting time for female patients to have their gynecologic examination. Next, set up the suture tray. Third, clean and restock the examination room.

español SPANISH TERMINOLOGY

Voy a examinarle.
  I am going to examine you.
Voy a reviser sus orejas.
  I am going to check your ears.
Voy a reviser su boca.
  I am going to check your nose.
Saque la lengua.
  Stick out your tongue.
Voy a reviser su piel.
  I am going to examine your skin.
Voy a reviser su abdomen (vientre).
  I am going to examine your abdomen.
Voy a reviser su espalda.
  I am going to examine your back.

MEDIA MENU

- **Student CD**
  - **CMA/RMA Certification Exam Review**
- **Premium Online Course**
  http://thePoint.lww.com/Kronenberger3e
- **Internet Resources**

LiveAdvise Online Tutoring & Competency Training
http://thePoint.lww.com/LiveAdvise

American Academy of Family Physicians
www.aafp.org

American Academy of Family Physicians
www.familydoctor.org

American College of Physicians—Internal Medicine
www.acponline.org

CDC Screen for Life: National Colorectal Cancer Action Campaign
www.cdc.gov/cancer/screenforlife/

American Cancer Society
www.cancer.org

National Breast Cancer Foundation
www.nationalbreastcancer.org

PROCEDURE 20-1: Assisting With the Adult Physical Examination

Purpose: Prepare the room and patient for the general physical examination, assist the physician during the examination, assist the patient as needed after the examination, and clean up the examination room
Equipment: A variety of instruments and supplies, including the stethoscope, ophthalmoscope, otoscope, penlight, tuning fork, nasal speculum, tongue blade, percussion hammer, gloves, water-soluble lubricant, an examinations light, and patient gown and draping supplies
Standard: This procedure should take 15 minutes.

Steps	Reasons
1. Wash your hands.	Hand washing aids infection control.
2. Prepare the examination room and assemble the equipment.	A clean room that is free of contamination prevents transfer of microorganisms. **Step 2.** The examination room should be clean, neat, and orderly.
3. Greet the patient by name and escort him or her to the examining room. 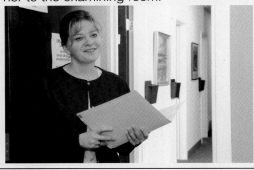	Identifying the patient by name prevents errors. **Step 3.** Identify the patient and escort him or her to the exam room.
4. Explain the procedure.	Explaining the procedure reduces anxiety and may help to ensure compliance.
5. Obtain and record the medical history and chief complaint.	
6. Take and record the vital signs, height, weight, and visual acuity.	The vital signs and other measurements give the physician an overall picture of the patient's health. **Step 6.** Taking the patient's vital signs is an important part of the physical exam.

(continued)

PROCEDURE 20-1:   **Assisting With the Adult Physical Examination** *(continued)*

Steps	Reasons
7. If the physician requires it, instruct the patient to obtain a urine specimen and escort him or her to the bathroom (refer to Chapter 43 for more information on obtaining a urine specimen).	Even if a urine specimen is not part of the physical examination, an empty bladder makes abdominal and/or pelvic examinations more comfortable.
8. Once inside the examination room, instruct the patient in disrobing including directions on how to put the gown on (open in the front or back). Leave the room unless the patient needs assistance.	The gown must open in the direction that provides accessibility for the examination. Elderly and disabled persons may need help disrobing and putting on the gown.
9. Help the patient sit on the edge of the examination table and cover the lap and legs with a drape. 	The sitting position is often the first position used by the physician. **Step 9.** The patient should be draped appropriately.
10. Place the medical record outside the examination room and notify the physician that the patient is ready. 	Make sure the patient's name on the medical record is facing inward to maintain confidentiality from anyone passing by the room. Alerting the physician helps prevent delays. **Step 10.** Place the medical record with identifying information turned away from the hallway.

(continued)

PROCEDURE 20-1: **Assisting With the Adult Physical Examination** *(continued)*

Steps	Reasons
11. Assist the physician by handing him or her the instruments as needed and positioning the patient appropriately.	Anticipating the physician's needs promotes efficiency and saves time. Only the parts of the body being examined should be exposed. Always preserve patients' privacy and keep them covered as much as possible. Tissues may be used to wipe off excess lubricant.

A. Begin by handing the physician the instruments necessary for examining the following:

- Head and neck — Stethoscope
- Eyes — Ophthalmoscope, penlight
- Ears — Otoscope, tuning fork
- Nose — Penlight, nasal speculum
- Sinuses — Penlight
- Mouth — Tongue blade, penlight. Hand the tongue blade to the physician by holding it in the middle. When it is returned to you, grasp it in the middle again so that you do not touch the end that was in the patient's mouth.
- Throat — Glove, tongue blade, laryngeal mirror, Penlight

B. Help the patient drop the gown to the waist for examination of the chest and upper back. Hand the physician the stethoscope.

C. Help the patient pull the gown up and remove the drape from the legs so that the physician can test the reflexes. Hand the physician the percussion hammer.

D. Help the patient to lie supine, opening the gown at the top to expose the chest again. Place the drape to cover the waist, abdomen, and legs. Hand the physician the stethoscope.

E. Cover the patient's chest and lower the drape to expose the abdomen. Hand the physician the stethoscope.

F. Assist with the genital and rectal examinations. Hand the patient tissues following these examinations.

For females:

- Assist the patient to the lithotomy position and drape appropriately.
- For examination of the genitalia and internal reproductive organs, provide a glove, lubricant, speculum, microscope slides or liquid prep solution, and Ayres spatula or brush.
- For the rectal examination, provide a glove lubricant, and fecal occult blood test slide.

(continued)

PROCEDURE 20-1: Assisting With the Adult Physical Examination *(continued)*

For males
- Help the patient stand and have him bend over the examination table for a rectal and prostate examination.
- For a hernia examination, provide a glove.
- For a rectal examination, provide a glove, lubricant, and fecal occult blood test slide
- For a prostate examination, provide a glove and lubricant.

G. With the patient standing, the physician can assess the legs, gait, coordination, and balance.

12. Help the patient sit at the edge of the examination table.	The physician often discusses findings with the patient at this time and may provide instructions.
13. Perform any follow-up procedures or treatments.	
14. Leave the room while the patient dresses unless he or she needs assistance.	Leaving the room provides privacy for the patient.
15. Return to the examination room when the patient has dressed to answer any questions, reinforce physician instructions, and provide patient education.	Compliance depends on full understanding of the treatment plan. Patient education is the responsibility of all health care workers, including the medical assistant.
16. Escort the patient to the front desk.	You can clarify appointment scheduling or billing issues.
17. Properly clean or dispose of all used equipment and supplies. Clean the room with a disinfectant and prepare for the next patient.	All instruments, supplies, and equipment that came into direct contact with the patient must be appropriately decontaminated or disposed of.
18. Wash your hands and record any instructions from the physician. Also note any specimens and indicate the results of the test or the laboratory where the specimens are being sent for testing.	Procedures and instructions are considered not to have been done if they are not recorded.

Charting Example:

01/19/08 1:30 PM CC: Annual physical exam complete per Dr. Smith. ECG done; results given to Dr. Smith. Blood drawn and sent to Acme lab for CBC, electrolytes, and liver panel. Pt. instructed to return to office in 2 weeks to discuss laboratory results. Pt. given written and verbal instructions for 1800-calorie, low-sodium diet as ordered. Pt. verbalized understanding.

—J. Bohr, CMA

- Your role as a medical assistant during the physical examination is to assist both the physician and the patient.
- Efficiency, accuracy, and attention to detail are crucial as you assist the physician and anticipate what will be needed in the examination.

- Assessing the patient's needs, developing a good interpersonal relationship, and providing support to the patient are important to help the patient have a pleasant office visit.

Warm Ups   for Critical Thinking

1. During the physical examination, the physician asks the patient to walk across the room. What can be determined about the patient's health from observing the patient's gait?

2. After the physical examination, a patient asks you, "Why did the physician hit my chest with his fingers while listening?" How do you explain to the patient what the doctor was doing?

3. Why is it possible for the physician to assess vascular health by checking the interior eye with the ophthalmoscope?

4. How can you anticipate what instruments or supplies the physician may need during the physical examination? Why is this important?

5. When checking the ophthalmoscope for working condition, you discover that it is not working. What do you think might be the problem? How would you handle this situation?

Answers   to Checkpoint Questions

1. Although there are some basic instruments and supplies found in most medical offices, the exact equipment used from one office to the next may vary according to the preference and specialty of the physician.

2. The tuning fork and audioscope are used to test hearing. The otoscope is used to assess the internal structures of the ear.

3. The anoscope is the shortest and is used to inspect the anal canal. The proctoscope is longer than the anoscope and is used to visualize the rectum and the anus. The sigmoidoscope is the longest of the three and is used to inspect the rectum and sigmoid colon.

4. The examination technique that requires the use of the hands or fingers is palpation.

5. The working condition of equipment that may be used during patient examinations should be checked at the beginning of each work day to increase efficiency and improve patient care.

6. The clinical medical assistant is responsible for preparing the examination room, preparing the patient, assisting the physician, and cleaning the examination room and equi

CHAPTER 21

Sterilization and Surgical Instruments

Outline

Principles and Practices of Surgical Asepsis
Sterilization
Surgical Instruments
Forceps

Scissors
Scalpels and Blades
Towel Clamps
Probes and Directors
Retractors

Care and Handling of Surgical Instruments
Storage and Record Keeping
Maintaining Surgical Supplies

Learning Objectives

Upon successfully completing this chapter, you will be able to:

1. Spell and define the key terms
2. Describe several methods of sterilization
3. Categorize surgical instruments based on use and identify each by its characteristics
4. Identify surgical instruments specific to designated specialties

5. State the difference between reusable and disposable instruments
6. Explain how to handle and store instruments, equipment, and supplies
7. Describe the necessity and steps for maintaining documents and records of maintenance for instruments and equipment

Performance Objectives

Upon successfully completing this chapter, you will be able to:

1. Sanitize equipment and instruments (Procedure 21-1)

2. Properly wrap instruments for autoclaving (Procedure 21-2)
3. Perform sterilization techniques and operate an autoclave (Procedure 21-3)

Competencies

CAAHEP

- Wrap items for autoclaving
- Perform sterilization techniques
- Practice standard precautions

ABHES

- Wrap items for autoclaving
- Perform sterilization techniques
- Practice standard precautions

autoclave	hemostat	ratchet	scissors
disinfection	needle holder	sanitation	serration
ethylene oxide	obturator	sanitize	sound
forceps	OSHA	scalpel	sterilization

The goal of surgical asepsis is to free an item or area from all microorganisms, including pathogens and other microorganisms (see Chapter 17). The practice of surgical asepsis, also known as sterile technique, should be used during any office surgical procedure, when handling sterile instruments to be used for incisions and excisions into body tissue, and when changing wound dressings. Surgical asepsis prevents microorganisms from entering the patient's environment; medical asepsis prevents microbes from spreading to or from patients.

In a medical office, your responsibilities may include assisting with minor surgical procedures while maintaining surgical asepsis. To manage this responsibility, you must do the following:

- Become familiar with many types of surgical instruments
- Understand the principles and practices of surgical asepsis
- Understand and use **disinfection** and **sterilization** techniques
- Use equipment designed for sterilization, treatment, and diagnostic purposes
- Maintain accurate records and inventory of purchases related to surgical equipment and supplies

The physician expects you to understand sterile technique and to be able to maintain sterility throughout procedures. Any break in sterile technique, no matter how small, can lead to infection the body cannot fight. Even small infections can delay the patient's recovery and are physically, mentally, and financially costly to the patient.

Principles and Practices of Surgical Asepsis

As a medical assistant, you are responsible for preventing infection in accordance with the principles and practices of asepsis as it relates to items used during minor office surgical procedures. Surgical asepsis requires the absence of microorganisms, infection, and infectious material on instruments, equipment, and supplies. Disinfection, or medical asepsis, is different from sterilization (Table 21-1). By becoming familiar with the

manufacturer's recommendations for processing instruments according to the purposes for which the items will be used, you will be able to determine the appropriate level of asepsis.

Sterilization

While **sanitation** and disinfection are adequate for maintaining medical asepsis in the medical office, these practices are not sufficient to process instruments and equipment used during sterile procedures (see Chapter 17). Objects requiring surgical asepsis must be **sanitized** first and sterilized by either a physical or chemical process. Procedure 21-1 describes the procedure for sanitizing instruments in preparation for sterilization. Sterilization is the complete elimination or destruction of all forms of microbial life, including spore forms. Steam under pressure, dry heat, **ethylene oxide** gas, and liquid chemicals are principle sterilizing agents. Although in medical offices steam under pressure is the most frequently used method of sterilization, the method depends on the nature of the material to be sterilized and the type of microorganism to be destroyed. Table 21-2 describes the various methods of sterilization and the temperatures and time of exposure if applicable.

 CHECKPOINT QUESTION

1. How do sanitization, disinfection, and sterilization differ?

Sterilization Equipment

Several types of sterilization equipment are used in clinics and medical offices. As a clinical medical assistant, it is your responsibility to do the following:

- Become familiar with the uses and operation of each piece of equipment
- Schedule periodic preventive maintenance or servicing of the equipment
- Maintain adequate supplies for general operational needs

Table 21-1.	**Comparison of Medical and Surgical Asepsis**	
	Medical Asepsis	**Surgical Asepsis**
Definition	Destroys microorganisms after they leave the body	Destroys microorganisms before they enter the body
Purpose	Prevents transmission of microbes from one person to another	Prevents entry of microbes into the body in invasive procedures
When Used	During contact with a body part that is not normally sterile	During contact with a normally sterile part of the body
Differences in Handwashing Technique	Hands and wrists are washed for 1–2 minutes	Hands and forearms are washed for 5–10 minutes with a brush

The Autoclave

The most frequently used piece of equipment for sterilizing instruments today is the **autoclave** (Fig. 21-1). The autoclave has two chambers: an outer one where pressure builds and an inner one where the sterilization occurs. Distilled water is added to a reservoir, where it is converted to steam as the preset temperature is reached. The steam is forced into the inner chamber, increasing the pressure and raising the temperature of the steam to 250°F or higher, well above the ordinary boiling temperature of water (212°F or 100°C). The pressure has no effect on sterilization other than to increase the temperature of the steam. The high temperature allows for destruction of all microorganisms, including viruses and spores.

An air exhaust vent on the bottom of the autoclave allows the air in the chamber to be pushed out and replaced by the pressurized steam. When no air is present, the chamber seals and the temperature gauge begins to rise. Most automatic autoclaves can be set to vent, time, turn off, and exhaust at preset times and levels. Older models may require that the steps be advanced manually. All manufacturers provide instructions for operating the machine and recommendations for the times necessary to sterilize different types of loads. These instructions should be posted in a prominent place near the machine.

Sterilization is required for surgical instruments and equipment that will come into contact with internal body tissues or cavities that are considered sterile. The autoclave is commonly used to sterilize minor surgical instruments, surgical storage trays and containers, and some surgical equipment, such as bowls for holding sterile solutions. Instruments or equipment subject to damage by water should not be sterilized in the autoclave. These items can be sterilized with gas. Items that are not subject to water damage but may be destroyed by heat can be cold-sterilized or soaked for a prescribed amount of time in a liquid such as glutaraldehyde or

Table 21-2	**Sterilization Methods**	
Methods	**Concentration or Level**	
Heat		
Moist heat (steam under pressure)	250°F or 121°C for 30 min	
Boiling	212°F or 100°C for ≥ 30 min	
Dry heat	340°F or 171°C for 1 hour 320°F or 160°C for 2 hours	
Liquids		
Glutaraldehyde	Follow manufacturer's recommendations or OSHA requirements and guidelines	
Formaldehyde	Follow manufacturer's recommendations or OSHA requirements and guidelines	
Gas		
Ethylene oxide	450–500 mg/L 50°C	

OSHA, Occupational Safety and Health Administration.

A

B

Figure 21-1 (**A**) An autoclave that may be found in the medical office; note the clearly marked dials and gauges. (**B**) The interior of the autoclave.

formaldehyde. Always follow the manufacturer's recommendations for sterilizing instruments or equipment and for using any chemical products for sterilization. Procedure 21-2 describes preparation of instruments for sterilization in the autoclave.

 CHECKPOINT QUESTION

2. Why is the properly working autoclave more effective at sterilizing equipment compared to boiling water?

Sterilization Indicators

Tape applied to the outside of the material used to wrap instruments or supplies for the autoclave indicates that the items have been exposed to steam, but the tape cannot ensure the sterility of the contents (Box 21-1 and Fig. 21-2). Sterilization indicators placed inside the packs register that the proper pressure and temperature were attained for the required time to allow steam to penetrate the inner parts of the pack (Fig. 21-3). Improper wrapping, loading, or operation of the autoclave may prevent the indicator from registering properly.

Types of indicators include those that change colors at high temperatures. Specially designed tubes containing wax pellets are also used to indicate that the required temperature was reached, as evidenced by the melted wax. Although most types of sterilization indicators work well, the best method for determining effectiveness of sterilization is the culture test. Strips impregnated with heat-resistant spores are wrapped and placed in the center of the autoclave between the packages in a

BOX 21-1

AUTOCLAVE INDICATOR TAPE

Autoclave tape is designed to change color in the presence of heat and steam. In extreme instances, the tape may change appearance when stored too close to heat sources. Most tapes have imprinted lines that darken after exposure, but sterilization of the package contents is not ensured by a color change on the autoclave tape. Proper sterilization can be assumed only if accompanying sterilization indicators have registered that all elements of the sterilization process (time and temperature) have been achieved.

Figure 21-3 Sterilization indicators and autoclave indicator tape. Gas indicator tape (left) and steam indicator tape (right).

Figure 21-2 The stripes on autoclave indicator tape change color, indicating that the pack has been exposed to steam.

designated load, such as the first load of the day. The strips are removed from their packets and placed in a broth culture to be incubated according to the instructions of the manufacturer. At the end of the incubation period, the culture is compared to a control to determine that all spores have been killed. If sterilization was not achieved, the load must be reprocessed.

 CHECKPOINT QUESTION

3. What is the difference between a sterilization indicator and autoclave tape?

Loading the Autoclave

Load the autoclave loosely to allow steam to circulate. If too many items are packed into the autoclave, steam will not penetrate the items in the center. Place empty wrapped containers or bowls on their sides with the lids wrapped separately. If containers are upright in the autoclave, air, which is heavier than steam, will settle into the interior of the container and keep steam from circulating to the inner surfaces. Place all packs on their sides to allow for the maximum steam circulation and penetration (Fig. 21-4).

Operating the Autoclave

All components of autoclaving—temperature, pressure, steam, and time—must be correct for the items to reach sterility. Follow the instruction manual carefully. All machines use the same principles, but operation varies. Become familiar with the function of the machine in your facility. Instructions may be covered in plastic or laminated and posted beside the machine for easy reference.

The autoclave has a reservoir tank that should be filled with distilled water only. Tap water contains chemicals and minerals that would coat the interior chamber, clog the exhaust valves, and hinder the overall operation of the autoclave. When filling the internal chamber of the autoclave with distilled water from the reservoir, be

Figure 21-4 Properly loaded autoclave.

sure the water level is at the fill line. If too much water is added to the chamber, the steam will be saturated and may not be efficient, and too little water will not produce the required amount of steam. Procedure 21-3 outlines the general steps for operating an autoclave.

The temperature, pressure, and time required vary with the items being sterilized. In most cases, 250°F at 15 pounds of pressure for 20 to 30 minutes will be sufficient, but you should follow the manufacturer's instructions for the load content. Solid or metal loads take slightly less time than soft, bulky loads. The timer should not be set until the proper temperature has been attained. Some microorganisms, such as spores, are killed only if exposed to high enough temperature for a specific amount of time.

When the items have been in the autoclave at the right temperature for enough time, the timer will sound, indicating that the cycle is finished. Be sure to vent the autoclave to allow the pressure to drop safely. After the pressure has dropped to a safe level, open the door of the autoclave slightly to allow the temperature to drop and the load to cool and dry. Newer autoclaves vent automatically. Do not handle or remove items from the autoclave until they are dry because bacteria from your hands would be drawn through the moist coverings and contaminate the items inside the wrapping. Once the items are dry, remove the packages and store them in a clean, dry, dust-free area. Packs that are sterilized on site in the autoclave are considered sterile for 30 days and must be sterilized again after this period. Always store recently autoclaved items toward the back of the cabinet, rotating the previously autoclaved items to the front. In addition, you are responsible for performing maintenance on the autoclave at regular intervals. Post a schedule for this maintenance near the machine; allow for cleaning the lint trap, washing out the interior of the chamber with a cloth or soft brush, and checking the function of all components. This schedule can remind and document the service with space for initialing or signing after the maintenance has been done.

 CHECKPOINT QUESTION

4. Why is it important to set the timer on the autoclave during a cycle only after the correct temperature has been reached?

Surgical Instruments

You must be able to identify surgical instruments according to their design and function. A surgical instrument is a tool or device designed to perform a specific function, such as cutting, dissecting, grasping, holding, retracting, or suturing. Surgical instruments are designed to perform specific tasks based on their shape; they may be curved, straight, sharp, blunt, serrated, toothed, or smooth. Many are made of stainless steel and are reusable; others are disposable. It is your responsibility to know the proper use and care of the surgical instruments in your clinical setting.

Most instruments used in office procedures can be identified by carefully examining the instrument. The most widely used surgical instruments are **forceps**, **scissors**, **scalpels**, and clamps. Table 21-3 shows the most commonly used instruments and equipment by specialty.

TABLE 21-3	Commonly Used Instruments and Equipment by Specialty	
	Instrument	**Use**
Obstetrics, Gynecology	Vaginal speculum	Open vagina to view vaginal walls, cervical os; perform procedures; sized; may be reusable metal or disposable plastic
	Tenaculum	Grasping and holding tissue with hook-like tips
	Uterine **sounds**	Assess depth of uterus; graduated in inches or centimeters
	Uterine dilator	Widens cervical os; usually 3–18 mm
	Curet	Blunt or sharp; for scraping endometrium
	Biopsy forceps	Secure pieces of tissue for microscopic study

Gynecology instruments: (A) Graves vaginal speculum. (B) Pederson vaginal speculum. (C) Duplay tenaculum forceps. (D) Schroeder tenaculum forceps. (E) Sims uterine sound. (F) Simpson uterine sound, malleable. (G) Hand uterine dilator. (H) Hegar uterine dilator. (I) Thomas uterine curets. (J) Sims uterine curets.

Orthopedics	Cast saw Cutters or spreaders	Remove cast

Orthopedic instruments: (A) Oscillating plaster saw. (B) Stille plaster shears. (C) Hennig plaster spreader.

(continued)

TABLE **21-3**	**Commonly Used Instruments and Equipment by Specialty** *(continued)*

	Instrument	Use
Urology	Urethral sounds	Explore bladder depth, direction; dilate urethral meatus in stenosis; sized Fr 8–26
	Prostate biopsy	Removes tissue for microscopic study

Urology instruments: (**A**) Otis-Dittel urethral sound. (**B**) Dittel urethral sound.

	Instrument	Use
Proctology	Anoscopes, proctoscopes	Visualize lower intestinal tract; most have **obturator** for ease of insertion
	Sigmoidoscope	Visualize lower sigmoid colon; rigid or flexible, with fiber optic light; some have suction device
	Punch biopsy	Remove small piece of tissue via small circular hole
	Alligator biopsy	Jaws grasp and excise tissue

Proctology instruments: (**A**) Ives rectal speculum (Fansler). (**B**) Pratt rectal speculum. (**C**) Hirschman anoscope.

	Instrument	Use
Otology, rhinology	Nasal or ear forceps	Insert or remove materials from nose or ear canal
	Nasal speculum	Opens, extends nostrils for visualization of nasal passages
	Curet	Remove cerumen from deep ear canal

Otology and rhinology instruments: (**A**) Wilde ear forceps. (**B**) Lucae bayonet forceps. (**C**) Buck ear curet. (**D**) Vienna nasal speculum.

(continued)

TABLE **21-3**	**Commonly Used Instruments and Equipment by Specialty** *(continued)*	
	Instrument	**Use**
Ophthalmology	Eye loop, lid retractor	Hold eyelids open for removal of foreign bodies
	Tonometer	Measure intraocular pressure to diagnose glaucoma

Ophthalmology instruments: **(A)** Desmarres lid retractor. **(B)** Bailey foreign body remover. **(C)** Schiotz tonometer.

Dermatology	Punch biopsy	Removes small circular sections of skin for microscopic studies; sized 2–8 mm, disposable or reusable
	Comedone extractor	Removes blackheads, opens pustules

Dermatology instruments: **(A)** Keyes cutaneous punch. **(B)** Schamberg comedone extractor.

Forceps

Forceps are surgical instruments used to grasp, handle, compress, pull, or join tissue, equipment, or supplies. The types of forceps include the following:

- **Hemostat:** A surgical instrument with slender jaws used for grasping blood vessels and establishing hemostasis.
- **Kelly clamp:** A curved or straight forceps or hemostat; those with long handles are widely used in gynecologic procedures.
- **Sterilizer forceps:** Used to transfer sterile supplies, equipment, and other surgical instruments to a sterile field. May also be called sterile transfer forceps.
- **Needle holder:** Used to hold and pass a needle through tissue during suturing.
- Spring or thumb forceps: Used for grasping tissue for dissection or suturing, such as tissue forceps and splinter forceps.

A variety of forceps can be seen in Figure 21-5. All forceps are available in many sizes, with or without

serrations or teeth, with curved or straight blades, and with ring tips, blunt tips, or sharp tips. Many have **ratchets** in the handles to hold the tips tightly together; these are notched mechanisms that click into position to maintain tension. Some have spring handles that are compressed between the thumb and index finger to grasp objects.

Physicians use a variety of forceps. You should study the names and purposes of each type to assist the physician when a specific instrument is requested.

 CHECKPOINT QUESTION

5. What are the most common instruments used in a medical office?

Scissors

Scissors are sharp instruments composed of two opposing cutting blades held together by a central pin at the pivot. Scissors are used for dissecting superficial, deep,

Figure 21-5 Forceps: **(A)** Rochester-Pean forceps. **(B)** Rochester-Ochsner forceps. **(C)** Adson forceps. **(D)** Bozeman forceps. **(E)** Crile hemostat. **(F)** Kelly hemostat. **(G)** Halsted mosquito hemostat. **(H)** Allis forceps. **(I)** Babcock forceps. **(J)** DeBakey forceps. **(K)** Allis tissue forceps. **(L)** Duplay tenaculum forceps. **(M)** Crile-Wood needle holder. **(N)** Ballenger sponge forceps. **(O)** Fine-point splinter forceps. **(P)** Adson dressing forceps. **(Q)** Potts-Smith dressing forceps. (Courtesy of Sklar Instruments, West Chester, PA).

or delicate tissues and for cutting sutures and bandages. Scissors have blade points that are blunt, sharp, or both, depending on the use of the instrument. The types of scissors include the following:

- Straight scissors cut deep or delicate tissue and sutures.
- Curved scissors dissect superficial and delicate tissues.
- Suture scissors cut sutures; they have straight top blades and curved-out, or hooked, blunt bottom blades to fit under, lift, and grasp sutures for snipping.

- Bandage scissors remove bandages; this type has a flattened blunt tip on the bottom longer blade that safely fits under bandages; most common type is the Lister bandage scissors.

Figure 21-6 shows various types of scissors.

Scalpels and Blades

A scalpel is a small surgical knife with a straight handle and a straight or curved blade. A reusable steel scalpel handle can hold different blades for different surgical procedures. Straight or pointed blades are used for incision and drainage procedures, while curved blades are used to excise tissue. Reusable handles are used only with disposable blades. Many offices use disposable handles and blades packaged as one sterile unit. Figure 21-7 shows various scalpels and blades.

Towel Clamps

Towel clamps are used to maintain the integrity of the sterile field by holding the sterile drapes in place, allowing exposure of the operative site (Fig. 21-8). A sterile field is a specific area that is considered free of all microorganisms.

Probes and Directors

Before entering a cavity or site for a procedure, the physician may first probe the depth and direction of the operative area. A probe shows the angle and depth of the operative area, and a director guides the knife or instrument once the procedure has begun (Fig. 21-9).

Retractors

Retractors hold open layers of tissue, exposing the areas beneath. They may be plain or toothed; the toothed retractor may be sharp or blunt. Retractors may be designed to be held by an assistant or screwed open to be self-retaining. Figure 21-10 shows several types of retractors.

 CHECKPOINT QUESTION

6. What types of instruments are used to remove tissue during a biopsy?

Care and Handling of Surgical Instruments

To ensure that surgical instruments always function properly, follow these guidelines:

1. Do not toss or drop instruments into a basin or sink. Surgical instruments are delicate, and the blade or tip is easily damaged by improper handling. Should you drop an instrument accidentally, carefully inspect it for damage. Damaged instruments can usually be repaired and should not be discarded unless repair is not feasible.
2. Avoid stacking instruments in a pile. They may tangle and be damaged when separated.
3. Always store sharp instruments separately to prevent dulling or damaging the sharp edges and to prevent accidental injury. Disposable scalpel blades should be removed from reusable handles and placed in puncture-proof sharps biohazard containers. If a disposable scalpel is used, the whole unit is discarded into the sharps container. Syringes with needles attached and suture needles should also be discarded in a sharps container and never in the trash or with other instruments for processing. Delicate instruments, such as scissors or tissue forceps or those with lenses, are kept separate to be sanitized and sterilized appropriately.
4. Keep ratcheted instruments open when not in use to avoid damage to the ratchet mechanism.
5. Rinse gross contamination from instruments as soon as possible to prevent drying and hardening, which makes cleaning more difficult. Always wear gloves and follow **OSHA** standards to prevent contact with possibly infected blood or body fluids.
6. Check instruments before sterilization to ensure that they are in good working order, and identify instruments in need of repair.

Figure 21-6 Scissors: **(A)** Straight-blade operating scissors. *Left to right:* S/S, S/B, B/B. **(B)** Curved-blade operating scissors. *Left to right:* S/S, S/B, B/B. **(C)** Spencer stitch scissors. **(D)** Suture scissors. **(E)** Lister bandage scissors. S/S, sharp/sharp; S/B, sharp/blunt; B/B, blunt/blunt. (Courtesy of Sklar Instruments, West Chester, PA.)

Figure 21-7 Scalpels: (**A**) Scalpel handles. (**B**) Surgical blades. (**C**) Complete sterile disposable scalpel. (Courtesy of Sklar Instruments, West Chester, PA.)

A. Blades or points should be free of bends and nicks.
B. Tips should close evenly and tightly.
C. Instruments with box locks should move freely but should not be too loose.
D. Instruments with spring handles should have enough tension to grasp objects tightly.
E. Scissors should close in a smooth, even manner with no nicks or snags. (Scissors may be checked by cutting through gauze or cotton to be sure there are no rough areas).
F. Screws should be flush with the instrument surface. They should be freely workable but not loose.
7. Use instruments only for the purpose for which they were designed. For instance, never use surgical scissors to cut paper or open packages, because this may damage the cutting edges.
8. Sanitize instruments before they are sterilized so that sterilization will work effectively.

 CHECKPOINT QUESTION

7. What should you do if you drop a surgical instrument accidentally?

Storage and Record Keeping

When using and maintaining sterile instruments, equipment, and supplies, staff are responsible for correctly

Figure 21-8 Towel clamps: (**A**) Backhaus towel clamp. (**B**) Jones cross-action towel clamp. (Courtesy of Sklar Instruments, West Chester, PA.)

Figure 21-9 Probes: (**A**) Director and tongue tie. (**B**) Double-ended probe. (**C**) Probe with eye. (Courtesy of Sklar Instruments, West Chester, PA.)

Figure 21-10 Retractors: **(A)** Volkman retractor. **(B)** Lahey retractor. **(C)** Senn retractor. (Courtesy of Sklar Instruments, West Chester, PA.)

storing these items, keeping accurate records of warranties and maintenance agreements, and keeping reordering information on hand. You should be familiar with the manufacturer's recommendations for each instrument or piece of equipment. Most offices have specific storage or supply areas for keeping sterile and other instruments and equipment. This area should be kept clean and dust free and should be close to the area of need. Clean and sterile supplies and equipment must be separated from soiled items and waste.

Medical assistants are also responsible for keeping accurate records of sterilized items and equipment. Information that must be recorded includes maintenance records and load or sterilization records. These records should include the following:

- Date and time of the sterilization cycle
- General description of the load
- Exposure time and temperature
- Name or initials of the operator
- Results of the sterilization indicator
- Expiration date of the load (usually 30 days)

The maintenance records include service provided by the manufacturer's representative and daily or recommended maintenance to keep the equipment in optimum working condition.

 CHECKPOINT QUESTION

8. What six items should be included on a sterilization record?

Maintaining Surgical Supplies

As a clinical medical assistant, you should keep an up-to-date master list of all supplies, including purchases

and replacements. Generally, one person is responsible for maintaining inventory, keeping maintenance schedules, and placing orders. If too many staff are involved, these tasks may be overlooked, or efforts may be duplicated. Instruction manuals for all equipment should be kept on file and consulted when ordering supplies for replacement or maintenance. Equipment records for each item should include the following:

- Date of purchase
- Model and serial numbers of the equipment
- Time of recommended service
- Date service was requested
- Name of the person requesting the service
- Reason for the service request
- Description of the service performed and any parts replaced
- Name of the person performing the service and the date the work was completed
- Signature and title of the person who acknowledged completion of the work

Warranties and guarantees should be kept with the equipment records, along with the name of the manufacturer's contact person. A tickler file should be kept to remind the staff of the need for manufacturer service and concurrent or periodic maintenance by the staff.

Parts and supplies for items that are vital to the operation of the facility should always be kept on hand. The shelf life of the item, the storage space available, and the time required to order and receive an item should be considered when deciding what items to keep in inventory. If a piece of equipment cannot function without all of its components or if some of those components have a short life, replacements must be readily available. For example, an ophthalmoscope without a light is virtually useless.

TRIAGE

While you are working in a medical office, the following three situations arise:

A. You need to wrap instruments for the autoclave that were sanitized earlier in the day.

B. A 45-year-old woman who just had a mole removed needs postoperative instructions before discharge, and the treatment room where the procedure was done is in need of cleaning for the next patient.

C. A load in the autoclave that ran earlier is finished. The sterilized packs have to be put away.

How do you sort these tasks? What do you do first? Second? Third?

The patient in situation B should be taken care of first. You should take time to explain any postoperative instructions and follow-up care clearly as indicated by the physician. Once the patient is discharged, the treatment room should be cleaned, and any used surgical equipment should be discarded appropriately or prepared for sanitation according to appropriate standard precautions. The next task includes wrapping the sanitized instruments in preparation for the autoclave. After unloading the autoclave and putting the sterilized packs away, the clean wrapped instruments can be placed in the autoclave for sterilization.

 WHAT IF?

Your medical office has one designated room for minor office surgical procedures, and two physicians in your office have scheduled minor office procedures for the same day and time. What should you do?

It is your responsibility to anticipate what the physician needs and address any concerns immediately. Upon discovering that two patients are scheduled for procedures on the same day and time, you should advise both physicians of the situation immediately. In some cases, the patient may have been told not to eat or drink anything on the morning of the procedure, and if this is the case and it is agreeable with both physicians, it would be most appropriate to schedule the patient who is NPO earliest in the day. Once the physicians determine who should use the room first, you should then call the patient who will need to be scheduled at a later time, using this opportunity to remind them of any preoperative orders if necessary. Always allow plenty of time between procedures for disinfecting the room, restocking the room with equipment and supplies, and sanitizing and sterilizing any equipment that was used and may be needed for the following procedure.

 LEGAL TIP
THE RIGHT TO KNOW

OSHA and state regulations have defined a specific law to protect you from hazardous materials. The law, The Right to Know, requires that all companies, including medical offices, using hazardous materials have material safety data sheets (MSDS) available to their employees. MSDS are prepared by the chemical manufacturer and clearly state how to handle and dispose of the chemical. These forms also include a list of possible health hazards to workers and identify the safety equipment needed for using the chemical. Never handle any type of chemical spill without first reading the MSDS. You are required to add to the MSDS binder any MSDS that accompany any supplies or equipment containing hazardous materials. This notebook should be placed in a stationary area where it can be easily consulted in case of an emergency involving hazardous materials.

MEDIA MENU

- **Student CD**
  - **CMA/RMA Certification Exam Review**
- **Premium Online Course**
  http://thePoint.lww.com/Kronenberger3e
- **Internet Resources**

LiveAdvise Online Tutoring & Competency Training
http://thePoint.lww.com/LiveAdvise

Medical Resources New and Reconditioned Equipment: Midmark and Ritter Autoclaves
www.medicalresources.com

Amsco Autoclaves and Sterilizers: Alfa Medical
www.sterilizers.com

Sklar Surgical Instruments
www.sklarcorp.com

Glutaraldehyde Guidelines for Safe Use and Handling in Health Care Facilities
www.state.nj.us/health/eoh/survweb/glutar.pdf

Occupational Safety and Health Administration (OSHA)
www.osha.gov

PROCEDURE 21-1: Sanitizing Equipment for Disinfection or Sterilization

Purpose: Properly sanitize instruments in preparation for disinfection or sterilization
Equipment: Instruments or equipment to be sanitized, gloves, eye protection, impervious gown, soap and water, small hand-held scrub brush

Steps	Reasons
1. Put on gloves, gown, and eye protection.	These devices protect against splattering and prevent contamination of your clothes. **Step 1.** Always wear PPE when a splash may occur.

(continued)

PROCEDURE 21-1: **Sanitizing Equipment for Disinfection or Sterilization** *(continued)*

Steps	Reasons
2. Take any removable sections apart. If cleaning is not possible immediately, soak the instrument or equipment to prevent the parts from sticking together.	
3. Check for operation and integrity of the equipment. Defective equipment should be repaired or discarded appropriately according to office policy.	
4. Rinse the instrument with cool water.	Hot water cooks proteins on, making the contaminants more difficult to remove.
5. After the initial rinse, force streams of soapy water through any tubular or grooved instruments to clean the inside as well as the outside.	
6. Use a hot, soapy solution to dissolve fats or lubricants on the surface. Use the soaking solution indicated by office policy.	
7. After soaking for 5–10 minutes, use friction with a soft brush or gauze to wipe down the instrument and loosen transient microorganisms. Abrasive materials should not be used on delicate instruments and equipment. Brushes work well on grooves and joints. Open and close the jaws of scissors or forceps several times to ensure that all material has been removed.	**Step 7.** Use a brush to loosen microorganisms on instruments.
8. Rinse well.	Proper rinsing removes soap or detergent residue and any remaining microorganisms.
9. Dry well before autoclaving or soaking in disinfectant.	Excess moisture decreases the effectiveness of the autoclave by delaying drying, and it dilutes the disinfectant.
10. Any items (brushes, gauze, solution) used in sanitation are considered grossly contaminated and must be properly disinfected or discarded.	

PROCEDURE 21-2: Wrapping Instruments for Sterilization in an Autoclave

Purpose: Properly prepare and wrap instruments for sterilization in the autoclave
Equipment: Instruments or equipment to be sterilized, wrapping material, autoclave tape, sterilization indicator, black or blue ink pen

Steps	Reasons
1. Assemble the equipment and supplies. Check the instruments being wrapped for working order.	Any instruments found to be defective, broken, or otherwise needing repair should not be wrapped or autoclaved.
2. Be sure that the wrapping material has these properties: • Permeable to steam but not contaminants • Resists tearing and puncturing during normal handling • Allows for easy opening to prevent contamination of the contents • Maintains sterility of the contents during storage 	The wrap may be double layers of cotton muslin, special paper, or appropriately sized instrument pouches. **Step 2. (A and B)** Autoclave pouches are convenient and come in a variety of sizes.
3. Tear off one or two pieces of autoclave tape. On one piece, indicate in ink the contents of the pack or the name of the instrument that will be wrapped, the date, and your initials.	After the item is wrapped, the contents cannot be seen. Also, dating the package allows the user to determine the quality of the contents based on the amount of time (usually 30 days) that sterilized contents are considered sterile.
4. When using autoclave wrapping material made of cotton muslin or special paper, begin by laying the material diagonally on a flat, clean, dry surface. Place the instrument in the center of the wrapping material with the ratchets or handles open. Include a sterilization indicator. 	The ratchets should be left open during autoclaving to allow steam to penetrate and sterilize all surfaces. **Step 4.** The ratchets are open.

(continued)

PROCEDURE 21-2: Wrapping Instruments for Sterilization in an Autoclave (continued)

Steps	Reasons
5. Fold the first flap at the bottom of the diagonal wrap up and fold back the corner, making a tab.	Making a tab allows for easier opening of the pack without contaminating the contents.

Step 5. Make a tab with the corner.

6. Fold the left corner of the wrap and then the right corner, each making a tab for opening the package. Secure the package with autoclave tape.

Step 6. The bottom, left, and right corners of the wrap are folded.

7. Fold the top corner down, making the tab tucked under the material.

A

B

Step 7. (A) The top corner is folded down. **(B)** Secure the wrapped instrument package with autoclave tape.

PROCEDURE 21-3: Operating an Autoclave

Purpose: Safely sterilize instruments or equipment using an autoclave
Equipment: Sanitized and wrapped instruments or equipment, distilled water, autoclave operating manual

Steps	Reasons
1. Assemble the equipment, including the wrapped articles and the sterilization indicator in each package according to office policy. **Step 1.** Properly wrapped items.	Some offices want a separately wrapped indicator autoclaved with the load for checking that the procedure was performed properly without opening a pack.
2. Check the water level of the autoclave reservoir and add more if needed.	Use only distilled water in the reservoir tank.
3. Add water to the internal chamber of the autoclave to the fill line.	Too little water makes too little steam; too much water may cause saturated steam, extending drying time, and may wick microorganisms into the damp packages.
4. Load the autoclave: A. Place trays and packs on their sides 1–3 inches apart. B. Put containers on their side with the lid off. C. In mixed loads, place hard objects on the bottom shelf and softer packs on the top racks.	Air circulation is not possible if items are tightly packed. Vertical placement forces out heavier air rather than pooling in the containers. Air can circulate in containers on their side with the lid off. Hard objects may form condensation that will drip onto softer items and wet them.
5. Read the instructions and close the machine. Most machines follow the same protocol: A. Close the door and secure or lock it. B. Turn the machine on. C. When the temperature gauge reaches the point required for the contents of the load (usually 250°F), set the timer. Many autoclaves can be programmed for the required time. D. When the timer indicates that the cycle is over, vent the chamber. E. After releasing the pressure to a safe level, crack the door of the autoclave to allow additional drying. Most loads dry in 5–20 minutes. Hard items dry faster than soft ones.	

(continued)

PROCEDURE 21-3:   Operating an Autoclave (continued)

Steps	Reasons
6. When the load has cooled, remove the items.	
7. Check the separately wrapped sterilization indicator, if used, for proper sterilization.	If the indicator registers that the load was properly processed, the items in the additional packs are considered sterile; if not, the items should be considered not sterile, and the load must be re-processed.
8. Store the items in a clean, dry, dust-free area for 30 days.	After 30 days, reprocessing is necessary. The pack need not be rewrapped, but the autoclave tape should be replaced with new tape with the current date.
9. Clean the autoclave per manufacturer's suggestions, usually by scrubbing the interior chamber with a mild detergent and a soft brush. Attention to the exhaust valve will prevent lint from occluding the outlet. Rinse the machine thoroughly and allow it to dry.	Always follow the manufacturer's recommendations for cleaning the autoclave.

Chapter Summary

- Most areas of the medical office require medical asepsis to maintain cleanliness and prevent the spread of infection to the patients and staff.
- When body tissues need repair or must be opened surgically, sterile technique or surgical asepsis is required.
- You are responsible for maintaining surgical asepsis, which necessitates that you understand the principles and practices of medical and surgical asepsis.
- You will need to know disinfection and sterilization techniques commonly used in the medical office in-

cluding the equipment used to sterilize and disinfect items.
- It will be your responsibility to keep accurate records and adequate supplies on hand.
- In addition, your responsibilities include being familiar with instruments used in office surgical procedures, which is the content of the next chapter, Chapter 22.

1. As the clinical medical assistant at Dr. Will's office, you have been asked to orient new employees to various aspects of the practice and develop an orientation booklet for all staff members. Design a booklet that contains the following information:
   - A basic explanation of the surgical equipment commonly used in the practice
   - The procedures for sanitizing, disinfecting, and sterilizing instruments
   - The operating instructions for the autoclave
2. Create a record that can be used to document sterilization using the autoclave.
3. Research the various types of commercial cold chemical sterilization solutions. Design a step-by-step procedure for using the solution to disinfect and sterilize. Note any hazards or safety precautions that should be followed when working with the chemical.
4. The physician is scheduled to perform a minor office surgical procedure this afternoon, and you realize the instrument she needs for the procedure is broken. How would you handle this situation? What can you do to prevent this situation in the future?
5. When checking the biologic sterilization indicator as required to be done weekly by your office policy, you discover that the autoclave has not been reaching the appropriate temperature sufficient to kill all microorganisms and their spores. The logbook indicated that the check last week found the autoclave to be in good working order. Can you be sure that all items autoclaved this past week are sterilized? What would you do?

1. Sanitation is maintenance of a healthful, disease-free environment by removing organic matter and other residue. Disinfection is destruction of pathogenic microorganisms but not their spores. Sterilization destroys all microorganisms and their spores on an item or instrument.
2. Boiling water will reach a temperature of 212°F, which is not hot enough to destroy all microorganisms including viruses and spores. An autoclave increases the temperature of boiling distilled water converted to steam by increasing the pressure in the chamber, raising the temperature to 250°F or higher.
3. Autoclave tape is used on the outside of a wrapped instrument or pack to identify the contents of the pack, the date the item was autoclaved, and the initials of the person who wrapped the pack. After exposure to steam, dark brown or black stripes will appear on the tape, acknowledging that the pack has been processed in the autoclave or exposed to steam. Sterilization indicators are placed inside the pack to indicate sterility of the contents.
4. The time indicated for sterilization should be started only after the appropriate temperature has been reached, since the temperature and time are both important for destruction of microorganisms and their spores. Items that have been exposed to the high temperature for less time than indicated by the manufacturer of the autoclave may not be sterile.
5. The most widely used surgical instruments in the medical office are forceps, scissors, scalpels, and clamps.
6. The physician may use forceps to remove tissue for biopsy.
7. Because surgical instruments are delicate, improper handling may easily damage sharp blades or pointed tips. If you do drop an instrument, inspect it carefully for damage. Many instruments are expensive, but damaged instruments can usually be repaired.
8. The six items to include on a sterilization record are: (1) date and time of the cycle, (2) a general description of the load, (3) time and temperature, (4) name or initials of the operator, (5) results of the sterilization indicator, and (6) load expiration date.

Outline

Preparing and Maintaining a Sterile Field
Sterile Surgical Packs
Sterile Transfer Forceps
Adding Peel-Back Packages and Pouring Sterile Solutions
Preparing the Patient for Minor Office Surgery
Patient Instructions and Consent

Positioning and Draping
Preparing the Patient's Skin
Assisting the Physician
Local Anesthetics
Wound Closure
Specimen Collection
Electrosurgery
Laser Surgery
Postsurgical Procedures
Sterile Dressings

Cleaning the Examination Table and Operative Area
Commonly Performed Office Surgical Procedures
Excision of a Lesion
Incision and Drainage
Assisting With Suture and Staple Removal

Learning Objectives

Upon successfully completing this chapter, you will be able to:

1. Spell and define key terms

2. List your responsibilities before, during, and after minor office surgery

3. Identify the guidelines for preparing and maintaining sterility of the field and surgical equipment during a minor office procedure

4. State your responsibility in relation to informed consent and patient preparation

5. Explain the purpose of local anesthetics and list three commonly used in the medical office

6. Describe the types of needles and sutures and the uses of each

7. Describe the various methods of skin closure used in the medical office

8. Explain your responsibility during surgical specimen collection

9. List the types of laser surgery and electrosurgery used in the medical office and explain the precautions for each

10. Describe the guidelines for applying a sterile dressing

Upon successfully completing this chapter, you will be able to:

1. Open sterile surgical packs (Procedure 22-1)
2. Use sterile transfer forceps (Procedure 22-2)
3. Add sterile solution to a sterile field (Procedure 22-3)
4. Perform skin preparation and hair removal (Procedure 22-4)
5. Apply sterile gloves (Procedure 22-5)
6. Apply a sterile dressing (Procedure 22-6)
7. Change an existing sterile dressing (Procedure 22-7)
8. Assist with excisional surgery (Procedure 22-8)
9. Assist with incision and drainage (Procedure 22-9)
10. Remove sutures (Procedure 22-10)
11. Remove staples (Procedure 22-11)

CAAHEP

- Dispose of biohazardous materials
- Practice standard precautions
- Prepare patient for and assist with procedures, treatments, and minor office surgeries
- Document appropriately

ABHES

- Prepare patients for procedures
- Assist physician with examinations and treatments
- Dispose of biohazardous materials
- Practice standard precautions
- Document accurately

approximate	coagulate	electrode	preservative
atraumatic	cryosurgery	fulgurate	purulent
bandage	dehiscence	keratosis	swaged needle
cautery	dressing	lentigines	traumatic

As a clinical medical assistant, you will have many responsibilities when minor surgery is performed in the physician's office. These include the following:

1. Reinforcing the physician's instructions to the patient regarding preparation for surgery, including at-home skin preparation as directed, fasting from food or fluids, bowel preparation, and other preparations that may be ordered.
2. Identifying the patient and gathering the proper equipment and supplies before the physician is ready to do the procedure.
3. Obtaining and witnessing the informed consent document if instructed to do so by the physician.
4. Preparing the treatment room, instruments, supplies, and equipment.
5. Assisting the physician during the procedure.
6. Applying a **dressing** and **bandage** to the surgical wound.
7. Instructing the patient about postoperative wound care, including observing the wound for changes that indicate infection or problems with healing.
8. Assisting the patient as needed before, during, and after the procedure.
9. Assisting with postoperative instructions such as prescriptions, medications, and scheduling return visits.

10. Removing and caring for instruments, equipment, and supplies, including properly disposing of disposable items, sharps, and contaminated or unused supplies.

11. Preparing the room for the next patient.

Although the types of surgery performed in the medical office vary with the type of medical specialty, the procedure for preparing the patient and setting up the supplies and equipment will require the same process, known as sterile technique. Procedures performed in many general practice offices include suture insertion and removal, incision and drainage, and sebaceous cystectomy. Some gynecologic procedures and urinary procedures also require sterile technique.

Preparing and Maintaining a Sterile Field

Minor office surgery involves procedures that penetrate the body's normally intact surface. Whenever a patient has an open wound, surgical asepsis must be maintained to prevent pathogens from entering the body tissues and causing an infection. Follow the following guidelines to maintain sterility before and during a sterile procedure:

1. Do not let sterile packages get damp or wet. Microorganisms can be drawn into the package by wicking, or absorption of the liquid along with the pathogens in it. If a package sterilized in the medical office gets moist, it must be repackaged in a clean, dry wrapper and sterilized again. Damp or wet disposable packages must be discarded.

2. Always face a sterile field to ensure that the area has not been contaminated. If you must leave the area or work with your back to the sterile field, the field must be covered with a sterile drape using sterile technique.

3. Hold all sterile items above waist level. When sterile items are not in your field of vision, you must presume that they have become contaminated.

4. Place sterile items in the middle of the sterile field. A 1-inch border around the field is considered contaminated.

5. Do not spill any liquids, even sterile liquids, onto the sterile field. Remember, the surface below the field is not sterile, and moisture will allow microorganisms to be wicked up into the surgical field.

6. Do not cough, sneeze, or talk over the sterile field. Microorganisms from the respiratory tract can contaminate the field.

7. Never reach over the sterile field. Dust or lint from clothing can contaminate the sterile field.

8. Do not pass soiled supplies, such as gauze or instruments, over the sterile field.

9. If you know or suspect that the sterile field has been contaminated, alert the physician. Sterility must be re-established before the procedure can continue.

Sterile Surgical Packs

Preparing the treatment or examination room for a surgical procedure is usually the responsibility of the medical assistant. Many medical offices keep a box with index cards or a loose-leaf binder listing the surgical procedures that are commonly performed in the office, including the items needed for setup. Some medical offices prepackage sterile setups in a suitable wrapper and prepare them in the office by autoclave sterilization (Fig. 22-1). These setups are labeled according to the type of procedure (e.g., lesion removal, suture setup) and contain the general instruments for that procedure. Some basic supplies (e.g., gauze sponges, cotton balls, and towels) may also be included before autoclaving.

To reduce the time and effort of sterilizing packs on site, many offices use commercially packaged disposable surgical packs. Disposable surgical packs have become increasingly popular because they are convenient and come with an almost infinite variety of contents. They may contain one sterile article (such as a 4 × 4 sterile dressing) or a complete sterile surgical setup. Many of the supplies are packaged in peel-apart wrappers with two loose flaps that can be pulled apart, and the sterile items can be dropped carefully onto the operative field. The insides of the wrappers may be opened out and used as a sterile field. Some packages are enclosed in plastic and wrapped inside a barrier material that can be used as a sterile field.

Directions for opening are clearly marked on the outside of sterile packs and should be read carefully before opening. If the surgical pack is opened improperly, the contents will be contaminated and cannot be used. Commercially prepared sterile packs are generally more expensive than packages prepared at the medical office, so care must be taken to avoid waste. Labels on commercially prepared packs list the contents in the pack item by item; site-prepared packs usually only state the type of setup. You should check the expiration date on the package; if the pack has expired, it must not be used

Figure 22-1 A wrapped sterile surgical package.

because sterility is in question. Procedure 22-1 describes the steps for opening sterile surgical packs.

As discussed in Chapter 21, a sterilization indicator should be put inside each surgical package to show that it has been properly sterilized. Tapes, strips, and packaging with indicator stripes or dots on the outside of the packs do not guarantee sterility. In the autoclave, sterility is achieved only by the right combination of temperature, pressure, steam, and time. In addition, improperly packing the autoclave can impede steam penetration to the articles. Therefore, sterilization indicators should be packaged within each pack and must be checked before beginning the surgical procedure. When you open a package of sterile objects, the procedure is the same whether the items are sterilized at the office or commercially prepared. For all sterile packs or supplies, keep the following in mind:

1. Clean hands are used to open the sterile items or packages. The unsterile area is the outside surface of the outside wrapper.
2. The sterile area includes the inside surface of the outside wrapper, the inside wrapper if any, and the contents of the package. These areas or items must not come into contact with any surface, including the hands, or they are considered contaminated and must be replaced.
3. Items are considered contaminated and should be repackaged and sterilized again:
   A. When moisture is present on the pack
   B. If the items are dropped outside the sterile field
   C. If the date on the outside of the package is beyond 30 days for site-prepared packages or it is past the posted expiration date on commercially prepared packages
   D. If the sterilization indicator inside the pack has not changed color
   E. If the wrapper is torn, damaged, or wet
   F. When any area is known or thought to have been touched by a contaminated item

 CHECKPOINT QUESTION

1. What are the nine guidelines that must be followed to maintain a sterile field?

Sterile Transfer Forceps

Setting up the sterile field requires clean hands and careful technique to avoid contaminating the contents inside the sterile area or field. In the event that sterile items must be manipulated or placed on the sterile field, sterile transfer forceps or sterile gloved hands must be used, since the hands can never be sterilized. The tips of the forceps and the articles being transferred must both remain sterile (Fig. 22-2). The handles, however, are considered medically aseptic, not sterile, because these are touched by the bare

Figure 22-2 Sterile transfer forceps may be used to add or move items on the sterile field.

hands of the person using them. Sterile transfer forceps are stored in a dry sterile container, in a wrapped sterile package, or in a sterile solution in a closed container system, such as the Bard Parker, which helps protect the tips of the forceps from contamination. In a closed dry container system, the forceps and container must be sanitized and autoclaved daily. In a closed sterile solution system, the forceps and the container are sterilized at least every day, and fresh sterilization solution is added daily. Only one forceps should be stored in a container to decrease the chance of contamination. After using the sterile transfer forceps without contaminating, place the forceps back in the container for use throughout the procedure or in other procedures scheduled that day. Follow office policy for sterilizing the forceps. Proper use of sterile transfer forceps requires that certain guidelines be followed (Procedure 22-2).

Adding Peel-Back Packages and Pouring Sterile Solutions

Procedure packages are frequently prepared with supplies (e.g., cotton balls and gauze squares) to eliminate the need to add more at the time of setup. However, patient assessment at the time of surgery may suggest the need for additional items. These small supplies are usually provided commercially in peel-apart packages. These packages may contain small or single items to be added to the surgical field. The package has an upper edge with two flaps that are used to open the package in a manner that maintains the sterility of the contents. To properly open a package, use both hands with the thumbs just inside the tops of the edges. Separate the flaps using a slow, outward motion of the thumbs and flaps (Fig. 22-3). Keep in mind that the inside of the sealed package and the contents are sterile but will be contaminated if touched by anything that is not sterile, such as your fingers, or if talking, coughing, or sneezing occurs as you open the package. There are three ways to add the contents of peel-back packages to the sterile field:

1. *Sterile transfer forceps.* Peel the edges apart with a rolling motion as described earlier. Holding down the two edges, lift the contents up and away with the forceps (Fig. 22-4).

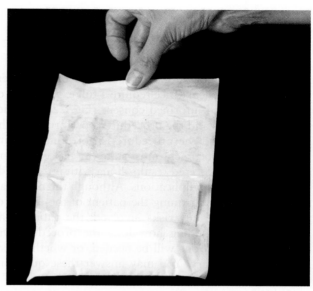

Figure 22-3 (A) Open sterile packets by grasping the edges and rolling the thumbs outward. (B) Opening the packet properly forms a sterile field.

2. *Sterile gloved hand.* This method requires two persons, usually the medical assistant, who opens the package, and the physician, who removes the contents with a sterile gloved hand. You must carefully hold the edges to avoid contaminating the physician's gloves (Fig. 22-5).

3. *Flip of the contents onto a sterile field.* To do this, you step back from the sterile field to prevent your hands and the outer wrapper, which is not sterile, from crossing it. Pull the edges down and away from the package contents and carefully toss or flip the item onto the middle of the sterile field without touching the 1-inch border around the sterile field. This 1-inch area is considered not sterile.

In most cases, items in presterilized peel-back envelopes cannot be sterilized after being opened and must be discarded even if not used. Because such items are relatively expensive, they should not be opened unnecessarily. A supply of items that might be needed during the procedure should be placed conveniently close to the area and added only if needed.

Whether site prepared or commercially prepared, trays are not processed or stored with liquids in open containers. Solutions must be added as needed at the time of setup. Some procedures require sterile water or saline, while others require an antiseptic solution, such as Betadine. These will be poured into sterile containers added to the sterile field with sterile transfer forceps (Procedure 22-3).

 CHECKPOINT QUESTION

2. What are three ways that contents of peel-back packages can be added to the sterile field?

Figure 22-4 The physician may use sterile forceps to remove small supplies from peel-back packages.

Figure 22-5 Sterile gloved hands may be used to remove sterile items.

Preparing the Patient for Minor Office Surgery

Patient Instructions and Consent

Many of the minor surgical procedures that are performed in the medical office require a full explanation of the procedure and informed consent (Fig. 22-6). Either the patient agrees and the procedure is performed or the patient refuses and the procedure is not done. The informed consent document must state the procedure and its purpose and expected results along with possible side effects, risks, and complications. Although the physician is responsible for informing the patient of the details of the procedure and any risks involved, the patient may ask questions, including how long the procedure will last, what preparations will be needed, or whether fasting will be necessary. You may answer these questions after verifying the information with the physician.

It is always a good practice to give specific written instructions to the patient for any preparations to be made before arriving at the office so that the procedure can be done on schedule and with no preventable risk to the patient. The physician may prescribe medication for the patient to take at home before the procedure. As with any patient instructions, you should notify the physician if the patient seems confused or does not understand the instructions. Encourage the patient to call the office if questions arise later. Of course, the instructions should be documented in the medical record.

LEGAL TIP

INFORMED CONSENT

In today's litigious society, physicians routinely obtain signed informed consent forms even for minor office procedures. Printed forms are available, or the office may have its own form. Such forms may be used for procedures requiring legal witnessed signatures. Other more generic ones have blank spaces to add information relevant to the procedure to be performed. All forms should have spaces for the date and signatures of the patient, physician, and witness or witnesses. The medical assistant is not responsible for informing the patient but often witnesses the signing of the document by the patient. It is the physician's legal responsibility to inform the patient before the consent form is signed by the patient or legal guardian.

Positioning and Draping

Before positioning the patient for a minor surgical procedure, ask the patient to void; this helps prevent discomfort during the procedure. Offer to help the patient remove whatever clothing is necessary to expose the operative site. Expose only the area necessary for the procedure to ensure the patient's privacy. An air-conditioned office may be uncomfortably cool for patients. You may provide additional sheets or a blanket for comfort.

Assist the patient to assume a comfortable position on the examining table that offers exposure of and access to the operative site. Provide pillows for comfort and support. Do not make the patient maintain an uncomfortable position, such as the lithotomy or knee-chest, while waiting for the physician. Position the patient only when the physician is ready to begin the procedure. At the end of the procedure, assist the patient from the table, allowing as much time as needed. Often patients who did not need help removing clothing will require help dressing following minor office surgery. Be aware of this and assist as necessary.

The type of procedure and the patient's position determine the type of drapes used to expose the operative site and cover the patient. Disposable paper drapes are most commonly used in the medical office. They come in many sizes and shapes, each suited for specific uses. Paper drapes can be used alone, in combination, or with separate drape sheets and towels. Fenestrated drapes have an opening to expose the operative site while covering adjacent areas. Fenestrated drapes may be small, such as those used for suture insertion, or large, such as those used to cover the legs and lower abdomen but expose the perineal area. Some sterile drapes are combined with adhesive-backed clear plastic, which sticks to the patient's skin and eliminates the need for towel clamps. Sterile drapes are applied by picking up the drape on the 1-inch border (no gloves needed), lifting over the surgical area without contaminating the drape, and laying the drape on the patient from farthest away to closest (Fig. 22-7). This ensures that you do not reach over the drape after it is placed on the patient.

When removing contaminated drapes from the patient following a procedure, put on clean examination gloves and carefully roll the items away from the body, keeping the contaminated areas innermost (Fig. 22-8). This helps to surround the dirtier areas of the sheet with the cleaner area and helps prevent contaminating your clothing. Because the sheets, towels, or drapes may be contaminated with blood or other body fluids, follow standard precautions (see Chapter 17).

Preparing the Patient's Skin

The goal of preoperative skin preparation is to remove as many microorganisms as possible from the skin to decrease the chance of wound contamination. Skin preparation may be simply applying an antiseptic solution to the area or may include removing gross contaminants and hair from the operative area. Hair can be re-

---

SPECIAL CONSENT TO OPERATION OR OTHER PROCEDURE(S)

PATIENT _____ PATIENT NUMBER _____

DATE _____ TIME _____

1. I HEREBY AUTHORIZE DOCTOR _____ AND/OR SUCH ASSIS-
   TANTS AS MAY BE SELECTED BY HIM, TO PERFORM THE FOLLOWING PROCEDURE(S):

   ON _____
   (NAME OF PATIENT OR MYSELF)

2. THE PROCEDURE(S) LISTED ABOVE HAVE BEEN EXPLAINED TO ME BY DR.
   AND I UNDERSTAND THE NATURE AND THE CONSEQUENCES OF THE PROCEDURE(S).

3. I RECOGNIZE THAT, DURING THE COURSE OF THE OPERATION, UNFORESEEN CONDI-
   TIONS MAY NECESSITATE ADDITIONAL OR DIFFERENT PROCEDURES THAN THOSE SET
   FORTH. I FURTHER AUTHORIZE AND REQUEST THAT THE ABOVE NAMED SURGEON, HIS
   ASSISTANTS, OR HIS DESIGNEES PERFORM SUCH PROCEDURES AS ARE IN HIS PRO-
   FESSIONAL JUDGMENT NECESSARY AND DESIRABLE, INCLUDING, BUT NOT LIMITED TO,
   PROCEDURES INVOLVING PATHOLOGY AND RADIOLOGY. THE AUTHORITY GRANTED
   UNDER THIS PARAGRAPH SHALL EXTEND TO REMEDYING CONDITIONS NOT KNOWN TO
   DR. _____ AT THE TIME THE OPERATION IS COMMENCED.

4. I AM AWARE THAT THE PRACTICE OF MEDICINE AND SURGERY IS NOT AN EXACT SCI-
   ENCE AND I ACKNOWLEDGE THAT NO GUARANTEES HAVE BEEN MADE TO ME AS TO THE
   RESULTS OF THE OPERATION OR PROCEDURE.

5. TISSUE REMOVED DURING SURGERY SHALL BE SENT TO PATHOLOGY TO BE EXAMINED
   AND DISPOSED OF IN ACCORDANCE WITH THE RULES AND REGULATIONS OF THE MED-
   ICAL STAFF OF THE SURGERY CENTER.

Procedure has been discussed with patient. (Surgeon's Signature)   SIGNATURE OF PATIENT

PATIENT IS UNABLE TO SIGN BECAUSE   ☐ HE (SHE) IS A MINOR _____ YEARS OF AGE

☐ OTHER (SPECIFY) _____

WITNESS   PERSON AUTHORIZED TO SIGN FOR PATIENT

                                     RELATIONSHIP OF ABOVE TO PATIENT

Figure 22-6 Sample consent form.

moved with depilatory creams but often requires shaving the skin (Procedure 22-4).

 CHECKPOINT QUESTION

3. What is a fenestrated drape?

Assisting the Physician

Local Anesthetics

When office surgery of any kind is performed, the site is first anesthetized (numbed) with a local anesthetic to minimize the pain and discomfort felt by the patient. Occasionally, when a wound contains embedded debris that must be removed prior to repair, the local anesthetic will be injected before preparing the wound site to facilitate wound cleaning. Lidocaine (Xylocaine) and lidocaine with epinephrine (0.5–2%) are two of the many local anesthetics commonly used in medical offices. Others are lidocaine (Baylocaine), mepivacaine (Carbocaine), and bupivacaine (Marcaine). Epinephrine is added to local anesthetics to cause vasoconstriction and to slow absorption by the body and lengthen the anesthetic's effectiveness. It may be used when the physician anticipates a long procedure, but anesthesia

Figure 22-7 Applying a sterile drape.

with epinephrine should never be used on the tips of the fingers, toes, nose, or penis, since the vasoconstriction may cause death of tissue in these areas.

Two methods may be used to administer local anesthesia. In one method, you draw the anesthetic for the physician into a syringe, keeping the vial beside the syringe for the physician's approval. In this case, the anesthetic is usually given to the patient before the physician puts on sterile gloves, since the outside of the syringe and needle unit are not sterile.

The second method is used if the physician puts on sterile gloves before administering the anesthetic. In this case, a sterile syringe and needle are included on the sterile field setup. When the physician is ready to administer the anesthetic, you show the physician the label on the vial, clean the rubber stopper of the vial with an alcohol swab, and hold the vial while the physician draws the required amount into the syringe. There are many methods of holding the vial securely while the physician withdraws the medication; however, the most common way is for you to hold the vial with one hand while supporting your wrist with the other hand (Fig. 22-9). You and the physician together develop a method to maintain surgical asepsis.

Figure 22-8 Removing a contaminated drape.

Wound Closure

Many types of wounds require closure to ensure rapid healing with minimal scarring. This is accomplished by bringing the edges of the wound as close together as possible in their original position (approximation). Sutures are used to close wounds and incisions and to bring tissue layers into close approximation. Skin closures are performed after cyst or tissue sample removal, to close lacerations, or any time skin surfaces require assistance for healing. Supplies used to suture skin include needles and suture material. Skin staples are sometimes used to close large incisions over areas where **dehiscence** can occur, such as the knee, hip, or abdomen, but these are not usually inserted in the medical office.

Needles and Sutures

Needles used in minor office surgery are chosen for the type of surgery to be performed. Needles are classified as follows:

- By shape: curved or straight
- By point: tapered or cutting
- By eye: **atraumatic** (swaged) or **traumatic** (with an eye)

Round straight needles are called domestic needles, and straight cutting needles are called Keith needles. Curved needles used in surgical procedures are usually clamped in a needle holder before being handed to or used by the physician. Straight needles are not clamped in a needle holder but are handed to the physician with the point up. Straight needles are rarely used in medical offices.

Cutting needles are used on tough tissues, such as skin. Round or tapered (noncutting) needles are used on subcutaneous tissue, peritoneum, and muscle. Atraumatic needles, or **swaged needles**, have suture material that has been mechanically attached to the needle by the manufacturer and do not require threading. These are called atraumatic because they cause less trauma than threaded needles as they pass through the tissues. Unlike atraumatic or swaged needles, threaded needles have an eye with a double thickness of suture that must be pulled through tissues. The double thickness of this suture makes a larger and therefore more traumatic opening in the tissues than a swaged suture.

In medical offices, curved swaged needles are used far more often than any other type. Swaged needles are selected for a procedure according to the size and length of the suture material and the attached needle gauge clearly marked on the packaging material. When a suture must be threaded through an eyed needle, both needle gauge and suture size must be selected. The physician usually selects the suture and needle, but you should know your physician's preferences and antici-

Figure 22-9 Hold the vial containing the anesthetic downward, supporting that wrist with the other hand.

pate needs whenever possible. Sutures, needles, and suture–needle combinations are contained in peel-apart packages that are sterile on the inside so that they can be added to the sterile field (Fig. 22-10). This may be done by sterile transfer forceps, by a sterile gloved hand, or by carefully flipping them onto the sterile field.

Sutures come in various gauges (diameters) and lengths. Very thick sutures are numbered 1 to 5, with 5

Figure 22-10 Suture material and needles are supplied in see-through packages with the size of the suture material and the type of needle listed on the packet. The inside of the packet is sterile.

being the thickest. Sutures smaller than size 1 are expressed with added zeros. Small sutures, which become progressively smaller, range from 1-0 to 10-0 or smaller (i.e., 1-0, 2-0, 3-0, and so forth). A very fine 10-0 suture, which is about the diameter of a human hair, is generally used in microsurgery. When a fine suture is needed, such as on the face and neck, 23-0 and 24-0 sutures are commonly used. A very fine suture decreases scarring and gives a better cosmetic result.

Sutures also come in absorbable and nonabsorbable forms. Absorbable sutures, or catgut (made from the intestines of sheep or cattle), are readily broken down in the body and usually do not have to be removed. The two forms of absorbable gut suture are chromic, which is chemically treated to delay absorption for several days, and plain, which is not treated and is more quickly absorbed. Absorbable sutures are used most frequently in hospitals during surgery on deep tissues.

Nonabsorbable sutures are available in a great variety of brands, sizes, lengths, and swaged needles; they are the most versatile. Nonabsorbable sutures either remain in the body permanently or are removed after healing. Nonabsorbable sutures are used on the skin, intestines, or bone; to ligate larger vessels; and to attach heart valves and various artificial and natural grafts. Nonabsorbable sutures are made of fibers such as silk, nylon, Dacron, or cotton or stainless steel wire.

Skin Staples

Another form of nonabsorbable suture is the metal skin clip or staple. These are commonly made of stainless steel, but some very specialized types are made of sterling silver for use in neurosurgery and other procedures. When nonabsorbable sutures or staples are used to close skin wounds, they must be removed when the wound has healed completely. Depending on the location of the skin wound, nonabsorbable sutures or staples remain in place for varying lengths of time; the head and neck may require 3 to 5 days due to increased blood supply to these areas. Sutures in the arms and legs may require 7 to 10 days.

CHECKPOINT QUESTION

4. How do swaged needles differ from threaded ones?

Adhesive Skin Closures

Adhesive skin closures are used to **approximate** the edges of a small wound if sutures are not needed. They are appropriate where there is little tension on the skin edges. The strips are placed transversely across the line of the wound to bring the wound edges in close approximation (Fig. 22-11). In most instances, the strips are

Figure 22-11 Adhesive skin closures. (**A**) These lightweight lengths of porous tape are used for closing small wounds. (**B**) Strips are placed transversely across a wound.

left in place until they fall off. However, in some cases, the physician may want them removed or replaced if soiled with drainage. When removing these strips, carefully lift the edges distal to the wound and pull gently toward the wound. Never pull the strips away from the wound because tension on the wound site may disrupt the healing process.

Specimen Collection

Many minor office surgical procedures yield specimens that must be sent to a laboratory to be examined by a pathologist. Specimens include samples of tissue, wound exudate, foreign bodies, and so on. The medical assistant must choose the proper container with the appropriate **preservative** (substance that delays decomposition) for the type of procedure being performed. The laboratory where the specimen is sent usually provides the appropriate containers with preservative, and you should have a stock of them on hand. Hold the open container steady to avoid touching the sides as the physician drops the specimen into the preservative (Fig. 22-12).

You are responsible for attaching a label to the specimen container with the patient's name and the date

Figure 22-12 Tissue samples are placed in the preservative by the physician.

written clearly on the label, and you must complete a laboratory request form to send with the specimen. These forms require information such as the patient's name, age, sex, and identification number or social security number; date; type of specimen; type of examination; and the physician's name or laboratory contract number. Specimens obtained during a minor surgical procedure must be transported to the pathology laboratory as quickly as possible.

Electrosurgery

Electrosurgery uses high-frequency alternating electric current to destroy or cut and remove tissue. It is used to **coagulate**, or clot, small bleeding vessels. Electrosurgery is considered an alternative to traditional office surgery and is rapidly gaining favor for many procedures. An advantage of electrical surgery is the **cautery** produced by the electricity that seals small bleeding vessels and coagulates nearby cells to reduce bleeding and loss of cell fluid. Electrosurgical units use disposable **electrodes** with tips of various sizes and shapes to deliver the desired amount of electric current to the tissues (Fig. 22-13). The following procedures are considered electrosurgery:

- *Fulguration* destroys tissue with controlled electric sparks. As the physician holds the electrode tip 1 to 2 mm from the site, a series of sparks destroys the superficial cells at the site.
- *Electrodesiccation* dries and separates tissue with an electric current. The electrode is placed directly on the site.
- *Electrocautery* causes quick coagulation of small blood vessels with the heat created by the electric current. Electrocautery is commonly referred to as electrocoagulation.
- *Electrosection* is used for incision or excision of tissue. Bleeding is minimal with this type of procedure, but more damage can occur to surrounding tissues.

Medical offices frequently use electrosurgery to remove moles, cysts, warts, and certain types of skin and

Figure 22-13 A disposable electrosurgical unit. The blade is designed either to cut or to cauterize.

cervical cancers. Electrosurgical equipment includes various electrode tips, such as blades, needles, loops, and balls, each with specific uses.

During electrosurgery, your responsibilities are to ensure the safety and comfort of the patient and to pass the electrode to the physician as needed. As with all instruments, the electrode must be passed in its functional position. The electrode is handed to the physician with the tip down.

Because electric current is delivered to the tip by the electrosurgical machine, great care should be exercised to prevent injuries. Although the physician activates the device, it is possible to cause injury to the patient, physician, or yourself by careless handling of the device. Take care to ground the patient before electrosurgery. Metal conducts electricity and can cause serious burns. When assisting with electrosurgery, follow these safety measures:

- Ensure that all working parts are in good repair. The electrical current is carefully regulated; if the machine is defective, serious injury to the patient may occur.
- Ensure that all metal is removed from the patient. The patient must be asked about any metal implants or a cardiac pacemaker. Metal conducts electricity and can cause burns. Metal implants may become very hot, and pacemakers may malfunction during the procedure.
- Ensure that the patient is grounded with a pad supplied by the manufacturer. Attach it to the patient at a site recommended by the manufacturer (some recommend placing the pad far from the operative site; others suggest placing it near the site). Improper placement can result in injury.
- Place the grounding pad firmly and completely against the patient's skin. Apply a conducting gel to the pad and to the patient's skin, or use an adhesive-backed pad to facilitate conduction through the grounding pad. Areas of skin against the pad that are not well connected will result in hot spots and may burn the patient.

Although disposable tips are usually used today, reusable tips are still used in some offices. Reusable tips are disinfected and processed in the autoclave according to the manufacturer's directions. Reusable tips may be polished with steel wool if they become dull. Disposable tips should be discarded after use. Electrosurgical machines should be inspected periodically to ensure proper working order. The operating manual states the periodic maintenance to be performed by office staff and routine inspections to be performed by trained technicians. Surfaces should be kept clean and dry; machines should be kept covered when not in use.

 CHECKPOINT QUESTION

5. Which type of electrosurgery is used for incision or excision of tissue?

Laser Surgery

Lasers are devices that focus high-intensity light in a narrow beam to create extreme heat and energy. In medicine, lasers can be used to cut tissue and coagulate small bleeding vessels. There are many types of lasers, each with fairly specific applications in medicine. The following are the most common types of lasers encountered in the medical office:

- Argon laser: used for coagulation
- Carbon dioxide laser: used for cutting tissue
- Nd:YAG laser: used for coagulation and to separate warts and moles from surrounding tissues

Light from the laser is not usually visible. Colored filters are used to illuminate the laser's target, enabling the physician to direct the laser beam to the affected area. As with other electronic devices, attention to care and handling of the laser helps ensure that it is in good working order when it is needed. It is important to read and follow the manufacturer's recommended maintenance procedures as described in the instruction manual.

Everyone who is in the room, including the patient, during the laser procedure is required to wear goggles for eye protection. Health care workers are recommended to complete a training program before assisting with laser procedures to ensure that safety precautions are followed.

 CHECKPOINT QUESTION

6. What is one important safety feature worth noting when assisting with a laser procedure?

Postsurgical Procedures
Sterile Dressings

Sterile dressings are items such as 4 × 4–inch absorbent gauze sponges and nonadhering dressings that have been processed for use on open wounds. Sterile dressings are generally prepackaged in small numbers but may come in bulk containers. They are manufactured in various sizes and shapes, each for a specific use and chosen according to the size of the wound and the amount of drainage. Dressings should be handled with sterile technique. A sterile dressing may be secured by various bandages (sling, cravat, roller, tubular gauze) to hold the dressing in place, protect the injured part, or restrict movement. Chapter 27 describes bandaging techniques. Procedure 22-5 describes putting on sterile gloves, Procedure 22-6 describes applying a sterile dressing to a surgical wound, and Procedure 22-7 describes changing an existing dressing on a wound.

A sterile dressing is considered contaminated if it is damp or outdated, if its wrapper is damaged, or if it is improperly removed from its wrapper. Sterile dressings are used directly over a wound for the following reasons:

1. To cover and protect from contamination
2. To absorb drainage such as blood, serum, or pus
3. To exert pressure on an open wound to control bleeding
4. To hide disfigurement during healing
5. To hold medications against a wound to facilitate healing

When you remove a sterile dressing or change an existing one, always wear clean examination gloves and carefully observe for any drainage or exudates, noting this in the patient's chart. The terminology for describing wound drainage is outlined in Box 22-1. Immediately following the closure of a wound, it is normal to see serous or serosanguineous drainage in scant or moderate amounts, depending on the extent of the wound or incision. **Purulent** drainage, or drainage with color other than pink, is a sign of infection. Notify the physician when the wound is uncovered so that it can be examined and a decision can be made regarding how well healing is progressing. Box 22-2 describes the types and phases of wound healing.

 CHECKPOINT QUESTION

7. What is the difference between a dressing and a bandage?

Cleaning the Examination Table and Operative Area

In preparation for the next patient, all used equipment must be discarded properly or transported to the equipment room for sanitizing before sterilization. The examination room must be cleaned as part of the procedure using standard precautions. Because of the possibility of

---

BOX 22-1

WOUND DRAINAGE

When observing wound drainage, be sure to note:

Color

- Serous (clear)
- Sanguineous (blood tinged)
- Serosanguineous (pinkish or clear and red mixed)
- Purulent (white, green, or yellow-tinged drainage; usually accompanied by an unpleasant odor characteristic of infection)

Amount

- Copious (large amount)
- Medium (moderate amount)
- Scant (small amount)

The amount can also be quantified by indicating the size of the drainage (e.g., 2-inch diameter, entire 4 × 4 dressing saturated) or the size of the dressing.

 LEGAL TIP

PROTECTED HEALTH INFORMATION

Often, patients who are seen in the medical office for minor surgical procedures must have a note from the physician in order to return back to work or to school. Some offices have a standard form that can be filled out and signed by the physician indicating very generally that the patient has had a procedure and should return back to school or work on a specific day. Unless you have the patient's written consent, you should never indicate the type of procedure on these notes or answer specific questions via the telephone should employers or school personnel call the office for information. Giving information without the patient's written consent would be a violation of the privacy laws included in HIPAA.

---

biohazardous materials, you should remove papers and sheets in a rolling movement so outside surfaces cover the interior of the bundle. Do not let table covers and sheets come into contact with your clothing. Discard the sheets and covers appropriately. After applying gloves, wipe down the examination table, surgical stand, sink, counter, and other surfaces used during the procedure

BOX 22-2

THE HEALING PROCESS

Types of Wound Healing

Healing by Primary Intention: This simplest form of healing occurs in wounds whose edges are closely approximated, allowing the entrance of little or no bacteria to complicate the process. The edges of the wound lie closely together, new cells form quickly to bind the site, and capillaries expand themselves across the tissue break to restore circulation to the tissues. Scarring is usually minimal.

Healing by Secondary Intention: Granulation of tissue is present in the wound, and the edges of the wound join indirectly. Because the skin edges are not closely approximated, additional new cells are required to fill spaces in the lesion. Capillaries may not be able to reach across the gap to restore full circulation. Nerves may not rejoin, which results in diminished nerve stimulus through the area. A large scab forms to protect the area while healing goes on below it. Scarring is more severe than with primary intention healing.

Healing by Tertiary Intention: The wound initially is left open if there is the possibility that the wound may already be contaminated with microorganisms and closing it would only trap the microorganisms, increasing the potential for an infection. The wound is left open to fill in with granular tissue. There is considerable scar formation.

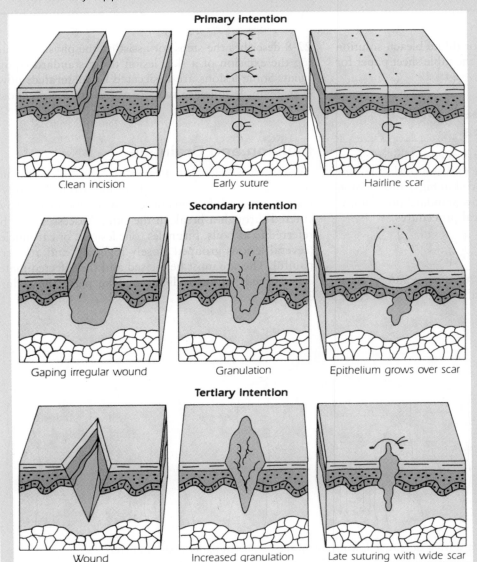

Types of wound healing. *(Top)* Primary intention. *Left to right:* Clean incision; early suture; hairline scar. *(Center)* Secondary intention. *Left to right:* Gaping irregular wound; granulation; epithelium grows over scar. *(Bottom)* Tertiary intention. *Left to right:* Wound; increased granulation; late suturing with wide scar.

(continued)

BOX 22-2 *(continued)*

Phases of Wound Healing

Phase I (inflammatory, lag, or exudative phase): This phase usually lasts from 1 to 4 days. The body attempts to heal itself by increasing the circulation to the part and by beginning to reroute or repair the supplying vessels. The increased circulation brings with it more white blood cells to mount a defense against pathogens. Serum and red blood cells brought by the additional blood form a glue-like fibrin to plug the wound. As the fibrin dries, it pulls the edges of the wound closer together and forms a scab. Signs that this phase is working are edema from the tissue fluid, warmth from the extra blood, redness from the vasodilation, and pain from the pressure on the nerve endings caused by the edema.

Phase II (proliferative, healing, or granulation phase): This phase may last from several days to several weeks. The vessels continue to repair themselves and may reroute if damage is severe. The scab from phase I continues to dry and to pull the edges of the wound as closely together as possible.

Phase III (remodeling, maturation, or scarring phase): This phase may take from weeks to years, depending upon the severity of the wound. Fibroblasts build scar tissue to guard the area.

---

with an approved disinfectant or dilute bleach solution and allow them to dry. Replace the table sheet paper for the next patient.

Commonly Performed Office Surgical Procedures

Two of the most frequently performed minor surgeries in the general medical office are excision of skin lesions (moles, **lentigines**, **keratoses**, and skin tags) and incision and drainage of abscesses. Follow standard precautions when assisting with these surgical procedures.

Excision of a Lesion

Physicians may excise lesions with electrocautery, laser, **cryosurgery**, or standard surgical equipment. Procedure

22-8 describes the steps for assisting the physician during the excision of a skin lesion using standard equipment. Some lesions are desiccated or **fulgurated**; however, many lesions are sent to pathology for diagnosis after excision.

Incision and Drainage

An abscess is a local collection of pus in a cavity surrounded by inflamed tissue. It results from the body's response to an infectious process when pathogens have entered through a break in the skin. Abscesses may be referred to as boils, furuncles (one lesion), or carbuncles (several lesions grouped closely together) and are very painful. The site must be incised and the infected material drained before healing can take place (Procedure 22-9).

Figure 22-14 Clean a wound outward from the site following any of the numbered patterns shown here.

Assisting With Suture and Staple Removal

In many instances, you will be required to remove sutures from a wound. Patients should understand that they might feel a pulling sensation during suture removal but should not feel pain. First, cleanse the area with an antiseptic solution. Either wearing sterile gloves or using sterile transfer forceps with clean hands, clean the area in a circular motion away from the wound or in straight wipes away from the suture line (Fig. 22-14). The wipe is discarded after each sweep, and a new one is used for the next sweep across the area. Either a sterile disposable suture removal kit, which contains all of the equipment needed for suture removal (Fig. 22-15), or sterile reusable equipment may be used (Procedure 22-10).

Following hospital surgery, some incisions are closed with metal staples rather than sutures. Patients often leave the hospital before the staples can be removed safely and return later to the physician's office to have them removed. Frequently, it will be your responsibility to remove the staples. Most offices use staple removal kits similar to the kits supplied for suture removal. Included in the staple removal kit is a special instrument for removing the staples instead of suture scissors. Procedure 22-11 describes the process for removing staples.

 CHECKPOINT QUESTION

8. What methods may be used to excise lesions in the medical office?

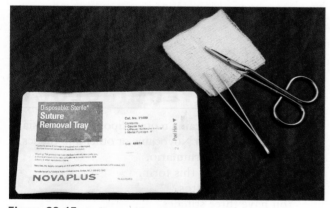

Figure 22-15 A disposable suture removal kit.

 PATIENT EDUCATION

POSTOPERATIVE INSTRUCTIONS

After any surgical procedure, the patient should receive written and verbal discharge instructions, including how to care for the postoperative wound, taking prescribed medications correctly, and returning to the office for follow-up visits, dressing changes, and suture removal as ordered by the physician. The patient should be informed of the signs and symptoms of infection and should be instructed to report the following conditions:

- Excessive bleeding from the wound (additional teaching should include how to stop any excessive bleeding by applying direct pressure or elevating the body area).
- Redness, red streaks, or excessive swelling around the surgical site.
- Fever.

Tell the patient to call the office if these symptoms arise. In addition, you will tell the patient the following:

- When to return to the office to have the dressing or bandage changed or how and when to change the bandage or dressing at home.
- The need for follow-up visits. Have the patient schedule the appointment or appointments before leaving and provide an appointment card for each appointment.
- After speaking with the physician, tell the patient when he or she can take a shower or bath and whether the surgical wound can get wet. (Whether the wound may get wet depends on location and depth of the wound and the surgeon's preference.)
- If a specimen was taken for a pathology test, tell the patient when the results will be available.
- Answer any questions about postoperative experience and always encourage patients to call the office at any time if a problem or concern arises.

TRIAGE

The physician has just performed a needle biopsy for a lesion on Mr. Smith's lower back. You have to do the following three tasks:

A. Label the specimen and complete the laboratory requisition form.
B. Apply a dressing to Mr. Smith's lower back.
C. Help Mr. Smith get dressed and into a wheelchair.

How do you sort these tasks? What do you do first? Second? Third?

The correct order is A, B, C. All specimens must be immediately labeled. Incorrectly labeled specimens or poorly completed requisition forms may result in the laboratory not being able to test the specimen. It is appropriate to apply a dressing to the wound and then assist the patient to get dressed and into a wheelchair.

MEDIA MENU

• **Student CD**

• **CMA/RMA Certification Exam Review**

• **LWW's Medical Assisting Skills DVD**

• **Procedures 22-5, 22-6, 22-7, 22-10, 22-11**

• **Premium Online Course**
http://thePoint.lww.com/Kronenberger3e

• **Internet Resources**

LiveAdvise Online Tutoring & Competency Training
http://thePoint.lww.com/LiveAdvise

American Society of Plastic Surgeons
www.plasticsurgery.org

American Society for Dermatologic Surgery
www.asds-net.org

Center for Laser Surgery
www.lasersurgery.com

The Association for the Advancement of Wound Care
www.aawconline.org

WHAT IF?

What if you accidentally cut your finger while cleaning up after a minor office surgical procedure?

Remove your gloves and immediately wash your hands with an antiseptic solution. Then have the physician evaluate the wound. The physician will suggest that you wash the wound by performing a handwashing procedure, and antibiotics may be prescribed. The patient should be asked for permission to take a blood sample to test for hepatitis B, hepatitis C, and HIV. State laws vary regarding the legality of health care workers demanding a blood sample for testing. After blood from the patient is examined for the hepatitis B surface antigen, you may be given hepatitis B immunoglobulin (HBIG) and/or hepatitis B vaccine. You should consider obtaining the vaccine for hepatitis now. Many states require that health care workers be immunized at their employer's expense. Finally, be sure to notify your supervisor of any work-related injury so that it may be appropriately documented. The Needlestick Safety and Prevention Act requires that a sharps injury log be maintained and that it include the type and brand of device involved in the incident, the area in which the incident occurred, and a description of the incident. The name of the employee should not be recorded in the injury log. Preventing accidental exposure to contaminated blood or body fluids requires being alert and working without distractions.

español
SPANISH TERMINOLOGY

Es alergico a la Novcaina u otros tipos de anesthesia?
   Are you allergic to Novocaine or other anesthetics?
Debe firmar esta formulario.
   You need to sign this form.
Usted tiene tres puntos.
   You have three stitches.
Le duelen los puntos?
   Do your stitches hurt?
Vuelva a la oficina el lunes.
   Return to the office on Monday.

PROCEDURE 22-1:   Opening Sterile Surgical Packs

Purpose: Open sterile packages without contaminating the contents
Equipment: Surgical pack, surgical or Mayo stand

Steps	Reasons
1. Wash your hands.	Handwashing aids in infection control. Your hands should be clean for this procedure.
2. Verify the procedure to be performed and remove the appropriate tray or item from the storage area. Check the label for contents and expiration date. Check the package for tears and moisture.	Packages that have passed the expiration date should not be used. Moist or torn areas contaminate the contents of the package.
3. Place the package, with the label facing up, on a clean, dry, flat surface such as a Mayo or surgical stand.	Although the field will be protected by a barrier undersurface, microorganisms must be kept at a minimum by using an area as free of pathogens as possible. The surgical stand makes it easy to move the field for the physician's convenience.
4. Without tearing the wrapper, carefully remove the sealing tape. With commercial packages, carefully remove the outer protective wrapper.	Many disposable packages are wrapped in clear plastic film that will become the sterile field when properly opened. Packages prepared in the office are sealed with autoclave tape, which should clearly indicate that the package has been through the autoclave.
5. Loosen the first flap of the folded wrapper by pulling it up, out, and away; let it fall over the far side of the table or stand. **Step 5.** Open the first flap away from you.	This prevents you from having to reach across the sterile field again
6. Open the side flaps in a similar manner, using your left hand for the left flap and your right hand for the right flap. Touch only the unsterile outer surface; do not touch the sterile inner surface. **Step 6.** Open the side flaps.	This method minimizes your movement over the sterile areas of the package.

(continued)

PROCEDURE 22-1: Opening Sterile Surgical Packs (continued)

Steps

Reasons

7. Pull the remaining flap down and toward you by grasping the outside surface only. The outer surface of the wrapper is now against the surgical stand; the sterile inside of the wrapper forms the sterile field.

Step 7. Pull the remaining flap down and toward you.

8. Repeat Steps 5 to 7 for packages with a second or inside wrapper. This wrapper also provides a sterile field upon which to work. The field is now ready for the procedure to begin.

9. If you must leave the area after opening the field, cover the tray and its contents with a sterile drape. Without leaving or turning your back on the sterile setup area, open the sterile drape and carefully lift it out of the package by the edges without contaminating it. Carefully lay the drape over the sterile field, working from your body out so that your arms do not cross the uncovered sterile field but do cross the drape that has been placed over the tray.

Step 9. Place the drape over the sterile tray without putting your arms over the uncovered tray.

PROCEDURE 22-2:   **Using Sterile Transfer Forceps**

Purpose: Use sterile transfer forceps without contamination during a sterile setup
Equipment: Sterile transfer forceps in a container with sterilization solution, a sterile field, sterile items to be transferred

Steps	Reasons
1. Slowly lift the forceps straight up and out of the container without touching the outside of the container or its inside above the level of the solution.	The area above the soaking solution and the rim are considered not sterile.
2. Hold the forceps with the tips down at all times.	This prevents the solution from running toward the unsterile handles and then back to the grasping blades and tips, which would contaminate them. **Step 2.** The tips of the forceps should be held in a downward position.
3. Keep the forceps above waist level.	This prevents accidental and unnoticed contamination.
4. With the forceps, pick up the articles to be transferred and drop them onto the sterile field, but do not let the forceps come into contact with the sterile field.	The forceps may be moist from the soaking solution, which may wick microorganisms from the surface below onto the sterile field. Note: Transfer forceps that have been wrapped and autoclaved may be placed with tips on the sterile field and handles extending beyond the 1-inch border that is considered contaminated. Doing this allows you to move objects around the field for the physician's convenience.
5. Carefully place the forceps back in the sterilization solution.	The sterilization solution in the forceps container keeps the tips of the forceps sterile for future use. The solution should be changed at least daily or according to office policy. **Step 5.** Put the forceps into the container without contaminating.

PROCEDURE 22-3: Adding Sterile Solution to a Sterile Field

Purpose: Pour a sterile solution into a container on the sterile field without contamination
Equipment: Sterile setup, container of sterile solution, sterile bowl or cup

Steps	Reasons
1. As with any drug or medication, identify the correct solution by carefully reading the label. If necessary, use the sterile transfer forceps and place the sterile bowl or cup on the sterile field.	The label should be checked three times to prevent errors: when taking the container from the shelf, before pouring the solution, and when returning the container to the shelf.
2. Check the expiration date on the label; do not use the solution if it is out of date, if the label cannot be read, or if the solution appears abnormal. Sterile water and saline bottles must be dated when opened and must be discarded if not used within 48 hours.	Out-of-date solutions may have changed chemically or deteriorated and are not considered sterile.
3. If you are adding medication, such as lidocaine, to the solution, show the medication label to the physician now.	This allows for verification of the contents.
4. Remove the cap or stopper. Hold the cap with your fingertips, with the cap opening down to prevent contamination of the inside of the cap. If you must put the cap down, place it on a side table (not the sterile field) with the open end up. If you are pouring the entire contents onto the sterile field, discard the cap. Retain the bottle to keep track of the amount added to the field and for charting later. It can then be discarded.	If the cap becomes contaminated and is returned to the bottle, the contents are considered contaminated. Placing the cap on a surface with the opening up prevents contamination of the interior of the cap. **Step 4.** Hold the cap facing downward to prevent contamination of the inside.
5. Grasp the container with the label against the palm of your hand (known as palming the label).	If solution runs down the side of the bottle in this position, it will not obscure the label. **Step 5.** Hold the bottle of sterile solution with the label in your palm.
6. Pour a small amount of the solution into a separate container or waste receptacle.	The lip of the bottle is considered contaminated; pouring off this small amount cleanses the lip.

(continued)

PROCEDURE 22-3:   **Adding Sterile Solution to a Sterile Field**
(continued)

Steps	Reasons
7. Without reaching across the sterile field, carefully and slowly pour the desired amount of solution into the sterile container from not less than 4 inches and not more than 6 inches above the container. The bottle of solution should never touch the sterile container or tray, as this will cause contamination.	Pouring the solution slowly reduces the chance of splashing and overfilling. Solution poured too fast or from an improper height may splash. Touching the container to objects on the sterile field contaminates the field. If the solution splashes onto the field, wicking will cause contamination from the surface below.
8. After pouring the desired amount of solution into the sterile container, recheck the label for the contents and expiration date and replace the cap carefully, without touching the bottle rim with any unsterile surface of the cap.	This ensures accuracy. Careful replacement of the cap ensures that the contents remain sterile.
9. Return the solution to its proper storage area or discard the container after checking the label again.	You will have checked the solution label a total of three times to avoid errors.

PROCEDURE 22-4: Performing Hair Removal and Skin Preparation

Purpose: Prepare the skin by removing any hair and applying an antiseptic solution before a surgical procedure

Equipment: Nonsterile gloves; shave cream, lotion, or soap; new disposable razor; gauze or cotton balls; warm water; antiseptic; sponge forceps

Steps	Reasons
1. Wash your hands.	Handwashing aids infection control.
2. Assemble the equipment.	This ensures that all supplies are available. A new razor must be used for each patient to prevent the transmission of pathogens and to ensure the closest possible shave.
3. Greet and identify the patient. Explain the procedure and answer any questions.	This prevents errors in treatment, helps gain compliance, and eases anxiety.
4. Put on gloves and prepare the patient's skin: A. For shaving, apply shaving cream or soapy lather to the area. Pull the skin taut and shave by pulling the razor across the skin in the direction of hair growth. Repeat this procedure until all hair is removed from the operative area. Rinse and thoroughly pat the shaved area dry with a gauze square. B. If the patient's skin is not to be shaved, wash and rinse the skin with soap and water and dry the skin thoroughly.	Gloves must be worn when contact with blood or body fluids is possible. Shaving cream or soapy lather on the skin reduces friction and helps prevent scratching. Shaving in the direction of hair growth gives the closest shave while reducing the chance of nicking the skin. Rinsing removes soap residue and hair from the shaved area. Pat dry rather than rub to prevent abrasions. Using gauze squares for drying picks up stray hairs that might have been left behind during rinsing.
5. Apply antiseptic solution of the physician's choice to the skin surrounding the operative area using sterile gauze sponges, sterile cotton balls, or antiseptic wipes. Holding the gauze or cotton ball in the sterile sponge forceps, wipe the skin in circular motions starting at the operative site and working outward. Discard each sponge after a complete sweep has been made. If the area is large or circles are not appropriate, the sponge may be wiped straight outward from the operative site, then discarded and the procedure repeated until the entire area has been thoroughly cleaned. At no time should a wipe that has passed over the skin be returned to the cleaned area or to the antiseptic solution.	Discarding sponges after each stroke prevents contamination of the wound by microorganisms brought back to the area from the surrounding skin.
6. Holding dry sterile gauze sponges in the sponge forceps, thoroughly pat the area dry. In some instances, the area may be allowed to air dry.	Moist skin may moisten the sterile drapes, causing wicking and contaminating the site.
7. Instruct the patient not to touch or cover the prepared area.	This avoids contaminating the operative site, which would require repeating the procedure.
8. Inform the physician that the patient is ready for the procedure. Drape the prepared area with a sterile drape if the physician will be delayed for more than 10 or 15 minutes.	

PROCEDURE 22-5: Applying Sterile Gloves

Purpose: Apply prepackaged sterile gloves without contamination
Equipment: One package of sterile gloves in the appropriate size

Steps	Reasons
1. Remove rings and other jewelry.	Rings may pierce the gloves and contaminate the procedure.
2. Wash your hands.	Wearing gloves is not a substitute for handwashing but must be done in addition to it.
3. Place the prepackaged gloves on a clean, dry, flat surface with the cuffed end toward you.	Sterile gloves are packaged for ease of application in this fashion.

A. Pull the outer wrapping apart to expose the sterile inner wrap.
B. With the cuffs toward you, fold back the inner wrap to expose the gloves.

Step 3. (A) Pull the outer wrapping apart to expose the sterile inner wrap. **(B)** With the cuffs toward you, fold back the inner wrap.

4. Grasping the edges of the outer paper, open the package out to its fullest.	The inner surface of the package is a sterile field.

Step 4. (A and B) Grasp the edges and open the packages.

(continued)

PROCEDURE 22-5:   Applying Sterile Gloves *(continued)*

Steps	Reasons
5. Using your nondominant hand, pick up the dominant hand glove by grasping the folded edge of the cuff and lifting it up and away from the paper. The folded edge of the cuff is contaminated as soon as it is touched with the ungloved hand. Be very careful not to touch the outside surface of the sterile glove with your ungloved hand.	Lift it up and away to avoid letting the fingers of the glove brush an unsterile surface.

Step 5. Using your nondominant hand, lift the cuff of the glove for the dominant hand, touching only the inner surface of the cuff. Curl your thumb inward as you insert your hand.

Steps	Reasons
6. Curl your fingers and thumb together and insert them into the glove. Then straighten your fingers and pull the glove on with your nondominant hand still grasping the cuff.	This prevents accidental touching of the outside surface of the glove.
7. Unfold the cuff by pinching the inside surface that will be against your wrist and pulling it toward the wrist.	This ensures that only the unsterile portions are touched by the hands.

Step 7. Pull the glove snugly into place, touching only the inside surface of the cuff.

Steps	Reasons
8. Place the fingers of your gloved hand under the cuff of the remaining glove, lift the glove up and away from the wrapper, and slide your ungloved hand carefully into the glove with your fingers and thumb curled together.	This prevents the sterile glove from accidentally touching an unsterile surface and ensures that the fingers will not brush the sterile surface of the glove.

Step 8. With your thumb curled, slip the gloved dominant hand into the cuff of the remaining glove.

(continued)

PROCEDURE 22-5: Applying Sterile Gloves *(continued)*

Steps	Reasons
9. Straighten your fingers and pull the glove up and over your wrist by carefully unfolding the cuff.	At all times, sterile must touch sterile only. Folding the cuffs out to their fullest allows the greatest area of sterility.
	Step 9. Unfold the cuff and pull the glove on snugly
10. Settle the gloves comfortably onto your fingers by lacing your fingers together and adjusting the tension over your hands.	The gloves should fit snugly without wrinkles or areas that bind the fingers.
	Step 10. Adjust the fingers for a comfortable fit.
11. Remove contaminated sterile gloves exactly as you would remove contaminated nonsterile gloves and discard them appropriately.	If removed correctly, one glove will be balled into the other with no opportunity to touch the soiled area of either glove.

PROCEDURE 22-6: Applying a Sterile Dressing

Purpose: Using sterile dressings and sterile technique, apply a sterile dressing to a surgical wound without contamination
Equipment: Sterile gloves, sterile gauze dressings, scissors, bandage tape, any medication to be applied to the wound if ordered by the physician

Steps	Reasons
1. Wash your hands and assemble the necessary supplies.	Handwashing aids infection control.
2. Assemble the equipment and supplies.	This ensures that all of the supplies are available before beginning the procedure.
3. Greet and identify the patient. Ask about any tape allergies before selecting tape. With the size of the dressing in mind, cut or tear lengths of tape to secure the dressing. Set the tape aside in a convenient place.	Patients must be identified to prevent errors in treatment. Some patients are sensitive to certain tape adhesives. Many types of hypoallergenic tape are available. Having tape cut and prepared saves time and may prevent the dressing from slipping while tape is cut after the dressing is applied.

(continued)

PROCEDURE 22-6: Applying a Sterile Dressing *(continued)*

Steps	Reasons
4. Explain the procedure and instruct the patient to remain still during the procedure and to avoid coughing, sneezing, and talking until the procedure is complete.	Unexpected movements by the patient may result in contamination of the sterile supplies and the wound. Talking, coughing, and sneezing release droplets of moisture containing microorganisms from the respiratory tract that may contaminate the sterile field and the wound.
5. Open the dressing pack to create a sterile field, leaving the sterile dressing on the inside of the opened package. Observe the principles of surgical asepsis. Many packets are designed to be peeled apart. 	Sterile technique ensures sterility of the dressing after it is open. Packages of dressings are sterile on the inside; if opened properly, the inner surface may be used as a sterile field. **Step 5.** Open the sterile dressing pack or packs.
6. To maintain sterility: A. If sterile gloves are to be used, open the appropriate package of gloves. Using sterile technique, put on the gloves before touching any sterile items. B. If using sterile transfer forceps to apply the dressing (the no-touch method), use sterile technique to arrange the dressing on the wound, and do not touch the dressing or the site with the hands.	
7. Apply to the sterile dressing that will directly cover the wound any topical medication ordered by the physician, being careful not to touch the end of the medication bottle or tube to the dressing. 	The outside end of the medication bottle or tube may not be sterile. **Step 7.** Apply medication if ordered without touching the end of the container on the dressing.
8. Using the already opened sterile dressings and sterile technique, apply the number of dressings necessary to cover and protect the wound. Sterile dressings must be carefully placed on the wound and not allowed to drag over the skin. 	If the dressing is dragged over the skin, it will be contaminated by microorganisms from the surrounding skin and may cause infection. **Step 8. (Left)** Using sterile gloves. **(Right)** Using sterile forceps.

(continued)

PROCEDURE 22-6: Applying a Sterile Dressing (continued)

Steps	Reasons
9. Apply the previously cut lengths of tape over the dressing to secure it, but avoid overuse of tape. When the wound is completely covered, you may remove your gloves or keep them on while you tape the dressing. Discard the gloves in the proper receptacle.	Tape is used only to keep the dressing in place. It should allow observation of any bleeding or drainage. Too much tape can cause perspiration that will dampen the dressing and compromise sterility. Tape should not obstruct blood circulation. Excessive tape also must later be removed, which may hurt. A bandage may be applied over the dressing to hold it in place, add support, or immobilize the area.

Step 9. (A) Securing a dressing with tape. **(B)** Securing a dressing with a bandage.

Steps	Reasons
10. When the patient is to change dressings at home, provide appropriate instructions. Dressings should be kept clean and dry and changed when wet or soiled. Otherwise, dressings should be changed as instructed by the physician. Make sure patients understand the signs of infection, such as redness, swelling, pain, or undue warmth at the site, and instruct them to call the office at once if these appear. Also say what to do in case of excessive bleeding or drainage and how to manage any drains.	Microorganisms may be transported to the wound by capillary action if the dressing is wet or soiled.
11. Wearing clean examination gloves, properly dispose of or care for equipment and supplies. Disposable articles contaminated with wound drainage or blood go into a biohazard container. Clean the work area, remove your gloves, and wash your hands.	Follow standard precautions.
12. Return reusable supplies (unopened sterile gloves or dressings, tape) to their appropriate storage areas; all others should be discarded correctly.	Unopened supplies should be returned to the appropriate storage areas for reuse. Discarding uncontaminated reusables is wasteful.
13. Record the procedure.	Procedures are considered not to have been done if they are not recorded in the patient's medical record.

Charting Example:

10/14/2008 4:45 PM DSD applied to surgical wound (L) anterior forearm. No bleeding from incision, edges well approximated with 4 sutures intact. Pt. given verbal and written instructions on dressing change and wound care at home. To RTO in 5 days for suture removal

—L. Hicks, CMA

PROCEDURE 22-7: Changing an Existing Sterile Dressing

Purpose: Carefully remove an existing dressing from a wound and cover it with a sterile dressing using sterile technique

Equipment: Sterile gloves; nonsterile gloves; sterile dressing; prepackaged skin antiseptic swabs or sterile antiseptic solution in a sterile basin and sterile cotton balls or gauze; tape; approved biohazard container

Steps	Reasons
1. Wash your hands and assemble the necessary supplies.	Handwashing aids infection control.
2. Assemble the equipment and supplies.	This ensures that all supplies are available before you begin the procedure.
3. Greet and identify the patient. Explain the procedure and answer any questions.	This prevents errors in treatment, helps gain compliance, and eases anxiety.
4. Prepare a sterile field, including opening sterile dressings. If using a sterile container and solution, open the package containing the sterile basin and use the inside of the wrapper as the sterile field for the basin. Flip the sterile gauze or cotton balls into the basin and appropriately pour in the antiseptic solution. If using prepackaged antiseptic swabs, carefully open an adequate number for the size of the wound and set them aside without contaminating them.	Opening sterile supplies after applying sterile gloves will cause contamination of your gloves and your supplies.
5. Instruct the patient not to talk, cough, sneeze, laugh, or move during the procedure.	Respiratory droplets may contaminate the sterile field. Movement may cause accidental contamination of the field.
6. Wearing clean gloves, carefully remove the tape from the wound dressing by pulling it toward the wound. Remove the old dressing. Note: If the dressing is difficult to remove because of dried blood, it may be soaked with sterile water or saline for a few minutes to loosen it. Gently pull the edges of the dressing toward the center. Never pull on a dressing that does not come off easily. If this procedure does not sufficiently loosen the dressing or causes undue discomfort to the patient, immediately notify the physician.	Tape pulled away from the direction of the wound may pull the healing edges of the wound apart. **Step 6.** Pull the tape toward the wound.
7. Discard the soiled dressing into a biohazard container. Do not pass it over the sterile field.	The dressing will be soiled with blood and body fluids and must be considered hazardous. Dressings passed over the sterile field will shed microorganisms and contaminate the area.

(continued)

PROCEDURE 22-7:   Changing an Existing Sterile Dressing (continued)

Steps	Reasons
8. Inspect the wound for degree of healing, amount and type of drainage, appearance of wound edges, and so on.	The wound is inspected now because wound cleaning removes most exudate. Make a mental note for charting when the procedure is complete.
9. Observing medical asepsis, remove and discard your gloves. The physician may want to inspect the wound before you remove exudate or drainage to determine whether healing is proceeding as expected. If a culture is ordered, the specimen must be taken before the wound is cleaned to ensure the most reliable findings.	
10. Using proper technique, put on sterile gloves. Clean the wound with the antiseptic solution ordered by the physician. Clean in a straight motion with the cotton or gauze or the prepackaged antiseptic swab. Discard the wipe (cotton ball, swab) after each stroke and use a fresh sterile one to continue. Never return the wipe to the antiseptic solution or to the skin after one sweep across the area.	The wound must be cleaned before fresh dressings are applied. Returning the wipe to the wound area or solution brings microorganisms from the surrounding skin to the open lesion.
11. Remove your gloves and wash your hands.	Your hands must be washed before you apply the sterile dressing with sterile gloves or sterile forceps.
12. Change the dressing using the procedure for sterile dressing application and using sterile gloves or sterile transfer forceps (Procedure 22-6).	
13. Record the procedure.	Procedures are considered not to have been done if they are not recorded.

Charting Example:

11/23/2008 11:30 AM Dressing to (R) lower leg changed, small amount of yellow purulent drainage noted—Dr. Blake aware. Wound culture for C&S obtained and sent to Acme laboratory. Wound cleansed with Betadine as ordered; DSD reapplied. Moderate amount of redness and swelling at wound site; edges well approximated. Instructed to RTO in 2 days for C&S results and dressing change

—B. Lamont, CMA

PROCEDURE 22-8: Assisting With Excisional Surgery

Purpose: Prepare for and assist with excisional surgery while maintaining sterile technique
Equipment: At the side: sterile gloves, local anesthetic, antiseptic wipes, adhesive tape, specimen container with completed laboratory request. On the field: basin for solutions, gauze sponges and cotton balls, antiseptic solution, sterile drape, dissecting scissors, disposable scalpel, blade of physician's choice, mosquito forceps, tissue forceps, needle holder, suture and needle of physician's choice.

Steps	Reasons
1. Wash your hands and assemble the necessary supplies.	Handwashing aids infection control.
2. Assemble the equipment.	This ensures that all supplies are available.
3. Greet and identify the patient. Explain the procedure and answer any questions.	This prevents errors in treatment, helps gain compliance, and eases anxiety.
4. Set up a sterile field on a surgical stand with the at-the-side equipment close at hand. Cover the field with a sterile drape until the physician arrives.	
5. Position the patient appropriately.	The required position depends on the location of the lesion.
6. Put on sterile gloves or use sterile transfer forceps and cleanse the patient's skin as described in Procedure 24-4. Some physicians prefer to do this themselves after gloving, using supplies on the field. The physician's preference always takes precedence over any outlined procedure.	The antiseptic discourages the entrance of microorganisms into the wound. After cleansing the skin, remove the gloves, if used, and wash the hands.
7. The physician will perform the procedure; you may be asked to assist. This usually involves adding supplies as needed, watching closely for opportunities to assist the physician, and comforting the patient.	It is not necessary for you to wear sterile gloves during the procedure unless the physician requires you to handle sterile instruments or supplies.
8. If the lesion is to be referred to pathology for analysis, you will be required to assist with collecting the specimen in an appropriate container.	Always follow standard precautions, wearing examination gloves when handling specimens. Have the container ready to receive the specimen.
9. At the end of the procedure, wash your hands and dress the wound using sterile technique (Procedure 22-6).	The wound must be covered to protect the incision from contamination.
10. Thank the patient and give appropriate instructions for care of the operative site, changing the dressing, postoperative medications, and follow-up visits as ordered by the physician.	Courtesy encourages the patient to have a positive attitude about the physician's office.

(continued)

PROCEDURE 22-8:	**Assisting With Excisional Surgery** *(continued)*

Steps	**Reasons**
11. Wearing gloves, clean the examining room in preparation for the next patient. Discard all used disposables in appropriate biohazard containers. Return unused items to their proper places. Remove your gloves and wash your hands.	Standard precautions must be followed. **Step 11.** Discard any disposable sharps items such as a scalpel into the appropriate biohazard container.
12. Record the procedure.	

Charting Example:

09/19/2008 8:45 AM Mole to posterior (L) shoulder removed per Dr. Snider. Specimen sent to Acme lab. T 98.4 (O), P 96, R 20, BP 134/78 (R) sitting. 4 × 4 DSD applied to surgical incision; minimal sanguineous drainage noted. Pt. given verbal and written instructions on wound care, postop antibiotics, pain medication, and follow-up visits. Verbalized understanding. To RTO ×2 days for drsg change

—B. Cole, CMA

PROCEDURE 22-9:	**Assisting With Incision and Drainage (I & D)**

Purpose: Prepare for and assist with an incision and drainage procedure while maintaining sterile technique
Equipment: At the side: sterile gloves; local anesthetic; needle and syringe if not placed on sterile field; antiseptic wipes; adhesive tape; sterile dressings; packing gauze; culture tube if the wound may be cultured. On the field: basin for solutions; gauze sponges and cotton balls; antiseptic solution; sterile drape; syringes and needles for local anesthetic; commercial I & D sterile setup or scalpel, dissecting scissors, hemostats, tissue forceps; sterile 4 × 4 gauze sponges; sterile probe (optional).

Steps

The steps for this procedure are similar to those in Procedure 22-8. Specifically, you are expected to prepare the surgical field and the patient's surgical area as instructed or preferred by the physician. After the procedure, the wound must be covered to avoid further contamination and to absorb drainage. The exudate is a hazardous body fluid requiring standard precautions. Although a culture and sensitivity may be ordered on the drainage from the infected area, no other specimen is usually collected.

Charting Example:

04/15/2008 11:30 AM Postop VS T 100.4 (O), P 88, R 24, BP 128/88 (R) sitting. 4 × 4 DSD applied to surgical wound on (L) posterior neck. Given verbal and written instructions on wound care, dressing changes, and follow-up. Verbalized understanding

—E. Black, CMA

PROCEDURE 22-10: Removing Sutures

Purpose: Using aseptic technique, remove sutures from a wound
Equipment: Skin antiseptic; clean exam gloves; sterile gloves; prepackaged suture removal kit OR thumb forceps, suture scissors, and 2 × 2 gauze

Steps	Reasons
1. Wash your hands and apply clean examination gloves.	Handwashing aids infection control.
2. Assemble the equipment.	This ensures that all supplies are available.
3. Greet and identify the patient. Explain the procedure and answer any questions.	This prevents errors in treatment, helps gain compliance, and eases anxiety.
4. If dressings have not been removed, remove them and properly dispose of them in the biohazard container. Remove your gloves and wash your hands if a soiled dressing was removed.	
5. Put on clean examination gloves and cleanse the wound with an antiseptic, such as Betadine, using a new antiseptic gauze for each swipe down the wound and removing any old drainage or blood.	The wound must be as free of pathogens as possible before removal of the sutures to prevent contamination of the wound.
6. Open the suture removal packet using sterile asepsis or set up a field for on-site sterile equipment. Put on sterile gloves.	Suture removal is a sterile procedure.
7. The knots will be tied so that one tail of the knot is very close to the surface of the skin; the other will be closer to the area of suture that is looped over the incision.	

Step 7. (A) With the hemostat or thumb forceps, lift the stitch up and away from the skin. **(B)** Cut the stitch near the skin. **(C)** Using the forceps, pull the freed stitch up and out.

A. With the thumb forceps, grasp the end of the knot closest to the skin and lift it slightly and gently up from the skin.

B. Cut the suture below the knot as close to the skin as possible.

B. Cutting below the knot and close to the skin frees the knot at an area that has not been ex posed to the outside surface of the body. The only part of the suture that will pull through the tissues will be the suture that was under the skin surface.

C. Use the thumb forceps to pull the suture out of the skin with a smooth, continuous motion, at a slight agnle in the direction of the wound.

C. This prevents tension on the healing tissue.

(continued)

PROCEDURE 22-10:   Removing Sutures *(continued)*

Steps	Reasons
8. Place the suture on the gauze sponge. Repeat the procedure for each suture to be removed.	This helps in counting the number removed; if six sutures were inserted and are now to be removed, there should be six sutures on the gauze sponge at the end of the procedure.
9. Clean the site with an antiseptic solution, and if the physician has so indicated, cover it with a sterile dressing.	Some wounds still need to be protected; some have healed well enough to be left uncovered.
10. Thank the patient and properly dispose of the equipment and supplies. Clean the work area, remove your gloves, and wash your hands.	Standard precautions must be followed. Courtesy encourages a positive attitude about the physician's office.
11. Record the procedure, including the time, location of sutures, number removed, and condition of the wound.	Procedures are considered not to have been done if they are not recorded.

Charting Example:

06/26/2009 3:30 PM ×6 sutures removed from (L) ring finger. Wound well approximated, no drainage

—J. Rose, RMA

PROCEDURE 22-11:   Removing Staples

Purpose: Using aseptic technique, remove staples from a wound
Equipment: Antiseptic solution or wipes, gauze squares, sponge forceps, prepackaged sterile staple removal instrument, examination gloves, sterile gloves

Steps	Reasons
1. Wash your hands.	Handwashing aids infection control.
2. Assemble the equipment.	This ensures that all supplies are available.
3. Greet and identify the patient. Explain the procedure and answer any questions.	This prevents errors in treatment, helps gain compliance, and eases anxiety.
4. If the dressing is still in place, put on clean examination gloves and remove it. Dispose of the dressing in a biohazard container.	The dressing is contaminated and must be handled with standard precautions. Remove gloves and wash your hands.
5. Clean the incision with antiseptic solution. Pat dry with sterile gauze sponges.	The incision must be cleaned before removing the staples to avoid infection. If exudate is present, the staples may not be easy to see.
6. Put on sterile gloves.	Staple removal is a sterile procedure.

(continued)

PROCEDURE 22-11: Removing Staples (continued)

Steps	Reasons
7. Gently slide the end of the staple remover under each staple to be removed. Press the handles together to lift the ends of the staple out of the skin.	The remover is designed to open the staple so that the ends will lift free and minimize discomfort.
	Step 7. Slide the end of the staple remover under each staple. Press the handles together to lift the ends of the staple out of the skin.
8. Place each staple on a gauze square as it is removed.	This helps in counting the staples at the end of the procedure.
9. When all staples are removed, gently clean the incision as instructed for all procedures. Pat dry and dress the site if ordered to do so by the physician.	The area should be cleaned and dried before any new dressing is applied to avoid wicking microorganisms. Healing may be far enough along to allow the wound to remain uncovered.
10. Thank the patient and properly care for or dispose of all equipment and supplies. Clean the work area, remove your gloves, and wash your hands.	Standard precautions must be followed.
11. Record the procedure.	Procedures are not considered to have been done if they are not recorded.

Charting Example:

3/17/2008 10:30 AM ×15 staples removed from (L) knee incision; edges well approximated, no redness or drainage noted. Wound left open to air as ordered by Dr. Perez

—B. Daniels, CMA

- With the spiraling costs of health care, many procedures that were once performed only in hospitals are now being performed in medical offices.
- As a medical assistant, you will be required to become more proficient in minor surgical procedures as offices change to meet the needs of the patients. Continuing education, research, and on-the-job training will keep you current on the changes in the field of surgery and in the new equipment that is used during minor office surgical procedures.
- No matter how technical or sophisticated the surgical procedure or equipment, however, you must not forget the feelings of apprehension many patients have. Although it is your responsibility to prepare the treatment room and assist the physician, you are also obligated to instruct the patient accurately on any presurgical preparations, obtain third-party authorization if necessary, reassure the patient during the procedure, and give the patient accurate information about postsurgical care as ordered by the physician.
- After the procedure, you must disinfect the examination room and prepare it for future patients.

Warm Ups for Critical Thinking

1. Dr. Brown has just informed Mrs. Levine that she should return tomorrow for office surgery. While you are alone with the patient, Mrs. Levine begins to cry and expresses great concern about the procedure. What should you do?

2. Refer to an anatomy book and review the anatomy of a hair follicle. Why are skin nicks more likely if the hair is shaved in the opposite direction of its natural growth?

3. Why is it preferable for infected wounds to heal with delayed or unclosed surface edges?

4. Prepare a patient education sheet outlining postoperative wound care.

5. This morning, you are assisting Dr. Patrick with an ingrown toenail removal. When the patient arrives, you notice that the consent form has not been signed. The patient agrees to sign the consent form but indicates that he has some questions about the risks involved. Should you let him sign the consent? Why or why not? What would you do?

Answers to Checkpoint Questions

1. To maintain a sterile field, you must keep sterile packages dry, face the sterile field, keep sterile items above waist level, keep items in the middle of the field, avoid spills, not cough or sneeze near the field, never reach over the field, not pass contaminated items over the field, and alert the physician if the field becomes contaminated.

2. Contents of a peel-back package can be added to the sterile field with sterile forceps or a sterile gloved hand or by flipping them onto the field.

3. A fenestrated drape has an opening to expose the treatment site while covering adjacent areas.

4. Swaged (atraumatic) needles have the appropriate size suture material attached by the manufacturer. Threaded needles have an eye with a double thickness of suture that must be pulled through the tissues.

5. Electrosection is the type of electrosurgery used for incision or excision of tissue.

6. When assisting with laser procedures, everyone present must protect their eyes by wearing goggles.

7. Dressings are used to cover and protect a wound, absorb drainage, exert pressure, hide disfigurement, and hold medications against the skin. Bandages are placed over dressings to hold the dressing in place, protect the injured part, or restrict movement.

8. Electrocautery, laser, cryosurgery, and standard surgical procedures are methods that may be used to excise skin lesions in the medical office.

Pharmacology

Outline

Medication Names
Legal Regulations
  Food and Drug Administration
  Drug Enforcement Agency
  Inventory, Storage,
    Dispensation, and Disposal
    of Medications

Sources of Drugs
Drug Actions
  Pharmacodynamics
  Pharmacokinetics
  Drug Interactions
  Side Effects and Allergies

Sources of Information
Prescriptions
  Refilling Prescriptions

Learning Objectives

Upon successfully completing this chapter, you will be able to:

1. Spell and define key terms

2. Describe basic principles of pharmacology

3. Identify chemical, trade, and generic drug names

4. Name the regulations and branches of government that impact prescription medications and controlled substances

5. Explain the various drug actions and interactions including pharmacodynamics and pharmacokinetics

6. Describe the difference between medication side effects and allergies

7. Name the sources for locating information on pharmacology

Competencies

CAAHEP

- Apply pharmacology principles to prepare and administer oral and parenteral (excluding IV) medications

- Perform within legal and ethical boundaries

- Demonstrate knowledge of federal and state health care legislation and regulations

ABHES

- Follow established policy in initiating or terminating medical treatment

- Dispose of controlled substances in compliance with government regulations

480

allergy	contraindication	pharmacodynamics	side effect
anaphylaxis	drug	pharmacokinetics	synergism
antagonism	generic name	pharmacology	trade name
chemical name	interaction	potentiation	

As a clinical medical assistant, you may be responsible for administering medications under the supervision of the physician. It is important that you acquire knowledge of medications, their uses and potential abuses, range of dosages, methods of administration, and adverse effects. **Pharmacology** is the term given to the study of drugs and their actions, dosages, and side effects. A **drug** is a chemical substance that affects body function or functions. Medications are available in many forms and are administered in various ways to produce therapeutic effects.

Medication Names

Most medications have a **chemical name**, a **generic name,** and a **trade name** (Box 23-1). The chemical name is the first name given to any medication. It identifies the chemical components of the drug. The generic name is assigned to the medication during research and development. When the drug is available for commercial use and distribution by the original manufacturer, it is given a brand, or trade, name. The trade name is registered by the US Patent Office and has the official trademark symbol (™) after its name. After the patent expires, any other company that manufactures the medication may assign its own trade name to the generic equivalent. The first letter of a trade name is always capitalized; generic names begin with lowercase letters.

Drugs can be classified according to their actions and effects on the body. Table 23-1 lists some commonly used drugs, prescription and nonprescription, and their classifications.

BOX 23-1

DRUG NAMES

Chemical Name	7-chloro-1,3-dihydro-1-methyl-5-phenyl-2H-1,4-benzodiax-epin-2-one
Trade Name	Valium
Generic Name	Diazepam

CHECKPOINT QUESTION

1. What is the difference between a drug's chemical name and trade name?

Legal Regulations

Food and Drug Administration

Consumers in the United States are protected by federal regulations regarding the production, prescribing, or dispensing of medications. In 1906, the Pure Food and Drug Act was passed. After being amended in 1938, it required that the safety of a drug be proved before distribution to the public. The amended law was renamed the Federal Food, Drug, and Cosmetic Act. In 1952, the Durham-Humphrey Amendment banned many drugs from being dispensed without a prescription. The Kefauver-Harris Amendment of 1962 required testing of prescription and nonprescription medications for effectiveness before their release for sale. The Food and Drug Administration (FDA) was established to regulate the manufacture and distribution of drugs and food products and to ensure accuracy in the ingredients listed on the labels of food and drug products.

Drug Enforcement Agency

In 1970, the Controlled Substances Act was passed to regulate the manufacture and distribution of drugs whose use may result in dependency or abuse. This act also requires that anyone who manufactures, prescribes, administers, or dispenses controlled substances register with the United States Attorney General under the Bureau of Narcotics and Dangerous Drugs (BNDD). The Drug Enforcement Agency (DEA) is a branch of the Department of Justice (DOJ) and is designated to exercise strong regulatory control over all drugs listed by the BNDD. This authority extends to prescribing, refilling, and storing controlled substances in the medical office. The DEA is concerned with controlled substances only; medications not subject to abuse are not regulated by this agency.

As a medical assistant, you may be responsible for maintaining or reminding the physician about professional records and licensure, including registration with

TABLE 23-1   Classifications of Drugs

Therapeutic Classification	Effect or Action/Uses	Common Examples
Adrenergic blocking agents	Affect the alpha receptors of adrenergic nerves	Metoprolol tartrate (Lopressor), propranolol hydrochloride (Inderal)
Adrenergics	Mimic the activity of the sympathetic nervous system	Epinephrine (Adrenaline), ephedrine sulfate
Analgesics	Used to relieve pain	Aspirin, acetaminophen (Tylenol), codeine
Antacids	Neutralize or reduce the acidity of the stomach carbonate (Tums)	Magnesia (Milk of Magnesia), calcium
Anthelmintics	Kills parasitic worms	Piperazine citrate, mebendazole (Vermox)
Antianginal agents	Promote vasodilation	Nitroglycerine, diltiazem hydrochloride (Cardizem)
Antianxiety agents	Act on subcortical areas of the brain to relieve symptoms of anxiety	Alprazolam (Xanax), chlordiazepoxide (Librium), diazepam (Valium)
Antiarrhythmics	Various actions and effects	Disopyramide (Norpace), procainamide hydrochloride (Pronestyl), esmolol (Brevibloc)
Antibiotics	Destroy, interrupt, or interfere with the growth of microorganisms	Penicillin, ampicillin, cefaclor, tetracycline
Anticoagulants and thrombolytics	Used to prevent the formation of blood clots or dissolve blood clots	Heparin sodium, streptokinase (Streptase)
Anticonvulsants	Reduce the excitability of the brain	Phenobarbital, phenytoin (Dilantin)
Antidepressants	Various actions	Amitriptyline hydrochloride (Elavil), fluoxetine hydrochloride (Prozac)
Antidiarrheals	Decrease intestinal peristalsis	Loperamide hydrochloride (Imodium A-D)
Antiemetic agents	Prevents nausea and vomiting	Dimenhydrinate (Dramamine), promethazine hydrochloride (Phenergan)
Antifungals	Destroy or retard the growth of fungi	Ketoconazole (Nizoral), miconazole nitrate (Monistat 3 or 7)
Antihistamines	Counteracts the effects of histamine on body organs and structures	Chlorpheniramine maleate (Chlor-Trimeton), diphenhydramine hydrochloride (Benadryl)

(continued)

TABLE 23-1	Classifications of Drugs *(continued)*	
Therapeutic Classification	**Effect or Action/Uses**	**Common Examples**
Antihypertensives	Increase the size of arterial blood vessels	Chlorpheniramine maleate (Aldomet), prazosin (Minipres)
Anti-inflammatory agents	Reduce irritation and swelling of tissues	Aspirin, ibuprofen (Motrin); naproxen (Naprosyn)
Antineoplastic agents	Slow the rate of tumor growth	Cyclophosphamide (Cytoxan)
Antipsychotics	Exact mechanism not understood; used to treat psychoses	Thorazine, Haldol
Antipyretics	Decrease body temperature	Aspirin, Tylenol
Antitussives, mucolytics, and expectorants	Relieve coughing, loosen respiratory secretions, or aid in the removal of thick secretions	Codeine sulfate, Benylin, Entex
Antivirals	Inhibit viral replication	Acyclovir (Zovirax), AZT
Bronchodilators	Dilate the bronchi	Albuterol sulfate (Ventolin), Alupent
Cardiotonics	Increase the force of the myocardium	Digoxin (Lanoxin), Primacor
Cholinergic blocking agents	Affect the autonomic nervous system	Atropine sulfate, scopolamine hydrobromide
Cholinergics	Mimic the activity of the parasympathetic nervous system	Neostigmine (Prostigmin), pilocarpine hydrochloride
Decongestants	Reduce swelling of nasal passages	Pseudoephedrine hydrochloride (Sudafed)
Diuretics	Increase the secretion of urine by the kidneys	Furosemide (Lasix), chlorothiazide (Diuril)
Emetics	Promote vomiting	Ipecac syrup
Histamine H2 antagonists	Inhibit the action of histamine at the H2 receptor cells of the stomach	Cimetidine (Tagamet), ranitidine
Hormones, female	Used to prevent symptoms of menopause	Estradiol (Estraderm), medroxyprogesterone acetate (Provera)
Hormones, male	Androgen therapy to treat testosterone deficiency	Halotestin
Immunologic agents (vaccines)	Stimulate the immune response to create protection against disease	Pneumococcal vaccine, influenza virus vaccine, diphtheria and tetanus toxoid
Insulin and oral hypoglycemics	Used to control diabetes	NPH and Ultralente insulin, Orinase, Glucotrol

(continued)

TABLE 23-1	Classifications of Drugs (continued)	
Therapeutic Classification	**Effect or Action/Uses**	**Common Examples**
Sedatives and hypnotics	Sedatives relax and calm; hypnotics induce sleep	Butabarbital sodium, Restoril
Stimulants	Increase activity of the central nervous system	Doxapram hydrochloride (Dopram), amphetamine Sulfate
Thyroid and antithyroid agents	Used to increase or decrease the amount of thyroid hormone produced	Levothyroxine sodium (T4), Levothroid

Summarized from Scherer JC, Roach SS. Introductory Clinical Pharmacology, 5th ed. Philadelphia: Lippincott-Raven Publishers, 1996.

the DEA. When the physician registers with the US Attorney General under the BNDD, a registration number (DEA number) is issued. Physicians are registered for 3 years after application and acceptance. The DEA does not take responsibility if the physician's registration expires. The registration retires with the physician; it does not stay with the medical office.

The DEA is also responsible for revising the list of drugs in the Schedule of Controlled Substances (Table 23-2). These substances have been identified as having a potential for abuse and dependency. Drug dependence, sometimes referred to as addiction, can be either psychological, physical, or both. A patient who has developed physical dependence on a drug will have mild to severe physiologic symptoms that gradually decrease in intensity after the drug is stopped. Patients who are psychologically dependent have acquired a need for the feeling brought on by the drug. Patients who are pre-

TABLE 23-2.	Controlled Substances	
Schedule	**Description**	**Examples**
I	These drugs have the highest potential for abuse and have no currently accepted medicinal use in the US. There are no accepted safety standards for use of these drugs or substances even under medical supervision, although some are used experimentally in carefully controlled research projects.	Opium, marijuana, lysergic acid diethylamide (LSD), peyote, mescaline
II	These drugs have a high potential for abuse. They have a current accepted medicinal use in the US, but with severe restrictions. Abuse of these drugs can lead to dependence, either psychological or physiologic. Schedule II drugs require a written prescription and cannot be refilled or called into the pharmacy by the medical office. Only in extreme emergencies may the physician call in the prescription. A handwritten prescription must be presented to the pharmacist within 72 hours.	Morphine, codeine, cocaine, Seconal, amphetamines, Dilaudid, Ritalin
III	These drugs have a limited potential for psychological or physiologic dependence. The prescription may be called in to the pharmacist by the physician and refilled up to five times in a 6-month period.	Paregoric, Tylenol with codeine, Fiorinal
IV	These drugs have a lower potential for abuse than those in Schedules II and III. They can be called into the pharmacist by a medical office employee and may be filled up to five times in a 6-month period.	Librium, Valium, Darvon, phenobarbital
V	These drugs have a lower potential for abuse than those in schedules I, II, III, and IV.	Lomotil, Dimetane, Expectorant DC, Robitussin-DAC

Five schedules, or categories, of controlled substances were established by the Bureau of Narcotics and Dangerous Drugs. Medications in the five schedules may be revised periodically after review.

scribed controlled substances must be monitored closely for signs of physical or psychological dependence.

Controlled substances in Schedule II are received from suppliers using a Federal Triplicate Order Form DEA 222. Schedules III, IV, and V do not require triplicate forms, but invoices for receipts of the substances must be maintained for 2 years. Box 23-2 describes how to handle inventory of controlled substances.

If controlled substances are prescribed and not administered at the office, some states require only that the information be recorded in the patient's chart; others require a separate file of prescription copies of controlled substances. Law enforcement officials recommend that the DEA number not be preprinted on the prescription. Officials at regional DEA offices are available to answer any questions regarding the drugs under its control. As a medical assistant, you should make sure the physician's office is on the DEA's periodic mailing list to keep abreast of changes.

 CHECKPOINT QUESTION

2. What information must be documented when a controlled substance is administered in the medical office?

 WHAT IF?

Bob Sandler, a 38-year-old accountant, was first seen in the office 2 weeks ago for a back injury that occurred after doing some home repair work the previous weekend. At the initial visit, the physician prescribed an opioid pain medication and a muscle relaxant. Today, Mr. Sandler tells you that his medications were stolen, and he would like a refill for both. What if both drugs had a high potential for abuse and were often purchased illegally on the street? Would you suspect that the patient was selling his medication? How could you be sure that this was not occurring?

While the medical assistant must be an advocate for the patient, he or she must also be vigilant about the possibility of drug abuse in the patient population and the community at large. It is imperative that the medical assistant gather as much information as possible about "lost" or "stolen" medications and report any illegal activities to the proper authorities. Patients who have had medications stolen that have a high abuse potential will want to report the theft to the police. Some physicians want to see a police report before issuing another prescription.

 LEGAL AND ETHICAL TIP

REPORTING SUSPECTED ABUSE OF CONTROLLED SUBSTANCES IN THE MEDICAL OFFICE

If you suspect that a physician or any other health care professional is illegally diverting controlled substances, you have a legal and ethical responsibility to report this suspicion. Gather and document evidence and the reasons you suspect diversion of substances. You should have a clear and compelling case to present to the proper authorities, usually the local police. In addition, if a physician is involved, report this evidence to the Drug Enforcement Agency and the American Medical Association (AMA). You should also notify the state medical society. If the suspected health care worker is not a physician, report it to the appropriate supervisor or superior. Most states have programs to assist health care professionals in obtaining appropriate psychological help to deal with addiction or dependency issues. In most instances, you will remain anonymous.

Inventory, Storage, Dispensation, and Disposal of Medications

Most medical offices store medications in the office for use during office hours or to give to patients for use at home. Often, pharmaceutical company sales representa-

BOX 23-2

HANDLING INVENTORY OF CONTROLLED SUBSTANCES

1. When you receive controlled substances, make sure that both you and a second employee sign the receipt.
2. List all controlled substances on the appropriate inventory form (Fig. 23-1).
3. When a controlled substance leaves the medical office inventory, record the following information: drug name, patient, dose, date, ordering physician, and employee who handled the procedure.
4. Keep all controlled substance inventory forms for 2 years.
5. Ensure that controlled substances are kept in a locked safe or in a secure locked box.
6. Notify the local law enforcement agency immediately if these drugs are lost or stolen.

Controlled Substance:		Meperidine (Demerol) 50mg Injection			
Amount Ordered:		50 mg vials/ampules			Date:

Date	Patient Name	Ordering Physician	Dose Given	Amount Discarded	Employee Signature

Figure 23-1 Controlled substance inventory form.

tives will leave medication samples specifically for you to dispense at the direction of the physician. In either situation, it will be your responsibility to maintain an inventory of these medications, including the amount of each drug being stored and a written record of medications taken for administration in the office or dispensed to the patient for use at home (Fig. 23-1). Medications kept in the medical office should be stored away from patients or other visitors who may come to the office. Ideally, the medication area should be locked and accessible only by authorized clinical staff. It will be your responsibility to keep this medication area clean, neat, and organized.

When disposing of medications other than controlled substances, you should follow the office policy and procedure manual. In some cases, the appropriate pharmaceutical representative may need to be notified and may advise you to place any expired medications into a container to be picked up and disposed of by the company. Never dispose of expired medications in regular trash containers. For controlled substances that need to be disposed, a witness should watch the disposal, and both parties will be required to sign appropriate DEA forms noting the name of the drug and the amount disposed.

Sources of Drugs

Drugs are available from numerous natural sources, such as plants, minerals, and animals. They may also be synthetic (prepared in the laboratory by artificial means). Table 23-3 lists a number of commonly prescribed drugs and their sources.

Drug Actions and Interactions

Pharmacodynamics

Pharmacodynamics is the study of the ways drugs act on the body, including the actions on specific cells, tissues, and organs. All drugs cause cellular change (drug action) and some degree of physiologic change (drug effect). An action of a local drug, such as an ointment or lotion applied to the skin, is limited to the area where it is administered. A drug administered for a systemic effect is absorbed into the blood and carried to the organ or tissue on which it will act. An example of this is antibiotic therapy for a urinary tract infection. The antibiotic tablets are taken orally, but once they are absorbed, the action takes place in the urinary bladder, where the drug destroys any microorganisms. A systemic effect can be produced by administering drugs orally (by mouth), sublingually (under the tongue), rectally, by injection, transdermally (through the skin), or by inhalation (through the lungs). A number of factors can influence a drug's action in the body including:

- *Age:* Elderly people have slower metabolic processes. Age-related kidney and liver dysfunctions also extend the break down and excretion times in these patients,

TABLE **23-3**	Common Drugs and Their Sources	
Source	**Drug**	**Use**
Plants		
Cinchona bark	Quinidine	Antiarrhythmic
Purple foxglove	Digitalis	Cardiotonic
Opium poppy	Paregoric	Antidiarrheal
	Morphine	Analgesic
	Codeine	Antitussive, analgesic
Minerals		
Magnesium	Milk of Magnesia	Antacid, laxative
Silver	Silver nitrate	Placed in eyes of newborns to kill *Neisseria gonorrhoeae*; chemical cautery of lesions
Gold	Solganal	Arthritis treatment
Animal Proteins		
Porcine or bovine pancreas	Insulin	Antidiabetic hormone
Porcine or bovine stomach acids	Pepsin	Digestive hormone
Animal thyroid glands	Thyroid, USP	Hypothyroidism
Synthetics		
	Demerol	Analgesic
	Lomotil	Antidiarrheal
	Gantrisin	Sulfonamide
Semisynthetic		
Escherichia coli bacteria and altered DNA molecules	Humulin	Antidiabetic hormone

so it is necessary to monitor the cumulative effects of drugs in the elderly. Children may have a more immediate response to drugs and, therefore, must be assessed frequently.

- *Weight*: Many drug dosages are calculated and administered according to the patient's weight. As a general rule, the larger the patient, the greater the dose; however, individual sensitivity to the effects of drugs should be taken into consideration.
- *Sex*: Women may react differently to certain drugs than men because of the ratio of fat to body mass or fluctuating hormone levels.
- *Existing Pathology*: If the body is compromised by a disease process, absorption, distribution, metabolism, and excretion may be altered.
- *Tolerance*: Some medications given over a long period of time may cause the body to become resistant to their effects, requiring larger doses to achieve the desired response.

Medical assistants should always administer medications under the direct order of a physician. Under no circumstance should the dosage be adjusted or altered unless specifically instructed to do so by the physician.

Pharmacokinetics

Pharmacokinetics is the study of the action of drugs within the body based on the route of administration, rate of absorption, duration of action, and elimination from the body. Specifically, the processes included in pharmacokinetics include absorption (getting the drug into the bloodstream), distribution (movement of the drug from the bloodstream into the cells and tissues), metabolism (the physical and chemical breakdown of drugs by the body, including the liver), and excretion (byproducts sent to the kidneys to be removed from the body). In the presence of hepatic disease, the liver may not be able to break down the drug properly, and the patient may undergo toxic effects caused by an accumulation of the drug in the liver or the bloodstream. In this situation, the drug may be noted as contraindicated by the manufacturer, or not recommended for use, in patients with a history of liver disease. Some drugs reach the kidneys relatively unchanged; these drugs can be detected in the urine during excretion, when the waste products of drug metabolism are eliminated from the body. However, if the kidneys are compromised by disease, medication may not be properly eliminated, adding to the danger of a cumulative, or building, effect and possible toxicity or poisoning.

 CHECKPOINT QUESTION

3. Why should pharmacokinetics be taken into consideration before administering medications?

Drug Interactions

When two or more drugs are taken simultaneously, one drug may increase, decrease, or cancel the effects of the other. These **interactions** may occur with prescribed drugs, over-the-counter medications, herbal or other natural supplements, and alcohol consumption. These **interactions** must always be taken into account when prescribing medications, administering medications, obtaining a medication history, or educating a patient about taking medications. Types of interactions include **synergism** (two drugs working together), **antagonism** (an effect in which one drug decreases the effect of another), and **potentiation** (occurs when one drug prolongs or multiplies the effect of another drug). Physicians prescribing two or more drugs may be using these drug interactions to cause a desired effect. An example of this is use of a muscle relaxant and a pain medication to reduce the pain associated with an injury to a muscle or muscle group. However, some drug interactions produce undesirable effects. For example, antacids taken to relieve symptoms of indigestion may prevent absorption of antibiotics, such as tetracycline (antagonism), while sedatives and barbiturates taken together can cause central nervous system depression (synergism). Table 23-4 lists other important drug-related terms you should know.

Side Effects and Allergies

When gathering a patient's medical history, you must always ask about allergies of any sort, particularly allergies to medications. A drug **allergy** is a reaction such as hives, dyspnea, or wheezing. In addition, the allergic reaction **anaphylaxis** can be life threatening. Allergic reactions can be immediate or delayed 2 hours or longer, depending on the route of administration; however, many allergic reactions occur within minutes if the medication

 PATIENT EDUCATION

FOOD–DRUG INTERACTION

Many medications interact with food. Some medications are best absorbed when taken on an empty stomach. Two such medications are the antibiotics ampicillin and nafcillin (Unipen). Other medications should be taken with food to decrease the potential for stomach upset. These include ibuprofen (Motrin), an analgesic and anti-inflammatory); amoxicillin, an antibiotic; and verapamil (Calan), a heart medication. Certain medications interact with specific types of food. For example, green leafy vegetables can interact with Coumadin, an anticoagulant, and make the patient's bleeding time increase. Also, grapefruit juice interacts with atorvastatin (Lipitor), a medication used to lower blood cholesterol levels, to reduce its efficacy. It is important for patients to know about any food–drug interaction that may affect them. Information about food and drug interactions can be found in most pharmacology books. You will need to learn as much as you can about the medications that are commonly prescribed by the physician with whom you are working.

is administered by injection. The medical assistant must interview the patient carefully about symptoms of allergies and note in the medical record the names of any medications that produce true allergic symptoms. Drug allergies should always be noted prominently on the front of the patient's medical record and on each page of the medication record. Because of the possibility of an anaphylactic reaction, patients should never be given medications that they have had an allergic reaction to in the past. You should always check the chart and ask the patient before administering any medications in the medical office as an additional safety measure.

Many patients state that they have an allergy to certain medications when in fact the reaction was a **side effect**. Side effects are reactions to medications that are predictable (as noted by the manufacturer of the medication) and that occur in some patients who take the medication. For example, some medications may cause nausea unless taken with food, and in this case, nausea may be listed by the manufacturer as a side effect. Other medications may cause drowsiness or dryness of the mouth. While side effects are often annoying, they are not life threatening and should not be noted on the patient's allergy list.

If a patient is receiving allergy medications or any medication that has a high incidence of allergic reactions (e.g., penicillin), the patient should wait for 20 to 30 minutes and be rechecked before leaving the office. Some

TABLE 23-4	Drug-Related Terms to Know
Term	**Meaning**
Therapeutic classification	States purpose for the drug's use (e.g., cardiotonic, anti-infective, antiarrthymic).
Teratogenic category	Relates the level of risk to fetal or maternal health. These rank from Category A through D, with increasing danger at each level. Category X indicates that the particular drug should never be given during pregnancy.
Indications	Gives diseases for which the particular drug would be prescribed.
Contraindications	Indicates conditions or instances for which the particular drug should not be used.
Adverse reactions	Refers to undesirable side effects of a particular drug.
Hypersensitivity	Refers to an excessive reaction to a particular drug; also known as a drug allergy. The body must build this response; the first exposures may or may not indicate that a problem is developing.
Idiosyncratic reaction	Refers to an abnormal or unexpected reaction to a drug peculiar to the individual patient; not technically an allergy.

offices require all patients receiving injections to wait for a specific amount of time (15 to 20 minutes) before leaving the office. Always follow the policies of the medical office with regard to administering medications.

 CHECKPOINT QUESTION

4. How does synergism differ from antagonism?

Sources of Information

The *Physician's Desk Reference* (PDR) is widely used as a reference for drugs in current use. It is intended for physicians, but since the medical assistant must know about various medications administered in the office, the PDR is a valuable resource for anyone, including the medical assistant, to use before administering medications (Fig. 23-2). This resource is clearly written to iden-

tify a drug's chemical name, brand name or names, and generic name. It also lists the properties, indications, side effects, **contraindications**, dosages, and so on. One section of the PDR contains pictures of various medications. This book is sometimes distributed to physicians free of charge; however, it is also available for use in libraries and for purchase in bookstores.

The *United States Pharmacopeia Dispensing Information* (USPDI) consists of two paperback volumes providing drug information for the health care provider. It defines drug sources, chemistry, physical properties, tests for identity, storage, and dosage. The USPDI does not contain photographs of the medications and must be purchased by the physician.

The *American Hospital Formulary Service* (AHFS), which is distributed to practicing physicians, contains concise information arranged according to drug classifications. The *Compendium of Drug Therapy* is published annually and is also distributed to physicians. It includes photographs of the drugs and phone numbers of major pharmaceutical companies and poison control centers.

Prescriptions

Medications may be administered (given in the office), dispensed (a supply given for later use), or prescribed (a written order to be filled by a pharmacist). You may be permitted to complete the prescription form and obtain the physician's signature if directed to do so by the physician. An established protocol and traditional form must be followed when filling out prescriptions:

Line 1. *Date.* Prescriptions must be filled within 6 months of the date of issuance.

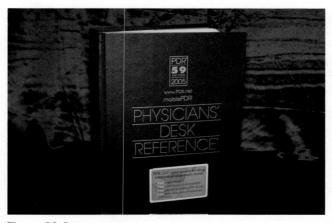

Figure 23-2 The PDR.

Line 2. *Patient's name and address.* The pharmacist needs this information to fill the prescription.

Line 3. *Superscription.* The symbol Rx is found at the top left of the blank prescription pad. Literally it means recipe, or "take thou."

Line 4. *Inscription.* This includes the name of the medication, the desired form (e.g., liquid, tablet, capsule), and the strength (e.g., 250 mg, 500 mL).

Line 5. *Subscription.* This states the amount to be dispensed (e.g., 60 tablets, 120 mL).

Line 6. *Signature.* This section notes any instructions for taking the medication (e.g., with meals, three times a day, four times a day).

Line 7. *Refills.* The number of times a prescription can be refilled should be indicated on the prescription and is generally no more than 5 times within 6 months. If no refills are indicated, the word none should be circled, or 0 should be written in.

Line 8. *Physician's signature.* The physician is responsible for prescriptions written in his or her office and should check and sign all prescriptions.

Line 9. *Generic.* Some physicians and insurance companies allow generic substitutes for some medications but not others. Note on the prescription whether generic substitutions can be made. If the physician does not want a specific medication substituted with a generic drug, "DAW" can be written on the prescription, which means "dispense as written."

All prescribed medications must be documented in full in the patient's record (Fig. 23-3). Prescriptions that are called or faxed to the pharmacist must also be documented. The chart is a legal document and may be called into court in the event of legal action. If the medication order is not recorded, it will be presumed that the medication was never ordered. Figure 23-4 shows a sample prescription form.

Refilling Prescriptions

In most situations, a patient needing one or more prescriptions refilled will be required to make an appointment to see the physician, especially if the medications are controlled substances. Occasionally, a patient may phone the office requesting an emergency refill for a medication that is prescribed to be taken daily but has no additional refills noted on the bottle by the pharmacist. You should pull the patient's chart and check with the physician before calling any prescriptions into the pharmacy. This is also true if the pharmacist calls the medical office requesting the refill for the patient. Always check with the physician before authorizing the refill of any medication.

Some drugs, such as digoxin, have a cumulative effect and may become toxic if blood levels are not monitored closely. For this reason, it is important that you be familiar with the medications prescribed by the physician and promptly schedule any laboratory tests ordered by the physician. In addition, you should be vigilant about notifying the physician with the results of any patient laboratory blood tests that may be ordered to monitor the effects of medications. Patients who request phone refills for medications that need blood monitoring should be encouraged to comply with the physician's recommendations for such laboratory tests. It will be your responsibility to help patients understand the importance of maintaining therapeutic blood levels of these medications.

CHECKPOINT QUESTION

5. What does the superscription on the prescription indicate, and how does it differ from the subscription?

DATE	TIME	ORDERS
7/5/XX	1000	Prescription for ampicillin 250 mg, p.o., qid X 7 days as ordered by Dr. Smith
		Sally Smith, CMA

Figure 23-3 Documentation of a prescribed medication in a patient record.

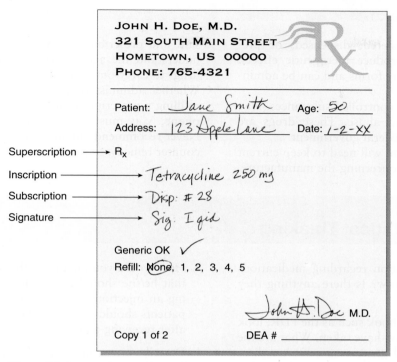

JOHN H. DOE, M.D.
321 SOUTH MAIN STREET
HOMETOWN, US 00000
PHONE: 765-4321

Patient: Jane Smith   Age: 50

Address: 123 Apple Lane   Date: 1-2-XX

Superscription → R$_x$

Inscription → Tetracycline 250 mg

Subscription → Disp. # 28

Signature → Sig. I qid

Generic OK ✓
Refill: None, 1, 2, 3, 4, 5

John H. Doe M.D.

Copy 1 of 2   DEA # _____

Figure 23-4 Prescription form.

TRIAGE

Three patients have called the office asking you for prescription refills. It is 10 AM What is the correct priority order for looking at the patient's medical record and calling the pharmacy for a refill?

A. A 52-year-old patient says she went to take her methyldopa (Aldomet) this morning but was out of it. She takes it every morning at 9:00 for her blood pressure.

B. A mother says her 3-year-old son spilled the bottle of ampicillin on the floor. The next dose is due at 2:00 this afternoon.

C. A 66-year-old patient says she is out of her sleeping pills. She wants a refill for temazepam (Restoril).

How do you sort these patients? Which prescription should be called in to the pharmacy first? Second? Third?

Important: Before calling any medication refill into the pharmacy, you must look at the patient's medical record and be sure there are refill orders on the chart. Also, you must follow your office's policy on prescription refills.

 Patient A should be done first; it is important that blood pressure medications be taken at the same time every day. Patient B is next so that the 2:00 PM dose is not missed. Patient C's prescription should be handled last.

MEDIA MENU

- **Student CD**
  - **Case Study**
    Clinical Interactive Case Study 2: Vital Signs, Patient Education, and Refusal of Treatment
  - **Animations**
    Drug Absorption; Drug Distribution; Drug Binding; Drug Excretion
  - **CMA/RMA Certification Exam Review**
- **Premium Online Course**
  http://thePoint.lww.com/Kronenberger3e
- **Internet Resources**

  The Food and Drug Administration
  www.fda.gov/medwatch

  The *Physician's Desk Reference*
  www.pdr.net

  MedlinePlus, National Institutes of Health
  http://medlineplus/gov/

  National Center of Complementary and Alternative Medicine
  http://nccam.nih.gov

  MedicineNet
  www.MedicineNet.com

  American Hospital Formulary Service
  http://ashp.org

- Medications are administered, dispensed, or prescribed to patients to produce therapeutic effects. They are available in many forms and can be administered in various ways.
- Some medications, called controlled substances, may result in dependency and abuse. These drugs are strictly regulated by the federal government.
- As a medical assistant, you will need to keep current on the legal regulations concerning the manufacture, sale, and prescribing of medications. You must also understand the actions, effects, and interactions of drugs to carry out a physician's medication orders.
- Whether administering medications in the office or refilling a prescription order to a pharmacy over the phone, you must always have a physician order. Never recommend any medication, even an over-the-counter remedy, to a patient.

Warm Ups   for Critical Thinking

1. What type of information regarding medications do patients need to know? Is there anything they do not need to know?

2. Using a drug reference book such as the PDR, look up a medication that you have taken. What are the medication's trade and generic names? Are there any side effects or contraindications? Explain what you learned about this medication that you did not already know.

3. How would you interact with a patient who insists that he/she should leave immediately after receiving an injection when the office policy states that patients should remain in the office for 15 minutes after receiving an injection?

4. Describe how you could keep prescription pads secure during the typical day working in the medical office.

Answers   to Checkpoint Questions

1. A drug's chemical name identifies the chemical components of the drug; the trade name is the name under which the manufacturer distributes the drug commercially.

2. When a controlled substance is administered, you must document the drug name, patient, dose, date, ordering physician, and your name as the employee who administered the drug.

3. Before giving any medication, you should be familiar with the drug, including the actions of the medication and specific patient responses to the medication. Pharmacokinetics is based on the route of administration, rate of absorption, duration of action, and how the drug is eliminated from the body.

4. Synergism refers to an interaction between two drugs or other substances in which the action of one is enhanced by the other. Antagonism is an interaction in which one drug or substance decreases the effects of another.

5. The superscription indicates the medication name, desired form, and strength. The subscription indicates the amount of medication to dispense.

CHAPTER 24

Preparing and Administering Medications

Outline

Medication Administration Basics
Safety Guidelines
Seven Rights for Correct Medication Administration
Systems of Measurement

Routes of Medication Administration
Oral, Sublingual, and Buccal Routes
Parenteral Administration
Other Medication Routes

Principles of Intravenous (IV) Therapy
Intravenous Equipment
Troubleshooting Problems

Learning Objectives

Upon successfully completing this chapter, you will be able to:

1. Spell and define the key terms

2. List the safety guidelines for medication administration

3. Explain and demonstrate how to correctly calculate an adult medication dosage

4. Explain the differences between various parenteral and nonparenteral routes of medication administration

5. Describe the parts of a syringe and needle and name those parts that must be kept sterile

6. List the various needle lengths, gauges, and preferred site for each type of injection

7. Compare the types of injections and locate the sites where each may be administered safely

8. Describe principles of intravenous (IV) therapy

Performance Objectives

Upon successfully completing this chapter, you will be able to:

1. Administer oral medications (Procedure 24-1)

2. Prepare injections (Procedure 24-2)

3. Administer an intradermal injection (Procedure 24-3)

4. Administer a subcutaneous injection (Procedure 24-4)

5. Administer an intramuscular injection (Procedure 24-5)

6. Administer an intramuscular injection using the Z-track method (Procedure 24-6)

7. Apply transdermal medications (Procedure 24-7)

8. Obtain and prepare an intravenous site (Procedure 24-8)

CAAHEP

- Apply pharmacology principles to prepare and administer oral and parenteral (excluding IV) medications
- Maintain medication and immunization records
- Document appropriately
- Practice standard precautions
- Dispose of biohazardous materials
- Perform within legal and ethical boundaries

ABHES

- Prepare and administer medications as directed by physician
- Maintain medication records
- Document accurately
- Practice standard precautions
- Dispose of biohazardous materials

Key Terms

ampule
apothecary system of measurement
buccal
diluent

gauge
induration
infiltration
Mantoux
metric system

nebulizer
ophthalmic
otic
parenteral

sublingual
topical
vial

Medication Administration Basics

Before administering any medications in the medical office, you should be familiar with the medication ordered by the physician and the procedures necessary to administer the drug accurately and safely. As a clinical medical assistant, you must look up any drugs you are not familiar with to determine the drug classification, the usual dosage, and the route of administration. In addition, you should be thoroughly familiar with the terminology, abbreviations, symbols, and signs used in prescribing, administering, and documenting medications. The abbreviations listed in Table 24-1 are most commonly used and should be memorized. The abbreviations listed in red have been identified as potentially dangerous to use by the Joint Commission on the Accreditation of Health Organizations and may result in medication errors.

Safety Guidelines

To ensure safety when administering medications, follow these guidelines:

1. Know the policies of your office regarding the administration of medications.
2. Give only the medications that the physician has ordered in writing. Do not accept verbal orders.

3. Check with the physician if you have any doubt about a medication or an order.
4. Avoid conversation and other distractions while preparing and administering medications. It is important to remain attentive during this task.
5. Work in a quiet, well-lighted area.
6. Check the label when taking the medication from the shelf, when preparing it, and when replacing it on the shelf or disposing of the empty container. This is known as the three checks for safe administration.
7. Place the order and the medication side by side to compare for accuracy.
8. Check the strength of the medication (e.g., 250 versus 500 mg) and the route of administration.
9. Read labels carefully. Do not scan labels or medication orders.
10. Check the patient's medical record for allergies to the actual medication or its components before administering.
11. Check the medication's expiration date. Outdated medications should be discarded according to office policy and should never be administered to a patient.
12. Be alert for color changes, precipitation, odor, or any indication that the medication's properties have changed. If the medication has changed in consistency, color, or odor, discard it appropriately.

TABLE 24-1 Abbreviations

The abbreviations noted in red are considered unsafe and should be avoided.

Abbreviation	Meaning	Abbreviation	Meaning
ac	before meals	NS	normal saline
ad lib	as desired	OD	right eye
AM, am, A.M.	morning	OS	left eye
amp	ampule	OU	both eyes
amt	amount	oz	ounce
AD	right ear	p	after
AS	left ear	pc	after meals
AU	both ears	PM, pm, P.M.	afternoon or evening
aq	aqueous	po, PO	by mouth
bid	twice a day	prn, PRN	whenever necessary
c̄	with	q	every
cap	capsule	qd	every day
cc	cubic centimeter	qh	every hour
DC, disc, d/c	discontinue	q2h	every 2 hours
disp	dispense	q3h	every 3 hours
dl, dL	deciliter	qid	four times a day
elix	elixir	qod	every other day
et	and	qs	quantity sufficient
ext	extract	qt	quart
fl, fld	fluid	R	right, rectal
g, gm	gram	Rx	take, prescribe
gr	grain	s̄	without
gt(t)	drop(s)	SC, subcu, S/Q, SQ	subcutaneously
h, hr	hour	Sig	label
hs, HS	hour of sleep	SL	sublingual
Id, ID	intradermal	ss	one-half
IM	intramuscular	stat, STAT	immediately
IV	intravenous	supp	suppository
Kg	kilogram	syr	syrup
L, l	liter	tab	tablet
lb	pound	T, tb, tbs, tbsp	tablespoon
mcg, μg	microgram	t, tsp	teaspoon
mEq	milliequivalent	tid	three times a day
ml, mL	milliliter	tinc	tincture
NaCl	sodium chloride	u	units
NKA	no known allergies	ung	ointment
NPO	nothing by mouth		

The abbreviations in red have been identified as potentially dangerous to use by the Joint Commission on the Accreditation of Health Organizations and may result in medication errors.

13. Measure exactly. There should be no bubbles in liquid medication.
14. Have sharps containers as close to the area of use as possible.
15. Put on gloves for all procedures that might result in contact with blood or body fluids.
16. Stay with the patient while he or she takes oral medication. Watch for any reaction and record the patient's response.
17. Never return a medication to the container after it is poured or removed.
18. Never recap, bend, or break a used needle.
19. Never give a medication poured or drawn up by someone else.
20. Never leave the medication cabinet unlocked when not in use.
21. Never give keys for the medication cabinet to an unauthorized person. Limit access to the medication cabinet by limiting access to the cabinet keys.
22. Never document medication given by someone else, and do not ask someone else to document medication that you have administered.

 CHECKPOINT QUESTION

1. When are the "three checks" for safe medication administration performed?

When the physician writes a prescription for a medication, you will often be the health care provider who gives this prescription to the patient and records that this medication was ordered on the medication record in the patient health record (see Legal Tips box). In some cases, the physician may ask you to dispense a sample of the prescribed medication provided by the pharmaceutical representative to the patient until the prescription can be filled later at the pharmacy. Once the patient takes the prescription to the pharmacy, the pharmacy will fill the prescription according to the physician orders. In addition, the pharmacist will give the patient written information about taking the medication and any side effects that might be encountered. Also, the pharmacist will note any specific instructions and warnings on the medication container. Patients should always be encouraged to contact the office for any questions or problems concerning medications ordered by the physician.

Seven Rights for Correct Medication Administration

Medication errors should not occur during careful preparation or administration. By observing the seven rights during medication administration, you will eliminate the potential for many errors. The seven rights are as follows:

1. Right patient. Ask the patient to state his or her name. Some patients will answer to any name, so simply saying the name is not assurance that you have the correct patient.
2. Right time. Most medications ordered to be given in the office are to be given before the patient leaves. Some patients may have to be told when the next dose is due.
3. Right dose. Check doses carefully. Many medications come in various strengths.
4. Right route. Some medications are prepared for administration by a variety of routes. Is it oral, **parenteral, otic, ophthalmic,** or **topical**?
5. Right drug. Many medication names are very much alike; for instance Orinase and Ornade may be confused if you are not careful. Always look up unfamiliar medications in a drug reference book such as the *Physician's Desk Reference* (PDR).
6. Right technique. Check how the medication is to be given, such as orally and with or without food. Intramuscular, subcutaneous, and intradermal injections should be given only after carefully choosing a site and with the correct procedure.
7. Right documentation. The medical record is a legal document. Make sure that the medication is documented after it is administered (not before) and that you have documented it in the correct medical record. All medications given in the medical office must be documented immediately with the name of the medication, the dose, route, and site (if injected), and the documentation must be signed by the medical assistant. The patient's response should be charted as well, when appropriate.

 CHECKPOINT QUESTION

2. What information should be recorded in the patient's medical record after administering any medication?

 LEGAL TIP
MEDICATION ERRORS

Even if you are extremely careful, you may make an error when administering a medication. It is imperative that you report the error to the physician and that intervention measures start immediately. The error and all corrective actions must be documented thoroughly in the patient's medical record. An incident report should be completed for the error and filed in the medical office as verification that all possible precautions were taken for the patient.

Systems of Measurement

The most common system of measurement used in the medical office is the **metric system**; however, the **apothecary system of measurement** may still used by some physicians. The household system of measurement is most often used by patients (Box 24-1). Both the apothecary and the household systems of measurement should be avoided in the medical setting, since the measurements are not as accurate as in the metric system. While working in the clinical setting, you may find it necessary to convert from one system to another. In addition, you may be required to calculate a dose in one system of measurement using mathematical equations. It is necessary to master the elements of the systems of measurement before attempting to calculate dosages.

Metric, Household, and Apothecary

The metric system is used in the United States and throughout the world. Because the metric system is based on multiples of 10, decimals, not fractions, are used in calculating and recording dosages. In the metric system, the base unit of *length* is the *meter* (m). The base unit of *weight* is the *gram* (g or gm), and the liter (L or l) is used to measure fluid and gas volume. Prefixes used in the metric system show a fraction or multiple of the base. The following prefixes are often used:

- Micro- (0.000001)
- Milli- (0.001)
- Centi- (0.01)
- Deci- (0.1)
- Kilo- (1000.0)

For example, using the base unit of a gram, fractional measurements are as follows:

- Microgram (mcg, μg), one-millionth of a gram (×0.000001)
- Milligram (mg), one-thousandth of a gram (×0.001)
- Kilogram (kg), 1000 grams (×1000.0)

Decagrams and centigrams are not used in medication administration.

With the base unit of a liter (1 L = approximately 1.06 quarts), fractional measurements in milliliters (ml, mL) are commonly used in medication administration. Also, 1 cubic centimeter (cc) is equivalent to 1 mL, and therefore, the measures are used interchangeably at times.

The apothecary system is used less frequently now than in the past and is gradually being replaced by the metric system. In the apothecary system, liquid measurements include drop (gt) or drops (gtt), minim (min, m), fluid dram (fl dr), fluid ounce (fl oz), pint (pt), quart (qt), and gallon (gal). Measurements for solid weights include grain (gr), dram (dr), ounce (oz), and pound (lb). Roman numerals are used for smaller numbers, and fractions may be used when necessary. Decimals are never used in the apothecary system.

The household system of measurement includes measures such as the teaspoon (tsp), tablespoon (tbsp), ounce (oz), cup (c), pint (pt), quart (qt), and pound (lb). While this system is not used in the medical office for calculating doses, patients may need to be instructed on the proper household measurement for taking medications ordered in the metric system (e.g., 5 mL is equivalent to 1 tsp). Table 24-2 lists commonly used equivalents in the metric, apothecary, and household systems of measurement.

CHECKPOINT QUESTION

3. What are three systems of measurement? Which is the most commonly used in the medical office?

Converting Between Systems of Measurement

Apothecary or Household to Metric

To convert from one system to another system, use the following rules:

- To change grains (apothecary system) to grams (metric system), divide the number of grains ordered by 15. Example: gr 30 ÷ 15 = 2 g.
- To change grains (apothecary system) to milligrams (metric system), multiply the grains by 60. Use this rule with less than 1 grain. Example: gr 1/4 × 60 = 15 mg.

BOX 24-1

HOUSEHOLD MEASURES

Household measurements include cups, medicine droppers, teaspoons, and tablespoons. Some of the approximate equivalents to household measurements are:

1 teaspoon = 1 fluid dram = 5 mL
1 tablespoon = ½ fluid ounce = 4 fluid drams = 15 mL
2 tablespoons = 1 fluid ounce = 30 mL

Caution patients who will be using household measurements to avoid using table flatware and regular cups. Standard measuring spoons and cups are more accurate.

TABLE 24-2 Most Commonly Used Approximate Equivalents

Metric	Apothecary	Household
60 mg	gr i	
0.06 mL	minim i	1 drop
1.0 g	gr xv	
1.0 mL	minim xv	1/5 tsp
5.0 mL	1 dram	1 tsp
15 mL	¹/₂ oz	1 tbsp
30 mL	1 oz	2 tbsp
500 mL	6 oz	1 pint
1000 mL	2 oz	1 quart

There are many discrepancies among these approximate equivalents. For example, 30 mL is the accepted equivalent for 1 oz, but 29.57 mL is the exact equivalent. Such discrepancies are inevitable when equivalencies between the two systems are not exact. The discrepancies are within a 10% margin of error, which usually is acceptable in pharmacology.

Reprinted with permission from Taylor C, Lillis C, Le Mone P. Fundamentals of Nursing: The Art and Science of Nursing Care, ed 2. Philadelphia: Lippincott, 1993:1347.

- To change ounces (household) to milliliters (metric system), multiply the ounces by 30. Example: 4 oz × 30 = 120 mL.
- To change milliliters (metric system) to fluid ounces (household system), divide the milliliters by 30. Example: 150 mL ÷ 30 = 50 oz.
- To change kilograms (metric system) to pounds (household system), multiply the kilograms by 2.2. Example: 50 kg × 2.2 = 110.0 lb.
- To change pounds to kilograms (metric system), divide the pounds (household system) by 2.2. Example: 44 lb ÷ 2.2 = 20 kg.

Metric to Metric

In the metric system, it is sometimes necessary to convert measurements using the same unit of measure. For example, the physician may order 0.5 grams of medication, and the medication label reads 500 mg. To convert within the metric system, use the following rules:

- To change grams to milligrams, multiply grams by 1000 or move the decimal point three places to the right. Example: 0.5 g × 1000 = 500 mg.
- To change milligrams to grams, divide the milligrams by 1000 or move the decimal point three places to the left. Example: 500 mg ÷ 1000 = 0.5 g.
- To change milligrams to micrograms, multiply the milligrams by 1000 or move the decimal point three places to the right. Example: 5 mg × 1000 = 5000 μg.

- To change micrograms to milligrams, divide the micrograms by 1000 or move the decimal point three places to the left. Example: 500 μg ÷ 1000 = 0.5 mg.
- To change liters to milliliters, multiply the liters by 1000 or move the decimal point three places to the right. Example: 0.01 L × 1000 = 10 mL.
- To change milliliters to liters, divide the milliliters by 1000 or move the decimal point three places to the left. Example: 100 mL ÷ 1000 = 0.1 L.

There is no conversion necessary when changing cubic centimeters to milliliters; they are approximately the same.

Calculating Adult Dosages

Administration of medication is an exact science; errors in calculation can kill the patient. Although the physician will order the amount of medication to be administered to the patient, you may have to calculate the amount of medication to withdraw into a syringe or pour into a medicine cup. In addition to the physician's order, you must also be aware of the label on the medication container (Fig. 24-1) since both the physician's order and the information on the medication label are used to calculate the amount given. There are two methods by which doses are most frequently calculated for adults: the ratio method and the formula method. Measurements must be in the same system (preferably metric) and unit before a calculation can be made. For example, if the medication is ordered in the apothecary or household system but is packaged in the metric system, you must first convert the order (apothecary or household) to the metric system. If the medication is ordered in grams but is packaged in milligrams, the ordered dose must be converted to milligrams before any calculations can be made. When using the metric system, be careful to keep the decimal point in the correct place during calculations and be sure to convert fractions to decimals.

Ratio and Proportion

When using the ratio method to calculate doses, you must use the amount of medication ordered and the information on the medication label to create a ratio. Once the ratio has been determined, the proportion, or relationship between the two ratios, can be calculated to give you the amount of medication to administer. To calculate a dose using the ratio and proportion method, set up the problem as follows:

Dose on hand : Known quantity = Dose desired : Unknown quantity

Example 1. The physician orders erythromycin 250 mg. The label on the package reads erythromycin 100 mg/mL. The equation can be written as:

100 mg : 1 mL = 250 mg : X

Figure 24-1 Medication labels include the name of the medication and the dose per unit such as (**A**) 0.25 mg per tablet or (**B**) 250 mg per 5 mL.

Multiply the extremes (first and fourth terms) = 100X

Multiply the means (second and third terms) = 250

Write the proportion as follows: 100X = 250

Divide both sides of the equal sign by 100 to solve for X.

$$250 \div 100 = 2.5$$

Therefore, you administer 2.5 mL of erythromycin for the patient to receive the 250 mg ordered by the physician. *Note*: When you document the medication after administration, the amount given is the amount ordered by the physician in milligrams, not the amount in milliliters administered.

Example 2. The physician orders phenobarbital 25 mg. On hand are 12.5-mg tablets. State the equation:

$$12.5 \text{ mg} : 1 \text{ tablet} = 25 \text{ mg} : X$$

Multiply the extremes = 12.5X

Multiply the means = 25 mg

$$25 = 12.5X$$

Divide both sides by 12.5

$$25 \div 12.5 = 2 \text{ tablets}$$

In this example, you administer two tablets of phenobarbital to the patient and record that 25 mg was given.

The Formula Method

The formula method is written as follows:

$$(\text{Desired} \div \text{On hand}) \times \text{Quantity} = \text{Dose}$$

Example 1. The physician orders ampicillin 0.5 g. On hand, you have ampicillin 250-mg capsules. How much ampicillin should be administered? Remember, both doses must be in the same unit of measure. Convert grams in the physician's order to milligrams by multiplying the grams by 1000 (or move the decimal point three places to the right). The answer is 0.5 g equals 500 mg. With this information, you may set up your problem:

$$500 \text{ mg (desired)} \div 250 \text{ mg (on hand)} \times$$
$$1 \text{ (quantity)} = 2 \times 1 = 2$$

In this example, the quantity (one capsule) is how the medication (ampicillin 250 mg) comes supplied. You administer two capsules and chart that 0.5 g or 500 mg was given to the patient.

Example 2. The physician orders 0.35 g of a medication, and you have on hand a liquid form of the medication that is labeled 700 mg/mL. How many milliliters do you prepare to administer? Remember, measurements must be in equivalent units, so 0.35 g must be changed to 350 mg before setting up the formula.

$$(350 \text{ mg} \div 700 \text{ mg}) \times 1 \text{ mL} = 0.5 \text{ mL} = 0.5 \text{ mL}$$

CHECKPOINT QUESTION

4. Before calculating a dose, what must be done with the measurements if the physician orders the medication in milligrams and the medication is supplied in grams?

Calculating Pediatric Dosages

Although several formulas may be used to calculate children's doses, one method uses the body surface area (BSA) and is considered to be the most accurate method for children up to 12 years of age or adults who are below normal percentiles for body weight. A scale known as a nomogram (Fig. 24-2) is used to estimate the BSA in square meters according to the patient's height and weight. A straight line is drawn from the patient's height in inches or centimeters in column 1 to the patient's weight in kilograms or pounds in column 3

(Fig. 24-3). The line intersects on the BSA column (column 2) to give the BSA of the child. Once the BSA is determined, the following formula is used to calculate the medication dosage:

$$(BSA \times Adult\ dose) \div 1.7 = Child's\ dose$$

Other rules for calculating pediatric doses include Young's rule, Clark's rule, and Fried's rule. Young's rule is used to calculate doses for children aged 12 months to 12 years. This method requires that you determine the age of the child in years and divide by the age of the child in years plus 12. This number is multiplied by the adult dose.

$$Pediatric\ dose = \times Adult\ dose$$

Clark's rule is more accurate than Young's rule because it allows for variations in body size and weight for different ages. Using Clark's rule, the weight of the child is divided by 150 (presumed weight of average adult) and multiplied by the average adult dose to determine the pediatric dose.

$$Pediatric\ dose = \times Adult\ dose$$

Height		Surface Area	Weight	
Feet	Centimeters	Square Meters	Pounds	Kilograms

Figure 24-2 Nomogram for estimating surface area of infants and young children. To determine the surface area of the patient, draw a straight line between the point representing the height on the left vertical scale and the point representing the weight on the right vertical scale. The point at which this line intersects the middle vertical scale represents the patient's surface area in square meters.

Height		Surface Area	Weight	
Feet	Centimeters	Square Meters	Pounds	Kilograms

Figure 24-3 Using the nomogram, the child who is 32 inches tall and weighs 40 pounds has a BSA of 0.6 m².

Fried's rule, which is used for calculating doses for infants less than 2 years of age, bases the dose on the age of the child in months. In this case, 150 used in calculations is the age in months of a 12.5-year-old child, presuming that a child of that age would be eligible for an adult dose. Using Fried's rule, the child's age in months is divided by 150 and then multiplied by the average adult dose.

$$\text{Pediatric dose} = \times \text{Adult dose}$$

Some medications that require careful calibration are dosed per kilogram of body weight. Instructions for calculation are included in the package insert that comes with the medication or in the *Physician's Desk Reference.* For instance, the insert may state to give adults and children over 25 kg (55 lb) 500 mg of a particular medication and use the formula 25 mg/kg for children who weigh less than 25 kg. If the child weighs 20 lb, this weight must be converted to kilograms before any calculations are made. Since 1 kg is equal to 2.2 lb, the child who weighs 20 lb also weighs 9 kg. The equation for calculating the child's dosage would be set up as follows:

$$25 \text{ mg} \times 9 \text{ kg} = 225 \text{ mg}$$

Therefore, the physician will use this calculation to determine how much medication (225 mg) is appropriate for the child who weighs 20 lb (9 kg).

 CHECKPOINT QUESTION

5. When calculating how much medication to prescribe for an infant or child, which method for calculating pediatric dosages is most often used?

 WHAT IF?

A child is brought to the medical office having difficulty breathing and needing emergency medications? How does the physician have time to calculate the dose for the child's body weight?

In such a situation, the physician does not have the time to perform the calculations and instead may rely on a printed graph that lists precalculated emergency drug doses or on medication reference books. There is also computer software that is available that will automatically calculate and print a list of pediatric emergency medications and their doses. In this situation, it is important to remain calm and notify emergency services as directed by the physician since these trained professionals will have the knowledge and equipment required to resuscitate a child should the emergency situation deteriorate.

Routes of Medication Administration

Medication can be administered in many ways and is chosen by the physician after considering many factors. Sometimes the route is chosen because of cost, safety, or the speed by which the drug will be absorbed into the body. Certain drugs may be administered by only one route, while others may be administered in a variety of ways. Some drugs may be toxic if given by a certain route, some may be effective only if given by a specific route, and sometimes absorption will occur only through one particular route.

Oral, Sublingual, and Buccal Routes

Of all of the medication routes, the oral route is most preferred by patients and is the easiest to administer. However, medications taken orally, or by mouth, are usually slow to take effect, and this route cannot be used for unconscious patients, those with nausea and vomiting, or those who are ordered to take nothing by mouth. Drugs given orally may be administered as tablets, capsules, pills, or liquids (Procedure 24-1). Most are absorbed through the walls of the gastrointestinal tract. Drugs given orally in the medical office usually come in unit dose packs that contain the amount of the drug for a single dose (Fig. 24-4). These may be left by pharmaceutical sales representatives to be given as samples to patients. Unit dose packages are labeled with the trade name, generic name, precautions, instructions for storage, and an expiration date. Table 24-3 lists common solid and liquid forms of oral medications.

The physician may also order medications to be taken by either the **sublingual** or **buccal** routes. Medication taken sublingually is placed under the patient's tongue; it must not be swallowed. The drug is

Figure 24-4 Unit dose packages.

TABLE 24-3	**Forms of Oral Medications**
Form	**Description**

Solids

Form	Description
Buffered Caplet	Agents are added to decrease or counteract the medication's acidity to prevent gastric irritation.
Capsule	Powdered or granulated medication is enclosed in a gelatin capsule designed to dissolve in gastric enzymes or high in the small intestines.
Enteric Coated Tablet	A compressed dry form of a medication coated to withstand the gastric acidity and dissolve in the intestines. These may be medications that would be destroyed by the gastric enzymes or might be damaging to the gastric mucosa. Never crush or break enteric coated tablets.
Gelcap	An oil-based medication enclosed in a soft gelatin capsule.
Lozenge	A firm, compressed form of medication, usually for a local effect in the mouth or throat. Caution patients to let lozenges dissolve slowly and avoid drinking any fluids for a period of time after using the lozenge.
Powder	A finely ground form of medication; may be difficult for some patients to swallow.
Spansule or Time-Release Capsule	Gelatin capsules are filled with forms of the medication that will dissolve over a period of time rather than all at once. Never open spansules unless this is recommended by the manufacturer.
Tablet	Medication is formed into many shapes and colors for easy identification. Tablets usually dissolve high in the gastrointestinal tract. These may be broken into halves only if they have been scored for that purpose.

Liquids

Form	Description
Elixer	Medication is dissolved in alcohol, and flavoring is added. These are less sweet than syrups and are usually preferred by adults. They should not be used with alcoholics or diabetics.
Emulsion	Medication is combined with water and oil. Emulsions must be thoroughly shaken to disperse the medication evenly.
Extract	This is a very concentrated form of medication made by evaporating volatile plant oils. Extracts may be administered as drops and are usually given in a liquid to disguise their strong taste.
Gel	Medication is suspended in a thin gelatin or paste base.
Suspension	Particles are dissolved in a liquid that must be shaken well before administered.
Syrup	This very sweet form of medication is used frequently for children's medications and is usually flavored in addition to having a high sugar content.

dissolved by the saliva in the mouth and is absorbed directly into the bloodstream through the oral mucosa covering the sublingual vessels. Caution the patient not to eat or drink until the medication has totally dissolved.

Medication given by the buccal route is placed in the pouch between the cheek and gum at the side of the mouth. Buccal absorption of medication occurs through the vascular oral mucosa. Although few medications are manufactured for this route, the patient must not eat or drink until the medication is completely absorbed if this method is used to administer medications.

 CHECKPOINT QUESTION

6. What are the disadvantages of the oral route for medication administration?

Parenteral Administration

If a patient cannot take medications orally, if the drug cannot be absorbed through the gastrointestinal system, or if rapid absorption of the drug is desired, the parenteral route is used. Parenteral administration refers not only to injections but to all ways drugs are administered other than via the gastrointestinal tract. Administration by injection is the most efficient method of parenteral drug administration, but it can also be the most hazardous. While the effects may be quite rapid, the medication cannot be retrieved once injected, and because the skin is broken, it is possible for infection to develop if strict aseptic technique is not followed (Box 24-2)..

Equipment for Injections

Ampules, Vials, Cartridges

Medications used for injections are supplied in **ampules, vials,** and cartridges (Fig. 24-5). Ampules are small glass containers that must be broken at the neck so that the solution can be aspirated into the syringe. When the ampule is opened, all medication in it must be either used or discarded. It must not be saved for later use because once the ampule is broken, sterility cannot be maintained.

Vials are glass or plastic containers sealed at the top by a rubber stopper. They may be single-dose or multiple-dose containers. The contents of vials may be in solution or in powder, which requires reconstitution with a specific amount and type of **diluent** (diluting agent), usually sterile water or saline. Certain drugs, such as phenytoin (Dilantin), require a special diluent supplied by the manufacturer. When a powdered drug is reconstituted in a multiple-dose vial, the following must be written on the label:

1. Date of reconstitution
2. Initials of the person who reconstituted the drug
3. Diluent used

To reconstitute dry medication, withdraw the diluent using aseptic technique, add the diluent to the vial containing the powder, and roll the bottle between your palms to dissolve the medication completely. Shaking the vial may cause unnecessary bubbles. When the powder has completely dissolved, calculate the dose based on the amount of diluent added to the powder. The instructions from the manufacturer of the drug usually indicate how much diluent to add to the powder and the

Figure 24-5 Ampules, vials, prefilled cartridges, and holders.

resulting concentration of the mixture necessary for calculating dosages. You should always check the vial label or manufacturer's instructions before adding the diluent to determine the resulting dosage.

Vials intended for multiple doses may hold up to 50 mL and may be used repeatedly by inserting a needle through the self-sealing rubber stopper to remove a portion of the solution. Unit dose vials usually contain 1 to 2 mL, and all of the solution is removed for a single injection.

Prefilled syringes contain a premeasured amount of medication in a disposable cartridge with a needle attached. The prefilled cartridge and needle are placed in a holder for administration (Fig. 24-6). Examples of prefilled cartridges and holders are the Tubex and the Carpuject. After a prefilled cartridge and holder are used, only the used cartridge should be discarded in a sharps biohazard container. The holder is reusable.

Needles and Syringes

The choice of needle and syringe used for an injection depends on the type of injection and the size of the patient. The 1-mL and 3-mL hypodermic syringe are the sizes most commonly used for injections. In the medical office, syringes designed to hold 5 mL or more are usually used for irrigation only, not for injections. All syringes consist of a plunger, body or barrel, flange, and tip (Fig. 24-7). Types of syringes used for parenteral administration include tuberculin, or 1-mL, syringes, 3-mL syringes, and insulin syringes that are calibrated in units and are used for insulin only (Fig. 24-8).

Needle lengths vary from 3/8 inch to $1^{1}/_{2}$ inch for standard injections. **Gauge** refers to the diameter of the needle lumen. Needle gauge varies from 18 (large) to 30 (small); the higher the number, the smaller the gauge. Medical supply companies package hypodermic needles separately in color-coded packages (Fig. 24-9) or in color-coded envelopes with the syringe attached. The sizes are also written on the package. Choose the package with a needle length and gauge appropriate for the

BOX 24-2

INJECTIONS: MAINTAINING STERILITY

The following parts of a hypodermic setup must be kept sterile:

- Syringe tip
- Inside of barrel
- Shaft of plunger
- Needle

Figure 24-6 Prefilled syringes. **(A)** Prefilled medication cartridges and injector devices. **(B)** Inserting the cartridge into the injector device. **(C)** Ready for injection.

route of the injection. For example, an intramuscular injection for an adult requires a needle length of 1 to 1 ¹/₂ inches, depending on the size of the patient and the fat to muscle ratio. The needle gauge varies from 20 to 25 depending on the thickness of the medication to be administered. Thick medications, such as penicillin and hormones, are difficult to draw into a syringe using a small-gauge needle, such as a 25 or 27, and equally difficult to inject into the patient. Subcutaneous injections are generally given using a short, small-gauge needle: 23 to 25 gauge, 5/8 inch to ¹/₂ inch.

All hypodermic syringes are marked with 10 calibrations per milliliter on one side of the syringe. Each small line represents 0.1 mL. The other side of the syringe may be marked in minims (m), which are rarely used today. The tuberculin (TB) syringe is narrow and has a total capacity of 1 mL. There are 100 calibration lines

Figure 24-7 Parts of a syringe and needle. (Reprinted with permission from Cohen BJ. Medical Terminology: An Illustrated Guide. Philadelphia: Lippincott Williams & Wilkins, 2003.)

marking the TB 1-mL syringe, with each line representing 0.01 mL. Every tenth line is longer than the others to indicate 0.1 mL. TB syringes are used for newborn and pediatric doses, for intradermal skin tests, and any time small amounts of medication (less than 1 mL) are to be given.

The insulin syringe is used strictly for administering insulin subcutaneously to diabetic patients. It has a total capacity of 1 mL; however, the 1-mL volume is marked as 100 units (U) to represent the strength of 100 U insulin per milliliter when full. Each group of 10 U is divided by five small lines, and each line represents 2 U.

Figure 24-8 Syringes (*from top to bottom*): 10 mL, 3 mL, tuberculin or 1 mL, insulin, and low-dose insulin.

Figure 24-9 Needles. (**A**) Different gauges and lengths. (**B**) Parts of a needle.

Most of the insulin used today is U-100, which means that it has 100 U of insulin in each milliliter. The insulin syringe must be marked U-100 to match the insulin used. Procedure 24-2 describes the steps required for preparing an injection.

 CHECKPOINT QUESTION

7. What are ampules and vials, and how do they differ?

Types of Injections
Intradermal Injections

Intradermal medications are administered into the dermal layer of the skin by inserting the needle at a 10° to 15° angle, almost parallel to the skin surface (Fig. 24-10). When an intradermal injection is administered correctly, the needle tip and lumen are slightly visible under the skin, and a small bubble, known as a wheal, is raised in the skin. Recommended sites for intradermal injections include the anterior forearm and the back. Intradermal injections are used exclusively to administer skin tests for tuberculosis screening, the **Mantoux** test, and allergy testing. Procedure 24-3 describes the steps for giving an intradermal injection.

The tine test is another skin test used for routine screening of tuberculosis, but it is not considered as diagnostic as the Mantoux test. Both methods use purified protein derivative (PPD) from a live tuberculin bacillus culture to test for the presence of tuberculin antibodies. The tine applicator contains small tines impregnated with PPD. After cleansing the forearm, press the tine applicator firmly into the intradermal layer of the skin (Fig. 24-11). A positive tine test is usually followed by a Mantoux test. Both the tine test and the Mantoux test must be read within 48 to 72 hours. A positive Mantoux reaction has **induration**, a hard raised area over the in-

jection site, larger than 10 mm. This positive reaction indicates the possibility of exposure to tuberculosis; however, it does not indicate that the patient has active tuberculosis (see Chapter 30). A complete medical history and further testing by sputum culture and radiography are required for a definitive diagnosis. Redness over the intradermal injection site should not be considered induration. An induration of less than 10 mm in a patient with no known risk factors, such as previous tuberculosis or HIV infection, is considered negative.

Figure 24-10 Comparison of the angles of insertion for intramuscular, subcutaneous, and intradermal injections. (Reprinted with permission from Cohen BJ. Medical Terminology: An Illustrated Guide. Philadelphia: Lippincott Williams & Wilkins, 2003.)

Figure 24-11 Administering the tine test for tuberculosis screening.

Subcutaneous Injections

Subcutaneous (SQ or SC) injections are given into the fatty layer of tissue below the skin by positioning the needle and syringe at a 45° angle to the skin (see Fig. 24-10). The subcutaneous route is chosen for drugs that should not be absorbed as rapidly as through the intramuscular or intravenous (IV) route. Common sites include the upper arm, thigh, back, and abdomen. Procedure 24-4 describes the steps for administering a subcutaneous injection.

Intramuscular Injections

Intramuscular (IM) injections are given by positioning the needle and syringe at a 90° angle to the skin (see Fig. 24-10). Absorption of IM medications is fairly rapid because of the rich vascularity of muscle. If slower absorption is desired, the medication is mixed with an oil base rather than saline or water to prolong absorption time. A 1-inch to 1 1/2–inch needle is required to administer an intramuscular injection to an adult. The length of the needle depends on the muscle chosen for injection and the size of the patient.

Recommended muscles used for IM injections include the deltoid (Fig. 24-12), dorsogluteal (Fig. 24-13), ventrogluteal (Fig. 24-14), and vastus lateralis (Fig. 24-15). The rectus femoris (Fig. 24-16) can also be used when the other sites are contraindicated. It is recommended that no more than 1 mL be injected into the deltoid muscle and no more than 3 mL be injected into the other muscles in an adult. Children less than 2 years of age should never receive injections in the gluteal muscle, since this muscle is not well developed until the child is walking. The muscle chosen for the injection depends on the preference of the medical assistant, the patient, and the amount of medication to be administered. Also, some pharmaceutical companies recommend specific sites for medications to be injected intramuscularly, and the medical assistant should use these sites as indicated.

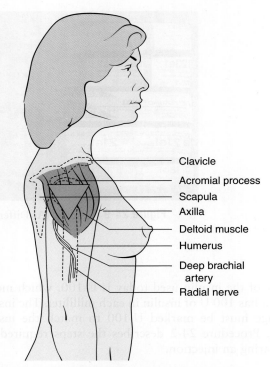

Figure 24-12 The deltoid muscle site for intramuscular injection is located by palpating the lower edge of the acromial process. At the midpoint, in line with the axilla on the lateral aspect of the upper arm, a triangle is formed. Medications are administered within this triangle.

Clavicle
Acromial process
Scapula
Axilla
Deltoid muscle
Humerus
Deep brachial artery
Radial nerve

Gold sodium thiomalate, a medication used to treat arthritis, and some vaccines are examples of medications that have specific guidelines for administration set forth by the manufacturer. Procedure 24-5 describes the steps for administering an intramuscular injection.

Z-Track Method of Intramuscular Injections

This method is used for IM administration of medications that may irritate or damage the tissues if allowed to leak back along the line of injection. An example of a medication that should be administered using this technique is iron dextran, which is used to treat iron deficiency anemia. The Z-track method prevents leakage by sealing off the layers of skin along the route of the needle (Fig. 24-17). If the medication is extremely caustic, directions may include changing the needle after drawing up the solution. An additional precaution may include drawing up to 0.5 mL of air into the syringe after the medication has been aspirated into the syringe. When the medication is injected at a 90° angle, the additional air rises to the top of the syringe and is injected after the medication. This clears the needle and the path of the injection (Fig. 24-18). Procedure 24-6 describes the steps for administering an intramuscular injection using the Z-track method.

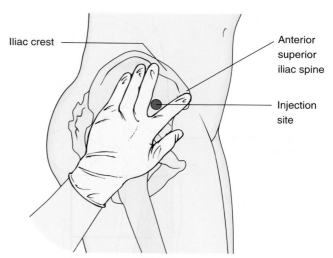

Figure 24-14 The ventrogluteal site is located by placing the palm on the greater trochanter and the index finger toward the anterior superior iliac spine. The middle finger is then spread posteriorly away from the index finger as far as possible. A "V" or triangle is formed by this maneuver. The injection is made in the middle of the triangle.

Figure 24-13 The dorsogluteal site for administering an intramuscular injection is lateral and slightly superior to the midpoint of a line drawn from the trochanter to the posterior superior iliac spine. Correct identification of this site minimizes the possibility of accidentally damaging the sciatic nerve.

 CHECKPOINT QUESTION

8. Name the types of injections and the possible sites for each type.

Other Medication Routes

Rectal Administration

Rectal medications are packaged in the form of suppositories or liquids administered as a retention enema (Fig. 24-19). They can provide a local effect or be absorbed through the rectal mucosa for a systemic effect. Rectal medications may be used for patients who are NPO (allowed nothing by mouth) or who have nausea and vomiting, but they are never used for patients who have diarrhea. Suppositories have a cocoa butter or glycerin base that melts at body temperature. They should be stored in the refrigerator to prevent melting. Rectal medications are rarely administered in the medical office, but you may be required to instruct the patient in the proper technique for administration at home. Both retention enemas and rectal suppositories should be retained by the patient for about 20 to 30 minutes before elimination.

 PATIENT EDUCATION

ADMINISTERING RECTAL MEDICATIONS AT HOME

Some medications have to be administered rectally. You should teach the patient or family member to perform this procedure if the medication is to be taken at home. Here are some key points to discuss:

- Gloves should be worn.
- A small amount of a lubricant should be added to the suppository for easy insertion. The lubricant maybe supplied with the suppository, or it can be purchased separately at the pharmacy.
- Advise the patient to remain lying on the bed for about 15 minutes after the suppository is inserted.
- The suppository should be inserted past the anal sphincter.

Vaginal Administration

Vaginal medications include creams, tablets, cocoa butter–based suppositories, and solutions for douches. Examples include hormonal creams and antibiotic or antifungal preparations (Fig. 24-20). Very few medications other than those for local effects are prescribed for vaginal administration. Instruct the patient to remain lying for a while after the insertion of vaginal medications.

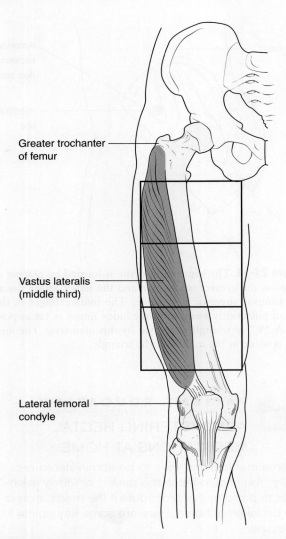

Figure 24-15 The vastus lateralis site for intramuscular injections is identified by dividing the thigh into thirds horizontally and vertically. The injection is given in the outer middle third.

For comfort, the patient may have to wear a light pad to absorb any drainage.

Transdermal Administration

Dermal medications, which are applied to the skin, include topical creams, lotions, ointments, and transdermal medications. **Topical** medications (creams, ointments, sprays, and lotions) produce local effects, while transdermal medications produce systemic effects. Medication administered transdermally is delivered to the body by absorption through the skin. Delivery is slow and maintains a steady, stable level of medication. You should never cut a transdermal patch, since doing so alters the rate of absorption. Dermal patches are placed on the skin, usually on the chest or back, upper

Figure 24-16 The rectus femoris site for intramuscular injections is used only when other sites are contraindicated.

arm, or behind the ear (for medications that prevent motion sickness). Procedure 24-7 describes the steps for applying transdermal medications.

Inhalation

Inhalation is administration of medication, water vapor, or gas by inspiration of the substance into the lungs. Medication administered by inhalation is absorbed quickly through the alveolar walls into the capillaries, but a disease condition may make absorption difficult to predict. Patients with chronic pulmonary disease or disorder may self-administer certain medications with a handheld **nebulizer** or inhaler, both producing a fine spray of medicated mist that is inhaled directly into the lungs (see Chapter 30).

 CHECKPOINT QUESTION

9. How are medications given by the inhalation route absorbed?

Principles of Intravenous (IV) Therapy

With the IV route, a sterile solution of a drug is injected through a catheter or needle that has been inserted into a

Figure 24-17 The Z-track technique is used to administer medications that are irritating to subcutaneous tissue. The skin is pulled to one side, the needle is inserted, and the solution is injected after careful aspiration. When the needle is withdrawn and the displaced tissue is allowed to return to its normal position, the solution is prevented from escaping from the muscle tissue.

vein by a procedure known as venipuncture (refer to Chapter 41). IV medication has the quickest action because it enters the bloodstream immediately. In most cases, the physician administers IV medications, but some ambulatory care centers expect medical assistants to be proficient at setting up the equipment and fluids for an IV, performing the venipuncture, and regulating the IV fluids as directed by the physician. Only drugs intended for IV administration should be given by this route.

Intravenous Equipment

The equipment necessary for starting an IV includes the fluids (determined by the physician), the IV catheter (angiocatheter), and the tubing and valve that connect the IV fluids to the catheter and regulate the flow of fluids into the patient (Fig. 24-21). Once the intravenous line

 TRIAGE

While you are working in a medical office setting, the following three situations arise:

A. A 50-year-old man is complaining of dyspnea, and the doctor has ordered a nebulizer treatment.
B. A 65-year-old woman needs her first dose of an antibiotic.
C. A 47-year-old woman slipped on the ice in the parking lot and is having moderate pain in the right ankle. The doctor has ordered a pain medication injection.

How do you sort these patients? Who do you see first? Second? Third?

Patient A should be treated first; any patient with chest pain or shortness of breath should be treated as a number 1 priority. Patient C should be medicated for pain control. Last, patient B should be given the antibiotic. Remember, you must closely monitor this patient for 30 minutes for signs of an allergic reaction. All three of these patients need to be closely evaluated after receiving their medications. Ask yourself, is the patient breathing better? Is the pain better? Communicate your findings with the physician.

is started, the fluids are administered through the vein either to replace fluids lost by the patient or to administer medications through special ports on the tubing.

Examples of fluids that come prepackaged for use in IV therapy are Ringer's lactate (RL), dextrose 5% and water (D_5W), 0.9% normal saline, 0.45% normal saline, or a combination (D_5NS, D_5RL). The physician chooses the type and amount of fluid to be administered. An administration set (tubing) is used, with one end (the end with the drip chamber) inserted into the IV fluid bag and the other end inserted into the IV catheter after it is in the vein (Procedure 24-8). After securing the IV catheter and attaching the administration set tubing, adjust the flow of fluids by adjusting the roller clamp and carefully watching the fluids drip into the drip chamber. Carefully count the drops per minute so you can adjust the flow of fluids to the exact rate desired. The amount of fluid to be administered is ordered by the physician in terms of milliliters per hour (e.g., 125 mL/hour). Using this physician order, determine how fast to run the solution following this procedure:

• Determine the drop factor (number of drops needed to deliver 1 mL of fluid) as noted on the administra-

Air above medication

Medication

Air lock

Figure 24-18 An air bubble added to the syringe after the medication has been accurately measured helps to expel solution that is trapped in the shaft of the needle when the injection is given. It also helps to trap the injected solution in the intramuscular tissue.

tion set tubing package (macrodrip systems deliver 10 or 20 drops per milliliter, and microdrip systems deliver 60 drops per milliliter.)

- The physician order will include the type of fluid (e.g., RL, D_5W), the amount (e.g., 125 mL), and the time frame (e.g., per hour).
- Use the following formula to calculate the number of drops per minute necessary to deliver the amount of fluid:

(Volume in milliliters ÷ Time in minutes) ×
Drop factor (gtt/min) = Drops per minute

For example, if the physician orders an IV of RL at 100 mL/hour and the administration set delivers 10 gtt/mL, the formula would be set up as follows:

(100 mL ÷ 60 minutes) = 1.67

1.67 × 10 gtt/mL = 17 gtt/min
(16.7 rounded up to nearest tenth = 17)

In this situation, you would regulate the roller clamp so that 17 drops per minute flow into the drip chamber to deliver 100 mL/hour as ordered by the physician. If the

physician would like the patient to have an intravenous line available, but not necessarily for administering fluids, a to-keep-open (TKO) or keep-vein-open (KVO) rate will be ordered. The flow of fluids into the vein to prevent clotting may be 15 to 30 mL/hour as determined by the physician. The same formula is used to calculate this rate: (rate = volume ÷ time × drop factor).

Troubleshooting Problems

The medical assistant must be vigilant about watching the IV fluids and the site of venipuncture. **Infiltration** occurs when IV fluid infuses into the tissues surrounding the vein, usually because the catheter has been dislodged. Carefully securing the IV catheter and the administration tubing usually prevents infiltration. In case of infiltration, stop the flow of fluids, remove the catheter, and notify the physician. Infiltration is characterized by the following:

- Swelling and pain at the IV site
- A slow or absent flow rate into the drip chamber of the administration set with the roller clamp open

A

B

Figure 24-19 (**A**) These are examples of suppositories. (**B**) Rectal suppositories should be introduced into the anus well beyond the internal sphincter.

A

B

Figure 24-20 (**A**) Vaginal suppository and applicator. (**B**) Insertion of vaginal cream using applicator.

• No blood return or backup into the tubing when the fluid bag is below the level of the heart

Phlebitis may occur when the intravenous catheter has caused inflammation in the vein or when there is an infection present. Often the irritation or infection occurs at the insertion site and is characterized by redness, swelling, and tenderness. There may also be a red streak starting at the insertion site and following the vein upwards on the extremity. Although the IV may be flowing without difficulty, signs of infection or inflammation indicate that the IV line should be removed and reinserted as ordered by the physician.

Regardless of the reason for reinserting an IV, you must use either the other arm or a site above the level of infiltration or infection. Procedure 24-8 outlines the steps for the initial insertion or reinsertion of an intravenous line.

 CHECKPOINT QUESTION

10. How would you explain an IV that is not flowing even with the roller clamp open?

Figure 24-21 IV equipment including the fluid and tubing.

PROCEDURE 24-1: **Administering Oral Medications**

Purpose: Accurately administer oral medications
Equipment: Physician's order, oral medication, disposable calibrated cup, glass of water, patient medical record

Steps	Reasons
1. Wash your hands.	Handwashing aids infection control.
2. Review the physician's medication order and select the correct medication. Compare the label to the physician's instructions. Note the expiration date. Check the label three times: when taking it from the shelf, while pouring, and when returning it to the shelf.	Carefully dispensing medications helps prevent errors. Outdated medication should not be administered but should be discarded appropriately.
3. Calculate the correct dosage to be given if necessary.	
4. If using a multidose container, remove the cap from the container, touching only the outside of the lid. Single, or unit-dose, medications come individually wrapped in packages that may be opened by pushing the medication through the foil backing or peeling back a tab on one corner.	The inside of the lid of a multidose bottle will be contaminated if touched.

5. According to your calculations and the label, remove the correct dose of medication.
A. For solid medications:
  (1) Pour the capsule or tablet into the bottle cap to prevent contamination.
 	
  (2) Transfer the medication to a disposable cup.
 	
B. For liquid medications:
  (1) Open the bottle and place the lid on a flat surface with the open end up to prevent contamination of the inside of the cap.
	
	Step 5 A (1). Pour the tablet into the bottle cap.
	
	Step 5A (2). Transfer the medication into a disposable cup.

(continued)

PROCEDURE 24-1: | **Administering Oral Medications** *(continued)*

Steps	Reasons

(2) Palm the label to prevent liquids from dripping onto the label and possibly damaging it or making it illegible.

Step 5 B (2). Palm the label of the container when pouring liquids.

(3) With the opposite hand, place your thumbnail at the correct calibration on the cup. Holding the cup at eye level, pour the proper amount of medication into the cup, using your thumbnail as a guide.

Steps	Reasons
6. Greet and identify the patient. Explain the procedure. Ask the patient about medication allergies that might not be noted on the chart.	Identifying the patient prevents errors. Explaining the procedure helps ease anxiety and may improve compliance. The medical record should be checked for allergies, but the patient should also be asked, since allergies may not have been noted.
7. Give the patient a glass of water to wash down the medication unless contraindicated and administer the medication by handing the patient the disposable cup containing the medication.	Water helps the patient swallow the medication, but water is contraindicated for medications intended for a local effect (such as cough syrup or lozenges) and for buccal or sublingual medications.
8. Remain with the patient to be sure that all of the medication is swallowed. Observe any unusual reactions, report them to the physician, and enter them in the medical record.	You cannot assume that the patient swallowed the medication unless you observe it.
9. Thank the patient and give any appropriate instructions.	
10. Wash your hands.	
11. Record the procedure in the patient's medical record, noting the date, time, name of medication, dose administered, route of administration, and your name.	Procedures are considered not to have been done if they are not recorded.

Charting Example:

12/14/2008 8:45 AM Ampicillin 125 mg PO given to pt. NKA

—*T. Jones, CMA*

PROCEDURE 24-2: Preparing Injections

Purpose: Accurately prepare a medication by injection
Equipment: Physician's order, medication for injection (ampule or vial), antiseptic wipes, needle and syringe of appropriate size, small gauze pad, biohazard sharps container, patient's medical record

Steps	Reasons
1. Wash your hands.	Handwashing aids infection control.
2. Review the medication order and select the correct medication. Compare the label to the physician's instructions. Note the expiration date. Check the label three times: when taking it from the shelf, while drawing it up into the syringe, and when returning it to the shelf.	Carefully dispensing medications helps prevent errors. Outdated medication should not be administered to a patient but should be discarded appropriately.
3. Calculate the correct dosage to be given if necessary.	
4. Choose the needle and syringe according to the route of administration, type of medication, and size of the patient.	
5. Open the needle and syringe package. Assemble if necessary. Make sure the needle is firmly attached to the syringe by grasping the needle at the hub and turning it clockwise onto the syringe. 	Needles and syringes often are preassembled, or they may be purchased separately. A needle that is not firmly attached may be detached during the procedure. **Step 5.** Grasp the needle at the hub and turn it clockwise.

6. Withdraw the correct amount of medication:
A. From an ampule:
  (1) With the fingertips of one hand, tap the stem of the ampule lightly to remove any medication in or above the narrow neck.
  (2) Wrap a piece of gauze around the ampule neck to protect your fingers from broken glass. Grasp the gauze and ampule firmly with the fingers. Snap the stem off the ampule with a quick downward movement of the gauze. Be sure to aim the break away from your face. Dispose of the ampule top in a biohazard sharps container to prevent injury.
 	
	Step 6 A (2). Grasp the gauze and ampule firmly.

(continued)

PROCEDURE 24-2:   Preparing Injections (continued)

Steps	Reasons
(3) After removing the needle guard, insert the needle lumen below the level of the medication. Withdraw the medication by pulling back on the plunger of the syringe without letting the needle touch the contaminated edge of the broken ampule. Withdraw the desired amount of medication and dispose of the ampule in a biohazard sharps container.	
(4) Remove any air bubbles by holding the syringe with the needle up and gently tapping the barrel of the syringe until the air bubbles rise to the top. Draw back on the plunger to add a small amount of air, then gently push the plunger forward to eject the air out of the syringe. Be careful not to eject any medication if the required dosage has been drawn up.	
B. From a vial:	
(1) Using the antiseptic wipe, cleanse the rubber stopper of the vial to avoid introducing bacteria into the medication.	**Step 6 B (1).** Clean the rubber stopper with an antiseptic wipe.
(2) Remove the needle guard and pull back on the plunger to fill the syringe with an amount of air equal to the amount of medication to be removed from the vial.	**Step 6 B (2).** Pull back on the plunger, sucking air into the syringe.
(3) Insert the needle into the vial through the center of the cleansed vial top. Inject the air from the syringe into the vial above the level of the medication to avoid producing foam or bubbles in the medication. Injecting an equal amount of air into the vial will prevent	

(continued)

PROCEDURE 24-2: Preparing Injections (continued)

Steps	Reasons

a vacuum from forming in the vial, which would make withdrawal of the medication difficult.

(4) With the needle inside the vial, invert the vial, holding the syringe at eye level. Aspirate, or withdraw, the desired amount of medication into the syringe.

(5) Displace any air bubbles in the syringe by gently tapping the barrel of the syringe with the fingertips. Remove the air by pushing the plunger slowly and forcing the air into the vial.

Step 6 B (3). Insert the needle through the rubber stopper.

Step 6 B (4). Invert the vial.

Step 6 B (5). Tap the barrel gently to remove air bubbles from the medication.

---

7. Carefully recap the needle by placing the needle guard on a hard, flat surface, and without contaminating the needle, insert the needle into the cap and scoop up the cap with one hand.

Recapping the needle protects the sterility of the needle until the medication can be administered. Recapping with two hands should be avoided to prevent needle sticks, especially after giving an injection

PROCEDURE 24-3: Administering an Intradermal Injection

Purpose: Accurately prepare and administer a medication by intradermal injection
Equipment: Physician's order, medication for injection (ampule or vial), antiseptic wipes, needle and syringe of appropriate size, small gauze pad, biohazard sharps container, clean exam gloves, patient's medical record

Steps	Reasons
1. Wash your hands.	Handwashing aids infection control.
2. Review the order and select the correct medication Compare the label to the physician's instructions. Note the expiration date. Check the label three times: when taking it from the shelf, while drawing it up into the syringe, and when returning it to the shelf or discarding the unit dose vial or ampule.	Carefully dispensing medications helps prevent errors. Outdated medication should not be administered to a patient but should be discarded appropriately.
3. Prepare the injection according to the steps in Procedure 24-2.	
4. Greet and identify the patient. Explain the procedure and ask the patient about medication allergies that might not be noted on the medical record.	Correctly identifying the patient prevents errors.
5. Select the appropriate site for the injection. Recommended sites are the anterior forearm and the middle of the back.	
6. Prepare the site by cleansing with an antiseptic wipe using a circular motion starting at the anticipated injection site and working toward the outside. Do not touch the site after cleaning.	The site must be prepared by first removing microorganisms from the area. Wiping in a circular motion will carry the microorganisms away from the site.
7. Put on gloves.	Standard Precautions must be followed for protection against potential exposure to blood.
8. Remove the needle guard. Using your non-dominant hand, pull the patient's skin taut.	Stretching the skin allows the needle to enter the skin with less resistance and secures the patient against movement.
9. With the bevel of the needle facing upward, insert the needle at a 10° to 15° angle into the upper layer of the skin. When the bevel of the needle is under the skin, stop inserting the needle. The needle will be slightly visible below the surface of the skin. It is not necessary to aspirate when performing an intradermal injection.	The needle should be inserted almost parallel to the skin to ensure that penetration occurs within the dermal layer. The bevel of the needle facing up will allow the wheal to form. If the bevel faces downward, no wheal will be formed.

Step 9. Insert the needle at a 10° to 15° angle.

(continued)

PROCEDURE 24-3:   Administering an Intradermal Injection
(continued)

Steps	Reasons
10. Inject the medication slowly by depressing the plunger. A wheal will form as the medication enters the dermal layer of the skin. Hold the syringe steady for proper administration.	Moving the needle once it has penetrated the skin will cause discomfort to the patient.
	Step 10. A wheal is formed when the medication is injected under the skin in an intradermal injection.
11. Remove the needle from the skin at the angle of insertion. Do not use an antiseptic wipe or gauze pad when withdrawing the needle. Do not press or massage the site. Do not apply an adhesive bandage.	Pressure on the wheal may press the medication into the tissues or out of the injection site. Any redness or swelling produced by applying an adhesive bandage could result in an inaccurate reading of the test.
12. Do not recap the needle. Dispose of the needle and syringe in an approved biohazard sharps container. The sharps container should be placed where you have easy access to it after the injection is given.	Discarding the needle and syringe without recapping helps reduce the risk of an accidental needle stick.
13. Remove your gloves and wash your hands.	

14. Depending upon the type of skin test administered, the length of time required for the body tissues to react, and the policies of the medical office, perform one of the following:
  A. Read the test results. Inspect and palpate the site for the presence and amount of induration.
  B. Tell the patient when to return (date and time) to the office to have the results read.
  C. Instruct the patient to read the results at home. Make sure the patient understands the instructions. Have the patient repeat the instructions if necessary.	

15. Document the procedure, site, results, and any instructions given to the patient.	Procedures are considered not to have been done if they are not recorded.

Charting Example:

05/04/2008 10:35 AM Mantoux test, 0.1 mL PPD ID, (L) anterior forearm. Pt. given verbal and written

instructions to RTO in 48–72 hrs to have results read. Pt. verbalized understanding

—P. King, CMA

| **PROCEDURE 24-4:** | **Administering a Subcutaneous Injection** |

Purpose: Accurately prepare and administer a medication by subcutaneous injection
Equipment: Physician's order, medication for injection (ampule or vial), antiseptic wipes, needle and syringe of appropriate size, small gauze pad, biohazard sharps container, clean exam gloves, adhesive bandage, patient's medical record

Steps	Reasons
1. Wash your hands.	Handwashing aids infection control.
2. Review the medication order and select the correct medication. Compare the label to the physician's instructions. Note the expiration date. Check the label three times: when taking it from the shelf, while drawing it up into the syringe, and when returning it to the shelf.	Carefully dispensing medications helps prevent errors. Outdated medication should not be administered to a patient but should be discarded appropriately.
3. Prepare the injection according to the steps in Procedure 24-2.	
4. Greet and identify the patient. Explain the procedure and ask the patient about medication allergies that may not be noted on the medical record.	Correctly identifying the patient prevents errors.
5. Select the appropriate site for the injection. Recommended sites include the upper arm, thigh, back, and abdomen.	
6. Prepare the site by cleansing with an antiseptic wipe using a circular motion starting at the anticipated injection site and working toward the outside. Do not touch the site after cleaning.	The site must be prepared by first removing microorganisms from the area. Wiping in a circular motion will carry the microorganisms away from the site.
7. Put on gloves.	Standard Precautions must be followed for protection against exposure to blood.
8. Remove the needle guard. Using your nondominant hand, hold the skin surrounding the injection site in a cushion fashion.	Holding the skin up and away from the underlying muscle will ensure entrance into the subcutaneous tissues. Proper technique will help ensure that the subcutaneous tissue, not the muscle, is entered.

Step 8. Cushion the tissue between your fingers for the SQ injection.

Steps	Reasons
9. With a firm motion, insert the needle into the tissue at a 45° angle to the skin surface. Hold the barrel between the thumb and the index finger of the dominant hand and insert the needle completely to the hub.	A quick, firm motion is less painful to the patient. Full insertion ensures that the medication is inserted into the proper tissue.

Step 9. Insert the needle at a 45° angle for a subcutaneous injection.

(continued)

PROCEDURE 24-4: Administering a Subcutaneous Injection *(continued)*

Steps	Reasons
10. Remove your nondominant hand from the skin.	
11. Holding the syringe steady, pull back on the syringe gently. If blood appears in the hub or the syringe, a blood vessel has been entered. If this occurs, do not inject the medication. Remove the needle and prepare a new injection.	If medication intended for subcutaneous administration is administered into a blood vessel, the medication can be absorbed too quickly, producing undesirable results.
12. Inject the medication slowly by depressing the plunger.	If medication is injected too rapidly, pressure is created, which will cause patient discomfort and may cause tissue damage.
13. Place a gauze pad over the injection site and remove the needle at the angle at which it was inserted. Gently massage the injection site with the gauze pad with one hand while discarding the needle and syringe into the sharps container with the other hand. Do not recap the used needle. Apply an adhesive bandage if needed.	Discarding the needle and syringe without recapping helps reduce the risk of an accidental needle stick. Massaging helps to distribute the medication so that it can be more completely absorbed.
14. Remove your gloves and wash your hands.	
15. An injection given for allergy desensitization requires that the patient remain in the office for at least 30 minutes for observation of any reaction. If the patient experiences any unusual reaction after any injection, notify the physician immediately.	
16. Document the procedure, site, results, and instructions if given.	Procedures are considered not to have been done if they are not recorded.

Charting Example:

03/04/2008 9:30 AM Regular insulin 5 units SQ (R) posterior upper arm

—M. Collins, CMA

PROCEDURE 24-5:   Administering an Intramuscular Injection

Purpose: Accurately prepare and administer a medication by intramuscular injection
Equipment: Physician's order, medication for injection (ampule or vial), antiseptic wipes, needle and syringe of appropriate size, small gauze pad, biohazard sharps container, clean exam gloves, adhesive bandage, patient's medical record

Steps	Reasons
1. Wash your hands.	Handwashing aids infection control.
2. Review the order and select the correct medication. Compare the label to the physician's instructions. Note the expiration date. Check the label three times: when taking it from the shelf, while drawing it up into the syringe, and when returning it to the shelf.	Carefully dispensing medications helps prevent errors. Outdated medication should not be administered to a patient but should be discarded appropriately.
3. Prepare the injection according to the steps in Procedure 24-2.	
4. Greet and identify the patient. Explain the procedure and ask the patient about medication allergies that might not be noted on the medical record.	Correctly identifying the patient prevents errors.
5. Select the appropriate site for the injection. Recommended sites include the deltoid, vastus lateralis, dorsogluteal, and ventrogluteal areas; however, the site should be chosen based on the medication and age and size of the patient.	Skill and accuracy are crucial when locating intramuscular injection sites since major blood vessels and nerves may lie near the muscles.
6. Prepare the site by cleansing with an antiseptic wipe using a circular motion starting at the anticipated injection site and working toward the outside. Do not touch the site after cleaning.	The site must be prepared by first removing microorganisms from the area. Wiping in a circular motion will carry the microorganisms away from the site.
7. Put on gloves. A B	Standard Precautions must be followed for protection against potential exposure to blood. **Step 8 (A).** Hold the skin taut for an average size person. **Step 8 (B).** Bunch the muscle in a thin person.
8. Remove the needle guard. Using your nondominant hand, hold the skin surrounding the injection site taut with the thumb and index fingers or grasp the muscle in a small person with little body fat.	Holding the skin taut in an average or overweight adult will allow for easier insertion of the needle. Bunching the muscle produces a deeper mass in a very thin person.

(continued)

PROCEDURE 24-5: **Administering an Intramuscular Injection** *(continued)*

Steps	Reasons
9. While holding the syringe like a dart, use a quick, firm motion to insert the needle into the tissue at a 90° angle to the surface. Hold the barrel between the thumb and the index finger of the dominant hand and insert the needle completely to the hub.	A quick, firm motion is less painful to the patient. Full insertion at 90° ensures that the medication is inserted into the proper muscle tissue.
	Step 9. Insert the needle at a 90° angle to the hub
10. Remove your nondominant hand from the skin and gently pull back on the plunger while holding the syringe steady. If blood appears in the hub or the syringe, a blood vessel has been entered. If this occurs, do not inject the medication. Remove the needle and prepare a new injection.	If medication intended for intramuscular administration is administered into a blood vessel, the medication can be absorbed too quickly, producing undesirable results.
11. Inject the medication slowly by depressing the plunger.	If medication is injected too rapidly, pressure is created, which will cause patient discomfort and may cause tissue damage.
12. Place a gauze pad over the injection site and remove the needle at the same angle at which it was inserted. Gently massage the injection site with the gauze pad with one hand while discarding the needle and syringe into the sharps container with the other hand. Do not recap the used needle. Apply an adhesive bandage if needed.	Discarding the needle and syringe without recapping helps reduce the risk of an accidental needle stick. Massaging helps to distribute the medication into the tissues so that it can be more completely absorbed.
13. Remove your gloves and wash your hands.	
14. Observe the patient for any unusual reactions. If the patient experiences any unusual reaction after any injection, notify the physician immediately.	
15. Document the procedure, the site, results, and instructions if given.	Procedures are considered not to have been done if they are not recorded.

Charting Example:

05/06/2008 2:00 PM Solu-Medrol 20 mg IM (L) DG
—O. Campbell, CMA

PROCEDURE 24-6: Administering an Intramuscular Injection Using the Z-Track Method

Purpose: Accurately prepare and administer a medication by Z-track intramuscular injection
Equipment: Physician's order, medication for injection (ampule or vial), antiseptic wipes, needle and syringe of appropriate size, small gauze pad, biohazard sharps container, clean exam gloves, adhesive bandage, patient's medical record

Steps	Reasons
1. Follow Steps 1 through 7 as described in Procedure 24-5 (Administering an Intramuscular Injection). NOTE: The ventrogluteal, vastus lateralis, and dorsogluteal sites work well for the Z-track method; the deltoid does not.	
2. Remove the needle guard. Rather than pulling the skin taut or grasping the tissue as you would for an intramuscular injection, pull the top layer of skin to the side and hold it with the nondominant hand throughout the injection. **Step 2.** Pull the top layer of skin to one side using the edge of your nondominant hand.	
3. While holding the syringe like a dart, use a quick, firm motion to insert the needle into the tissue at a 90° angle to the skin surface. Hold the barrel between the thumb and the index finger of the dominant hand and insert the needle completely to the hub. Continue to hold the skin to one side with the nondominant hand.	A quick, firm motion is less painful to the patient. Full insertion at 90° ensures that the medication is inserted into the proper muscle tissue.
4. Aspirate by withdrawing the plunger slightly. If no blood appears, push the plunger in slowly and steadily. Count to 10 before withdrawing the needle.	If medication intended for intramuscular administration is administered into a blood vessel, the medication can be absorbed too quickly, producing undesirable results. Counting to 10 before removing the needle allows time for the tissues to begin absorbing the medication.
5. Remove the needle at the same angle at which it was inserted while releasing the skin. Do not massage the area. Discard the needle and syringe into the sharps container. Apply an adhesive bandage if needed.	Discarding the needle and syringe without recapping helps reduce the risk of an accidental needle stick.

(continued)

PROCEDURE 24-6:   Administering an Intramuscular Injection Using the Z-Track Method (continued)

Steps	Reasons
6. Remove your gloves and wash your hands.	
7. Observe the patient for any unusual reactions. If the patient experiences any unusual reaction after any injection, notify the physician immediately.	
8. Document the procedure, the site, the results, and the instructions if given.	Procedures are considered not to have been done if they are not recorded.

Charting Example:

07/11/2008 3:30 PM Imferon 25mg IM Z-track (R) DG

—E. Edwards, CMA

PROCEDURE 24-7:   Applying Transdermal Medications

Purpose: Accurately prepare and administer a transdermal medication
Equipment: Physician's order, medication, clean exam gloves, patient's medical record

Steps	Reasons
1. Wash your hands.	Handwashing aids infection control.
2. Review the order and select the correct medication. Compare the label to the physician's instructions. Note the expiration date. Check the label three times: when taking it from the shelf, while drawing it up into the syringe, and when returning it to the shelf.	Carefully dispensing medications helps prevent errors. Outdated medication should not be administered to a patient but should be discarded appropriately.
3. Greet and identify the patient. Explain the procedure and ask the patient about medication allergies that might not be noted on the medical record.	Correctly identifying the patient prevents errors.
4. Select the appropriate site and perform any necessary skin preparation. The sites are usually the upper arm, the chest or back surface, or behind the ear. These sites should be rotated. Ensure that the skin is clean, dry, and free from any irritation. Do not shave areas with excessive hair; trim the hair closely with scissors	Shaving may abrade the skin and cause the medication to be absorbed too rapidly.
5. If there is a transdermal patch already in place, remove it carefully while wearing gloves. Discard the patch in the trash container. Inspect the site for irritation.	Touching the medication with bare hands may cause it to be absorbed into your skin, causing undesirable reactions.

(continued)

PROCEDURE 24-7: Applying Transdermal Medications (continued)

Steps	Reasons
6. Open the medication package by pulling the two sides apart. Do not touch the area of medication.	**Step 6.** Open the transdermal medication by pulling the wrapper apart.
7. Apply the medicated patch to the patient's skin following the manufacturer's directions. Press the adhesive edges down firmly all around, starting at the center and pressing outward. If the edges do not stick, fasten with tape.	Starting at the center eliminates air spaces that may prevent contact with the skin.
8. Wash your hands.	
9. Document the procedure and the site of the new patch in the medical record.	Procedures are considered not to have been done if they are not recorded.

Charting Example:

09/06/2008 8:30 AM Transdermal nitroglycerin 0.2mg/hr patch to (L) anterior chest

—R. Evans, RMA

PROCEDURE 24-8: Obtaining and Preparing an Intravenous Site

Purpose: Accurately start a peripheral IV line

Equipment: Physician's order including the type of fluid to be used and the rate, intravenous solution, infusion administration set, IV pole, blank labels, IV catheter (Angiocath), antiseptic wipes, tourniquet, small gauze pad, biohazard sharps container, clean exam gloves, bandage tape, adhesive bandage, patient medical record

Steps	Reasons
1. Wash your hands.	Handwashing aids infection control.
2. Review the physician's order and select the correct catheter, solution, and administration set. Compare the label on the infusion solution to the physician's order. Note the expiration dates on the infusion solution and the administration set.	Carefully checking the order and the solution helps prevent errors. Outdated solutions or equipment should not be used but should be discarded appropriately.
3. Prepare the solution by attaching a label to the solution indicating the date, time, and name of the patient, and hang the solution on an IV pole. Remove the administration set from the package and close the roller clamp. 	Although there may be other clamps on the administration set, close only the roller clamp, since this is the primary clamp that will be used to adjust the flow rate. **Step 3.** Close the roller clamp on the administration set.
4. Remove the end of the administration set by removing the cover on the spike (above the drip chamber). Remove the cover from the infusion port (on the bottom of the bag) and insert the spike end of the administration set into the IV fluid.	Maintain sterility of the end of administration set and the port on the infusion solution bag at all times. **Step 4.** The spike on the administration set tubing will be inserted completely into the port on the IV solution bag.

(continued)

PROCEDURE 24-8:   **Obtaining and Preparing an Intravenous Site** *(continued)*

Steps	Reasons
5. Fill the drip chamber on the administration set by squeezing the drip chamber until it is about half full.	Do not fill the drip chamber completely. You must observe the flow of drops into this chamber to determine the rate.

Step 5. Fill the drip chamber about half full.

Steps	Reasons
6. Open the roller clamp and allow fluid to flow from the drip chamber through the length of the tubing, displacing any air. Do not remove the cover protecting the end of the tubing. Close the roller clamp when the fluid has filled the tubing and no air is noted. Drape the filled tubing over the IV pole and perform a venipuncture.	
7. Greet and identify the patient. Explain the procedure and ask the patient about medication allergies that might not be noted on the medical record.	Correctly identifying the patient prevents errors.
8. Prepare the IV start equipment by tearing or cutting two to three strips of tape that will be used to secure the IV catheter after insertion. Also, inspect each arm for the best available vein.	After inserting the IV, you will not be able to let go of the catheter to tear or cut tape without the danger of the catheter falling out or being pulled out by the weight of the tubing.
9. Wearing gloves, apply the tourniquet 1 to 2 inches above the intended venipuncture site. The tourniquet should be snug but not too tight. Ask the patient to open and close the fist of the selected arm to distend the veins.	Standard Precautions must be followed for protection against potential exposure to blood. Making a fist raises the vessels out of the underlying tissues and muscles.

Step 9. Pull tourniquet snugly around the arm.

Steps	Reasons
10. Secure the tourniquet by using the half-bow. Make sure the ends of the tourniquet extend upward to avoid contaminating the venipuncture site.	
11. Select a vein by palpating using your gloved index finger to trace the path of the vein and judge its depth. Release the tourniquet after palpating the vein if it has been left on for more than 1 minute.	

(continued)

CHAPTER 24

PROCEDURE 24-8: **Obtaining and Preparing an Intravenous Site** *(continued)*

Steps   **Reasons**

12. Prepare the site by cleansing with an antiseptic wipe using a circular motion starting at the anticipated venipuncture site and working outward. Do not touch the site after cleaning.

Step 12. Prepare the venipuncture site by working outward from the center.

13. Place the end of the administration set tubing on the exam table for easy access after venipuncture. Anchor the vein to be punctured by placing the thumb of the nondominant hand below the intended site and holding the skin taut.

14. Remove the needle cover from the IV catheter. Using the dominant hand, insert the needle and catheter unit directly into the top of the vein with the bevel of the needle up at a 15° to 20° angle for superficial veins and while holding the catheter by the flash chamber, not the hub of the needle. Watch for blood in the flash chamber located next to the catheter hub during insertion of the catheter into the vein.

Holding the catheter by the hub may prevent you from seeing problems during insertion of the catheter. A blood flashback indicates that the needle, not necessarily the catheter, has been correctly inserted into the vein. A "pop" may be felt when the vein has been entered.

15. When the blood flashback is observed, lower the angle of the needle until flush with the skin and slowly advance the needle and catheter unit about ¹/₄ inch.

Step 15. After needle and catheter unit has been inserted into the vein, slowly advance the unit about ¹/₄ inch and then stop.

16. Once the needle and catheter unit have been inserted slightly into the lumen of the vein, hold the flash chamber of the needle steady with the nondominant hand and slide the catheter (using the catheter hub) off of the needle and into the vein with the dominant hand. The catheter should be advanced into the vein up to the hub.

(continued)

PROCEDURE 24-8: **Obtaining and Preparing an Intravenous Site** *(continued)*

Steps	Reasons
17. With the needle partly occluding the catheter, release the tourniquet. Remove the needle and discard into a biohazard sharps container. Connect the end of the administration tubing to the end of the IV catheter that has been inserted into the vein. Open the roller clamp and adjust the flow according the physician's order.	A sterile 2 × 2 gauze pad may be placed under the catheter hub to absorb blood that will flow back out of the catheter after the needle has been completely removed before the tubing is attached.
18. Secure the hub of the IV catheter with tape by placing one small strip, sticky side up, under the catheter and crossing one end over the hub and adhering onto the skin on the opposite side of the catheter. Cross the other end of the tape in the same fashion and adhere to the skin on the opposite side of the hub. A transparent membrane adhesive dressing can then be applied over the entire hub and insertion site.	Avoid placing tape directly over the insertion site so that signs of infection or other problems can be observed readily. **Step 18.** Tape the catheter in place carefully and apply an adhesive dressing over the entire hub and insertion site.
19. Make a small loop with the administration set tubing near the IV insertion site and secure with tape.	This will prevent the catheter from being pulled if the tubing should be pulled or tugged.
20. Remove your gloves, wash your hands, and document the procedure in the medical record indicating the size of the IV catheter and the location, type of infusion solution, and rate.	Procedures are considered not to have been done if they are not recorded.

Charting Example:

05/11/2008 11:45 AM IV started with #22 Angiocath, (L) anterior forearm, 1000 mL RL solution at
TKO rate

—J. Partin, CMA

MEDIA MENU

- **Student CD**

  - **Case Study**
    Clinical Interactive Case Study 1: Triage in an Emergency Situation, Communication and Documentation

  - **Animations**
    Intramuscular Injection; Intravenous Injection

  - **CMA/RMA Certification Exam Review**

- **LWW's Medical Assisting Skills DVD**

  - **Procedures 24-1, 24-2, 24-3, 24-4, 24-6, 24-7**

- **Premium Online Course**
  http://thePoint.lww.com/Kronenberger3e

- **Internet Resources**

  LiveAdvise Online Tutoring & Competency Training
  http://thePoint.lww.com/LiveAdvise

  Medwatch
  http://www.fda.gov/medwatch/

  Physician's Desk Reference
  http://www.pdr.net/home/pdrHome.aspx

  eMedguides
  http://www.emedguides.com/index.jsp

  National Center for Complimentary and Alternative Medicine
  http://nccam.nih.gov/

  Institute for Healthcare Improvement
  http://www.ihi.org/IHI/

  Patient Safety and Quality Healthcare
  http://www.psqh.com/index.html

Chapter Summary

- The administration of medication is one of the most challenging and exacting procedures performed in the medical office.
- Few other procedures require such intense concentration and attention to detail or include such potential for danger to the patient.
- You will be asked to practice interpersonal skills, such as tact and diplomacy, to make these procedures acceptable to the patient and to allay the anxiety felt by almost all patients during the administration of medications.
- It is also your responsibility to be familiar with and follow the laws in your state regarding the administration of medications.

1. Design a patient education brochure that will teach patients about administering rectal medications at home.

2. After inserting the needle while giving an intramuscular injection, you aspirate by pulling back slightly on the plunger. As you do this, blood appears in the syringe. What has happened? What should you do?

3. Another coworker has just given an oral medication to a patient in the office. She asks you to document the procedure. How would you handle this situation?

4. When preparing a medication for injection, you become distracted and forget how much medication you need to draw up into the syringe. What should you do?

Answers | to Checkpoint Questions

1. The three checks are performed when the medication is taken from the shelf, when it is poured, and when it is put back on the shelf.

2. The name of the medication and the dose, route, and site (if injected) should be noted in the medical record after administering any medication. In addition, the entry should be signed by the medical assistant who gave the medication, and any adverse patient reaction or response should be noted.

3. The three systems used to measure medications are the metric, apothecary, and household systems. The metric system is the most commonly used system in the medical office.

4. Medications supplied must be in the same system of measurement and the same unit of measurement as the medication being ordered. If the physician orders a medication in milligrams and the medication is supplied in grams, either the medication ordered must be changed to grams OR the medication supplied must be changed to milligrams.

5. A method commonly used to calculate medication dosages for children up to 12 years of age uses the body surface area (BSA) of the child. This method is also considered to be the most accurate.

6. Oral medication typically takes effect slowly. Also, the oral route cannot be used for patients who are unconscious, for those with nausea and vomiting, and for those who are NPO.

7. Ampules and vials are medication containers. An ampule is a glass container with a narrow neck that must be broken to obtain the medication. A vial is a glass or plastic container sealed with a rubber stopper. Vials may contain medication in either solution (liquid) form or dry form.

8. Types of injections include intradermal, subcutaneous, and intramuscular. Sites for intradermal injections include the anterior forearm and the back. Sites for subcutaneous injections include the upper arm, thigh, back, and abdomen. Sites for intramuscular injections include the deltoid, ventrogluteal, and vastus lateralis.

9. Medication administered through the inhalation route will be absorbed through the alveolar walls into the capillaries in the lungs.

10. An intravenous line that has the roller clamp open but is not running may have a twist in the tubing or the IV catheter or a needle may be infiltrated. An infiltrated IV should be discontinued and restarted.

Diagnostic Imaging

Outline

Principles of Radiology
 X-Rays and X-Ray Machines
 Outpatient X-Rays
 Patient Positioning
 Examination Sequencing
 Radiation Safety
Diagnostic Procedures
 Mammography
 Contrast Medium Examinations
 Fluoroscopy

Computed Tomography
Sonography
Magnetic Resonance Imaging
Nuclear Medicine
**Interventional Radiologic
 Procedures**
Radiation Therapy
**The Medical Assistant's Role in
 Radiologic Procedures**
 Calming the Patient's Fears

Assisting With Examinations
Handling and Storing
 Radiographic Films
**Transfer of Radiographic
 Information**
 Teleradiology

Learning Objectives

Upon successfully completing this chapter, you will be able to:

1. Spell and define the key terms

2. Explain the theory and function of x-rays and x-ray machines

3. State the principles of radiology

4. Describe routine and contrast media, fluoroscopy, computed tomography, sonography, magnetic resonance imaging, nuclear medicine, and mammographic examinations

5. Explain the role of the medical assistant in radiologic procedures

Performance Objectives

Upon successfully completing this chapter, you will be able to:

1. Assist with x-ray procedures (Procedure 25-1)

Competencies

CAAHEP

- Prepare patient for and assist with procedures, treatments, and minor office surgeries
- Perform within legal and ethical boundaries
- Document appropriately

ABHES

- Prepare patients for procedures
- Assist physician with examinations and procedures
- Document accurately

Key Terms

cassette
contrast medium
film
fluoroscopy
magnetic resonance

imaging
nuclear medicine
radiograph
radiography
radiologist

radiology
radiolucent
radionuclide
radiopaque
teleradiology

tomography
ultrasound
x-rays

Principles of Radiology

The discovery of **x-rays** in the late nineteenth century forever changed the practice of medicine. Routine x-ray imaging, computed tomography (CT), sonography, **magnetic resonance imaging**, and **nuclear medicine** are now commonly used diagnostic and therapeutic procedures. Advances in radiation therapy continue to be at the forefront of the treatment for cancer.

Radiology continues to evolve through technologic changes that provide ever-increasing diagnostic information to physicians. As the technology advances, the need to teach patients becomes even more important. Medical assistants are often directly involved in preparing patients for outpatient radiographic procedures, performing basic radiographic procedures in the medical office, and assisting in the general educational process.

X-Rays and X-Ray Machines

X-rays are high-energy waves that cannot be seen, heard, felt, tasted, or smelled and that can penetrate fairly dense objects, such as the human body. This penetrating ability is what allows x-rays to be powerful diagnostic and therapeutic tools. Diagnostically, these penetrating waves create two-dimensional shadowlike images on **film** that is similar to photographic film. Unprocessed film must be protected from light and kept in a special holder called a **cassette** before use. Once the film inside the cassette has been exposed to x-rays, the cassette is placed in a special machine that removes the film and processes it. The processed film containing a visible image is called a **radiograph** (Fig. 25-1). The process by which these films are produced is called **radiography**.

Electricity of extremely high voltage in the x-ray tube produces x-rays. The x-rays leave the tube in one primary direction as a beam, through a device used to control the size of the beam. The light that shines on the patient is not part of the beam but is a positioning aid that illuminates the area covered by the beam. A patient may hear noises coming from the tube area during an

Figure 25-1 Radiograph of chest.

exposure, but these are made by the equipment, not the x-rays.

Today, x-ray machines are sophisticated and technologically advanced. Many are designed to work with computers to produce digital images of the body. Fluoroscopic units can reveal motion within the body. Most permanently installed radiographic units include a special table, some of which can be electronically rotated from the horizontal to the vertical. In this situation, the radiographic film is placed in a cassette that slides into a slot or opening on the table.

Images are formed on the x-ray film as the rays either pass through or are absorbed by the tissues of the body. **Radiolucent** tissues, such as air in the lungs, permit the passage of x-rays, while **radiopaque** tissues, such as bone, do not permit the passage of x-rays. Because bone is dense and absorbs much of the radiation beam, these structures appear white on a radiograph. Air is not dense and does not absorb much radiation. Therefore, air in a structure shows up dark on a radiograph. Other body tissues, such as muscle, fat, and fluid, show as varying shades of gray because of the way each tissue absorbs the x-rays. Physicians who specialize in interpreting the images on the processed film are **radiologists**.

Outpatient X-Rays

The medical community is making a conscious effort to have as much treatment as possible done on an outpatient basis, and thus, some medical offices have on-site x-ray equipment. Outpatient diagnostic imaging centers have also been created to offer these services. Some companies specialize in providing minimal x-ray services to patients in long-term care facilities or the patients' homes.

In some states, you may be permitted to take and process simple images such as bone or chest radiographs. The training for medical assistants varies, but most curricula include a formal course in the theory of radiography and a written examination offered by the state radiographic association for the general operator. In other states, only licensed radiographers may take and process radiographs. You should be familiar with your state laws and comply with any regulations.

 CHECKPOINT QUESTION

1. How would you describe x-rays to a patient?

Patient Positioning

The x-ray exposure on film is a two-dimensional image. Because the human body is a three-dimensional structure, x-ray examinations usually require a minimum of two exposures taken at 90° to each other. For instance,

a chest radiographic examination requires one exposure from the back and another from the side (Fig. 25-2). Other examinations necessitate three or more exposures at different angles. These different angles of exposure are the basis for standard positioning for x-ray examinations (Box 25-1).

Examination Sequencing

Most radiographic procedures can be performed in any order of convenience, but certain procedures must follow certain sequences in specific situations. For example, patients with gallbladder symptoms may go through a series of procedures, progressing from the simple noninvasive oral cholecystogram (an x-ray of the gallbladder after the ingestion of a **contrast medium** orally) to the more complex operative cholangiogram (x-ray of the bile ducts after injection with a contrast medium during a surgical procedure).

Another example is barium studies, the name given to examinations performed after administration of barium sulfate. A patient with gastrointestinal (GI) symptoms may undergo a series of barium studies to assist the physician in diagnosis. Because of the nature of the barium studies and the length of time required to eliminate the barium from the digestive tract, barium enemas are usually scheduled after upper GI examinations. If an endoscopic study, such as an esophagogastroscopy, is ordered, it is imperative that these be scheduled before any procedure involving barium to avoid having the barium obstruct or interfere with the visualization of internal structures.

The barium study that requires filling only the large intestine with barium is the barium enema. Because this procedure involves the last part of the GI tract, this barium can be eliminated fairly quickly so that other examinations can be performed. If an upper GI examination, commonly referred to as an upper GI or barium swallow, is performed first, it may be several days before all of the barium is out of the patient's system. Any residual barium in the GI tract can obscure vital structures in subsequent procedures, preventing them from contributing diagnostic information. The proper sequencing of scheduling the barium enema first and the upper GI last will usually provide diagnostic information in a shorter time.

 CHECKPOINT QUESTION

2. Why is it important to schedule a barium enema before an upper GI or barium swallow?

Radiation Safety

Of primary concern to all radiation workers and patients is the proper and safe use of radiant energy. The

Anteroposterior projection

Posteroanterior projection

Right lateral projection

Left lateral projection

Left posterior oblique projection

Right posterior oblique projection

Left anterior oblique projection

Right anterior oblique projection

Figure 25-2 Standard positions.

hazards of radiation have been known for many decades, and warnings about x-ray radiation are usually posted in appropriate areas (Fig. 25-3). X-rays have the potential to cause cellular or genetic damage to the body, and the results of this damage may not manifest for several years after exposure. The adverse effects are most extreme for rapidly reproducing cells. Pregnant women, children, and reproductive organs of adults are at the highest risk because of their rapid cell division and growth.

Radiation safety procedures for patients include the following:

1. Minimizing exposure amounts.
2. Avoiding unnecessary examinations.
3. Limiting the area of the body exposed.
4. Shielding sensitive body parts, such as the gonads and the thyroid gland.
5. Evaluating the pregnancy status of female patients before performing examinations.

Safety procedures for clinical staff working around x-ray equipment include the following:

1. Limiting the amount of time exposed to x-rays.
2. Staying as far away from the x-rays as possible dur-

TRIAGE

While working in a medical office setting, the physician has asked you to call the hospital and schedule Mrs. Roberts for the following three tests.

A. An esophagogastroduodenoscopy (EGD)
B. Barium enema
C. Barium swallow

What is the correct order for scheduling these tests to be performed?

The correct order is the EGD, the barium enema, and finally the upper GI series or barium swallow. It is important that these procedures be scheduled in this order to ensure optimal results.

ing exposure, preferably standing behind a barrier such as a wall lined with lead.
3. Using available shielding for protection, such as lead aprons and gloves (Fig. 25-4).
4. Avoiding holding patients during exposures. For children requiring assistance, a parent wearing a lead apron may be recruited during the procedure.
5. Wearing individual dosimeters, which are small devices that contain radiographic film clipped to the outside of the uniform, to record the amount of radiation, if any, to which the worker has been exposed (Fig. 25-5). These badges are provided by the employer and are obtained from companies that specifically monitor any radiation exposure of individual health care providers.
6. Ensuring proper working condition of the equipment by scheduling routine maintenance.

For both patients and medical assistants working around radiation, these concerns can be summed up in what is called the ALARA concept: doing whatever is necessary to keep radiation exposure *as low as reasonably achievable.*

Diagnostic Procedures

Routine radiographic examinations require little or no preparation of the patient and are the most commonly performed examinations. These procedures are most readily accepted by the patient and are named for the part of the body involved in the radiographic procedure (Table 25-1). These studies are performed for viewing primarily bone structure or abnormalities.

BOX 25.1

STANDARD TERMINOLOGY FOR POSITIONING AND PROJECTION

Radiographic View
Describes the body part as seen by an x-ray film or other recording medium, such as a fluoroscopic screen. Restricted to the discussion of a *radiograph* or *image.*

Radiographic Position
Refers to a specific body position, such as supine, prone, recumbent, erect, or Trendelenburg. Restricted to the discussion of the *patient's physical position.*

Radiographic Projection
Restricted to the discussion of the *path of the central ray.*

Positioning Terminology
Lying Down

1. *Supine*, lying on the back
2. *Prone*, lying face downward
3. *Decubitus*, lying down with a horizontal x-ray beam
4. *Recumbent*, lying down in any position

Erect or Upright

1. *Anterior position*, facing the film
2. *Posterior position*, facing the radiographic tube
3. *Oblique position*, (erect or lying down)
   A. Anterior, facing the film
      i. *Left anterior oblique*, body rotated with the left anterior portion closest to the film
      ii. *Right anterior oblique*, body rotated with the right anterior portion closest to the film
   B. Posterior, facing the radiographic tube
      i. *Left posterior oblique*, body rotated with the left posterior portion closest to the film
      ii. *Right posterior oblique*, body rotated with the right posterior portion closest to the film

From The American Registry of Radiologic Technologists ® "Content Specifications for The Examination in Radiography." Publication date: July 2004.

 CHECKPOINT QUESTION

3. How does the dosimeter protect you from radiation?

Figure 25-3 X-ray warning sign.

Mammography

Mammography, x-ray examination of the breast, is used as a screening tool for breast cancer (Box 25-2). Each breast is compressed in a specialized device to even the thickness, allowing for an optimal diagnostic image. Needle localization studies using the information gained from the mammogram allow the physician to withdraw small amounts of cells from suspicious areas in a minimally invasive procedure. Mammography has become a vital adjunct to biopsy (Fig. 25-6).

Contrast Medium Examinations

Within the abdomen, many structures having similar radiation absorption rates are superimposed on each other. This makes differentiating structures difficult. The use of a radiopaque contrast medium helps differentiate between body structures by artificially changing the absorption rate of a particular structure. For example, barium sulfate absorbs radiation and shows white on a radiograph (Fig. 25-7). There are many contrast media for various applications. Iodinated compounds are used in many areas of the body, including the kidneys and blood vessels, and in some CT scans. Patients who may have an intestinal perforation may be given an iodinated contrast medium instead of barium because that material spilling into the peritoneum is much less troublesome to the patient than barium would be.

Radiographic examinations using contrast media are performed to evaluate not only a structure but also its function. For example, patients having excretory urography have a contrast medium injected, and the anatomic structure of each kidney is evaluated as the medium passes through the urinary tract. Contrast media may be introduced into the body in several ways, including by mouth, intravenously, or through a catheter, depending on the material and area of the body being examined. It is important that you ask the patient about allergies, especially shellfish allergies. Usually, patients allergic to shellfish are actually allergic to the high iodine content

Figure 25-4 X-ray protection equipment.

Figure 25-5 Dosimeter badge.

of the shellfish, and because injectable contrast media are iodine based, this information needs to be relayed to the radiology center before the patient is scheduled. Another concern for patients undergoing radiographic procedures requiring contrast media is the preparation they must undergo before some of these procedures, especially barium studies. Preparation of the patient for a barium study might include the following:

- Liquid diet only for the evening meal on the day before the examination.
- Laxatives the day preceding the examination to help clean the intestinal tract.
- Nothing by mouth (NPO) after midnight the day before the examination. This usually includes no gum chewing or cigarette smoking because both activities increase gastric secretions that may interfere with the ability of the contrast medium to coat the wall of the intestine.

This general preparation applies to any contrast examination of the abdominal structures. Although this type of radiographic procedure is not performed in the medical office, you must ensure that the patient has proper instructions for preparing for the procedure and is notified of the scheduled time and facility. If patients are not properly prepared for contrast studies, they may have to be rescheduled for another time and day and must undertake the preparations again. Explaining the importance of the preparation can be one of the most important contributions you can make to the patient's care in contrast examinations.

 CHECKPOINT QUESTION

4. How does contrast media aid in differentiating between body structures?

Fluoroscopy

Fluoroscopy, or fluoro studies, use x-rays to observe movement within the body. The movement may be of a contrast medium, such as barium sulfate through the digestive tract or iodinated compounds showing the beating of the heart or blood flow through specific blood vessels. Fluoroscopy is also used as an aid to other types of treatments, such as reducing fractures and implanting devices such as pacemakers.

Computed Tomography

Tomography is a procedure in which the x-ray tube and film move in relation to one another during the exposure, blurring out all structures except those in the focal plane. CT uses a combination of x-rays from a tube circling the patient and computers that analyze the x-rays to create cross-sectional images of the body. CT may be done with or without contrast medium. In addition, some CT units can create three-dimensional images so that organs can be viewed from all angles (Fig. 25-8).

 CHECKPOINT QUESTION

5. What procedures would require the use of fluoroscopy?

Sonography

Ultrasound, or sonography, uses high-frequency sound waves, not x-rays, to create cross-sectional still or real-time (motion) images of the body, usually with the help

Table 25-1	Routine Radiographic Examinations by Body Region
Region	**Patient Preparation**
Trunk	Disrobing of the area: chest, ribs, sternum, shoulder, scapula, clavicle, abdomen, hip, pelvis, sternoclavicular, acromioclavicular, sacroiliac joints
Extremities	Removing jewelry or clothing that might obscure parts of interest: fingers, thumb, hand, wrist, forearm, elbow, humerus, toes, foot, os calcis, ankle, lower leg, knee, patella, femur
Spine	Disrobing of the appropriate area: cervical, thoracic, or lumbar spine; sacrum; coccyx
Head	Removing eyewear, false eyes, false teeth, earrings, hairpins, and hairpieces: skull, sinuses, nasal bones, facial bones and orbits, optic foramen, mandible, temporomandibular joints, mastoid and petrous portion, zygomatic arch

BOX 25-2

AMERICAN CANCER SOCIETY (ACS) AND CENTERS FOR DISEASE CONTROL AND PREVENTION (CDC) GUIDELINES FOR BREAST CANCER SCREENING

The American Cancer Society recommends mammography for women yearly starting at the age of 40. However, women with known risk factors such as a family history of breast cancer may have mammography screenings earlier than the age of 40 years. The CDC recommends the following cancer screening for women with no symptoms:

- Mammography over the age of 40 every 1 to 2 years.
- Clinical breast exam, or breast exam by a physician or nurse, yearly to palpate the presence of lumps or other changes.
- Breast self-exam monthly to check for the presence of lumps, changes in the size or shape of the breast, or any other changes in the breasts or underarm.

Figure 25-7 Barium-filled large intestine.

of a computer. This application is often used to demonstrate heart function or abdominal or pelvic structures. It is commonly used in prenatal testing to visualize the developing fetus. Many obstetricians routinely schedule at least one sonogram before the fourth month of pregnancy (Fig. 25-9).

Magnetic Resonance Imaging

Magnetic resonance imaging (MRI) uses a combination of high-intensity magnetic fields, radio waves, and computer analysis to create cross-sectional images of the body. MRI does not use x-rays. The image depends on the chemical makeup of the body. MRI is commonly used for a variety of studies, including the central nervous system and joint structure. Some MRI studies are performed with contrast. Typically, the patient must be prepared for a long procedure snugly enclosed in a machine that makes numerous knocking and whirring noises. Some facilities use open MRI, which does not make a patient feel as claustrophobic as the closed MRI (Fig. 25-10). Patients with a fear of enclosed places may require a mild sedative before closed MRI.

Nuclear Medicine

Nuclear medicine entails the injection of small amounts of **radionuclides**, which are radioactive materials with short life spans, designed to concentrate in specific areas of the body. Sophisticated computer cameras detect the radiation and create an image. This technique is commonly used to study the thyroid, brain, lungs, liver, spleen, kidney, bone, and breast. These examinations are commonly called scans.

A sophisticated nuclear medicine study, *positron emission tomography* (*PET*), uses specialized equipment to

Figure 25-6 Mammography machine.

Figure 25-8 A computed tomography (CT) scanner.

Figure 25-10 An open MRI.

produce detailed sectional images of the body's physiologic processes. Another procedure, *single photon emission computed tomography (SPECT)*, is a nuclear study that produces sectional images of the body as detectors move around the patient. Both of these procedures are useful in the early diagnosis of physiologic and cellular abnormalities, such as those associated with cancerous tumors.

 CHECKPOINT QUESTION

6. Which diagnostic imaging technique would most likely be ordered for diagnosing cancer in the early stages?

Interventional Radiologic Procedures

Interventional radiologic techniques are designed to treat specific disease conditions. For some patients, these ther-

Figure 25-9 A sonogram.

apeutic techniques are so effective that there is no need for surgery. Some interventional procedures may be life-saving. The following are some types of techniques:

- *Percutaneous transluminal coronary angioplasty (PTCA)*, also known as balloon angioplasty, is used to enlarge the lumen of a coronary artery with a balloon-tipped catheter. Using fluoroscopy, the catheter is placed at a point of partial occlusion or stenosis. The balloon is then briefly inflated, compressing the plaque against the sides of the vessel. After the balloon is deflated, the catheter is removed, and the lumen of the vessel remains larger, allowing for improved blood flow through the blood vessel. Balloon angioplasties may be performed in almost any blood vessel.
- *Laser angioplasties* use laser beams to remove deposits in vessels using fluoroscopy.
- *Vascular stents* (plastic or wire tubes) may be inserted into the stenosed, or constricted, area of a vessel to maintain its patency. Fluoroscopy is used to guide placement of the stent.
- *Embolizations* artificially stop active bleeding from a blood vessel or reduce blood flow to a diseased area of an organ.

Radiation Therapy

A major force in the fight against cancer for many years has been radiation therapy. The use of high-energy radiation to destroy cancer cells may not only prolong the lives of many patients but also saves lives. Used in conjunction with surgery, chemotherapy, or both, radiation is possibly the best-known treatment for cancer. Because the radiation is intense enough to destroy cancer cells, it may also damage adjacent normal cells. Therefore, treatments must be planned carefully and precisely by a radiologist, a physician who specializes in radiology.

PATIENT EDUCATION

ADVANCEMENT IN SURGICAL PROCEDURES

Today, many surgeries that once required large abdominal incisions and extended hospital stays are performed in outpatient ambulatory surgical centers through small incisions and a laparoscope. For example, gallstones are removed with a laparoscope guided by an interventional radiologist, and the patient returns home the same day of surgery. Abdominal aortic aneurysms are treated with a similar procedure, resulting in shorter hospital admissions and less pain. You need to stay current regarding new procedures and surgical techniques so that you can be informed and reassure patients and their families who may not be as aware of the advances made in health care.

WHAT IF?

What if your patient asks you to give him the results of a recently taken chest x-ray?

Many patients are anxious to find out test results including the results of radiology procedures. Often, these patients will ask you for the results before the physician has had an opportunity to read any radiology reports or to look at the actual radiograph. You should tell this patient that the physician would prefer to talk to him about the results and any questions can be answered at that time by the physician. Although you may have access to radiology reports, it is not appropriate to discuss the results with the patient unless the physician has given you permission to do so.

Treatment consists of a precise, carefully planned regimen of therapy, including the frequency and amount of radiation to be used and the number of exposures during a given period. The area of the body to be exposed must be defined exactly so that each treatment is identical. The therapy consists of placing the patient in a position described by the treatment plan and having the exact amount of radiation administered by a radiology technician. Usually the patient has little to do but lie still.

The patient's prognosis varies with the situation. Most patients have some side effects, which may include hair loss, weight loss, loss of appetite, skin changes, and digestive system disturbances. Once the treatment plan is carried out, most of the side effects disappear.

 CHECKPOINT QUESTION

7. What type of health care practitioner is responsible for prescribing and monitoring the effects of radiation therapy for the treatment of cancer?

The Medical Assistant's Role in Radiologic Procedures

Because professional medical assistants have a variety of responsibilities in patient care, they often are in an ideal position to help alleviate patients' anxiety regarding radiology. Anxiety may be relieved by giving patients information about examinations they do not understand, by making patients feel comfortable enough to ask questions, and by answering questions in terms the patient can understand.

Calming the Patient's Fears

Some patients who have experience with the medical system have learned to overcome their anxieties and to find answers to their questions. No matter how much they have been through before, however, there is always something new or something they do not understand that may make them feel as if they have lost control of their situation. Being sensitive to patients' feelings is one of the greatest talents anyone in medicine can possess and should be an important part of your training and personality.

Unfortunately, many patients must undergo procedures they do not understand and do not know enough about to be able to ask relevant questions. Many feel like spectators rather than participants in their own care. Medical assistants can affect a patient's emotional response to a radiologic procedure by explaining what to expect in simple, everyday language, not technical medical terms. The technical aspects of radiology make it difficult for patients to understand. The key to success in explaining radiology procedures to patients is simplicity, leaving the details to the physician.

As noted earlier, explaining the preparations for examinations and their importance is vital to the success of many procedures. Equally important may be an explanation of what to do after the procedure. A barium enema, for instance, can lead to constipation if the patient does not drink enough fluids after the examination. This simple direction can save the patient much distress.

Assisting With Examinations

As a medical assistant, you may be expected to assist with radiologic examinations in the following ways:

• Tell the patient what clothing to remove or assist with clothing removal as needed.

WHAT IF?

A patient has been scheduled for a barium study at a local outpatient facility but calls your office to ask what to do if he ate breakfast this morning. What should you do?

As a medical assistant, you must understand the reason for fasting before certain diagnostic procedures. In this situation, the patient should be instructed to call the diagnostic facility for further instructions, which will include rescheduling the procedure. Emphasize to the patient the importance of following all instructions carefully since not doing so will interfere with the procedure and/or the results. Not following instructions will result in further inconvenience of the patient and delay of a possible diagnose, further delaying treatment and outcomes for the patient.

- Help the patient take the position for the procedure, emphasizing the importance of remaining still and following breathing directions.
- Perform specific radiologic procedures, such as bone or chest radiography, as permitted by your state's laws and your education and training.
- Place film in an automatic processor and reload new film into the cassette.
- Distribute or file radiographs and reports appropriately.

Procedure 25-1 details the procedure for assisting with x-ray procedures.

Handling and Storing Radiographic Films

Advancing technology and the need for quality control have led to automated processing and developing of film to eliminate human error. Automated processing machines produce a film usually in less than 2 minutes. Because processors vary by manufacturer, you need to be proficient in the operation of your particular facility's equipment.

Unexposed film must be protected from moisture, heat, and light by storage in a cool, dry place, preferably in a lead-lined box. Film packets, exposed or unexposed, must be opened in a darkroom using only the darkroom light for illumination. The film is placed in a cassette for use in any area outside the darkroom. Intensifying screens in the cassette are used to reduce the amount of exposure required. Special sleeves or envelopes of various sizes are available for storing the film that has been

labeled with the name of the patient (Fig. 25-11). Film must be protected and stored in a cool, dry area.

 CHECKPOINT QUESTION

8. How can the medical assistant help with radiologic examinations?

Transfer of Radiographic Information

Radiographic images obtained on site for use by the physician remain part of the patient's permanent record. Digital images can be saved on a computer diskette or compact disk. In many cases, however, radiographic studies are performed at one site for consultation or referral at another site. X-ray films belong to the site where the study was performed. The examining physician or radiologist generally writes a summary of the examination to the referring physician. You may need the patient's permission to have the summary of findings sent to the office physician.

With a short-term referral, the examining physician usually returns the films to the referring physician. Patients who have ongoing concerns or who change physicians may request the information contained in their records after submitting written consent. In addition, the patient may obtain copies of the original radiographs if necessary.

Teleradiology

The use of computed imaging and information systems, **teleradiology**, is providing new benefits in medicine. Many institutions use a picture archiving and communication system (PACS) in which computers store and

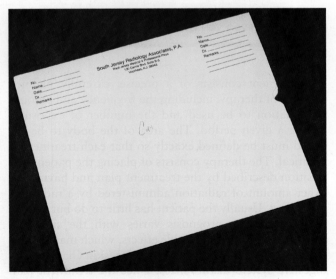

Figure 25-11 An x-ray envelope.

transmit images. Digital images from CT, for instance, can be transmitted via telephone lines to distant locations. This allows consultation with experts on a difficult case within a matter of minutes. Previously unavailable expertise can be brought to rural areas for greatly improved patient care. The result is improved patient care over large geographic areas, not just in specific locations. The term teleradiology is often used to describe this radiology over a great distance.

 CHECKPOINT QUESTION

9. If digital images are taken, how are these records stored?

PROCEDURE 25-1: Preparing a Patient for an X-Ray

Purpose: Prepare the patient for general x-ray procedure
Equipment: Patient gown and drape.
Standard: This procedure should take 5 minutes.

Steps	Reasons
1. Wash your hands.	Hand washing aids infection control.
2. Greet the patient by name, introduce yourself, and escort him or her to the room where the x-ray equipment is maintained.	Identifying the patient by name prevents errors.
3. Ask female patients about the possibility of pregnancy. If the patient is unsure or indicates pregnancy in any trimester, consult with the physician before proceeding with the x-ray procedure.	Fetal exposure to x-rays may be damaging to developing organs and tissues.
4. After explaining what clothing should be removed, if any, give the patient a gown and privacy.	For a chest x-ray, you will have the patient remove all clothing from the waist up. Jewelry such as necklaces may also have to be removed since these will show up on the x-ray and may obscure the images the physician needs to view for diagnosis.
5. Notify the x-ray technician or physician that the patient is ready for the x-ray procedure. Stay behind the lead-lined wall during the x-ray procedure to avoid exposure to x-rays during the procedure.	Depending on state law, you may or may not be permitted to be trained to perform x-ray procedures.
6. After the x-ray, ask the patient to remain in the room until the film has been developed and checked for accuracy and readability.	On occasion, the x-ray will need to be repeated for clarity or adjusted patient position.
7. Once you have determined that the exposed film is adequate for the physician to view for diagnosis, have the patient get dressed and escort him or her to the front desk.	At that time, you can explain any further physician instructions or billing procedures.
8. Document the procedure in the medical record.	Procedures are considered not to have been done if they are not recorded.

Charting Example:

10/19/2008 AP Chest x-ray obtained per x-ray tech. Radiograph placed on viewbox—Dr. Jones notified for review

—S. Smith, CMA

MEDIA MENU

- **Student CD**
  - **CMA/RMA Certification Exam Review**
- **Premium Online Course**
  http://thePoint.lww.com/Kronenberger3e
- **Internet Resources**

  LiveAdvise Online Tutoring & Competency Training
  http://thePoint.lww.com/LiveAdvise

  Radiology Info: The radiology information resource for patients
  http://www.radiologyinfo.org/

  Virtual Hospital: A digital library of health information
  http://www.vh.org/

  American Society of Radiologic Technologists
  http://www.asrt.org

  Access Excellence Resource Center: The Living Skeleton
  http://www.accessexcellence.org/RC/VL/xrays/index.html

español
SPANISH TERMINOLOGY

Tiene que estar en ayunas antes de la prueba.
  You must not eat or drink anything before the test.
Debe comer una comida ligera la noche antes de la prueba.
  You may eat a light supper the night before the test.
Debe seguir estas instrucciónes al pie de la letra.
  You must follow these directions exactly.
Tengo que tomarle una placa.
  I have to take an x-ray.

Chapter Summary

- Radiology is continually evolving as a tool to diagnose and treat disease. As a medical assistant:
- You must understand the common types of diagnostic and therapeutic radiologic procedures that may be ordered by the physician.

- You may also be responsible for teaching patients about these procedures in general and about any particular preparations required.
- When assisting the physician, you must always follow radiation safety precautions carefully for the protection of yourself and your patient.

1. While preparing a female patient for an x-ray procedure, she explains to you that she might be pregnant. How would you handle this situation?

2. Create a poster for your office summarizing the key points of radiation safety.

3. Constipation is a common problem among patients who have barium studies. How can patient education diminish this problem?

4. An elderly woman is concerned about having an ultrasound of her gallbladder and states that she does not want to have any more x-rays. Based on what you know about sonography, how would you respond to this patient?

5. Explain the importance of patient privacy laws (HIPAA) and teleradiology. What is your role in maintaining privacy in using teleradiology?

Answers | to Checkpoint Questions

1. X-rays are invisible, high-energy waves that travel at the speed of light. These waves penetrate the body, making an impression on a piece of film placed behind or in front of the area of the body being examined. While taking an x-ray is not painful, the x-rays may be harmful to certain internal organs. A lead-lined blanket may be placed over those areas of the body to protect internal organs.

2. Barium enemas fill only the large intestine with barium. Because the large intestine is the last part of the GI tract, this barium can be eliminated quickly. If an upper GI examination is performed first, it may be days before barium can be eliminated, which may delay other examinations.

3. A dosimeter does not protect you from radiation but will monitor your exposure, if any, to x-rays in the environment.

4. Contrast media artificially change the absorption rate of x-rays in the structures that contain this media. This change in absorption rate allows the structures to be seen clearly instead of blending in with adjacent structures. For example, barium sulfate in the large intestine absorbs radiation and shows up as white areas on a radiograph, allowing this structure to be easily examined on an exposed x-ray film.

5. Fluoroscopy is useful for x-rays that require the ability to observe movement within the body, such as the movement of barium through the digestive tract or blood flow through a blood vessel.

6. The PET scan or SPECT scan in nuclear medicine would most likely be ordered by the physician to diagnose physiologic and cellular abnormalities such as those found in cancer.

7. The radiologist, a physician who specializes in radiology, is usually responsible for prescribing and monitoring radiation therapy for the treatment of cancer.

8. Medical assistants can help with radiologic examinations by providing instruction to patients, positioning patients, handling x-ray film, and distributing or filing radiographs and reports. In some states, the medical assistant may take simple x-rays.

9. Digital images can be saved and stored on a computer diskette or compact disk.

Outline

Medical Office Emergency Procedures
  Emergency Action Plan
  Emergency Medical Kit
  The Emergency Medical
    Services System
Patient Assessment
  Recognizing the Emergency
  The Primary Assessment

The Secondary Assessment
Types of Emergencies
  Shock
  Bleeding
  Burns
  Musculoskeletal Injuries
  Cardiovascular Emergencies
  Neurologic Emergencies

Allergic and Anaphylactic
  Reactions
Poisoning
Heat- and Cold-Related
  Emergencies
Behavioral and Psychiatric
  Emergencies

Learning Objectives

Upon successfully completing this chapter, you will be able to:

1. Spell and define key terms

2. Describe the role of the medical assistant in an emergency

3. Identify the five types of shock and the management of each

4. Describe how burns are classified and managed

5. Explain the management of allergic reactions

6. Describe the management of poisoning and the role of the poison control center

7. List the three types of hyperthermic emergencies and the treatment for each type

8. Discuss the treatment of hypothermia

9. Describe the role of the medical assistant in managing psychiatric emergencies

Performance Objectives

Upon successfully completing this chapter, you will be able to:

1. Administer oxygen (Procedure 26-1)

2. Perform cardiopulmonary resuscitation (Procedure 26-2)

3. Use an automatic external defibrillator (AED) (Procedure 26-3)

4. Manage a foreign body airway obstruction (Procedure 26-4)

5. Control bleeding (Procedure 26-5)

CAAHEP

- Practice Standard Precautions
- Prepare patient for and assist with routine and specialty examinations
- Prepare patient for and assist with procedures, treatments, and minor office surgeries
- Document appropriately
- Instruct individuals according to their needs

ABHES

- Prepare patients for procedures
- Recognize emergencies
- Perform first aid and CPR
- Assist physician with examinations and treatments
- Document accurately

Key Terms

allergen	heat cramps	hypovolemic shock	burn
anaphylactic shock	heat exhaustion	infarction	seizure
cardiogenic shock	heat stroke	ischemia	septic shock
contusion	hematoma	melena	shock
ecchymosis	hyperthermia	neurogenic shock	splint
full-thickness burn	hypothermia	partial-thickness	superficial burn
frostbite			

Medical Office Emergency Procedures

Emergency medical care is the immediate care given to sick or injured persons. When properly performed, it can mean the difference between life and death, rapid recovery and long hospitalization, and temporary disability and permanent disability. Emergency medical care in the medical office entails identifying the emergency, delivering basic first aid, and furnishing temporary assistance or basic life support until a rescue squad and advanced life support can be obtained.

An emergency can occur anywhere and to anyone. For example, a patient who is being seen for a routine examination may have a heart attack, collapse, and require immediate cardiopulmonary resuscitation (CPR). A diabetic patient or co-worker may lapse into a diabetic coma (refer to Chapter 36 for diabetic emergency procedures). A patient may fall down a flight of stairs and receive trauma to the head or limbs. In a life-threatening situation, the well-prepared medical assistant can obtain important information and perform lifesaving procedures before the ambulance or rescue squad arrives, increasing the patient's chance for survival. Medical assistants should be certified in CPR and removing foreign body airway obstructions. Currently, the American Association of Medical Assistants (AAMA) requires certified medical assistants (CMAs) to demonstrate proof of current CPR certification to recertify their credential. This training may be provided by

the American Red Cross, American Heart Association, American Safety and Health Institute, or National Safety Council. You should contact one of these agencies for specific information regarding training and certification. This chapter is not meant to provide a comprehensive study of all aspects of emergency care; instead, it briefly reviews the information in such a training course.

Emergency Action Plan

Every medical office should have an emergency action plan, including the following:

- The local emergency rescue service telephone number (usually 911)
- Location of the nearest hospital emergency department
- Telephone number of the local or regional poison control center
- Procedures for various emergencies
- List of office personnel who are trained in CPR
- Location and list of contents of the emergency medical kit or crash cart

Whether confronted with a cardiac emergency or psychiatric crisis, medical assistants must be able to coordinate multiple ongoing events while rendering patient care. Contributing to the complexity of a medical emergency are such factors as panicky family members, the arrival of emergency personnel, and possibly language barriers. You must be able to remain calm in these situations while reacting competently and professionally.

Emergency Medical Kit

Proper equipment and supplies should be readily available in a medical emergency. Although the office's equipment and supplies vary with the medical specialty, emergency equipment and supplies are fairly standard. This equipment should be kept in a designated location that is accessible to all staff. Standard supplies for a medical emergency kit are listed in Box 26-1. Although items used during an emergency should be replaced as soon as possible, a medical assistant or other staff member should check the contents of the emergency kit or crash cart regularly, perhaps weekly, to verify that contents are available and that no item has gone beyond the expiration date. If so, the expired items should be replaced immediately.

The Emergency Medical Services System

The initial element of any emergency medical services (EMS) system is citizen access. The availability of rapid, systematic intervention by personnel specifically trained in providing emergency care is an integral part of the EMS system. Most communities have a 911 system to report emergencies and summon help by telephone. The communications operator at the local EMS station will answer the call, take the information, and alert the EMS, fire, or police department as needed. In communities without a 911 system, emergency calls are usually made directly to the local ambulance, fire, or police department. You should know the emergency system used in your community. Emergency phone numbers should be prominently displayed by all telephones in the medical office.

Some communities have an enhanced 911 system that automatically identifies the caller's telephone number and location. If the telephone is disconnected or the caller loses consciousness, the communications operator can still send emergency personnel to the scene. In the medical office, an emergency requiring notification of the EMS includes situations that are life threatening or have the potential to become life threatening, such as the symptoms of a heart attack, **shock**, or severe breathing difficulties. In each of these cases, the medical assistant provides immediate care to the patient, including CPR if necessary, while directing another staff member to notify the physician. During assessment of the emergency by the physician, the medical assistant should continue to provide first aid or be prepared to assist the physician in administering first aid while another staff member notifies the EMS. The staff member who calls EMS should be able to describe the emergency to the

---

BOX 26-1

EMERGENCY MEDICAL KIT AND EQUIPMENT

The following are standard supplies that can be used to make up an emergency medical kit:

- Activated charcoal
- Adhesive strip bandages, assorted sizes
- Adhesive tape, 1- and 2-inch rolls
- Alcohol (70%)
- Alcohol wipes
- Antimicrobial skin ointment
- Chemical ice pack
- Cotton balls
- Cotton swabs
- Disposable gloves
- Elastic bandages, 2- and 3-inch widths
- Gauze pads, 2 × 2– and 4 × 4–inch widths
- Roller, self-adhesive gauze, 2- and 4-inch widths
- Safety pins, various sizes
- Scissors
- Syrup of ipecac
- Thermometer
- Triangular bandage
- Tweezers

In addition to these contents, the following equipment should be available:

- Blood pressure cuff (pediatric and adult)
- Stethoscope
- Bag-valve mask device with assorted size masks
- Flashlight or penlight
- Portable oxygen tank with regulator
- Oxygen masks
- Suction unit and catheters

Additional equipment that may be available includes:

- Various sizes of endotracheal tubes
- Laryngoscope handle and various sizes of blades
- Automatic external defibrillator
- Intravenous supplies (catheters, administration set tubing, assorted solutions)
- Emergency drugs including atropine, epinephrine, and sodium bicarbonate

---

communications operator. The operator will then know what level of emergency personnel and rescue equipment to send. Excellent communication skills and cooperation between health care team members is essential during a medical office emergency.

Documentation in the medical record is an important responsibility in all patient care, including emergency care. EMS personnel depend on accurate and complete information regarding the patient's symptoms, the nature of the emergency, and any treatment performed prior to their arrival. This information should be placed in the patient's record in chronological order as events occurred or treatments were performed. Any vital signs taken during the emergency should also be recorded. Emergencies that involve visitors or staff must also be documented, and in this case, a blank paper or progress note page will be sufficient to record the details and outline the care provided. Information should include but not be limited to the following:

1. Basic identification, including name, age, address, and location of the patient's emergency contact if known
2. The chief complaint if known
3. Times of events, beginning with recognition of the emergency, management techniques, and changes in patient's condition
4. The patient's vital signs
5. Specific emergency management rendered in the office, such as CPR, bandaging, splinting, and medications administered before and after the emergency
6. Observations of the patient's condition, including any slurred speech, lethargy, confusion, and so on
7. Any medical history, allergies, or current medications if known

When the EMS personnel arrive, assist them as necessary. Let them examine the patient and take over the emergency care. You can also help by removing any obstacles to removal of the patient by stretcher and keeping family members in the reception area or a private room.

 CHECKPOINT QUESTION

1. What should you document before the ambulance arrives in an emergency?

Patient Assessment

The two primary objectives in assessment of the patient are to identify and correct any life-threatening problems and provide necessary care. Each step of the assessment must be managed effectively before proceeding to the next. For example, airway, breathing, and circulation must be intact before you take a history. In addition, survey the scene quickly to identify hazards or clues to the patient's condition. For example, an elderly person found at the bottom of a stairway will likely have head or neck injuries and should be treated in such a way as to avoid moving the head, neck, or spinal column. Emesis found near a person that resembles coffee grounds may be a clue to bleeding in the gastrointestinal system that may result from peptic ulcer disease and hemorrhage.

Recognizing the Emergency

When providing emergency care, do not assume that the obvious injuries are the only ones. Less noticeable or internal injuries may also have occurred during an accident. You should look for the causes of the injury, which may provide a clue to the extent of physical damage. For example, the elderly patient who fell down the stairs may have a noticeable bump on the forehead; this is obvious, but perhaps the patient has an injury in the cervical spine that is not as readily noticeable. In the case of an injury to the head or back when spinal fracture is possible, be especially careful not to move the victim any more than necessary and avoid rough handling.

The Primary Assessment

Once you are at the victim's side, an initial survey of the patient is the first step in emergency care. This is a rapid evaluation, usually done in less than 45 seconds. The purpose of the primary assessment is to identify and correct any life-threatening problems. Quickly assess the following aspects of the patient:

- Responsiveness
- Airway
- Breathing
- Circulation

Checking for responsiveness means noting whether the patient is conscious or unconscious. If the patient is unconscious, attempt to awaken the patient by speaking and touching the shoulder. If no response occurs, assess the patient's airway by using the head tilt–chin lift method. Patients who may have neck injuries should have the airway opened using the jaw thrust method to avoid further injury to the spinal cord (Figs. 26-1 and 26-2). An unconscious patient who is supine is likely to have a partial or total airway obstruction caused by the tongue falling back into the oropharynx, producing snoring respirations or total airway obstruction. Opening the patient's airway may be necessary to allow adequate respirations. In the event of a foreign body airway obstruction, it will be necessary to clear the airway to perform effective rescue breathing.

Once the airway is open, evaluate the patient's breathing by watching for movement of the chest up or down while listening and feeling over the mouth and nose for signs of adequate ventilation. If the patient is not breathing, artificial respiration must be started im-

Figure 26-1 The head tilt–chin lift technique for opening the airway. The head is tilted backward with one hand (down arrow). while the fingers of the other hand lift the chin forward (up arrow).

mediately. A face mask with a one-way valve or a bag–valve–mask device is recommended when performing rescue breathing and should be used if available (Fig. 26-3). Respirations that are too fast, too slow, or irregular also require medical intervention. Immediate intervention for these conditions may include breathing into a mask or paper bag for respirations that are too fast (hyperventilation) or administering oxygen as directed by the physician. Any obvious noises, such as stridor or wheezes, are noted and reported to the physician (see Chapter 30).

Evaluate circulation in adults and children by checking the carotid pulse (Fig 26-4). The brachial pulse is

Figure 26-3 Using a mask with a one-way valve, begin rescue breathing if no breathing is noted in the primary survey.

used to evaluate circulation in infants. If no pulse is found, begin cardiopulmonary resuscitation chest compressions immediately (Fig. 26-5). Some medical offices may have an automatic external defibrillator (AED) as part of the emergency medical kit (Fig. 26-6). Training to use the AED is included in most CPR classes. Many public places such as airports and shopping malls have AED units available for use by those individuals trained appropriately. Procedure 26-1 describes the procedure for administering oxygen in the medical office, while Procedures 26-2, 26-3, and 26-4 explain cardiopulmonary resuscitation, the use of the AED, and managing a patient with a foreign body airway obstruction.

During the primary assessment, also check for any hemorrhage, and if found, control the bleeding quickly (Procedure 26-5). Evaluate perfusion, or blood flow through the tissues, by checking the temperature and moisture of the skin.

Figure 26-2 The jaw thrust technique for opening the airway. The hands are placed on either side of the head. The fingers of both hands grasp behind the angle of the jaw, bringing it up (arrow).

Figure 26-4 Check for circulation by palpating the carotid pulse.

CHECKPOINT QUESTION

2. What is the purpose of the primary assessment?

 PATIENT EDUCATION

CHOKING

While the danger of choking is always present with small children, many adults choke to death each year. Here are some important tips to prevent choking in adults:

- Always chew food carefully before swallowing. Focus on eating by avoiding eating and driving a car at the same time..
- Avoid excessive alcohol consumption, especially while eating.
- Laughter and talking increase your chance of choking. Do not talk with food in your mouth.
- Older adults who wear dentures should go for an annual dental evaluation to make sure dentures fit snugly.
- With age, saliva production decreases, making it more difficult to swallow. Encourage older patients to take smaller bites and chew food longer, sipping liquids as needed.

The Secondary Assessment

After conducting a primary assessment and assessing that the patient's airway, breathing, and circulation are adequate, a secondary assessment can be performed. The secondary assessment includes asking the patient questions to obtain additional information and performing a more thorough physical evaluation to find less obvious problems than those noted in the primary assessment. To

Figure 26-5 Chest compressions should be started if no signs of circulation, including a pulse, are present.

Figure 26-6 The automatic external defibrillator (AED) can be used to defibrillate a life-threatening heart rhythm.

gain an accurate impression during the secondary assessment, the following four areas are assessed:

1. *General appearance.* The patient's skin color and moisture, facial expression, posture, motor activity, speech, and state of alertness provide important clues about the mental and physical condition. Check for a medical bracelet or necklace. Medicine bottles in a pocket or purse can also be helpful.
2. *Level of consciousness.* By the time you have completed the primary survey and noted the patient's general appearance, the level of consciousness may be apparent. A decrease in oxygen to the cells of the brain, neurologic damage from a cerebrovascular accident (stroke), and intracranial swelling are just some of the conditions that may alter a patient's level of consciousness. The AVPU system uses a common language to describe the patient's level of consciousness:

- A, *A*wake and alert
- V, responds to *V*oice
- P, responds only to *P*ain
- U, *U*nresponsive or unconscious

3. *Vital signs.* After noting the general appearance and determining the level of consciousness, assess the vital signs, including the pulse and respiratory rates and blood pressure. Assessment of temperature is important for patients who have altered skin temperature or have been exposed to environmental temperature extremes. Patients with a history of infection, chills, or fever and children with **seizures** should always have their temperature taken.
4. *Skin.* An initial evaluation of the temperature and moisture of skin should have been noted during the primary survey. A more thorough look should now

be taken. Skin is normally dry and somewhat warm. Moist, cool skin may indicate poor blood flow to the tissues and possibly shock. The color of the skin should be noted as an indication of the circulation near the surface of the body and oxygenation of the tissues.

The Physical Examination

A head-to-toe survey that includes examination of the head and neck, chest and back, abdomen, and extremities in this sequence should be done only after completing the primary and secondary surveys. Although the physician usually performs this examination, you must be prepared to assist as needed while continuing to reassure the patient.

Head and Neck

If a cervical spine injury is suspected, immediately immobilize the spine and avoid manipulating the neck during examination of the head. Inspect the face for edema, bruising, bleeding, and drainage from the nose or ears. Examine the mouth for loose teeth and dentures. The condition and severity of a neurologic injury or patient with altered consciousness can be assessed by checking the pupils with a flashlight or penlight. The pupils should be checked for several characteristics:

- Equality in size
- Dilation bilaterally in darkness or dim light
- Rapid constriction to light in both eyes
- Equal reaction to light

To evaluate the pupils for these qualities, shade both eyes from the light and use a flashlight or small penlight at an angle 6 to 8 inches from each eye. The conscious patient should not look directly into the light. Report the findings to the physician.

Chest and Back

The anterior chest is evaluated to some degree when the patient's respiratory status is evaluated. A further inspection of the chest should be done after removing clothing from a patient with trauma or abnormal vital signs. Patients with cardiac or respiratory complaints should also have their chest more thoroughly evaluated. Palpation of the chest and back may reveal the possibility of rib fractures.

Abdomen

The abdomen of all patients is evaluated, but it is particularly important for those with GI symptoms or suspicion of blood or fluid loss as seen in vaginal bleeding, vomiting, or **melena** (blood in the stool). The abdomen is inspected for scars, bruises, and masses. A distended abdomen may indicate hemorrhage in the abdominal cavity.

WHAT IF?

What if your patient has a cervical fracture?

Fractures to the cervical spine can be life threatening or seriously disabling. There are seven cervical vertebrae in the neck, and fractures to the first cervical vertebra (C-1), the most superior vertebra, tend to be fatal unless immediately and aggressively treated by emergency services personnel before transport to a trauma center. Fractures to the second and third cervical vertebrae (C-2 and C-3) often result in permanent or long-term respiratory dependency on a mechanical ventilator since the involuntary respiratory center of the brain is affected. Vertebrae fractures of the fourth to seventh cervical vertebrae (C-4 to C-7) will result in various levels of paralysis and motor impairment. If you suspect a patient has a cervical fracture or other vertebral fracture, keep the head and neck of the patient still and call for emergency personnel. Never move the patient unless the patient is in immediate danger. The emergency medical technicians will properly immobilize the head and neck of the patient for transport to the hospital, where radiographic tests will diagnose the extent of the injury.

Arms and Legs

An examination of the arms and legs is the last step of the head-to-toe survey. Inspect the arms and legs for swelling, deformity, and tenderness. Also note any tremors in the hands. To determine the neurologic status of the arms and legs, assess strength, movement, range of motion, and sensation, including comparing one side of the body with the other. Muscle strength in the upper extremities is checked by having the patient squeeze both of your hands at the same time. Leg strength may be determined by having the patient push each foot against your hand, again at the same time, while noting any weakness in one side or the other. Assess sensation by using a safety pin or other tool to determine the patient's response to pain. Throughout the examination, you must note the comparison of both sides, including any weakness or decreased sensation in one side or the other. Again, the physician will most likely be performing this examination, but you must be prepared to assist as needed.

CHECKPOINT QUESTION

3. What diagnostic signs are evaluated in the secondary assessment?

Types of Emergencies

Shock

Shock is lack of oxygen to the individual cells of the body, including the brain, as a result of a decrease in blood pressure. Although the cause of the low blood pressure varies, the body initially adjusts for any type of shock by increasing the strength of the heart contractions and the heart rate while constricting the blood vessels throughout the body. As shock progresses, the body has more difficulty trying to adjust, and eventually tissues and body organs have such severe damage that the shock becomes irreversible and death ensues. The signs and symptoms of shock include:

- Low blood pressure
- Restlessness or signs of fear
- Thirst
- Nausea
- Cool, clammy skin
- Pale skin with cyanosis (bluish color) at the lips and earlobes
- Rapid and weak pulse

Types of Shock

Hypovolemic shock is caused by loss of blood or other body fluids. If the cause is blood loss, it is hemorrhagic shock. Dehydration caused by diarrhea, vomiting, or profuse sweating can also lead to hypovolemic shock.

Cardiogenic shock is an extreme form of heart failure that occurs when the function of the left ventricle is so compromised that the heart can no longer adequately pump blood to body tissues. This type of shock may follow death of cardiac tissue during a myocardial infarction (heart attack).

Neurogenic shock is caused by a dysfunction of the nervous system following a spinal cord injury. Normally, the diameter of all blood vessels is controlled by the involuntary nervous system and smooth muscles surrounding the vessels. After a spinal cord injury, the nervous system loses control of the diameter of the blood vessels, and vasodilation ensues. Once the blood vessels are dilated, there is not enough blood in the general circulation, so that blood pressure falls and shock ensues.

Anaphylactic shock is an acute general allergic reaction within minutes to hours after the body has been exposed to an offending foreign substance. You must carefully observe patients for this type of shock after giving medications and during allergy testing (see later section on anaphylaxis).

Septic shock is caused by a general infection of the bloodstream in which the patient appears seriously ill. It may be associated with an infection such as pneumonia or meningitis, or it may occur without an apparent source of infection, especially in infants and children. Initially, a fever is present, but the body temperature falls, a clinical sign suggestive of sepsis.

Management of the Patient in Shock

Because shock can result from many types of medical situations or trauma, you should always be prepared to treat the patient for shock in any emergency situation that occurs in the medical office. After performing the primary and secondary assessments, the following list of general guidelines for managing a patient in shock should be observed:

1. Observe the patient for and maintain an open airway and adequate breathing.
2. Control bleeding.
3. Administer oxygen as directed by the physician.
4. Immobilize the patient if spinal injuries may be present.
5. Splint fractures.
6. Prevent loss of body heat by covering the patient with a blanket, especially if the patient is cold.
7. Assist the physician with starting an intravenous line as ordered (refer to Chapter 24).
8. Elevate the feet and legs of a patient with low systemic blood pressure.
9. Transport the patient to the closest hospital as soon as possible by notifying the EMS as directed by the physician.

 CHECKPOINT QUESTION

4. What does it mean when a patient is in shock?

Bleeding

Soft tissue injuries involve damage to the skin and/or underlying musculature.

When a blunt object strikes the body, it may crush the tissue beneath the skin. Although the skin does not always break, severe damage to tissue and blood vessels may cause bleeding within a confined area. This is called a closed wound. Types of closed wounds include **contusions, hematomas,** and crush injuries. A contusion is a bruise or collection of blood under the skin or in damaged tissue (Fig. 26-7). The site may swell immediately or 24 to 48 hours later. As blood accumulates in the area, a characteristic black and blue mark, called **ecchymosis,** is seen.

A blood clot that forms at the injury site, generally when large areas of tissue are damaged, is a hematoma. As much as a liter of blood can be lost in the soft tissue when a large bone is fractured. Crush injuries are usually caused by extreme external forces that crush both

Figure 26-7 A closed wound; contusion.

tissue and bone. Even though the skin remains intact, underlying organs may be severely damaged. Regardless of the type of swelling in a closed wound, the treatment includes the application of ice to reduce and prevent additional swelling to the area (refer to Procedure 28-2 in Chapter 28, Orthopedics).

In an open wound, the skin is broken, and the patient is susceptible to external hemorrhage and wound contamination. An open wound may be the only surface evidence of a more serious injury, such as a fracture. Open wounds include abrasions, lacerations, major arterial lacerations, puncture wounds, avulsions, amputations, and impalements (Fig. 26-8). When managing any patient with an open wound, follow standard precautions to protect yourself against disease transmission and to protect the patient from further contamination. An open injury to these tissues is a wound. Box 26-2 describes common soft tissue injuries and wounds.

BOX 26-2

TYPES OF SOFT TISSUE INJURIES

- **Abrasion**, the least serious type of open wound, is little more than a scratch on the surface of the skin. All abrasions, regardless of size, are painful because of the nerve endings involved.
- **Laceration** results from snagging or tearing of tissues that leaves a freely bleeding jagged wound. Skin may be partly or completely torn away, and the laceration may contain foreign matter that can lead to infection. A wound caused by a broken bottle or a piece of jagged metal is a laceration.
- **Major arterial laceration** can cause significant bleeding if the sharp or jagged instrument cuts the wall of a blood vessel, especially an artery. Uncontrolled major arterial bleeding can result in shock and death.
- **Puncture wounds** can result from sharp, narrow objects like knives, nails, and ice picks. Punctures also can be caused by high-velocity penetrating objects, such as bullets. A special case of the puncture wound is the *impaled object wound*, in which the instrument that caused the injury remains in the wound. The object can be anything—a stick, arrow, piece of glass, knife, steel rod—that penetrates any part of the body.
- **Avulsion** is a flap of skin torn loose; it may either remain hanging or tear off altogether. Avulsions usually bleed profusely. Most patients who present with an avulsion work with machinery. Home accidents with lawn mowers and power tools are common causes of avulsion.
- **Amputation** is caused by the ripping, tearing force of industrial and automobile accidents, often great enough to tear away or crush limbs from the body.

Figure 26-8 An open wound; laceration.

Management of Bleeding and Soft Tissue Injuries

Management of open soft tissue injuries includes controlling bleeding by applying direct pressure (Procedure 26-5). Sterile gauze should be used to cover the wound if possible to avoid introducing microorganisms into the wound. Management of an amputated body part includes controlling the bleeding but also preserving the severed part for possible reattachment later. To preserve the severed body part:

- Place the severed part in a plastic bag.

- Place this bag in a second plastic bag. This second bag will provide added protection against moisture loss.
- Place both sealed bags in a container of ice or ice water, but do not use dry ice.

An impaled object should not be removed but requires careful immobilization of the patient and the injured area of the body (Fig. 26-9). Because any motion of the impaled object can cause additional damage to the surface wound and underlying tissue, you must stabilize the object without removing it by placing gauze pads around the object and securing with tape. The immobilized impaled object can be carefully removed after transportation to the hospital.

 CHECKPOINT QUESTION

5. How should an open wound that is bleeding be treated?

Burns

The four major sources of burn injury are thermal, electrical, chemical, and radiation. *Thermal burns*, also called heat burns, result from contact with hot liquids, solids, superheated gases, or flame. *Electrical burns* are caused by contact with low- or high-voltage electricity. Lightning injuries are also considered electrical burns. *Chemical burns* result when wet or dry corrosive substances come into contact with the skin or mucous membranes. The amount of injury with a chemical burn depends on the concentration and quantity of the chemical agent and the length of time it is in contact with the skin. *Radiation burns* are similar to thermal burns and can occur from overexposure to ultraviolet light or from any extreme exposure to radiation.

Classification of Burn Injuries

Classification of burn injuries depends on the depth, or tissue layers involved. Factors that determine the depth of the burn include the agent causing the burn, the temperature, and the length of time exposed. Burns are classified according to the depth of injury: **superficial** (first degree), **partial thickness** (second degree), or **full thickness** (third degree).

Calculation of Body Surface Area Burned

The extent of body surface area (BSA) injured by the burn is most commonly estimated by a method called the rule of nines. This method calculates the percentage of total body surface of individual sections of the body. With the rule of nines for an adult, 9% of the skin is estimated to cover the head and another 9% for each arm, including front and back (Fig. 26-10). Twice as much, or 18%, of the total skin area covers the front of the trunk, another 18% covers the back of the trunk, and 18% covers each lower extremity. The area around the genitals is the additional 1% of the BSA. In infants and children, the percentages are the same except that the head is 18% and each lower extremity is 13.5% of the total BSA. Usually, the emergency room physician determines the percentage of body burned using this rule, not the medical assistant.

Figure 26-9 An impaled object.

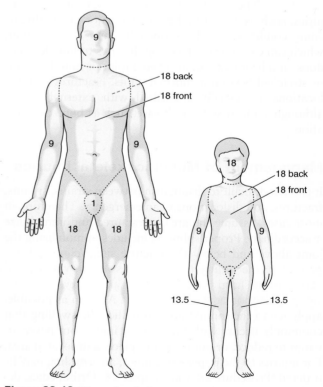
Figure 26-10 The rule of nines.

Management of the Burn Victim

Follow these guidelines for managing burn patients in the medical office:

1. Eliminate the source of the burn, if necessary, by washing the area with cool water.
2. Have someone notify the physician, and take the patient immediately to an examination or treatment room.
3. Continually assess the patient's airway, breathing, and circulation. Begin CPR if necessary.
4. Remove all jewelry and clothing as necessary to evaluate the extent of the burn.
5. Administer oxygen as instructed by the physician.
6. Treat the patient for shock and accompanying low blood pressure.
7. Notify the EMS as directed by the physician.
8. Document the time and type of treatments given.
9. Assist with the necessary procedures for transporting the patient to the hospital.

 CHECKPOINT QUESTION

6. What are the four major sources of burn injuries?

Musculoskeletal Injuries

Injuries to muscles, bones, and joints are some of the most common problems encountered in providing emergency care. The seriousness varies widely, from simple injuries, such as a fractured finger, to major or life-threatening conditions, such as open fracture to the femur, which can cause severe bleeding. Injuries to muscles, tendons, and ligaments occur when a joint or muscle is torn or stretched beyond its normal limits. Fractures and dislocations are usually associated with external forces, although some arise from disease, such as bone degeneration.

Management of Musculoskeletal Injuries

It is often difficult to distinguish between strains, sprains, fractures, and dislocations in an emergency. Therefore, in most cases, assume the area is fractured and immobilize it accordingly. Proper splinting includes immobilizing the joint above and below the fracture site. Splinting helps prevent further injury to soft tissues, blood vessels, and nerves from sharp bone fragments and relieves pain by stopping motion at the fracture site. As soon as possible, apply ice to the injured area to reduce the swelling that commonly occurs with this type of injury, but never attempt to reduce, or put back into place, a dislocated area. For injuries to the upper extremities, an arm sling may be ordered (Procedure 28-1 in Chapter 28, Orthopedics, describes how to apply an arm sling).

Types of Splints

Any device used to immobilize a sprain, strain, fracture, or dislocated limb is a **splint**. Splinting material may be soft or rigid and can be improvised from almost any object that can provide stability. Commercial types include traction, air, wire ladder, and padded board splints (Fig. 26-11). Regardless of the type of splint, once applied, you must examine the extremity for signs of impaired circulation. To check the circulation of an extremity:

- Observe the skin color and nail beds of the affected extremity. A pale or cyanotic color indicates that the circulation is impeded.
- Locate a pulse in the artery distal to the affected extremity. A weak or absent pulse also indicates that circulation is decreased to the area.
- Watch for increased swelling of the extremity. Although this may not indicate that the circulation is impaired, the swelling itself can reduce circulation.

If the circulation is impaired with the splint in place, it must be removed or loosened immediately to provide for adequate blood flow, or tissue **ischemia** (decrease in oxygen) and **infarction** (death) may occur.

 CHECKPOINT QUESTION

7. What is the purpose of applying a splint?

Cardiovascular Emergencies

Cardiovascular disease accounts for nearly 1 million deaths each year in the United States. The most common problem is coronary artery disease. Approximately two-thirds of sudden deaths from coronary artery disease occur out of the hospital, and most occur within 2 hours of the onset of symptoms. As coronary artery disease progresses, less and less oxygen can get to the car-

Figure 26-11 Types of splints.

diac muscle, which leads to tissue ischemia and eventual infarction of the cardiac tissue. The early symptoms of a myocardial infarction (heart attack) include the following:

- Chest pain not relieved by rest
- A complaint of pressure in the chest or upper back
- Nausea or indigestion
- Chest pain that radiates up into the neck and jaw or down one arm
- Anxiety

Early treatment, including basic life support, early defibrillation, and advanced life support, can prevent many of these deaths. If cardiopulmonary resuscitation is initiated promptly and the patient is rapidly and successfully defibrillated, the patient's survival chances improve. As noted earlier, an automatic external defibrillator, or AED, may be available in your medical office and should be used as soon as possible after it is determined that the victim does not have a pulse. When applied to the patient's chest, the AED will analyze the rhythm and advise the operator to shock, or defibrillate, the patient by simply pressing a button.

Neurologic Emergencies

A seizure is caused by an abnormal discharge of electrical activity in the brain. During a seizure, erratic muscle movements, strange sensations, and a complete loss of consciousness can occur. A seizure is not a disease but a manifestation or symptom of an underlying disorder. Epilepsy, head injury, and drug toxicity can cause seizures. A thorough patient history is important when assessing these patients. It should include the following:

- Information about previous seizure disorders
- Frequency of seizures if recurrent
- Prescribed medications
- Any history of head trauma
- Alcohol or drug abuse
- Recent fever
- Stiff neck (as seen in meningitis)
- A history of heart disease, diabetes, or stroke.

In managing a patient having a seizure, you must give priority to assessing the patient's responsiveness, airway, breathing, and circulation. In certain types of seizures, the patient loses consciousness and, therefore, cannot protect the airway. During the seizure, the muscles of the body, including those of the face, will contract tightly. If you attempt to force an object between the teeth to prevent the patient from biting the tongue, the result will most likely be injury to you or the patient. Frequently, patients vomit during the seizure and lose bowel or bladder control. Particular attention and care are necessary to clear and maintain the airway without causing injury to yourself or the patient. Assisting the

patient into the recovery position (on one side) will help secretions such as blood or vomit drain from the mouth (Fig. 26-12). Secretions may be removed from the mouth using a suction machine if available.

The most important thing you can do for a patient during a seizure is protect the patient from injury. If the patient lost consciousness and fell at the beginning of the seizure, care will be necessary to protect the neck and cervical spine until immobilization can occur.

 CHECKPOINT QUESTION

8. What are some causes of seizure activity in a patient?

Allergic and Anaphylactic Reactions

A severe allergic reaction called anaphylaxis causes most emergency department visits related to allergies. An allergic reaction is a generalized reaction that can occur within minutes to hours after the body has been exposed to a substance recognized by the immune system as foreign and to which it is oversensitive. The systemic signs and symptoms of anaphylaxis are more severe than for a simple allergic reaction, but repeated

Figure 26-12 Patient in recovery position.

exposure to a substance that produces allergic reactions may ultimately lead to an anaphylactic reaction and should be avoided.

Common Allergens

An **allergen** is a substance that gives rise to hypersensitivity or allergy. The allergen may be a drug, insect venom, food, or pollen and may be injected, ingested, inhaled, or absorbed through the skin or mucous membranes. A person may have symptoms within seconds after exposure to an allergen, or the reaction may be delayed for several hours. You must ask every patient about allergies at every visit and indicate them on the front of the patient's chart and the medication record. Check the patient's medical record and ask about allergies *before* administering any medications in the office; this is essential to prevent allergic reactions or anaphylaxis in patients with known hypersensitivity.

Although the exact incidence of anaphylactic reactions is difficult to pinpoint, it is estimated that 1% to 2% of patients who receive penicillin in the United States have some form of allergy to the drug and that one in 50,000 injections of penicillin results in death from anaphylaxis. However, you must be alert to the signs and symptoms of allergic reactions after administering any medication, not just penicillin. Patients with moderate to severe allergy symptoms often receive frequent injections of specific allergens to reduce the symptoms associated with allergies. These patients should be monitored especially closely for anaphylaxis, and they should not be permitted to leave the office for a prescribed amount of time, often 20 to 30 minutes after the injection. When documenting that an injection was given, you should also note the condition of the patient upon discharge.

Signs and Symptoms

The initial signs and symptoms of an allergic reaction may include severe itching, a feeling of warmth, tightness in the throat or chest, or a rash. The primary rule for any exposure is that the sooner the symptoms occur after the exposure, the more severe the reaction is likely to be. Be observant and ready to treat any patient who has these symptoms, since airway obstruction, cardiovascular collapse, and shock can occur if the situation worsens. Since the primary cause of death in an anaphylactic reaction is swelling of the tissues in the airway, leading to airway obstruction, observe the patient closely for signs of airway involvement, including wheezing, shortness of breath, and coughing. Choking or tightness in the neck and throat may signal this danger. Tachycardia, hypotension, pale skin, dryness of the mouth, diaphoresis (profuse sweating), and other signs of shock may also be present.

Management of Allergic and Anaphylactic Reactions

The patient having a severe allergic reaction will often be anxious. Some allergic reactions are mild, without respiratory problems or signs of shock. These simple reactions can be managed by administering oxygen or medications such as antihistamines to relieve symptoms as directed by the physician. If respiratory involvement occurs without signs of shock, the physician may order that epinephrine (1:1000) be given subcutaneously. The patient with a severe anaphylactic reaction who is in shock needs more aggressive therapy, including additional medications, an intravenous line, and monitoring of the cardiac rhythm. The primary goal when treating a patient having an anaphylactic reaction is restoring respiratory and circulatory function. The following steps are required for managing allergic reactions, including anaphylaxis:

- Do not leave the patient, but have another staff member request that the physician immediately evaluate the patient and bring the emergency kit or cart, including oxygen.
- Assist the patient to a supine position.
- Assess the patient's respiratory and circulatory status by obtaining the blood pressure, pulse, and respiratory rates.
- Observe the skin color and warmth.
- If the patient complains of being cold or is shivering, cover him or her with a blanket.
- Upon the direction of the physician, start an intravenous line (refer to Chapter 24) and administer oxygen.
- As ordered by the physician, administer medications as ordered.
- Document vital signs and any medications and treatments given, noting the time each set of vital signs is taken or medications are administered.
- Communicate relevant information to the EMS personnel, including copies of the progress notes or medication record as needed.

 CHECKPOINT QUESTION

9. What is the primary cause of death in anaphylaxis?

Poisoning

The likelihood that one will be exposed to toxins in the home or workplace is increasing. In addition to over-the-counter and prescription medications often found in the home, household chemicals are an additional hazard and are often designed to have a pleasant odor and color. Industrial chemicals offer another possibility of poisoning. These chemicals may affect a single victim or many victims in the event of a hazardous materials incident. Most toxic exposures occur in the home, and almost 50% occur in children aged 1 to 3 years (Fig. 26-13). Although about 90% of reported poisonings are accidental, intentional exposures usually affect adolescents and adults, and they tend to have a higher death rate. Fortunately, deaths from drug overdoses and poisoning are rare, but you must know how to respond if a patient comes to the office or telephones with a possible poisoning.

TRIAGE

While working in a busy medical urgent care center, the following three patients arrive at the same time:

A. A 4-year-old child arrives, carried in by his mother who states that he has had vomiting and diarrhea for approximately 2 days but has recently become "sleepy and hard to arouse."

B. A 36-year-old female comes in complaining of pain in her hand after spilling a cup of hot coffee on it. You notice that the palm of her left hand is red and has several small blisters on it.

C. A 40-year-old man had cut his thumb while using a box cutter at work. He has a towel on it and notes that the bleeding has "stopped," but he still would like to have it evaluated by the physician.

How do you sort these patients? Who do you see first? Second? Third?

Anytime there is change in anyone's mental status, it should be treated as a priority. See patient A first since he may be dehydrated and headed for hypovolemic shock. Patient B should be seen next. She has a first- and second-degree burn, and although these may be painful, she is not in immediate danger of shock. Patient C should be seen last. The patient is capable of holding pressure to the site to control bleeding, but he may need sutures to close the wound as well as a tetanus injection.

Poison Control Center

The American Association of Poison Control Centers (AAPCC) has established standards and regional poison control centers throughout the country. These centers are staffed by physicians, nurses, and pharmacists. When information about a poisoning or drug overdose is not readily available, the poison control center is a valuable resource, and the phone number should be posted near all phones in the medical office. The profes-

Figure 26-13. Advise adults to store cleaning products out of the reach of small children.

sionals at the poison control center can usually evaluate a potential or known toxic exposure, instruct the caller in the use of syrup of ipecac to induce vomiting if indicated, and check on the patient's progress by follow-up telephone calls.

Management of Poisoning Emergencies

Exactly how and when a poison control center is consulted should be part of the medical office's protocol. Few toxic substances have specific antidotes, so the management of the poisoning is aimed at treating the signs and symptoms and assessing the involved organ systems. The patient may go to the medical office after the poisoning, or more commonly, the patient or caregiver telephones the office requesting information. In either situation, you must obtain the following information *before* making the call to poison control:

• The nature of the poisoning (ingested, inhaled, skin exposure)
• The age and weight of the victim
• The name of the substance
• An estimate of the amount of poison
• When the exposure occurred
• The patient's present signs and symptoms

Once the poison control center has been notified and instructions given, you must be prepared to treat the patient as directed and notify the EMS to transport the patient to the hospital. Never give a patient syrup of ipecac or otherwise induce vomiting unless directed to do so by the professionals at the poison control center.

 CHECKPOINT QUESTION

10. Why is it important to have the phone number of the poison control center near the telephone in the medical office?

Heat- and Cold-Related Emergencies

Environmental temperature is one of the many variables to which the body normally adjusts, maintaining equilibrium. Human beings depend on the ability to control core body temperature within a range of several degrees. Measured rectally, this core temperature is 37.6°C (99.6°F). The peripheral temperature is usually lower (98.6°F orally). Several conditions can disrupt the normal heat-regulating mechanisms of the body. These are divided into two main categories: **hyperthermia** and **hypothermia**.

Hyperthermia

Hyperthermia is the general condition of excessive body heat. Correct management depends on assessment of the underlying cause. The first type of hyperthermia includes **heat cramps**, which is muscle cramping that follows a period of heavy exertion and profuse sweating in a hot environment. While sweat is primarily water, it also contains the electrolyte sodium, which is needed for muscle function. Heavy sweating, which is a normal compensatory mechanism to cool the body, will result in a sodium deficit, which compromises muscle function and produces muscle cramps. A patient with heat cramps often complains of cramping in the calves of the legs and in the abdomen. Cramping may also occur in the hands, arms, and feet. Mental status and blood pressure usually remain normal, although an increased pulse rate is common.

Heat cramps signal the need for cooling and rest. In uncomplicated cases, the patient is encouraged to take fluids by mouth, but nausea may make intravenous infusion necessary. If the patient is able to take fluids by mouth, give a commercial electrolyte solution such as Gatorade, or salt can be added to water or fruit juice at 1 teaspoon per pint. Cramps can sometimes be prevented entirely with similar oral intake before physical exertion and every 20 minutes during exercise. Salt tablets are not recommended because they may cause nausea.

Heat exhaustion results most often from physical exertion in a hot environment without adequate fluid replacement. Body temperature usually remains normal or slightly above normal. Patients have central nervous system symptoms such as headache, fatigue, dizziness, or syncope (fainting). Although the skin is typically moist and the pulse rate is high, skin color, blood pressure, and respiratory rate vary with the degree to which the body is able to hold off the distress. Patients in late stages of heat exhaustion have pale skin, low blood pressure, and rapid respiration.

Heat stroke is a true emergency. The body is no longer able to compensate for the rapid rise in body temperature (past 105°F) and may undergo brain damage or death. Heat stroke victims can deteriorate quickly to coma, and many patients have seizures. The skin is classically hot, flushed, and dry. Vital signs are elevated initially but may drop, with ensuing cardiopulmonary arrest. Heat stroke demands rapid cooling of the body. After alerting the physician, follow office policy for the management of hyperthermia and heat stroke, which will include these steps:

- Move the patient to a cool area.
- Remove clothing that may be holding in the heat.
- Place cool, wet cloths or a wet sheet on the core surface areas of the body where the ability to cool the central blood is the greatest: the scalp, neck, axilla, and groin.
- Administer oxygen as directed by the physician and apply a cardiac monitor.
- Notify the EMS for transportation to the hospital as directed by the physician.

Hypothermia

The body's core temperature can drop several degrees without loss of normal body function. The body usually tolerates a 3° to 4°F drop in temperature without symptoms; hypothermia is an abnormally low body temperature, below 35°C (95°F). Internal metabolic factors and significant heat loss to the external environment can lead to hypothermia. Very cold air and immersion in cold water can cause a rapid drop in core temperature. The following are the signs and symptoms of hypothermia:

- Cool, pale skin
- Lethargy and mental confusion
- Shallow, slow respirations
- Slow, faint pulse rate

Basic management of hypothermia includes handling the patient gently, removing wet clothing, and covering the patient to prevent further cooling. If there is evidence of rewarming (skin warm, respirations approaching normal, no shivering) and the patient is alert and able to swallow, give warm fluids by mouth. Avoid drinks that constrict peripheral blood vessels, such as those that contain caffeine (coffee and tea). Fluids that cause dilation of the blood vessels, such as alcohol, should also be avoided. Warm beverages with sugar, such as hot chocolate, can be given to begin replacement of the fuel that the body needs to restore normal heat production. No fluids should be given by mouth to patients who have a diminished or changing level of consciousness.

Frostbite

Windy subfreezing weather creates the greatest risk for **frostbite**. Small body parts with a high ratio of surface area to tissue mass (fingers, toes, ears, and nose) are most vulnerable to frostbite, although larger areas of the extremities are also vulnerable during profound cooling. Exposure to cold can cause tissues to freeze, and the frozen cells will die.

The type and duration of contact are the two most important factors in determining the extent of frostbite injury. Touching cold fabric, for example, is not nearly as dangerous as coming into direct contact with cold metal, particularly if the skin is wet or even damp. The combination of wind and cold is dangerous. *Superficial frostbite* appears as firm and waxy gray or yellow skin in an area that loses sensation after hurting or tingling. Prolonged exposure can lead to blistering and eventually *deep frostbite*, which most often affects the hands and feet. No warning symptoms appear after the initial loss of feeling. Freezing progresses painlessly once the nerve endings are numb. Skin becomes inelastic and the entire area feels hard to the touch. Deep frostbite results in tissue death, and the affected tissue must be removed surgically or amputated.

Superficial frostbite can be managed by warming the affected part with another body surface, for example placing an ungloved hand over the nose or ears. Management for more than superficial frostbite is rapid rewarming after any system-wide hypothermia has been corrected. Deep frostbite should be managed only in the hospital to prevent further damage to the tissue. You may be asked to do the following as directed by the physician:

- Immerse the frozen tissue in lukewarm water (418C, 1058F) until the area becomes pliable and the color and sensation return.
- Do not apply dry heat.

- Do not massage the area; massage may cause further tissue damage.
- Avoid breaking any blisters that may form.
- Notify the EMS for transportation to a hospital.

If rewarming is not attempted, bandage the frostbitten part with dry sterile dressings. Frostbitten tissue is similar to burned tissue in that it is vulnerable to infection. Take care to keep the affected part as clean as possible. All frostbite victims should be assessed for hypothermia. Clothing offers good protection against weather only if it is loose enough to avoid restricting circulation. Tight gloves, cuffs, boots, and straps add to the danger.

CHECKPOINT QUESTION

11. What is the difference between heat exhaustion and heat stroke?

Behavioral and Psychiatric Emergencies

Psychological distress may be mild, moderate, or severe. The degree of intensity determines the type and amount of intervention necessary. A psychiatric emergency is different from an emotional crisis, and you must know how to differentiate between the two. A psychiatric emergency is any situation in which the patient's moods, thoughts, or actions are so disordered or disturbed that harm or death may result for the patient or others if no intervention occurs. An emotional crisis, on the other hand, is a situation with much less intensity. While it may be distressing to the patient, in most cases, it is not likely to end in danger, harm, or death without immediate intervention. However, if neglected entirely, an emotional crisis may escalate to a full psychiatric emergency.

A true behavioral emergency, like a medical emergency, carries a serious threat. Urgent behavioral situations usually require some form of professional psychological evaluation and intervention and require transportation to the hospital. The following guidelines are useful for handling a psychiatric emergency:

- Notify the physician and the EMS as directed.
- Offer reassurance and general support to the patient and any caregivers or family members who may be present.
- Accurately document information, including vital signs and the patient's behavior.

PROCEDURE 26-1: Administer Oxygen

Purpose: Administer oxygen according to the physician's order
Equipment: Oxygen tank with regulator, oxygen delivery system (nasal cannula, mask)

Steps	Reasons
1. Wash your hands.	Handwashing aids infection control.
2. Check the physician order for the amount of oxygen and the delivery method (nasal cannula, mask).	
3. Assemble the equipment.	**Step 3.** An oxygen tank and nasal cannula.
4. Greet and identify the patient. Explain the procedure.	Identifying the patient prevents errors. Explaining the procedure helps ease anxiety and may improve compliance.
5. Connect the distal end of the tubing on the oxygen delivery method (nasal cannula or mask) to the adapter on the regulator, which is connected to the oxygen tank..	**Step 5.** Connect the distal end of the oxygen tubing to the regulator.
6. Place the oxygen delivery system (nasal cannula or mask) on the patient. A B	**Step 6. (A)** Place the nasal cannula into the patient's nares, or **(B)** secure the mask over the nose and mouth.

(continued)

PROCEDURE 26-1: **Administer Oxygen** *(continued)*

7. Turn the regulator dial to the appropriate number of liters per minute as ordered by the physician.

Step 7. Turn on the oxygen by rotating the dial on the oxygen tank regulator.

8. Record the procedure in the patient's medical record.	Procedures are considered not to have been done if they are not recorded.

Charting Example:

12/23/2008 2:15 PM Oxygen applied per nasal cannula at 4L/min as ordered

—*J. Leigh, CMA*

PROCEDURE 26-2: **Perform Cardiopulmonary Resuscitation (Adult)**

Purpose: Perform rescue breathing and chest compressions (cardiopulmonary resuscitation) on an adult
Equipment: CPR mannequin for practice, mouth-to-mouth barrier device, gloves
NOTE: Demonstration of competency depends upon the individual student and the structured educational protocol by certified trainers for the American Heart Association, American Red Cross, or the National Safety Council.

Steps	Reasons
1. Determine unresponsiveness by shaking the patient and shouting "Are you okay?"	Establishing unresponsiveness prevents rescue measures being taken for a patient who does not need them.
2. If the patient does not respond, assess for airway patency and respiratory effort using the head tilt–chin lift maneuver with the patient in a supine position. Instruct another staff member to get the physician and the emergency medical cart. If gloves are easily accessible, put clean gloves on both hands. Otherwise, put them on when the emergency medical cart arrives.	If you suspect a neck injury, use the jaw thrust maneuver to open the airway after rolling the patient carefully to the back without twisting or moving the neck.

(continued)

PROCEDURE 26-2: Perform Cardiopulmonary Resuscitation (Adult) *(continued)*

Steps	Reasons
3. After opening the airway, assess for breathing by placing your face 2 to 3 inches in front of the patient's mouth to feel for air movement while observing the chest, looking for the rise and fall of the chest. 	Using these methods to determine the presence of respiratory effort will avoid giving respirations to a patient who is breathing. **Step 3.** Watch the chest for movement while feeling for air movement from the mouth or nose.
4. If the breathing is adequate, place the patient in the recovery position until the patient regains consciousness or the physician instructs you to call emergency medical services (EMS).	The recovery position includes the patient lying on his or her side, which facilitates respirations and prevents aspiration of emesis in the event that the patient vomits.
5. If the patient is not breathing adequately, begin rescue breathing by placing a barrier device over the patient's mouth and nose and giving two slow breaths, causing the chest to rise without overfilling the lungs.	The physician will probably want EMS notified at this point since quick access to advanced care will increase the patient's chance for survival. Giving slow breaths will provide oxygen without overfilling the lungs. Overfilling the lungs with air will cause gastric distention and vomiting.
6. After giving two breaths, check for cardiac function by feeling for a pulse using the carotid artery on the side of the patient's neck.	
7. If a pulse is present, but inadequate respiratory effort is present, continue rescue breathing as needed.	During rescue breathing, you will need to check for a pulse periodically and be prepared to begin chest compressions if needed. If the patient resumes adequate breathing, place the patient into the recovery position.
8. If no pulse is present, follow the protocol for chest compressions according to the standards of the training provided by the American Heart Association, the American Red Cross, or the National Safety Council.	During chest compressions, avoid pressing directly on the xiphoid process at the bottom of the sternum to prevent injury to internal structures.
9. After about 1 minute of chest compressions, check the carotid pulse. If no pulse is present, continue chest compressions and rescue breathing. If the pulse returns but respirations do not, continue with rescue breathing. Continue CPR until relieved by another health care provider or EMS arrives.	

(continued)

PROCEDURE 26-2: Perform Cardiopulmonary Resuscitation (Adult) *(continued)*

NOTE: In the clinical situation, respiratory barrier devices and gloves will be available to protect you from the patient's oral secretions and should be used appropriately.

All health care professionals should receive training for proficiency in CPR in an approved program. The procedure described here is not intended to substitute for proficiency training with a mannequin and a structured protocol.

Charting Example:

10/14/ 2008 10:30 AM Pt arrived c/o chest pain. Skin diaphoretic, color pale. Pulse 125 and regular, BP 88/54 (L). Collapsed in exam room, Dr. Barton notified. Pulse and respirations absent, CPR started. EMS notified per Dr. Barton
—S. Pencil, CMA

10/14/2008 10:40 AM CPR continued per EMS, pt. unresponsive. Transported to General Hospital. Patient's wife, Helen, notified of transport
—S. Pencil, CMA

PROCEDURE 26-3: Use an Automatic External Defibrillator (AED) (Adult)

Purpose: Correctly apply and use an AED on an adult patient
Equipment: Practice automatic external defibrillator, chest pads with connection cables appropriate for the AED machine, scissors, dry gauze pads, gloves, and mannequin

Steps	Reasons
1. Determine unresponsiveness by shaking the patient and shouting, "Are you okay?"	Establishing unresponsiveness prevents rescue measures being taken for a patient who does not need them.
2. Follow the procedure for assessing airway patency and respirations, giving two rescue breaths and checking for the presence of a carotid pulse (see Procedure 26-2). Instruct another staff member to notify the physician and obtain the emergency cart and AED.	
3. Begin CPR if there is no pulse or adequate respirations.	

(continued)

PROCEDURE 26-3: Use an Automatic External Defibrillator (AED) (Adult) (continued)

Steps	Reasons
4. When the AED is available, continue CPR while a second rescuer removes the patient's shirt and prepares the chest for the AED electrodes. This second rescuer will be in control of operating the AED.	If the patient's skin is wet, use a dry towel or cloth to dry the chest. If the patient is wearing a transdermal medication patch on the chest, remove the patch and wipe any excess medication off of the chest. If there is excessive hair on the patient's chest, use a disposable razor to remove any hair over where the chest electrode pads will be placed. **Step 4.** The first rescuer continues CPR while the second rescuer prepares the AED.
5. After removing the sticky paper backing on the AED electrode pads, apply the chest electrodes onto the patient's chest, one on the upper right chest and the other on the lower left chest.	**Step 5.** Place the AED pads on the upper right chest and the lower right chest.
6. Once the electrodes are in place, connect the wire from the electrodes to the AED unit and turn the AED on.	**Step 6.** Connect the AED electrode wires to the AED machine.
7. Follow the instructions given by the AED as the heart rhythm is being analyzed. Do not touch the patient during the analysis, including doing CPR. If no shock is necessary, the AED will indicate this nd instruct you to resume CPR. Begin CPR by checking the patient for respirations and a carotid pulse. If these are not present, resume CPR.	The AED machine will verbally tell you what to do. Listen for all instructions and follow the directions given by the machine.

(continued)

PROCEDURE 26-3: Use an Automatic External Defibrillator (AED) (Adult) *(continued)*

Steps	Reasons
8. If the AED instructs you that an electrical shock is necessary, the second rescuer will operate the machine, making sure that no person is touching the patient or the exam table (if the patient is on a table) before pressing the appropriate button on the AED to deliver the electrical shock.	If another person is touching the patient or the exam table when an electrical shock is delivered, the shock will be transferred to that person as well as the patient.
	Step 8. The second rescuer delivers the electrical shock if indicated.
9. After delivering the shock, the AED will again analyze the patient's heart rhythm. The patient must not be touched during this process.	If a shock is not advised and CPR is resumed, the AED will ask you to stop CPR periodically to reanalyze the rhythm. Do not touch the patient while the AED is analyzing the heart rhythm.
10. Continue to follow the instructions given by the AED, which will include either reshocking the patient or resuming CPR. Always assess the patient's respirations and carotid pulse before resuming CPR.	Continue this pattern until EMS arrives and takes over the emergency procedure.

NOTE: All health care professionals should take an approved training course in CPR and use of an AED. This procedure is not intended to substitute for proficiency training with a mannequin in a structured educational protocol.

Charting Example:

11/15/2008 3:15 PM Pt. became unresponsive while waiting in reception area; no pulse or respiratory effort. Dr. Barton notified, CPR started
—*J. Crete, CMA*

11/15/2008 3:18 PM AED applied, 2 electrical shocks delivered, pulse returned, no respiratory effort. Rescue breathing resumed
—*J. Crete, CMA*

11/15/2008 3:25 PM EMS here. Pt. transported to General Hospital
—*J. Crete, CMA*

PROCEDURE 26-4: **Manage a Foreign Body Airway Obstruction (Adult)**

Purpose: Respond appropriately to an adult (conscious and unconscious) with a foreign body airway obstruction

Equipment: Mouth-to-mouth barrier device, gloves, CPR mannequin

Steps	Reasons
1. For a conscious patient, ask, "Are you choking?" If the patient can speak or cough, the obstruction is not complete. Observe the patient for increased distress and assist as needed, but do not perform abdominal thrusts.	The patient who is coughing or speaking can breathe and may be able to remove the obstruction without assistance. Performing abdominal thrusts on a patient who is not in need of assistance may cause injury.
2. If the patient cannot speak or cough and is displaying the universal sign of distress (grasping the throat with both hands), follow these steps to perform abdominal thrusts and have a co-worker notify the physician: A. Stand behind the patient and wrap your arms around his or her waist. B. Make a fist with your nondominant hand, with the thumb side against the patient's abdomen between the navel and the xiphoid process. **Step 2 B.** Make a fist, with the thumb side against the abdomen. C. Grasp your fist with your dominant hand and give quick upward thrusts. Completely relax your arms between each thrust and make each thrust forceful enough to dislodge the obstruction in the airway.	
3. Repeat the thrusts until the object is expelled and the patient can breathe or the patient becomes unconscious.	Several thrusts may be necessary to expel the object.
4. If the patient is unconscious OR becomes unconscious, perform a tongue-jaw lift followed by a finger sweep to remove the object if possible.	Before performing the tongue-jaw lift and finger sweep, apply clean examination gloves to avoid contact with the patient's oral secretions.
5. Open the airway and try to give the patient two rescue breaths (see Procedure 26-2)	Repositioning the patient's head ensures that the airway obstruction is not caused by improper head position.
6. If rescue breaths are obstructed, begin abdominal thrusts: A. Straddle the patient's hips.	

(continued)

PROCEDURE 26-4: | **Manage a Foreign Body Airway Obstruction (Adult)** *(continued)*

Steps	Reasons

B. Place the palm of one hand between the patient's navel and the xiphoid process.

C. Lace your fingers with the other hand against the back of the properly positioned hand.

---

7. Give five abdominal thrusts, and then repeat the tongue-jaw lift and finger sweep maneuver. Attempt to give rescue breaths. If rescue breaths adequately ventilate the patient, continue rescue breaths until the patient resumes breathing OR EMS arrives, as indicated by the physician. While you are performing rescue breathing, periodically check for a carotid pulse and be prepared to start CPR if necessary.

---

8. If no object is removed after the finger sweep or the lungs cannot be inflated during the attempted rescue breaths, continue the cycle of abdominal thrusts, tongue-jaw lift, finger sweep, and rescue breaths until EMS arrives.

NOTE: Obese or pregnant patients require chest thrusts rather than abdominal thrusts. Children over the age of 8 years are considered to be adults for the purpose of foreign body airway obstruction.

All health care professionals should take an approved training course in CPR, use of an AED, and managing a foreign body airway obstruction in an approved program. This procedure is not intended to substitute for proficiency training with a mannequin in a structured educational protocol.

Charting Example:

07/09/2008 2:15 PM Pt. choked on a throat lozenge in the examination room. Abdominal thrusts x6
administered; lozenge removed. Dr. Kramer notified. Pulse 104, respirations 26, BP 160/98 (R)
—R. Lent, CMA

PROCEDURE 26-5:   Control Bleeding

Purpose: Adequately control external bleeding to prevent further hemorrhage and shock
Equipment: Gloves, sterile gauze pads

Steps	Reasons
1. Identify the patient and determine, if possible, what type of accident caused the external bleeding. Immediately escort the patient to an examination room and have someone notify the physician.	Injuries that are due to the use of a weapon will require reporting to the local law enforcement authorities.
2. Obtain clean examination gloves and an adequate supply of sterile gauze pads, preferably 4 × 4–size pads.	The gloves will protect you from the patient's blood, whereas the sterile gauze pads will prevent microorganisms from entering the open wound. If sterile gauze pads are not immediately available, the use of nonsterile gauze pads to control bleedings is appropriate until sterile pads can be obtained.
3. Apply the exam gloves and quickly open two to three packages of gauze pads. Instruct the patient to lie down on the exam table if he/she has not already done so.	Having the patient lie down reduces the risk of fainting.
4. Using the sterile gauze pads, apply direct pressure to the wound. Maintain pressure until the bleeding stops. Hold pressure for at least 20 minutes without removing the gauze to check for bleeding.	Lifting the gauze to check for continued bleeding may remove any clots that are beginning to form, causing the bleeding to resume or worsen. **Step 4.** Apply direct pressure to the wound.
5. If the bleeding continues or seeps through the gauze, do not remove it. Apply additional gauze on top of the saturated gauze while continuing to apply direct pressure.	
6. As directed by the physician, apply direct pressure to the artery delivering blood to the area while continuing to apply direct pressure to the wound.	Pressure points include the brachial artery, the radial artery, the femoral artery, and the popliteal artery.
7. Once the bleeding is controlled, be prepared to assist the physician with a minor office surgical procedure to close the wound OR notify EMS for transport to the hospital as directed by the physician.	Always monitor the patient for signs of shock and be prepared to treat the patient appropriately.

Charting Example:

01/20/2008 1:45 PM Pt. presented with laceration to left hand due to hand saw accident at home. Wound approximately 4 inches across palm of hand and bleeding profusely. Direct pressure applied. Dr. Smith notified
—S. Jones, CMA

01/20/2008 1:50 PM Bleeding controlled after direct pressure to brachial artery per Dr. Smith. Wound bandaged, pt. transported to General Hospital emergency room per EMS
—S. Jones, CMA

MEDIA MENU

- **Student CD**
  - **Case Studies**
    Interactive Case Study 2: Managing a
    Medical Office Emergency
    Interactive Case Study 1: Triage in an
    Emergency Situation, Communication,
    and Documentation
  - **CMA/RMA Certification Exam Review**
- **LWW's Medical Assisting Skills DVD**
  - **Procedure 26-1**
- **Premium Online Course**
  http://thePoint.lww.com/Kronenberger3e
- **Internet Resources**

  **LiveAdvise Online Tutoring & Competency
  Training**
  http://thePoint.lww.com/LiveAdvise

  **American Association of Poison Control
  Centers**
  www.aapcc.org

  American Heart Association
  www.americanheart.org

  American Red Cross
  www.redcross.org

  American Safety and Health Institute
  www.ashinstitute.com

  National Safety Council
  www.nsc.org

español
SPANISH TERMINOLOGY

Tiene dolor?
  Do you have pain?
Tiene dificultad para respirar?
  Are you having any problem breathing?
Cuando ocurrio el accidente?
  When did the accident happen?
Calmese, por favor. La ambulancia esta en camino.
  Calm down, please. The ambulance is on the way.

Chapter Summary

Dealing with a medical emergency in the office will require you to:

- Communicate clearly and calmly.
- Recognize the need for immediate medical intervention.
- Perform emergency procedures immediately and competently.
- Provide first aid and life support measures that can mean the difference between life and death.
- Reassure the patient and family members.
- Work with the physician and other health care team members efficiently and with confidence.

1. When an emergency occurs, the patient's family members may become anxious and emotionally distraught. How can you help to calm an anxious family member?

2. Investigate the Good Samaritan law in your state. Prepare a poster describing the laws in your state.

3. While obtaining a chief complaint, your patient complains of shortness of breath. His respiratory rate is 36, and his skin is cool and clammy. What should be your next steps? Why?

4. The mother of a 15-year-old boy calls the office and tells you that her son has just been stung by a bee. She says he has never been stung before, and she is concerned about the amount of swelling around the site of the sting on his arm. However, you hear him coughing in the background. Are there any questions that you might want to ask the mother? How would you handle this call?

5. On a hot summer day, the mail carrier comes into your office to deliver the mail and collapses on the floor in the reception area. You notice that his skin is flushed and hot to touch. Should you move this person to an exam room? What could be the possible cause for his symptoms? How would you treat this patient?

Answers   to Checkpoint Questions

1. Before the ambulance arrives, you should document basic identification, the chief complaint, times that specific events occurred, vital signs, techniques used to treat the patient, and any observations.

2. The purpose of the primary assessment is to identify and correct any life-threatening problems.

3. The diagnostic signs of the secondary assessment are general appearance, level of consciousness, vital signs, and skin appearance.

4. Shock is defined as lack of oxygen to individual cells resulting from low blood pressure. The patient in shock will have a variety of signs including low blood pressure, a rapid and weak pulse, cool and clammy skin, and pale skin with cyanosis.

5. Treat an open wound that is bleeding by applying direct pressure until the bleeding has been controlled. If an item is impaled, immobilize the impaled object, but do not remove it.

6. The four major types of burn injuries are thermal, electrical, chemical, and radiation.

7. Splinting helps prevent further injury to soft tissues, blood vessels, and nerves from sharp bone fragments and relieves pain by stopping motion at the fracture site.

8. Epilepsy, head injury, and drug toxicity can cause seizure activity in a patient.

9. The primary cause of death from anaphylaxis is airway obstruction.

10. The poison control center staff can assist with evaluating a potential or known toxic exposure and instruct you on procedures to follow including possibly administering syrup of ipecac to induce vomiting if indicated.

11. Heat exhaustion is caused by physical exertion in a hot environment while the body temperature remains normal or slightly above normal. Heat stroke is characterized by a rapid rise in body temperature, often above 105°F. Heat stroke is a true medical emergency.

FUNDAMENTALS OF CLINICAL MEDICAL ASSISTING
(CHAPTERS 16–26)

1. While checking today's schedule in the family practice office where you work, you notice the following patients are scheduled for this morning:

   • A biopsy of a suspicious mole at 9:00 AM

   • A routine adult physical examination at 10:00 AM for an established patient.

   • An incision and drainage of a furuncle at 8:00 AM

   • Four new patients are being seen throughout the morning before lunch at 12:00 PM

   A. What instruments and sterile supplies will the physician need to perform the biopsy and incision and drainage procedures? (knowledge)

   B. Explain how you will prepare each of the minor office surgical patients for the procedures to be performed today. (comprehension)

   C. One of the new patients being seen today is elderly and has arthritis of the fingers, which are obviously deformed. She is unable to hold a pen or pencil to fill out the new patient paperwork. How would you solve this problem? What safety issues might apply to this patient in the medical office? (application)

   D. How would you plan your morning based on this schedule? (analysis)

   E. What could happen if one of the new patients becomes light-headed and faints while having blood taken for some routine tests? (synthesis)

   F. Based on what you know, what judgment would you make about the absence of a surgical consent form for the patient having the incision and drainage procedure? (evaluation)

2. The physician in your office has asked you to schedule and give the patient information about having a barium swallow and a barium enema at a local outpatient facility.

   A. How would you explain these procedures to the patient who is concerned about having too many x-rays? (knowledge)

   B. What digestive organs will the barium swallow allow the physician to visualize, and what will be visualized during the barium enema? (comprehension)

   C. Explain what preparation is necessary for the patient for each of these radiographic procedures. (application)

   D. Which of these two procedures should be scheduled first, and why? (analysis)

   E. What would happen, if anything, if the patient did not follow the proper procedure for preparing for either of these x-rays? (synthesis)

   F. Describe how you could support the patient while giving instructions to the patient who needs to have these two procedures performed? (evaluation)

3. During a busy afternoon at your medical office, you have been notified by the receptionist that a patient in the waiting area is complaining of difficulty breathing. The physician is currently with another patient in an examination room.

   A. Why did the receptionist alert you about this patient? (knowledge)

   B. Explain the various reasons why a patient may complain of difficulty breathing. (comprehension)

   C. After going to the reception area and bringing the patient to an examination room, what questions would you ask the patient? (application)

   D. Would it be appropriate to obtain vital signs on this patient? Why or why not? (analysis)

   E. Suppose the patient collapsed and stopped breathing in the reception area. How would you react? (synthesis)

   F. How would you justify starting cardiopulmonary resuscitation including chest compressions for a patient who has collapsed and stopped breathing? (evaluation)

4. The physician has ordered you to administer an intradermal injection TB test on the patient in your office who will be starting a new job next week. You are also to give an antibiotic intramuscular injection to another patient.

   A. Where would you administer the TB test? (knowledge)

   B. Compare the supplies (needles, syringes) used for these two types of injections. Explain the similarities and the differences. (comprehension)

   C. How would you choose the muscle to use to administer the intramuscular antibiotic? (application)

D. What questions would you ask either patient before administering these injections? (analysis)

E. How could you adapt this situation for the patient who does not speak English? (synthesis)

F. What is the value or importance of wearing gloves while administering injected medications? (evaluation)

5. While taking the vital signs of an established patient who complains of nausea, your adult patient suddenly grabs the waste basket in the examination room and vomits into the trash can. His skin is pale and moist, and he seems "shaky."

A. What medical terminology could you use to describe this patient in the medical record? (knowledge)

B. Can you explain why the patient is shaky and pale? (comprehension)

C. In addition to obtaining the vital signs, what questions could you ask the patient to assist the physician in making an accurate diagnosis? (application)

D. What interference can you make abou the patient's blood pressure based on his skin color and condition? (analysis)

E. How would you adapt this situation to avoid the patient from having to use the exam room trash can to vomit? (synthesis)

F. Would you recommend that this patient lie down? Why or why not? (evaluation)

CHAPTER

27

Dermatology

Outline

Common Disorders of the Integumentary System
Skin Infections
Inflammatory Reactions
Disorders of Wound Healing
Disorders Caused by Pressure
Alopecia

Disorders of Pigmentation
Skin Cancers
Diagnostic Procedures
Physical Examination of the Skin
Wound Cultures
Skin Biopsy

Urine Melanin
Wood's Light Analysis
Bandaging
Types of Bandages
Bandage Application Guidelines

Learning Objectives

Upon successfully completing this chapter, you will be able to:

1. Spell and define key terms

2. Describe common skin disorders

3. Explain common diagnostic procedures

4. Prepare the patient for examination of the integument

5. Assist the physician with examination of the integument

6. Explain the difference between bandages and dressings and give the purpose of each

7. Identify the guidelines for applying bandages

Performance Objectives

Upon successfully completing this chapter, you will be able to:

1. Apply a warm or cold compress (Procedure 27-1)

2. Assist with therapeutic soaks (Procedure 27-2)

3. Apply a tubular gauze bandage (Procedure 27-3)

Competencies

CAAHEP

• Practice standard precautions

• Prepare patient for and assist with routine and specialty examinations

• Document appropriately

• Instruct individuals according to their needs

• Provide instruction for health maintenance and disease prevention

Competencies *(continued)*

ABHES

- Prepare patients for procedures
- Practice standard precautions
- Assist physician with examinations and treatments
- Document accurately

Key Terms

alopecia	erythema	macule	seborrhea
bulla	folliculitis	neoplasm	urticaria
carbuncle	furuncle	pediculosis	verruca
cellulitis	herpes simplex	pruritus	vesicle
dermatophytosis	herpes zoster	psoriasis	
eczema	impetigo	pustule	

Common Disorders of the Integumentary System

The skin, or integument, is the largest organ of the body. Clear skin glowing with health indicates a good general state of wellness; pallor, cyanosis, or dry, scaly skin indicates poor general health. Although it has many functions, including maintaining homeostasis, one of the most important functions of the integumentary system is to protect the underlying tissues and organs from the external environment. Figure 27-1 shows a cross-section of the normal anatomy of the skin and accessory structures. Unbroken skin provides a protective barrier that prevents the entrance of microorganisms and is the body's first line of defense against infection. In addition, the skin protects the body from mechanical injury, damaging substances, and the ultraviolet rays of the sun. The study of the skin is dermatology, and a physician who specializes in disorders of the skin is a dermatologist. The general practice physician may diagnose diseases of the integumentary system or may refer patients to the dermatologist.

 CHECKPOINT QUESTION

1. How does the skin help to prevent infectious microorganisms from entering the body?

Skin Infections

Many integumentary disorders are manifested by lesions or abnormalities in skin tissue (Fig. 27-2). These lesions may be primary or secondary to primary lesions. When working with a patient who may have a skin infection, you should always wear protective equipment, such as examination gloves, since the drainage from any lesions may be infective.

Bacterial Infections
Impetigo

Impetigo is a contagious bacterial infection of the skin that is common in young children. It may be caused by *Staphylococcus* or *Streptococcus* microorganisms. Lesions appear on exposed areas, such as the face and neck. Terms used to describe many skin lesions, not just those seen in a patient with impetigo, include the following:

Macule: small, flat skin discoloration (Fig. 27-2A).
Vesicle: small fluid-filled sac (Fig. 27-2D).
Bulla: large fluid-filled sac (Fig. 27-2E).
Pustule: pus-filled sac (Fig. 27-2F).

Initially, impetigo may appear as an area of **erythema**; however, patches of vesicles that produce honey-colored drainage and crusts follow the redness (Fig. 27-2K). These vesicles leave red areas when the crusts are removed. Treatment is washing the area two or three times a day and applying a topical antibiotic as ordered by the physician. Oral antibiotics may also be prescribed for severe cases. Scratching must be discouraged to prevent the spread of the infection, and patients must be instructed to wash towels, washcloths, and bed linens daily. Individuals at risk for developing impetigo are those in poor health, those with conditions such as anemia or malnutrition, and those with poor hygiene; however, any person handling contaminated laundry or otherwise exposed to the infectious material should be

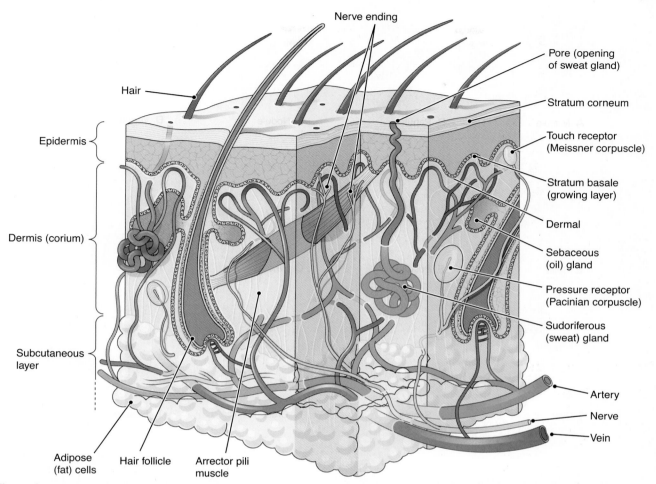

Figure 27-1 Cross section of the skin. (Reprinted with permission from Cohen BJ. Memmler's The Human Body in Health and Disease. Philadelphia: Lippincott Williams & Wilkins, 2005.)

encouraged to practice frequent medical asepsis such as handwashing.

Folliculitis

Folliculitis is a superficial infection of a hair follicle (Fig. 27-2N). It is characterized by itching, burning, and the formation of a pustule. Treatment is aimed at promoting drainage and healing. Saline soaks or compresses (Procedures 27-1 and 27-2) may be ordered for 15 minutes twice a day followed by application of an anti-infective ointment or cream and a dressing to absorb any drainage. If folliculitis is left untreated, it may lead to the formation of an abscess. An abscess is formed when a small sac of pus, or purulent material, accumulates at the site of inflammation. The causative agent of these infections is often *Staphylococcus*.

Furuncle

A **furuncle**, more commonly known as a boil, is a deep-seated infection of a hair follicle or gland (Fig. 27-2O). Friction and pressure at the site may contribute to its formation. A hard, painful nodule forms (Fig. 27-2C),

enlarges for several days, and then erupts, with pus oozing from the site. The cause of the infection is often *Staphylococcus*. Treatment of a furuncle includes application of moist heat to assist in ripening it, or bringing it to a head, and antibiotic therapy. Often a minor surgical procedure known as incision and drainage (I & D) is performed to remove the purulent material and facilitate healing. (Chapter 22 discusses incision and drainage in detail.)

Carbuncle

A **carbuncle** consists of infection in an interconnected group of hair follicles or several furuncles joined together in a mass (Fig. 27-2P). The subcutaneous tissue in the surrounding area is also involved, and *Staphylococcus* is often responsible. Carbuncles are hard, round, extremely painful swellings that enlarge over several days to a week. Eventually they soften and erupt, discharging pus from several sites. When the skin sloughs away, a scarred cavity remains. The patient often has a fever.

Treatment of a carbuncle is with systemic antibiotics, moist heat (Procedures 27-1 and 27-2), and inci-

Figure 27-2 Skin lesions. Primary lesions: (**A**) Macule. Flat, circumscribed discoloration. (**B**) Papule. Palpable elevated solid lesion smaller than 1 cm; colors vary. (**C**) Nodule. Raised solid lesion larger than 1 cm. (**D**) Vesicle. Small elevation filled with clear fluid. (**E**) Bulla. Vesicle or blister larger than 1 cm. (**F**) Pustule. Lesion containing pus. (**G**) Wheal. Transient elevation of the skin caused by edema of the dermis and surrounding capillary dilation. (**H**) Plaque. Elevated solid lesion on skin or mucosa; larger than 1 cm. (**I**) Cyst. Tumor that contains semisolid or liquid material. Secondary lesions: (**J**) Scales. Heaped-up horny layer of dead epidermis. (**K**) Crust. Covering formed from serum, blood, or pus drying on the skin. (**L**) Fissures. Cracks in the skin. (**M**) Ulcer. Lesion formed by local destruction of the epidermis and part of the underlying dermis. Other lesions: (**N**) Superficial folliculitis. Local infection of a hair follicle. (**O**) Furuncle. Acute inflammation deep within hair follicle. (**P**) Carbuncle. Infection involving subcutaneous tissues around several hair follicles.

sion and drainage once the lesion has matured. A topical anti-infective agent and loose bandages are also applied to the area. The site may require a wick, or sterile gauze packing, to remain in the cavity for several days to facilitate healing.

Cellulitis

When an existing wound is infected and the infection spreads to the surrounding connective tissue, **cellulitis** results. The skin becomes hot, red, and edematous (Fig.

27-3). If it is not treated, the underlying tissue may be destroyed or develop an abscess. A systemic anti-infective, such as an antibiotic, usually provides rapid and successful treatment.

CHECKPOINT QUESTION

2. Which of the listed bacterial infections develop in the hair follicles?

Figure 27-3 Cellulitis infection.

Viral Infections
Herpes Simplex

Herpes simplex infections produce lesions commonly known as cold sores or fever blisters. The lesions, which appear on the lips, mouth, face, and nose, are small vesicles grouped on a red base. They eventually erupt, leaving a painful ulcer and then a crust. The infection may be precipitated by other infections, such as upper respiratory infections, or by menstruation, fatigue, trauma, stress, or exposure to the sun.

The causative agent is herpes simplex virus I (HSVI). Herpes simplex II is responsible for the sexually transmitted disease known as genital herpes. Typically, HSVI infections are recurrent, and no effective treatment eliminates or controls the disease. During an outbreak, the lesions appear and demonstrate the characteristics noted earlier and should be considered infectious. Antiviral drugs, such as valacyclovir or acyclovir, have been shown to decrease the severity of the outbreaks in some people, but they do not offer a cure. Treatment is aimed at relieving discomfort with topical anesthetic ointment to relieve the pain until the lesions heal, usually in 5 to 7 days.

Herpes Zoster

Herpes zoster, or shingles, is caused by the same virus that causes chickenpox. It is believed that, after an initial infection with the varicella virus, the virus lies dormant in the nervous system for years. Herpes zoster usually occurs in adults and may become active in times of physical or emotional stress or immunodepression. When reactivated, the virus spreads down a nerve to the skin, causing redness, swelling, and pain. After about 48 hours, a band of lesions develops (Fig. 27-4). They begin as papules, which are small, red solid elevations on the skin (Fig. 27-2B). Shingles commonly appear on

Figure 27-4 Herpes zoster (shingles).

the face, back, and chest and are frequently unilateral. These lesions progress to vesicles and pustules and then dry crusts and may last for 2 to 5 weeks. Scarring and alterations in pigmentation are common. Pain often remains after the lesions have disappeared, in some cases for several months.

The treatment of a herpes zoster breakout includes an opioid analgesic for the discomfort or nerve block for severe pain. Locally, calamine lotion may be used for itching. The area must be protected from air and the irritation of clothing. Acyclovir is sometimes used to alleviate the severity of the disease.

Verruca

A **verruca** is a wart, or squamous cell papilloma (benign skin tumor), that appears as a rough, raised lesion with a pitted surface. Verruca may occur singly or in groups and may be found anywhere on the skin or mucous membranes. They commonly appear on the fingers, hands, or feet and may vary in size, shape, and appearance. The causative agents include papilloma viruses, and the treatment is removal. Removing a wart may be achieved with keratolytic agents, which cause softening and shedding of the skin; liquid nitrogen, which freezes and destroys the affected tissue; podophyllum resin, a caustic agent found in many over-the-counter wart medications; laser therapy, which removes the affected tissue using radiation of the visible infrared spectrum of light; or surgical excision. They may also disappear spontaneously.

 CHECKPOINT QUESTION

3. How can viral skin infections be prevented?

Fungal Infections

Fungal infection of the skin (**dermatophytosis**) is caused by a group of molds called dermatophytes. The group of fungal diseases called tinea is collectively known as ringworm; its members are named according to the area of the body infected. All tinea infections are considered contagious.

There are several types of dermatophytes, but the treatment is similar, including the application of topical antifungal powders, creams, or shampoos. Antifungal medications such as griseofulvin may be prescribed orally for severe cases. Inflamed lesions may be treated with wet compresses or soaks.

Tinea Capitis

Tinea capitis affects the scalp. It is contagious and appears most frequently in children. It is characterized by round gray scaly patches (dried skin flakes) and areas of **alopecia** (baldness). There are usually no symptoms except light itching.

PATIENT EDUCATION

FUNGAL INFECTIONS

Because fungi thrive in moist conditions, a general measure for treating fungal infections and preventing the spread of infection is to keep the infected area clean and dry. Instruct patients diagnosed with fungal infections to wear loose-fitting clothing and launder clothing daily. Socks and underclothing should be changed frequently, and clothing should not be shared with others. Shower shoes should be worn in public showers and pools since these areas are usually wet, providing an optimum environment for the fungus to grow on floors and be transmitted directly to the feet.

Tinea Corporis

Tinea corporis (also known as tinea circinata) manifests on hairless portions of the body. It is characterized by itchy red rings that are clear in the center with a scaly border (Fig. 27-2J). It is frequently found on the face and arms but may also be found on the trunk (Fig. 27-5).

Tinea Cruris

Tinea cruris, known in lay terms as jock itch, is found on the skin in the groin area and the gluteal folds. The lesions, which cause marked itching, are red macules with clear centers and scaly borders.

Tinea Pedis

Tinea pedis, or athlete's foot, is characterized by itching, burning, and stinging between the toes and on the soles

Figure 27-5 Tinea corporis (ringworm) fungal infection.

of the feet. The lesions may appear as red, weepy vesicles, as chronic dry scales, or as fissures (crack-like lesions) between the toes (Fig. 27-2L).

Tinea Unguium

Also known as onychomycosis, tinea unguium causes thickening, discoloration, and crumbling of the nails, most often the toenails. It is difficult to cure and often requires months of local antifungal preparations. In severe cases, an oral antifungal medication, griseofulvin, is prescribed.

Tinea Versicolor

Tinea versicolor, also known as pityriasis versicolor, is a fungal infection; however, it is not caused by dermatophytes. It is not known exactly what sort of fungus is the causative agent. The disease causes a multicolor rash, generally over the upper trunk. It is most common in young people during warm weather, and it is chronic. Its lesions vary from macular to raised, round, or oval; vary from darkly pigmented to depigmented; and are slightly scaly. There are usually no symptoms. Diagnosis of tinea versicolor is determined with a Wood's light, an ultraviolet light used in a darkened room to show abnormalities in the skin as fluorescent. Treatment includes the use of selenium sulfide for 7 days along with topical antifungal cream or lotion.

 CHECKPOINT QUESTION

4. Why should you avoid direct contact with skin lesions?

Parasitic Infections
Scabies

Scabies is a contagious skin disorder caused by the itch mite *Sarcoptes scabiei*. It is spread by direct contact and produces small vesicles or pustules between the fingers and at the inner wrist, elbows, axillae, waist, and groin.

The itching caused by the mite is worst at night, when the female burrows under the epidermis to lay her eggs.

Treatment for scabies is aimed at disinfestation. For adults, an antiparasitic such as 1% lindane cream is applied from the neck down at bedtime. One application of 5% permethrin, or Elimite, cream is effective and is the drug of choice for children. All bedding and clothing for the entire family should be laundered daily until the infestation is resolved.

Pediculosis

Pediculosis is an infestation of the skin with a parasite known commonly as lice. Three types of the louse *Pediculus humanus* infest the body: *P. humanis var. capitis* infests the scalp (pediculosis capitis) and the eyelashes or eyelids (pediculosis palpebrarum); and *P. humanis var. corporis* or *var. vestimenti* is found on the body (pediculosis corporis) and the pubic hairs (pediculosis pubis). Wherever they are found, itching is intense, and the skin often becomes secondarily infected from scratching. Lice feed on human blood and lay eggs (nits) on body hair or clothing fibers. Nits may be seen on hair shafts close to the skin or in seams of clothing.

Pediculosis is common among populations with overcrowding, such as head lice in schools, and poor hygiene. The infestation is transmitted through physical contact with an infested person, by sitting on an infested toilet seat, or by sharing a comb, brush, clothing, or bedding that is infested. Benzene hexachloride creams, lotions, or shampoos are used for all types of pediculosis. All clothing and linen must be dry cleaned or washed in hot water and ironed. Sealing items in plastic bags for 30 days or heating them to 140°F will kill lice on items that cannot be laundered.

 CHECKPOINT QUESTION

5. How are parasitic skin infections spread?

Inflammatory Reactions

Eczema

Eczema is an inflammatory skin disorder usually involving only the epidermal layer of the skin. It is more common in children than adults and is characterized by itching and lesions that generally begin as red patches, proceed to weepy vesicles, and end up as dry scaly crusts (Fig. 27-6). They appear on the face, neck, bends of the knees and elbows, and the upper trunk. It is not clear why some patients develop this disorder, which is chronic and may have periods of remission and exacerbation. Possible causes of eczema depend on the individual and may include the following:

- Food allergies to fish, eggs, and milk products
- Medication or chemical allergies

Figure 27-6 Eczema.

- Sensitivity to irritating soaps, household cleaning products, deodorants, and perfumes
- Inhalants such as pollen, dust, or animal dander
- Poor circulation to a body part
- Ultraviolet rays

Treatment is removing the cause and promoting healing of the lesions. The causative agent should be avoided if it is known. The patient should maintain good hydration and keep the skin well moistened with emollients. A humid environment is recommended. Warm, not hot, baths should be taken daily with a nondrying soap. The skin should be dried immediately, and scratchy clothing should be avoided.

Exudative lesions are treated with soaks, baths, or wet dressings for 10 to 30 minutes three or four times daily. Domeboro, Aveeno, or bicarbonate is good for these purposes. In addition, the physician may order the following treatments:

- Topical corticosteroid lotion, cream, or ointment to be used twice a day
- Bandages at night to protect against scratching
- Antihistamines for severe **pruritus** (itching)
- For scales, a topical steroid ointment. Systemic corticosteroids, such as prednisone, may be ordered in severe cases.

Seborrheic Dermatitis

Seborrheic dermatitis (skin inflammation), also known as **seborrhea**, is an overproduction of sebum. It is a chronic disorder resulting in greasy yellow scales primarily on the scalp, where it is called seborrheic dandruff. Underlying redness and pruritus may be present. The eyelids, face, chest, back, umbilicus, and body folds may also be affected. It is thought that seborrhea is caused by a genetic predisposition and a combination of hormones, nutrition, infection, or stress. It is treated with shampoo and topical corticosteroid lotion.

Urticaria

Urticaria, or hives, is an acute inflammatory reaction of the dermis. It begins with itching, followed by erythema and swelling. The wheals (Fig. 27-2G) have a pale center with a red edge. They resemble a mosquito bite and appear in clusters anywhere on the body. Hives are self-limiting, lasting from a few days to a few weeks. The most common causes include contact with these substances:

• Foods, including shellfish, strawberries, tomatoes, citrus fruits, eggs, and chocolate
• Inhalants, including feathers or animal dander
• Chemicals, cosmetics, and medications
• Sunlight
• Insect bites or stings
• Heat, cold, or pressure on the skin
• Infection
• Stress

Treatment of urticaria is reduction of the inflammatory response. The cause should be avoided if known. Antihistamines are usually given to reduce itching and swelling, and a short course of prednisone is sometimes ordered. Starch or Aveeno baths twice a day may be ordered to make the patient more comfortable. Epinephrine is given if the symptoms of urticaria develop rapidly and are associated with dyspnea. These symptoms are indicative of anaphylaxis, a severe life-threatening emergency (see Chapter 26).

Acne Vulgaris

Acne vulgaris is an inflammatory disease of the sebaceous glands. Its cause is not known in all cases, and it may occur in any adult, but it commonly occurs during adolescence as a result of the increase in hormone production. It is characterized by pimples, comedones (blackheads), cysts (fluid-filled sacs beneath the skin) (Fig. 27-2I), and scarring. The lesions may occur on the face, neck, upper chest, back, and shoulders. Overactive sebaceous glands produce excessive sebum that gets trapped in a follicle, producing a dark substance that results in a blackhead. Leukocytes accumulate, producing pus.

Treatment for acne includes a regimen of tretinoin (Retin-A), benzoyl peroxide, and tetracycline. Sunlamp treatments are sometimes used to dry the lesions.

Psoriasis

Psoriasis is a chronic inflammatory skin disorder characterized by bright red plaques (Fig. 27-2H) covered with dry, silvery scales. Although the cause is unknown, it is a chronic disorder and often difficult to treat. Psoriasis is usually found on the scalp, elbows, knees, base of the spine, palms, soles, and around the nails (Fig. 27-7). There are usually no vesicles, and itching varies from mild to severe. Exacerbations are common during cold weather, stress, and pregnancy. Treatment includes tar preparations and topical steroid cream or

Figure 27-7 Psoriasis.

ointment. Exposure to ultraviolet light three times a week may also be prescribed.

 CHECKPOINT QUESTION

6. How are eczema and psoriasis different?

Disorders of Wound Healing

Keloids

Keloids, an overproduction of scar tissue, occur as a complication of wound healing. The scar tissue forms as a result of excessive collagen accumulation. A raised nodule forms and does not resolve with time. The cause is unknown. It occurs most frequently in young women, especially during pregnancy, and is particularly common in African Americans. The most common sites are the neck and shoulders. Injections of cortisone are sometimes effective in treating keloids.

Disorders Caused by Pressure

Callus and Corn

A callus, sometimes called a callosity, is a raised painless thickening of the epidermis. It is caused by pressure or friction on the hands and feet. A corn is a hard, raised thickening of the stratum corneum on the toes. It results from chronic friction and pressure, especially from poorly fitting shoes. The pressure compresses the dermis, making it thin and tender and causing pain and inflammation. Soft corns can form between the toes.

The treatment for calluses and corns begins with relieving the pressure. Shoes should be made of soft leather and fit properly. Liners may be inserted in shoes to relieve pressure. Bandages and corn pads also help correct the problem. In some cases, the physician recommends surgical intervention or use of a keratolytic agent to cause chemical peeling.

Decubitus Ulcers

Decubitus ulcers are also called pressure sores and are caused by prolonged pressure to an area of the body, usually over a bony prominence (Fig. 27-2M). The pressure impairs blood supply, oxygen, and nutrition to the area, which results in an ulcerative lesion and eventual tissue death. The most common sites are over the sacrum and hips, but these ulcers may also occur on the back of the head, ears, elbows, heels, and ankles. They are most common in aged, debilitated, and immobilized patients. Bedridden and wheelchair-bound patients are at risk for developing decubiti unless they are repositioned frequently, every 2 hours, to relieve pressure. Special mattresses, pads, and pillows are useful in preventing pressure sores.

Decubitus ulcers are graded, or staged, according to the degree of tissue involvement (Table 27-1). Treatment consists of topical antibiotic powder and adhesive absorbent bandages and dressings. Deep infections may require systemic antibiotics and possibly surgical debridement.

WHAT IF?

An elderly patient comes into the office with multiple decubitus ulcers. What should you do?

The elderly are always at risk for developing skin ulcerations; however, the physician must assess the situation to determine whether the patient is receiving adequate care at home. Patients who arrive in the medical office with multiple ulcers in different stages of healing may be abused or neglected. Elder abuse is less often identified, but some experts believe it is as common as child abuse. If you suspect elder abuse, contact your local department of social services. The investigation may substantiate the abuse (requiring referral to law enforcement) or may identify ways to alleviate the situation (caregiver education, respite care) without removing the patient from home. In some states, the law requires reporting elder abuse. The physician who fails to do so can be fined or be subject to other penalties.

Intertrigo

Intertrigo is a disorder of skin breakdown that occurs in the body folds of obese persons. The combination of heat, moisture, and friction of the skin against itself in these areas causes the skin to break down. Humid climates and poor hygiene often aggravate the condition. Erythema and skin fissures result, and the affected area itches, stings, and burns.

Treatment for intertrigo is proper hygiene and an attempt to keep the area clean and dry. Talcum powder or cornstarch is often recommended. Antibacterial or antifungal lotion or powder is necessary if secondary infection is present.

 CHECKPOINT QUESTION

7. What patients are most at risk for developing decubitus ulcers?

Alopecia

Alopecia, or baldness, may be the result of physical trauma, systemic disease, bacteria or fungal infection, chemotherapy, excessive radiation, hormonal imbalance, or genetic predisposition. Baldness caused by scarring and inherited male pattern baldness are permanent and cannot be reversed; however, the drug minoxidil may be recommended by the physician to stimulate hair growth in male pattern baldness. For other causes of baldness, treatment of the underlying disorder often results in new hair growth.

Disorders of Pigmentation

Albinism

Albinism is a genetically determined condition of partial or total absence of the pigment melanin in the skin, hair, and eyes. The skin is pale, the hair is white, and the irises of the eyes appear pink (Fig. 27-8). The skin will not tan and is prone to sunburn. Because no pigment is present to protect the underlying eye structures from the ultraviolet rays of the sun, eye problems may develop as a result of this disorder. Albinism has no treatment.

TABLE 27-1	Staging or Grading for Decubitus Ulcers
Stage	**Description**
I	Red skin does not return to normal when massaged or when pressure is relieved.
II	Skin is blistered, peeling, or cracked superficially.
III	Skin is broken, with loss of full thickness; subcutaneous tissue may be damaged; serous or bloody drainage may be present.
IV	Deep, crater-like ulcer shows destruction of subcutaneous tissue; fascia, connective tissue, bone, or muscle may be exposed and may be damaged.

Figure 27-8 Albinism.

Vitiligo

Vitiligo is a progressive chronic destruction of melanocytes, which are cells in the epidermis that produce melanin, a skin pigment. This disorder is thought to be an autoimmune disorder in patients with an inherited predisposition. The depigmented areas occur as white patches that sometimes have a hyperpigmented border. It usually occurs in exposed areas of the skin.

There is no effective treatment for vitiligo. Patients are advised to protect the areas from the sun because they are prone to sunburn in the absence of melanin. Waterproof cosmetics may be used to cover the area.

Leukoderma

Leukoderma is a permanent local loss of skin pigment that results from damage caused by skin trauma. It is particularly common in African Americans. Causes of leukoderma include contact with caustic chemicals and the sequela of burns or infection.

Nevus

A nevus, also known as a birthmark or mole, is a congenital pigmented skin blemish. It is usually circumscribed and may involve the epidermis, connective tissue, nerves, or blood vessels. Nevi are usually benign, not cancerous, but may become malignant (cancerous). Patients should be cautioned to watch for changes in the

color, size, and texture of any nevus. Bleeding and itching should also be reported (Box 27-1).

 CHECKPOINT QUESTION

8. Which of the disorders of pigmentation are inherited?

Skin Cancers

Basal Cell Carcinoma

Basal cell carcinoma is a slow-growing cancer that appears most commonly on exposed areas of the body, usually the face, but may also occur on the shoulders or chest. The lesion has a waxy appearance with a depressed center and a rolled edge where blood vessels may be apparent. Metastasis (spreading to other areas of the body) almost never occurs, but if left untreated, the lesions will grow locally and may ulcerate and damage surrounding tissues (Fig. 27-9). The most common treatment for basal cell carcinoma is surgical removal, and this may be done in the physician's or dermatologist's office. Radiation therapy and cryosurgery, or removal using a cold agent such as liquid nitrogen, are alternative treatments.

BOX 27-1

WHEN IS A SKIN LESION ABNORMAL?

Most melanomas, a type of skin cancer, are pigmented, elevated skin lesions that frequently develop from a new or existing mole. The key to treatment of this potentially deadly cancer is early detection of changes in size, color, shape, elevation, texture, or consistency of any pigmented area, old or new, or of any spot or bump. Being familiar with what is normal for you will help you notice what is abnormal.

The eventual outcome of melanoma is governed by how deeply it has invaded the skin, which also determines how aggressively the cancer will be treated. A cancer prevention message first used in Australia and currently being promoted in the United States is "Slip! Slop! Slap! Wrap!" which may help individuals to remember: Slip on a shirt, Slop on sunscreen, Slap on a hat, and put on Wrap-around sunglasses to protect your eyes and the skin around them.

Figure 27-9 Basal cell carcinoma. (Reprinted with permission from Goodheart HP. Goodheart's Photoguide of Common Skin Disorders. Philadelphia: Lippincott Williams & Wilkins, 2003.)

Squamous Cell Carcinoma

Squamous cell carcinoma is slightly less common than basal cell carcinoma and occurs in any squamous (scaly) epithelial area of the body, such as the lungs, cervix, or anus, but is most frequently found on the skin (Fig. 27-10). This type of skin cancer is a slow-growing, malignant **neoplasm** (tumor). The lesions are firm, red, horny or prickly, and painless, and they range widely in size. Those on exposed areas are thought to result from exposure to the sun. Other areas not normally exposed, such as mucous membranes, are thought to be affected as the result of frequent irritation. Treatment is the same as for basal cell carcinoma. Although basal cell carcinoma is not generally metastatic, squamous cell carcinoma will spread readily through underlying and surrounding tissues.

Figure 27-10 Squamous cell carcinoma. (Reprinted with permission from Goodheart HP. Goodheart's Photoguide of Common Skin Disorders. Philadelphia: Lippincott Williams & Wilkins, 2003.)

Malignant Melanoma

Malignant melanoma is a cancer of the skin that forms from melanocytes. Lesions vary from macules to nodules and often have an irregular border and a variety of colors (Fig. 27-11). Mixtures of white, blue, purple, and red are the most common. The tumor grows both in radius and in depth into the dermis. In about 30% to 35% of cases, it grows in a pre-existing nevus.

Malignant melanoma, which is thought to be caused by excessive exposure to sunlight, is the leading cause of death due to skin disease. It is the ninth most common cancer. The incidence is one in 105 individuals in the United States. Those at highest risk for developing the disease have blond or red hair, fair skin, blue eyes, and a tendency to sunburn and spend a lot of time out of doors (Box 27-2).

Treatment of malignant melanoma is surgical removal after a biopsy, possibly including removal of lymph tissue. The patient's prognosis depends on the depth of the tumor. Tumors over 1.5 mm often metastasize to the lymph nodes, liver, lungs, and brain and are often fatal.

 CHECKPOINT QUESTION

9. Which is more likely to metastasize, basal cell or squamous cell carcinoma?

 PATIENT EDUCATION

PLAYING IT SAFE IN THE SUN

During the summertime, many teenagers enjoy lying on the beach and acquiring a tan, while others are exposed to the sun by working outdoors in jobs such as lifeguarding. These two habits can lead to long-term skin problems. As a medical assistant, you can help educate teenagers about these risks. The following patient education tips

(continued)

1 cm   1 cm

A   **B**

Figure 27-11 Malignant melanoma. **(A)** Left: Superficial melanoma. **(B)** Right: Nodular melanoma.

are useful reminders for any patient who is exposed to excessive sunlight:

- The powerful rays of the sun can injure your eyes. Always wear sunglasses.
- Even one sunburn can increase your potential for developing skin cancer.
- A hat can prevent sunburn on the scalp. Also, a hat can help keep the sun away from the face.
- Use the highest level of sun block that is available. Apply it frequently.
- Do not apply oil to the skin to tan faster.
- Avoid lying on the beach during peak sun hours. Enjoy beach activities during the early morning or late afternoon.

Diagnostic Procedures

Physical Examination of the Skin

Examination of the skin is performed primarily by inspection. Many lesions can be diagnosed by the characteristic size, shape, and distribution on the skin; however, laboratory studies may be necessary to confirm a diagnosis. As the medical assistant, you may assemble the equipment as directed by the physician, verify that an informed consent has been obtained for surgical procedures, and properly direct specimens to the appropriate laboratories. Observe standard precautions when handling any specimens, including those obtained from the skin.

Before the examination, prepare the examination room and the patient. Use a gown and draping appropriate to the patient's symptoms and area to be examined. During the examination, aid the physician by ensuring

---

BOX 27-2
EFFECTS OF SUNLIGHT ON THE SKIN

In addition to sunburn and premature aging, exposure to the sun's ultraviolet rays is the major cause of skin cancers. Primary prevention of skin cancer consists of limiting exposure to ultraviolet light by wearing proper clothing and using sunscreen. Exposure to the sun is not recommended during the 5 peak hours of the day: 10:00 AM to 3:00 PM. A sunscreen with at least a 15 SPF (sun protective factor) is considered good protection in blocking ultraviolet rays. Although many sunscreens contain PABA (aminobenzoic acid), which may cause allergy in some people, a number of PABA-free sunscreens are available. Exposure to ultraviolet rays through the use of sunlamps and tanning beds should also be discouraged.

---

that the lighting is adequate and directed properly, assisting in obtaining wound cultures, maintaining asepsis, and applying topical medications, sterile dressings, and bandages. Protect skin lesions from further infection by using medical or surgical asepsis as indicated.

After the dermatologic examination, reinforce the physician instructions about caring for the skin condition at home, including:

- Keeping bandages clean and dry
- Returning to the office to have sutures or staples removed
- How long to avoid getting the area wet
- Applying topical medications

When the patient has left the office, clean and disinfect the examination room according to the office policy.

Wound Cultures

Obtain a wound culture by getting a sample of wound exudate (drainage) using a sterile swab, applying the specimen to a growth medium, and allowing the microorganisms to grow. A sample of the culture is placed on a slide in the laboratory and observed under a microscope to diagnose the type of the bacterial or fungal infection. Chapter 44 describes the specific procedure for collecting a wound specimen.

 CHECKPOINT QUESTION

10. What are the responsibilities of the medical assistant regarding diagnosing skin lesions?

Skin Biopsy

The purpose of a skin biopsy is to remove a small piece of tissue from a lesion so that it may be examined under a microscope to determine whether it is a benign or malignant growth. A local anesthetic is injected by the physician, and sterile asepsis is used throughout the procedure (see Chapter 22). The three types of skin biopsy performed by the physician are excision, punch, and shave. In an excision biopsy, the entire lesion is removed for evaluation. When a punch biopsy is done, a small section is removed from the center of the lesion. A shave biopsy cuts the lesion off just above the skin line. Regardless of the method used to obtain the skin biopsy, samples of tissue are sent to the laboratory for analysis.

Urine Melanin

Melanin is not normally present in the urine unless the patient has malignant melanoma. A urine test to detect the presence of melanin is done with a random sample of urine from the patient. The specimen is sent to the laboratory, allowed to sit for 24 hours, and then examined under a microscope for the presence of melanin.

Wood's Light Analysis

Wood's light is an ultraviolet light that is used to detect fungal and bacterial infections, scabies, and alterations in pigment. When it is directed 4 to 5 inches from the patient's skin in a darkened room, certain abnormalities in the skin and hair appear as fluorescent colors that can be diagnosed by the physician and treated accordingly.

 CHECKPOINT QUESTION

11. Why are skin biopsies performed?

Bandaging

Bandages are strips of woven materials, typically absorbent, that are used for many purposes, such as:

1. Applying pressure to control bleeding
2. Holding a dressing in place
3. Protecting dressings and wounds from contamination
4. Immobilizing an injured part of the body
5. Supporting an injured part of the body

Types of Bandages

- *Roller bandages* are soft woven materials packaged in a roll. Roller bandages are available in various lengths and widths from 1 inch to 6 or more inches (Fig. 27-12). The bandage size used depends on the part being bandaged and the desired thickness of the completed bandage. Most bandages are made of a porous, lightweight material and may be either sterile or clean. Gauze bandages conform easily to angular surfaces of the body. A crepe-like stretchy gauze is made to adjust to various body contours and resists unrolling much better than plain roller gauze. Kling and Conform are two frequently used brands.
- *Elastic bandages*, such as the Ace brand, are special bandage rolls with elastic woven throughout the fabric (Fig. 27-13). They are generally brownish-tan. Unlike other types of roller gauze, elastic bandages can be given to the patient to take home to be washed and reused many times. Because of the elastic fibers, great care must be exercised when applying the bandage to prevent compromising circulation and still provide support to the injured part. Elastic bandages should be applied without wrinkling in concentric or overlapping layers. Bandages should fit snugly but not too tightly. Adjust the bandage if it seems too loose or if the patient says it is uncomfortable or tight. Some elastic bandages have an adhesive backing, which helps keep the layers in place and provides a secure, snug, and comfortable fit. To avoid applying it too tightly, never stretch or pull on the elastic

Figure 27-12 Gauze roller bandage.

bandage during application. Ask the patient how tight the bandage feels as it is being applied, and instruct the patient on signs of impaired circulation by checking the extremity distal to the bandage for the following indications:
A. Increased swelling or pain
B. Pale skin
C. Cool skin compared to the other extremity
- *Tubular gauze bandages* are used to enclose rounded body parts. The bandage resembles a hollow tube and is very stretchy (Fig. 27-14). It is used to enclose fingers, toes, arms, and legs and even the head and trunk. Tubular gauze bandages are available in various widths to fit any part of the body from $\frac{1}{2}$ inch to 7 inches. Tubular gauze is applied using a metal or plastic tubular frame-like applicator. The applicator is available in various sizes and should be slightly larger than the body part to be covered. This enables the gauze to slide easily over the body part. Applicators are marked according to a size number that corresponds to different sizes of tubular gauze. Procedure 27-3 describes the specific steps for applying a tubular gauze bandage.

Figure 27-13 An elastic bandage.

Figure 27-14 A tubular bandage.

Bandage Application Guidelines

When properly applied, bandages should feel comfortably snug and should be fastened securely enough to remain in place until removed. Bandages can be fastened with safety pins, adhesive tape, or clips. You gain the patient's confidence when you apply a bandage that is comfortable and neat looking and that stays in place. Patients become understandably upset when bandages fall off during normal activities. The following are general guidelines for applying bandages:

1. Observe the principles of medical asepsis, including handwashing, to prevent the transfer of pathogens. Surgical asepsis is not necessary. The bandage may be used to cover a sterile dressing or may be used alone if there is no open wound.
2. Keep the area to be bandaged and the bandage itself dry and clean because moisture may wick bacteria into the wound. A moist bandage encourages the growth of pathogens and is uncomfortable for the patient.
3. Never place a bandage directly over an open wound. Apply a sterile dressing first, and cover it with a bandage for protection. The bandage should extend approximately 1 to 2 inches beyond the edge of the dressing.
4. Never allow skin surfaces of two body parts to touch each other under a bandage. Wound healing may cause opposing surfaces to adhere and result in scar tissue formation. For example, burned fingers must be dressed separately but may be bandaged together.
5. Pad joints and any bony prominence to help prevent skin irritation caused by the bandage rubbing against the skin over a bony area.
6. Bandage the affected part in the normal position: joints should be slightly flexed to avoid muscle strain, discomfort, and pain. Muscle spasms may occur if the part is made to assume an unnatural position.
7. Apply bandages beginning at the distal part and extending to the proximal part of the body. Bandage turns that extend distal to proximal aid in return of venous blood to the heart and help make the bandage more secure.
8. Always talk with the patient during the bandaging. If the patient complains that it is too tight or too loose, adjust the bandage. Instruct the patient to do the same at home. The bandage should fit snugly, but if it is too tight, it may impair circulation. If it is too loose, it may fall off.
9. When bandaging hands and feet, leave the fingers and toes exposed whenever possible to make it easier to check for circulatory impairment. If the skin feels cold or looks pale, the nail beds look cyanotic, or the patient complains of swelling, numbness, or tingling of the toes or fingers, remove the bandage immediately and reapply it correctly.

Figure 27-15 illustrates various techniques for wrapping bandages.

 TRIAGE

While working in a medical office setting, the following three situations occur:

A. The physician has asked you to apply a new dressing to a 24-year-old man who lacerated his finger today and just had four sutures inserted by the physician.
B. The receptionist informs you that a patient has arrived and signed in but is complaining of a rash that is "itching." The receptionist is concerned that the scratching patient may be contagious, and she would like him put into an examination room right away.
C. A 32-year-old woman is waiting in the procedure room to have a suspicious mole removed from her back. You need to set up the sterile tray for this minor office surgical procedure.

How do you sort these patients? Who do you see first? Second? Third?

Patient B should be taken directly to an examination room since the cause for the patient's symptom (itching) is not known. If you will be expected to assist the physician with the minor surgical procedure, it would be best to take care of patient A because applying a dressing should take only a few minutes. After applying the dressing and discharging the patient, then you can set up for the surgical procedure and assist the physician. However, if your physician does not usually require you to assist during minor procedures, it might be more logical to set up for the procedure then apply the dressing to patient A, allowing plenty of time for wound care instructions if necessary.

Figure 27-15 The six basic techniques for wrapping a roller bandage. **(A)** A *circular turn* is used to anchor and secure a bandage when it is started and ended. Hold the free end of the rolled material in one hand and wrap it about the area and back to the starting point. **(B)** A *spiral turn* partly overlaps a previous turn. The overlapping varies from half to three-fourths of the width of the bandage. Spiral turns are used to wrap a cylindrical part of the body like the arms and legs. **(C)** A *spiral reverse turn* is a modification of a spiral turn. The roll is reversed halfway through the turn. This works well on tapered body parts, such as the forearm and wrist. **(D)** A *figure-of-8 turn* is best used when an area spanning a joint, like the elbow or knee, requires bandaging. It is made by making oblique turns that alternately ascend and descend, simulating the number 8. **(E)** A *spica turn* is a variation of the figure-of-8 turn. It differs in that the wrap includes a portion of the trunk or chest. **(F)** The *recurrent turn* is made by passing the roll back and forth over the tip of a body part. Once several recurrent turns have been made, the bandage is anchored by completing the application with another basic turn like the figure-of-8. A recurrent turn is especially beneficial when wrapping the stump of an amputated limb.

PROCEDURE 27-1:   Applying a Warm or Cold Compress

Purpose: Apply warm or cold compresses according to a physician's order
Equipment: Warm compresses: appropriate solution (water with possible antiseptic if ordered) warmed to 110°F or recommended temperature, bath thermometer, absorbent material (cloth, gauze), waterproof barriers, hot water bottle (optional), clean or sterile basin, gloves; Cold compresses: appropriate solution, ice bag or cold pack, absorbent material (cloth, gauze), waterproof barriers, gloves

Steps	Reasons
1. Wash your hands.	Handwashing aids in infection control.
2. Check the physician's order and assemble the equipment and supplies.	
3. Pour the appropriate solution into the basin. For hot compresses, check the temperature of the warmed solution. **Step 3.** Check hot solution with a bath thermometer.	The solution must not be hot enough to injure the patient.
4. Greet and identify the patient. Explain the procedure.	Identifying the patient prevents errors in treatment. Explaining the procedure helps ease anxiety and ensure compliance
5. Ask patient to remove clothing as appropriate and to put on a gown. Drape as appropriate.	Privacy must always be provided.
6. Protect the examination table with waterproof barrier.	Wet surfaces are uncomfortable for the patient and may cause chilling.
7. Place absorbent material or gauze in the prepared solution. Wring out excess moisture.	Compresses should be moist but not dripping; avoid wetting the patient.
8. Lightly place the compress on the patient's skin and ask about the temperature for comfort. Observe the skin for changes in color.	Always ask the patient whether the temperature of the compress is causing pain or discomfort.
9. Gently arrange the compress over the area and contour the material to the area. Insulate the compress with plastic or other waterproof barrier. **Step 9.** Place a waterproof barrier over the compress material.	Unless the material is against the skin, temperature will not be transferred to the area of concern. Insulating the area with the waterproof barrier will retard temperature loss and avoid getting the rest of the patient wet.

(continued)

PROCEDURE 27-1: **Applying a Warm or Cold Compress**
(continued)

Steps	Reasons
10. Check the compress frequently for moisture and temperature. Hot water bottles or ice packs may be used to maintain the temperature. Rewet absorbent material as needed.	The temperature should stay fairly constant. If the material dries, benefits will be lost.
11. After the prescribed amount of time, usually 20 to 30 minutes, remove the compress, discard disposable materials, and disinfect reusable equipment.	Equipment should be available for the next use. Cross-contamination must be avoided.
12. Remove your gloves and wash your hands.	
13. Document the procedure, including duration of treatment, type of solution, temperature of solution if a warm compress was used, skin color after treat-|ment, assessment of the area, and the patient's response.	Procedures are considered not to have been done if they are not recorded

Note: If the compress is being applied to an area with an open lesion, sterile technique is required. Warm compresses will speed suppuration to increase healing. Cold compresses will slow bleeding and decrease inflammation.

Charting Example:

10/16/2008 10:45 AM Hot compress applied to the left ankle ×20 min. Skin pink after treatment; no broken areas or blisters noted on the skin

—B. Barth, CMA

PROCEDURE 27-2: Assisting With Therapeutic Soaks

Purpose: Perform a therapeutic soak as directed by the physician
Equipment: Clean or sterile basin or container in which to place the body part comfortably, solution and/or medication, dry towels, bath thermometer, gloves

Steps	Reasons
1. Wash your hands.	Handwashing aids in infection control.
2. Assemble the equipment and supplies, including a basin or container of the appropriate size. Pad surfaces of container.	If the container is uncomfortably small, soaking the body area will be difficult and may cause muscle spasms. Surfaces should be padded for comfort.
3. Fill the container with solution and check the temperature with a bath thermometer. The temperature should be below 110°F to avoid blood pressure changes caused by vasodilation.	Assessing the temperature will prevent burning or injuring tissues.
4. Greet and identify the patient. Explain the procedure.	Identifying the patient prevents errors in treatment. Explaining the procedure helps ease anxiety and ensure compliance.
5. Slowly lower the area to be soaked into the container and check the patient's reaction. Arrange the part comfortably. Check for pressure areas and pad the edges as needed for comfort.	Immersing the part too quickly can shock the patient. If the patient is not comfortable, muscle spasms or strain may result
	Step 5. The basin should be large enough to immerse the entire body area.
6. While soaking, check the temperature of the solution every 5 to 10 minutes. If additional water or solution must be added to maintain the temperature, remove some of the solution and then add warmed solution while holding your hand between the patient and the stream of the solution being poured. Mix or swirl the soak to ensure constant, even temperature.	The proper temperature must be maintained for maximum benefit. Avoid pouring the solution or water directly against the patient's skin.
	Step 6. Shield the patient's skin when adding warm solution to the soak.
7. Soak for the prescribed amount of time, usually 15 to 20 minutes. Remove the part from the solution and carefully dry the area with a towel.	The area may be sensitive to brisk rubbing but must be dried to prevent chilling the patient or causing discomfort.
8. Properly care for the equipment; appropriately dispose of single-use supplies.	

(continued)

PROCEDURE 27-2: **Assisting With Therapeutic Soaks**
(continued)

Steps	Reasons
9. Document the procedure, including duration of treatment, type and temperature of solution, skin color after treatment, assessment of the area, including the condition of any lesions, and the patient's response.	Procedures are considered not to have been done if they are not recorded.

Charting Example:

4/19/2008 12:20 PM Left great toe soaked in Betadine solution ×15 min. Mod. amount of tan drainage from edges of toenail noted after soak

—*J. Brighton, RMA*

PROCEDURE 27-3: **Applying A Tubular Gauze Bandage**

Purpose: Apply tubular gauze bandage to a digit or extremity
Equipment: Tubular gauze, applicator, tape, scissors

Steps	Reasons
1. Wash your hands.	Handwashing aids in infection control.
2. Greet and identify the patient. Explain the procedure.	This prevents error in treatment, helps gain the patient's compliance, and eases anxiety.
3. Choose the appropriate size tubular gauze applicator and gauze width according to the size of the area to be covered. Manufacturers of tubular gauze supply charts with suggestions for the appropriate size for various body parts.	The applicator and gauze should slip easily over the body part. Choose an applicator slightly larger than the part to be covered. The gauze designed to fit the chosen applicator will provide a secure fit.
4. Select and cut or tear adhesive tape in lengths to secure the gauze ends.	Tape ensures that the gauze will not slip off. Having it at hand before beginning the procedure saves time and effort.
5. Place the gauze bandage on the applicator in the following manner: A. Be sure the applicator is upright (open end up) and placed on a flat surface. B. Pull a sufficient length of gauze from the stock box; do not cut it yet. C. Open the end of the length of gauze and slide it over the upper end of the applicator; estimate and push the amount of gauze that will be needed for this procedure onto the applicator.	

Step 5 C. Place the applicator upright and slide the end of the gauze over the applicator.

(continued)

PROCEDURE 27-3: Applying A Tubular Gauze Bandage *(continued)*

Steps	Reasons
D. Cut the gauze when the required amount of gauze has been transferred to the applicator.	
6. Place the applicator over the distal end of the affected part (finger, hand, toe, leg) and begin to apply the gauze by pulling it over the applicator onto the skin. Hold it in place as you move to Step 7.	The applicator should begin distally and work proximally.
7. Slide the applicator up to the proximal end of the affected part. Holding the gauze at the proximal end of the affected part, pull the applicator and gauze toward the distal end. 	This keeps the bandage from slipping. If the bandage is not held in place at the early stages of application, it may not completely cover the part **Step 7.** Hold the gauze at the proximal end of the affected part and pull the applicator toward the distal end.
8. Continue to hold the gauze in place at the proximal end. Pull the applicator 1 to 2 inches past the end of the affected part if the part is to be completely covered. Sometimes the gauze need not extend beyond a limb but covers only the area around the wound. 	The bandage will be secured at the distal end if the part is to be completely covered. If the distal portion of the limb is not to be covered, the bandage must extend at least 1 inch beyond the wound site to ensure adequate coverage. **Step 8.** Pull the applicator 1 to 2 inches past the affected area.
9. Turn the applicator one full turn to anchor the bandage.	The bandage will be securely held in place by the twist.
10. Move the applicator toward the proximal part as before. 	**Step 10.** Move the applicator toward the proximal part.

(continued)

PROCEDURE 27-3: Applying A Tubular Gauze Bandage
(continued)

Steps	Reasons
11. Move the applicator forward about 1 inch beyond the original starting point. Anchor the bandage again by turning it as before.	Anchoring provides a secure fit.
	Step 11. Move the applicator forward about 1 inch beyond the starting point.
12. Repeat the procedure until the desired coverage is obtained. The final layer should end at the proximal part of the affected area. Any extra length of gauze can be cut from the applicator. Remove the applicator.	The part should be adequately covered to protect the wound.
13. Secure the bandage in place with adhesive tape, or cut the gauze into two tails and tie them at the base of the tear. Tie the two tails around the closest proximal joint. Use the adhesive tape sparingly to secure the end if not using a tie.	The bandage must be securely fastened to keep it in place until it is changed.
	Step 13. Secure the bandage with adhesive tape.
14. Properly care for or dispose of equipment and supplies. Clean the work area. Wash your hands.	Standard precautions must be followed.
15. Record the procedure.	Procedures are considered not to have been done if they are not recorded.

Charting Example:

02/08/2008 9:15 AM Sterile dressing change to right index finger, tubular bandage applied and secured over dressing

—*T. Matthews, CMA*

MEDIA MENU

- **Student CD**
  - **Animations**
    Wound Healing
  - **CMA/RMA Certification Exam Review**
- **LWW's Medical Assisting Skills DVD**
  - **Procedure 27-3**
- **Premium Online Course**
  http://thePoint.lww.com/Kronenberger3e
- **Internet Resources**

  LiveAdvise Online Tutoring & Competency Training
  http://thePoint.lww.com/LiveAdvise

  American Cancer Society
  www.cancer.org

  American Academy of Dermatology
  www.aad.org

  American Board of Dermatology
  www.abderm.org

  American Society of Dermatology
  www.asd.org

  Dermatology Image Atlas, Johns Hopkins University
  http://dermatlas.med.jhmi.edu

español
SPANISH TERMINOLOGY

¿Cuán largo ha tenido usted ese lunar?
  How long have you had that mole?
He tenido este lunar durante 5 años.
  I have had this mole for 5 years.
Esta ampolla es dolorosa.
  This blister is painful.

Chapter Summary

- The skin and its accessories make up the largest and most visible organ of the body.
- Assessment of the integument offers the first glimpse into a person's total state of health.
- The medical physician who treats disorders of the skin is called a dermatologist; however, the medical assistant working in other offices will also be exposed to various types of integumentary system disorders.
- A responsibility of the medical assistant includes assisting the physician in correctly identifying and treating various forms of skin lesions.

- Typically, the medical assistant will be responsible for applying sterile dressings directly over a skin lesion or wound and should always remember to follow sterile technique.
- Always provide patient instruction during and after bandaging, alerting the patient to the signs and symptoms of impaired circulation.
- Bacterial skin infections may be contagious, and you should follow standard precautions, including good handwashing, after being with any patient with a skin disorder that may be infectious.

1. Sunlight or ultraviolet rays are needed to convert vitamin D, which is necessary for calcium and phosphorous absorption. Why is it important that children be exposed to sunlight regularly during their growing years?

2. After considering the factors needed for any microorganism to thrive, explain why molds and fungi thrive in a public shower or pool.

3. Create a patient information sheet describing the difference between eczema and psoriasis.

4. Using a drug reference book, research the usual dosage, side effects, and contraindications of the drug minoxidil, which is used to treat alopecia.

5. How would you respond to a patient who complains that his friend has recently been diagnosed with vitiligo and he is worried that he might also get this disease?

Answers | to Checkpoint Questions

1. Intact skin helps prevent invasion by microorganisms into underlying tissue.

2. Folliculitis, furuncle, and carbuncle are bacterial skin infections that develop in the hair follicles. Folliculitis is infection of one hair follicle. A furuncle is an infection deep within the hair follicle. A carbuncle is an infection of subcutaneous tissue around several hair follicles.

3. Many viral skin infections can be prevented by avoiding direct contact with skin lesions and maintaining a healthy immune system.

4. Often, the diagnosis of a skin lesion or rash is not known right away. Avoiding direct contact or wearing gloves if contact is necessary will decrease the chances of you acquiring a contagious skin infection such as a tinea infection.

5. Parasitic skin infections occur when the organism is transmitted through physical contact with an infested person. Sitting on an infested toilet seat and sharing combs, brushes, clothing, or bedding that is infested are also sources of infestation.

6. Both eczema and psoriasis are inflammatory skin disorders. While eczema is characterized by lesions that begin as red patches, proceed to vesicles, and eventually become scaly crusts, psoriasis is characterized by red plaques covered with dry, silvery scales.

7. The patients most at risk for developing decubitus ulcers include people who are elderly, immobilized, or debilitated, especially those who are bedridden or wheelchair bound.

8. The skin disorders of pigmentation that are inherited include albinism, nevus, and possibly vitiligo.

9. Squamous cell carcinoma will spread through underlying and surrounding tissue.

10. Your responsibilities regarding diagnosing skin lesions will include preparing the examination room and patient for any procedures that the physician will perform to make an accurate diagnosis. In addition, you will be responsible for giving any patient instructions and educating the patient on preventing the spread of any contagious skin infections.

11. A skin biopsy is used to examine a lesion for benign and malignant cells.

Outline

The Musculoskeletal System and Common Disorders
Sprains and Strains
Dislocations
Fractures
Bursitis
Arthritis
Tendonitis
Fibromyalgia
Gout
Muscular Dystrophy
Osteoporosis
Bone Tumors

Spine Disorders
Abnormal Spine Curvatures
Herniated Intervertebral Disc
Disorders of the Upper Extremities
Rotator Cuff Injury
Adhesive Capsulitis, or Frozen Shoulder
Lateral Epicondylitis, or Tennis Elbow
Carpal Tunnel Syndrome
Dupuytren Contracture

Disorders of the Lower Extremities
Chondromalacia Patellae
Plantar Fasciitis
Common Diagnostic Procedures
Physical Examination
Diagnostic Studies
The Role of the Medical Assistant
Warm and Cold Applications
Ambulatory Assist Devices

Learning Objectives

Upon successfully completing this chapter, you will be able to:

1. Spell and define key terms

2. List and describe disorders of the musculoskeletal system

3. Compare the different types of fractures

4. Identify and explain diagnostic procedures of the musculoskeletal system

5. Discuss the role of the medical assistant in caring for the patient with a musculoskeletal system disorder

6. Describe the various types of ambulatory aids

Upon successfully completing this chapter, you will be able to:

1. Apply an arm sling (Procedure 28-1)
2. Apply cold packs (Procedure 28-2)
3. Use a hot water bottle or commercial hot pack (Procedure 28-3)
4. Measure a patient for axillary crutches (Procedure 28-4)
5. Instruct a patient in various crutch gaits (Procedure 28-5)

Competencies

CAAHEP

- Practice standard precautions
- Prepare patient for and assist with routine and specialty examinations
- Document appropriately
- Instruct individuals according to their needs

ABHES

- Prepare patients for procedures
- Assist physician with examinations and treatments
- Document accurately

Key Terms

ankylosing spondylitis	callus	goniometer	phonophoresis
arthrogram	contracture	iontophoresis	prosthesis
arthroplasty	contusion	kyphosis	reduction
arthroscopy	electromyography	lordosis	scoliosis
bursae	embolus	Paget's disease	

The Musculoskeletal System and Common Disorders

Muscles allow movement of the body through contraction and relaxation. Bones support the body and respond to the contractions and relaxations (Fig. 28-1). Because the two systems depend on each other to function, they are often referred to as a single system—the musculoskeletal system. Within this system are joints, areas where two or more bones are held together by connective tissue and cartilage. The integrity of the entire system is required for normal body support and movement (Fig. 28-2).

When there is a problem with the musculoskeletal system, orthopedists and physical therapists often provide appropriate treatment and rehabilitation. However, medical assistants working in other specialties, such as family practice or urgent care centers, also care for patients with musculoskeletal disorders. The most common disorders of the musculoskeletal system are sprains, dislocations, fractures, joint disruptions, and degeneration. The musculoskeletal system reacts to injury or disease with pain (Box 28-1), swelling, inflammation, deformity, and/or limitation of range and function.

Sprains and Strains

Injury to a joint capsule and its supporting ligaments is called a sprain, and injury to a muscle and its support-

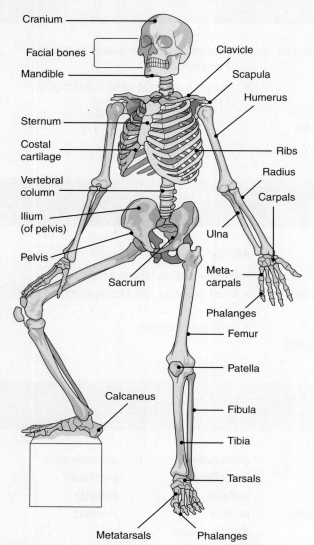

Cranium

Facial bones

Mandible

Clavicle

Scapula

Humerus

Sternum

Costal cartilage

Ribs

Vertebral column

Radius

Carpals

Ilium (of pelvis)

Ulna

Pelvis

Meta-carpals

Sacrum

Phalanges

Femur

Patella

Calcaneus

Fibula

Tibia

Tarsals

Metatarsals   Phalanges

Figure 28-1 The axial skeleton is shown in yellow; the appendicular skeleton is shown in blue. (Reprinted with permission from Cohen BJ. Memmler's The Human Body in Health and Disease. Philadelphia: Lippincott Williams & Wilkins, 2005.)

ing tendons is called a strain. Damage to a muscle, ligament, or tendon may result in joint instability. If the ligament is completely torn, it cannot efficiently stabilize the joint. Common symptoms are inflammation and pain. Applying ice at the time of injury helps reduce swelling and pain. For mild sprains, treatment includes exercise to prevent joint stiffness and muscle atrophy. Therapeutic devices and compression wraps reduce swelling. Moderate sprains must be treated with care to prevent further injury because the ligaments are weakened and healing may take 6 to 8 weeks. Severe sprains often require surgery, and the recovery may take longer than 8 weeks.

In the spine, a sprain to the facet joint (the area between vertebrae) can cause pain not only at the point of difficulty, but also radiating into an extremity (radicular pain) as a result of impingement on the nerve root that passes close to the joint. For example, an injury to the facet joint between vertebrae of the lower back often causes pain in the back that radiates down one leg or the other. An injury to the anterior cruciate ligament in the knee greatly compromises the joint's stability. The knee becomes swollen, painful, and unstable and has limited motion. Complete tears in the ligaments of the knee require surgery and extensive rehabilitation. An injury to the Achilles tendon in the lower posterior leg is extremely painful and limits the ability to walk. A tear in this tendon requires surgery followed by immobilization.

Dislocations

Dislocation of a joint, also called a luxation, occurs when the end of the bone is displaced from its articular surface. It can be caused by trauma or disease, or it may be congenital. Common sites of dislocations include the shoulders, elbows, fingers, hips, and ankles. A subluxation is a partial dislocation in which the bone is pulled out of the socket but all joint structures maintain their proper relationships. Partial dislocations can result from weakness, decreased muscle tone, gravity, or neurologic deficit. The muscles bear most of the responsibility for preventing subluxation. Common symptoms of dislocations include pain, pressure, limited movement, and deformity. Numbness and loss of a pulse in the affected extremity can also occur. Treatment includes realigning the bones and immobilization of the joint. The patient may have to do exercises to strengthen supporting muscles to avoid recurrences.

CHECKPOINT QUESTION

1. How does a luxation differ from a subluxation?

Fractures

A fracture is a break or disruption in a bone caused by falls, other trauma, disease, tumors, or unusual stress. There are many types of fractures, each with its own set of problems (Table 28-1). However, all fractures have one symptom in common: pain. Other manifestations may include swelling, hemorrhage, lack of movement or unusual movement, **contusions**, and deformity of the body part involved.

Treatment is **reduction** (realigning the bones) by placing the broken ends into proper alignment. Casting, splinting, wrapping, and taping are means of maintaining and immobilizing a closed reduction while the bone heals. If it is not possible to obtain proper alignment by a closed reduction, surgery is required; this open reduc-

Figure 28-2 Normal range of motion of selected joints: flexion/extension; pronation/supination; abduction/adduction; circumduction; dorsiflexion/plantar flexion; inversion/eversion; and rotation. (Reprinted with permission from Cohen BJ. Memmler's The Human Body in Health and Disease. Philadelphia: Lippincott Williams & Wilkins, 2005.)

tion may require the insertion of pins, a plate, or other hardware to maintain alignment of the bones. Fractures in the shoulder are serious because the immobilization necessary for healing may cause scar tissue (adhesions) to form in the capsule, resulting in a severe loss of motion and function. These patients require extensive physical therapy to regain complete use of the involved arm.

Casts

Fractures must be immobilized to facilitate healing of the bone in the proper alignment. In most instances, both proximal and distal joints are included in the cast to ensure that movement is restricted. Box 28-2 describes various types of casts. The casting material is ei-

ther plaster or fiberglass. Traditional plaster casts are bandages impregnated with calcium sulfate crystals and are supplied as rolls of material in widths appropriate to a variety of sites. After water is added to the dry rolls of bandage and the wet material is applied to the extremity, a chemical reaction generates heat that may be uncomfortable to the patient for a short time, usually less than 30 minutes. This chemical reaction is necessary to produce a rigid dressing when dry. The bandage will mold smoothly to the casting site as it is applied.

A plaster cast is rather soft until it is fully dry, which can take as long as 72 hours. Patients must be cautioned not to exert pressure on the drying cast so as to avoid pressure sores from indentations. Plaster casts must be kept dry at all times.

BOX 28-1

MUSCULOSKELETAL PAIN

Rest, immobilization, or both may be needed to relieve pain in acute soft tissue strains, sprains, and inflammations. Because painful movement may cause further damage to the injured tissue, restriction of movement may also be required. This can be accomplished by rest and by the use of a cast, brace, sling, splint, collar, elastic wrap, or corset. If weight bearing is painful or inadvisable because of fracture or musculoskeletal pathology, an ambulatory aid (e.g., cane, walker, or crutches) may be used.

The use of hot moist packs, a heating pad, or warm baths can help increase circulation, relax spasms, and ease sore muscles. Ice packs help prevent swelling, decrease inflammation, and reduce contusions, which may follow a direct blow on a muscle.

With contusions, the capillaries (small blood vessels) rupture and bleed into the tissue. Swelling and inflammation may result. Reduction of the bleeding is crucial; it is accomplished by applying cold packs and a pressure bandage. Immobilization to prevent further injury is also important. Within a few days, pain-free exercises and heat applications should be introduced to begin healing.

Generally, movement should begin as soon as possible after a soft tissue injury to maintain a healthy joint and resilient muscles. Gentle active or passive movement in the pain-free range, mild joint immobilization, traction, or exercise can be effective in maintaining normal range, function, and strength.

Because of its lighter weight, water resistance, and durability, fiberglass is often used for casting. While the application is similar to the plaster cast, the polyurethane additives harden in minutes, eliminating the extended drying time. After the cast has set, the material will not soften when wet but must be dried to prevent skin lesions. The fabric has a more open weave than plaster, which helps maintain skin integrity.

Assisting With Plaster or Fiberglass Cast Application

After positioning the patient comfortably before the procedure begins, drape the patient to expose only the part to be casted, avoiding unnecessary exposure and protecting other skin areas from the casting material. The part to be casted should be clean and dry; apply a bandage or dressing to any lesions before casting. Assemble the following items:

- Tubular soft fabric stocking material large enough to encircle the limb
- Roller padding, also called sheet wadding
- Casting material
- Bucket of cool or tepid water
- Plaster or cast knife
- Utility gloves

The limb is covered first with the soft knitted tubular material with extra fabric above and below the projected casting length to allow for a padded fold at each end. The soft roller padding is applied in fairly thick layers over bony prominences (Fig. 28-3). The limb is wrapped from the distal end to the proximal end with the soaked casting material. You may be responsible for soaking the material until bubbles no longer form around the rolls. The rolls should be pressed, not wrung, until they are wet through but not dripping. Wear utility gloves to protect your hands from the material. When the site is adequately covered, rough edges are trimmed with the plaster knife, and the knitted fabric is folded back to form cuffs at each end. The skin outside the cast is cleansed of casting material to avoid discomfort and skin breakdown.

Because of the unsupported weight an arm cast may put on the shoulder muscles, a sling is ordered to relieve and redistribute the weight. Slings are also used when casting is not necessary but the arm must be immobilized to facilitate healing. Procedure 28-1 describes the steps for applying a sling; however, many commercially made slings are now available that adjust easily depending on the size of the patient.

Plaster or Fiberglass Cast Removal

To remove a plaster or fiberglass cast, cuts are made in the cast through its length on opposite sides, dividing it into halves. An electric oscillating circular saw known as a cast cutter is used (Fig. 28-4). Assure the patient that this will not cut the skin. Wear safety goggles to protect your eyes from flying particles and caution the patient also. The cast will be split apart with a cast spreader, and the padding will be cut with utility scissors. The patient should be warned that the skin will be pale and dry and the muscle will be weak and shrunken from disuse. Also explain that the skin may be sensitive to touch and temperature. Creams and lotions help alleviate the dryness, and physical therapy and exercise will restore the muscle tone.

 CHECKPOINT QUESTION

2. Why is it important to not touch plaster casts until completely dry?

TABLE 28-1	Types of Fractures
Type	**Description**
Simple or closed	Does not protrude through the skin; usually treated with a closed reduction
Compound or open	Broken end protrudes through the skin; infection a major concern; surgery often required
Spiral	Occurs with torsion or twisting injuries; appears to be S-shaped on radiographs
Impacted	One bone segment driven into another
Greenstick	Common injury in children; partial or incomplete break in which only one side of a bone is broken, like a green stick
Transverse	At right angles to axis of bone; generally caused by excessive bending force or direct hit on bone
Oblique	Slanted across axis of bone
Comminuted	Bone is fragmented, usually by much direct force; difficult to reduce because many pieces of bone must be held in proper alignment; more complicated to treat if articular surface if involved, so surgery usually required; severe soft tissue damage common because of the force necessary to cause the fracture
Compression	Damage from application of strong force against both ends, such as a fall; vertebrae susceptible to compression fractures, especially in elderly
Depressed	Fracture of flat bones (usually skull), causing fragment to be driven below surface of bone
Avulsion	Caused by strong force applied to bone by sharp twisting, pulling motion of attached ligaments or tendons resulting in a tearing away of bone fragments
Pathologic	Usually result of disease process such as osteoporosis (brittle bones), **Paget's disease** (a chronic skeletal disease in the elderly with bowing of the long bones), bone cysts, tumors, or cancers

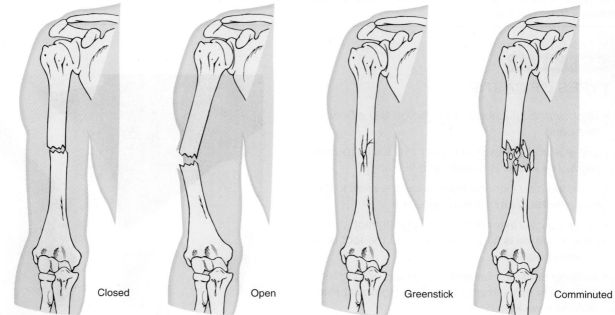

Closed   Open   Greenstick   Comminuted

A

(**A**) Types of fractures: closed, open, greenstick, comminuted.

(continued)

TABLE 28-1 **Types of Fractures** *(continued)*

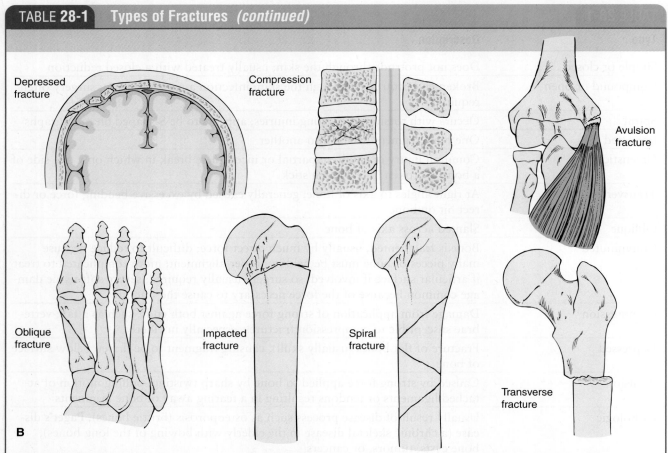

Depressed fracture

Compression fracture

Avulsion fracture

Oblique fracture

Impacted fracture

Spiral fracture

Transverse fracture

B

(B) Types of fractures: depressed fracture, compressed fracture, avulsion fracture, oblique fracture, impacted fracture, spiral fracture, transverse fracture.

BOX 28-2

TYPES OF CASTS

- *Short arm cast* extends from below the elbow to mid palm.

- *Long arm cast* extends from the axilla to mid palm. The elbow is usually at a 90° angle.

- *Short leg cast* extends from below the knee to the toes; the foot is in a natural position.

- *Long leg cast* extends from the upper thigh to the toes; the knee is slightly flexed, and the foot is in a natural position.

- *Walking cast* may be either short leg or long leg; the cast is extra strong to bear weight and may include a walking heel.

- *Body cast* encircles the trunk, usually from the axilla to the hip.

- *Spica cast* encircles part of the trunk and one or two extremities.

Figure 28-3 Applying a roller bandage before the casting material.

Figure 28-4 A cast cutter and saw. (Courtesy of M-PACT Worldwide, Eudora, KS.)

LEGAL TIP

ASSESSING CIRCULATION AFTER A CAST APPLICATION

A cast that is applied improperly can lead to nerve and vascular damage, resulting in permanent loss of function to the extremity. In extreme situations, a surgical amputation may be required. To ensure proper care and to avoid lawsuits, it is essential that distal extremity circulation be assessed and documented before and after reductions and casting. Also, the patient should be taught to watch for and report signs of impaired circulation.

Healing of Fractures

The most important criterion for successful healing of a fracture is an adequate blood supply. The blood secretes an important glue-like substance known as **callus**, which is deposited around the break. Callus holds the ends of the bones together; with time, the callus turns to bone. The bone cells mold the callus and smooth the fracture site to close to its original size. Immobilization of the fracture site allows successful molding and reshaping. The elderly may heal slowly, and prosthetic joint replacement may be necessary if bone restructuring is inadequate (Box 28-3).

If the blood supply is inadequate to the healing bone or tissue, union may be delayed or absent. If damage is sufficient or if severe trauma, disease, tumor, or complications are involved, amputation may be necessary. Amputation is a drastic measure that is performed only when all other avenues are exhausted. A **prosthesis** enables the amputee to resume functional activities such as walking, grasping, and holding.

PATIENT EDUCATION

CAST CARE

Instruct patients with casts to do the following:

- Be aware of the initial warmth of the drying cast; this will diminish in 20 to 30 minutes.
- Keep a plaster cast dry.
- Avoid indentations by allowing the cast to dry completely before handling or propping it on a hard surface.
- Note that the fingers and toes are left uncovered to check for color, swelling, numbness, and temperature; report any impairment to the physician immediately.
- Report odors, staining, or undue warmth of the cast.
- Prevent swelling by elevating the limb for at least 24 hours after casting and as often as possible after that time.
- Never insert any object under the cast to scratch beneath it. Breaks in the skin may become infected and require that the cast be removed prematurely.

BOX 28-3

BONE HEALING IN THE ELDERLY

A fractured femur in the elderly raises special concerns. Bone-repairing osteoblasts are less able to use calcium to restructure bone tissue at any site in the elderly, but the neck of the femur, the most common fracture site, is especially vulnerable to delayed or imperfect healing because the blood supply is poor. Fractures through this area, involving the femoral head or neck or just inferior to the greater trochanter, may require hip arthroplasty or total hip replacement.

Most hip joint replacement prostheses are metal or polyethylene molded to conform to the joints they are designed to replace. Total hip replacement, usually used for degenerative joint disease or rheumatoid arthritis, replaces the head and neck of the femur and the acetabular surface. Knee replacement replaces both the head of the tibia and the distal epiphysis of the femur.

Early repair and return to mobility prevent contractures and atrophy of the supporting muscles. Postoperative walking prevents many of the complications associated with prolonged confinement in the elderly, such as pathologic fractures, static pneumonia, and renal calculi.

(continued)

BOX 28-3 *(continued)*

Hip and knee replacement: acetabular (pelvic) component; femoral (proximal) component; femoral (distal) component; tibial component.

A potentially life-threatening complication of a fracture is a fat **embolus**. This type of embolus results from the release of fat droplets from the yellow marrow of the long bones. If the embolus lodges in the coronary or pulmonary vessels or in a large vessel in the brain, it can block the vessel, causing an infarction and death.

 CHECKPOINT QUESTION

3. What is the difference between an open and closed reduction of a fracture?

PATIENT EDUCATION

HELPING ELDERLY PATIENTS AVOID HIP FRACTURES

Older patients are particularly likely to fall and fracture bones, and when this happens, one of the most common bones broken is the head of the femur. These fractures take a long time to heal and often result in the patient being admitted to a skilled nursing facility for rehabilitation. Therefore, it is important for you to teach older patients fall prevention techniques. Here are some important tips:

* Always wear shoes with good, solid tie strings.
* Be sure that lighting is adequate, both inside and outside the home.
* Remove scatter rugs inside the home.
* Place grab bars throughout the home where extra assistance may be needed in getting out of chairs or off of the toilet.

Advise the patient that one-floor living is best, and teach the patient ways to reorganize the home to avoid climbing stairs.

Bursitis

Bursae, small pad-like sacs filled with a clear synovial fluid, surround some joints in areas of excessive friction, such as under tendons and over bony prominences. Their primary purposes are to reduce friction between moving parts and to prevent damage. The subdeltoid bursa in the shoulder between the deltoid muscle and the joint capsule is the most common site of bursitis, an inflammation of the bursa. Other frequent sites include the olecranon process at the elbow, the trochanter at the hip, the prepatellar bursae at the knee, and the heel.

The most common symptom of bursitis is pain during range-of-motion movement (see Fig. 28-2). In subdeltoid bursitis, pain occurs in the midrange of abduction but not at the beginning or end of the range. Pain occurs in the shoulder and arm when the inflamed bursa is pinched between the head of the humerus and the clavicle during abduction.

Treatment for bursitis usually consists of anti-inflammatory medications, rest, heat or cold applications, ultrasound to promote healing, and activities within the pain-free range. Physical therapy for range-of-motion exercises may also be ordered by the physician.

CHECKPOINT QUESTION

4. What is the most common site of bursitis?

Arthritis

Osteoarthritis, or degenerative joint disease, is caused by wear and tear on the weight-bearing joints. As the articular cartilage degenerates, the ends of the bones enlarge, causing an intrusion of bone into the joint cavity. The patient has pain and restricted movement in the affected joint. Treatment of osteoarthritis includes administration of anti-inflammatory medications and intra-articular corticosteroid injections to control the pain and inflammation. Patients may also require the use of an ambulatory aid such as a cane, walker, or crutches to decrease joint stress.

Rheumatoid arthritis is a systemic autoimmune disease that attacks the synovial membrane lining of the joint. Ultimately it leads to inflammation, pain, stiffness, and crippling deformities. It usually begins in non–weight-bearing joints such as the fingers but eventually may affect many joints, including the hands, wrists, elbows, feet, ankles, knees, and neck.

Marie-Strumpell disease, or **ankylosing spondylitis,** is rheumatoid arthritis of the spine. It is characterized by extreme forward flexion of the spine and tightness in the hip flexors. Rheumatoid arthritis in children is known as Still's disease.

The treatment for rheumatoid arthritis is similar to the treatment for osteoarthritis: anti-inflammatory medications orally and corticosteroid or gold injections into the affected joint, heat and cold applications, and protection of painful joints with splints or braces. In severe cases, the joint may be surgically replaced with an artificial one.

 CHECKPOINT QUESTION

5. How does osteoarthritis differ from rheumatoid arthritis?

Tendonitis

Muscles are attached to bones by tendons, which aid the body's mobility and stability. Tendonitis is inflammation of these structures. This disorder usually occurs after strains, sprains, overuse, or overstretching of the tissue. Although pain does not occur with passive movement, active movement is painful, and resistance to movement is intensely painful because the tissue must contract during active and resisted movement. Local tenderness is usual. The most common site of tendonitis is at the supraspinatus tendon in the shoulder, one of the rotator cuff muscles. Palpation over the tendon will elicit exquisite pain. Sometimes tendonitis is caused by calcium deposits, and this type is called calcific tendonitis.

The treatment for tendonitis consists of oral anti-inflammatory medications, rest, heat or cold applications, ultrasound, **iontophoresis** (electrical transfer of ions), massage, and transverse friction massage (deep massage across the fibers of the tendons). Usually the patient is referred to a licensed massage therapist for the massage or transverse friction massage.

Fibromyalgia

Fibromyalgia causes multiple and often nonspecific symptoms including widespread pain in specific body areas, muscular stiffness, fatigue, and difficulty sleeping. This disorder varies from person to person, and the symptoms can be intermittent, making diagnosis difficult. Although the exact cause of this disorder is not known, some evidence suggests abnormalities in the immune system, perhaps resulting from a viral infection. Although it does not lead to other serious diseases, fibromyalgia tends to be chronic and is diagnosed by ruling out all other diseases and disorders with similar symptoms.

Treatment for fibromyalgia is based on relieving the symptoms with nonsteroidal anti-inflammatory medications, exercise, rest, and personal counseling, as indicated for the clinical depression that often accompanies this disorder because it is chronic.

 CHECKPOINT QUESTION

6. What is the usual cause of tendonitis?

Gout

Gout, a metabolic disease of overproduction of uric acid, is a form of arthritis caused by the deposit of uric acid crystals into a joint, usually in the great toe. Although the cause of gout is unknown, the patient may have a history of injury to the joint, obesity, and a high-protein diet, especially a diet high in purines (alcoholic beverages, turkey, sardines, trout, bacon, and organ meats). The patient with gout complains of a painful, hot, inflamed joint; symptoms worsen unless treated. Periods of remission and exacerbation may occur. Gout may become chronic and can lead to multiple joint involvement with chronic pain, degeneration, and deformity. Symptoms are relieved by taking nonsteroidal anti-inflammatory medications and by avoidance of purine-rich foods and alcohol. Medication to prevent uric acid formation or foster its excretion from the body may also be prescribed.

 CHECKPOINT QUESTION

7. What foods should be avoided in the patient with gout?

Muscular Dystrophy

The congenital disorders collectively known as muscular dystrophy are characterized by varying degrees of progressive wasting of skeletal muscles. There is no neurologic involvement, but the skeletal muscles waste and weaken. Some forms of the disease affect the heart and other organs. The most common type of muscular dystrophy, Duchenne, is apparent in males in early childhood and is usually fatal by young adulthood as respiratory and cardiac muscles fail. Several forms, such as facioscapulohumeral and limb girdle dystrophy, progress slowly from a childhood onset and result in varying degrees of disability. Duchenne, facioscapulohumeral, and limb girdle dystrophies are genetically transmitted.

Diagnosis of muscular dystrophy is based on family and patient history. The characteristic signs are frequently the most obvious diagnostic indicators of the disease. They include muscle weakness, clumsiness, frequent falling, and muscle spasms. **Electromyography** and muscle biopsy are used to rule out nervous system involvement. There is no known cure for any form of muscular dystrophy; however, exercise, physical therapy, and the use of splints or braces can relieve the symptoms. As mobility decreases, the use of a cane, walker, or wheelchair may be useful in maintaining independence.

Osteoporosis

Porous bones, or osteoporosis, is a condition in which the bones are deficient in calcium and phosphorus, making them brittle and vulnerable to fractures. The cause may be dietary, with general deficiencies in calcium, vitamin D, or phosphorus, or it may be primary progressive inability to metabolize calcium brought on by estrogen deficiency in elderly women or sedentary lifestyle, alcoholism, liver disorder, or rheumatoid arthritis.

There are few signs of osteoporosis other than a gradual loss of stature or height, progressive kyphosis (or dowager's hump), and spontaneous, nontraumatic fractures. Diagnosis includes bone scan, densitometry (a test that measures the density of the bones), thyroid and parathyroid studies, and serum calcium and phosphorus determinations. Treatment is preventing fractures by increasing appropriate levels of exercise to strengthen the bones. Hormone therapy with estrogen or a combination of estrogen and progesterone may be prescribed for postmenopausal women to prevent loss of minerals from the bones that occurs with the natural decrease in these hormones during menopause. Calcium and vitamin D supplements are beneficial to arrest the progression but will not cure the underlying degenerative factors once osteoporosis has begun.

Bone Tumors

Bone tissue is rarely the primary site for malignancies but is frequently a site of metastasis. Primary osteosarcomas occur most often in young men, although they may occur at any age in either sex. Osteogenic sarcomas originate in the bony tissue, while nonosseous tumors seed to the bones from other sites. Ewing sarcoma, originating in the marrow and invading the shaft of the long bones, is common in young adults, especially adolescent boys.

There is no known cause of malignant skeletal tumors, but one hypothesis is that rapid development of bone tissue during growth spurts is a predisposing factor. Bone pain is the most common early sign. The pain is most intense at night, is usually dull and centered at the site, and is not relieved by resting the body part. Depending on the site, the mass may be palpable through the skin and muscles. Biopsy is the definitive diagnostic test after a bone scan suggests the need. Surgical treatment includes excision of the tumor, including a large margin of surrounding bone structure and nearby lymph nodes, or amputation if the tumor is in an extremity. Chemotherapy and radiation are usually indicated also.

 CHECKPOINT QUESTION

8. Why is exercise used to treat or prevent osteoporosis?

Spine Disorders

The vertebral column (Fig. 28-5) is made up of 33 vertebrae and numerous joints. The cervical, thoracic, and lumbar vertebrae are separated from each other by 23 intervertebral discs; the vertebrae of the sacrum and coccyx are fused, with no discs separating the bones. These vertebrae and their discs absorb and transmit the shock of running, walking, and jumping and keep the spine flexible for a high degree of mobility. Many strong ligaments and structures support and protect the spine, including the anterior and posterior longitudinal ligaments and the four natural curves in the spine. However, back injuries are common and are a leading cause of work-related injury among health care professionals. Box 28-4 offers some suggestions for avoiding back strain, and patients can use these general guidelines as well.

Abnormal Spine Curvatures

Exaggerated or abnormal curvatures of the spine affect the posture and the alignment of the shoulders and hips. An abnormally deep lumbar curve is **lordosis**, or swayback. Abnormal thoracic curvature, particularly of the upper portion, is called **kyphosis**, or hunchback. A side-to-side or lateral curvature is called **scoliosis**; it is commonly screened for in school children, especially girls, and if severe enough, it is surgically corrected during adolescence (Fig. 28-6).

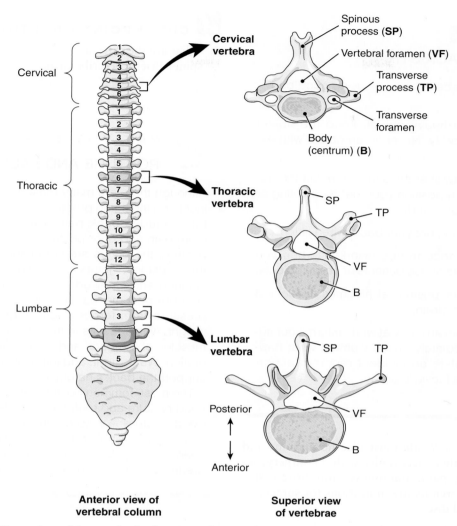

Figure 28-5 (Left) Front view of the vertebral column. (Right) Vertebrae from above. (Reprinted with permission from Cohen BJ. Memmler's The Human Body in Health and Disease. Philadelphia: Lippincott Williams & Wilkins, 2005.)

Treatment of abnormal spinal curvatures entails the use of bracing to straighten the curve to a normal position. Transcutaneous muscle stimulation devices cause the muscles on one side to contract and draw the spine into its proper position. When necessary, orthopedic surgery is performed to straighten the spinal column.

Herniated Intervertebral Disc

The lumbar spine is one of the most frequently injured parts of the body because it absorbs the body's full weight and the weight of anything that is carried. Because most of the movement in the lumbar spine occurs at the L-4 to L-5 and L-5 to S-1 segments, most herniated discs are seen at these levels, but injury can occur in any disc in the spine.

A disc herniates when its soft center, known as the nucleus, ruptures through its tough outer layer to protrude into the spinal canal, sometimes pressing on the spinal cord. It is usually caused by severe trauma, degenerative change, or strenuous strain. Common symptoms include severe back pain, numbness in one or both extremities, spasms, weakness, and limitation of movement. Flexion radiates pain into the extremities, and extension is restricted and causes pain at the spinal segment. Having the patient raise one leg from the supine position (known as the straight leg raise test) indicates whether the back pain is from a disc. A positive sign includes back pain with the leg at 45° to 60°. A flattened lumbar curve and a lateral shift of the spine are fairly common. Radiography may show a narrowed disc space.

Because bone strength throughout the body is diminished during confinement or inactivity, total bed rest is no longer a common treatment for most musculoskeletal disorders, including herniated discs, although pain limits activity. The treatment for herniated discs may include physical therapy for traction, massage, and mild

BOX 28-4

AVOIDING BACK STRAIN

You can prevent back strain by using good body mechanics:

- When lifting a heavy object, keep the object close to your body. Never lift an object with extended arms..

- Never lift and twist at the same time. Lift the object, and then reposition your feet by pivoting or taking two steps to turn.

- Bend your knees, not your back, when lifting.

- Ask for assistance from co-workers when you must lift or move obese patients or heavy objects.

- Maintain proper posture at all times; slouching causes muscle strain.

- If you do sustain an injury at work, inform your supervisor immediately and document what happened. Complete an incident report in accordance with the facility's policy.

extension exercises. While most disc herniations and bulges can be treated successfully without surgery, severe, unremitting pain, numbness, and progressive weakness of an extremity are indications for surgery to remove the injured disc.

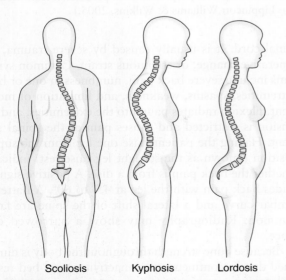

Scoliosis   **Kyphosis**   **Lordosis**

Figure 28-6 Abnormalities of the spinal curves. (Reprinted with permission from Cohen BJ. Memmler's The Human Body in Health and Disease. Philadelphia: Lippincott Williams & Wilkins, 2005.)

 CHECKPOINT QUESTION

9. What are the three abnormal curvatures of the spine? Briefly describe each.

 PATIENT EDUCATION

POSTURE AND BACK PAIN

Although there are many reasons for poor posture including the aging process, the result of poor posture includes back pain, which often results in more pain and poor posture. In patients with poor posture, the bones are not aligned properly, and the muscles, joints, and ligaments become strained and stressed. As the discs between the vertebra become less resilient, there is increased pressure from forces such as gravity and body weight, which results in the loss of flexibility in the muscles of the back and spine and spine degeneration. Weak, tight, and inflexible muscles cannot support the back's natural curves.

The most common posture faults are the forward head posture and rounded shoulders. Maintaining good posture—or correcting poor posture—can help reduce a bulging disc or relieve the biomechanical stress caused by poor skeletal alignment, greatly aiding musculoskeletal system functioning.

Disorders of the Upper Extremities

The structures of the upper extremity include the shoulder, elbow, wrist, and hand. Movement of the shoulder occurs in a ball-and-socket joint, which is the most mobile joint in the body. The elbow, a hinge joint, is made up of the articulation of the humerus with the radius (lateral) and the ulna (medial) and allows movement in one direction only.

The complex structure of the wrist allows for a variety of movements, including flexion, extension, ulnar deviation, radial deviation, and circumduction. However, the most intricate and specialized movements of the musculoskeletal system occur in the hand. The thumb, the first digit, accounts for 50% of hand function. The muscles that control the precision movements and fine motor activities of the hand are known as intrinsic muscles because they have both of their attachments, origin (the end of the muscle that stays relatively stationary or fixed) and insertion (the more movable end of the muscle), in the hand.

Rotator Cuff Injury

The rotator cuff is formed by the tendons of four muscles that hold the joint surfaces together during joint motion. Injury to the rotator cuff muscles in the shoulder can cause severe pain, weakness, and loss of function. Surgical intervention for rotator cuff injury is often necessary because the tendons do not heal quickly on their own. An extended period of postoperative rehabilitation and physical therapy is usually needed to increase range of motion and strength and to regain the use of the shoulder. Professional athletes, particularly baseball pitchers, are prone to rotator cuff injuries.

Adhesive Capsulitis, or Frozen Shoulder

Frozen shoulder, a shortening of the muscles and joint structures known as a **contracture**, affects the entire shoulder joint and its capsule. It usually results from a fracture or disease process that prevents movement; however, anything that causes pain or restricts motion (e.g., tendonitis, bursitis, nerve damage, stroke, sprain, or strain) can lead to a frozen shoulder.

Contractures develop when the joint is immobilized, allowing the collagen fibers to stick to each other and thereby limiting the movement in the joint. Adhesions and additional collagen are produced in response to injury, which results in a painful, tight, and constricted capsule. The shoulder movements most restricted are abduction and external rotation. Because full active range of motion is not possible, weakness and atrophy ensue.

Treatment consists of administration of anti-inflammatory medications and heat or cold applications. The physician may also prescribe physical therapy to include ultrasound, mobilization or manipulation, and stretching exercises. Recovery is slow and typically painful. Contractures in the joints are often preventable with proper management and by moving the joint through a full range of motion each day.

Lateral Epicondylitis, or Tennis Elbow

Lateral epicondylitis, often called tennis elbow, is a common elbow injury involving a sprain or strain of the tendons of origin of the wrist and finger extensor muscles. Symptoms include extreme pain with extension of the wrist, such as when trying to lift a cup or glass. Resistance to wrist extension and supination are the diagnostic tests for tennis elbow because both movements greatly increase the pain.

Treatment consists of ice applications, **phonophoresis** (ultrasound with cortisone) or iontophoresis, avoiding movements that cause the pain, use of a forearm strap just distal to the elbow to take the pressure off the tendon, transverse friction massage, and gentle passive exercise to maintain mobility. In prolonged, extreme cases, surgery may be indicated.

 CHECKPOINT QUESTION

10. Which of the disorders of the upper extremities may result from decreasing movement of the arm and shoulder?

Carpal Tunnel Syndrome

A repetitive motion injury, carpal tunnel syndrome occurs when the carpal bones and transverse carpal ligaments compress the median nerve at the wrist. Symptoms include numbness in the thumb and index and middle fingers and pain and weakness in the affected hand and wrist. Often pain awakens the patient at night.

Diagnostic tests for carpal tunnel syndrome include Phalen's test, in which holding the wrist in flexion reproduces the symptoms; Tinel's test, in which the wrist is held in hyperextension and the transverse carpal ligament is thumped, causing tingling in the hand and fingers; and nerve conduction tests.

Treatment of carpal tunnel syndrome can be conservative, with anti-inflammatory medications and immobilization of the wrist with a brace or splint. If surgical intervention is necessary, it consists of release of the transverse carpal ligament.

Dupuytren Contracture

Dupuytren contracture results in flexion deformities of the fingers, most often the ring and little fingers. It is caused by contractures of the fascia in the palm of the hand due to the proliferation or overgrowth of fibrous tissue (Fig. 28-7). As the fibrous tissue grows thicker,

Figure 28-7 A Dupuytren contracture.

PATIENT EDUCATION

LIVING WITH CARPAL TUNNEL SYNDROME

Patients with carpal tunnel syndrome should be questioned regarding their work environment. This syndrome is common among typists, computer operators, assembly line workers, and other professions that demand frequent grasping, twisting, and flexion of the wrist. Caution a patient who does a lot of word processing or typing to maintain good body alignment at all times in a properly proportioned and well-constructed chair. Palm supports for computer keyboards decrease the degree of wrist flexion. Advise the patient to take breaks and, if possible, to alternate computer work with other tasks. A physical therapist may offer range-of-motion exercises that the patient can do throughout the day to alleviate wrist tension. An occupational therapist can evaluate the work area and make suggestions for changes. Always consult the physician before making referrals.

function is lost because the fingers cannot be straightened. Dupuytren contracture is easily diagnosed by inspection and palpation. Surgery is often required to release the contractures. Although no medications are available to treat this disorder, corticosteroid injections may temporarily improve function in the hand. Stretching of the tight structures in the early stages may slow the progression.

 CHECKPOINT QUESTION

11. What is the treatment for carpal tunnel syndrome?

Disorders of the Lower Extremities

The musculoskeletal structures of the lower extremities include the hip, knee, ankle, and feet. The hip, a ball-and-socket joint, is important for weight bearing and walking. The acetabulum, the socket of the hip joint, is deep enough to hold most of the femoral head and is surrounded by three strong ligaments.

The largest joint in the body, however, is the knee. Locking the knee into extension allows one to stand for long periods without using the muscles. An integral part of the knee is the patella, which lies inside the quadriceps tendon and protects the hinge joint. Two important sets of ligaments, the collateral and cruciate ligaments, stabilize the knee. The knee is often injured because it is sup-

ported entirely by muscles and ligaments and because it is one of the most stressed joints, lying as it does between the two longest bones in the body.

Chondromalacia Patellae

Chondromalacia patellae is a degenerative disorder affecting the cartilage that covers the back of the patella, or kneecap. It usually occurs in young women and in athletes who perform activities that stress the knee, such as running, jumping, and bicycling. A common complaint is pain when walking down stairs or getting out of a chair. Rest, physical therapy, bracing or taping the knee, anti-inflammatory medications, ice therapy, and exercises to strengthen the quadriceps muscles can help to relieve the symptoms. If these treatments are not effective, an endoscope may be used to examine the joint and surrounding tissue for further problems (**arthroscopy**) (Fig. 28-8). In severe and chronic cases, a surgical procedure, **arthroplasty**, may be performed to repair or remove damaged cartilage.

Plantar Fasciitis

Plantar fasciitis, inflammation of the plantar fascia ligament that stretches across the bottom of the foot, is the most frequent cause of pain in the bottom of the foot. Although the cause of plantar fasciitis is not always known, repetitive activities that stress the plantar fascia ligament, such as running and walking for extended periods on hard surfaces, may cause it. Factors that may aggravate it include wearing improperly fitted shoes and being overweight. Diagnosis includes a history of pain in the foot and heel when getting out of bed or after sitting for long periods. Deep palpation over the plantar (sole) surface of the heel bone will elicit pain. Radiography of the foot may be ordered to identify stress fractures, bone

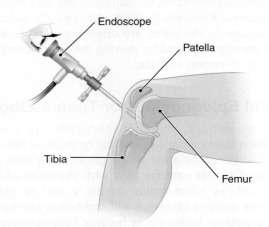

Figure 28-8 An arthroscopic examination of the knee. (Reprinted with permission from Cohen BJ. Medical Terminology: An Illustrated Guide. Philadelphia: Lippincott Williams & Wilkins, 2003.)

cysts, or heel spurs; however, ligaments do not show up clearly on radiographs, which are not routinely ordered to diagnose plantar fasciitis.

The treatment of choice for plantar fasciitis is a foot orthotic device (splint or heel pad) to support the arch and distribute the weight evenly. Physical therapy to stretch the ligament, ice therapy, massage, ultrasound, and nonsteroidal anti-inflammatory medications may also relieve the pain. Chronic planter fasciitis may necessitate wearing a night splint, which holds the affected foot at a 90° angle, preventing shortening and tightening of the plantar fascia during the night. Surgery is rarely done because of the high incidence of recurrence.

Common Diagnostic Procedures

Physical Examination

The physician's evaluation of the musculoskeletal system usually includes an assessment of structure and function, movement, and pain. An important part of the evaluation is the history, which includes the patient's description of the events and circumstances that led to the decision to seek medical help.

The physician observes the patient's overall physical state by noting how the patient walks, sits, stands, and moves. Concentrating on the area of concern, the physician evaluates the problem by visual inspection, palpation, and diagnostic tests. Pain and limited or compromised functions are warning signals. Strength also affects function and is a part of any musculoskeletal evaluation. Other important considerations are skin color, temperature, tone, and tenderness; abnormal findings may indicate underlying disease.

Diagnostic Studies

The most frequently used tools for detecting disorders of the musculoskeletal system are radiology and diagnostic imaging, which are used to diagnose fractures, dislocations, and degeneration or diseases of the bones and joints. Other radiographic studies include **arthrograms**, x-ray studies of the joints that may show joint disease, and myelograms, which help detect intervertebral disc conditions. A bone scan analyzes bone growth, density, tumors, and other pathology.

Computed tomography (CT) and magnetic resonance imaging (MRI) may reveal soft tissue disease, such as tumor, metastatic lesions, and ruptured or bulging discs. Electromyography and nerve conduction velocity tests measure the health and fitness of the nerves as they relate to conduction of nerve impulses and muscle function.

Goniometry is measurement of the amount of movement available in a joint by a protractor-like device called a **goniometer** (Fig. 28-9). A bone or muscle biopsy is also a valuable diagnostic tool. It allows intense ex-

Figure 28-9 A goniometer. (Reprinted with permission from Weber J, Kelley J. Health Assessment in Nursing. Philadelphia: Lippincott Williams & Wilkins, 2003.)

amination of the tissue under a microscope to determine cell damage, neoplasms (tumor or growth), or other types of diseases.

 CHECKPOINT QUESTION

12. What procedures can be used to diagnose musculoskeletal disorders?

The Role of the Medical Assistant

Warm and Cold Applications

Because of the time necessary for warm or cold applications, these procedures are not often done in the office. However, your responsibility may include instructing the patient in administering the treatments at home. Patients should understand the purpose of the procedure, how to perform it, the expected results, and any precautions or danger signs. Table 28-2 discusses the types of heat and cold applications and the purposes of each. Procedure 28-2 describes the steps for applying a cold pack, and Procedure 28-3 describes a hot pack application.

Precautions

When exposed to cool or warm temperatures, the body quickly adapts. For example, the water in a swimming pool feels cool at first, but after a short while, the body becomes used to the temperature, and it no longer feels

TABLE 28-2	Heat and Cold Treatments: Types and Purposes	
Dry Heat	**Moist Heat**	**Purposes**
Hot water bottle Heating pad Thermal pad Disposable heat pack Heat lamp	Compresses Warm soaks	Relieve muscle spasms or tension; relieve pain; hasten healing by increasing blood flow to an area; provide local or systemic warming
Dry Cold	**Moist Cold**	**Purposes**
Ice bag Ice collar Disposable ice pack	Compresses Cold soaks	Limit initial edema by decreasing capillary permeability (caution: cold retards edema by decreasing blood flow to the area); decrease bleeding or hemorrhage; decrease inflammation; relieve pain by numbing nerve pathways; provide local or systemic cooling

cool. The body has adapted. Using this reasoning, patients should be instructed that the benefits of heat or cold therapy are continuing even though they may not be able to feel the initial temperature change.

The body responds to extremes of temperature for extended periods by exerting an opposite effect called the rebound phenomenon. For example, heat applied to an area will cause dilation of the blood vessels, or vasodilation. However, if heat is applied beyond 30 minutes, vasoconstriction will occur as the body attempts to compensate for the heat. Therefore, applications left on longer than recommended by the physician will have an opposite effect to the one intended.

Some areas of the body with thin skin and few nerve receptors, such as the abdomen, are more sensitive to heat than areas such as the palms of the hands. When applying heat, remember that the very young, the elderly, the confused or disoriented patient, and patients with circulatory disorders or diabetes are particularly subject to burns. Box 28-5 provides additional guidelines for the proper use of heat and cold.

Generally, the temperature should be kept within the following guidelines:

- Warm: tepid, 95° to 98°F, to very warm, 115°F
- Cold: neutral, 93° to 95°F, to very cold, 50°F

In general and after checking with the physician, you should caution patients as follows:

Do not use heat:

- Within 24 hours after an injury, because it may increase bleeding
- For noninflammatory edema, because increased capillary permeability will allow additional tissue fluid to build up

- In cases of acute inflammation, because increased blood supply will increase the inflammatory process
- In the presence of malignancies, because cell metabolism will be enhanced
- Over the pregnant uterus
- On areas of erythema or vesicles, because it will compound the existing problem
- Over metallic implants, because it will cause discomfort

Do not use cold:

- On open wounds, because decreased blood supply will delay healing
- In the presence of already impaired circulation, because it will further impair circulation

 CHECKPOINT QUESTION

13. How does the body respond to prolonged exposure to temperature extremes?

Ambulatory Assist Devices

Patients may lose their ability to move normally because of an accident or injury, disease process, neurologic or muscular defect, or degeneration. Patients who require assistance to maintain mobility may use crutches, a cane, a walker, or a wheelchair. Medical assistants often are responsible for teaching patients how to use these ambulatory aids safely. Remind the patient to:

- Check the rubber tips frequently and replace worn tips immediately. (Most ambulatory aids require rubber tips, although some walkers have rollers.)

PATIENT EDUCATION

HEATING PADS

Heating pads are not often used in the office, but a heating pad may be ordered by the physician for the patient to use at home. The patient must be aware of the potential for injury if strict guidelines are not followed. Share these safety tips with your patient:

1. Most heating pads are equipped with a cover to ensure comfort and safety. If one is not provided, wrap the pad in a soft cover before applying to the skin.
2. Do not fold or bend the pad; wires may break and form an electrical short if not kept in alignment.
3. Do not use safety pins on the heating pad. Pins may cause malfunction if they come into contact with the wiring inside the pad.
4. Never place heating pads under the body; heat may build up as it is reflected from the surface below and cause burns.
5. Set the temperature to be comfortably warm at first touch (usually the low or medium setting); do not turn the temperature up to high as the body adjusts to the temperature.
6. Keep to the recommended time for heat treatments and allow circulation to return to normal at intervals.

- Check screws and bolts frequently; tighten as needed.
- Remove scatter rugs and small pieces of furniture that may cause falls.
- Use caution on wet surfaces to avoid falling.
- To avoid damage to the axillary nerve, do not place the axillary bars against the axilla.
- Avoid back and neck strain by standing straight and looking ahead.

Crutches

Crutches may be made of wood or tubular aluminum and may be ordered for short-term use or when the patient will need assistance long term for several months or years. Axillary crutches are the most common form and extend from just under the patient's axillae to the floor with hand grips to distribute weight to the palms. These crutches are typically prescribed for short-term conditions when the patient cannot bear weight on one extremity. The Lofstrand, or Canadian, crutch is usually aluminum and reaches just to the forearms, with a metal cuff to maintain its position on the arms and a covered hand grip to distribute the weight (Fig. 28-10). Lofstrand crutches allow the patient to release and use the hands without losing the crutches. These work well

A   **B**

Figure 28-10 Types of crutches. (**A**) Axillary crutches. (**B**) Lofstrand crutches (also known as Canadian or forearm crutches).

for patients who will need crutches for a long period or for those who have poor coordination. Procedure 28-4 explains the steps necessary for measuring and fitting a patient with axillary crutches, and Procedure 28-5 explains how to teach a patient the proper gait techniques.

PATIENT EDUCATION

TIPS FOR CRUTCH WALKING

To go up stairs:

- Stand close to the bottom step.
- With the body's weight supported on the hands, step up on the first step with the unaffected leg.
- Bring the affected side and the crutches up to the step at the same time.
- Resume balance before proceeding to the next step.
- *Remember:* The good side goes up first!

To descend stairs:

- Stand close to the edge of the top step.
- Bend from the hips and knees to adjust to the height of the lower step. Do not lean forward (leaning forward may cause a fall).

(continued)

- Carefully lower the crutches and the affected leg to the next step before moving the other extremity.
- Next, lower the unaffected leg to the lower step and regain balance.
- *Remember:* The affected foot goes down first!

To sit:

- Back up to the chair until you feel its edge on the back of your legs.
- Move both crutches to the hand on the affected side and reach back for the chair with the hand on the unaffected side.
- Lower yourself slowly into the chair.

Canes

A cane is used when the patient needs extra support and stability but requires only a small measure of assistance with weight bearing. The standard cane may be used when the patient needs very slight assistance. The tripod (three legs) or quad cane (four legs) is useful when the patient needs greater stability (Fig. 28-11). Tripod and quad canes can stand alone when patients need to use

their hands or have other support. They tend to be bulkier and heavier than standard canes, but because they offer greater stability and safety, they are good for patients who need more support than the standard cane affords.

To measure for proper cane length, have the patient stand erect. The cane should be level with the patient's greater trochanter, and the patient's elbow should be bent at a 30° angle. To walk with a cane, the patient should:

1. Position the cane on the unaffected side about 4 to 6 inches to the side and about 2 inches ahead of the foot.
2. Advance the cane and the affected leg together.
3. Bring the unaffected leg forward to a position just ahead of the cane.
4. Repeat the steps.

Walkers

A walker is a comfortable aid for the elderly and others with conditions that cause weakness or poor coordination. A walker is a lightweight aluminum frame shaped like three sides of a rectangle; however, because walkers are somewhat bulky, maneuvering in close quarters can be difficult. The walker frame should be level with the patient's hip, and the patient's elbow should be bent at about a 30° angle (Fig. 28-12). To use a walker:

1. Stand erect and move the walker ahead about 6 inches.

Figure 28-11 Three types of canes. (**A**) Single-ended canes with half-circle handles are recommended for patients requiring minimal support. (**B**) Single-ended canes with straight handles are recommended for patients with hand weakness. (**C**) Three- or four-prong canes are recommended for patients with poor balance.

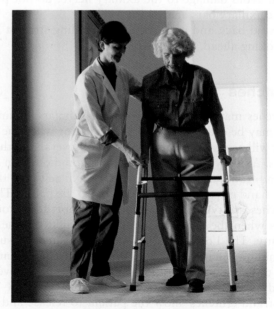

Figure 28-12 A properly adjusted walker.

2. Using an easy walking gait with hands on the walker grips, step into the walker.
3. Move the walker ahead again.
4. Repeat the steps.

 CHECKPOINT QUESTION

14. On which side of the body is the cane positioned?

 TRIAGE

While working in a medical office setting, the following three situations occur:

A. You need to teach a 78-year-old patient how to use a walker.
B. A 47-year-old woman just arrived in the office complaining of pain in her left wrist. She fell in the parking lot. You have been instructed to apply a cold pack to her wrist.
C. A 12-year-old patient needs a sling applied to her right arm.

How do you sort these patients? Who do you see first? Second? Third?

Patient B should be attended first. A cold pack should be applied to the injured wrist as soon as possible to help control the swelling and decrease the pain. Patient C should be seen next. Applying a sling will take less time than teaching patient A how to use the walker. Teaching an older patient may take extra time, skill demonstration, and return demonstration. In addition, a detailed patient education instruction pamphlet about the use of the walker should be given to the patient and explained in detail.

 MEDIA MENU

- **Student CD**
  - **Animations**
    Muscle Contraction
  - **CMA/RMA Certification Exam Review**
- **LWW's Medical Assisting Skills DVD**
  - **Procedures 28-4, 28-5**
- **Premium Online Course**
  http://thePoint.lww.com/Kronenberger3e
- **Internet Resources**

  LiveAdvise Online Tutoring & Competency Training
  http://thePoint.lww.com/LiveAdvise

  Arthritis Foundation
  http://www.arthritis.org

  Muscular Dystrophy Association
  http://www.mdausa.org

  About.com: What you need to know about orthopedics
  http://www.orthopedics.about.com

  American Association of Neurological Surgeons
  http://www.neurosurgerytoday.org/what/patient_e/carpal.asp

  Podiatry Online
  http://www.podiatryonline.com/main.cfm

español
SPANISH TERMINOLOGY

Voy a ponerle una tabilla en la pierna.
  I am going to put a splint on the leg.
Voy a examiner la pierna.
  I am going to examine your leg.
Doble las rodillas, no la espalda.
  Bend your knees, not your back.
Le duelen las articulaciónes?
  Do you have pain in your joints?

PROCEDURE 28-1: Apply an Arm Sling

Purpose: Correctly apply an arm sling
Equipment: A canvas arm sling with adjustable straps

Steps	Purpose
1. Wash your hands.	Handwashing aids infection control.
2. Assemble the equipment and supplies. Greet and identify the patient and explain the procedure.	Identifying the patient prevents errors in treatment. Explaining the procedure helps ease anxiety and ensure compliance.
3. Position the affected limb with the hand at slightly less than a 90° angle so that the fingers are a bit higher than the elbow.	This position helps reduce swelling of the hand and fingers
4. Insert the arm into the pouch end of the sling with the elbow fitting into the pocket corner.	

Step 4. Insert elbow into pocket of sling.

| 5. Bring the strap across the back and over the opposite shoulder to the front of the patient. | |

Step 5. Bring strap across back and to front of patient.

6. Secure the velcro end of the strap by inserting the end of it under the loop on the sling. Pull the strap through the loop an adequate amount so that the arm and hand inside the sling continue to be slightly elevated at a 90° angle.

(continued)

PROCEDURE 28-1:   **Apply an Arm Sling** *(continued)*

Steps	Purpose

Step 6. Bring strap through loop.

Steps	Purpose
7. Press the velcro ends together and check the patient's comfort and distal extremity circulation.	

Step 7. Check circulation.

Steps	Purpose
8. Document the appliance in the patient's chart.	Procedures are considered not to have been done if they are not recorded.

Charting Example

10/28/2008 11:15 AM Arm sling applied to (R) arm as ordered. Fingers to (R) hand warm and pink, no swelling. To RTO in 4 days
—T. Burton, RMA

PROCEDURE 28-2: Apply Cold Packs

Purpose: Apply a cold pack appropriately according to the physician's order
Equipment: Ice bag and ice chips or small cubes or a disposable cold pack, small towel or cover for the ice pack, gauze or tape

Steps	Purpose
1. Wash your hands.	Handwashing aids infection control.
2. Assemble the equipment and supplies, checking the ice bag for leaks. If using a commercial cold pack, read the manufacturer's directions.	Avoid wetting and chilling the patient. Small bits of ice help the bag to conform to the patient's contours better than large pieces.
3. Fill a reusable ice bag about two-thirds full. Press it flat on a surface to express air from the bag. Seal the container.	If the bag is too full of ice or air, it will not conform easily to the patient's contours.
4. If using a commercial chemical ice pack, activate it according to the manufacturer's instructions.	
5. Cover the bag in a towel or other suitable cover.	The cover will absorb condensation and make the procedure more comfortable for the patient. **Step 5.** Place the ice pack in a protective cover.
6. Greet and identify the patient. Explain the procedure.	Identifying the patient prevents errors in treatment. Explaining the procedure helps ease anxiety and ensures compliance.
7. After assessing the skin for color and warmth, place the covered ice pack on the area.	The area must be assessed for the documentation before treatment begins. The cold pack should not come into direct contact with the skin.
8. Secure the ice pack with gauze or tape.	The ice pack should lie securely against the patient's skin for the greatest benefit. Pins may puncture the ice bag. **Step 8.** Secure the ice pack with gauze or tape.
9. Apply the treatment for the prescribed amount of time and no longer than 30 minutes.	Longer than the prescribed time or 30 minutes may cause an adverse rebound effect, causing increased blood flow and swelling.

(continued)

PROCEDURE 28-2: Apply Cold Packs *(continued)*

10. During the treatment, assess the skin under the pack frequently for mottling, pallor, or redness. Remove the ice pack at once if these appear.	These signs indicate an adverse reaction and should be reported to the physician immediately after removing the ice pack.
11. Properly care for or dispose of equipment and supplies. Wash your hands.	If the equipment is reusable, it should be prepared for the next patient by disinfecting according to office policy. If it is disposable, discard it appropriately.
12. Document the procedure, site of the application, results including the condition of the skin after the treatment, and the patient's response.	Procedures are considered not to have been done if they are not recorded.

Charting Example

11/22/2008 10:45 AM *Ice bag applied to (L) anterior thigh as ordered ✕20 minutes. Skin before treatment swollen, with large contusion noted, no break in skin. After treatment, area pale and cool to touch, swelling decreased. Verbal and written instructions given for application qid at home; pt. verbalized understanding*

—*B. Barry, CMA*

PROCEDURE 28-3: Apply a Hot Water Bottle or Commercial Hot Pack

Purpose: Apply a hot pack appropriately according to the physician's order
Equipment: A hot water bottle or commercial hot pack, towel or other suitable covering for the hot pack

Steps	Purpose
1. Wash your hands.	Handwashing aids infection control.
2. Assemble equipment and supplies, checking the hot water bottle for leaks.	Checking for leaks avoids wetting the patient.
3. Fill the hot water bottle about two-thirds full with warm (110°F) water; place the bottle on a flat surface with the opening up and press out the excess air.	Excess air will prevent the bottle from conforming to the patient's contours.

Step 3. Express air from the bottle before capping.

(continued)

PROCEDURE 28-3: **Apply a Hot Water Bottle or Commercial Hot Pack** *(continued)*

Steps	Purpose
4. If using a commercial hot pack, follow the manufacturer's directions for activating it.	
5. Wrap and secure the pack or bottle before placing it on the patient's skin. **Step 5.** Wrap and secure the bag before placing on the patient's skin.	Covering the bag will increase the patient's comfort and prevent burning the skin.
6. Greet and identify the patient. Explain the procedure.	Identifying the patient prevents errors in treatment.
7. After assessing the color of the skin where the treatment is to be applied, place the covered hot pack on the area.	The area must be assessed for documentation before the treatment begins. The hot pack should not touch the skin. Heat therapy should be used cautiously in patients with circulatory disorders, diabetics, and the elderly.
8. Secure the hot pack with gauze or tape.	It should be securely against the patient's skin for the greatest benefit. Pins may puncture the hot pack.
9. Apply the treatment for the prescribed amount of time but for no longer than 30 minutes.	Longer than the prescribed time or 30 minutes may cause an adverse rebound effect and decreased blood flow to the area.
10. During the treatment, assess the skin every 10 minutes for pallor (rebound), excessive redness (pack too hot), and swelling (tissue damage). If you see any of these signs, immediately remove the hot pack.	These signs indicate an adverse reaction and should be reported to the physician immediately after you remove the hot pack.
11. Properly care for or dispose of equipment and supplies. Wash your hands.	Reusable equipment should be disinfected for the next patient. Disposables should be discarded appropriately.
12. Document the procedure, site of the application, results including condition of the skin after treatment, and the patient's response.	Procedures are considered not to have been done if they are not recorded.

Charting Example

7/11/2008 3:00 PM Hot pack to (L) shoulder ×30 minutes as ordered. Skin pink before treatment, slightly reddened after treatment. Pt. stated pain in upper back and shoulder relieved. Oral and written instructions given for applications at home qid, Pt. verbalized understanding

—*S. Rose, CMA*

PROCEDURE 28-4:   Measure a Patient for Axillary Crutches

Purpose: Accurately measure a patient for axillary crutches
Equipment: Axillary crutches with tips, pads for the axilla, and hand rests as needed

Steps	Purpose
1. Wash your hands.	Handwashing aids infection control.
2. Assemble the equipment, including crutches of the correct size.	Axillary crutches must always be fitted to the height of the patient.
3. Greet and identify the patient.	This helps avoid errors in treatment.
4. Ensure that the patient is wearing low-heeled shoes with safety soles.	Low-heeled shoes with good soles assist with adjusting the crutches to the patient's height and help prevent falls. While using the crutches, patients should wear shoes with the same heel height to avoid an improper crutch fit.
5. Have the patient stand erect. Support the patient as needed.	
6. While standing erect, have the patient hold the crutches naturally with the tips about 2 inches in front of and 4 to 6 inches to the sides of the feet. This is called the tripod position, and all crutch gaits start from this position.	
7. Using the tools as needed, adjust the central support in the base so that the axillary bar is about two finger-breadths below the patient's axillae. Tighten the bolts for safety at the proper height.	If the axillary bar presses on the axillae, nerve damage may occur. If it is too low, the crutches will be difficult to manage and will cause poor posture and back strain.
	Step 7. (A) Adjust the crutches to the patient's height by removing the wing nut and bolt and moving the extension. **(B)** Tighten the bolt securely.
8. Adjust the hand grips by raising or lowering the bar so that the patient's elbow is at a 30° angle when the bar is gripped. Tighten bolts for safety	Hand grips that are too high or too low will compromise safety and may cause nerve pressure.

(continued)

PROCEDURE 28-4: Measure a Patient for Axillary Crutches (continued)

Steps	Purpose
	Step 8. (A) Adjust the hand grips by raising or lowering along the shaft of the crutch. **(B)** Crutches are properly adjusted when the patient's elbow is at a 30° angle and two fingers can be inserted under the axilla on top of the crutch axillary bar.
9. If needed, pad axillary bars and hand grips with soft material, such as large gauze pads or small towels and secure with tape to prevent friction.	If padding is used on the axillary bars, make sure the padding is not touching the axilla; this is to avoid pressure and damage to the axillary nerve.
10. Wash your hands and record the procedure.	Procedures are considered not to have been done if they are not recorded.

Charting Example

> 3/17/2008 4:40 PM Pt. measured for axillary crutches as ordered; no pressure to axilla, elbows at a 30° angle. Given oral and written instructions for crutch safety and the 3-point and swing-through gaits. Demonstrated both gaits without difficulty. Verbalized understanding of instructions. Reinforced physician order for no weight bearing on (L) leg ×3 days, to return to office in 4 days
>
> —B. Daye, RMA

PROCEDURE 28-5: Instruct a Patient in Various Crutch Gaits

Purpose: Properly instruct a patient in various gaits using axillary crutches
Equipment: Axillary crutches measured appropriately for a patient

Steps	Purpose
1. Wash your hands.	Handwashing aids infection control.
2. Have the patient stand up from a chair, holding both crutches on the affected side, then sliding to the edge of the chair. The patient pushes down on the chair arm on the unaffected side, then pushes to stand. With one crutch in each hand, he or she rests on the crutches until balance is restored.	

(continued)

PROCEDURE 28-5: **Instruct a Patient in Various Crutch Gaits** *(continued)*

Steps	Purpose
3. Assist the patient to the tripod position.	To ensure safety and proper balance, crutches should be in this position before proceeding with any gait.

4. Depending on the patient's weight-bearing ability, coordination, and general state of health, instruct the patient in one or more of the following gaits:

4 POINT GAIT	2 POINT GAIT	3 POINT GAIT	SWING TO	SWING THROUGH
• Partial weight bearing both feet • Maximal support provided • Requires constant shift of weight	• Partial weight bearing both feet • Provides less support than 4 point gait • Faster than a 4 point gait	• Non weight-bearing • Requires good balance • Requires arm strength • Faster gait • Can use with walker	• Weight bearing both feet • Provides stability • Requires arm strength • Can use with walker	• Weight bearing • Requires arm strength • Requires coordination/balance • Most advanced gait
4. Advance right foot	4. Advance right foot and left crutch	4. Advance right foot	4. Lift both feet/ swing forward / land feet next to crutches	4. Lift both feet / swing forward / land feet in front of crutches
3. Advance left crutch	3. Advance left foot and right crutch	3. Advance left foot and both crutches	3. Advance both crutches	3. Advance both crutches
2. Advance left foot	2. Advance right foot and left crutch	2. Advance right foot	2. Lift both feet / swing forward / land feet next to crutches	2. Lift both feet / swing forward / land feet in front of crutches
1. Advance right crutch	1. Advance left foot and right crutch	1. Advance left foot and both crutches	1. Advance both crutches	1. Advance both crutches
Beginning stance	Beginning stance	Beginning stance	Beginning stance	Beginning stance

Crutch gaits.

(continued)

PROCEDURE 28-5: Instruct a Patient in Various Crutch Gaits *(continued)*

Steps	Purpose

A. Three-point gait, most commonly used for crutch training. For use when only one leg can bear weight or only partial weight bearing is allowed on the affected leg. Used by amputees, those with injury to one leg, and leg or foot surgery patients. Requires coordination and upper body strength.
  (1) Move both crutches forward with the unaffected leg bearing weight.
  (2) Supporting weight on hand grips, bring unaffected leg past crutches.
  (3) Repeat.
B. Two-point gait requires partial weight bearing and good coordination. Two points are raised, and two points are always on the floor.
  (1) Move right crutch and left foot forward.
  (2) As these points rest, move right foot and left crutch forward.
  (3) Repeat.
C. Four-point gait, slowest and safest of the gaits. At least three points are on the ground at all times. The affected leg must bear partial weight. Used by patients with degenerative diseases, spasticity, or poor coordination.
  (1) Move right crutch forward.
  (2) Move left foot just ahead of left crutch.
  (3) Move left crutch forward.
  (4) Move right foot just ahead of right crutch.
  (5) Repeat.
D. Swing-through gait.
  (1) Move both crutches forward.
  (2) With weight on hands, swing body ahead of crutches, with both legs leaving the floor together.
  (3) Move crutches ahead.
  (4) Repeat.
E. Swing-to gait.
  (1) Move both crutches forward.
  (2) With weight on hands, swing body even with crutches, with both legs leaving the floor.
  (3) Move crutches ahead.
  (4) Repeat.	

5. Wash your hands and record the procedure.	Procedures are considered not to have been done if they are not recorded.

Charting Example

See Charting Example for Procedure 28-4.

Chapter Summary

- The musculoskeletal system has many functions including:
  - Providing support and protection for vital organs
  - Allowing movement and mobility
  - Providing a frame (the skeleton) on which muscles are attached and the bones are held together at the joints
  - Providing stability and flexibility of the body
- Although the orthopedic physician specializes in the diagnosis and treatment of these conditions, you should expect to see patients with disorders of the musculoskeletal system in various medical offices, including pediatrics and family practice. In this chapter, you learned:

- Common disorders of the musculoskeletal system including the upper and lower extremities.
- Diagnostic procedures including x-ray procedures that may be ordered by the physician to assist in diagnosing disorders of the musculoskeletal system.
- Various types of ambulatory assist devices that may be necessary for patients who have mobility problems related to disorders of the musculoskeletal system including canes and crutches.
- Your role in working with patients in the medical office who may have disorders of the musculoskeletal system.

Warm Ups for Critical Thinking

1. Create a patient education brochure for the use of ambulatory aids. Be sure to include a brief description of the purpose of each aid along with the procedure steps.

2. The youth baseball league playoffs are coming to your town, and you are asked to staff the first aid station. What kinds of orthopedic injuries do you expect to see, and why? Develop a list of the first aid supplies that you want to have available and explain the reasons for your selections.

3. How would you respond to a patient with impaired circulation who tells you that he often uses a heat-ing pad to relieve the pain in his legs although the physician has warned him not to do so?

4. Your patient with plantar fasciitis asks you why the pain is worse in the morning when first getting out of bed. Describe how you could explain this condition to a patient with limited understanding of human anatomy.

5. Using a drug reference book, look up several anti-inflammatory medications (naproxen sodium, ibuprofen). What gastrointestinal disorders may result from taking these medications, and how can these side effects be avoided?

Answers to Checkpoint Questions

1. Luxation is a complete dislocation; subluxation is a partial dislocation.

2. It is important not to touch a wet plaster cast since pressure sores may develop on the skin from indentations made inadvertently in the wet cast from the fingers.

3. An open reduction includes surgery; a closed reduction does not.

4. The most common site of bursitis is in the area of the subdeltoid bursa in the shoulder between the deltoid muscle and the joint capsule.

5. Osteoarthritis is a degenerative joint disease caused by wear and tear on the weight-bearing joints in which the articular cartilage degenerates and the ends of the bones enlarge. Rheumatoid arthritis is a systemic autoimmune disease that attacks the synovium of the joint, ultimately leading to inflammation, pain, stiffness, and crippling deformities. It usually begins in the non–weight-bearing joints but eventually affects most of the joints of the appendicular skeleton.

6. Typically, tendonitis is due to inflammation caused from strains, sprains, overuse, or overstretching of these tissues.

7. Since foods high in purine may cause gout, patients should be discouraged from consuming alcoholic beverages, turkey, sardines, trout, bacon, and organ meats.

8. Exercise strengthens the bones and may help to prevent fractures that often result from osteoporosis.

9. Abnormal spinal curvatures include scoliosis (lateral curve), kyphosis (hunchback), and lordosis (swayback).

10. Injuries or disorders that limit movement of one or both arms may result in adhesive capsulitis.

11. The treatment for carpal tunnel syndrome consists of treating the inflammation with anti-inflammatory medications and immobilization of the wrist with a splint or brace. However, in some cases, surgery is necessary to release the transverse carpal ligament.

12. Procedures that may be ordered by the physician to diagnose musculoskeletal disorders include the physical examination, computed tomography, magnetic resonance imaging, electromyography, nerve conduction velocity, goniometry, arthrography, myelography, bone scan, and radiography.

13. After long exposure to temperature extremes, the body exerts the opposite effect. For example, heat applications lasting longer than 30 minutes will cause vasoconstriction rather than the intended vasodilation. This is called the rebound phenomenon, or rebound effect.

14. The cane is positioned on the unaffected side of the body.

CHAPTER
29

Ophthalmology and Otolaryngology

Outline

Common Disorders of the Eye
Cataract
Sty or Hordeolum
Conjunctivitis
Corneal Ulcer
Retinopathy
Glaucoma
Refractive Errors
Strabismus
Color Deficit
Diagnostic Studies of the Eye
Visual Acuity Testing
Color Deficit Testing
Tonometry and Gonioscopy
Therapeutic Procedures for the Eye
Instilling Eye Medications

Common Disorders of the Ear
Ceruminosis
Conductive and Perceptual
   Hearing Loss
Ménière's Disease
Otitis Externa
Otitis Media
Otosclerosis
Diagnostic Studies of the Ear
Visual Examination
Audiometry and
   Tympanometry
Tuning Fork Tests
Therapeutic Procedures for the Ear
Irrigations and Instillations

Common Disorders of the Nose and Throat
Allergic Rhinitis
Epistaxis
Nasal Polyps
Sinusitis
Pharyngitis and Tonsillitis
Laryngitis
Diagnostic Studies of the Nose and Throat
Visual Inspection
Therapeutic Procedures for the Nose and Throat
Throat Culture

Learning Objectives

Upon successfully completing this chapter, you will be able to:

1. Spell and define key terms

2. List and define disorders associated with the eye and identify commonly performed diagnostic procedures

3. List and define disorders associated with the ear and identify commonly performed diagnostic procedures

4. List and define disorders associated with the nose and throat and identify commonly performed diagnostic procedures

5. Describe patient education procedures associated with the eye, ear, nose, and throat

Upon successfully completing this chapter, you will be able to:

1. Measure distance visual acuity with a Snellen chart (Procedure 29-1)
2. Measure color perception with an Ishihara color plate book (Procedure 29-2)
3. Instill eye medication (Procedure 29-3)
4. Irrigate the eye (Procedure 29-4)
5. Irrigate the ear (Procedure 29-5)
6. Administer an audiometric hearing test (Procedure 29-6)
7. Instill ear medication (Procedure 29-7)
8. Instill nasal medication (Procedure 29-8)

CAAHEP

- Practice standard precautions
- Prepare patient for and assist with routine and specialty examinations
- Prepare patient for and assist with procedures, treatments, and minor office surgeries
- Document appropriately

ABHES

- Practice standard precautions
- Prepare patients for procedures
- Assist physician with examinations and treatments
- Perform selected tests that assist with diagnosis and treatment
- Document accurately

astigmatism
cerumen
decibel (db)
fluorescein angiography
hyperopia

intraocular pressure
myopia
myringotomy
ophthalmologist
ophthalmoscope
optician

optometrist
otolaryngologist
otoscope
presbycusis
presbyopia
refraction

retinal degeneration
tinnitus
tonometry
upper respiratory infection

Medical assistants working for **ophthalmologists**, who specialize in disorders of the eyes, or **otolaryngologists**, who specialize in disorders of the ears, nose, and throat (also known as ENT physicians), are expected to perform basic procedures associated with these body systems. Medical assistants working in general family practice and pediatric offices also encounter patients with eye or ear disorders and are expected to perform basic procedures associated with the eyes, ears, nose, and throat in these settings as well. This chapter describes the various disorders, diagnostic tests, and treatment modalities that are included in the eye, ear, nose, or throat examination.

Common Disorders of the Eye

Light waves are reflected off of all objects and are transmitted through various structures of the eye including the cornea, lens, and retina (Fig. 29-1). These impulses are transmitted via the optic nerve to the occipital lobe of the cerebral cortex in the brain. When the rays of light are bent, or refracted, by the curvature of the cornea and

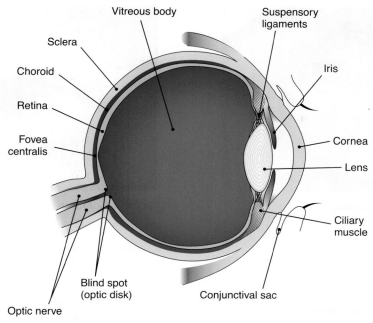

Figure 29-1 The eye. (Reprinted with permission from Cohen BJ. Memmler's The Human Body in Health and Disease. Philadelphia: Lippincott Williams & Wilkins, 2005.)

lens, the occiput recognizes whether the objects are in or out of focus. If the objects are out of focus to the occiput, impulses are sent to change the shape of the lens or the position of the extrinsic muscles to sharpen the image.

While the eye is a complex, highly developed organ, any of its many components may malfunction or become infected or diseased. The most common eye disorders that you may encounter in a medical office are described in the following sections. In addition, Box 29-1 describes guidelines for assisting sight-impaired patients in a medical office.

Cataract

A cataract is an opacity, or clouding, of the lens that leads to decreased visual acuity. Most commonly, cataracts are bilateral and seen in the elderly. A rare condition in infancy can result from maternal exposure to the rubella virus. This condition is known as congenital cataracts. Occasionally, trauma to the lens or chemical toxicity causes clouding of the lens.

The symptoms include gradual blurring and loss of vision over months as the clouding of the lens slowly progresses. The observer may see a milky opacity at the pupil rather than the normal black opening (Fig. 29-2). An examination with an **ophthalmoscope** reveals the white area behind the pupil if the cataract has not advanced to the point where it can be seen unassisted.

The treatment for cataracts is surgical removal of the opaque lens. This surgery is beneficial in 95% of patients and is usually an outpatient procedure. After the

cloudy lens has been removed, an intraocular lens is implanted, or the patient's vision is corrected by contact lenses or special glasses.

BOX 29-1

ASSISTING SIGHT-IMPAIRED PATIENTS

Follow these tips to assist a sight-impaired patient:

- Ask patients how you can help, and follow their requests and suggestions. Many sight-impaired patients know best what they need.
- When escorting the patient, offer your arm. Tell the patient the approximate length of the hallway and advise the patient of any turns, such as, "It should be about 20 steps and then we'll take a right." Avoid stairs if possible, but if you must assist a sight-impaired patient up or down stairs, advise the person of the number of steps. Many patients prefer to hold the railings for balance.
- If the patient has a guide dog, do not approach the dog without first speaking to the patient and receiving approval.
- If the patient needs extensive teaching on a particular subject, suggest using a tape recorder to record the instructions.

Figure 29-2 An eye with a cataract.

Figure 29-3 Conjunctivitis.

Sty or Hordeolum

A sty, or hordeolum, is an infection of any of the lacrimal glands of the eyelids, causing redness, swelling, and pain. The causative infectious organism is often *Staphylococcus aureus*, a microorganism commonly found on the skin. Warm compresses will hasten suppuration of the infection, and topical antibiotic drops or ointments attack the microorganism. You may be responsible for teaching the patient the procedure for applying warm compresses and instilling ophthalmic drops or ointment.

 CHECKPOINT QUESTION

1. What are the symptoms of a cataract?

Conjunctivitis

Conjunctivitis, an infection of the mucous membrane covering the sclera and cornea (conjunctiva) of the eye, is caused by several species of bacteria or viruses. Additional causes of conjunctivitis include allergens or irritants without an infectious process. Many pathogens cause unilateral conjunctivitis, but allergic conjunctivitis is almost always bilateral.

Signs and symptoms of conjunctivitis include tearing and occasionally exudates and pain (Fig. 29-3). Bacterial and viral conjunctivitis, or pink eye, is highly contagious and can rapidly spread through schools and day care centers. It is spread by contact; for example, an infectious child rubs the eyes, handles objects such as toys or books, and spreads the infection to the next child who comes into contact with the contaminated object. The infected child should not go to school or day care until the infection is treated and has been resolved. Good hygiene, including handwashing, helps prevent the spread of infectious conjunctivitis. Antibiotic ophthalmic drops or ointment are prescribed by the physician if the cause of the con-

junctivitis is bacterial. To prevent the spread of conjunctivitis, you should instruct the patient to do the following:

- Avoid rubbing the eyes to prevent spreading the infection to the other eye or to other people.
- Discard all eye makeup that may be infectious.
- Wash all towels, washcloths, and pillowcases after use.

Corneal Ulcer

A corneal ulcer is erosion of the surface of the cornea, leaving scar tissue that may lead to visual disturbances or blindness. Corneal ulcers are caused by several types of bacteria, fungi, viruses, and protozoa or by trauma, allergen, or toxin. Signs and symptoms include tearing, pain on blinking, and sensitivity to light. A visual examination with a penlight shows an irregular corneal surface. A fluorescein dye is administered by placing a strip gently in the sulcus of the eye; this stains the perimeter of the ulcer to confirm the diagnosis. Treatment includes rest and antibiotic therapy.

 CHECKPOINT QUESTION

2. Explain the difference between a sty and conjunctivitis.

Retinopathy

Retinopathy is a general term for disease or disorder affecting the retina. A decrease in the blood supply to the highly vascular retina will cause **retinal degeneration,** pathologic changes in cell structure that impair or destroy the retina's function. The causes include atherosclerosis that impedes blood flow to the retina, the microcirculatory changes associated with diabetes (diabetic retinopathy), and vascular changes resulting from long-term hypertension. Depending on the cause, the patient's loss of vision may be sudden or gradual. Loss of vision may be preceded by small intraocular hemorrhages, night blindness, or loss of the central visual field. If small vessels rupture and scar, they may pull against the retina and cause retinal detachment that results in blindness.

Diagnosis of retinopathy is made by a thorough eye examination and **fluorescein angiography**. This procedure involves injection of fluorescent dye into one of the veins of the arms and photographing the blood vessels of the eye as the dye moves through it. The treatment of retinopathy is based on treating the underlying cause. Although some forms of retinopathy respond well to treatment, others progress to full blindness.

Glaucoma

Glaucoma describes a group of disorders that result in increased **intraocular pressure**, or pressure within the eye. As aqueous humor is formed in the posterior chamber just in front of the lens, it flows through the pupil to the anterior chamber just behind the cornea. It eventually filters into the canal of Schlemm. Any pathology that impedes the outflow of aqueous humor (genetics, vasoconstriction) will increase the pressure, either very gradually or quite suddenly. The gradual form of glaucoma (open-angle glaucoma) may present with mild or no pain, visualizing halos around lights, and loss of peripheral vision. Most adult glaucoma patients have this type of glaucoma. Angle-closure glaucoma, an acute and sudden blockage, is characterized by severe eye pain, blurred vision, headache, nausea, and vomiting. Blindness may result within days of the onset of acute glaucoma unless the condition is diagnosed and treated quickly.

Treatment for chronic glaucoma includes medication, often a diuretic, to decrease intraocular pressure by slowing the formation of aqueous humor within the eyes or by improving the flow. Acute glaucoma may necessitate an iridectomy, or removal of part of the iris, to increase the outflow of the humor. Frequent eye examinations, including **tonometry**, may detect glaucoma and facilitate treatment before visual deficiencies and blindness result.

Refractive Errors

Errors of **refraction** are the most common of all eye problems. The primary types of refractive errors are **hyperopia, myopia, astigmatism,** and **presbyopia.** Hyperopia, also known as farsightedness, occurs in an eyeball that is too short from front to back to allow the lines of vision to reflect distinctly on the fovea centralis. The person with hyperopia cannot focus on objects near the face.

Myopia, also known as nearsightedness, results when the eyeball is too long. The lines of vision converge before they reach the fovea centralis and begin to diverge again at the fovea. Objects must be near the face for the image to be focused far back on the retina.

Astigmatism is unfocused refraction of light rays on the retina resulting from lens or corneal irregularities. If the cornea is not smooth, images refracted through it will not project sharply onto the retina; the effect is much like peering through wavy glass.

Presbyopia is vision change resulting from loss of lens elasticity with age. The lens normally adjusts to refract light from near or far. As a person ages, the ciliary bodies that hold and adjust the lens and the lens itself lose elasticity and no longer accommodate near vision; far vision may be unaffected. Symptoms usually begin gradually around age 40. Most adults are affected to some degree by age 50.

All refractive errors are treated with either corrective lenses or reshaping the lens with laser surgery (Fig. 29-4, Box 29-2). An **optometrist** is a trained specialist who measures errors of refraction and prescribes lenses. An **optician** is a trained specialist who grinds lenses to fulfill corrective prescriptions written by either an optometrist or an ophthalmologist, a medical doctor who treats eye disorders or performs surgical corrections.

CHECKPOINT QUESTION

3. What are the four common refractive errors? Briefly explain each.

Strabismus

Strabismus is a misalignment of eye movements, usually caused by muscle incoordination. Although most newborns are born with some degree of strabismus, coordination improves as the infant grows and the eye muscles strengthen. However, the strabismus does not resolve in some cases and requires medical intervention. Strabismus may take any of the following forms (Fig. 29-5):

- Esotropic, also known as cross eyes or convergent eyes
- Exotropic, also known as wall eyes or divergent eyes
- Hypotropic, deviation downward
- Hypertropic, deviation upward
- Concomitant, with both eyes moving together
- Nonconcomitant, with the two eyes moving independently

Treatment may require only patching, or covering, the unaffected eye to force the affected eye's muscles to strengthen. In some cases, surgery is required to correct the deviant muscle or muscles.

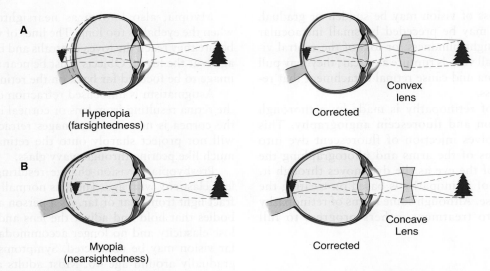

Figure 29-4 Errors of refraction. (**A**) The hypertrophic eye with convex corrective lens. (**B**) The myopic eye with concave corrective lens. (Reprinted with permission from Cohen BJ. Memmler's The Human Body in Health and Disease. Philadelphia: Lippincott Williams & Wilkins, 2005.)

BOX 29-2

LASER SURGERY TO CORRECT ERRORS OF REFRACTION

A procedure that is popular among patients to correct myopia, hyperopia, and astigmatism is a surgical procedure called LASIK, which stands for laser in-situ keratomileusis. An ophthalmologist uses a laser to reshape the cornea, allowing the light to properly focus on the retina and correcting these errors of refraction. Advantages of this procedure include:

* It is an outpatient procedure that takes very little time to perform.
* The vision of most people is corrected within 24 hours.
* There is a quick recovery time with very little pain.
* There is no need for glasses or contacts in most patients after the procedure.

Disadvantages include:

* The procedure is expensive.
* Changes made to the cornea cannot be reversed.
* Some side effects, such as dry eyes, may be experienced by some patients.

Patients wanting to know more about this procedure should be referred to an ophthalmologist.

Color Deficit

Color deficit is an absence of or a defect in color perception. Red, green, or blue perception may be impaired or absent. The term *color deficient* or *color deficit* is commonly used rather than referring to the disorder as color blindness.

This disorder is usually inherited on the X chromosome and affects more men than women. Occasionally, color deficit results from damage to the cones by medications or other substances that are toxic to the color-receptive nerve cells. Color deficit has no cure or correction.

 CHECKPOINT QUESTION

4. How is strabismus corrected?

Diagnostic Studies of the Eye

In most medical offices, the basic examination equipment includes the **ophthalmoscope**, a lighted instrument used to examine the inner surfaces of the eye. In many instances, visually examining the interior structures of the eyes can alert the physician to a number of vascular and hypertensive conditions because the blood vessels of the eye and the inner structures, such as the retina, are easily viewed (Fig. 29-6).

Visual Acuity Testing

Visual acuity, or clearness, is commonly assessed in the medical office using the Snellen eye chart. These charts are hung 20 feet from the patient at eye level in an area

Figure 29-5 Forms of strabismus. (**A**) Esotropic. (**B**) Exotropic. (**C**) Hypotropic. (From Weber J, Kelley J. Health Assessment in Nursing. 2nd ed. Philadelphia: Lippincott Williams & Wilkins, 2003.)

with good lighting and few distractions (Procedure 29-1). Normal vision (20/20) means the patient can see at 20 feet what the normal eye sees at 20 feet. The figures on the charts—letters, numbers, a series of E's, or common symbols—become progressively smaller to test

Figure 29-6 Examination of the eye with an ophthalmoscope. (Reprinted with permission from Willis MC. Medical Terminology: A Programmed Learning Approach to the Language of Health Care. Baltimore: Lippincott Williams & Wilkins, 2002.)

levels of perception (Fig. 29-7). For patients who cannot read or who do not speak English, the E chart may be used. A patient who can see only the line (letters or E's) on the chart at the 20/40 level has visual acuity at 20 feet equivalent to what a person with normal vision can see at 40 feet. The patient should wear any corrective lenses for the test unless the physician requests that the examination be done without them. Each eye is tested separately, with the opposite eye covered but not closed.

The picture chart is used for children. If a child is to be tested, first spend a few moments familiarizing the child with the objects on the chart. For example, if the picture is of a dog and the child has never seen one, the illustration may not be recognized as a dog. If necessary, enlist a parent or co-worker to help with the eye cover.

 CHECKPOINT QUESTION

5. When is the E chart used to test visual acuity?

Color Deficit Testing

The Ishihara method is used to test for color deficits (Procedure 29-2). It consists of 14 color plates with

Figure 29-7 Snellen charts used to assess distant vision. The charts on the left and right are used for young children and illiterate adults.

many four-colored dots forming a number, a letter, or a pattern of contrasting color in arrangement of dots (Fig. 29-8). Patients with deficient color perception are unable to see the design, numbers, or letters on plates 1 to 11, depending on the color deficiency. Although there is no cure or treatment for color deficits, knowledge of the deficit may help the patient with regard to coordinating clothing or choosing colors for decorating.

Tonometry and Gonioscopy

Using a tonometer, the physician measures the intraocular pressure or tension in the eye. The anterior eye is anesthetized with eye drops, and the instrument is moved against the cornea to measure the pressure required to produce an indentation or to flatten a small area of the cornea. This test is an important part of the eye examination to diagnose glaucoma. Although it is not routinely performed at the general practice medical office, tonometry is painless and done regularly at the ophthalmologist's or optometrist's office.

Gonioscopy, also performed at the ophthalmologist's or optometrist's office, is use of a special instrument (gonioscope) to measure the angle of the anterior

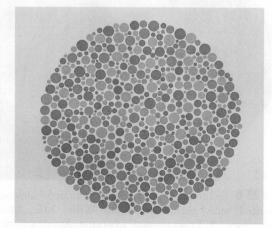

Figure 29-8 Ishihara color plate. (Courtesy of B. Proud. Copyright.)

chamber between the iris and the cornea. This test is useful to the physician in determining the cause of the increased intraocular pressure.

 CHECKPOINT QUESTION

6. Why is it important to have the pressure of the eye measured with a tonometer?

 PATIENT EDUCATION
PREVENTATIVE EYE CARE

Preventive care of the eye is a vital component of patient education. Regular eye checkups, proper care of contact lenses, control of diabetes and hypertension, annual tonometer checks for glaucoma yearly after age 40, and proper attention to eye injuries are important aspects of eye health maintenance.

Advise patients to wear sunglasses with ultraviolet protection during any sun exposure to avoid damage to the eyes. Children should also be fitted for sunglasses to protect their eyes against sun damage.

Advise patients not to rub their eyes. This can spread infection from person to person and can damage the cornea if a small foreign object is in the eye. Wearing goggles or safety glasses at appropriate times can prevent disease transmission and injury caused by foreign bodies.

Therapeutic Procedures for the Eye

Instilling Eye Medications

Medical assistants frequently have the responsibility of instilling ophthalmic medications and teaching patients about the procedure for home use. Instillations are used to treat infection or irritation, to dilate the pupil for retinal examination, and to apply anesthetic for treatment or testing (Procedure 29-3). Eye irrigations may also be ordered by the physician, usually to remove foreign bodies. Procedure 29-4 describes the steps for an eye irrigation.

 TRIAGE

You have the following three tasks:

A. Patient A is on the phone asking for advice on pain and blurred vision in his left eye after wearing his contact lens through the night.
B. Patient B is waiting in an examination room for you to complete a visual acuity and Ishihara test required for a pre-employment physical exam.
C. A pharmacist telephones with a question about a patient's prescription for glaucoma medication.

How do you sort these tasks? What do you do first? Second? Third?

After asking the receptionist to take a message from the pharmacist calling regarding patient C, address patient A since he will need an appointment to be seen right away. Wearing contact lens longer than prescribed can scratch the cornea, and the patient should be seen as soon as possible to avoid further damage. Next, complete and record the eye examinations for patient B's physical examination. Once these situations are resolved, call the pharmacist and answer any questions, clarify concerns, or refer the matter to the physician.

Common Disorders of the Ear

The ear is divided into three sections: the external ear, the middle ear, and the inner ear (Fig. 29-9). When sound waves hit the tympanic membrane, the vibrations pass through structures in the middle and inner ear. The auditory, or eustachian, tube connects the middle ear with the nasopharynx, and during swallowing, pressure is equalized in the middle ear. This equalization through the eustachian tube prevents pressure from building up in the middle ear and rupturing the tympanic membrane.

Patients who have problems with the ear or hearing are often referred to an otolaryngologist. Medical assistants in general practices also encounter patients with various disorders of the ears because pain and hearing loss are a frequent outcome of certain diseases and can occur at any age. Box 29-3 describes guidelines for assisting hearing-impaired patients in a medical office.

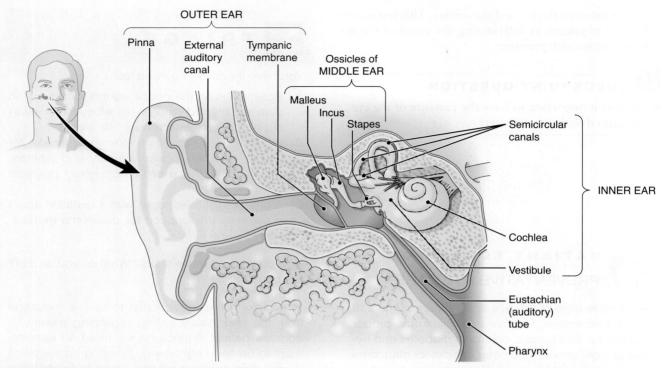

Figure 29-9 The ear, showing the outer, middle, and inner subdivisions. (Reprinted with permission from Cohen BJ. Memmler's The Human Body in Health and Disease. Philadelphia: Lippincott Williams & Wilkins, 2005.)

Ceruminosis

Ceruminosis, or impacted earwax, is a frequent reason for diminished hearing. **Cerumen** is usually soft and moist and leaks out in such small amounts that it is unnoticed. Occasionally, the cerumen becomes hard and dry or excessive hair in the ear holds the wax in the ear canal, causing it to build up against the tympanic membrane.

BOX 29-3

ASSISTING HEARING-IMPAIRED PATIENTS

Follow these tips to assist a hearing-impaired patient:

- Speak normally; do not yell or raise your voice. Doing so will not facilitate the hearing capabilities of the patient.
- Get the patient's attention before speaking and make sure he or she can see your lips while you talk.
- Speak clearly, but remember that the patient is hearing impaired, not mentally challenged.
- If the patient is deaf and requires an interpreter, speak to the patient, not the interpreter.

The presenting symptoms may be a gradual hearing loss or **tinnitus**, an extraneous noise heard in one or both ears. An examination of the ear canal with an **otoscope** shows the obvious reason. The wax may be softened by warm ear drops or hydrogen peroxide and removed by an ear curet or by gently washing with an irrigating device using water at room temperature (Procedure 29-5).

Conductive and Perceptual Hearing Loss

Conductive and perceptual hearing loss are the two categories of hearing impairment. In conductive loss, sound waves are not appropriately transmitted to the level of the cochlea. In perceptual, or sensorineural, loss, transmission from the oval window to the receptors in the brain is impaired. Many patients present with both, a condition called mixed deafness.

Causes of hearing loss include heredity, infection, trauma, ototoxic drugs, some neurologic diseases, exposure to loud noises, and **presbycusis**. Presbycusis usually results from a hardening of the joints between the ossicles (three small bones in the middle ear), which occurs with aging.

Diagnosis of hearing loss of any type is done by testing the hearing using an audiometer (Fig. 29-10) in the medical office. Procedure 29-6 describes the steps for performing a hearing test using the audiometer.

Figure 29-10 The audiometer.

Treatment is aimed at addressing the underlying cause of the hearing loss if possible. A stapedectomy may be performed for otosclerosis, with a replacement for the impaired joint. Cochlear implants are gaining favor for those whose hearing loss is caused by impairment in the cochlear receptors. Conductive hearing loss can be treated successfully in most instances with hearing aids; perceptual loss is far more difficult to correct.

 CHECKPOINT QUESTION

7. What is the difference between conductive and perceptual hearing loss?

 WHAT IF?

What if your patient asks you if a hearing aid could help her?

Hearing aids help many people, but they do not fully restore the ability to hear. The purpose of the aid is to amplify sound waves. Not all patients with hearing loss are good candidates for hearing aids. For example, patients who have permanent nerve damage generally do not have significant improvement with standard hearing aids.

The two basic types of aids are bone conduction receivers, which sit behind the ear and press against the skull, and air conduction receivers, which fit into the auditory canal. The size and type of hearing aid depends on the patient's specific condition and need. Binaural (both ears) aids are available and often can be fitted into eyeglasses for inconspicuous appearance.

Patients must understand that a hearing aid will improve their hearing, not correct it. Teach patients about maintenance requirements so they can keep the device in good working condition, and explain how to adjust the volume control. Have the patient speak to the physician regarding any concerns about purchasing and using a hearing aid.

Ménière's Disease

Ménière's disease, a degenerative condition of unknown cause, affects the inner ear and upsets the body's ability to maintain equilibrium in addition to causing loss of hearing. The symptoms include vertigo, sensorineural hearing loss, and tinnitus. Severe symptoms may lead to nausea and vomiting. Periods of remission are followed by exacerbation. Although there is no cure, many of the symptoms can be treated with palliative medication. If the symptoms persist or increase and become incapacitating, it may be necessary to destroy the organs of the inner ear. The result of this drastic measure is immediate relief of symptoms, but the patient is irreversibly deaf.

Otitis Externa

Also known as swimmer's ear, otitis externa is an inflammation or infection of the external ear. It is common in summer and is caused by any number of pathogens that grow in the warm, moist ear canal. The presenting symptoms include pain on movement of any adjoining structures around the ear, jaw, and auricle. Otoscopy reveals a red, swollen ear canal (Fig. 29-11). Although the physician may order that debris (pus or excessive cerumen) be gently washed from the area, otitis

Figure 29-11 The red, swollen ear canal of a patient with otitis externa. (From Bickley LS, Szilagyi P. Bates' Guide to Physical Examination and History Taking. 8th ed. Philadelphia: Lippincott Williams & Wilkins, 2003.)

externa is best treated by an antibiotic, either topical (Procedure 29-7) or systemic, warm compresses, and medication to relieve pain.

Applying an alcohol solution after swimming can help prevent this problem. Encourage patients who are prone to otitis externa to wear earplugs while swimming and to avoid using objects such as swabs or hairpins to clean inside the ear canal.

PATIENT EDUCATION
OTOLOGIC DISORDERS

Teach patients to recognize symptoms of otologic disorders (hearing loss, pain, drainage) and to report them promptly to the physician. Proper attention at the early stage of an infection or injury can often prevent serious or irreversible damage.

Instruct patients that it is acceptable to clean the external ear with a cotton-tipped applicator but that they should not put the applicator inside the ear canal. This drives cerumen deeper into the ear and creates more impaction than may already be present.

Tell children not to put small objects such as beans, peas, or small parts of toys in their ears because they may become lodged and removal may require surgery. Caution parents to complete all antibiotic treatment for children's ear infections even though the symptoms subside. The infection may linger after the patient is asymptomatic. Ear recheck appointments should be kept as scheduled to ensure that the child is free of infection.

Otitis Media

Otitis media, an inflammation or infection of the middle ear, is frequently caused by an **upper respiratory infection**. Pathogens responsible for pharyngitis, nasopharyngitis, and the common cold frequently travel through the warm, moist eustachian tube to the middle ear. As the infection increases, the mucous membranes of the eustachian tubes swell, closing off the opening to the middle ear. With no way to drain, fluid builds up as a response to the infection and causes pain and pressure on the flexible tympanic membrane. If pressure is sufficient, the membrane may tear or perforate spontaneously to relieve the pressure.

This disorder is common in infants and children because of the relatively horizontal position of the eustachian tube between the nasopharynx and middle ear. Children have very short, almost horizontal eustachian tubes, which can be problematic if microorganisms from the nasopharynx are forced into the

middle ear by coughing. The problem is compounded for children who are put to bed with a bottle of milk or formula. The milk acts as a hospitable medium for bacteria.

Symptoms include severe pain, fever of varying degrees, and mild to moderate hearing loss. Infants may be fussy and tug at their ears. Any elevation in a child's temperature should be a warning to check for otitis media. Diagnosis is usually made by otoscopy, which may reveal a reddened, bulging tympanic membrane (Fig. 29-12). Bubbles can sometimes be seen behind the thin membrane. Treatment is an antibiotic for bacterial infection and an analgesic for pain relief. A decongestant may reduce some of the swelling. In severe chronic cases, a **myringotomy** (surgical incision into the tympanic membrane) may be performed to relieve pressure. Tubes may be inserted through the tympanic membrane and remain for several months to equalize the pressure if the problem persists.

 CHECKPOINT QUESTION

8. What are the symptoms of otitis media in an infant?

Otosclerosis

Otosclerosis is a disorder of the ossicles of the inner ear, especially the stapes bone. This disorder, thought to be hereditary, results from ossification or hardening of the bones causing loss of hearing of low tones. The treatment for otosclerosis is hearing aids or microsurgical implantation of a stapedial prosthesis to replace the sclerotic joint and allow movement of the bones.

Otitis media

Figure 29-12 A bulging tympanic membrane of a patient with otitis media. (From Moore KL, Dalley AF II. Clinical Oriented Anatomy. 4th ed. Baltimore: Lippincott Williams & Wilkins, 1999.)

Diagnostic Studies of the Ear

Visual Examination

Using an otoscope, the physician can view the auditory canal and eardrum (Fig. 29-13). Disposable otoscopes are available; reusable otoscopes use disposable speculum covers that are changed between patients. Some reusable otoscopes use the same base as an ophthalmoscope.

Audiometry and Tympanometry

An audiometer can be used to detect hearing loss (Procedure 29-6). Audiometers produce pure tones of various **decibel (dB)** levels and frequencies heard through earphones or an instrument that resembles an otoscope. The decibel is a unit for measuring the intensity of sound. Speech audiometry uses voice tones rather than pure tones to assess hearing.

Impedance audiometry evaluates tympanic membrane and ossicle mobility. A probe is inserted into the auditory meatus and emits tones of various intensity levels that bounce back to the probe receiver. If the tympanic membrane and ossicles are normal, the movement is transmitted and rebound is picked up by the receiver to produce a curve on the graph. If the tympanic membrane and ossicles are less mobile than normal, much of the sound transmitted bounces back and is reflected to the instrument to produce a distinct curve on the graph. Tympanometry works like the audiometer but uses air pressure rather than tones to produce the graph.

 CHECKPOINT QUESTION

9. Which of the tests described allows the physician to visualize the ear canal and tympanic membrane?

Figure 29-13 Examination of the ear with an otoscope. (Reprinted with permission from Willis MC. Medical Terminology: A Programmed Learning Approach to the Language of Health Care. Baltimore: Lippincott Williams & Wilkins, 2002.)

Tuning Fork Tests

Two tests that may be performed using the tuning fork are the Rinne test and the Weber test. The Rinne test entails lightly tapping the tuning fork, placing the end of it on the mastoid bone, and then moving it to the external auditory meatus to determine conductive hearing loss. In normal hearing, the sound is louder through the external auditory meatus than the bone. The Weber test entails gently tapping the tuning fork and placing it on the midline of the forehead to differentiate between conductive and sensorineural hearing loss. In conductive loss, the sound is louder in the affected ear; in sensorineural loss, the sound is louder in the unaffected ear. Although the physician most likely is the one who performs the tuning fork tests, you should ensure that the tuning fork is available and assist as needed.

Therapeutic Procedures for the Ear

Irrigations and Instillations

Ear irrigations are performed to relieve pain, to remove debris or foreign objects, or to apply medication solutions. Ear instillations may include a local anesthetic for the relief of pain associated with otitis externa or otitis media or a topical antibiotic for otitis externa. These medications include the words "for otic use" on the label. For medication irrigations and instillations, observe the principles of medication administration, including checking the medication label for the expiration date.

Common Disorders of the Nose and Throat

Allergic Rhinitis

Allergic rhinitis is inflammation of the mucous membranes of the nasal passages usually resulting from exposure to an allergen. Symptomatic treatment with antihistamine medication is usually offered to relieve the symptoms. It is also known as hay fever or seasonal allergic rhinitis when it appears in response to seasonal plant pollens. If the symptoms are present year round, it is perennial allergic rhinitis and is usually a reaction to household irritants, such as dust mites and pet dander. The signs are obvious, with paroxysmal sneezing, intense rhinorrhea (nasal drainage), congestion, and watery reddened eyes.

Diagnosis usually entails history and differential diagnosis. Mucous secretions may reveal an increase in immunoglobulin E in response to the allergens. An allergist may isolate the offending protein by skin testing. Allergy treatment entails exposure to the allergen in minute doses to desensitize the immune reaction.

Middle turbinate
Inferior turbinate

Figure 29-14 Physical examination of the nose with a nasal speculum. (Reprinted with permission from Nettina SM. The Lippincott Manual of Nursing Practice. Philadelphia: Lippincott Williams & Wilkins, 2001.)

Epistaxis

Commonly known as nosebleed, epistaxis generally occurs from trauma to the nasal membranes, but it may be secondary to another disorder, such as hypertension, malignancy, polyps, or the fragile capillaries associated with pregnancy. Diagnosis necessitates a history and inspection of the nasal mucosa with a nasal speculum (Fig. 29-14). The initial therapy for simple epistaxis is having the patient sit upright with the head slightly forward to avoid postnasal drainage that may lead to nausea. Compress the nares against the septum for 5 to 10 minutes with either ice or a cold, wet compress. Advise the patient to remain still and not to blow the nose until the physician concludes that all danger is past.

Bleeding that continues more than 10 minutes after treatment begins is considered severe. For severe epistaxis, the physician may insert nasal packing or a balloon catheter that may remain in place several hours to several days. For secondary bleeding, treatment of the underlying cause may be indicated. Cautery to an exposed blood vessel helps if that is the only cause.

 CHECKPOINT QUESTION

10. What factors may contribute to epistaxis?

Nasal Polyps

Nasal polyps are small pendulous tissues that obstruct breathing. Polyps usually occur in the mucous membranes of the nasal passages as a response to long-term allergies. Symptoms include a feeling of fullness or congestion and occasionally a nasal discharge. Diagnosis requires direct examination with a nasal speculum or radiography of the nasal structures. Treatment may be corticosteroids applied either topically or by injection directly into the polyps. The underlying allergy must be treated to prevent recurrence of polyps. If conservative treatment is not effective, conventional or laser surgery is required.

Sinusitis

Sinusitis, or inflammation of one or more of the sinus cavities, can be either acute or chronic. Acute sinusitis is usually the result of an upper respiratory infection and is fairly easily resolved. Chronic sinusitis is more persistent and more difficult to control. Either form is particularly common when microorganisms are forced into the moist sinus cavities during hard nose blowing.

Symptoms of sinusitis include the obvious signs of an upper respiratory infection, with the addition of a purulent nasal discharge and facial pain over the sinus areas. Diagnosis requires direct visualization using a nasal speculum, radiography of the sinuses, needle puncture of the sinuses to withdraw a specimen for culture, and ultrasound.

Serious complications in the brain and middle ear may occur if sinusitis is not treated promptly with antihistamines or ephedrine nose drops to shrink mucosal tissue and relieve pressure. Steroidal nasal sprays may also be prescribed. Procedure 29-8 describes the steps for instilling nasal medication. If the cause of the sinusitis is a bacterial infection, antibiotics are prescribed by the physician and effectively relieve symptoms within 7 to 10 days. Chronic sinusitis may require treatment for 4 to 6 weeks. Total blockage of the sinus cavity may result if the disorder is not treated; this may require surgery to puncture the wall between the nose and the involved sinus cavity to allow drainage.

 CHECKPOINT QUESTION

11. What is the usual cause of a sinus infection?

 PATIENT EDUCATION

NASAL DISORDERS

Patients need to be alert for any changes in their breathing pattern. The early symptoms of any nasal disorder must be treated as soon as possible to prevent complications. Instruct children not to put small pieces of food or toys in the nose.

Instruct patients about the rebound phenomena of nasal sprays and drops. If used without the advice of a physician, these medications may become addictive. After frequent use, the nasal mucosa responds to withdrawal of the medication with congestion. Nasal preparations should never be used more than four times a day for 3 days unless specified by the physician.

Pharyngitis and Tonsillitis

Inflammation of the epithelial tissues of the throat and of the tonsils produces similar symptoms of sore throat and difficulty swallowing. Examination of the throat reveals red, swollen tissues and possibly pustules on the tonsils or in the throat (Fig. 29-15). You may be asked to obtain a throat specimen from these patients for transportation to an outside laboratory for a culture, or you may be required to perform a rapid strep test on the specimen in the office (Chapter 44 describes the steps for collecting throat specimens.) Treatment of a sore throat may include gargles, an analgesic, and an antibiotic, especially if the throat culture reveals a bacterial infection. Tonsillitis may be treated with an antibiotic, or if the problem is chronic, the tonsils may be surgically removed—a tonsillectomy. This procedure usually includes removal of both pharyngeal tonsils (adenoids) and palatine tonsils.

Laryngitis

Inflammation of the larynx can result from an infection, irritation, or overuse of the voice. The result is hoarseness, cough, and difficulty speaking. Diagnosis is made after a thorough history and visual inspection of the pharynx for redness and signs of infection. Laryngitis may be treated with an antibiotic if it is thought to be caused by a bacterial infection, but more often, it is left to resolve on its own. The patient is told to rest the voice and speak as little as possible. A cool-mist humidifier may be helpful in soothing the throat.

 CHECKPOINT QUESTION

12. Describe the symptoms of a patient with laryngitis.

Figure 29-15 Pharyngitis with swollen tonsils. (From The Wellcome Trust, National Medical Slide Bank, London, United Kingdom.)

 LEGAL TIP

A patient calls the office at 4:45 PM complaining of a sore throat. Scheduled appointments are running 1 to 2 hours behind. Because it is the middle of flu season, you think it is safe to tell the patient that he has a virus and can be seen in the morning. During the night, the patient's throat closes because of the infection and obstructs his airway. The patient dies, and the autopsy report shows a tonsillar abscess. Could the patient's family sue you? Yes! As a medical assistant, you cannot presume to diagnose medical conditions. You made a medical decision and diagnosed the patient when you decided that the symptoms indicated a virus. Only the physician can make a diagnosis. Always follow office policy regarding telephone advice, and document all phone conversations after bringing them to the physician's attention

Diagnostic Studies of the Nose and Throat

Visual Inspection

Examination of the nose and throat entails visually inspecting the nose using a nasal speculum or viewing the throat using a penlight and tongue depressor. The physician may order radiography and culture to identify infectious microorganisms. The physician may also palpate the lymph nodes in the neck and other neck structures related to the upper airway. You may be responsible for preparing the patient and assisting during the examination.

Therapeutic Procedures for the Nose and Throat

Throat Culture

A throat culture in cases of suspected pharyngitis or tonsillitis can help determine what microorganism is causing the problem. The patient's throat is gently swabbed with a sterile culture swab to obtain the specimen. A sterile swab is necessary to avoid culturing microorganisms not in the throat. After the specimen is obtained, it is either processed in the office with a commercially prepared test kit such as those that check for streptococcal bacteria or sent to a laboratory for analysis. If the specimen is sent to the laboratory, it must be placed in a culture medium, labeled, and sent in a biohazard bag with the appropriate laboratory request. (Chapter 44 describes the steps for collecting throat specimens.)

CHECKPOINT QUESTION

13. Why is it necessary to use a sterile swab to obtain the throat culture specimen?

español
SPANISH TERMINOLOGY

el ojo
 The eye
los oidos
 The ears
la nariz
 The nose
la garganta
 The throat
Cuando fue la ultima vez que se hizo un examen de la vista?
 When was the last time you had a vision test?
Padece de dolor de oido?
 Do you have earaches?

MEDIA MENU

- **Student CD**
  - **CMA/RMA Certification Exam Review**
- **Premium Online Course**
  http://thePoint.lww.com/Kronenberger3e
- **Internet Resources**
  LiveAdvise Online Tutoring & Competency Training
  http://thePoint.lww.com/LiveAdvise

  American Academy of Otolaryngology, Head and Neck Surgery
  www.entnet.org

  Vision Connection
  www.visionconnection.org

  Journal of Pediatric Ophthalmology and Strabismus
  www.journalofpediatricophthalmology.com

  American Foundation for the Blind
  www.afb.org

  Foundation Fighting Blindness
  www.blindness.org

  Prevent Blindness America
  www.preventblindness.org

  American Optometric Association
  www.aoa.org

  Self-help for the hard-of-hearing
  www.shhh.org

PROCEDURE 29-1: Measuring Distance Visual Acuity

Purpose: To assess and document the distance visual acuity of a patient in both eyes, with or without corrective lenses
Equipment: Snellen eye chart, paper cup or eye paddle

Steps	Purpose
1. Wash your hands.	Handwashing aids infection control.
2. Prepare the examination area. Make sure the area is well lighted, a distance marker is placed exactly 20 feet from the chart, and the chart is at eye level.	All distance visual acuity testing is done at 20 feet for consistency of results.
3. Greet and identify the patient. Explain the procedure.	Patients who understand the procedure are likely to be compliant and produce an accurate test result.
4. Position the patient at the 20-foot marker.	The patient may stand or sit as long as the chart is at eye level and the patient is 20 feet from it.

(continued)

PROCEDURE 29-1:   **Measuring Distance Visual Acuity** *(continued)*

Steps	**Purpose**
5. Observe whether the patient is wearing glasses. If not, ask the patient about contact lenses and mark the results of the test accordingly.	The visual acuity examination is usually performed with patients wearing their corrective lenses, if they have them. If the patient wears his or her corrective lenses, then the record must indicate that the lenses were worn for the test.
6. Have the patient cover the right eye with the paper cup or the eye paddle. Instruct the patient to keep both eyes open during the test.	The test starts with the right eye covered for consistency. The hand should not be used to cover the eye, since pressure against the eye or peeking through the fingers affects the results. Closing one eye will cause squinting of the other, which changes the vision and skews the findings.

Step 6. Have the patient cover the right eye.

Steps	**Purpose**
7. Stand beside the chart and point to each row as the patient reads aloud the indicated lines, starting with the 20/200 line. This number is on the right side of the chart next to each line.	It is generally best to start at about the second or third row to judge the patient's response. If these lines are read easily, move down to smaller figures. If the patient has difficulty reading the larger lines, notify the physician.
8. Record the smallest line that the patient can read with either one or no errors, according to office policy. If the patient reads line 5 with one error with the left eye, it will be recorded as OS (ocularis sinistra) 20/40–1. If no errors are read at the 20/40 line, it is recorded as OS 20/40. Your physician may prefer that only lines read without any error be counted as correct.	
9. Repeat the procedure with the left eye covered and record as in Step 8, using OD (ocularis dexter). If the patient squints or leans forward while testing either eye, record this observation on the patient record.	
10. Wash your hands and document the procedure.	Procedures are considered not to have been done if they are not recorded.

Charting Example:

01/16/2008 4:30 PM *Visual acuity OD 20/40–1 OS 20/20 with correction. Dr. Smart aware*

—*C. Mayers, CMA*

PROCEDURE 29-2: Measuring Color Perception

Purpose: To assess and document color perception
Equipment: Ishihara color plates, gloves

Steps	Purpose
1. Wash your hands, put on gloves, and get the Ishihara color plate book.	Handwashing aids infection control. Gloves in this case are to protect the plates, not the patient or health care worker. Oils from the hands can alter the colors and interfere with the test results.
2. Identify the patient and explain the procedure. Ensure that the patient is seated comfortably in a quiet, well-lighted room. Indirect sunlight is best. (Sunlight should not shine directly on the plates; the colors fade with exposure to bright lights.) Patients who wear glasses or contact lenses should keep them on.	The Ishihara tests color perception, not visual acuity. Corrective lenses do not interfere with accurate test results.
3. After opening the book, hold the first plate in the book about 30 inches from the patient and ask if he or she can see the number in the dots on the plate.	The first plate should be obvious to all patients and serves as an example. **Step 3.** Hold the first plate about 30 inches from the patient.
4. Record the results of the test by noting the number or figure the patient reports on each plate, using the plate number followed by the response. If the patient cannot distinguish the pattern, record as the plate number followed by the letter X. The patient should not take more than 3 seconds to read the plates and should not squint or guess. These indicate that the patient was unsure and are recorded as X.	

(continued)

PROCEDURE 29-2:	Measuring Color Perception *(continued)*

Steps	Purpose
5. Record the results for plates 1 to 10. Plate 11 requires the patient to trace the winding bluish-green line between the two x's. Patients with a color deficit will not be able to trace the line.	If 10 or more of the first 11 plates are read correctly without difficulty, the patient does not have a color deficit. Plates 12, 13, and 14 are usually used to detect the degree of deficiency in patients with red–green color deficiencies. Procedures are considered not to have been done if they are not recorded.
6. Store the book in a closed, protected area away from light to safeguard the integrity of the colors. Remove your gloves and wash your hands.	

Charting Example:

12/22/2008 10:30 AM *Ishihara color deficit testing performed:*

Plate 1	12	Plate 7	X *(normal 45)*
Plate 2	8	Plate 8	X *(normal 2)*
Plate 3	5 *(normal 2)*	Plate 9	2 *(normal X)*
Plate 4	X	Plate 10	X *(normal 16)*
Plate 5	21 *(normal 74)*	Plate 11	X *(traceable)*
Plate 6	X *(normal 7)*		

—*B. Cotton, CMA*

PROCEDURE 29-3:	Instilling Eye Medications

Purpose: Instill and document ophthalmic medications as ordered by the physician
Equipment: Physician's order and patient record, ophthalmic medication, sterile gauze, tissues, gloves

Steps	Purpose
1. Wash your hands.	Handwashing aids infection control.
2. Obtain the patient's medical record, including the physician's order, correct medication, sterile gauze, and tissues.	The medication must specify ophthalmic use. Check the label three times before administering the ophthalmic solution or ointment. Medications formulated for other uses may be harmful if used in the eyes.
3. Greet and identify the patient. Explain the procedure. Ask the patient about any allergies not recorded in the chart.	Identifying the patient prevents errors in treatment.
4. Position the patient comfortably.	The patient may lie or sit with the head tilted slightly back and the affected eye slightly lower to avoid the medication running into the unaffected eye.

(continued)

PROCEDURE 29-3:   Instilling Eye Medications (continued)

Steps	Purpose
5. Put on gloves and pull down the lower eyelid with sterile gauze while asking the patient to look up. **Step 5.** Pull the lower eyelid down and ask the patient to look up.	Since there is potential for contact with secretions from the eye, you must wear gloves. Pulling down the lower lid exposes the conjunctival sac to receive the medication. If the patient is looking up and away from the medication, the blink reflex may not be triggered.
6. Instill the medication: A. Ointment: Discard the first bead of ointment from the container onto a tissue without touching the end of the medication tube to the tissue. Place a thin line of ointment across the inside of the lower eyelid, moving from the inner canthus outward. Release the ointment by twisting the tube slightly. Do not touch the tube to the eye. B. Drops: Hold the dropper close to the conjunctival sac (about half an inch away) but do not touch the patient. Release the proper number of drops into the sac. Discard any medication left in the dropper.	The first bead of ointment is considered contaminated. Placing the ointment in the sac avoids touching the eye with the tip of the ointment tube. Twisting the tube releases the ointment. Discarding the remaining medication prevents contaminating the remainder of a multiple dose container.
7. Release the lower lid and have the patient gently close the eye and roll it to disperse the medication.	
8. Wipe off any excess medication with the tissue. Instruct the patient to apply light pressure to the puncta lacrimalis for several minutes.	Pressing the puncta prevents the medication from running into the nasolacrimal sac and duct.
9. Properly care for or dispose of equipment and supplies. Clean the work area and wash your hands.	
10. Record the procedure.	Procedures are considered not to have been done if they are not recorded.

Charting Example:

10/14/2008 8:45 AM *Garamycin ophthalmologic ointment applied to OS*

—*B. Marker, CMA*

PROCEDURE 29-4:   Irrigating the Eye

Purpose: Irrigate the eye as ordered by the physician and document the procedure
Equipment: Physician's order and patient record, small sterile basin if sterile solution is used, irrigating solution (water) and medication (if ordered), protective barrier or towels, emesis basin, sterile bulb syringe, tissues, gloves

Steps	Purpose
1. Wash your hands and put on gloves.	Handwashing aids infection control. You must wear gloves when you may be exposed to body fluids
2. Assemble the equipment, supplies, and medication if ordered. Check the label three times as recommended for medication administration, and make sure the label indicates ophthalmic use. Note: If both eyes are to be treated, use separate equipment (solution and bulb syringe) to avoid cross-contamination.	Unless water is ordered for the eye irrigation, solutions for the eye must be sterile and must be formulated for ophthalmic use.
3. Greet and identify the patient. Explain the procedure.	Identifying the patient prevents errors in treatment. Patients who understand the procedure are generally cooperative and compliant.
4. Position the patient comfortably, either with the head tilted and the affected eye lower or lying with the affected eye down.	With the affected eye down, there is little chance of contamination running into the unaffected eye
5. Drape the patient with the protective barrier or towel to avoid wetting the clothing.	
6. Place the emesis basin against the upper cheek near the eye with the towel under the basin. With clean gauze, wipe the eye from the inner canthus outward to remove debris from the lashes.	Debris from the lashes may be washed into the eye.
7. Separate the lids with the thumb and forefinger of your nondominant hand. To steady your hand, you may lightly support your dominant hand, holding the syringe with solution on the bridge of the patient's nose parallel to the eye.	

Step 7. Separate the eyelids with the thumb and forefinger.

(continued)

PROCEDURE 29-4: **Irrigating the Eye** *(continued)*

Steps	Purpose
8. Gently irrigate from the inner to the outer canthus, holding the syringe 1 inch above the eye. Use gentle pressure and do not touch the eye. The physician will order the time or amount of solution to be used. Debris from the lashes may be washed into the eye.	The solution must flow from the inner to the outer canthus to avoid washing pathogens into the punctum. With the syringe 1 inch above the eye, there is little chance of touching the eye and causing discomfort

Step 8. Hold the syringe 1 inch above the eye.

Steps	Purpose
9. Use tissues to wipe any excess solution from the patient's face.	This prevents the spread of microorganisms.
10. Properly dispose of equipment or sanitize as recommended and remove your gloves. Wash your hands.	
11. Record the procedure in the patient's record, including the amount, type, and strength of the solution; which eye was irrigated; and any observations.	Procedures are considered not to have been done if they are not recorded.

Charting Example:

04/16/2008 11:30 AM OD irrigated with 500 mL sterile NS, return clear

—J. Penta, CMA

PROCEDURE 29-5: **Irrigating the Ear**

Purpose: : Irrigate the ear as ordered and document the procedure
Equipment: Physician's order and patient's record, emesis or ear basin, waterproof barrier or towels, otoscope, irrigating solution (water), bowl for solution, gauze

Steps	Purpose
1. Wash your hands.	Handwashing aids infection control.
2. Assemble the equipment and supplies.	Ear irrigation is not a sterile procedure.
3. Greet and identify the patient. Explain the procedure.	Identifying the patient prevents errors in treatment. Ear irrigations are not usually painful, but the flow of the solution may be uncomfortable. The patient may be more cooperative if this is understood

(continued)

PROCEDURE 29-5: Irrigating the Ear (continued)

Steps	Purpose
4. Position the patient comfortably erect.	
5. View the affected ear with an otoscope to locate the foreign matter or cerumen. A. Adults: Gently pull ear up and back to straighten the auditory canal. B. Children: Gently pull ear slightly down and back to straighten the auditory canal.	The area of treatment must be visualized before irrigation begins. If debris from the external auricle is not removed, it may be washed into the canal **Step 5.** The shape of the ear canal changes with growth. To allow good inspection, position the ear as illustrated.
6. Drape the patient with a waterproof barrier or towel.	Wet clothing would be uncomfortable for the patient
7. Tilt the patient's head toward the affected side.	Tilting the head will facilitate the flow of solution
8. Place the drainage basin under the affected ear. **Step 8.** Place the basin under the ear.	
9. Fill the irrigating syringe or turn on the irrigating device.	
10. Gently position the auricle as described, using your nondominant hand.	The canal must be straight for visualization and treatment.
11. With your dominant hand, place the tip of the syringe in the auditory meatus and direct the flow of the solution gently up toward the roof of the canal.	Directing the flow against the upper surface prevents pressure against the tympanic membrane and facilitates the outflow of solution.
12. Continue irrigating for the prescribed period or until the desired result (cerumen removal) is obtained.	If the patient complains of pain or discomfort, stop the irrigation and notify the physician.
13. Dry the patient's external ear with gauze. Have the patient sit for awhile with the affected ear down to drain the solution.	Solution left in the ear is uncomfortable.
14. Inspect the ear with the otoscope to determine the results.	It may be necessary to repeat the procedure, and it is always necessary to inspect the area to record the results.

(continued)

PROCEDURE 29-5: Irrigating the Ear *(continued)*

Steps	Purpose
15. Properly care for or dispose of equipment and supplies. Clean the work area. Wash your hands.	This prevents the spread of microorganisms.
16. Record the procedure in the patient's chart.	Procedures are considered not to have been done if they are not recorded.

Note: If the tympanic membrane appears to be perforated, do not irrigate without checking with the physician; solution may be forced into the middle ear through the perforation. Remove any obvious debris at the entrance of the canal before beginning the irrigation.

Charting Example:

03/17/2008 3:30 PM AD irrigated with 500 mL sterile water; return clear with 2 large pieces of yellow-brown cerumen noted

—*S. Stark, CMA*

PROCEDURE 29-6: Audiometry Testing

Purpose: To accurately assess and document a hearing test using audiometry
Equipment: Audiometer, otoscope

Steps	Purpose
1. Wash your hands.	Handwashing aids infection control.
2. Greet and identify the patient. Explain the procedure. Take the patient to a quiet area or room for testing.	Patients who understand the procedure are likely to be compliant, producing accurate results. A quiet room allows for accurate results without distraction. Determine the signal (raising the hand, saying yes) to indicate that the tones are heard.
3. Using an otoscope or audioscope with a light source, visually inspect the ear canal and tympanic membrane before the examination.	Looking into the ear canal verifies that there are no obstructions, such as cerumen, to interfere with the test. If you see an obstruction, notify the physician.
4. Choose the correct size tip for the end of the audiometer. Attach a speculum to fit the patient's external auditory meatus, making sure the ear canal is occluded with the speculum in place.	The design of the tip or speculum obviates bulky ear phones. The tip should block any environmental noise during the test.
5. With the speculum in the ear canal, retract the pinna: up and back for adults; down and back for children.	Pulling the pinna up and back for adults and down and back for children straightens the ear canal

(continued)

PROCEDURE 29-6: Audiometry Testing *(continued)*

Steps	Purpose

Step 5. Pull the pinna down and back for children. (Courtesy of Welch-Allyn.)

Steps	Purpose
6. Turn the instrument on and select the screening level. There is a pretest tone for practice if necessary. Press the start button and observe the tone indicators and the patient's responses.	The signal (raising the hand, saying yes) was determined before you began the test. The audiometer will proceed down each tone with a light indicator.

A

B

Step 6. (A) Place the audiometer tip in the patient's ear. (B) The patient should give a signal when each tone is heard. (Courtesy of Welch-Allyn.)

Steps	Purpose
7. Screen the other ear.	
8. If the patient fails to respond at any frequency, rescreening is required.	If the patient does not hear a specific tone, a second opportunity should be given.
9. If the patient fails rescreening, notify the physician.	A patient who fails to hear one or more tones may be referred to an audiologist.
10. Record the results in the medical record.	Procedures are considered not to have been done if they are not recorded.

Charting Example:

02/14/2008 9:00 AM Audiometry testing performed AU, results in chart

—S. Smythe, RMA

PROCEDURE 29-7:   Instilling Ear Medication

Purpose: Instill otic medication as ordered and document the instillation
Equipment: Physician's order and patient's record, otic medication with dropper, cotton balls
Standard: This procedure should take 5 minutes.

Steps	Purpose
1. Wash your hands.	Handwashing aids infection control.
2. Check the medication label three times as specified for medication administration. The label should specify otic preparation.	Medication for otic instillation is formulated for that purpose.
3. Greet and identify the patient. Explain the procedure.	Identifying the patient prevents errors in treatment. Patients who understand the procedure are generally compliant.
4. Have the patient seated with the affected ear tilted upward.	The medication must be allowed to flow through the canal to the tympanic membrane.
5. Draw up the ordered amount of medication.	
6. Straighten the canal. A. Adults: Pull the auricle slightly up and back. B. Children: Pull the auricle slightly down and back.	
7. Insert the tip of the dropper without touching the patient's skin and let the medication flow along the side of the canal.	Touching the patient will contaminate the dropper. The medication should flow gently to avoid discomfort.

Step 7. Insert the tip of the dropper without touching the ear.

Steps	Purpose
8. Have the patient sit or lie with the affected ear up for about 5 minutes after the instillation.	The medication should rest against the tympanic membrane for as long as possible.
9. If the medication is to be retained in the ear canal, insert a moist cotton ball into the external auditory meatus without force.	A slightly moist cotton ball will keep the medication in the canal and not wick it out. Forcing the cotton ball into the ear canal could be painful to the patient.
10. Properly care for or dispose of equipment and supplies. Clean the work area. Wash your hands.	This prevents the spread of microorganisms.
11. Record the procedure in the patient record.	Procedures are considered not to have been done if they are not recorded.

Charting Example:

06/15/2008 12:30 PM Neosporin otic solution, 2 gtt instilled into AS as ordered

—D. Barth, CMA

PROCEDURE 29-8:   Instilling Nasal Medication

Purpose: Instill nasal medication as ordered and document the instillation
Equipment: Physician's order and patient's record, nasal medication, drops or spray, tissues, gloves

Steps	Purpose
1. Wash your hands.	Handwashing aids infection control.
2. Assemble the equipment and supplies. Check the medication label three times.	Medications for use in the nasal passages must be formulated for these surfaces.
3. Greet and identify the patient. Explain the procedure and ask the patient about any allergies not documented.	Identifying the patient prevents errors in treatment. Nasal instillations are uncomfortable but should not be painful; patients will be more cooperative if they understand the procedure.
4. Position the patient comfortably recumbent. Extend the patient's head beyond the edge of the examination table or place a pillow under the shoulders. Support the patient's neck to avoid strain as the head tilts back. **Step 4.** Tilt the patient's head back.	The patient must be properly positioned if the medication is to reach the upper nasal passages.
5. Administer the medication. A. Hold the dropper upright just above each nostril and dispense one drop at a time without touching the nares. Keep the patient recumbent for 5 minutes. B. Place the tip of the bottle at the naris opening without touching the patient's skin or nasal tissues and spray as the patient takes a deep breath.	Touching the dropper to the nostril would contaminate the dropper. For effective treatment, the patient must allow the medication to reach the upper nasal passages. The medication must reach the upper passages; if the patient breathes out while the medication is being sprayed, the medication is exhaled and does not reach the nasal passages.
6. Wipe any excess medication from the patient's skin with tissues.	Excess medication around the nares is uncomfortable.
7. Properly care for or dispose of equipment and supplies. Clean the work area. Remove your gloves and wash your hands.	This prevents the spread of microorganisms.
8. Record the procedure in the patient's chart.	Procedures are considered not to have been done if they are not recorded.

Charting Example:

06/15/2008 12:00 PM Oxymetazoline hydrochloride 0.05% nasal spray, 2 sprays to each nostril as ordered per Dr. Greene

—D. Pratt, CMA

Although not all patients who have disorders of the eyes or ears need a referral to an ophthalmologist or otolaryngologist, you will routinely encounter patients who need to have these conditions properly diagnosed and treated. Keep in mind that:

- Disorders of the eyes, ears, nose, and throat may affect any patient at any age

- Severe complications, such as an infection of the brain or hearing loss, can result in patients who are not receiving adequate attention or not following the physician's instructions for treatment.
- You will play a vital role by assisting with ear, nose, and throat examinations and educating patients regarding their treatment.

Warm Ups for Critical Thinking

1. The mother of a 10-month old boy explains to you that the baby has had a runny nose and has been fussy for the past 2 days. You notice that he is pulling at his right ear. What equipment do you anticipate that the physician will need for examining the child?

2. A 16-year-old girl complains of a sore throat. Her vital signs are T 102.8 (O), P 112, R 24, and BP 112/84. The physician examines her and tells you to obtain a throat specimen for a rapid strep test to determine whether the pharyngitis is due to an infection with streptococcal bacteria. The patient is reluctant to let you obtain a throat culture, saying it will make her gag and vomit. How do you handle this situation?

3. The school nurse at the local high school phones your office asking for information about a student who has been out of school the past 3 days with conjunctivitis. Specifically, she wants to know whether this student has been diagnosed with this condition or is simply truant. How do you handle this phone call?

4. An elderly patient is having difficulty hearing and would like you to explain why the physician wants you to irrigate his ears for ceruminosis. He is concerned that the procedure will be uncomfortable. What could you say to the patient to ease his anxiety?

5. You notice that another medical assistant working in the office is getting frustrated with an adult male during a visual acuity test using the Snellen eye chart. The patient doesn't seem to know the letters of the alphabet and you suspect that he is illiterate, but may have been embarrassed to tell the other MA before the examination started. Would you intervene? What would you say?

Answers to Checkpoint Questions

1. The symptoms of a cataract include gradual blurring and loss of vision that worsens as the clouding of the lens slowly progresses.

2. A sty is an infection of the glands of the eyelids; conjunctivitis is an infection of the conjunctiva, the mucous membrane that covers the sclera and cornea.

3. Four common refractive errors are hyperopia (farsightedness), myopia (nearsightedness), astigmatism (unfocused refraction of light rays on the retina), and presbyopia (age-related vision changes).

4. The treatment for strabismus includes covering the unaffected eye to force the affected eye's muscles to strengthen; however, surgery may be required.

5. The E chart is used for patients who cannot read or who do not speak English.

6. The pressure of the eye is measured with a tonometer to diagnose glaucoma.

7. Conductive hearing loss stops the flow of sound before the cochlea. Perceptual hearing loss stops the flow of nerve impulses from the cochlea to the brain.

8. The symptoms of otitis media in an infant include fussiness, tugging at the affected ear, and fever.

9. The otoscope allows the physician to visualize the ear canal and tympanic membrane.

10. Trauma, hypertension, malignancy, polyps, and the fragile capillaries associated with pregnancy contribute to epistaxis.

11. An upper respiratory infection may also result in sinusitis.

12. The symptoms of laryngitis include hoarseness, cough, and difficulty speaking.

13. A sterile swab is used to obtain the throat culture to prevent obtaining a culture of microorganisms not in the throat.

Outline

**Common Respiratory
Disorders**
Upper Respiratory Disorders
Lower Respiratory Disorders
**Common Cancers of the
Respiratory System**
Laryngeal Cancer
Lung Cancer

**Common Diagnostic and
Therapeutic Procedures**
Physical Examination of the
Respiratory System
Sputum Culture and Cytology
Chest Radiography

Bronchoscopy
Pulmonary Function Tests
Arterial Blood Gases

Learning Objectives

*Upon successfully completing this chapter, you
will be able to:*

1. Spell and define key terms

2. Identify the primary defense mechanisms of
the respiratory system

3. List and describe disorders of the respiratory system

4. Explain various diagnostic procedures of
the respiratory system

5. Describe the physician's examination of
the respiratory system

6. Discuss the role of the medical assistant
with regard to various diagnostic and therapeutic procedures

Performance Objectives

*Upon successfully completing this chapter, you
will be able to:*

1. Instruct a patient in the use of the peak
flowmeter (Procedure 30-1)

2. Administer a nebulized breathing treatment
(Procedure 30-2)

3. Perform a pulmonary function test
(Procedure 30-3)

Competencies

CAAHEP

- Practice standard precautions
- Perform respiratory testing
- Prepare patient for and assist with routine and specialty examinations
- Prepare patient for and assist with procedures, treatments, and minor office surgery
- Document appropriately
- Instruct individuals according to their needs

ABHES

- Prepare patients for procedures
- Assist physician with examinations and treatments
- Perform selected tests that assist with diagnosis and treatment
- Perform respiratory testing
- Document accurately

Key Terms

atelectasis	dyspnea	laryngectomy	thoracentesis
chronic obstructive pulmonary disease (COPD)	forced expiratory volume	palliative	tidal volume
	hemoptysis	status asthmaticus	tracheostomy

The respiratory system provides the body with the oxygen that all cells need to perform their functions (Fig. 30-1). It also eliminates carbon dioxide, a waste product, and water from the body. The respiratory system works closely with the cardiovascular system to deliver oxygen to every cell in the body. When a cell is too long deprived of oxygen, the cell dies, and when many cells die, so does the tissue.

The upper airways, tracheobronchial tree, and alveoli come into contact with air from the atmosphere or environment, which can contain dust, pathogenic microorganisms, and other irritants. In healthy individuals, defense mechanisms in the respiratory system help to protect the body from disease and illness caused by these environmental contaminants. Table 30-1 summarizes the major defense mechanisms of the respiratory system. Disease can occur, however, when these defenses are overwhelmed by cigarette smoke, air pollution, infectious organisms, or other irritants.

PATIENT EDUCATION

EFFECTS OF SMOKING ON THE AIRWAYS

Cigarette smoking has many harmful effects on the body. Smoke from a cigarette irritates the airways and causes the membrane to produce more mucus. This increased production of mucus, along with the increase in dust and debris that collects in the mucus, slows down the body's normal clearing processes. The smoke anesthetizes the cilia lining the respiratory tract so they stop waving the debris away. Over time, large amounts of thick, sticky mucus are retained in the lungs, blackening the lung tissue and sealing the alveolar sacs. This thick, tarry mucus causes the patient to cough frequently, especially in the mornings, and to be prone to bronchitis, both acute and chronic, as a result of the destruction of the protective mechanisms of the airway from the heat and tar inhaled in the smoke.

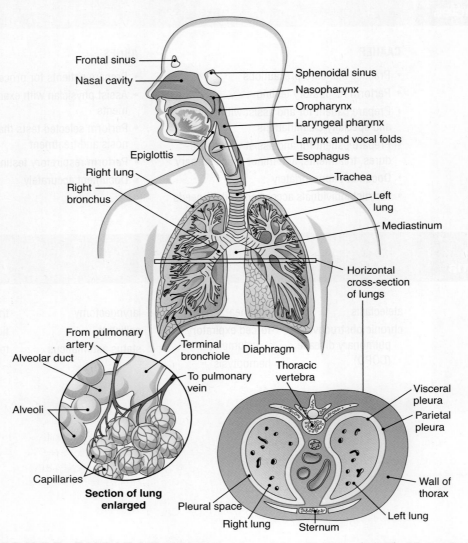

Figure 30-1 The respiratory system. (Reprinted with permission from Cohen BJ. Memmler's The Human Body in Health and Disease. Philadelphia: Lippincott Williams & Wilkins, 2005.)

TABLE **30-1**	Defenses of the Respiratory System
Defense	**Function**
Nasal hairs	Filter large dust particles from the air
Mucous membranes	Trap dust and other particles, add moisture
Turbinates in nose	Whirl air around to increase warming, humidifying, filtering
Epiglottis	Closes over trachea to prevent aspiration during swallowing
Airway reflexes	Trigger cough to clear irritants in pharynx, larynx, trachea
Airway smooth muscles	Constrict when irritation occurs to prevent entry of foreign substances
Macrophage in alveoli	Phagocytize ("eat") bacteria, other foreign cells, debris
Tonsils	Filter air moving through passageways to protect against bacterial invasion; aid in formation of white blood cells

Common Respiratory Disorders

Upper Respiratory Disorders

The most common problems of the upper respiratory tract are caused by infectious microorganisms and by allergic reactions that produce inflammation. Acute rhinitis, sinusitis, pharyngitis, tonsillitis, and laryngitis are described in Chapter 29; these are also considered upper respiratory disorders.

Lower Respiratory Disorders

Diseases of the lower respiratory tract may be acute (sudden in onset with relatively short duration) or chronic (progressing over time or recurring frequently). Acute diseases of the lower respiratory tract include bronchitis and pneumonia. Chronic diseases include asthma, chronic bronchitis, and emphysema. The last two diseases are usually grouped as chronic obstructive pulmonary disease because most patients have elements of both emphysema and chronic bronchitis.

Bronchitis

Bronchitis is an inflammation of the mucous membranes of the bronchi caused by infection or irritation that induces increased production of mucus in the trachea, bronchi, and bronchioles. The most prominent symptom of bronchitis is a productive cough. If a bacterial or viral infection is present, the sputum may change color from the normal white or clear to yellow, green, gray, or tan. If an infection is suspected, you may be asked to obtain a sputum specimen for culture and sensitivity to determine the causative microorganism and appropriate antibiotic therapy. (Chapter 44 outlines the procedure for collecting a sputum specimen.) In many cases, the physician bases a diagnosis of bronchitis on the history and symptoms of the patient without ordering a sputum culture.

The treatment of bronchitis generally includes an antibiotic for bacterial infection, smoking cessation, rest, and increased fluid intake. A cough suppressant may be prescribed, especially for use at night, but this is controversial because of the body's need to clear secretions from the airways. Retained secretions can become infected and lead to pneumonia.

Pneumonia

Pneumonia is a bacterial or viral infection in the alveoli, or tiny air sacs that are the site of gas exchange in the lungs. The buildup of fluid and congestion in the alveoli prevents effective gas exchange. Diagnostic testing usually includes analysis of a sputum specimen and chest radiography. Bacterial pneumonias tend to be sudden and severe in onset, causing a fever, cough, chills, and **dyspnea**. Infections caused by bacteria also tend to be local to one lobe or area of the lung. Treatment of bacterial pneumonia primarily includes an appropriate antibiotic, bed rest, and medication to relieve symptoms. Pneumonia caused by bacteria often requires hospitalization for administration of intravenous antibiotics and oxygen, especially in the elderly or debilitated patients.

Viral pneumonia is usually more gradual in onset but can be just as serious. Antibiotics are ineffective in treating viral pneumonia; however, the physician may order an antibiotic to prevent a secondary bacterial infection. Viral pneumonia tends to spread throughout the lung fields and often is marked by a fever and productive cough. Treatment may include bed rest or hospitalization.

CHECKPOINT QUESTION

1. What are the characteristics of bacterial and viral pneumonia?

Asthma

Asthma is a reversible inflammatory process involving primarily the small airways such as the bronchi and bronchioles. Asthma manifests as constriction of the smooth muscle lining the airways, spasms of the bronchi and bronchioles (bronchospasm), swelling of the mucous membranes of the airways, and increased mucus production with productive coughing. All three of these manifestations narrow the airways, making it difficult for the patient to move air into and out of the lungs.

The patient having an asthma attack may have dyspnea, coughing, wheezing, and, in severe cases, cyanosis. Patients with asthma usually have exacerbations, which are periods of frequent attacks, and remissions, which are periods when they are relatively symptom free. Attacks may be triggered by exposure to allergens, such as mold or dust; inhaled irritants, such as cigarette smoke; upper respiratory infections; psychological stress; cold air; or exercise. In some instances, the immediate cause of the asthma attack is unknown. While asthma is considered a chronic disorder that occurs in children or adults, many children with asthma outgrow it by adulthood.

Many medications are available to prevent or control the symptoms of asthma, but it is important that they be used properly. On days that the patient has no symptoms of asthma, he or she should use a device called a peak flowmeter (Fig. 30-2) to determine the amount of air moving into and out of the lungs (Procedure 30-1). Instruct the patient to use the peak flowmeter correctly and record the results on a chart or diary provided by the medical office. This record, known as the patient's personal best, assists the physician in establishing and maintaining a medication protocol.

Figure 30-2 The peak flowmeter.

Patients with symptoms of asthma, including wheezing and difficulty breathing, may be prescribed a nebulized breathing treatment with a bronchodilator, a medication to dilate the bronchi, such as albuterol (Procedure 30-2). After the bronchodilator is in the nebulizer administration setup, the machine is turned on and causes the liquid medication to break apart into a fine spray that is inhaled by the patient through a mouthpiece or mask. Since bronchodilator medications cause an increase in the heart rate, you should monitor the patient's pulse before, during, and after the treatment. If the patient becomes lightheaded, discontinue the treatment, have the patient lie down, obtain the vital signs, and notify the physician.

An asthma attack that does not respond to medication is an emergency known as **status asthmaticus.** Because such attacks can be fatal, the patient needs immediate emergency medical services and hospitalization.

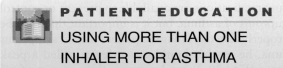

CHECKPOINT QUESTION

2. What factors may trigger an asthma attack?

PATIENT EDUCATION

USING MORE THAN ONE INHALER FOR ASTHMA

Asthmatics may use more than one inhaler. One medication is usually a bronchodilator to open the bronchioles and control bronchospasms. Another type of inhaler is a corticosteroid. Steroids help to control inflammation in the bronchioles and generally are prescribed only during a respiratory illness.

Teach the patient to use the bronchodilator first, wait 5 minutes, and then use the steroid. Using the steroid inhaler after the bronchodilator allows for more steroid medication to enter the lung tissue, making it more effective.

Some patients are prescribed two inhaled bronchodilators. One type is used daily to prevent asthma attacks, and the other is used as a rescue inhaler. The rescue inhaler should be used only when the asthma cannot be controlled with the daily regimen. Before teaching a patient about the correct pattern for using the inhalers, clarify the information with the physician. Each asthmatic responds differently and requires an individualized approach to care.

Chronic Obstructive Pulmonary Disease

Chronic bronchitis and emphysema are most commonly caused by cigarette smoking. As a result, patients who have smoked over a long period often exhibit signs and symptoms of both of these disorders. Chronic bronchitis is a chronic inflammation and swelling of the airways with excessive mucus production, obstruction of the bronchi, and trapping of air behind mucus plugs. The trapping of this air overinflates the alveoli. Chronic bronchitis is not usually an infectious process but, instead, is produced by chronic irritation of the airways by cigarette smoke or other pollutants. However, because of the increase in sputum and the difficulty these patients have in clearing their sputum, they are prone to develop respiratory infections.

Emphysema is a disease process in which the walls of the damaged alveoli stretch and break down after repeated exposure to irritants such as cigarette smoke and air pollution. The pulmonary capillaries also break down, and the tiny airways leading to each alveolus weaken and collapse. The end result is a sharp reduction in surface area for gas exchange, and once again, air is trapped in the enlarged air sacs that were once clusters of tiny alveoli.

The combination of these diseases, together called **chronic obstructive pulmonary disease (COPD),** produces characteristic symptoms. COPD is a likely cause of shortness of breath, chronic cough, sputum production, and wheezing in the patient with a history of smoking. The onset of these symptoms is usually slow and gradual over years, and the patient may go a long time without realizing that he or she has signs and symptoms of a disease. Many people with COPD have some of the signs and symptoms of asthma, and many of these patients take asthma medications.

Once a patient is diagnosed with COPD, the disease process is not usually reversible. Many patients have a hard time accepting that fact and insist that their physician provide a cure or restore the lungs to normal function. Although the disease is not curable, the progression of COPD can be slowed and the quality of life improved significantly through education about the disease, a prescribed exercise regimen, proper use of medications, good nutrition, and home oxygen therapy.

LEGAL TIP

Patients with chronic and irreversible diseases, such as COPD, must never be led to believe that the doctor can cure the disease. Avoid making statements such as "Everything will be okay" or "The doctor can help you," and also be careful not to indicate that the patient will return to normal function. Legally, the doctor is responsible for your actions, including promises, even if they are innocent and were said only to make the patient feel better. These statements may be taken as a guarantee, and if the results are not achieved, the patient may file a lawsuit on the grounds that a contract was broken and the promised results were not delivered.

PATIENT EDUCATION

LIVING WITH COPD

To improve the quality of life, encourage a patient diagnosed with COPD to follow these suggestions:

1. Quit smoking if you haven't already done so! Even though the lungs have been permanently damaged, further deterioration will be reduced if you stop smoking now.
2. Get a flu vaccination each fall and make sure you have had the pneumonia vaccine.
3. Avoid crowds, especially in the winter, when the viruses that cause colds and influenza are prevalent.
4. If pollution is high, stay indoors with the air conditioning on if possible.
5. Use your abdominal muscles instead of your shoulder and neck muscles to avoid strain and fatigue in these muscles.
6. Drink lots of fluids unless the physician has limited your fluid intake. Water is the best fluid. Good fluid intake is the best way to keep the

mucus in your airways thin so that it is easy to cough up.
7. Follow a healthy, balanced diet.
8. Avoid doing difficult physical tasks (e.g., vacuuming or mowing the lawn) all in one day. If you must do these chores, do them in short periods spaced throughout the day with frequent rest periods.
9. Organize your home to minimize standing, reaching, and lifting.

WHAT IF?

What if a patient requires home oxygen therapy?

Many patients with severe COPD or end-stage lung cancer are discharged from the hospital with oxygen to use at home. Most surgical supply companies and pharmacies can arrange to have oxygen therapy equipment delivered to the home. The oxygen is usually supplied by a machine called a concentrator that runs on electricity. The concentrator separates oxygen out of room air and concentrates it for delivery to the patient. Attached to the cylinder is a flowmeter, or regulator, that indicates the amount of oxygen being delivered. The patient should be instructed to leave the oxygen at the setting prescribed by the physician. Too much oxygen can be toxic for some patients, such as those with emphysema. A cannula (plastic tube with pronged openings that fit into the nares) is attached to the flowmeter and delivers oxygen to the patient's airways. The company supplying the oxygen should instruct the patient regarding safe home oxygen administration. Since oxygen is highly flammable, you should reinforce safety precautions during oxygen use, including avoiding open flames and sparks. In addition, the supplier should be available 24 hours a day for emergency oxygen maintenance.

Tuberculosis

Tuberculosis is an infectious disease spread by respiratory droplets from a person infected with *Mycobacterium tuberculosis*. The patient with active tuberculosis has signs and symptoms such as a productive cough, night sweats, and malaise. Although no tuberculosis vaccine is available, a screening test can be administered to detect a previous infection. However, a patient with a positive screening test for tuberculosis does not necessarily have active disease and therefore may not be contagious. The procedure for administering and reading the results of the screening tests (Mantoux and tine tests) for tuberculosis is described in Chapter 24. Patients with symptoms of tuberculosis should be treated as contagious and encouraged to wear a protective mask over the nose and mouth to prevent spreading the disease through infected droplets released into the air during speaking and coughing. In addition, you are required to report any diagnosis of tuberculosis to the local public health department. The treatment for tuberculosis includes a regimen of antibiotic therapy that lasts for months. You should provide emotional support for these patients, since the treatment lasts up to a year, and encourage compliance with the prescribed regimen at each office visit.

 CHECKPOINT QUESTION

3. What two disease processes are present in a patient with COPD?

Common Cancers of the Respiratory System

Laryngeal Cancer

Cancer of the larynx is seen most commonly in heavy smokers and alcoholics. The presenting symptoms are usually hoarseness that lasts longer than 3 weeks, a feeling of a lump in the throat, or pain and burning in the throat when drinking citrus juice or hot liquids. A patient with laryngeal cancer may be treated with radiation, surgery, or both. Surgery usually is a **laryngectomy,** or removal of the larynx, and formation of a permanent **tracheostomy** stoma (Fig. 30-3). Patients who have had a laryngectomy are unable to speak normally but can be trained to use esophageal speech or a prosthetic speech device.

Lung Cancer

Lung cancer is one of the most common causes of death in both men and women. Cigarette smoking is believed to be the most common cause; 80% of lung cancer pa-

Incision in trachea after retracting infrahyoid muscles and incising isthmus of thyroid

Deep cervical fascia

Tracheostomy tube

Pretracheal fascia

Esophagus

2nd and 4th tracheal rings

Figure 30-3 The patient with a tracheostomy. (From Moore KL, Dalley AF II. Clinical Oriented Anatomy. 4th ed. Baltimore: Lippincott Williams & Wilkins, 1999.)

tients are smokers. Prognosis is generally poor for patients with lung cancer, with only 8% of men and 12% of women surviving for 5 years. One of the reasons is that symptoms tend to present rather late in the disease, when it has already had a chance to metastasize, or spread to other organs. Also, many of the symptoms are nonspecific and are seen in most heavy smokers. These symptoms include chronic cough, wheezing, dyspnea, **hemoptysis**, and chest pain.

Diagnosis of lung cancer is made by chest radiography, sputum cytology, bronchoscopy, biopsy, or **thoracentesis**. Treatment is generally **palliative**, giving relief but not a cure, and usually includes surgery, radiation, and chemotherapy. These treatments may improve the patient's prognosis and prolong survival.

 CHECKPOINT QUESTION

4. What factor appears to contribute to both laryngeal cancer and lung cancer?

Common Diagnostic and Therapeutic Procedures

Physical Examination of the Respiratory System

The traditional examination of the chest consists of four parts: inspection, palpation, percussion, and auscultation. Each is briefly described in the following sections. For the physician to perform this examination efficiently, the patient should be sitting up, and all clothing should be removed from the waist up. The patient should be given a gown and draped appropriately (see Chapter 20).

Inspection

Inspection consists of a visual examination of the chest and the patient's respiratory pattern (Table 30-2).

During inspection, the physician looks for abnormal shape of the thorax, use of accessory muscles to breathe, surgical scars, cyanosis, and any other visible signs of previous or current respiratory disease.

Palpation

In palpation, the physician uses his or her hands to feel the patient's throat for lumps, areas of tenderness, and location of the trachea, which may be displaced by a tumor. The patient may be asked to say "99" while the physician feels the chest wall in different places to assess the vibrations produced. Solid masses (such as tumors) or fluids (as in pneumonia) increase vibrations, whereas increased air (as seen in emphysema) reduces the vibrations.

Percussion

Percussion is placing a finger (or fingers) on the chest and striking it with the fingers of the other hand. The physician listens for the sound to determine whether it is normal (resonant), like the sound produced by a drum. Dull or flat sounds are heard in patients with consolidation of pulmonary tissue, such as **atelectasis**, pneumonia, or a tumor. A hyperresonant sound is hollow and is heard in patients with emphysema. Children with cystic fibrosis (see Chapter 37, Pediatrics) often require chest percussion to loosen the thick respiratory secretions throughout the day.

Auscultation

Auscultation is listening to the patient's lungs and airway passages with a stethoscope. The physician systematically listens to each side of the chest in each area to compare the sounds bilaterally. The patient should breathe deeply, with an open mouth and the head turned away from the physician's face. The patient is encour-

TABLE 30-2	Abnormal Respiratory Patterns
Pattern	**Description**
Apnea	No respirations
Bradypnea	Slow respirations
Cheyne-Stokes	Rhythmic cycles of dyspnea or hyperpnea subsiding gradually into brief apnea
Dyspnea	Difficult or labored respirations
Hypopnea	Shallow respirations
Hyperpnea	Deep respirations
Kussmaul	Fast and deep respirations
Orthopnea	Inability to breathe except while sitting or standing
Tachypnea	Fast respirations

aged not to breathe too rapidly to avoid hyperventilation, which can cause dizziness. During auscultation, the physician listens for abnormal or adventitious sounds, such as crackles and wheezes, which may also indicate a disease process (Table 30-3).

 CHECKPOINT QUESTION

5. What are the four methods used to examine the respiratory system?

Sputum Culture and Cytology

Sputum cultures are obtained to aid with diagnosis and treatment decisions in patients with suspected pneumonia, tuberculosis, or other infectious diseases of the lower airway. A microbiology laboratory will culture and incubate the specimen to identify any pathogenic microorganisms. Sputum specimens obtained for cytology are analyzed in the laboratory for abnormal cells that may indicate precancerous or cancerous conditions of the lung or airway. In all cases, it is important to obtain a specimen that the patient has coughed up and expectorated from the lower airways, with minimal contamination by oral and pharyngeal secretions. The patient is asked to cough deeply and collect the specimen in a sterile container (see Chapter 44). After instructing the patient on coughing and collecting the specimen, you process the specimen and prepare the laboratory request for transportation to the laboratory for analysis.

Sputum collection for suspected cancer or for tuberculosis may be required over three consecutive mornings. The specimens should be brought into the office as soon as possible to avoid deterioration of the specimen. Most diagnostic specimens are obtained early in the morning, when the greatest volume of secretion has ac-

cumulated. If this is not possible, a specimen may also be collected after a nebulized breathing treatment with a bronchodilator. The patient may be weak from illness, thick mucus may be difficult to bring up, and coughing may exhaust the patient. A cool-mist humidifier may be ordered for use at home to help loosen thick secretions. It is vitally important that the patient understand that the specimen must be collected from the lung fields and not from the mouth. The difference between saliva and sputum should be explained to the patient at his or her level of understanding.

Chest Radiography

Chest radiography can help in the diagnosis of a large variety of pulmonary problems, including pneumonia, lung cancer, emphysema, tuberculosis, and pulmonary edema. Often the physician orders two views: a posteroanterior (PA) view and a lateral view. This gives the physician a three-dimensional view. If the procedure is performed at the hospital or other outpatient facility, you may have to schedule it and request the results after the radiographs are interpreted by the radiologist.

 CHECKPOINT QUESTION

6. What is being analyzed in a sputum specimen?

Bronchoscopy

Bronchoscopy is an endoscopic procedure in which a lighted scope is inserted into the trachea and bronchi for direct visualization. This procedure is considered invasive and requires the patient's written consent. It is usually performed in an outpatient surgical setting, and you may have to schedule it. Bronchoscopy can be used for

TABLE **30-3**	Abnormal Breath Sounds
Breath Sound	**Description**
Bubbling	Gurgling sounds as air passes through moist secretions in airways
Crackles (rales)	Crackling sound, usually inspiratory, as air passes through moist secretions in airways. Fine to medium crackles indicate secretions in small airways and alveoli. Medium to coarse crackles indicate secretions in larger airways.
Friction rub	Dry, rubbing or grating sound
Rhonchi	Low-pitched, continuous sound as air moves past thick mucus or narrowed air passages
Stertor	Snoring sound on inspiration or expiration; indicates a partial airway obstruction
Stridor	Shrill, harsh inspiratory sound; indicates laryngeal obstruction
Wheeze	High-pitched musical sound, either inspiratory or expiratory; indicates partial airway obstruction

many diagnostic purposes, such as obtaining sputum specimens, obtaining tissue for biopsy, and visually assessing airway changes caused by chronic pulmonary diseases such as COPD or asthma. It can also be used therapeutically, for example to clear out mucus plugs or to remove a foreign body.

Pulmonary Function Tests

Pulmonary function tests are performed with a spirometer that measures the amount of air a patient can move in and out of the lungs (Fig. 30-4). The patient breathes into a mouthpiece and performs several breathing maneuvers that you explain during the test. By measuring the patient's airflow and comparing the results with predicted values for the patient's height, weight, gender, age, and race, the physician gains valuable information concerning whether the patient has mild, moderate, or severe obstructive or restrictive disease. The patient's **tidal volume** and **forced expiratory volume** are two measurements that can be obtained during the pulmonary function test. Procedure 30-3 describes the steps for performing the pulmonary function test.

Arterial Blood Gases

Arterial blood gas (ABG) determinations measure the pH and pressures of oxygen and carbon dioxide in arterial blood. The results can indicate whether the patient's lungs are adequately exchanging gases. ABGs can also give information about metabolic acid-base problems, such as diabetic ketoacidosis. Drawing blood from an artery takes special training and is not routinely done in the medical office. However, you may be required to schedule a patient for an arterial puncture at a laboratory or hospital and record the results, which are usually phoned to the office.

Pulse Oximetry

Many medical offices have a pulse oximeter, which quickly and painlessly determines the percentage of oxygen saturation on a patient's capillary blood cells (Fig. 30-5). The pulse oximeter is small, fitting into the palm of the hand, and includes a digital display that notes the patient's pulse rate and oxygen saturation when a sensor cable is attached to the nail bed of the patient's index finger. Pulse oximeter readings should be obtained as a baseline for patients with chronic respiratory conditions and for patients with respiratory signs and symptoms, such as complaints of dyspnea or wheezing. The results should be recorded as a percentage; readings above 95% are considered normal. Although patients with chronic conditions such as emphysema may have readings of 90% or higher, readings below 90% should be reported to the physician immediately.

CHECKPOINT QUESTION

7. What are the ways the physician can obtain information to help diagnose respiratory disorders?

Figure 30-5 Pulse oximetry is used to measure oxygen saturation of arterial blood. (Reprinted with permission from Cohen BJ. Medical Terminology: An Illustrated Guide. Philadelphia: Lippincott Williams & Wilkins, 2003.)

Figure 30-4 A pulmonary function testing machine. (Courtesy of Spirometrics.)

TRIAGE

While working in a medical office, the following three situations occur this afternoon:

A. Patient A is an elderly male with emphysema who is wheezing. The doctor has ordered a nebulized treatment with a bronchodilator.

B. Patient B is a 34-year-old woman who is scheduled to have a pulmonary function test today as part of a pre-employment physical. She is anxious about getting the test "over with" so that she can pick up her children from school.

C. Patient C has been seen and discharged by the doctor but is waiting for you to schedule a bronchoscopy that the physician has ordered to be done later this week.

How do you sort these patients? Who do you see first? Second? Third?

Patient A should be seen first. Anyone who has trouble breathing or a respiratory problem must be treated as a priority. It is important to monitor this patient closely for any changes in condition before, during, and after treatment. Place patient B in an examination room and tell her that you will start the test within 10 minutes or advise her that she can reschedule the test for later this week. Inform patient C that you will schedule her procedure and notify her by phone of the exact date and time. Patients often become anxious about impending tests and can easily become upset with delays. Offer reassurance to the patient as needed.

 MEDIA MENU

- **Student CD**
  - **CMA/RMA Certification Exam Review**
- **LWW's Medical Assisting Skills DVD**
  - **Procedures 30-2, 30-3**
- **Premium Online Course**
  http://thePoint.lww.com/Kronenberger3e
- **Internet Resources**

LiveAdvise Online Tutoring & Competency Training
http://thePoint.lww.com/LiveAdvise

Centers for Disease Control and Prevention
http://www.cdc.gov

American Lung Association
http://www.lungusa.org

American Association of Respiratory Care
http://www.acr.org

American Thoracic Society
http://www.thoracic.org

American Cancer Society
http://www.cancer.org

 español
SPANISH TERMINOLOGY

Tose con flema?
　Do you cough up any phlegm?
De que color es la flema?
　What color is it?
Clara
　Clear
Blanca
　White
Amarilla
　Yellow
Verde
　Green
Oscura
　Dark

PROCEDURE 30-1: **Instructing a Patient on Using the Peak Flowmeter**

Purpose: Instruct the patient on the correct procedure for using and recording measurements using the peak flowmeter.

Equipment: Peak flowmeter, recording documentation form

Steps	Reasons
1. Wash your hands.	Handwashing aids infection control.
2. Assemble the peak flowmeter, disposable mouthpiece, and patient documentation form.	The flowmeter is used to instruct patients in performing a peak flow reading. A disposable mouthpiece should be used. In some offices, the patient is instructed in using a peak flowmeter that is given to him or her to take home and use. In this case, no disposable mouthpiece is necessary.
3. Greet and identify the patient and explain the procedure.	Identifying the patient prevents errors.
4. Holding the peak flowmeter upright, explain how to read and reset the gauge after each reading.	In the upright position, the meter is calibrated with numbers and contains a sliding gauge that should move freely up and down the meter next to the numbers.

Step 4. The peak flowmeter and sliding gauge.

Steps	Reasons
5. Instruct the patient to put the peak flowmeter mouthpiece in the mouth, forming a tight seal with the lips. After taking a deep breath, the patient should blow hard into the mouthpiece without blocking the back of the flowmeter.	The patient should close the lips around the mouthpiece without biting down. Blocking the back of the flowmeter will interfere with the movement of the gauge.
6. Note the number on the flowmeter corresponding to the level at which the sliding gauge stopped after the patient blew hard into the mouthpiece. Reset the gauge to zero.	A normal range provided with the flowmeter is based on the patient's age, height, and weight. Ideally, the patient's readings should be within this range.
7. Instruct the patient to perform this procedure three times consecutively, in the morning and at night, and to record the highest reading on the form.	The highest reading is the patient's best reading. Recording the readings on the form allows the patient to follow his or her progress based on medication therapy or exposure to allergens.

Step 7. A peak flowmeter documentation form.

(continued)

PROCEDURE 30-1: Instructing a Patient on Using the Peak Flowmeter *(continued)*

Steps	Reasons
8. Explain to the patient the procedure for cleaning the mouthpiece by washing with soapy water and rinsing without immersing the flowmeter in water.	Cleaning the mouthpiece is sanitary and prevents the spread of microorganisms.
9. Document the procedure. if they are not recorded.	Procedures are considered not to have been done if they are not recorded.

Charting Example

12/11/2008 3:30 PM Pt. instructed on using a flowmeter—return demonstration without difficulty, verbalized understanding. Given patient documentation form, instructed to record readings in morning and evening. Today's reading 400 LPM. No dyspnea, c/o wheezing or SOB

—E. Michael, RMA

PROCEDURE 30-2: Performing a Nebulized Breathing Treatment

Purpose: Set up and administer a nebulized breathing treatment in the medical office
Equipment: Physician order, patient's medical record, inhalation medication, saline for inhalation, nebulizer disposable setup, nebulizer

Steps	Reasons
1. Wash your hands.	Handwashing aids infection control.
2. Assemble the equipment and medication; check the medication label three times, as when administering any medications.	Checking the medication label three times prevents errors.
3. Greet and identify the patient and explain the procedure.	Properly identifying the patient will avoid errors. Explaining the procedure promotes understanding and compliance.
4. Remove the nebulizer treatment cup from the setup and add the exact amount of medication ordered by the physician.	The physician bases the amount of bronchodilator on the age and weight of the patient.

Step 4. The nebulizer medication cup.

(continued)

PROCEDURE 30-2:　**Performing a Nebulized Breathing Treatment** *(continued)*

Steps	Reasons
5. Add 2–3 mL of saline for inhalation therapy to the cup that contains the medication.	The bronchodilator must be mixed with saline before being administered to the patient.
6. Place the top on the cup securely, attach the T piece to the top of the cup, and position the mouthpiece firmly on one end of the T piece.	The top of the mouthpiece usually screws onto the bottom of the cup, providing a reservoir for the medication and saline.

Step 6. A nebulizer machine and disposable setup with mouthpiece.

Steps	Reasons
7. Attach one end of the tubing securely to the connector on the cup and the other end to the connector on the nebulizer machine.	
8. Ask the patient to put the mouthpiece in the mouth and make a seal with the lips without biting the mouthpiece. Instruct the patient to breathe normally during the treatment, occasionally taking a deep breath.	The patient may have difficulty breathing or be wheezing but should be encouraged to breathe as normally as possible. Breathing too rapidly may cause hyperventilation. Occasionally taking a deep breath will allow medication to be administered to deeper lung tissues.

Step 8. The T piece and medication cup.

Steps	Reasons
9. Turn the machine on. The medication in the reservoir cup will become a fine mist to be inhaled by the patient.	A fine mist will come from the opposite end of the T piece when the patient exhales.
10. Before, during, and after the breathing treatment, take and record the patient's pulse.	Most bronchodilators cause a slight increase in the heart rate. Notify the physician if the increase is significant or if the patient has symptoms such as dizziness.

(continued)

PROCEDURE 30-2: Performing a Nebulized Breathing Treatment *(continued)*

11. When the treatment is over and the medication cup is empty, turn the machine off and have the patient remove the mouthpiece.	The treatment typically takes about 15 minutes.
12. Disconnect the disposable treatment setup and dispose of all parts in a biohazard container. Properly put away the machine.	The setup equipment, including the mouthpiece, may be contaminated with hazardous microorganisms and should be handled and disposed of properly.
13. Wash your hands and document the procedure, including the patient's pulse before, during, and after the treatment.	Procedures are considered not to have been done if they are not recorded. Again, the bronchodilator used for nebulized treatments may cause the heart rate to increase, and the pulse should be noted and recorded during and after the treatment.

Charting Example

11/26/2008 9:15 AM Pt. given nebulized breathing treatment with albuterol 2 mg and 3 mL NS for inhalation—pulse before treatment 88, during treatment 100, and after treatment 110. Pt. states she is "breathing easier" after treatment, skin warm and dry, color pink

—J. Barker, CMA

PROCEDURE 30-3: Perform a Pulmonary Function Test

Purpose: Perform a pulmonary function test and record the procedure
Equipment: Physician order, patient's medical record, spirometer and appropriate cables, calibration syringe and log book, disposable mouthpiece, printer, nose clip

Steps	Reasons
1. Wash your hands.	Handwashing aids infection control.
2. Assemble the equipment, greet and identify the patient, and explain the procedure.	Identifying the patient prevents errors, and explaining the procedure promotes compliance.
3. Turn the pulmonary function test machine on, and if the spirometer has not been calibrated according to office policy, calibrate it using the calibration syringe according to the manufacturer's instructions. Record the calibration in the appropriate log book.	The spirometer must be calibrated daily to ensure accurate results.

Step 4. The calibration syringe used for checking the pulmonary function machine.

(continued)

PROCEDURE 30-3: **Perform a Pulmonary Function Test** *(continued)*

Steps	Reasons
4. With the machine on and calibrated, attach the appropriate cable, tubing, and mouthpiece according to the type of machine being used.	One cable is plugged into an electrical outlet, and another cable or tube is connected to the spirometer and the patient's mouthpiece.
5. Using the keyboard on the machine, enter the patient's name or identification number, age, weight, height, sex, race, and smoking history.	The spirometer automatically takes these parameters into consideration when providing the results.
6. Ask the patient to remove any restrictive clothing, such as a necktie, and show the patient how to apply the nose clip.	Restrictive clothing can stop the chest from fully expanding, causing an inaccurate result. The nose clip stops air from being expelled from the nose during the test.
7. Ask the patient to stand, breathe in deeply, and blow into the mouthpiece as hard as possible. The patient should continue to blow into the mouthpiece until the machine indicates that it is appropriate to stop blowing. A chair should be available in case the patient becomes dizzy or lightheaded. **Step 7.** The patient should blow into the mouthpiece as instructed.	Some machines signal to stop blowing with a buzz or beep; however, you may have to instruct the patient if the machine gives only a visual signal. Some patients become lightheaded during this procedure and should be observed closely for signs of difficulty or imbalance.
8. During the procedure, coach the patient as necessary to obtain an adequate reading.	Many patients feel that they have exhaled all air from the lungs when the machine is instructing them to continue. All air must be exhaled to obtain accurate results. The machine will indicate whether the reading or maneuver is adequate.
9. Continue the procedure until three adequate readings, or maneuvers, are performed.	Three maneuvers are usually required to obtain the patient's best result. The patient may rest between readings if necessary.
10. After printing the results, properly care for the equipment and dispose of the mouthpiece into the biohazard container. Wash your hands.	The mouthpiece may be contaminated and must be handled and discarded properly.
11. Document the procedure and place the printed results in the patient's medical record.	The three maneuvers will be recorded on one printout. Procedures are not considered to have been done if not properly recorded.

Charting Example

06/12/2008 3:00 PM PFT performed for employment physical as ordered by Dr. John. ×3 maneuvers obtained without difficulty. Dr. John notified of results in chart

—P. Hill, CMA

You can play an important role in helping the patient to maintain healthy lungs and in assisting the physician to diagnose and treat respiratory disease. It is important that you remember that:

- Because the air that we breathe is open to the atmosphere, the respiratory system is susceptible to infection and irritant injury.
- Disorders of the respiratory system can affect either the upper respiratory system or the lower respiratory system.

- Chronic disorders of the respiratory system include emphysema and asthma, while acute disorders include sinusitis and the common cold.
- The peak flowmeter is used by patients at home to assess breathing, while a pulmonary function test is done in the office and gives the physician more information about the health of the lungs.
- Diagnosis of infectious respiratory infections can be done through the sputum culture.

Warm Ups   for Critical Thinking

1. Why do you think it is better to inhale through the nose than through the mouth?

2. Mr. Gardner, aged 55, has been diagnosed with COPD and has many questions about his condition. Identify the characteristics of COPD. How do you explain this disease to Mr. Gardner?

3. Your patient has recently had an upper respiratory infection and was seen today for bronchitis. Why would the physician tell the patient to take the cough suppressant only at night? Use a drug reference book and look up some possible cough suppressants that might be ordered by the physician. Are there any precautions that the patient should be made aware of before taking these medications?

4. The mother of an 8-year-old child with asthma tells you that the child has tested positive for an allergy to cats. Unfortunately, their family owns two cats. The mother tells you that she is reluctant to give the cats away since her son will "probably outgrow his asthma" according to a family friend whose daughter also has asthma. How would you respond? Could the allergy to cats trigger an asthma attack?

5. Develop a patient brochure on the effects of smoking. Investigate the products available for smoking cessation and include these in your brochure.

Answers   to Checkpoint Questions

1. The onset of bacterial pneumonia is usually sudden and severe; symptoms include fever, cough, chills, and dyspnea. This type of pneumonia is typically local. In contrast, the onset of viral pneumonia is usually gradual; symptoms include fever and a hacking cough. Unlike bacterial pneumonia, viral pneumonia tends to be spread throughout the lung fields.

2. Factors that may trigger an asthma attack are environmental allergens, irritants, infection, stress, cold air, and exercise.

3. The two disease processes in a patient with COPD are chronic bronchitis and emphysema.

4. Cigarette smoking may contribute to both laryngeal cancer and lung cancer.

5. The four parts of the chest examination are inspection, percussion, palpation, and auscultation.

6. A sputum specimen is analyzed for abnormal cells that may be present in the sputum.

7. The methods of diagnosing respiratory disorders are physical examination, peak flowmeter readings, sputum cultures, chest radiography, bronchoscopy, pulmonary function testing, assessment of arterial blood gases, and pulse oximeter readings.

Outline

Common Disorders of the Cardiovascular System
Disorders of the Heart
Carditis
Congestive Heart Failure
Myocardial Infarction
Cardiac Arrhythmia
Congenital and Valvular Heart Disease
Disorders of the Blood Vessels
Atherosclerosis

Hypertension
Varicose Veins
Venous Thrombosis and Pulmonary Embolism
Cerebrovascular Accident
Aneurysm
Anemia
Common Diagnostic and Therapeutic Procedures
Physical Examination of the Cardiovascular System

Electrocardiogram
Holter Monitor
Chest Radiography
Cardiac Stress Test
Echocardiography
Cardiac Catheterization and Coronary Arteriography

Learning Objectives

Upon successfully completing this chapter, you will be able to:

1. Spell and define key terms

2. List and describe common cardiovascular disorders

3. Identify and explain common cardiovascular procedures and tests

4. Describe the roles and responsibilities of the medical assistant during cardiovascular examinations and procedures

5. Discuss the information recorded on a basic 12-lead electrocardiogram

6. Explain the purpose of a Holter monitor

Performance Objectives

Upon successfully completing this chapter, you will be able to:

1. Perform a basic 12-lead electrocardiogram (Procedure 31-1)

2. Apply a Holter monitor for a 24-hour test (Procedure 31-2)

CAAHEP

- Practice standard precautions
- Prepare patient for and assist with routine and specialty examinations
- Prepare patient for and assist with procedures, treatments, and minor office surgeries
- Perform electrocardiography
- Document appropriately
- Instruct individuals according to their needs

ABHES

- Prepare patients for procedures
- Assist physician with examinations and treatments
- Perform electrocardiograms
- Document accurately

Key Terms

aneurysm
angina pectoris
artifact
atherosclerosis
bradycardia
cardiomegaly
cardiomyopathy

cerebrovascular accident (CVA)
congestive heart failure
coronary artery bypass graft
electrocardiography

endocarditis
lead
myocardial infarction (MI)
myocarditis
palpitations

percutaneous transluminal coronary angioplasty
pericarditis
tachycardia
transient ischemic attack (TIA)

Cardiovascular disease is a major cause of illness and death. The cardiologist is a physician who specializes in disorders of the heart, and many patients with chronic cardiac conditions are referred to the cardiology office for treatment and follow-up. However, many of these patients are seen in internal medicine or family practice medical offices also. Because medical assistants see patients who have cardiovascular disorders regardless of the medical specialty, you must understand the cardiovascular system, associated disorders, and common tests and procedures that are ordered for diagnosis and treatment.

Common Disorders of the Cardiovascular System

The cardiovascular system consists of the heart (Fig. 31-1) and blood vessels, including the arteries, capillaries, and veins. The rhythmic contractions of the heart pump oxygen-rich blood from the lungs throughout the body to oxygenate and nourish the tissues and remove wastes for elimination. While the heart and blood vessels are a closed system for the flow of blood (Fig. 31-2), disorders anywhere in this system may adversely affect other body systems that depend on the cardiovascular system for delivery of oxygen and nutrients. Depending on the body system affected by the lack of oxygen and nutrients being delivered, the following can be symptoms of various heart disorders:

- Chest pain
- Dyspnea
- Fatigue
- Diaphoresis
- Nausea and vomiting
- Irregular heartbeat
- Changes in peripheral circulation
- Edema
- Skin ulcers that do not heal
- Pain that increases with walking and decreases with rest
- Changes in skin color

While some of these symptoms can indicate disorders not related to the heart or blood vessels, you should obtain an accurate history and chief complaint and communicate any finding to the physician through complete documentation.

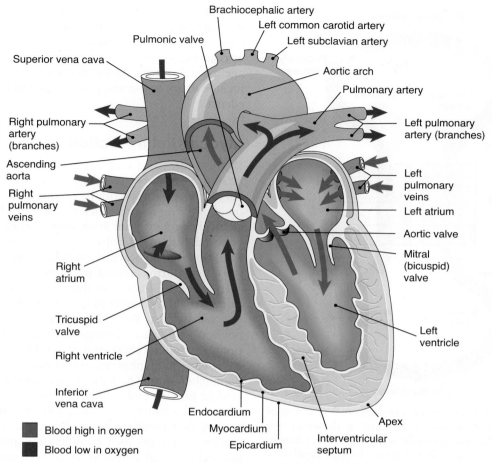

Figure 31-1 The heart and great vessels. (Reprinted with permission from Cohen BJ. Memmler's The Human Body in Health and Disease. Philadelphia: Lippincott Williams & Wilkins, 2005.)

Disorders of the Heart

Carditis

Cardiac inflammation, or carditis, may affect any of the layers of the heart muscle, and although other factors may be involved, it is usually the result of a systemic infection. **Pericarditis,** an inflammation of the sac that covers the outside of the heart, may be acute or chronic. It is caused by a pathogen, neoplasm, or autoimmune disorder, such as lupus erythematosus or rheumatoid arthritis. Other causes of pericarditis include certain chemicals, radiation, and uremia in patients with kidney failure. Signs and symptoms include a sharp pain in the same locations as with a **myocardial infarction (MI),** except that pain increases on inspiration and on lying down but decreases on sitting up and leaning forward. Dyspnea, tachycardia, neck venous distention, pallor, and hypertension are warning signs that serous fluid is compressing the heart and interfering with cardiac function. Treatment is relieving the symptoms and, if possible, correcting the underlying cause, including administering an antibiotic for bacterial infection.

Myocarditis may be diffused through the heart muscle or may be local to a focal point. Causes include radiation, chemicals, and bacterial, viral, or parasitic infection. Signs and symptoms of early acute episodes are usually nonspecific, such as fatigue, fever, and mild chest pain. Chronic cases may lead to heart failure with **cardiomegaly** (an enlarged heart muscle), arrhythmias, and valvulitis. Treatment is supportive care and medication as ordered by the physician to kill the responsible pathogen.

Chronic or acute **endocarditis** is infection or inflammation of the inner lining of the heart, the endocardium. The lining of the heart and its valves may gather clusters of platelets, fibrin, and white blood cells to trap the pathogens. These clusters, called vegetations, may break away to become emboli that travel to the spleen, kidneys, lungs, or nervous system. These formations may also scar the valves and erode the chordae tendinea, small tendons that attach the heart valves to the ventricles. The destruction of these structures may result in reflux, or backflow, of the valves or blood. Diagnosis of endocarditis requires a blood culture to identify the

Figure 31-2 Blood vessels form a closed system for the flow of blood. Blood high in oxygen (oxygenated) is shown in red; blood low in oxygen (deoxygenated) is shown in blue. Changes in oxygen content occur as blood flows through capillaries. (Reprinted with permission from Cohen BJ. Memmler's The Human Body in Health and Disease. Philadelphia: Lippincott Williams & Wilkins, 2005.)

causative agent. Treatment is directed at eliminating the infecting organism.

 CHECKPOINT QUESTION

1. How does the pain in pericarditis differ from pain of myocardial infarction?

Congestive Heart Failure

Congestive heart failure (CHF) is a condition in which the heart cannot pump effectively. Failure of the right ventricle causes congestion of the peripheral extremities, while failure of the left ventricle leads to pulmonary congestion. Many patients have failure of both sides of the heart; their signs and symptoms include edema of the lower extremities and dyspnea. As blood flow to organs such as the brain and kidneys decreases, patients may also have complaints related to the organs involved. Progressive heart failure results in damage to vital organs and death.

The causes of CHF include coronary artery disease, myocardial disease, valvular heart disease, and hypertension. While there is no cure for it, treatment is aimed at relieving symptoms and preventing permanent damage to vital organs. Medications given to CHF patients include drugs to increase cardiac function and decrease edema.

Myocardial Infarction

Death of any part of the heart muscle, called myocardial infarction (MI), occurs when one or more of the coronary arteries becomes totally occluded, usually by atherosclerotic plaques or by an embolism. An MI may occur suddenly without prior symptoms or in patients with diagnosed atherosclerotic coronary artery disease. Symptoms of myocardial infarction may be similar to those felt during **angina pectoris** in patients with ischemic heart disease, but this disorder is distinguished by pain that lasts longer than 20 to 30 minutes and is unrelieved by rest. Box 31-1 describes criteria that the physician will use to distinguish the chest pain of angina pectoris from the chest pain of MI. Other symptoms include nausea, diaphoresis, weakness, vomiting, and abdominal cramps. The patient may complain of feeling a viselike grip around the chest cavity. The skin may become cool, clammy, and pale, and the patient may feel anxiety or impending doom. Some patients have nonspecific symptoms such as indigestion and therefore do not seek medical attention. In 20% of patients, the MI may be silent, diagnosed only by routine **electrocardiography** (ECG). It is imperative not to ignore or dismiss complaints by patients with symptoms of MI or to accept the patient's own diagnosis that "It's only indigestion." Although the death of myocardial tissue that occurs during an MI cannot be reversed, early medical intervention may reduce the amount of tissue that dies and increase the patient's chances of survival. Procedures such as **percutaneous transluminal coronary angioplasty** (PTCA) and **coronary artery bypass graft** (CABG) are performed to increase blood flow to the cardiac muscle (Box 31-2).

 CHECKPOINT QUESTION

2. Why is it important to treat a patient with myocardial infarction as early as possible?

Cardiac Arrhythmia

When the electrical conduction system of the heart is not functioning normally, cardiac arrhythmias may develop and can be detected on the electrocardiography. Cardiac arrhythmia or dysrhythmia is an abnormal heart rhythm that may occur as a primary disorder or as a response to

BOX 31-1

IS IT ANGINA OR MYOCARDIAL INFARCTION?

The pain felt with angina and MI is brought about by myocardial anoxia, or increased need for oxygen to the heart muscle because of exertion, stress, or extremes of heat or cold. Typically, angina is relieved by rest or nitroglycerin, a vasodilator. However, pain from an MI is not relieved by these measures. The following is a brief comparison of these two disorders:

	Angina	**Myocardial Infarction**
Description	Moderate pressure deep in the chest; squeezing, suffocating feeling	Severe deep pressure not relieved by reducing stressors; crushing pressure
Onset	Pain gradual or sudden; subsides quickly, usually in less than 30 minutes; can be relieved by nitroglycerin, rest, or reducing stressors	Pain sudden; remains after stressors reduced or relieved; not relieved by nitroglycerin
Location	Mid-anterior chest, usually diffuse, radiates to back, neck, arms, jaw, and epigastric area	Mid-anterior chest with same radiating patterns
Signs and symptoms	Dyspnea, nausea, signs of indigestion, profuse sweating	Nausea, vomiting, fear, diaphoresis, pounding heart, palpitations

Any patient who calls the medical office complaining of chest pain must be examined immediately. The office should have an established protocol for handling these calls. The physician must be consulted to decide whether the patient should be directed to the nearest emergency department or come directly to the office.

---

a systemic problem. Arrhythmia may also be a reaction to a drug toxicity or an electrolyte imbalance. Normally, the sinoatrial (SA) node is the pacemaker of the heart (Fig. 31-3), initiating an electrical impulse in the adult at rest 60 to 100 times a minute. This is sinus rhythm. Arrhythmia may occur if the SA node initiates electrical impulses too fast or too slowly. If the SA node is damaged or the conduction pathway is blocked, the heart will beat too slowly to meet the body's demands. This type of arrhythmia, called **bradycardia**, is characterized by a heart rate less than 60 beats per minute. If the SA node initiates an electrical impulse faster than 100 times per minute, the arrhythmia is called **tachycardia**.

More serious arrhythmias occur when the ventricles beat too fast, a condition known as ventricular tachycardia (VT). This condition occurs when some of the electrical signals originate in the ventricles rather than in the SA node. Once the ventricles begin to beat at a very rapid rate, less blood is pumped out of the heart with each contraction, since the heart's chambers do not have time to fill with blood before the next contraction begins. As less blood is pumped into circulation, less oxygen is carried to the tissues. This lack of adequate blood and oxygen may cause dizziness, unconsciousness, or cardiac arrest.

Another arrhythmia is ventricular fibrillation. Ventricular fibrillation is a medical emergency that occurs when the heart is quivering rather than contracting in an organized fashion. In this condition, very little blood is pumped out of the heart, and the patient will fall unconscious and die very quickly unless a shock with a cardiac defibrillator is administered immediately to restore normal cardiac electrical activity. Automatic external defibrillators (AED) are now available in many medical offices and public places, such as airports and shopping malls. All professional medical assistants should receive certification in cardiopulmonary resuscitation (CPR) and use of the AED, which is relatively easy to operate (Box 31-3). Patients who require frequent defibrillation may benefit from the insertion of an implantable cardiac defibrillator that will automatically deliver an electrical shock to restore normal cardiac conduction. These devices should not be confused with cardiac pacemakers, which help to regulate the normal rhythm of the heart.

BOX 31-2

CORRECTIVE CARDIAC SURGERY

The least traumatic form of cardiac surgery is the *percutaneous transluminal coronary angioplasty* (*PTCA*). A double-lumen catheter with a balloon surrounding the upper portion is inserted into a vessel in the groin or axilla. This catheter is threaded into the coronary vessels, with the surgeon watching a fluoroscopic screen while performing the procedure. When the occlusion is found, the balloon is inflated to press the atherosclerotic plaque against the arterial walls and relieve the occlusion. A laser may be used to remove the plaque. A spring or mesh (called a stent) may be inserted and left in place within the vessel to maintain patency. This procedure is less invasive than bypass surgery, but occasionally the artery rebuilds plaque at the site, or the stent may fill with plaque and the artery may occlude again.

Coronary artery bypass graft (*CABG*) is performed by grafting a piece of vessel from another part of the body to the area beyond the occlusion and to the ascending aorta, providing a patent passage for the blood. The surgery requires a still field of surgery, so the heart must be stopped and the patient supported by a cardiopulmonary bypass machine for the length of the operation. The saphenous vein may be used for multiple bypasses; the internal mammary artery is used if the surgery is not extensive. Hospitalization may be as long as 5 to 7 days, and 20% of patients develop a repeat thrombus within 1 year.

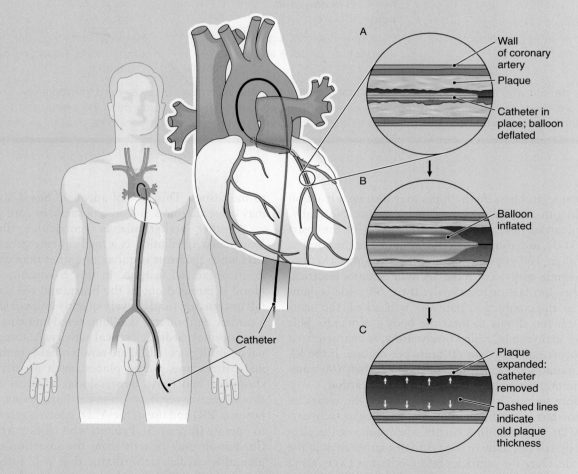

Percutaneous transluminal coronary angioplasty (PTCA). **(A)** *A guide is threaded into the coronrary artery.* **(B)** *A balloon catheter is inserted through the occlusion.* **(C)** *The balloon is inflated and deflated until plaque is flattened and the vessel is opened.*

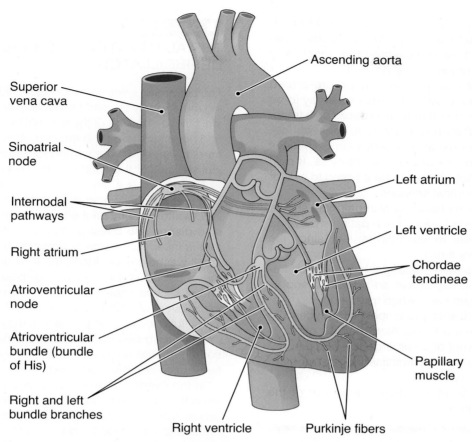

Superior vena cava

Sinoatrial node

Internodal pathways

Right atrium

Atrioventricular node

Atrioventricular bundle (bundle of His)

Right and left bundle branches

Right ventricle

Ascending aorta

Left atrium

Left ventricle

Chordae tendineae

Papillary muscle

Purkinje fibers

Figure 31-3 Conduction system of the heart. (Reprinted with permission from Cohen BJ. Memmler's The Human Body in Health and Disease. Philadelphia: Lippincott Williams & Wilkins, 2005.)

Artifical Pacemakers

When a patient's heart conduction system cannot maintain normal sinus rhythm without assistance, an electrical source can be implanted to assist or replace the sinoatrial node. The permanent or temporary artificial pacemaker is surgically implanted either between the chest wall and the rib cage or within the chest cavity. The pacemaker may be programmed to fire, or initiate an electrical charge, continuously at a predetermined rate or on demand, only when the patient's normal heart rate falls below a preset number.

Pacemaker programming initially occurs when the pacemaker is inserted in an outpatient or inpatient surgical facility. If additional programming or assessment is necessary, the pacemaker may be evaluated by telephone monitoring: the patient uses the telephone receiver to transmit the rate and function of the pacemaker to a physician at the receiving site. If battery function is failing and replacement is not possible or advisable, batteries can be recharged transdermally. A charging unit is placed over the implantation site and plugged into an ordinary electrical outlet. The power cell is recharged through the skin with no discomfort to the patient. Pacemakers are battery operated and usually are manu-

factured to retain their charge for up to 20 years. Recharging or changing the battery in an implanted pacemaker usually requires an outpatient surgical procedure under a local anesthetic.

CHECKPOINT QUESTION

3. Which two cardiac arrhythmias are emergencies requiring immediate intervention by the medical assistant?

PATIENT EDUCATION

NITROGLYCERIN

A medication commonly prescribed to increase blood flow to the cardiac muscle is nitroglycerin, a vasodilator. Vasodilators open the lumen of vessels, increasing blood supply to the heart muscle. Patient education should include the following instructions:

- Keep the medication in the dark bottle supplied by the pharmacy because nitroglycerin can be deactivated if exposed to light.

(continued)

- Be alert for any side effects, such as light-headedness, syncope, and hypotension. Caution patients not to drive or operate other machinery until these symptoms have passed.
- Be aware that nitroglycerin may be prescribed and dispensed as either tablets or a spray to be used as needed, or it may be ordered as a transdermal patch worn constantly to maintain vasodilation. The usual administration guidelines are for three doses at 5-minute intervals. If pain persists, the patient should be advised to call for emergency medical services.
- Patients with arthritis or visual impairment should use nitroglycerin spray. These patients may find the spray easier to use than tablets, since the tablets are very small.
- Check the expiration date of the medication frequently, and always have an adequate supply available at home and when traveling.
- Encourage patients prescribed nitroglycerin to obtain and wear a Medic Alert bracelet or necklace. In the event of an emergency, first responders can assist with administering this medication if necessary.
- Ensure that the medication is kept out of the reach of children.

Congenital and Valvular Heart Disease

Valvular disease is an acquired or congenital abnormality of any of the four cardiac valves. Valvular heart disease is characterized by stenosis and obstructed blood flow or by valvular degeneration and backflow of the blood against the course of the circulatory pathway. The valves in the left side of the heart are most often affected. The most common congenital valve diseases include atrial septal defect (ASD), ventricular septal defect (VSD), patent ductus arteriosus (PDA), coarctation of the aorta, aortic or pulmonic stenosis, bicuspid aortic valve, mitral valve prolapse, and tetralogy of Fallot (Table 31-1).

Rheumatic heart disease, an acquired valvular disease, presents clinically as a generalized inflammatory disease occurring 10 to 21 days after an upper respiratory infection caused by group A beta-hemolytic streptococci. It is characterized by inflammatory lesions of the connective tissues, particularly in the heart, joints, and subcutaneous tissues. The heart valves are damaged by an abnormal response of the immune system caused by the turbulence of the infected blood. This damage results in a systolic murmur. Although it usually attacks children aged 5 to 15, rheumatic heart disease has declined significantly since the 1940s.

BOX 31-3

THE AUTOMATIC EXTERNAL DEFIBRILLATOR

The automatic external defibrillator (AED) is becoming more widely supplied in public places and medical offices because of the minimal training required and potential to save the life of a patient with sudden cardiac arrest without waiting for emergency medical services or transportation to a hospital.

The device is a small defibrillator in a zippered bag that is usually orange or red with the acronym *AED* written clearly on the front. Inside the bag are also disposable chest pads connected to a cord that is inserted into the connection on the AED. A small washcloth for drying the skin before placing the chest pads if necessary, disposable razor to shave excess chest hair, and examination gloves in the event of possible exposure to blood or other body fluids during the procedure may be added to the AED bag because these items may be necessary to ensure adequate contact between the patient's skin and the chest pads.

In the event that an unconscious patient or victim is found with no pulse (refer to cardiopulmonary resuscitation criteria), the rescuer should apply the chest pads as trained, and using the pictures provided on the pads as a guide, connect the cable to the machine and turn the machine on. The machine has verbal commands to guide the user through the steps necessary to provide an electrical shock if necessary. Do not touch or move the patient while the machine is analyzing the patient's cardiac rhythm or when the machine determines that an electrical shock is necessary.

Mitral valve stenosis, a condition that occurs when the leaflet cusps of the mitral valve fuse and thicken, may result from rheumatic heart disease. When the valve cusps thicken and fuse, the result is an abnormally narrow valve; hence mitral regurgitation, or backflow, of blood from the left ventricle into the left atrium occurs. Patients with mitral stenosis often have dyspnea, or shortness of breath, and their ability to exert themselves physically may be limited. Pulmonary edema may also develop and cause symptoms such as dyspnea and a productive cough.

Treatment of valvular disease depends on the type and severity of the abnormality. Severe cases may require medication, low-sodium diet, and prophylactic antibiotic before surgery or dental work. If medication is not successful, surgical replacement of the involved valves may be necessary.

TABLE **31-1**	Diseases of the Cardiac Valves and Congenital Cardiac Defects	
Disorder	**Description**	**Treatment**
ASD	Abnormal opening between atria, allowing unoxygenated blood in right atrium to mix with oxygenated blood in left atrium; congenital	Surgery to close
VSD	Abnormal opening between ventricles, allowing unoxygenated blood in right ventricle to mix with oxygenated blood in left ventricle; congenital	Surgery to close
PDA	Abnormal opening between pulmonary artery and aorta; congenital	Surgery to close
Coarctation of the aorta	Narrowing of the aorta resulting in high blood pressure in upper extremities and low blood pressure in lower extremities; congenital	Surgery to increase diameter of aorta
Bicuspid aortic valve	Aortic valve having 2 cusps instead of 3, resulting in incomplete closure between aorta and left ventricle during systole and diastole; congenital	Surgical replacement of aortic valve
Aortic or pulmonic stenosis	Narrowing of aortic or pulmonary artery valve leaflets, causing overwork of cardiac muscle and hypertrophy of ventricles; as stenosis increases, valve becomes less flexible	Dilation of stenosed area or surgical replacement of valve
MVP	Drooping of one or both cusps of mitral (bicuspid) valve into left ventricle during systole, resulting in incomplete closure of valve and backflow of blood from left ventricle into left atrium	Usually benign; treatment is alleviating any symptoms (palpations, chest pain); prophylactic antibiotic may be ordered before dental procedures
Tetralogy of Fallot	Four defects: pulmonary stenosis, dextraposition of aorta, ventricular septal defect, and hypertrophy of right ventricle; congenital	Surgery to correct

CHECKPOINT QUESTION

4. What microorganism may be responsible for rheumatic heart disease and cardiac valvular damage?

Disorders of the Blood Vessels

Atherosclerosis

Diseases of blood vessels—arteries or veins—often begin with collection of fatty plaques made of calcium and cholesterol inside the walls of the vessels. These plaques narrow the lumen, or opening, of the blood vessels and impede blood flow. This condition, which is known as **atherosclerosis**, is problematic in arteries because oxygen and nutrients are prevented from reaching various tissues of the body. In addition to the occlusion that occurs with atherosclerosis, the plaques are rougher than the walls of a normal artery and may remain stationary as a thrombus or break away from the wall of the artery as an embolus (Fig. 31-4). Signs and symptoms of atherosclerosis usually result from ischemia to a body part

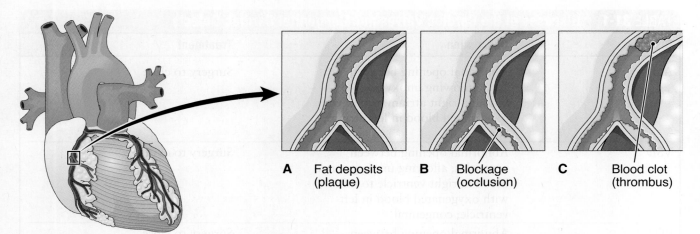

Figure 31-4 Coronary atherosclerosis. (**A**) Fat deposits narrow an artery, leading to ischemia. (**B**) Blockage of the coronary artery. (**C**) Formation of a blood clot (thrombus), leading to MI. (Reprinted with permission from Cohen BJ. Memmler's The Human Body in Health and Disease. Philadelphia: Lippincott Williams & Wilkins, 2005.)

and may include pain or numbness, loss of normal blood flow, or loss of a palpable pulse to the affected body area.

If the coronary arteries are involved, the condition is coronary artery disease (CAD), the most common type of heart disease and the leading cause of death in men and women in the United States. Patients with CAD may have the following symptoms:

- Angina pectoris (pain radiating to the arm, jaw, shoulder, back, or neck, usually felt on exertion and relieved by rest)
- Pressure or fullness in the chest, felt most severely during exertion and relieved by rest
- Syncope (fainting)
- Edema of the extremities, especially the legs
- Unexplained cough, generally without respiratory symptoms
- Excessive fatigue
- Dyspnea

Predisposing conditions for atherosclerosis and coronary artery disease (CAD) include a diet high in saturated fats and a family history of hypercholesterolemia. Other risk factors include cigarette smoking, diabetes mellitus, and hypertension. Consuming a diet low in cholesterol and saturated fats, participating in a moderate exercise program, maintaining normal body weight and blood pressure, and not smoking may minimize the chances for developing atherosclerosis and CAD or reduce the progression if a diagnosis has been made. If necessary, the physician may order lipid-lowering medication for patients whose blood cholesterol and triglyceride levels are not affected by dietary or other behavioral changes.

Diagnosis of atherosclerosis is often made by angiography to locate the occlusion and evaluate the de-

gree of obstruction (Fig. 31-5). In this procedure, a catheter is inserted into the blood vessel, and radiographic images are taken as a contrast medium is injected into the vessel. The radiographs are evaluated for the presence and amount of plaque buildup or the presence of a thrombus. Doppler ultrasonography, a test that uses sound waves to produce an image of the blood vessel, may also be ordered to detect atherosclerosis. Doppler ultrasonography, or echocardiography, can be used to determine the ability of the heart to fill and pump blood. This noninvasive test uses sound waves to

Figure 31-5 Atherosclerotic coronary occlusion. (Reprinted with permission from Rubin E, Farber JL. Pathology. Philadelphia: Lippincott Williams & Wilkins, 2005.)

produce a picture of the heart on a video monitor to detect areas of poor blood flow or damaged muscle.

A relatively new noninvasive test for CAD is cardiac calcium scoring using electron beam computed tomography (CT). In this procedure, CT of the coronary arteries using an electron beam identifies the amount of fat and calcium buildup within the coronary arteries. An elevated score indicates an increased risk for developing CAD, especially if other risk factors are present.

The treatment for atherosclerosis often includes lifestyle changes, as described earlier, to reverse or prevent further atherosclerotic formations. If the condition is severe, lipid-lowering medication may be prescribed. Surgery to remove the plaque or improve blood flow through an artery may also be indicated for some patients. Your responsibilities will include coordinating diagnostic procedures based on the physician's orders and insurance requirements and teaching patients about behaviors that can prevent atherosclerosis and CAD. Patients diagnosed with atherosclerosis and CAD require emotional support to encourage compliance with medication and lifestyle changes, such as diet and exercise.

 CHECKPOINT QUESTION

5. What are four predisposing factors for heart disease?

Hypertension

Patients with a resting systolic blood pressure above 140 mm Hg and a diastolic pressure above 90 mm Hg are said to be hypertensive. Hypertension cannot be diagnosed on the basis of one blood pressure measurement, since other factors, such as emotional upset or anxiety, may cause a temporary increase in blood pressure. Since many factors may affect the blood pressure, the physician often requires several blood pressure readings before making the diagnosis of hypertension. Once a diagnosis of hypertension is made, you may play a major role in assisting with the control of this condition by regularly monitoring the patient's blood pressure and medication prescriptions; teaching the patient about dietary and lifestyle changes, such as smoking cessation and weight loss; and recording complete and accurate information regarding the medical history each time the patient visits the office. Refer to Table 19-6 in Chapter 19 for more information regarding blood pressure readings and what constitutes normal, prehypertension, and hypertension I and II.

One type of hypertension, essential hypertension, is a major cause of stroke and renal failure and is a major consequence of atherosclerosis anywhere in the circulatory system. The long-term effects of essential hypertension may include weakening of the arteries throughout the body and enlargement of the left ventricle of the heart. Left ventricular hypertrophy, or enlargement, occurs gradually as the heart works harder to overcome the higher pressure in the arteries. Essential hypertension is often called a silent killer because the disease is gradual and frequently produces no symptoms in the patient, striking anyone regardless of age, race, sex, or ethnic origin.

Malignant hypertension is severe and sudden in onset and is most common in African-American men under age 40 years regardless of other risk factors. Patients with malignant hypertension have signs and symptoms including diastolic blood pressure greater than 120 mm Hg and blurred vision, headache, and possibly confusion. The physician should be notified immediately if these symptoms are present.

While the cause of essential hypertension may be unknown, its correlation with an elevated serum cholesterol level has been shown. After diagnosis, some patients can control the high blood pressure with a low-sodium, low-fat diet, an exercise program, weight reduction if needed, and antihypertensive and lipid-reducing medications. Diuretic medication may be prescribed to reduce the amount of sodium in the body, which in turn reduces the total fluid volume. The decrease in fluid volume reduces strain on the heart and blood vessels. Patients should also be informed of methods to reduce the cholesterol and triglycerides in their diet.

Patients who have been prescribed antihypertensive medications should be instructed to take that medication as prescribed. Many patients feel that because their blood pressure has reached a manageable level, they do not need to continue the prescribed medication. Explain that the medication is the cause of the lowered blood pressure and that discontinuing the treatment without consulting the physician may jeopardize their recovery.

 CHECKPOINT QUESTION

6. What two disorders may result from untreated hypertension?

Varicose Veins

Varicosities, the most common circulatory disease of the lower extremities, occur when the superficial veins of the legs swell and distend (Fig. 31-6). Eventually the valves in the veins fail to close properly, allowing blood to pool and stretch the walls of the veins. People who sit or stand for long periods without moving or contracting their leg muscles are predisposed to varicose veins. A hereditary weakness in the vein walls is also a predisposing factor. Varicosities may also be secondary to deep vein thrombosis. Signs and symptoms of varicose veins are swelling, aching, and a feeling of heaviness in the legs. Varicosities may also be asymptomatic. Many

Figure 31-6 Varicose veins of the lower extremities. (Reprinted with permissiosn from Bickley LS, Szilagy PG. Bates' Guide to Physical Examination and History Taking. Philadelphia: Lippincott Williams & Wilkins, 2003.)

patients consider varicose veins unattractive and seek treatment even without symptoms.

Treatment of varicose veins is usually conservative, with instructions to avoid standing or sitting for long periods to reduce symptoms and prevent the development of further varicosities. Other helpful measures that may be ordered by the physician include wearing elastic support stockings or wrapping the legs with elastic bandages and elevating the legs for specified periods. Surgery to remove the veins is usually the last approach. Another treatment technique is injection of a sclerosing agent into small varicose vein segments, but this is not suggested for large areas.

Venous Thrombosis and Pulmonary Embolism

Thrombi, or blood clots, in the peripheral or pulmonary veins commonly affect patients with underlying cardiovascular disease. Risk factors for developing thrombi may be either primary (inherited) or secondary (acquired). Primary causes include hemolytic anemia and sickle cell disease, and secondary factors include long-term immobility, chronic pulmonary disease, thrombophlebitis, varicosities, and defibrillation after cardiac arrest. Chemical contraceptives for women have also been implicated in a higher risk of developing thrombi in young women who have none of the usual predisposing factors. The risk increases in women who smoke. A thrombus in the peripheral venous circulatory system may dislodge and become an embolus. This embolus is dangerous to the patient,

since the blood clot can lodge in the pulmonary circulation (causing a pulmonary embolism), the cardiac circulation (causing MI), or the cerebral circulation (causing a **cerebrovascular accident [CVA]**).

Peripheral vascular occlusion may also lead to stasis ulcers, which are caused by breakdown of the skin and underlying tissue due to inadequate circulation to the area. These ulcers develop as deep red discolorations, itching, edema, and large areas of scaling skin leading to fissures and ulcers. Increasing circulation to the lower extremities with use of support stockings, weight reduction, and elevating the limbs may prevent formation of these ulcers.

A blood clot lodged in the pulmonary circulation is a pulmonary embolism. Signs and symptoms of a pulmonary embolism include dyspnea, syncope, and severe pleuritic chest pain with respiration. Diagnosis may include chest radiography, an electrocardiogram, a lung scan, or a pulmonary arteriogram. Doppler studies are used to diagnose deep vein thrombosis. Depending on the severity, treatment may include bed rest with elevation of the affected extremity, anticoagulant medication such as coumadin, or surgery.

 CHECKPOINT QUESTION

7. What disease occurs when the superficial veins in the legs become swollen and distended?

 PATIENT EDUCATION

ANTICOAGULANT THERAPY

Patients with certain types of cardiac problems are prescribed anticoagulant medications, commonly called blood thinners, which are used to decrease the risk of a thrombus or embolus developing. Coumadin is a common oral anticoagulant. Lovenox, another anticoagulant, is given as an injection. Teach patients who are prescribed anticoagulants as follows:

• Monitor the mouth, urine, and stool for any signs of bleeding.
• Use a soft-bristle toothbrush.
• Call the office if any signs of bleeding occur.
• Avoid injuries and falls while taking anticoagulant medications.
• Be aware that needlesticks from injections or venipuncture require prolonged application of pressure afterward to control bleeding and bruising.
• Comply with orders for blood work. Anticoagulant medications necessitate frequent tests for blood counts and bleeding times.

- Limit the intake of foods high in vitamin K (asparagus, cabbage, fish, broccoli, cheese, pork, spinach, cauliflower, and rice). These patients should be given a printed flyer on dietary restrictions.
- Avoid taking over-the-counter medications containing aspirin or ibuprofen without consulting the physician. These drugs may cause an increase in bleeding times, interfering with the actions of the anticoagulant.
- Take the medication at the same time every day. If a dose is missed, take it as soon as it is remembered that day, but do not take a double dose.

Cerebrovascular Accident

Cerebrovascular accident (CVA), sometimes called stroke, results suddenly when damage to the blood vessels in the brain occurs. The damage blocks the circulation, resulting in ischemia, or lack of oxygen, to that part of the brain. Brain tissue dies without adequate oxygen. A common cause of CVA is blockage of the cerebral artery by thrombus or embolus. Hemorrhage, atherosclerotic heart disease, and hypertension are additional causes of CVAs. Unfortunately, CVAs are the most common nervous system disorder in the elderly and one of the leading causes of death in the United States.

Patients who have CVAs usually have varying degrees of weakness or paralysis of one side of the body, with possible involvement of language and comprehension. Symptoms vary according to which artery and which part of the brain is affected. CVAs are fatal when vital centers of the brain are damaged. Once the brain tissue is damaged by a CVA, treatment is aimed at reducing further death of cerebrovascular tissue and assisting the patient to regain any affected function. Patients who have CVAs need many months of rehabilitation, including physical therapy, occupational therapy, and speech therapy. You must remember that, although these patients may not be able to communicate effectively with you, they are capable of understanding and should be treated with respect, dignity, and compassion.

Ischemia to small areas of the brain over short periods is known as **transient ischemic attack (TIA)**. TIA, or mini-stroke, should be considered a warning sign for a possible impending cerebrovascular accident. TIAs may be caused by atherosclerotic plaques narrowing the arteries supplying blood to the brain, a small embolus that reduces the flow of blood to an area, or spasms of the blood vessels. The symptoms vary according to the arteries affected but usually include the following:

- Mild numbness or tingling in the face or a limb
- Difficulty swallowing

- Coughing and choking
- Slurred speech
- Unilateral visual disturbance
- Dizziness

As many as 50% to 80% of patients who exhibit symptoms of TIAs progress to a stroke. The signs of a major stroke may begin as a TIA and progress to loss of consciousness, hyperpnea (deep, gasping breaths), anisocoria (unequal pupils), and hemiplegia (unilateral paralysis). Any patient who has the signs and symptoms of a TIA or a CVA should be sent to the emergency room following all physician instructions and office policies.

Aneurysm

Weakened blood vessel walls are predisposed to abnormal dilation. Dilation in the form of an **aneurysm** may occur in any vessel, but arteries are most often affected (Fig. 31-7). Because of the high pressure so close to the heart, the aorta is the most common site. The normally elastic vessel wall develops a ballooning effect in one or many forms, all of them dangerous:

- A *dissecting aneurysm* tears the inner walls of the artery and allows blood to leak into the lining of the vessel; the wall will eventually die and tear open.
- A *sacculated aneurysm* balloons from the arterial wall into a sac, which may burst.
- A *berry aneurysm* is usually a congenital defect in a cerebral artery.

Causes of aneurysms include trauma, hypertension, atherosclerosis, certain fungal infections, syphilis, and congenital defects. Symptoms include pain or pressure at the site. Death may occur quickly if the tear is not repaired. Diagnosis is based on a thorough history and examination, an arteriogram or aortogram, computed tomography, or magnetic resonance imaging. Surgical resection is the only option.

 CHECKPOINT QUESTION

8. What is the physiologic reason for a stroke?

Anemia

Deficiencies in hemoglobin or in the numbers of red blood cells result in anemia. Anemia is not considered a disease but is a symptom of an underlying disorder. Anemia can result from any of the following:

- Blood loss due to hemorrhage or slow internal bleeding
- A diet low in iron or a malabsorption condition (nutritional anemia)
- Suppressed (by chemotherapeutic medication) or diseased bone marrow, resulting in decreased blood cell formation (aplastic anemia)

- Vitamin B$_{12}$ deficiency due to a lack of intrinsic factor (pernicious anemia)
- Genetic abnormality (sickle cell anemia, thalassemia)
- Destruction of functioning red blood cells by various means, such as liver or spleen dysfunction or toxins (hemolytic anemia)

Symptoms of anemia may include cardiovascular alterations such as tachycardia and pallor, anorexia and weight loss, dyspnea on exertion, and fatigue. Treatment of anemia must address the cause; it can include increasing dietary iron, blood transfusions, and injection of vitamin B$_{12}$ (cyanocobalamin) on a regular basis. Aplastic anemia may require a bone marrow transplantation.

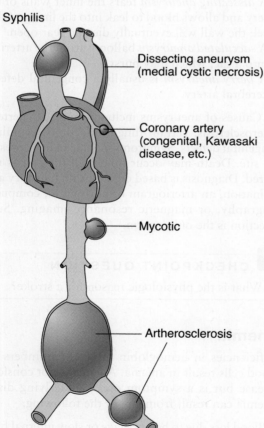

Figure 31-7 The locations of aneurysms. (Reprinted with permission from Rubin's Pathology: Clinicopathologic Foundations of Medicine. Philadelphia: Lippincott Williams & Wilkins, 2005.)

Unfortunately, genetic abnormalities, such as sickle cell anemia and thalassemia, cannot be corrected at this time.

Common Diagnostic and Therapeutic Procedures

Testing for cardiovascular disorders may be either invasive or noninvasive. Invasive techniques require entering the body by the use of a tube, needle, or other device. Noninvasive techniques do not require entering the body or puncturing the skin. Depending on the patient's symptoms, testing may be basic and can be done easily during the general physical examination by auscultating the heart and chest cavity. Additional tests the physician may order that you perform in the medical office can include chest radiography or 12-lead ECG. Sometimes initial findings indicate the need for a more sophisticated procedure, such as cardiac catheterization, which is performed at an outpatient surgical center or hospital.

Physical Examination of the Cardiovascular System

The cardiovascular examination is the most basic noninvasive procedure used to assess the heart and blood vessels. When preparing a patient for a cardiovascular examination, you will obtain vital information, including accurate determination of weight, blood pressure, heart and respiratory rates, body temperature, and cardiovascular history. It is also important to obtain a complete list of the patient's medications and current dosages, including any herbal and vitamin supplements and over-the-counter medications. A brief social and family history should include lifestyle and familial risk factors for cardiovascular disorders. The patient should be questioned regarding a history of smoking tobacco, alcohol intake, family history of heart disease, hypercholesterolemia, diet, and exercise. Specifically, you should ask the following questions to elicit important information from a patient with cardiovascular problems:

- Why are you seeing the cardiologist or physician today?
- What symptoms have you been having?
- How long have you had the pain, discomfort, distress, or unusual sensations? (Patients may not think of chest discomfort as a cardiac symptom.)
- Where is the pain or discomfort? Does it stay in one place or radiate in any direction?
- Is the pain associated with any other symptoms, such as shortness of breath, nausea, weakness, sweating, or dizziness?
- If you have been short of breath, does it restrict any of your activities or require you to sleep on additional pillows at night?
- Are you a smoker?
- Do you drink alcoholic beverages?

As you proceed with the interview, keep in mind that patients with cardiovascular problems are usually understandably anxious and concerned. They may bring with them family members who are also concerned or anxious. It is your responsibility to help ease apprehension and to offer reassurance and support when appropriate.

The physician or cardiologist usually begins the examination with a review of the patient's history and reason for the office visit. The physician also reviews the patient's vital signs and medications, noting any allergies to medications and other substances. The physician inspects the patient to evaluate the general appearance, noting the circulation and any swelling of the extremities, color of the skin, and jugular vein distention. Palpation is used to evaluate the efficiency of the circulatory pathways and peripheral pulses. Using auscultation with a stethoscope, the physician can evaluate the sounds made as blood flows through the heart and the valves open and close. Abnormal heart sounds, such as bruits and murmurs, may be detected (Box 31-4).

In addition to obtaining important information and data before the physician examines the patient, you must also provide instructions and materials for proper gown wearing and draping. After the examination, the physician may order an ECG, which you will perform and give to the physician for diagnosis.

 CHECKPOINT QUESTION

9. What is a heart murmur?

BOX 31-4

ABNORMAL HEART SOUNDS

Abnormal heart sounds, called *murmurs*, are sounds the blood makes as it courses through the heart valves. The sounds vary with the severity and location of the abnormality. For instance, they may blow, rasp, rub, bubble, whistle, whoosh, and/or click. A murmur is not a disease, but it may indicate organic heart disease.

Functional murmurs may only occur during elevations in body temperature or during times of physical stress and are not usually a cause for concern. *Organic murmurs* indicate structural abnormalities of varying degrees and are always present. A cardiologist evaluates the murmur by noting its location in the heart, when it occurs in the cardiac cycle, how long it lasts, and its characteristic sound.

Electrocardiogram

One of the most valuable diagnostic tools for evaluating the electrical pathway through the heart is the electrocardiogram, known by the acronym ECG or EKG. The ECG is the graphic record of the electrical current as it progresses through the heart. It can be performed as part of a routine physical examination or as needed for a patient with chest pain, discomfort, or other signs and symptoms of possible cardiac problems. During the ECG, you are responsible for explaining the procedure to the patient and applying combinations of electrodes, called **leads**, on the patient's limbs and precordial area (anterior chest). ECGs are used to assist in diagnosing ischemia, delays in impulse conduction, hypertrophy of the cardiac chambers, and arrhythmias. They are not used to detect anatomic disorders, such as heart murmurs.

The ECG tracing is printed on graph paper that is either blue or black with a heat-labile white coating. Graph lines are printed over the white coating, appearing as small blocks with thicker lines outlining every five small blocks. On standard ECG paper, each small block is 1 mm². The large blocks are 5 mm² (Fig. 31-8A). Some older ECG machines contain a stylus that heats and melts the white coating, exposing the dark background beneath to record the movement of the stylus as the electrical impulses are detected. Newer ECG machines dispense ink from a cartridge into the stylus to mark the ECG tracing paper. The ECG paper may be affected by pressure as well as heat and should be handled carefully to prevent extraneous markings. Each small horizontal block represents time (0.04 seconds), and the vertical small blocks represent voltage (0.1 millivolts). After the heart's electrical markings are traced on the paper, the heart rate and time required for the electrical impulses to spread through the heart can be determined (Fig. 31-8B).

ECG Leads

Over the years, a standard system of electrode placement has evolved, and nomenclature has been developed for the recordings from different electrode combinations. Each lead records the electrical impulse through the heart from a different angle. Viewing the conduction of the electrical impulses in these various angles gives the physician a fairly complete view of the entire heart. The standard ECG has 12 leads that produce a three-dimensional record of the impulse wave. Four wires are labeled and color-coded for the limb that the wire should be connected to, and six wires are labeled for connection to electrodes placed on the anterior chest (Box 31-5). The four limb electrodes should be positioned away from bony areas and on muscular areas, such as the calves, outer thighs, and above the elbow. Adjustments may be necessary for patients with amputations, surgery to the extremity, or trauma to the arms or legs.

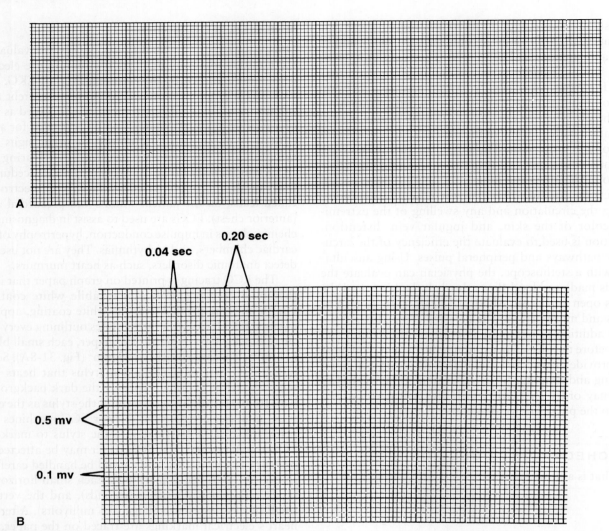

Figure 31-8 ECG graph paper. (**A**) Each small square is 1 mm × 1 mm. Each fifth line is marked darker to make a cube of 5 mm × 5 mm (acutal size). (**B**) Horizontally, the graph paper represents time in seconds. Each small square represents 0.04 seconds, and each large square represents 0.2 seconds. Five large squares = 1 second (5 × 0.2).

WHAT IF?

What if the physician asks you to perform an ECG on a child?

Although pediatric cardiac problems may not be encountered daily in the medical office, obesity, elevated cholesterol and triglyceride blood levels, and type 2 diabetes are conditions that are seen increasingly frequently in pediatric and family practice offices, and these conditions may require intervention, including electrocardiography. While the placement of the electrodes is similar to that for an adult, smaller electrodes for use on the smaller patient allow for easier placement. A standard ECG can be done on children over 8 or 9 years of age; however, for younger children, the sensitivity, or gain, on the machine should be changed according to the physician's orders or office policy and procedure manual. If the sensitivity or gain is changed, this must be noted on the ECG before it goes into the medical record.

BOX 31-5

ABBREVIATIONS USED IN PERFORMING ECGS

RA	right arm
LA	left arm
LL	left leg
RL	right leg
V_1–V_6	chest leads
aVR	augmented voltage right arm
aVL	augmented voltage left arm
aVF	augmented voltage left foot or leg

BOX 31-6

POSITIONING OF UNIPOLAR PRECORDIAL (CHEST) LEADS

- $LV_1 = (RA + LA + LL)$ to V_1: Fourth intercostal space at right margin of sternum
- $LV_2 = (RA + LA + LL)$ to V_2: Fourth intercostal space at left margin of sternum
- $LV_3 = (RA + LA + LL)$ to V_3: Midway between V_2 and V_4
- $LV_4 = (RA + LA + LL)$ to V_4: Fifth intercostal space at junction of midclavicular line
- $LV_5 = (RA + LA + LL)$ to V_5: Horizontal level of V_4 at left anterior axillary line
- $LV_6 = (RA + LA + LL)$ to V_6: Horizontal level of V_4 and V_5 at midaxillary line

The right leg (RL) electrode, the grounding lead, helps reduce alternating current (AC) interference and keeps the average voltage of the patient the same as that of the recording instrument. The other three limb leads attached to electrodes on the patient's left leg and arms make up the combinations necessary for the first six views of the heart in the 12-lead ECG. The first three combinations, which are standard bipolar leads also known as Einthoven leads, allow frontal visualization of the heart's electrical activity from side to side. Each lead provides specific measurements:

- Lead I measures the difference in electrical potential between the right arm (RA) and the left arm (LA).
- Lead II measures the difference in electrical potential between the right arm (RA) and the left leg (LL).
- Lead III measures the difference in electrical potential between the left arm (LA) and the left leg (LL).

The same limb electrodes provide measurement of the signal between one electrode and the average of the remaining two. These second three combinations, the augmented unipolar limb leads, allow visualization from a frontal view top to bottom:

- Lead aVR (LL 1 LA) to RA measures the potential at the right arm.
- Lead aVL (LL 1 RA) to LA measures the potential at the left arm.
- Lead aVF (RA 1 LA) to LL measures the potential at the left foot.

For a closer look at the electrical conduction through the heart, electrodes are placed directly on the anterior chest wall, but the limb electrodes must remain attached to the patient. The positioning of the chest electrodes must be precise for accuracy. These leads, the unipolar precordial (chest) leads, show the comparison of the chest electrode potential to the average of the three limb electrodes (Box 31-6). All electrodes must connect to the wires of the ECG machine. Each lead is clearly marked on the ECG paper as it is printed, or specific codes may be printed on the paper to denote each lead (Table 31-2). The recording of the ECG on paper varies from one machine to another, but the principles and techniques are universal (Procedure 31-1).

ECG Interpretation

The physician's interpretation of the standard 12-lead ECG includes an examination of various wave forms associated with the cardiac cycle (Fig. 31-9). Commonly measured components of an ECG tracing are discussed in the following sections.

PR Interval

The time from the beginning of the P wave to the beginning of the QRS complex is called the *PR interval*. This time interval represents depolarization of the atria and the spread of the depolarization wave up to and including the atrioventricular node.

TABLE **31-2**	Coding ECG Leads		
Lead	**Code**	**Lead**	**Code**
I	.	V1	-.
II	..	V2	-..
III	...	V3	-...
aVR	-	V4	-....
aVL	—	V5	-.....
aVF	—-	V6	-......

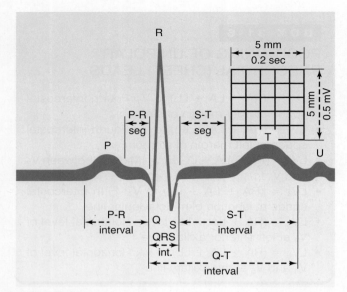

Figure 31-9 The cardiac cycle waves, segments, and intervals. (Reprinted with permission from Cohen BJ. Medical Terminology: An Illustrated Guide. Philadelphia: Lippincott Williams & Wilkins, 2003.)

PR Segment

The PR segment represents the period between the P wave and QRS complex.

ST Segment

The distance between the QRS complex and the T wave from the point where the QRS complex ends (J-point) to the onset of the ascending limb of the T wave is called the *ST segment*. On the ECG, this segment is a sensitive indicator of myocardial ischemia or injury.

Ventricular Activation Time

The time from the beginning of the QRS complex to the peak of the R wave, the *ventricular activation time*, represents the time necessary for the depolarization wave to travel from the inner surface of the heart (endocardium) to the outer surface of the heart (epicardium).

During the ECG, the paper speed on the machine should be set at 25 mm per second, which allows the electrical impulses (seen as waves) on the ECG to be measured using the blocks on the ECG paper as a reference (each small horizontal block is 0.04 seconds). Movement of the electricity through the atria is noted and measured on the ECG tracing as the PR interval (the normal PR interval is 0.12 to 0.20 seconds). Electrical movement through the ventricles is measured and noted on the ECG as the QRS complex, which is normally less

than 0.12 seconds. The following elements are taken into consideration:

- Rate: how fast the heart is beating
- Rhythm: regularity of cardiac cycles and intervals
- Axis: position of the heart and direction of depolarization, or electrical movement, through the heart
- Hypertrophy: size of the heart
- Ischemia: decrease in blood supply to an area of the heart
- Infarction: death of heart muscle resulting in loss of function

Under usual diagnostic conditions, the 12-lead ECG provides sufficient data. As the medical assistant, you are responsible for obtaining a good-quality ECG without avoidable **artifacts**. An artifact is an abnormal signal that does not reflect electrical activity of the heart during the cardiac cycle. Artifacts can be due to movement by the patient, mechanical problems with the ECG machine, or improper technique. Table 31-3 describes three types of artifacts and how to prevent them.

Sometimes the physician requests a rhythm strip along with the ECG. A rhythm strip is a long strip of a certain lead or a combination of leads. It may be used to define certain cardiac arrhythmias. While most ECG machines have a button that automatically records the 12 views in the 12-lead ECG, a rhythm strip must be obtained using the manual mode on the ECG machine.

 CHECKPOINT QUESTION

10. Which three waves represent a cardiac cycle on an ECG?

Holter Monitor

In many instances, an ECG that records the electrical activity of the heart for a brief moment in the medical office does not reveal cardiac problems. For diagnosis of intermittent cardiac arrhythmias and dysfunctions, a monitor that records for at least 24 hours is used. The Holter monitor is small and portable and can be worn comfortably for long periods without interfering with daily activities (Fig. 31-10). It may be set to record continuously or only when the patient presses a record button when feeling symptoms. This record button is also known as an incident or event button. When applying the Holter monitor, you must instruct the patient to keep a diary of daily activities. The physician will interpret the ECG tracing recorded by the Holter monitor and compare these findings with activities recorded in the diary to get an accurate view of what activities, if any, precipitate cardiac arrhythmias. Procedure 31-2 describes the steps for applying a Holter monitor.

PATIENT EDUCATION

The Holter Monitor Patient Diary

A patient with a Holter monitor must keep a diary of daily activities. When the patient has symptoms, he or she depresses an incident (or event) button on the machine and then records in the diary the activity that caused the incident, including the symptoms. At intervals, the patient also records daily activities such as working quietly at a desk, driving a car, eating a meal, watching television, and sleeping. All activities must be noted, including elimination, sexual intercourse, anger, laughter, and so on. Some monitors are equipped with small tape recorders so the patient can keep an audio diary instead of a written one.

Chest Radiography

Chest radiography provides valuable basic information about the anatomic location and gross structures of the heart, great vessels, and lungs. It also aids in the evaluation of such disorders as CHF and pericardial effusions. Many patients with CHF have an enlarged heart, especially the ventricles, and pericardial effusions appear as white markings around the heart on the film. Many patients with chronic cardiac conditions also have pulmonary problems, and the chest film can be used to assess the lungs. Any abnormal swelling or growth of the heart or great vessels (aorta, inferior vena cava, superior vena cava, pulmonary arteries) can also be assessed.

Figure 31-10 A Holter Monitor. (Courtesy of Welch Allyn.)

TRIAGE

While working in a medical office, the following three situations occur:

A. A 29-year-old woman has been seen by the physician, who orders application of a Holter monitor. She also needs instruction on the importance of completing the diary.

B. A 62-year-old woman needs an ECG. She is complaining of heaviness in her chest.

C. A 17-year-old patient and his mother have just arrived in the office with written orders from an orthopedic surgeon that he needs a "stat preop" ECG. The patient is scheduled for knee surgery in the morning.

How do you sort these patients? Who do you see first? Second? Third?

Do the ECG for patient B first. Her chest heaviness may be due to a cardiac problem, and the physician should assess this ECG immediately. See patient A next, since she has been waiting. After applying the Holter monitor and explaining the diary, do the ECG for patient C. Every surgeon has standard orders for various tests he or she wants completed before doing surgery. ECGs are commonly ordered and read by a cardiologist or internist before a surgical procedure. Although the written order is written as stat, the test can be done as soon as possible and convenient.

Cardiac Stress Test

To measure the response of the cardiac muscle to increased demands of oxygen, the physician may request a cardiac stress test. The heart is usually tested with the patient walking on a treadmill (Fig. 31-11) with periodic increases in the rate or angle of the walk or run, but it may also be done on a stationary bicycle. The patient is attached to an ECG monitor for constant tracing during the test, and the blood pressure is monitored before, during, and after the test. The test is performed according to the physician's orders, and the ECG is interpreted by the physician, but you may be responsible for attaching the electrodes, monitoring and recording the blood pressure, and assisting the physician in watching the patient for signs of light-headedness. Emergency resuscitation equipment should be available in case of cardiac or respiratory difficulties. This test may indicate the need for further cardiac testing. The cardiac stress test may be done as part of a routine physical examination in adults without symptoms or as a diagnostic tool for patients who have intermittent periods of angina pectoris or **palpitations**.

 CHECKPOINT QUESTION

11. What is the purpose of a cardiac stress test?

Echocardiography

An echocardiogram, or echo, uses sound waves generated by a small device called a transducer. These waves travel through the cardiac chambers, walls, and valves and are transmitted back to a screen, where they can be viewed and interpreted. Echocardiograms help the physician to diagnose suspected or known valvular disease in adults and children. Echocardiograms also aid in diagnosing the severity of heart failure and **cardiomyopathy**. In addition, this test can be used to detect injuries to the heart in patients with trauma. Only the most specialized cardiac medical offices have the equipment and personnel (ultrasonographers) to obtain echocardiographs. In most instances, your role is to schedule the outpatient procedure and give the patient any instructions required by the facility. Usually no patient preparations are required for echocardiography.

Cardiac Catheterization and Coronary Arteriography

Cardiac catheterization is a common invasive procedure used to help diagnose or treat conditions affecting the

TABLE **31-3**	Types of Artifacts

Wandering baseline, somatic muscle temor, and AC interference.

Artifact	Possible Cause	How to Prevent Problems
Wandering baseline	Electrodes too tight or too loose; electrolyte gel dried out; skin has oil, lotion, or excessive hair	Apply electrodes properly; apply new electrodes; prepare skin before applying electrodes
Muscle or somatic artifact	Patient cannot remain still because of tremors or fear	Reassure patient; explain procedure and stress the need to keep still; patients with disease may be unable to stay motionless
Alternating current artifact	Improperly grounded ECG machine	Check cables to ensure properly grounded machine before beginning test
	Electrical interference in room	Move patient or unplug appliances in immediate area
	Dangling lead wires	Arrange wires along contours of patient's body

coronary arterial circulation. It may be performed on patients with shortness of breath, angina, dizziness, palpitations, fluttering in the chest, rapid heartbeat, and other cardiovascular symptoms to determine the severity or cause of the problem. It is often indicated after a cardiac stress test or echocardiogram reveals an abnormality. This procedure is not done in the medical office, but the medical assistant may be responsible for scheduling diagnostic cardiac catheterizations at a local outpatient facility or hospital and giving the patient any instructions required by the outpatient facility. If the procedure is for treatment, it must be done at an inpatient facility that has immediate access to open heart surgical equipment and personnel in the event of an emergency.

During the catheterization, the physician, usually a cardiologist, inserts a flexible tube into a blood vessel in either the arm or the groin and gently guides it toward the heart. When the catheter is in place, coronary arteriography is performed by injecting contrast medium, revealing the heart's chambers, valves, great vessels, and coronary arteries on a monitor. If atherosclerotic plaques are found, an angioplasty may be performed or scheduled for later (see Box 31-2).

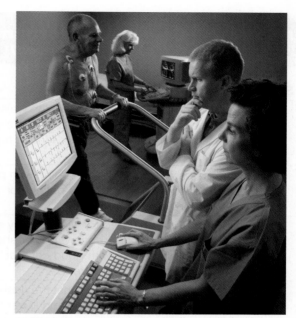

Figure 31-11 Walking on a treadmill while monitoring the heart's activity with an ECG maching is one way to determine the heart's ability to adapt to increased work during exercise. (Courtesy of Borgess Medical Center, Kalamazoo, MI.)

CHECKPOINT QUESTION

12. How is the echocardiography obtained?

PROCEDURE 31-1: Performing a 12-Lead Electrocardiogram

Purpose: Prepare a patient and obtain a 12-lead ECG that is free from artifacts
Equipment: Physician's order, patient record, ECG machine with cable and lead wires, ECG paper, disposable electrodes that contain coupling gel, gown and drape, skin preparation materials including a razor and antiseptic wipes

Steps	Reasons
1. Wash your hands.	Handwashing aids infection control.
2. **Step 2.** The ECG machine	
3. Greet and identify the patient. Explain the procedure.	This avoids errors in treatment and helps gain compliance.
4. Turn the machine on and enter appropriate data, including the patient's name and/or identification number, age, sex, height, weight, blood pressure, and medications.	This information will assist the physician in determining a proper diagnosis.

(continued)

PROCEDURE 31-1:	**Performing a 12-Lead Electrocardiogram** *(continued)*

Steps	Reasons
5. Instruct the patient to disrobe above the waist, and provide a gown for privacy. Female patients should also be instructed to remove any nylons or tights.	Clothing may interfere with proper placement of the leads. Patients wearing pants do not have to remove them if they can be pulled up to expose the lower legs.
6. Position the patient comfortably supine with pillows as needed for comfort. Drape the patient for warmth and privacy.	If the patient is uncomfortable, too cool, or improperly draped, movement is likely, which will result in artifact on the ECG tracing.
7. Prepare the skin as needed by wiping away skin oil and lotions with the antiseptic wipes or shaving any hair that will interfere with good contact between the skin and the electrodes.	Skin preparation ensures properly attached leads and helps avoid improper readings and lost time repeating the test.
8. Apply the electrodes snugly against the fleshy, muscular parts of the upper arms and lower legs according to the manufacturer's directions. Apply the chest electrodes, V_1–V_6.	Electrodes that are not snug against the skin or are on bony prominences may cause improper reading and artifact. In case of an amputation or otherwise inaccessible limb, place the electrode on the uppermost part of the existing extremity OR on the anterior shoulder (upper extremity) and groin (lower extremity).

A

B

Step 8. (A) Applying limb electrodes. **(B)** Applying chest electrodes.

9. Connect the lead wires securely according to the color-coded notations on the connectors (RA, LA, RL, LL, V_1–V_6). Untangle the wires before applying them to prevent electrical artifacts. Each lead must lie unencumbered along the contours of the patient's body to decrease the likelihood of artifacts. Double-check the placement.	Improperly placed leads will result in time lost to an inaccurate reading and retesting.

Step 9. The wires should lie along the contours of the patient's body.

(continued)

PROCEDURE 31-1: **Performing a 12-Lead Electrocardiogram**
(continued)

Steps	Reasons
10. Determine the sensitivity, or gain, and paper speed settings on the ECG machine before running the test. Set sensitivity or gain on 1 and paper speed on 25 mm/second.	A sensitivity setting of 1 and a paper speed of 25 mm/second are necessary to obtain an accurate ECG. These settings should not be changed without a direct order from the physician and the changes noted on the final ECG tracing.
11. Depress the automatic button on the ECG machine to obtain the 12-lead tracing. The machine will automatically move from one lead to the next without your intervention.	If the physician wants only a rhythm strip tracing, use the manual mode of operation and select the lead manually
12. When the tracing is complete and printed, check the ECG for artifacts and a standardization mark.	With sensitivity set on 1, the standardization mark should be 2 small squares wide and 10 small squares high. The standardization mark documents accuracy of operation and provides a reference point.

Normal Standard
Standardization mark
is 10 mm high
A

One-Half Standard
Standardization mark
is 5 mm high
B

Double Standard
Standardization mark
is 20 mm high
C

Step 12. (A) Normal standardization mark is 10 mm high. **(B)** One-half standardization mark is 5 mm high. **(C)** Double standardization mark is 20 mm high.

Steps	Reasons
13. If the tracing is adequate, turn off the machine and remove and discard the electrodes. Assist the patient to a sitting position and help with dressing if needed.	Some patients become dizzy while lying supine.
14. If a single-channel machine was used (each lead produced on a roll of paper, one lead at a time), carefully roll the ECG strip without using clips to secure the roll. This ECG must be mounted on 8 × 11–inch paper or a form before going into the medical record according to the office policy and procedure.	Folding the ECG tracing or applying clips may make marks on the surface, obscuring the reading. Special forms may be purchased specifically for mounting a single-channel ECG strip and placing it in the medical record.
15. Record the procedure in the patient's medical record.	Procedures are considered not to have been done if they are not recorded.
16. Either place the ECG tracing and the patient's medical record on the physician's desk or give it directly to the physician, as instructed.	

Charting Example:

12/02/2008 9:45 AM Pre-employment 12-lead ECG obtained and placed in chart
—A. Perez, CMA

PROCEDURE 31-2: Applying a Holter Monitor

Purpose: Prepare and instruct a patient on wearing a Holter monitor for continuous cardiac monitoring
Equipment: Physician's order, patient record, Holter monitor with appropriate lead wires, fresh batteries, carrying case with strap, disposable electrodes with coupling gel, adhesive tape, gown and drape, skin preparation materials including a razor and antiseptic wipes, diary
Standard: This procedure should take 10 minutes.

Steps	Reasons
1. Wash your hands.	Handwashing aids infection control.
2. Assemble the equipment.	
3. Greet and identify the patient. Explain the procedure, reminding the patient that it is important to carry out all normal activities for the duration of the test.	Identifying the patient and explaining the procedure avoids errors in treatment and helps gain compliance. A normal routine is essential to allow the physician to identify areas of concern.
4. Explain the purpose of the incident diary, emphasizing the need to carry it at all times during the test. Ask the patient to remove all clothing from the waist up and put on the gown, and drape appropriately for privacy.	The chest must be exposed for proper placement of the electrodes.
5. With the patient seated, prepare the skin for electrode attachment. Provide privacy. Shave the skin if necessary and cleanse with antiseptic wipes.	Shaving and cleansing the skin will improve adherence of the adhesive on the electrodes.

6. Expose the adhesive backing of the electrodes and follow the manufacturer's instructions to attach each firmly. Apply the electrodes at the specified sites:

   A. Right manubrium border

   B. Left manubrium border

   C. Right sternal border at the fifth rib

   D. Fifth rib at the anterior axillary line

   E. Right lower rib cage over the cartilage as a ground lead.

Step 6. (A) Sites for Holter electrodes. (B) Place the Holter electrodes as directed by the manufacturer.

(continued)

PROCEDURE 31-2:   **Applying a Holter Monitor** *(continued)*

Steps	Reasons
7. Check the security of the attachments.	
8. Position electrode connectors down toward the patient's feet. Attach the lead wires and secure with adhesive tape.	Application of adhesive tape over the connections will help ensure that the leads do not work loose during the day. **Step 8.** Securely tape each electrode. Tape the lead wires to the patient's body.
9. Connect the cable and run a baseline ECG by hooking the Holter to the ECG machine with the cable hookup.	Check for accurate function of the Holter.
10. Assist the patient to dress carefully with the cable extending through the garment opening. Clothing that buttons down the front is convenient.	This prevents pulling and strain on the leads.
11. Plug the cable into the recorder and mark the diary. If needed, explain the purpose of the diary to the patient again. Give instructions for a return appointment to evaluate the recording and the diary.	
12. Record the procedure in the patient's medical record.	Procedures are considered not to have been done if they are not recorded.

Charting Example:

11/28/2008 1:00 PM Holter monitor ordered and applied; baseline ECG done. Oral and written instructions given regarding care and use of monitor. Instructions for completion of diary also given. Pt. verbalized understanding of use of monitor and completion of diary. To RTO tomorrow PM for removal of the monitor
—R. Steele, CMA

MEDIA MENU

- **Student CD**
  - **Case Studies**
    Interactive Case Study 2: Managing a
    Medical Office Emergency
    Interactive Case Study 2: Vital Signs, Patient
    Education, and Refusal of Treatment
  - **Animations**
    Cardiac Cycle; Congestive Heart Failure;
    Hypertension; Myocardial Blood Flow; and
    Stroke
  - **CMA/RMA Certification Exam Review**
- **LWW's Medical Assisting Skills DVD**
  - **Procedures 31-1, 31-2**
- **Premium Online Course**
  http://thePoint.lww.com/Kronenberger3e
- **Internet Resources**

  **LiveAdvise Online Tutoring & Competency
  Training**
  http://thePoint.lww.com/LiveAdvise

  American Heart Association
  http://www.americanheart.org

  American Red Cross
  http://www.redcross.org

  National Safety Council
  http://www.nsc.org

  American College of Cardiology
  http://www.acc.org

  American Society of Hypertension, Inc.
  http://www.ash-us.org

  American Medical Association
  http://www.ama-assn.org

español SPANISH TERMINOLOGY

Tiene la presion alta?
  Do you have high blood pressure?
Tiene dolor en el pecho?
  Do you have chest pain?
Ha sentido dolor en el brazo izquierdo?
  Have you ever had pain in the left arm?
Tiene mareos?
  Do you have dizzy spells?

- The circulatory system is a closed transport system kept in motion by the force of the beating heart.
- Nutrients are delivered to cells, cellular wastes are picked up, hormones are directed to target cells, and disease-fighting mechanisms are transported to areas of concern.
- The patient with undiagnosed cardiac disease may complain of lethargy, shortness or breath, or swelling of the extremities.
- Your responsibility includes:
  - Obtaining a complete cardiac history from all patients.
- Assisting with the physical examination.
- Performing or assisting with diagnostic testing.
- Scheduling any cardiac procedures that are not performed in your medical office.
- Obtaining necessary referrals from third-party payers when the physician concludes that the patient should be evaluated by a cardiologist.
- Educating patients at every opportunity to prevent cardiac disease and offering support once a cardiac diagnosis has been made by the physician.

Warm Ups for Critical Thinking

1. Draw a diagram of the heart and a cardiac cycle as seen on the ECG. How would you explain an ECG to a patient? How would you assist the patient in relaxing for this procedure?

2. Compare and contrast the signs and symptoms of a CVA and a TIA. What kind of help does a patient need at home after a stroke? What language barriers might you encounter with the patient who has had a stroke, and how could you overcome these barriers?

3. Explain anemia and identify its symptoms. Why does anemia cause these symptoms? What dietary instructions should be given to a patient with iron deficiency anemia?

4. Prepare a patient education brochure that describes hypertension and its causes, symptoms, and possible treatments. In this brochure, explain why hypertension is often referred to as the silent killer.

5. Using a drug reference book, look up nitroglycerin. What is the usual dosage? How often can this drug be taken for the pain of angina?

6. Research the reason for why many patients with mitral valve disease are prescribed prophylactic anitbiotics before dental procedures. What would you say to a patient who does not want to take these antibiotics before a dental procedure?

Answers to Checkpoint Questions

1. With pericarditis, pain increases with inspiration and movement; pain during MI will not change with patient positioning.

2. It is important to treat a person suffering a myocardial infarction as soon as possible to decrease the amount of cardiac muscle damaged from lack of oxygen.

3. Two arrhythmias that require immediate intervention are ventricular tachycardia and ventricular fibrillation.

4. Rheumatic heart disease and cardiac valvular disease may be caused by an upper respiratory infection caused by group A beta-hemolytic streptococci.

5. Four predisposing factors for heart disease are history of elevated cholesterol, smoking, diabetes mellitus, and hypertension.

6. Stroke and renal failure may result from untreated hypertension.

7. Varicose veins occur when the superficial veins in the legs become swollen and distended.

8. The physiologic cause of a cerebrovascular accident, or stroke, is a decrease in oxygen to part of the brain due to a blockage in the artery from an embolism or hemorrhage. The part of the brain that does not receive oxygen dies.

9. A murmur is an abnormal heart sound caused by incomplete closing of one or more of the valves.

10. P, QRS, and T waves represent a cardiac cycle on an ECG.

11. A cardiac stress test measures the response of the myocardium to increased demands for oxygen.

12. Echocardiography uses sound waves.

CHAPTER

32 Gastroenterology

Outline

Common Gastrointestinal Disorders
Mouth Disorders
Esophageal Disorders
Stomach Disorders
Intestinal Disorders
Liver Disorders
Gallbladder Disorders

Pancreatic Disorders
Common Diagnostic and Therapeutic Procedures
History and Physical Examination of the GI System
Blood Tests

Radiology Studies
Nuclear Imaging
Ultrasonography
Endoscopic Studies
Fecal Tests

Learning Objectives

Upon successfully completing this chapter, you will be able to:

1. Spell and define key terms

2. Describe common disorders of the alimentary canal and accessory organs

3. Explain the purpose of various diagnostic procedures associated with the GI system

4. Discuss the role of the medical assistant in diagnosing and treating disorders of the GI system

Performance Objectives

Upon successfully completing this chapter, you will be able to:

1. Assisting with colon procedures (Procedure 32-1)

CAAHEP

- Practice standard precautions
- Prepare patient for and assist with routine and specialty examinations
- Prepare patient for and assist with procedures, treatments, and minor office surgeries
- Document appropriately
- Instruct individuals according to their needs

ABHES

- Prepare patients for procedures
- Assist physician with examinations and treatments
- Document accurately

Key Terms

anorexia	hepatomegaly	malocclusion	peristalsis
ascites	hepatotoxin	melena	sclerotherapy
dysphagia	insufflator	metabolism	stomatitis
guaiac	leukoplakia	obturator	turgor
hematemesis			

The gastrointestinal (GI) system, or tract, is responsible for the ingestion, digestion, transportation, and elimination of the food we eat (Fig. 32-1). Nutrients are broken down by the action of digestive enzymes into units that can be absorbed through the walls of the GI system into the circulatory and lymphatic systems. This process starts when something is put into the mouth, chewed, and mixed with the enzymes in saliva. Through **peristalsis**, food is pushed along the GI tract, further breaking it down into segments and mixing it with enzymes to hasten the breakdown into nutrients. **Metabolism** is the breakdown of food into usable units through these physical and chemical changes. Any unused food material is eliminated as waste from the GI system as feces.

Disorders of the GI system may affect the alimentary canal, also called the GI tract, or accessory organs such as the liver, gallbladder, and pancreas. This chapter describes common disorders of the GI system and the accessory organs, diagnostic procedures, and your role as a medical assistant working with patients with gastrointestinal disorders. Although the physician who specializes in disorders of the GI system is the gastroenterologist, medical assistants working in other offices, such as family practice and internal medicine, often encounter patients with disorders of this body system.

Common Gastrointestinal Disorders

Mouth Disorders

While disorders of the teeth, gums, and oral cavity are typically diagnosed and treated by the dentist, patients requiring a referral to a dentist or oral surgeon may be seen first in the medical office. Physicians and other health care professionals should be aware of these disorders and their importance to the nutrition, digestion, and overall health status of the patient. Your role includes taking an accurate medical history, including inquiring about the condition of the oral cavity and teeth, making referrals as ordered by the physician, and educating patients about the care of the gums and teeth to prevent health problems and loss of teeth.

Caries

Dental caries (tooth decay) is the most widespread disease of the oral cavity. Bacteria allowed to remain on the teeth erode the enamel and allow infection to reach the inner portions of the tooth. Factors that may contribute to the development of dental caries include a poor diet, inadequate dental hygiene, and **malocclusion**, which is

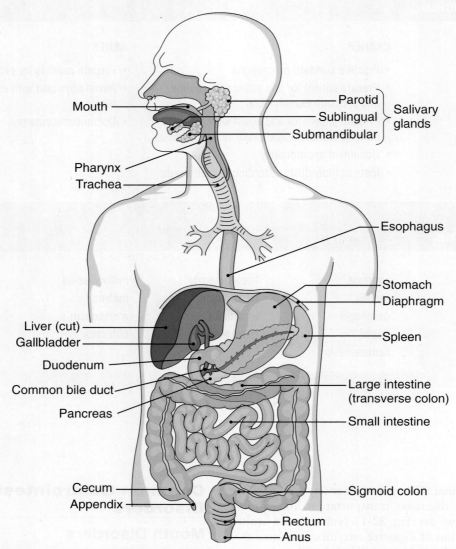

Mouth

Parotid
Sublingual
Submandibular
} Salivary glands

Pharynx
Trachea

Esophagus

Stomach
Diaphragm

Liver (cut)
Gallbladder
Duodenum
Common bile duct
Pancreas

Spleen

Large intestine
(transverse colon)

Small intestine

Cecum
Appendix

Sigmoid colon

Rectum
Anus

Figure 32-1 The digestive system. (Reprinted with permission from Cohen BJ. Memmler's The Human Body in Health and Disease. Philadelphia: Lippincott Williams & Wilkins, 2005.)

abnormal contact between the upper teeth and the lower teeth. Prevention of dental caries includes consuming a balanced diet low in sugars, good oral hygiene as prescribed by the dentist, and frequent professional dental care. Treatment may include drilling the dental caries and replacing the space with a filling or extraction of the affected teeth. Because dental caries can cause discomfort with chewing or biting, they may affect nutrition and ultimately digestion and the overall health of the patient.

Stomatitis

Stomatitis, an inflammation of the oral mucosa, may be caused by a virus, bacteria, or fungus. The two most common forms are herpetic stomatitis, caused by the herpes simplex virus, and candidiasis, caused by the fungus *Candida albicans.*

Herpes simplex is usually self-limiting after the initial exposure to the virus. The virus is usually transmitted hand to mouth, mouth to mouth, or by vector (e.g., shared drinking glasses or eating utensils). The infection presents as a painful sore on the mucosa of the mouth (commonly called a canker sore) or on the lips (commonly called a fever blister or cold sore). After the initial infection, the virus lies dormant for long periods, with exacerbations during illness, stress, overexposure to the sun, or other trigger. Although there is no cure for herpes simplex, palliative measures such as ointments or creams may be purchased over the counter to relieve the discomfort.

Candida albicans, formerly called *Monilia albicans,* is an opportunistic yeast or fungus. This organism is always present in the mouth but is kept in check by other normal microorganisms found in the mouth including bacteria. When the normal bacterial balance in the mouth is altered, *C. albicans* microorganisms multiply, causing an infection that appears as a white substance covering the oral cavity and tongue. Factors that can upset the balance of these microorganisms in the mouth include the use of broad-spectrum antibiotics that kill many bacteria throughout the body, including the mouth, allowing the opportunistic organisms to grow without control. In babies, the disease is called thrush and commonly is caused by a favorable environment for the growth of *C. albicans*, as milk changes the pH of the mouth. In adults or infants, treatment with an antifungal agent usually cures the disorder and restores the balance of microbes in the mouth.

 CHECKPOINT QUESTION

1. What are the two most common causes of stomatitis?

Gingivitis

Gingivitis is an inflammation of the gingiva, or gums. It may lead to periodontitis, or inflammation, and possible destruction of the supporting structures of the teeth, including the gingiva, periodontal ligament, and mandibular or maxillary bone. In Americans, more teeth are lost to gum disease than to tooth decay. Good oral hygiene and frequent dental care help prevent premature loss of teeth. Once diagnosed, gingivitis is usually treated with an antibiotic.

Oral Cancers

Cancers of the oral cavity are common, especially among individuals who use tobacco products. The con-stant irritation of the tobacco causes white spots or patches, called **leukoplakia**, to form on the oral mucosa, particularly the lips and tongue. These lesions have clearly defined borders and frequently become malignant. Treatment includes surgery or chemical agents such as radiation or chemotherapy. Although cancer of the lips usually responds well to radiation or surgery, cancers of the margins of the tongue metastasize quickly and are commonly difficult to treat effectively.

 CHECKPOINT QUESTION

2. How can gingivitis be prevented?

Esophageal Disorders

Hiatal Hernia

Hiatal hernia, or diaphragmatic hernia, occurs when the stomach protrudes up through the diaphragm through a weakened or enlarged cardiac sphincter at the bottom of the esophagus, allowing a portion of the stomach to slide up into the chest cavity. This type of hernia is a common condition that frequently affects people over age 40 years. Weight gain, either recent or prolonged, can be a contributing factor. Normally, the cardiac sphincter, a muscle that separates the end of the esophagus from the beginning of the stomach, prevents gastroesophageal reflux, or backflow of gastric acids from the stomach into the esophagus. The presence of a hiatal hernia enables the stomach acid to backflow into the esophagus, causing considerable discomfort, including indigestion and epigastric pain in the upper abdomen (Fig. 32-2).

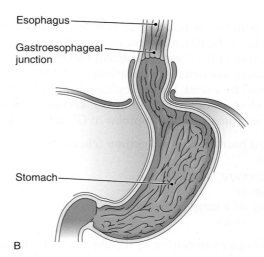

Figure 32-2 (**A**) Normal. (**B**) Hiatal hernia. The stomach protrudes through the diaphragm into the thoracic cavity, raising the level of the junction between the esophagus and the stomach. (Reprinted with permission from Cohen BJ, Wood DL. Memmler's The Human Body in Health and Disease. Philadelphia: Lippincott Williams & Wilkins, 2000.)

The symptoms of a hiatal hernia include abdominal pain and indigestion, especially after eating. Diagnosis is made by taking a careful medical history, chest radiographs, barium swallow, or endoscopy. Medical treatment is usually preferred to surgical intervention because surgically corrected hiatal hernias frequently recur. Medical interventions include diet modifications such as small, frequent meals with no food for at least 2 hours before bedtime. In addition, the physician may order antacids, weight loss, elevating the head of the bed when sleeping, and drug therapy to increase the tone of the cardiac sphincter.

Constant exposure to gastric acid from gastroesophageal reflux can lead to esophagitis, a condition that resembles abraded tissue along the lining of the esophagus. Constant irritation of the lining of the esophagus, also known as Barrett's esophagus, may lead to malignancy. Patients with Barrett's esophagus have a 30% to 40% chance of developing adenocarcinoma. If the source of irritation is gastroesophageal reflux, it will be diagnosed and treated much the same as a hiatal hernia.

Gastroesophageal Reflux Disease (GERD)

Patients who complain of any type of chest pain, including heartburn, should be assessed immediately because the chest pain of gastroesophageal reflux disease (GERD) may be similar to the chest pain of a patient having cardiac problems. In addition to the chest pain, signs and symptoms of myocardial involvement can include:

- Shortness of breath
- Nausea or vomiting
- Pain that spreads from the chest to the jaw, back, or arms

Chest pain that is not cardiac may be diagnosed by the physician as GERD, a chronic disorder characterized by discomfort in the chest (heartburn) due to the backflow of gastric contents into the esophagus. This disorder is caused by a weak lower esophageal sphincter that normally closes after food is swallowed, keeping the material in the stomach. The symptoms of GERD include:

- Frequent heartburn or indigestion relieved by antacids
- Hoarseness or laryngitis
- Sore throat
- A feeling of a lump in the throat
- Chronic cough

A thorough examination by the physician plus endoscopic and radiologic procedures are usually necessary to diagnose GERD. Once diagnosed, this disorder can be treated with appropriate medications. Untreated, GERD can lead to erosion of the esophagus and complications such as esophageal bleeding. GERD may also be the cause of esophageal cancers in some patients.

PATIENT EDUCATION
PREVENTING GASTRIC REFLUX

- Avoid spicy foods and chocolate, especially in the evening.
- Limit caffeine.
- Maintain optimum weight.
- Avoid overeating.
- Wait 1 hour after eating before exercising.
- Do not eat just before going to bed.
- Do not lie down just after eating.
- Stop smoking.
- Place blocks, bricks, or a stack of books under the legs of the bed to elevate the head, chest, and abdomen approximately 12 inches.
- See the physician if symptoms persist.

Esophageal Varices

Varicose veins (varices) of the esophagus result from pressure within the esophageal veins. This condition is commonly seen in patients diagnosed with cirrhosis of the liver. Since drainage from the portal vein is impaired by the liver damage, the veins of the esophagus become distended, resulting in varices. The most common and dangerous problem that results from esophageal varices is hemorrhaging if the distended veins rupture. Before a rupture occurs, the treatment of choice is **sclerotherapy**, which uses a chemical agent to cause fibrosing (hardening) of the area around the varices, preventing hemorrhaging. In the event of esophageal hemorrhage, the patient should be transported immediately to the emergency room, where pressure tubes can be applied directly to the varices to control the bleeding.

Esophageal Cancer

Cancer of the esophagus is most common among older men and is usually fatal. Predisposing factors for this type of cancer include chronic gastroesophageal reflux, smoking, and drinking alcohol. The malignancy narrows the lumen of the esophagus and causes **dysphagia** (difficulty swallowing). As the mass enlarges, swallowing solid food may become extremely painful. Vomiting and weight loss occur as the symptoms progress. A barium swallow with fluoroscopy outlines the lesion, and esophagoscopy with biopsy confirms the diagnosis. If the disease is local, surgical resection, chemotherapy, and radiation are the therapies of choice. No treatment has proven satisfactory, however, and the survival rates are very low.

CHECKPOINT QUESTION

3. What is a hiatal hernia, and how can it affect the esophagus?

Stomach Disorders

Gastritis

Gastritis, an inflammation of the lining of the stomach, can be acute or chronic. The most common causes include irritants such as alcohol and certain drugs, including aspirin and nonsteroidal anti-inflammatory medications (NSAIDs). The bacterium *Helicobacter pylori*, also often implicated, is presumed to enter the body through food contaminated with infected fecal material (fecal–oral route) or from eating or drinking from a utensil also used by someone who is infected with the bacteria (oral–oral route). It resides in the mucous lining of the stomach and secretes enzymes that attack the mucous membrane.

Gastritis can cause significant oozing of blood and may result in a positive test for occult (hidden) blood in the stool. In elderly patients, sufficient blood loss can result in anemia. Signs and symptoms of gastritis include evidence of GI bleeding, epigastric discomfort, nausea, and vomiting. Diagnosis is usually made by obtaining a careful and complete history and direct visualization of the gastric mucosa through an endoscopic procedure known as a gastroscopy. Treatment usually involves eliminating the irritant, restoring the proper gastric acidity, and administering antibiotics as prescribed by the physician.

Peptic Ulcers

Ulcers in the GI tract are erosions or sores left by sloughed tissues. These erosions can expose small blood vessels and produce bleeding and pain. Peptic ulcers occur from the exposure of the lining of the stomach and first part of the small intestine (duodenum) to hydrochloric acid (HCl), a caustic chemical produced and secreted by the lining of the stomach that may cause erosion if too much is excreted. As the mucosa erodes, the patient has abdominal pain that intensifies during peristalsis, especially after eating. As the erosions and mucosa become more irritated, the ulcers bleed. The bleeding may range from a slight oozing to life-threatening hemorrhage. Heavy bleeding will lead to **melena** (black tarry stools) or **hematemesis** (vomiting blood). Ulcers in the upper GI tract may perforate into the abdominal cavity with life-threatening consequences such as hypovolemic shock and peritonitis (Box 32-1). Chronic ulcerative conditions may also progress to malignancies.

The causes of peptic or gastric ulcers may include the use of chemicals that irritate the gastric mucosa, includ-

---

BOX 32-1

PERITONITIS

Peritonitis, an infection of the lining of the abdominal cavity, is a serious complication of several gastrointestinal disorders that may occur if contents of the intestines or other organs leak into the abdominal cavity. The patient will be acutely ill and will have a fever and elevated white blood cell count. In addition, the patient will be complaining of severe abdominal pain. Treatment of peritonitis requires hospitalization with intravenous antibiotics and continuous monitoring of the patient for signs of septic shock. This condition can quickly become fatal if not treated appropriately and aggressively.

---

ing aspirin, NSAIDs, and alcohol. Many gastric ulcers are also caused by an infection with *H. pylori*, which can be treated effectively with an antibiotic. Overproduction of gastric HCl also irritates the gastric mucosa and may produce erosions. Gastric acid production is under nerve and hormonal control and increases during times of emotional stress. Diagnosis of an ulcer is similar to the diagnosis of gastritis, including a thorough history and possibly endoscopic examination. The prescribed treatment for ulcers is avoiding the irritants causing the erosion, limiting the production of hydrogen by the gastric cells to neutralize the acid in the stomach, and an antibiotic as prescribed. Surgery to cut or disconnect the vagus nerve (vagotomy), which also reduces the secretion of HCl, may be performed if methods to decrease production of gastric acid are ineffective in treating the ulcer.

Gastric Cancer

Gastric cancer has no known cause, although smoking, excessive alcohol intake, ingesting foods high in preservatives, and genetic predisposition may contribute. Gastric cancer spreads rapidly to adjacent organs (the liver and pancreas) and throughout the peritoneal cavity. Signs and symptoms include chronic indigestion, weight loss, anorexia, anemia, and fatigue. The patient may have hematemesis with bright blood or coffee ground vomitus with dark blood. There may also be dark, bloody stools.

Diagnosis of gastric cancer requires an upper GI series with fluoroscopy, fiberoptic gastroscopy, and biopsy of the lesion or tumor. The extent of the disease can be determined by computed tomography (CT) and biopsy of the suspected metastatic sites, including adjacent organs. Surgery to remove the lesion may range from a subtotal gastric resection (removal of part of the stomach) to a total gastrectomy (removal of the entire stomach). If the cancer has metastasized, other organs may be removed, and radiation and chemotherapy may be necessary.

 CHECKPOINT QUESTION

4. What microorganism is found to be the cause of peptic ulcers in some patients?

Intestinal Disorders
Gastroenteritis

Gastroenteritis is general inflammation of the stomach, small intestine, and/or colon. This condition is caused by ingesting food or water that contains bacteria, viruses, parasites, or irritating agents such as spices. Food allergies and reactions to certain medications, such as antibiotics, may also inflame these organs. Symptoms include abdominal pain and cramping, nausea, vomiting, diarrhea, and fever.

The symptoms of gastroenteritis are self-limiting in most adults, usually lasting a few hours to a couple of days. However, because of the dehydration that can accompany the diarrhea and vomiting, gastroenteritis may be life threatening in the elderly, young children, and persons with diabetes mellitus. Treatment is palliative; it includes reducing the work of the GI tract by limiting food intake; treating the nausea, vomiting, and diarrhea; and maintaining the fluid balance by hydrating the body as needed. In severe cases, intravenous fluids must be administered to prevent dehydration and death, especially in the young and the elderly. If the cause of the inflammation is a bacterial or parasitic infection, an antibiotic or antiparasitic medication may be prescribed once the causative microorganism has been identified through a stool culture and analysis.

Duodenal Ulcers

Ulcerative lesions in the duodenum are often caused by exposure to highly corrosive gastric acid that is secreted by the stomach or other irritants that pass through the pylorus to the small intestine. Unlike the stomach, the duodenum has a normally alkaline pH, and the mucosa is not as well protected as the gastric mucosa. When food material passes through the pylorus and brings excessive acid or other irritants with it, an ulcer may form in the duodenum. As with the peptic ulcer, an overproduction of gastric acid may arise from ingestion of highly spicy foods or from overproduction of stress hormones, which also increases production of gastric acid. Treatment for duodenal ulcers is limiting or avoiding the irritating factors and reducing gastric acidity. If these measures are not successful, surgery may be an option. Ulcers in the duodenum left untreated may perforate the lining of the small intestine or may progress to cancerous lesions.

Malabsorption Syndromes

Malabsorption syndromes prevent the normal absorption of certain nutrients through the walls of the small intestines. Commonly, fat is not absorbed. A sign that a patient has a problem with malabsorption of fats includes stools that are frothy and pale. Because fat is necessary for the metabolism of vitamins A, D, E, and K, patients with this disorder require supplemental vitamin therapy.

Celiac sprue is a malabsorption syndrome marked by intolerance to gluten, a protein found in wheat and wheat byproducts. Celiac sprue can develop at any stage of life and often causes diarrhea high in fat. The cause of celiac sprue is not known, but it runs in families, suggesting a genetic factor.

Regardless of the nutrient involved in a patient with malabsorption syndrome, the patient is typically treated by addressing the suspected causes and avoiding or replacing the malabsorbed substances.

 CHECKPOINT QUESTION

5. How are peptic and duodenal ulcers different?

 PATIENT EDUCATION

GASTRIC BYPASS SURGERY TO TREAT OBESITY

Bariatrics is the study of morbid obesity. A popular surgical procedure to treat obesity is gastric bypass. Here are a few facts about this procedure:

- According to the American Society of Bariatric Surgery (www.asbs.org), candidates for the surgery must be severely obese and have failed to lose weight with other methods.
- Candidates for gastric bypass surgery must have either a body mass index greater than 40 (approximately 80–100 pounds over the ideal weight for height) or significant medical problems associated with being overweight.
- The abdomen is incised, and the stomach is reduced to about the size of a thumb. The large remainder of the stomach is bypassed, and the new, smaller stomach is attached directly to the small intestine.
- The surgery comes with risks and requires lifestyle changes. Anemia and nutritional deficiencies are long-term risks that must be monitored and prevented or corrected.
- Since weight reduction after this procedure is often quick and dramatic, patients should be encouraged to begin an exercise program following the surgery as indicated by the surgeon.

Crohn's Disease

Crohn's disease, also known as regional enteritis, is an inflammation of the deep lining of the bowel ranging from very mild to severe and debilitating. The cause of Crohn's disease is unclear, but it is thought to be an autoimmune disorder with a possible genetic link. Crohn's disease can affect the small bowel and the colon but is more common in the area of the ileocecal valve. The bowel walls become inflamed, and the lymph nodes enlarge, leading to edema of the bowel wall. When the lining of the bowel is swollen, the fluid from the intestinal contents cannot be absorbed, causing diarrhea and cramping, which may lead to more irritation and bleeding. Patients may also have periods of constipation, **anorexia**, and fever.

Although Crohn's disease is a chronic disorder, each episode of inflammation causes scarring. The scarring may lead to narrowing of the colon, obstructing the bowel. Bowel obstruction can be life threatening and is a medical emergency. Diagnosis of Crohn's disease necessitates a thorough history and analysis of the blood, which shows an increase in white blood cells and the erythrocyte sedimentation rate. A barium enema, or lower GI radiographic examination, if ordered by the physician, shows strictures alternating with normal bowel. Sigmoidoscopy and colonoscopy show patchy areas of inflammation within the bowel.

The treatment of Crohn's disease is symptomatic; it includes restoration of fluids and electrolytes, administering corticosteroids to reduce inflammation, rest, and a low-fiber diet. Surgery is performed in cases of perforation or hemorrhage. If the situation is severe, a colectomy with an ileostomy may be performed (Fig. 32-3).

Ulcerative Colitis

Like Crohn's disease, ulcerative colitis is an inflammatory bowel disease affecting the lining of the colon. It occurs most often in young women but may occur at any age and may affect men also. The cause is not known but is thought to be an abnormal GI immune reaction to foods or microorganisms. Ulcerative colitis is a chronic condition, and the symptoms can be mild or severe with periods of remission.

The tissue that lines the colon becomes congested and edematous, eventually sloughing off and leading to ulcers and bloody diarrhea. Sometimes pus and mucus are present in the stool. Malabsorption of fluids causes weakness, anorexia, nausea, and vomiting. Scarring can occur as the ulcers heal. The colon may produce pseudopolyps, which can be precancerous. Diagnosis may be determined by endoscopic examination or by a barium enema, and biopsy confirms the diagnosis. Colonoscopy is used to evaluate strictures caused by scarring and to assess the risk of cancer.

Figure 32-3 An ileostomy. The shaded portion indicates the section of the bowel that has been removed or is inactive. (Modified with permission from Cohen BJ. Medical Terminology: An Illustrated Guide. Philadelphia: Lippincott Williams & Wilkins, 2003.)

Treatment of ulcerative colitis requires controlling the inflammation and preventing the loss of fluids and nutrients during periods of exacerbation. If the disease is severe, a corticosteroid is prescribed to relieve the inflammation. Surgery is a last resort and usually involves a proctocolectomy with an ileostomy.

 CHECKPOINT QUESTION

6. Which of the inflammatory bowel diseases can lead to life-threatening bowel obstruction? How?

Irritable Bowel Syndrome

Patients with irritable bowel syndrome frequently complain of bouts of constipation alternating with diarrhea. Although the patient may have signs and symptoms resembling those of Crohn's disease or ulcerative colitis, irritable bowel syndrome usually does not result in weight loss, and the prognosis is good. However, this disorder can be debilitating because there is no warning for the bouts of diarrhea caused by the spastic colon. Women are more likely than men to have this chronic disorder, whose symptoms may range from mild to severe even though endoscopic examination shows no signs of disease. The origin of irritable bowel syndrome is thought to be psychogenic, a reaction to stress and emotions and the actions of the autonomic nervous system, which partly controls the colon. The consumption of specific food irritants may also precipitate an attack; however, the particular food item that triggers symptoms varies from person to person. Diagnosis requires a careful history, both physical and emotional. Other diseases are ruled out by testing. Treatment is stress management and identifying the offending food irritants. For severe flare-ups, the physician may order corticosteroids and antibiotics.

Diverticulosis

Diverticulosis is a chronic condition of thinning of the bowel wall, causing small out-pouches in the lining of the intestinal wall (Fig. 32-4). This disorder usually occurs in the sigmoid colon but may occur anywhere in the GI tract. The cause has been attributed to a diet deficient in roughage. While many people have diverticulosis without symptoms, the condition becomes more serious when the bowel wall becomes so thin that veins and arteries are exposed. Bleeding can occur when the wall is nicked by a piece of stool and may be severe enough to require surgery to stop the hemorrhage. A diet high in fiber and use of stool softeners may be ordered by the physician to prevent the signs and symptoms of this disorder.

Diverticulosis may progress to diverticulitis, or inflammation of these areas of weakness in the bowel wall. The inflammation is usually caused by fecal material becoming lodged in the thin pockets. The symptoms are fever and abdominal pain. As the bowel becomes swollen and distended, the diseased areas may rupture, exposing the peritoneum to fecal material and resulting in peritonitis. The pouches are visualized on films produced from a barium enema or directly through endoscopic studies. During the acute phase, treatment includes a bland diet and stool softeners until the inflammation has subsided.

Figure 32-4 Diverticulosis of the sigmoid colon. (Reprinted with permission from Neil Hardy, Westpoint, CT.)

PATIENT EDUCATION

MAINTAINING GOOD BOWEL HABITS

By following these guidelines, patients can prevent common problems of elimination:

- Eat a variety of foods, especially fresh fruits, vegetables, and whole grains. Limit the intake of highly processed foods.
- Drink eight glasses of water a day to keep the stools moist and easy to pass and to hydrate the tissues.
- Get some form of exercise daily. Even a walk around the block will aid muscle tone and help prevent sluggish metabolism.
- Make time for bowel movements when the stimulus is felt. Avoiding or delaying defecation results in loss of moisture from the stool and may make the bowel insensitive to the stimulus.
- Do not use laxatives or enemas. Frequent use may result in a lazy bowel that responds only to these chemical and physical stimuli.

The frequency of bowel elimination is an individual characteristic. If stools are passed only several times a week but are soft, formed, and passed with little effort, there should be no concern about constipation. However, constipation may be a problem if stools are passed daily but are hard, dry, and difficult to pass.

Polyps

Colon polyps are masses of benign mucous membrane lining the large intestine that are usually slow growing but may become cancerous. Polyps are usually discovered by a barium enema or during a colonoscopy. If the polyps are discovered at an early stage and removed, cancer of the colon may be prevented. Cancer of the colon may invade the muscle of the bowel and metastasize through the lymph system to other organs.

Hernias

The anterior abdominal wall is covered with various muscles that assist with movement and support and protect the internal structures of the abdomen. When these muscles weaken, the underlying organs or intestines may protrude through the weakened muscle wall, resulting in a hernia. Factors that may increase the risk for developing a hernia include a genetic predisposition to muscular weakness, lifting heavy objects, obesity, and pregnancy. The signs and symptoms of abdominal hernia include a protrusion or bulge over the area of the hernia. Specific types of abdominal hernias are named according to the area of the abdomen: the inguinal hernia occurs in right or left inguinal (groin) areas; the ventral hernia occurs in the front of the abdomen; and the umbilical hernia occurs over the umbilicus. The treatment for abdominal hernias includes surgically repairing the weakened muscle (herniorrhaphy) using grafting material as necessary. To prevent abdominal hernias, encourage the use of abdominal support and good body mechanics when lifting and weight reduction as prescribed by the physician.

 CHECKPOINT QUESTION

7. What has generally been noted as the cause of diverticulosis?

Appendicitis

The vermiform appendix, a small pouch of tissue protruding from the cecum or first part of the large intestine, is approximately 4 inches long. Although the function of this tissue is not clear, there is no direct involvement with the process of digestion. Appendicitis occurs when the vermiform appendix becomes infected and fills with bacteria, pus, and blood. Adolescents and young adult men are most commonly affected by this condition, but women and young children can also develop appendicitis. The symptoms include severe abdominal pain with tenderness over the right lower quadrant, vomiting, a fever, and an elevated white blood count. A thorough history should be obtained from any patient with these symptoms, and once the physician determines the diagnosis of appendicitis, it is necessary to make arrangements for immediate surgical removal of the infected appendix. If a diagnosis is not made quickly or the appendectomy is delayed, perforation of the appendix and peritonitis can result and make recovery more difficult for the patient.

Hemorrhoids

Hemorrhoids are external or internal dilated veins (varicosities) in the rectum. Internal hemorrhoids may enlarge and may bleed during defecation. A patient with external hemorrhoids may complain of rectal pain and itching and bleeding with bowel movements. Poor abdominal and pelvic floor muscle tone, poor dietary habits including a diet low in fiber, and chronic constipation may cause hemorrhoids. The diagnosis of external hemorrhoids is made by visual inspection, while internal hemorrhoids are diagnosed by anoscopy or proctoscopy. Treatment involves regulating the diet to control constipation, providing local pain relief, using a stool softener, and surgical ligation (hemorrhoidectomy) using standard surgical techniques, laser, or cryosurgery (freezing).

Colorectal Cancers

Cancer of the colon and rectum is often fatal, but the patient's chances for survival are better with early diagnosis and treatment. Although the cause of colorectal cancer is unknown, it has been linked to diets high in animal fats and low in fiber. It is commonly seen in patients with a history of ulcerative colitis or colorectal polyps and affects the first and last parts of the colon more often than other areas (Fig. 32-5). Early signs of colorectal cancer are vague abdominal pains with occasional bloody stools. Later signs depend on the section and amount of the colon involved and the degree of metastasis to other organs and tissues.

Many rectal cancers are discovered by a digital examination or an anoscopy, but sigmoidoscopy or colonoscopy is used to determine the extent of involvement. A barium enema with contrast air aids in the diagnosis. Laboratory tests include **guaiac** tests, such as the Hemoccult, which test for occult (hidden) blood in the stool. Surgical removal of the affected area, usually followed by chemotherapy and radiation, is the treatment of choice.

Functional Disorders

Functional disorders of the GI tract include the common disorders of constipation, diarrhea, and intestinal gas. Normally, peristalsis causes the products of digestion to move at a constant rate, not too slowly and not too quickly. Constipation occurs when the lower colon retains fecal material too long so that too much moisture is absorbed, making the stool hard and dry. Most con-

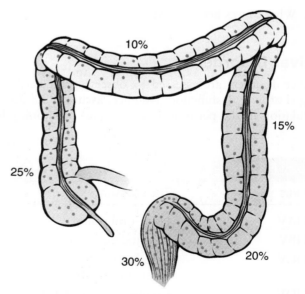

Figure 32-5 Percent distribution of cancer sites in the colon and rectum.

stipation is caused by poor bowel habits (avoiding defecation and overusing laxatives), low-fiber diet, and inadequate fluid intake. The quality of the stool is more important than the quantity. To avoid constipation, patients should be encouraged to increase oral fluid intake, eat foods high in fiber, such as raw vegetables and fruit, and maintain regular bowel habits. The physician may also prescribe a stool softener and an over-the-counter fiber product as needed.

When the fluid contents of the bowel are rushed through, as in diarrhea, the water and minerals are not reabsorbed into the system, and the stool is loose and watery. Bacterial or viral infection or a GI irritant causes the smooth muscles and mucous membranes to work to flush out the bowel as quickly as possible. The treatment for diarrhea includes medication to slow peristalsis, a bland diet, and increasing oral fluids to replace fluids and electrolytes lost in the stool.

Intestinal gas, produced by bacterial decomposition of proteins in the digestive tract, can lead to abdominal discomfort. Gas in the intestinal tract causes a feeling of fullness. The gas may be expelled from the stomach through the mouth (eructation, or belching) or from the intestines through the rectum (flatulence). The production of intestinal gas is due to intolerance of milk products, swallowing air through excessive talking or gum chewing, consuming gas-producing spicy or fatty foods, or slow emptying of the stomach and bowels. The problem can usually be relieved by avoiding the offending foods or behaviors. Various over-the-counter preparations and prescription medications can be used if the problem persists.

 CHECKPOINT QUESTION

8. What causes hemorrhoids?

Liver Disorders

Liver disorders are assessed by observing the cardinal signs of liver dysfunction: jaundice, **ascites** (fluid accumulation in the peritoneal cavity), and **hepatomegaly** (enlargement of the liver). It is vital to obtain a complete medical history from patients with a suspected liver disorder. Particular concern focuses on jaundice, anemia, splenectomy, alcohol use, travel to Third World countries, blood transfusions, use of **hepatotoxins** (drugs that are damaging to the liver), and abuse of controlled substances. Diagnostic tests for liver disorders include the following:

- Liver function tests, including prothrombin time and levels of bilirubin, alkaline phosphatase, albumin, and cholesterol
- Radiography and barium study
- Radioisotope liver scan
- Percutaneous peritoneoscopy and biopsy
- Surgical laparotomy and liver biopsy

Hepatitis

Hepatitis is an inflammation or infection of the liver that may lead to liver destruction and necrosis of hepatic cells. The five types of viral hepatitis are summarized in Table 32-1 and listed here:

- *Hepatitis A (HAV)*, the most common type of viral hepatitis, is also known as infectious hepatitis. HAV spreads in food and water contaminated with fecal material or seafood high in coliform bacteria. It is highly contagious, but the prognosis for recovery after an infection with hepatitis A is good.
- *Hepatitis B (HBV)*, also known as serum hepatitis, can be transmitted by contaminated blood and other body fluids. HBV may be so severe that death results, but the use of standard precautions will prevent spread. Fortunately, there is a vaccine to protect against HBV, and it is recommended for all health care workers.
- *Hepatitis C (HCV)*, also known as non-A, non-B hepatitis, can be transmitted via blood transfusion or percutaneous contamination. After the initial infection, HCV frequently progresses to chronic hepatitis that may be asymptomatic but is communicable. As with HBV, the use of standard precautions prevents spread.

TABLE **32-1**	**Types of Viral Hepatitis**	
Virus	**Transmission**	**Precautions**
HAV	Fecal–oral route	Handwashing
HBV	Sera and body fluids	Standard precautions; HBV vaccine
HCV	Blood transfusions Percutaneous contamination	Standard precautions
HDV	Coinfection with HBV	Standard precautions; HBV vaccine
HEV	Fecal–oral route	Handwashing; standard precautions

- *Hepatitis D (HDV)* occurs only in patients who have had HBV; it cannot survive without HBV.
- *Hepatitis E (HEV)* spreads in food or water contaminated with fecal material and ingested by the unsuspecting individual.

While the viruses responsible for the individual types of viral hepatitis are physically different, the symptoms of all types are similar. They may include fatigue, joint pain, flu-like symptoms with fever, jaundice, dark urine, and light stools. Complications of hepatitis include long-term impaired liver function, chronic hepatitis, liver cancer, and death.

Diagnosis of the various types of viral hepatitis is made by obtaining a complete medical history, blood analysis for hepatitis antibodies, and liver function studies. There is no cure once infection occurs, but the patient is encouraged to rest and take in a supportive diet. Interferon-alpha is given to some patients to assist the immune system in responding to viral hepatitis. Standard precautions must be observed to protect caregivers and health care workers from contracting hepatitis.

Another cause of hepatitis, toxic hepatitis, is exposure to chemical toxicants or hepatotoxic substances, including certain medications and alcohol. If the offending toxicant is eliminated early enough, the prognosis for recovery is good. The symptoms of toxic hepatitis resemble viral hepatitis, and the diagnosis is similar. A liver biopsy may identify the underlying pathology.

Cirrhosis or Fibrosis

Cirrhosis is a chronic disease characterized by destruction of liver cells and the formation of scar tissue or fibers throughout the liver, altering its function and efficiency. The causes of cirrhosis include a history of exposure to hepatotoxins, alcoholism, prolonged biliary obstruction, and a history of hepatitis. In the early stages, symptoms include vague GI discomfort. In the late stages, respiratory efficiency decreases because of ascites that forces the abdominal contents against the diaphragm. Bleeding tendencies result from the loss of clotting factors formed in the liver. Dermal pruritus (itching), jaundice, and hepatomegaly are usually present. Diagnosis is made by liver biopsy, liver scan, and blood work. Treatment includes avoiding the hepatotoxins or abstinence from alcohol to prevent further death of hepatic cells, a good diet, vitamin supplements, and supportive care. In cases of liver failure that accompanies increased destruction of liver tissue, the physician may recommend a liver transplantation.

✓ CHECKPOINT QUESTION

9. How does the cause of viral hepatitis differ from that of toxic hepatitis?

Liver Cancer

The liver is rarely a primary site for cancer but is frequently a target site of metastasis. This type of cancer is more common in men than in women and is rapidly fatal. There is no known cause, but primary liver cancers are thought to be due to exposure to carcinogenic chemicals, including hepatotoxins. Patients who have cirrhosis or hepatitis B are more likely than the general population to develop liver cancer.

In the early stages of the disease, patients usually complain of weight loss, weakness, and right upper quadrant pain. Jaundice may be present and will definitely develop as the disease progresses (Fig. 32-6). Diagnosis is confirmed by biopsy, liver function tests, and computed tomography (CT) or magnetic resonance imaging (MRI). If the lesion is small and local, resection is possible. Chemotherapy may be used in some instances. If there is no metastasis, a liver transplantation may be possible.

Gallbladder Disorders
Cholelithiasis and Cholecystitis

Cholelithiasis is the formation of gallstones made of cholesterol and bilirubin (Fig. 32-7). When the peristaltic action of the gallbladder is sluggish and bile pools in the sac, fluid is absorbed, leaving the solids to concentrate and solidify into stones. Cholecystitis is an acute or chronic inflammation of the gallbladder, usually resulting from an impacted stone in the duct. Cholecystitis or cholelithiasis usually causes pain as peristalsis presses bile against the blockage, especially after a fatty meal.

Signs and symptoms of any gallbladder disorder include acute right upper abdominal quadrant pain that

Figure 32-6 A patient with jaundice. (From Bickley LS, Szilagyi P. Bates' Guide to Physical Examination and History Taking. 8th ed. Philadelphia: Lippincott Williams & Wilkins, 2003.)

Figure 32-7 Cholelithiasis. The gallbladder has been opened to reveal numerous yellow cholesterol gallstones. (Reprinted with permission from Rubin E, Gorstein F, Rubin R, Schwarting R, Strayer D. Rubin's Pathology: Clinicopathologic Foundations of Medicine. Philadelphia: Lippincott Williams & Wilkins, 2005.)

may radiate to the shoulders, back, or chest; indigestion; nausea; and intolerance of fatty foods. Later in the illness, jaundice may appear as the ducts to the liver become blocked. Tests to determine the cause of the symptoms include cholecystography after the ingestion of a radiopaque dye, percutaneous transhepatic cholangiography, endoscopic retrograde cholangiopancreatography (ECRP), and duodenal endoscopy. Noninvasive procedures include ultrasound and CT. Flat plate radiographs are not especially accurate for evaluating gallbladder disorders. The treatment may be supportive or palliative, including pain medication and avoiding fatty foods; however, surgical removal of the stones (cholecystectomy) may be necessary, usually through endoscopic laparotomy. Lithotripsy (crushing the gallstones using sound waves) may also be used to break the stones into small pieces that can pass easily through the bile ducts and into the digestive system for elimination.

Gallbladder Cancer

Cancer of the gallbladder is rare and difficult to diagnose. Since the symptoms are similar to those of cholecystitis, this cancer is usually discovered during routine gallbladder tests performed to diagnose general gallbladder disease. The signs and symptoms include right upper quadrant pain, nausea and vomiting, weight loss, and anorexia. However, cholecystitis pain is usually sporadic, whereas pain due to malignancy is usually chronic and severe. The gallbladder may be palpable, and jaundice may be present. It is most common in older women and is rapidly fatal. The cause is not known, but theory suggests that cholelithiasis is a predisposing factor. Diagnosis includes liver function tests, CT, MRI, and cholecystography. Surgical cholecystectomy is the primary treatment, but survival rates are low.

 CHECKPOINT QUESTION

10. How are cholelithiasis and cholecystitis different?

Pancreatic Disorders

Pancreatitis

Pancreatitis is an inflammation of the pancreas that may be related to alcoholism, trauma, gastric ulcer, or biliary tract disease. Signs and symptoms include vomiting and steady epigastric pain radiating to the spine. Signs of progressive disease include abdominal rigidity and decreased bowel activity. Complications include diabetes mellitus, hemorrhage, shock, coma, and death as the digestive enzymes cause the organ to digest itself. Diagnostic blood tests show an increase in serum amylase and glucose levels. Ultrasound and CT are useful for diagnosis. Treatment includes pain relief and medication to reduce pancreatic secretions while the organ recovers. Prognosis depends on the extent and severity of damage to the pancreas.

Pancreatic Cancer

One of the deadliest malignancies is pancreatic cancer, which kills most patients within a year of diagnosis. There is no definitive cause of pancreatic cancer, but it occurs most often in middle-aged African-American men who smoke, who have a diet high in fats and proteins, or who are exposed to industrial chemicals for long periods.

Patients complain of weight loss, back and abdominal pain, and diarrhea. Commonly they are jaundiced. Diagnosis is made by laparoscopic biopsy, CT, MRI, endoscopic retrograde cholangiopancreatography (ERCP), and pancreatic enzyme studies. Surgical removal of the pancreas (pancreatotomy), chemotherapy, and radiation therapy are used to treat pancreatic cancer, but the survival rate is very low.

 CHECKPOINT QUESTION

11. What are some complications of pancreatitis?

Common Diagnostic and Therapeutic Procedures

History and Physical Examination of the GI System

Before beginning any patient's care, an adequate history must be obtained. The patient presenting with GI concerns will be assessed for signs (e.g., vomiting) and symptoms (e.g., nausea). From that base, the physician will determine the direction of the diagnostic testing to rule out or to confirm possible diagnosis. The history must include occupation, family history, recent travel to Third World countries, and current medications. Patients should also be required to complete a checklist of concerns, which may include heartburn, GI bleeding, weight gain or loss, history of alcohol use, and laxative and enema use.

The physician will assess skin **turgor** (elasticity), jaundice, edema, bruising, breath odor, size and shape of the abdomen, and presence and quality of bowel sounds. The physician will also palpate abdominal contents.

Blood Tests

Blood work ordered by the physician may include white and red blood cell counts. The red blood cells, hemoglobin, and hematocrit are used to assess possible anemia as the result of GI bleeding. White blood cell counts can help to detect infection, while the erythrocyte sedimentation rate is used to assess inflammatory processes, including inflammation of the GI system.

Blood may also be drawn and sent to the laboratory to determine liver function. Specifically, alkaline phosphatase, serum bilirubin, prothrombin time, and SGPT (serum glutamic pyruvic transaminase) levels are determined in a test collectively known as a liver panel. Pancreatic enzyme studies include evaluation of blood for levels of enzymes normally released by the pancreas, including trypsin, chymotrypsin, steapsin, and amylopsin. Results that fall outside of the normal ranges for these substances indicate pathology and necessitate further testing as determined by the physician.

Radiology Studies

Flat plate radiographs of the abdomen may be ordered for diagnosing GI problems, but without contrast medium, these radiographs are not so useful as contrast radiographs. Radiology studies of the stomach and intestines consist of instilling barium, a radiopaque liquid, into the GI tract orally or rectally to outline the organs and identify abnormalities. The radiographs include standard pictures taken at various intervals after the barium is administered by mouth or by enema. If a fluoroscope (special type of radiographic equipment) is used, movement of the chalky liquid barium is viewed while it fills the esophagus or colon, giving additional diagnostic information.

The barium swallow (also called an upper GI or UGI) series can reveal abnormal constrictions, masses, and obstruction in the esophagus, stomach, and duodenum. This examination requires that the patient have nothing by mouth (NPO) after midnight the night before the test. A small bowel series is an extension of the UGI that visualizes the barium flowing through the small intestine to diagnose abnormalities of the first part of the small intestine.

A barium enema, or lower GI study, provides an outline of the colon. It can reveal a blockage, cancerous growths, polyps, and diverticula. Since the lower GI study requires that the colon be empty of stool, the patient must be given specific instructions to follow before the examination. Box 32-2 outlines the standard preparation for a barium enema, which should be orally explained to the patient and given in written form.

Cholecystography is radiography of the gallbladder after the patient takes oral tablets containing a contrast material 12 hours prior to the procedure. The contrast medium is excreted from the liver into the gallbladder, and any abnormalities are viewed on the radiogram. After the initial films are taken, the patient is given a fatty meal that stimulates the contraction of the gallbladder to release bile and contrast medium into the bile ducts. Additional films may be taken to view any obstruction of these ducts by stones. The bile ducts may also be examined using percutaneous transhepatic

---

BOX 32-2

PATIENT PREPARATION FOR BOWEL STUDIES

Many bowel studies, such as barium enema and flexible sigmoidoscopy, require that the bowel be completely clear of fecal matter. With minor variations as directed by the physician, the bowel preparation usually includes the following:

- Liquid diet without dairy products for the full day before the procedure or a clear liquid evening meal
- A laxative or enema the evening preceding the procedure
- Nothing by mouth after midnight except water
- Rectal suppository, Fleet's enema, or cleansing enema the morning of the procedure

If inflammatory processes or ulcerations are suspected inside the bowel, only gentle cleansing will be used to avoid undue discomfort or possible perforation of lesions.

cholangiography, a test that entails injection of contrast material through a needle inserted through the skin into the hepatic duct. Once the dye is injected, radiography is performed for diagnosis by the physician.

The role of the medical assistant in radiographic procedures includes determining third-party payer (insurance) requirements for referrals or preauthorization, scheduling the procedure in an outpatient facility, and explaining to the patient the preparations for the examination as necessary. When the test is complete, the radiologist will submit a written report to the referring physician. Follow office policy and procedure for routing the report to the physician for review and advising the patient of the examination results.

 CHECKPOINT QUESTION

12. Why are contrast media used in radiography of the gastrointestinal organs?

Nuclear Imaging

Radionuclides, or radioactive elements, are often used in the diagnosis of disorders of the liver. After the elements are injected into the body, images are taken using a nuclear scanning device, and abnormalities can be detected and evaluated by the radiologist. The injected radionuclide remains radioactive for a short specific period, and there is usually very little, if any, patient preparation required for this test. The role of the medical assistant includes coordinating any third-party payer requirements such as preauthorization, scheduling the test at a nuclear imaging center or hospital, and following up with the patient when the results are returned to the medical office as indicated in the policy and procedure manual. Test results indicating abnormalities necessitate additional evaluation and testing as determined by the physician.

Ultrasonography

The use of high-frequency sound waves to diagnose disorders of internal structures is used in many specialties, including gastroenterology. Abnormalities in the structure of various digestive accessory organs, such as the liver and gallbladder, can be easily viewed using ultrasonography and require very little if any preparation by the patient. As with other diagnostic tests ordered by the physician, your role includes verifying third-party payer guidelines and obtaining preauthorization if needed. Although ultrasound does not use radiation or radiography, ultrasounds are scheduled in the imaging department of many outpatient or inpatient facilities. Your role includes scheduling the test, advising the patient of the date and time, following up after the test to obtain results if necessary, ensuring that the physician is aware

of the results, and notifying the patient with any findings or additional instructions as ordered by the physician.

Endoscopic Studies

Fiberoptic technology has enabled physicians to pass soft, flexible tubes down the esophagus into the stomach and small intestine or up into the colon for direct visualization of these organs. Supplemental laboratory specimens, including tissue biopsy samples; samples of secretions for gastric analysis, including pH; culture sample to check for bacteria; bile for crystals that may lead to the formation of stones; and cells for cytology, including cancerous or otherwise abnormal cells, can be obtained. Endoscopic examinations are also used to diagnose biliary disorders.

ERCP (endoscopic retrograde cholangiopancreatography) is used to visualize the esophagus, stomach, proximal duodenum, and pancreas with a flexible endoscope. When the endoscope is in place, dye is injected directly into the ducts of the gallbladder and pancreas, and radiographs are taken to determine patency and function of these structures and the biliary ducts (Fig. 32-8). This procedure is usually performed in an outpatient surgical center under anesthesia. Your role includes scheduling the procedure, advising the patient on any instructions prior to the test, and follow-up when the written report is sent by the gastroenterologist or radiologist.

Anoscopy, which may be performed in the medical office, is insertion of a metal or plastic anoscope into the rectal canal for visual inspection of the anus and rectum

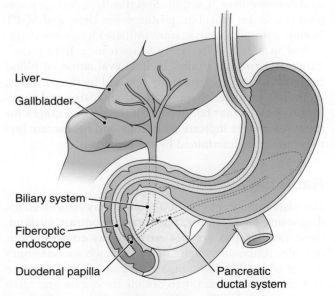

Figure 32-8 The ducts of the gallbladder and pancreas can be easily visualized during an ERCP. (From Cohen BJ. Medical Terminology. 4th ed. Philadelphia: Lippincott Williams & Wilkins, 2003.)

and to swab for cultures. The sigmoidoscopy examination provides a visual examination of the sigmoid colon using either a rigid sigmoidoscope or the more widely accepted flexible fiberoptic sigmoidoscope. The rigid sigmoidoscope is about 25 cm (10 inches) long. This instrument is supplied as reusable metal or disposable plastic and is calibrated in centimeters. An **obturator** in the lumen allows the instrument to be inserted with minimal discomfort and can be removed after insertion allowing for better visualization and obtaining specimens. The lens at the end magnifies the view for closer observation of the intestinal mucosa and can be moved aside to allow the physician to swab, suction, or sample the mucosa for biopsy. The handle contains the light source. The scope may be equipped with a hand bulb **insufflator**, a device for blowing air into the colon to expand the walls for easier visualization.

The flexible fiberoptic sigmoidoscope is more popular because it offers better visualization and is less uncomfortable for the patient (Fig. 32-9). The scope is very thin, can bend and maneuver curves, and can be inserted much farther than the rigid scope (Fig. 32-10). The instrument is 35 cm (about 14 inches) or 65 cm (about 26 inches). It usually includes an insufflator and suction in addition to the light source. Although smaller in diameter than the rigid scope, it can also be used to obtain samples and cultures.

Some physicians prefer that the bowel be as free of feces as possible and may order a light, low-residue meal the evening before the endoscopic examination. An evening laxative may also be ordered to be followed by a cleansing enema on the morning of the procedure. A light breakfast may be allowed but only if ordered by the physician. Other physicians prefer to view the mucosa as it normally appears, without preparation. Most medical offices note the preferred preparation in the policy and procedure manual. Your role includes informing the patient of the preferred preparation for the procedure, assisting the physician during the procedure, and offering

Figure 32-10 Sigmoidoscopy. The flexible scope is advanced past the proximal sigmoid colon and into the descending colon. (Reprinted with permission from Cohen BJ. Medical Terminology: An Illustrated Guide. Philadelphia: Lippincott Williams & Wilkins, 2003.)

reassurance and support to the patient. Procedure 32-1 describes the steps for assisting with colon procedures in the medical office.

 CHECKPOINT QUESTION

13. What does anoscopy involve, and how does it differ from sigmoidoscopy?

Fecal Tests

As part of the routine examination for adult patients, many physicians recommend testing a stool specimen for the presence of occult, or hidden, blood. A stool specimen may also be ordered to test for ova (eggs) and parasites if the physician suspects the patient has a parasite infection. You may be responsible for instructing the patient in the procedure for collecting these specimens, and in some cases, such as in testing the stool for occult blood, you may be responsible for testing the stool specimen after the patient returns it to the office. Chapter 44 discusses the procedure for instructing a patient to collect a stool specimen and for processing the specimens for occult blood.

Figure 32-9 A flexible sigmoidoscope.

TRIAGE

While you are working in a medical office, the following three situations occur:

A. A 44-year-old man is scheduled for a routine physical. However, he arrives in the office complaining of "heartburn" and is taken to an exam room where the physician has ordered an ECG.

B. An 18-year-old boy comes into the office with lower right abdominal pain. The physician wants blood drawn immediately to determine a white blood cell count and rule out appendicitis.

C. A 52-year-old woman has just seen the physician and needs to be scheduled for a colonoscopy at the local outpatient ambulatory surgical center.

How do you sort these patients? Who do you see first? Second? Third?

First, you should do the ECG on patient A. A feeling of indigestion or epigastric discomfort can be a sign of cardiac disease. Next draw patient B's blood, since an elevation in the white blood cell count indicates the need for additional tests and/or surgery for appendicitis. Finally, schedule the outpatient procedure for patient C after checking for appropriate insurance referrals.

Note: This sequence is the accepted triage standard; however, the physician may opt for the blood work to be done first if he or she considers that patient A's discomfort is probably due to gastric difficulties and has ordered the ECG as a prophylactic measure. This decision is based on the physical examinations of both patients. You and the physician must work as a team to achieve the best outcomes.

PROCEDURE 32-1: Assisting With Colon Procedures

Purpose: Prepare the patient and assist with endoscopic colon procedures
Equipment: Appropriate instrument (flexible or rigid sigmoidoscope, anoscope, or proctoscope), water-soluble lubricant, gown and drape, cotton swabs, suction (if not part of the scope), biopsy forceps, specimen container with preservative, completed laboratory requisition form, personal wipes or tissues, equipment for assessing vital signs, examination gloves

Steps	Reasons
1. Wash your hands.	Handwashing aids infection control.
2. Assemble the equipment and supplies. Write the name of the patient on the label of the specimen container and complete the laboratory requisition.	The name of the patient must be clearly marked on the container and the laboratory requisition form must be complete for accurate identification.
3. Check the light source if a flexible sigmoidoscope is being used. Turn off the power after checking for working order to avoid a buildup of heat in the instrument.	If heat is permitted to build up in the scope, the patient may be burned. If the rigid sigmoidoscope, anoscope, or proctoscope is being used, check the examination light for working order.

Step 3. Make sure the equipment, such as the sigmoidoscope, is in good working order.

| 4. Greet and identify the patient and explain the procedure. Inform the patient that a sensation of pressure or need to defecate may be felt during the procedure and that the pressure is from the instrument and will ease. The patient may also feel gas pressure when air is insufflated during | Identifying the patient prevents errors in treatment. Explaining the procedure helps ease anxiety and ensure compliance. |

(continued)

PROCEDURE 32-1:   **Assisting With Colon Procedures** *(continued)*

Steps	Reasons
sigmoidoscopy. Note: The patient may have been ordered to take a mild sedative before the procedure.	
5. Instruct the patient to empty the urinary bladder.	Pressure from the instrument may injure a full bladder. Urine in the bladder may increase discomfort.
6. Assess the vital signs and record them in the medical record.	Colon examination procedures may cause cardiac arrhythmias and a change in blood pressure in some patients. Baseline vital signs will allow you to detect variations from the patient's normal vital signs.
7. Have the patient undress completely from the waist down and put on a gown. Drape appropriately.	
8. Assist the patient onto the examination table. If the instrument is an anoscope or a fiberoptic device, Sims' position or a side-lying position is most comfortable. If a rigid instrument is used, the patient will assume a knee-chest position or be placed on a proctology table that supports the patient in a knee-chest position. Note: Do not ask the patient to assume the knee-chest position until the physician is ready to begin. The position is difficult to maintain. Drape the patient. **Step 8.** This patient is in the Sim's position.	These positions facilitate the procedure by moving the abdominal organs up into the abdominal cavity rather than the pelvis.
9. Assist the physician as needed with lubricant, instruments, power, swabs, suction, and specimen containers.	
10. During the procedure, monitor the patient's response and offer reassurance. Instruct the patient to breathe slowly through pursed lips to aid in relaxation if necessary.	
11. When the physician is finished, assist the patient into a comfortable position and allow a rest period. Offer personal cleaning wipes or tissues. Take the vital signs before allowing the patient to stand, and assist the patient from the table and with dressing as needed. Give the patient any instructions regarding care after the procedure and follow-up s ordered by the physician.	A drop in blood pressure on standing is common after lying in any of these positions for an extended period. If patients complain of dizziness or lightheadedness after sitting up, have them lie down. If any biopsy samples were taken, the patient may have slight rectal bleeding.
12. Clean the room and route the specimen to the laboratory with the requisition. Disinfect or dispose of the supplies and equipment as appropriate and wash your hands.	Follow standard precautions throughout the procedure.

(continued)

PROCEDURE 32-1: Assisting With Colon Procedures *(continued)*

Steps	Reasons
13. Document the procedure.	Procedures are considered not to have been done if they are not recorded.

Charting Example:

05/31/2008 12:45 PM T 98.6 (O), P 100, R 20, BP 144/86 (L). Sigmoidoscopy performed by Dr. Jacobs
and specimen obtained—pt. tolerated well. Specimen to Acme Lab, VS after procedure P 112, R 24, BP
146/86 (L). Pt. denied dizziness after procedure. Discharged per Dr. Jacobs.
—S. Clay, CMA

MEDIA MENU

- **Student CD**
  - **Case Studies**
    Interactive Case Study 1: Triage in an Emergency Situation, Communication and Documentation
  - **Animations**
    Cirrhosis
  - **CMA/RMA Certification Exam Review**
- **Premium Online Course**
  http://thePoint.lww.com/Kronenberger3e
- **Internet Resources**
  LiveAdvise Online Tutoring & Competency Training
  http://thePoint.lww.com/LiveAdvise

español SPANISH TERMINOLOGY

Padece de indigestion?
  Do you have indigestion?
Padece de estrenimiento?
  Are you constipated?
Tiene diarrea?
  Do you have diarrhea?
Ha notado sangre o mucosidad en las hecces fecales?
  Have you noticed any blood or mucus in the stools?

Chapter Summary

Information regarding the care of a patient with gastrointestinal disorders requires knowledge of the following:

- Any disruption of the processes of ingestion, absorption, or elimination is pathologic not only to the gastric system, but to other body systems and cells as well.
- Although the medical assistant working in the office of the gastroenterologist encounters many patients with disorders of the GI system, patients with gastric

disorders are commonly seen in other offices, including family practice, internal medicine, and pediatrics.
- A thorough history is essential for an accurate diagnosis of any gastrointestinal disorder.
- Assisting with various diagnostic procedures, such as colon examinations and stool testing, can also help the physician detect abnormalities in GI function.
- Patient education regarding diet and prevention of various gastric disorders is a critical aspect of the professional medical assistant's role and should be considered an ongoing process.

1. Review the preparation of the patient for an upper GI series and a barium enema. Create two handouts that include the following:

   • A description of each procedure

   • A list of reasons for the procedure

   • Preparations required to ensure reliable test results

2. Many endoscopic examinations require the patient to be in an uncomfortable and embarrassing position. How can you help alleviate the stress and anxiety?

3. Mrs. Barnes, a 43-year-old patient, was scheduled for a cholecystography at 11:00 AM today and was given all instructions and the oral contrast medium to take the morning of the examination. She calls the office at 10:30 AM and tells you that she forgot to take the dye tablets and wants to know whether she should take them now and go in for her test at the appointed time. What do you tell Mrs. Barnes?

4. Research the various surgeries used to treat obesity. In addition to the risks involved with having abdominal surgery, are there any side effects or risks with each procedure that may further affect the gastrointestinal system or other body systems?

5. Explain how a patient with gallstones can develop pancreatitis.

1. The two most common causes of stomatitis are infections with the herpes simplex virus and the fungus *Candida albicans*.

2. Gingivitis can be prevented through good oral hygiene and frequent dental care.

3. A hiatal hernia is caused by a defect in the diaphragm that lets part of the stomach slide up into the chest cavity. The stomach's cardiac sphincter and the diaphragmatic muscle tone normally prevent gastric acid reflux into the esophagus. Hiatal hernia permits the stomach acid to invade the esophagus, causing irritation.

4. *Helicobacter pylori*, or *H. pylori*, bacteria have been implicated in gastritis and some patients with peptic ulcers.

5. While the ulcerative lesions are similar in appearance and may be caused by the same factors, peptic ulcers are found on the lining of the stomach, and duodenal ulcers are in the first part of the small intestine (the duodenum).

6. Crohn's disease can lead to bowel obstruction. With each episode of inflammation, scarring may lead to narrowing of the colon and hence an obstruction.

7. Diverticulosis is believed to be caused by a diet deficient in roughage or bulk.

8. Hemorrhoids may be caused by poor abdominal and pelvic floor muscle tone, poor dietary habits including a diet low in fiber, and chronic constipation.

9. Viral hepatitis is caused by a virus; toxic hepatitis is a toxic reaction to chemical toxicants, certain medications, or alcohol.

10. Cholelithiasis is formation of stones in the gallbladder; cholecystitis is inflammation of the gallbladder, usually due to an impacted stone in the duct.

11. Complications of pancreatitis include diabetes mellitus, hemorrhage, shock, coma, and death as the digestive enzymes cause the organ to digest itself.

12. Contrast media are used to better visualize the organs of the gastrointestinal system that might not be easily seen in radiographs where contrast media are not used.

13. Anoscopy is insertion of an instrument into the rectal canal for visualization of the anus and rectum and to obtain swabs for culture. Sigmoidoscopy is visualization of the sigmoid colon using a rigid or flexible sigmoidoscope.

CHAPTER

33 Neurology

Outline

Common Nervous System Disorders
Infectious Disorders
Degenerative Disorders
Seizure Disorders
Developmental Disorders

Trauma
Brain Tumors
Headaches
Common Diagnostic Tests for Disorders of the Nervous System

Physical Examination
Radiologic Tests
Electrical Tests
Lumbar Puncture

Learning Objectives

Upon successfully completing this chapter, you will be able to:

1. Spell and define key terms

2. Identify common diseases of the nervous system

3. Describe the physical and emotional effects of degenerative nervous system disorders

4. List potential complications of a spinal cord injury

5. Name and describe the common procedures for diagnosing nervous system disorders

Performance Objectives

Upon successfully completing this chapter, you will be able to:

1. Assist with a lumbar puncture (Procedure 33-1)

CAAHEP

- Practice standard precautions
- Prepare patient for and assist with routine and specialty examinations
- Prepare patient for and assist with procedures, treatments, and minor office surgeries
- Document appropriately
- Instruct individuals according to their needs

ABHES

- Prepare patients for procedures
- Assist physician with examinations and treatments
- Document accurately

Key Terms

cephalalgia	dysphasia	meningocele	Queckenstedt test
concussion	electroencephalo-gram (EEG)	migraine	Romberg test
contusion		myelogram	seizure
convulsion	herpes zoster	myelomeningocele	spina bifida occulta
dysphagia			

Common Nervous System Disorders

The nervous system is the chief communication and command center for all parts of the body. The nervous system has two divisions: the central nervous system (CNS) and the peripheral nervous system (PNS). The CNS includes the brain and spinal cord (Fig. 33-1), and the PNS contains the nerves that transmit impulses. Nerves are found throughout the body and in the brain. The autonomic nervous system (ANS), a division of the PNS, functions without voluntary action. Together these divisions of the nervous system allow skeletal movement, maintain vital homeostatic functions such as breathing and heart rate, and promote thought processes including memory and logic. The complexity of the nervous system and its connections with the muscular system make it subject to many disorders that can be difficult to diagnose and treat effectively.

Neurology deals with study of the nervous system and its disorders, and the physician who specializes in this area is a neurologist. The medical assistant who works in a neurology office has many interesting and challenging patients. Also, the medical assistant who works in other medical specialties may also have patients with diseases or disorders of the nervous system. This chapter focuses on some of the common disorders of the nervous system and the role of the medical assistant who works with these patients.

LEGAL TIP

RISK MANAGEMENT

Risk management includes those activities performed in the medical office that may help reduce or eliminate litigation or lawsuits. A professional medical assistant can practice risk management by:

- Documenting concisely and accurately immediately following any patient encounter, either in person or on the telephone.
- Being familiar with the office policy and procedure manual and following the guidelines as written.
- Communicating clearly with patients and other health care providers while observing the laws regarding confidentiality.
- Maintaining compliance with state and federal laws with regard to filing insurance claims and billing procedures.
- Practicing within your scope of education and training.

Figure 33-1 Functional areas of the cerebral cortex. (Reprinted with permission from Cohen BJ. Memmler's The Human Body in Health and Disease. Philadelphia: Lippincott Williams & Wilkins, 2005.)

Infectious Disorders

Disorders of the nervous system range from minor inconveniences to lethal diseases. The following sections discuss the disorders in groups: infectious, degenerative, convulsive (**seizures**), developmental, traumatic, neoplastic (tumors), and headache.

Meningitis

Meningitis is characterized by inflammation of the meninges covering the spinal cord and the brain. The inflammation can result from either bacterial or viral infection. Viral meningitis is usually not life threatening and is often short lived, but bacterial meningitis is often severe and may be fatal. The infection is usually precipitated by an upper respiratory, sinus, or ear infection. Children are the age group most likely to develop meningitis. Meningitis can also result from head trauma when an open wound allows organisms to enter the cranium and nervous system.

Patients with meningitis have a variety of signs and symptoms, including nausea, vomiting, fever, headache, and a stiff neck. Patients may also complain of photophobia, or intolerance to light. A rash with small, reddish purple dots may appear on the body, and as patients become sicker, they may slip into a coma and have seizures.

To diagnose meningitis, the physician usually orders a complete blood count. If the white blood cell count is high, a lumbar puncture is performed, and cerebrospinal fluid (CSF) is sent to the laboratory for analysis to determine the infectious organism. The treatment of

meningitis depends on the organism causing the infection. The treatment for viral meningitis includes fluids and bed rest, and bacterial meningitis is treated with antibiotics and generally requires hospitalization. The local health department must be notified of the diagnosis, and some states require that an infectious disease form be filed. Check your office policy and procedure manual to determine who is responsible for obtaining, completing, and submitting these reports, keeping in mind that, in many offices, it is the medical assistant's responsibility. Depending on the type of meningitis, individuals (family, friends, co-workers, classmates) who have had contact with the patient may require prophylactic treatment.

Encephalitis

Encephalitis is an inflammation of the brain that frequently results from a viral infection following a varicella (chickenpox), measles, or mumps infection. A strain of the virus is transmitted by mosquitoes. This type is primarily seen on the East and Gulf coasts. Symptoms of all forms include drowsiness, headache, and fever. Seizures and coma may occur in later stages. Diagnosis is made via lumbar puncture and analysis of CSF.

Treatment of encephalitis requires hospitalization for intravenous fluid therapy and supportive care. The prognosis is usually good if the diagnosis is made early and treatment begins quickly. As with meningitis, the local health department should be notified to identify those who may have been exposed to the disease.

CHECKPOINT QUESTION

1. How does the treatment of viral meningitis differ from that of bacterial meningitis?

Herpes Zoster

Herpes zoster, or shingles, is caused by the virus that causes chickenpox and occurs only in those who have had a varicella infection (see Chapter 27). Herpes zoster usually occurs in adults, often in times of physical or emotional stress. The virus, which lies dormant after the initial infection, becomes reactivated and spreads down the length of a nerve, causing redness, swelling, and pain. After about 48 hours, a band of papules develops on the skin following the nerve pathway. These lesions commonly appear on the face, back, and chest and progress to vesicles, pustules, and then dry crusts similar to chickenpox lesions. The lesions may last for 2 to 5 weeks, and the patient may have pain after the lesions disappear.

The treatment of a herpes zoster breakout includes an analgesic or nerve block for pain. Calamine lotion may be applied to the skin to reduce itching. Antiviral medication, such as acyclovir, may be prescribed to alleviate the severity of the disease.

Poliomyelitis

Commonly called polio, this highly contagious and resistant virus affects the brain and spinal cord. The virus can live outside the body for several months, making it almost impossible to eliminate once it has appeared in a community. It is transmitted by direct contact, usually through the mouth. In the United States, its incidence has been greatly reduced by aggressive immunization programs. However, because not all children have received the proper schedule of immunizations and because some adults have not been immunized at all, concern about the disease still exists.

In the acute phase, the patient may complain of a stiff neck, fever, headaches, and a sore throat. Nausea, vomiting, and diarrhea may also occur. As the disease progresses, paralysis may develop. Muscle atrophy leads to eventual deformities. If the respiratory muscles are affected, the patient cannot breathe without artificial assistance.

A new dimension of the disease, postpoliomyelitis muscular atrophy (PPMA) syndrome, has been documented in some individuals who had polio as children. Many of these patients have signs and symptoms similar to those that signaled the onset of the original disease. They usually complain of muscle weakness and a lack of coordination. Typically, patients with PPMA are treated on an outpatient basis with supportive care. No cure is available.

During the acute stage of polio, treatment is palliative and supportive. After this acute stage has resolved, treatment of the patient is rehabilitation of the weakened extremities with a strong emphasis on physical and occupational therapy. To increase mobility, patients are fitted with mechanical supports such as braces and splints. Some patients must wear these devices indefinitely. Emotional support is important for these patients, particularly those with PPMA. Many need counseling to reconcile themselves to body image changes caused by the deformities and to allay fear of dependency.

Activities aimed at preventing polio are essential. You may be responsible for patient education regarding immunizations and keeping them current. The previously used oral polio vaccine contained a weakened form of the polio virus, but today's newer injectable form does not contain a live or weakened form of the virus. In the oral form, the virus could be shed in the stool of the immunized child, and caretakers who were not immunized could contract the disease. This is not possible with the newer form of the vaccine.

Tetanus

Tetanus, commonly called lockjaw, is an infection of nervous tissue caused by the tetanus bacillus, *Clostridium tetani*, which lives in the intestinal tract of animals and is excreted in their feces. The microorganism is also found in almost all soil. An infection occurs after the microbe enters the body through an open wound in the skin, often a puncture wound. Wounds caused by farm equipment involving manure are especially susceptible to a tetanus infection. All deep, dirty wounds should be treated as high risk for tetanus.

Tetanus has a slow incubation period. It may inhabit the body for up to 14 weeks before signs and symptoms appear. Initial symptoms include spasms of the voluntary muscles, restlessness, and stiff neck. As the disease progresses, seizures and **dysphagia** (difficulty swallowing) develop. The facial and oral muscles contract, leaving the mouth sealed with the teeth clenched tightly. Untreated, the respiratory muscles become paralyzed, and the disease is typically fatal.

Prevention is the best defense against tetanus. Wounds should be properly cleaned immediately. Dead tissue around the wound must be removed, and an antibiotic should be given if the wound appears infected. To obtain immunity early in life, immunizations are administered to infants and children on a schedule determined by the American Academy of Pediatrics and the Centers for Disease Control and Prevention. After the initial immunization schedule is complete, the vaccine must be given every 10 years for life. Patients who develop an infection with the tetanus microbe require immediate hospitalization and aggressive antibiotic therapy. The prognosis is guarded when tetanus has fully developed.

CHECKPOINT QUESTION

2. What are the initial signs of a tetanus infection?

Rabies

Rabies is caused by a virus that is commonly transmitted by animal saliva through a bite wound from an infected animal and spreads to the organs of the central nervous system. Animals that commonly transmit rabies are skunks, squirrels, raccoons, bats, dogs, cats, coyotes, and foxes. Children are at highest risk for rabies because they are most likely to be bitten by such animals.

The incubation period for rabies ranges from 10 days to many months, depending on the location of the bite. Initial symptoms include fever, general malaise, and body aches. As the disease progresses, mental derangement, paralysis, and photophobia develop. The patient's saliva becomes extremely profuse and sticky, and the throat muscles begin to spasm, making swallowing difficult or impossible, which causes profuse drooling. Muscle spasms of the throat occur at the sight of water or when attempting to drink water, resulting in hydrophobia. The progressive involvement of the tissues of the brain is often fatal.

Immediate treatment of a wound caused by an animal must be the first priority. After the wound is cleansed, the patient should receive an antibiotic and prophylactic vaccine therapy consisting of the human diploid cell vaccine and a rabies immune globulin vaccine. All animal bites must be reported to the city or county animal control center, and you may be responsible for completing and submitting the report. If possible, the animal should be quarantined and evaluated for behavioral changes. If the animal is domestic, a complete veterinary history must be obtained. A copy of the animal's rabies tag and certificate, if available, should be placed in the patient's chart.

Reye's Syndrome

Reye's syndrome, a devastating nervous system illness, typically occurs in children after a viral illness, commonly varicella (chickenpox). Studies have found that the use of aspirin in the presence of a viral illness increases the risk of developing Reye's syndrome. No other antipyretic agents have been implicated in this disorder. Reye's syndrome is not contagious.

While this disorder can affect all organs of the body, it most often affects the liver and the brain. Initial symptoms include vomiting and lethargy, and as the brain swelling continues, confusion, seizures, and coma may develop quickly. The signs and symptoms of Reye's syndrome should be treated as a medical emergency because early diagnosis and treatment increase the chances of recovering. The prognosis depends on the amount and severity of cerebral edema. Diagnosis is made by obtaining blood samples to determine liver function, including ammonia, aspartate aminotransferase, and alanine aminotransferase levels. Patients with Reye's syndrome require rapid hospitalization, aggressive antibiotic therapy to prevent secondary bacterial infection, and supportive care.

Degenerative Disorders
Multiple Sclerosis

The cause of multiple sclerosis (MS) is unknown, but possible origins include a viral infection, autoimmunity, immunologic response, and genetic predisposition. In MS, the myelin sheaths covering many neurons in the body degenerate and are replaced with plaque, which impairs nerve impulse conduction. Multiple sclerosis most commonly occurs in women aged 20 to 40 and is characterized by remissions and exacerbations. While there is no cure, the rate and severity of progression vary greatly among patients.

Typically, patients complain initially of progressive loss of muscle control. They may also complain of loss of balance, shaking tremors, and poor muscle coordination. Tingling and numbness can also be first signs of the disease. **Dysphasia** (difficulty speaking) may be another sign. As the disease progresses, bladder dysfunction and complaints of visual disturbances are common. Patients may also develop nystagmus (involuntary rapid movement of the eyeball in all directions).

Treatment of MS is palliative. Physical therapy is critical to limit the extent of muscle deterioration and to maintain existing muscle strength. As the disease progresses, the patient is often fitted for prosthetic appliances such as crutches to assist with mobility. Drug therapy includes muscle relaxants and steroids. Because this disease affects persons in the prime of life, patients with MS and their families require psychological support from all of their regular health care providers. Many support groups and counselors specialize in providing therapy for persons with debilitating diseases, including MS, and this information should be shared with patients and families as appropriate.

Amyotrophic Lateral Sclerosis

Commonly known as Lou Gehrig's disease, amyotrophic lateral sclerosis (ALS) causes a progressive loss of motor neurons. ALS is a terminal disease with no known cause, but a strong familial connection has been observed. It occurs most often in middle-aged men. It begins with loss of muscle mobility in the forearms, hands, and legs and then progresses to the facial muscles, causing dysphasia and dysphagia that worsen over time. Death usually occurs 3 to 5 years after the onset of symptoms.

Treatment of ALS consists of keeping the patient comfortable and educating the family. As the disease progresses, it becomes increasingly difficult for the patient to maintain an unobstructed airway. The family must be taught to prevent and manage choking. Often, the physician discusses advance directives, or end-of-life requests, with the family and the patient. Ideally, the medical assistant will be present for these discussions to provide emotional support.

Parkinson's Disease

This disease is most often seen in the elderly; however, it may begin in middle adulthood. Because the disease is a neurologic disorder affecting specific neurotransmitters, or chemicals, in the brain, the symptoms appear gradually and cause a decrease in muscle control. Common symptoms of this disease include rigid muscles, involuntary tremors, and difficulty walking. For more information about Parkinson's disease, refer to Chapter 38, Geriatrics.

 CHECKPOINT QUESTION

3. Should health care professionals worry that multiple sclerosis is contagious?

Seizure Disorders

Seizures, commonly called **convulsions**, are involuntary contractions of voluntary muscles caused by a rapid succession of electrical impulses through the brain. Seizures have many causes, including chemical imbalance, trauma, pregnancy-induced hypertension, tumor, and withdrawal from drugs or alcohol. However, many seizures are idiopathic (have no known cause).

Epilepsy is the most common form of seizure disorder. Epilepsy may appear in early childhood or at any life stage. Diagnosis is made through **electroencephalogram (EEG)** studies, blood tests, and radiologic tests. Epileptic seizures are characterized as either petit mal or grand mal. Petit mal seizures, also called absence seizures or partial seizures, are briefer than grand mal seizures and usually occur only in childhood. The child may appear to fall asleep or drift away momentarily. Some muscle twitching may occur. Then the child awakes and continues the interrupted

activity. Petit mal seizures may go undetected for many years.

Grand mal seizures, also called tonic-clonic seizures, are more involved than petit mal seizures. Generally, the patient will go through three phases:

1. The first phase is an aura, or warning that a seizure is impending. The aura may include tingling in the extremities, visual signs (such as flashing lights), or perception of a particular taste or odor. Not all patients have auras, but those who do usually perceive the same aural phenomena each time.
2. The second phase is complete loss of consciousness with extensive muscle twitching or contractions, which may be violent. The patient falls and usually loses control of bladder and bowel functions.
3. The third phase is the postictal phase. The patient slowly regains consciousness but remains drowsy for an extended time.

The primary treatment during the actual seizure is preventing injury to the patient (see Chapter 26). Epilepsy is treated with various pharmacologic agents that must be taken by the patient regularly to prevent seizure activity. Instruct patients to take their medication every day as prescribed by the physician, never missing a dose. Many epileptic patients who become stabilized and seizure free on medication decide they no longer need the medication. Remind these patients that stopping the medication may lead to the recurrence of seizures.

A patient who has seizures is usually permitted to have a driver's license, but each state has specific regulations requiring that patients be seizure free for a particular length of time. The patient may ask the physician to complete paperwork from the state issuing the driver's license, and you may be asked to assist with completion of these forms.

Febrile Seizures

Febrile (fever) seizures occur in a small number of children, most commonly aged 6 months to 3 years, with an elevated body temperature. Children with febrile seizures must have a complete physical and neurologic examination to rule out the possibility of organic origin of the seizures. Typically, children generally outgrow febrile seizures by age 6 or 7 and have no further seizure activity.

Treatment is gently returning the child's body temperature to a more manageable level. Cool compresses are preferable to ice baths or alcohol sponge baths, which may cause hypothermia. Because of the danger of Reye's syndrome, these children should not be given salicylates, or products containing aspirin, to reduce the temperature.

WHAT IF?

What if the mother of a 2-year-old child who recently had a febrile seizure tells you that she is scared that the child will have another seizure and that it will cause brain damage?

Because febrile seizures can be very scary for parents of small children, you can help them cope with these measures by doing the following:

- Reassure the parents that febrile seizures are common in young children and that they generally are not chronic.
- Allow the parents to be involved in the care of the child. If a seizure occurs in the medical office, urge the parents to hold and comfort the child after the seizure has subsided and the physician has evaluated the child.
- Provide easy-to-understand explanations for all procedures.
- Encourage parents to talk about their fears.
- Remain calm and demonstrate confidence in handling the situation.

Focal, or Jacksonian, Seizures

A focal seizure begins as a small local seizure that spreads to adjacent areas. For instance, the small seizure may begin in the fingers and spread to the hand and arm. The cause of focal seizures must be researched to prevent the progression to general seizures.

CHECKPOINT QUESTION

4. How do petit mal seizures differ from grand mal seizures?

Developmental Disorders
Neural Tube Defects

Many abnormalities may occur during the embryonic and fetal stages of development. As the embryo develops, the tissue over the neural tube (a tube-like section of the developing embryo) closes and evolves into the components of the CNS. If a developmental failure occurs on the proximal (upper) portion, anencephaly, or the absence of a brain, may result. An abnormality in development in the distal, or caudal, end of the neural tube results in spina bifida. **Spina bifida occulta** is the most benign form. In this condition, the posterior laminae of the vertebrae fail to close, typically at L-5 or S-1. There are usually no external signs of deformity, although there may be a skin dimple or dark tufts of hair over this area on the lower back. A **meningocele** occurs when the meninges protrude through the spina bifida. In spina bifida with **myelomeningocele**, the most severe form, the spinal cord and meninges protrude externally (Fig. 33-2). The main treatment is surgical intervention; prognosis is based on the extent of spinal cord involvement.

PATIENT EDUCATION
ALPHA-FETOPROTEIN

This blood test is routinely performed during the second trimester (weeks 16 to 18) of pregnancy to check for maternal serum levels of alpha-fetoprotein (AFP) and screen the fetus for defects in the neural tube. If this protein is found to be high, there may be nervous system disorders in the fetus such as spina bifida, whereas low levels may indicate trisomy 13 or Down syndrome. Because abnormal results may occur due to more than one fetus or incorrect due dates, high or low results indicate the need for further studies such as sonography or amniocentesis before a definitive diagnosis is made.

Hydrocephalus

Hydrocephalus occurs when the arachnoid and ventricular spaces of the brain contain excessive CSF. Although it occurs most commonly in infants and children as the result of a defect in CSF production or absorption, hydrocephalus sometimes occurs in adults as a result of tumor or trauma. Treatment is surgical insertion of a shunt, which reroutes the excessive CSF from the brain to the right atrium of the heart or the peritoneal cavity. The prognosis is usually good if hydrocephalus is treated aggressively in the early stages, before CNS damage.

Cerebral Palsy

Cerebral palsy describes a group of neuromuscular disorders that result from CNS damage during the prenatal, neonatal, or postnatal period. Although cerebral palsy is not progressive, the damage may become more obvious as developmental delays are discovered. Impairment may range from slight motor dysfunction to catastrophic physical and mental disabilities. Prognosis varies with the site of the damage and its severity. Treatment is supportive and rehabilitative. No cure exists.

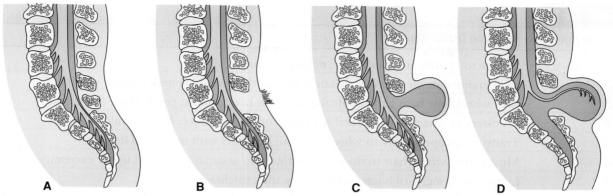

Figure 33-2 Spinal defects. (**A**) Normal spinal cord. (**B**) Spina bifida occulta. (**C**) Meningocele. (**D**) Meningomyelocele. (Reprinted with permission from Pillitteri A. Maternal and Child Health Nursing: Care of the Childbearing and Childrearing Family. 5th ed. Philadelphia: Lippincott Williams & Wilkins, 2007.)

 CHECKPOINT QUESTION

5. What is spina bifida, and how does it develop?

Trauma

Traumatic injuries are the most common causes of neurologic disorders and the leading killer of individuals aged 1 to 24 years. The trauma often is a preventable injury to the head that causes edema in the brain tissue or blows to the posterior neck and back, injuring the spinal cord. You can help prevent these types of injuries and the life-long impairments that accompany permanent damage to the CNS by encouraging parents to require their children to wear a helmet when bicycle riding, skating, skateboarding, and riding in a motor vehicle. Head trauma sustained in a motor vehicle accident often results from the passengers being tossed around the interior of the car or worse yet, ejected from the vehicle. Inexperienced teenage drivers should also be asked about the use of seat belts not just for themselves, but for their passengers as well.

Traumatic Brain Injuries

Children are at particularly high risk for head trauma. A child's head is large in proportion to the rest of the body; therefore, when children fall (as they frequently do), they often fall head first. Children are also prone to traumatic injuries because their reflex systems are immature. Traumatic injuries to the brain include **concussion, contusion,** and intracranial hemorrhage. A concussion is a nonlethal brain injury that results from blunt trauma. The patient may momentarily lose consciousness but promptly return to an awake and alert state. The treatment for concussion is rest and observation for signs of a more serious injury, contusion. A contusion is a focal alteration of cerebral circulation. Hemorrhages and ex-travasation, or pooling, of blood and fluid can result. Loss of consciousness results, and brain damage may occur. The patient may become confused and lethargic and have nausea and vomiting as the intracranial bleeding increases, causing pressure on the brain. Intracranial hemorrhage is bleeding of a vessel inside the skull due to trauma, congenital abnormality, or aneurysm.

Traumatic brain injuries are diagnosed with radiographic studies. Treatment for contusions and hemorrhages can be surgery, drug therapy, and supportive care. The prognosis for all brain injuries depends on the extent of damage and the location of the injury.

Spinal Cord Injuries

Spinal cord injuries are most common among individuals 15 to 35 years of age. Most spinal cord injuries are due to trauma from a motor vehicle accident, diving accident, or fall. A complete spinal cord injury is one in which the cord is transected and no neurologic abilities remain below the point of injury. An incomplete spinal cord injury is one in which the cord is injured or partially severed, causing minor to severe disability below the point of injury (Table 33-1). The higher in the spinal cord the injury is, the more serious the complications and paralysis for the patient. Table 33-2 describes the types of paralysis that a patient may have and the typical causes of each type.

In caring for patients who may have a spinal cord injury, the initial consideration is to prevent further damage. Accident victims with suspected spinal cord injuries must be kept immobile until proper emergency medical service personnel are present. Treatment in the emergency department is focused on stabilization, and patients usually require an extended hospitalization and rehabilitation, depending on the extent of the damage to the spinal cord.

In the physician's office, recovering trauma patients may receive follow-up treatment and evaluation. These

TABLE 33-1 | Spinal Cord Injuries

Level of Injury	Resulting Disabilities
C-1, C-2	Unable to breathe independently; no neck muscle control
C-3, C-4	May manipulate electric wheelchair with mouthpiece; some neck control possible
C-5	Uses wheelchair with hand controls; eats with hand splints; good elbow flexion
C-6	Transfers to wheelchair and bed with little or no assistance; good shoulder control
C-7	Transfers independently to wheelchair and bed; eats with no special devices
T-1, T-4	Moves from wheelchair to floor with little or no assistance; normal upper extremity function
T-5, L-2	Limited walking with bilateral leg braces and crutches
L-3, L-4	Walks with short leg braces with or without crutches
L-5, S-3	Walks independently with no equipment if foot strength is good

C = Cervical; L = Lumbar; S = Sacral; T = Thoracic.

patients are monitored for changes in their reflexes and evaluated for physical therapy and occupational therapy. The goal of long-term care is to prevent complications, which can include skin ulcerations (pressure ulcers), hypostatic pneumonia, bladder infection, muscle contractures, and psychological depression. Most of the physical complications are treated with physical therapy and good care either in the home or in the long-term rehabilitation facility. The mental and emotional complications require intensive therapy by counselors who specialize in treating patients with debilitating disorders.

 CHECKPOINT QUESTION

6. How does a complete spinal cord injury differ from an incomplete one?

Brain Tumors

A brain tumor may be either malignant or benign and may be a secondary or metastatic site. If the brain tumor is the primary site, it is named for the site of origin (e.g., glioma, meningioma, medulloblastoma). Both malignant and benign tumors can produce serious complica-

 PATIENT EDUCATION

SPINAL CORD AND TRAUMATIC BRAIN INJURIES

Spinal cord and traumatic brain injuries are common in young people. Both types of injuries can produce serious and even fatal results. As a medical assistant, you must take an active role in educating your community, patients, and friends about prevention of these injuries:

- Use seat belts in automobiles for all passengers.
- Secure infants and young children in approved car seats.
- Avoid alcohol when participating in sporting activities and driving.
- Obey traffic signs and speed limits.
- Avoid illicit drug use and any medication that impairs awareness.
- Wear a helmet while bicycling and riding a motorcycle.
- Never dive head first into water that is shallow or unclear.

TABLE 33-2 | Types of Paralysis

Type	Causes	Result
Hemiplegia	Cerebrovascular accident; trauma to one side of brain; tumors	Paralysis on one side of body, opposite the side of involvement
Paraplegia	Spinal cord trauma; spinal tumors	Paralysis of any part of the body below the point of involvement
Quadriplegia	Spinal cord trauma; spinal tumors	Paralysis of all limbs (usually cervical or high thoracic vertebra involvement)

tions for the patient because of the limited space inside the cranium. Generally, the patient has vague complaints of headaches, blurred vision, personality changes, or memory loss. In more advanced cases, seizures, blindness, and dysphagia may be evident. The type of tumor and its location affect the presenting symptoms, their severity and onset, and the prognosis.

Diagnosis is made primarily with radiologic studies. The treatment can include surgery, radiation therapy, chemotherapy, or a combination of radiation and chemotherapy.

Headaches

It is estimated that 70% of the population has **cephalagia**, or headaches. Headaches have a variety of origins, including stress, trauma, bone pathology, infection (e.g., sinus), or vascular disturbance. In many instances, the cause is never known.

Migraine headaches are one of the most common types. Migraine can be triggered by stress, high altitude, smoking, certain smells, or ingested chemicals (caffeine, alcohol, certain food additives), but in many situations, the cause is unknown. Many patients who have migraines have an aura, or sensory perception such as flashing lights or wavy lines, before onset. Once the migraine headache begins, the symptoms usually include a unilateral temporal headache, photophobia, diplopia (double vision), and nausea. Generally these headaches are treated with an analgesic, and the patient may be instructed to rest in a dark, quiet room. The physician may also prescribe medication to arrest the headache and symptoms when the migraine begins. These medications, sometimes called abortive headache medications, include the triptans (sumatriptan succinate [Imitrex] and naratriptan hydrochloride [Amerge]) or ergotamines (ergotamine titrate with caffeine [Cafergot] or dihydroergotamine mesylate [Migranal]).

Other common types of headaches include:

- *Tension headaches* are associated with contraction of the muscles of the neck and scalp due to stress. The treatment is a muscle relaxant, analgesic, and reversing the precipitating factors. Biofeedback techniques may also be useful to assist with coping with stress that cannot be avoided.
- *Cluster headaches* are similar to migraine headaches but typically occur at night. They are usually short lasting but may recur as often as 4 or 5 times a night for several weeks and then not again for weeks or months. Treatment is a muscle relaxant, analgesic, and stress relief techniques.

 CHECKPOINT QUESTION

7. What are some triggers for migraine headaches?

Common Diagnostic Tests for Disorders of the Nervous System

The physician may perform a variety of tests to evaluate a patient's neurologic status. These tests may be invasive or noninvasive and may include radiologic and electrical tests along with physical examination.

Physical Examination

The physical examination, a key component of diagnosis of nervous system disorders, includes the following evaluations:

- Mental status and orientation
- Cranial nerve assessment
- Sensory and motor functions
- Reflex assessment

The patient's mental status is evaluated by routine questioning to establish mental alertness and orientation. For example, the examiner may ask the patient to count to 10 and to state the president's name and the year.

Cranial nerves are assessed according to the methods described in Table 33-3. Visual acuity may be tested on a chart such as the Snellen eye chart, and the results can indicate a refractive error or a more serious neurologic disorder. Sensory function is tested with the pin versus soft brush method for spinal nerves and cranial nerves. The instrument commonly used is the Buck neurologic hammer (Fig. 33-3). With the patient's eyes closed, the physician uses the pin and brush to determine the patient's ability to distinguish between sensations. The physician evaluates sensory reception and determines whether there is a reception difference on either side of the body.

Motor functioning is tested by watching the patient walk. Many disorders can be detected by observing a patient's gait. Part of this assessment includes the **Romberg test**. The patient is asked to stand with feet together and with the eyes closed. A positive Romberg sign is noted if the patient sways or is unsteady.

The last part of the examination is reflex testing (Table 33-4). Figure 33-4 depicts the correct method for tendon reflex testing. Reflexes are scored on the following scale:

0 = No response
1+ = Diminished response
2+ = Normal
3+ = Brisker than normal
4+ = Hyperactive with clonus, which is the repetitive jerking of a muscle and indicates a neurologic disorder

Patients with weak or slow responses to stimuli applied during reflex testing may require additional testing

TABLE 33-3	Cranial Nerves and Assessment		
Nerve (Number)	**Type**	**Functions**	**Examination Methods**
Olfactory (I)	Sensory	Smell	Test each nostril for smell reception, interpretation
Optic (II)	Sensory	Vision	Test vision for acuity, visual fields
Oculomotor (III)	Motor	Pupil constriction, raise eyelids	Test papillary reaction to light, ability to open and close eyes
Trochlear (IV)	Motor	Downward, inward eye movement	Test for downward, inward eye movement
Trigeminal (V)	Motor	Jaw movements, chewing, mastication	Ask patient to open and clench jaws while palpating the jaw muscles
	Sensory	Sensation on face, neck	Test face and neck for pain sensations, light touch, temperature
Abducens (VI)	Motor	Lateral movement of eyes	Test ocular movement in all directions
Facial (VII)	Motor	Muscles of face	Ask patient to raise eyebrows, smile, show teeth, puff out cheeks
	Sensory	Sense of taste on anterior two-thirds of tongue	Test for taste sensation with various agents
Acoustic (VIII)	Sensory	Hearing	Test hearing ability
Glossopharyngeal (IX)	Motor	Pharyngeal movement and swallowing	Ask patient to say "ah," yawn to observe upward movement of soft palate; elicit gag response; note ability to swallow
	Sensory	Taste on lower third of tongue	Test for taste with various agents
Vagus (X)	Motor	Swallowing, speaking	Ask patient to swallow, speak; note hoarseness
Accessory (XI)	Motor	Movement of shoulder muscles	Ask patient to shrug against resistance
Hypoglossal (XII)	Motor	Movement, strength of tongue	Ask patient to protrude tongue, push tongue against cheek

to determine the source of the problem. Since the muscles require electrical impulses from the nervous system to contract, the physician must determine whether the

problem is with the muscles or if there is a disorder of the nervous system.

Radiologic Tests

The most common noninvasive radiologic tests include computed tomography (CT) and magnetic resonance imaging (MRI). These tests may be done with a contrast medium or dye. The contrast medium helps differentiate between the soft tissue areas of the nervous system and the tumors, lesions, or hemorrhages that may blend in with their supporting tissues.

A **myelogram** is an invasive radiologic test in which dye is injected into the cerebrospinal fluid. After the dye is injected, the spinal cord is filmed, and any abnormalities, such as tumors or damage from injury, can be detected. The blood vessels of the brain can be visualized

Figure 33-3 The Buck neurologic hammer.

TABLE 33-4	Reflex Testing		
Reflex	Method of Testing	Expected Response	Location
Brachioradialis	Tap styloid process of radius	Flexion of elbow	C-5, C-6
Biceps	Tap biceps tendon	Flexion of elbow	C-5, C-6
Triceps	Tap triceps	Extension of elbow	C-7
Patellar	Tap patellar tendon	Extension of leg	L-2, L-4
Achilles	Tap Achilles tendon	Plantarflexion of foot	S-1
Corneal	Light touch on corneoscleral corner	Closure of eyelid	CN V, VII

on radiographic film by injecting dye through a femoral artery catheter threaded up to the carotid artery in a test called cerebral angiogram.

Radiography of the skull may be used to rule out many possible disorders and is diagnostic for fractures.

Electrical Tests

The EEG is a noninvasive test that records electrical impulses in the brain. A variety of electrodes are placed on the patient's scalp, and tracings of brain wave activity are recorded. Typically, the patient is given a mild sedative to induce a quiet state. This test is used to assess hyperactive electrical responses in the brain as seen in patients with seizure disorders. In the inpatient acute care setting, EEG is used to determine brain activity in patients who are on life support but who may be brain dead and have no chance for recovery.

 CHECKPOINT QUESTION

8. What are the differences between a myelogram and an EEG?

Lumbar Puncture

A lumbar puncture is used to diagnose infectious inflammatory or bleeding disorders affecting the brain and spinal cord or as a means of injecting pain control medication into the spinal column near the nerves producing the pain. A needle is inserted into the subarachnoid space at L-4 to L-5, below the level of the spinal cord (Fig. 33-5). If CSF is removed and sent to the laboratory, it may be tested for glucose, protein, bacteria, cell counts, and red blood cells, which indicate intracranial bleeding. It may also be performed to evaluate intracranial pressure. An obstruction to CSF flow can be determined with the **Queckenstedt test**. For this test, you will be directed to press against the patient's jugular veins in the neck (right, left, or both) while the physician monitors the pressure of CSF. If CSF pressure increases when the jugular vein is compressed, the finding is normal. If no increase in pressure occurs, the flow of CSF is blocked.

If a lumbar puncture is performed in the medical office, your responsibility includes assisting the patient into a side-lying curled position or a supported forward-bending sitting position and maintaining sterility of the

Figure 33-4 Techniques for eliciting major tendon reflexes. (**A**) Biceps reflex. (**B**) Triceps reflex. (**C**) Patellar reflex. (**D**) Ankle or Achilles reflex.

Third lumbar vertebra

Dura mater

Subarachnoid space

Cauda equina

Figure 33-5 Technique for lumbar puncture. The L-3 to L-5 spaces are just below the line connecting the anterior and superior iliac spines. (Taylor C, Lillis CA, LeMone P. Fundamentals of Nursing. 2nd ed. Philadelphia: Lippincott, 1993:543.)

items used during the puncture (see Chapter 22). The physical position is uncomfortable and difficult to maintain, and you should help the patient to relax as much as possible by encouraging slow, deep breathing during the procedure. The steps for assisting the physician with a lumbar puncture are described in Procedure 33-1.

If CSF has been removed, the physician may require that the patient lie flat for 6 to 12 hours to prevent a spinal headache. In addition, the patient may require intravenous fluid and pain medication. For these reasons, the lumbar puncture is more commonly performed in outpatient clinics than in the medical office.

TRIAGE

While you are working in a medical office, the following three situations occur at the same time:

A. Patient A is a 35-year-old woman who came to the office with a severe migraine. She is sitting in the darkened examination room with an emesis basin because she has been nauseated and vomiting this morning. The physician has ordered an injection of sumatriptan succinate (Imitrex).

B. Patient B is a 46-year-old patient who came to the office for an injection of anesthetic into the spinal column to relieve chronic pain caused by an injury that occurred on the job 2 years ago.

C. Patient C is phoning about a bill received after an office visit last month. The patient is angry and demanding to speak to the physician immediately.

How do you sort these patients? Who do you see first? Second? Third?

Patient C should quickly be referred to the office manager or billing supervisor in a calm and professional manner. In most offices, the clinical medical assistant does not have enough information about the patient's account to determine the nature of the problem. Next, patient A should be given the injection and allowed to remain in the examination room until the medication has taken effect or she feels able to leave. While she is resting in the quiet, darkened room after the injection, you can prepare patient B and the treatment room.

español SPANISH TERMINOLOGY

Es buena su memoria?
  Is your memory good?
Le duele la cabezo?
  Have you any pain in the head?
Tiene usted vértigo?
  Do you feel dizzy?
Voltese a su lado izquierdo (derecho).
  Turn on your left (or right) side.

MEDIA MENU

- **Student CD**
  - **CMA/RMA Certification Exam Review**
- **Premium Online Course**
  http://thePoint.lww.com/Kronenberger3e
- **Internet Resources**

LiveAdvise Online Tutoring & Competency Training
http://thePoint.lww.com/LiveAdvise

Centers for Disease Control and Prevention
www.cdc.gov/ncidod/dvrd/rabies/

National Reye's Syndrome Foundation
www.reyessyndrome.org

National Institutes of Health
www.nlm.nih.gov/medlineplus/seizures.html

www.nlm.nih.gov/medlineplus/cerebralpalsy.html

North Pacific Epilepsy Research
www.seizures.net

Association for Spina Bifida and Hydrocephalus
www.asbah.org

Spina Bifida Association of America
www.sbaa.org

National Multiple Sclerosis Society
www.nationalmssociety.org

Amyotrophic Lateral Sclerosis Association
www.alsa.org

American Spinal Injury Association
www.asia-spinalinjury.org

PROCEDURE 33-1: Assisting With a Lumbar Puncture

Purpose: To prepare and assist the physician during a lumbar puncture

Equipment: Sterile and clean exam gloves, 3- to 5-inch lumbar needle with stylet (physician will specify gauge and length), sterile gauze sponges, sterile specimen container, local anesthetic and syringe, needle, adhesive bandages, fenestrated drape, sterile drape, antiseptic, skin preparation supplies (razor), biohazard sharps container, biohazard waste container

Steps	Purpose
1. Wash your hands.	Handwashing aids infection control.
2. Assemble the equipment, identify the patient, and explain the procedure.	Identifying the patient helps prevent errors in treatment. Explaining the procedure helps ease anxiety.
3. Check that the consent form is signed and in the chart. Warn the patient not to move during the procedure. Tell the patient that the area will be numb but pressure may still be felt after the local anesthetic is administered.	Because this is an invasive procedure, informed consent should be obtained and the form kept in the chart. Although there is little chance of damage to the spinal cord, movement may injure the patient and will probably contaminate the field.
4. Have the patient void. Direct the patient to disrobe and put on a gown with the opening in the back.	Emptying the bladder will decrease discomfort during the procedure. The back must be exposed for the procedure.
5. Prepare the skin unless this is to be done with sterile preparation. If the physician prefers to prepare the skin using sterile forceps after gloving, you may have to add sterile solution to the field. Assist as needed with administration of the anesthetic.	Before beginning, assess the lumbar region. If the site is hairy, it may be necessary to shave the skin before the procedure. Strict medical and surgical asepsis must be observed to reduce the risk of introducing microorganisms into the nervous system.

(continued)

PROCEDURE 33-1: **Assisting With a Lumbar Puncture** *(continued)*

Steps	Reasons
6. When the physician is ready, prepare the sterile field and assist with the initial preparations. Assist the patient into the appropriate position. A. For the side-lying position, stand in front of the patient and help by holding the patient's knees and top shoulder. Ask the patient to move so the back is close to the edge of the table.	These positions widen the space between the vertebrae to allow entrance of the needle. Your presence will help ensure that the patient does not move.

Step 6: The patient should be lying on the side with the knees drawn up, the head and neck down, and the back curled as much as possible.

Steps	Reasons
B. For the forward-leaning, supported position, stand in front of the patient and rest your hands on the shoulders as a reminder to remain still. Ask the patient to breathe slowly and deeply.	
7. Throughout the procedure, observe the patient closely for signs such as dyspnea or cyanosis. Monitor the pulse at intervals and record the vital signs after the procedure. Note the patient's mental alertness and any leakage at the site, nausea, or vomiting. Assess lower limb mobility. Assist the physician as necessary.	When the physician has the needle securely in place, the physician may ask you to help the patient to straighten slightly to ease tension and to allow a normal CSF flow.
8. If specimens are to be taken, put on gloves to receive the potentially hazardous body fluid. Label the tubes in sequence as you receive them. Label them also with the patient's identification and place them in biohazard bags.	Standard precautions must be followed.
9. If the Queckenstedt test is to be performed, you may be required to press against the patient's jugular veins in the neck (right, left, or both) while the physician monitors the pressure of CSF.	Normally, the pressure of CSF will rise and drop rapidly as the veins in the neck are compressed. If an obstruction is present, the rise and return to normal may be slow, or there may be no response to the external application of pressure.

(continued)

PROCEDURE 33-1:	Assisting With a Lumbar Puncture *(continued)*

Steps	Reasons
10. At the completion of the procedure, cover the site with an adhesive bandage and assist the patient to a flat position. The physician will determine when the patient is ready to leave the examining room and the office.	Some patients have headache after the procedure and must be monitored carefully during the recovery period.
11. Route the specimens as required. Clean the examination room and care for or dispose of the equi	Standard precautions must be followed throughout the procedure.

Charting Example:

02/12/08 8:30 AM *Patient positioned and draped for lumbar puncture. VS 120/80 (R), 86, 18. LP per formed by Dr. Alexander*

—B. Ryan, CMA

9:00 AM *LP complete. Pt. tolerated procedure well. CSF specimen to lab. Post LP VS 114/74 (R) 76, 16*

—B. Ryan, CMA

9:30 AM *Pt. denies discomfort. No n/v. No leakage at LP site. Bandage clean and dry. Pt and wife given discharge instructions. Verbalized understanding. Pt d/c per Dr. Alexander*

B. Ryan, CMA

Chapter Summary

- The nervous system is complex and works with both conscious and unconscious functions. Disorders of the nervous system can be grouped into several types:
  - Infectious
  - Degenerative
  - Convulsive
  - Developmental
  - Traumatic
  - Neoplastic
  - Headache
- Common diagnostic tests include:
  - Radiologic studies (e.g., CT, MRI)
  - EEG
  - Physical examination
  - Prenatal screening
  - Lumbar puncture
  - Radiography
- Your responsibilities when working with patients with neurologic disorders may include:
  - Assisting the physician with the neurologic examination
  - Scheduling patients for outpatient procedures
  - Providing emotional support to patients and their families or caregivers

1. Research and prepare a patient education fact sheet about migraine headaches, including the possible triggers, the causes, and the treatments (include abortive headache medications).

2. A 3-year-old girl comes to the office with varicella zoster (chickenpox). She has a fever, and the physician orders acetaminophen. The child's mother asks, "Why can't she have aspirin instead?" How do you respond?

3. Your patient, a 21-year-old man, was in a motor vehicle accident last year, and a spinal cord injury left him paraplegic. Explain how this injury has most likely affected his life, not just physically but emotionally and psychologically. How do you han-

dle any anger or apathy directed at you or the physician?

4. Prepare a presentation for a preschool class on safety, including riding bicycles or riding other toys outside, wearing helmets, and the importance of being in a booster seat while wearing a seatbelt in the car.

5. With cooperation from your instructor, schedule a presentation from a professional at the local health district to discuss communicable diseases such as meningitis and rabies in your community. What questions would you ask about diseases that affect the nervous system?

Answers to Checkpoint Questions

1. Viral meningitis is treated with fluids and bed rest, and bacterial meningitis requires antibiotic medication and hospitalization.

2. The initial symptoms of a tetanus infection include spasms of the voluntary muscles, restlessness, and a stiff neck.

3. MS results from the destruction of the myelin sheath that covers nerve cells by the patient's body. This is not a contagious disease.

4. Petit mal seizures are briefer than grand mal seizures. Grand mal seizures are more extensive than petit mal seizures and have three phases: an aura, or warning, of an impending seizure; complete loss of consciousness; and the postictal phase, during which the patient slowly regains consciousness.

5. Spina bifida results from an abnormality in the development of the distal end of the neural tube of the developing embryo.

6. A complete spinal cord injury is total transection of the spinal cord, with no neurologic abilities remaining below the point of injury. An incomplete spinal cord injury is one in which the cord is not completely severed, with minor to severe neurologic disabilities below the point of injury.

7. Although the cause may be unknown, some migraine headaches can be triggered by stress, high altitude, smoking, certain smells, or ingested chemicals (e.g., caffeine, alcohol, certain food additives).

8. An EEG is a noninvasive electrical test of brain waves. A myelogram is an invasive radiologic test in which dye is injected into the CSF to help detect abnormalities.

Outline

Common Urinary Disorders
Renal Failure
Calculi
Tumors
Hydronephrosis
Urinary System Infections
**Common Disorders of the
Male Reproductive System**
Benign Prostatic Hyperplasia
Prostate Cancer

Testicular Cancer
Hydrocele
Cryptorchidism
Inguinal Hernia
Infections
Impotence
**Common Diagnostic and
Therapeutic Procedures**
Urinalysis
Blood Tests

Cystoscopy or
    Cystourethroscopy
Intravenous Pyelogram and
    Retrograde Pyelogram
Ultrasound
Rectal and Scrotal
    Examinations
Vasectomy

Learning Objectives

Upon successfully completing this chapter, you will be able to:

1. Spell and define key terms

2. List and describe the disorders of the urinary system and the male reproductive system

3. Describe and explain the purpose of various diagnostic procedures associated with the urinary system

4. Discuss the role of the medical assistant in diagnosing and treating disorders of the urinary system and the male reproductive system

Upon successfully completing this chapter, you will be able to:

1. Perform a female urinary catheterization (Procedure 34-1)

2. Perform a male urinary catheterization (Procedure 34-2)

3. Instruct a male patient on the testicular self-examination (Procedure 34-3)

Competencies

CAAHEP

- Practice standard precautions
- Prepare patient for and assist with routine and specialty examinations
- Prepare patient for and assist with procedures, treatments, and minor office surgeries
- Document appropriately
- Instruct individuals according to their needs

ABHES

- Prepare patients for procedures
- Assist physician with examinations and treatments
- Document accurately

Key Terms

anuria	hematuria	nocturia	retrograde pyelogram
blood urea nitrogen	impotence	oliguria	specific gravity
catheterization	incontinence	prostate-specific anti-	ureterostomy
cystoscopy	intravenous pyelo-	gen	urinalysis
dialysis	gram (IVP)	proteinuria	urinary frequency
dysuria	lithotripsy	psychogenic	
enuresis	nephrostomy	pyuria	

The process of metabolism creates waste products that must be eliminated from the body. Several body systems contribute to preventing a buildup of the end products of metabolism, including the gastrointestinal system, the respiratory system, and the integumentary system. The urinary system also removes waste from the blood while regulating fluid volume, important electrolytes, blood pressure, and pH (acid-base) balance (Fig. 34-1). Disorders of the filters of the urinary system, the kidneys, are diagnosed through various urine and blood tests and radiographs. Patients with kidney problems are typically referred to a nephrolo-

gist, a physician who specializes in the physiology of the kidneys. Patients with disorders of the anatomy, or physical characteristics, of the urinary system are referred to another type of specialist, a urologist. Since the male reproductive system is so inextricably linked to the urinary system, disorders of the male reproductive system are also often referred to the urologist. This chapter does not review the anatomy and physiology of the urinary system but, instead, focuses on common disorders, diagnostic procedures, and treatments associated with the urinary and male reproductive systems.

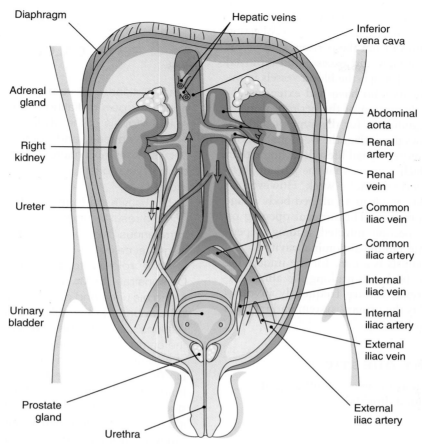

Figure 34-1 Urinary system with blood vessels. (Reprinted with permission from Cohen BJ. Memmler's The Human Body in Health and Disease. Philadelphia: Lippincott Williams & Wilkins, 2005.)

Common Urinary Disorders

Renal Failure

Renal failure is an acute or chronic disorder of kidney function manifested by the inability of the kidney to excrete wastes, concentrate urine, and aid in homeostatic electrolyte conservation. In acute renal failure, the patient has **oliguria** and a corresponding rise in nitrogen-containing wastes in the blood. The causes of acute renal failure include a serious loss of fluid due to severe burn or hemorrhage, trauma, toxic injury to the kidney, and an obstruction beyond the level of the collecting tubules.

Chronic renal failure is a gradual loss of nephrons with corresponding inability of the kidney to perform its functions. It may result from another disease process, such as systemic lupus erythematosus, diabetic neuropathy, radiation, or renal tuberculosis. The patient has general weakness, edema of the lungs and tissues, and neurologic symptoms such as confusion progressing to seizures and coma as the wastes, or toxins, not filtered by the kidneys build up in the blood.

Treatment for both acute and chronic renal failure may involve renal **dialysis** to remove nitrogenous waste products and excess fluid from the body. Dialysis dependence may be short term in an acute illness or long term in end-stage renal disease. Without functional nephrons, wastes must be filtered through membranes other than those in the renal tissues. Two methods are used: hemodialysis and peritoneal dialysis.

With hemodialysis, toxins are removed from the blood by routing the patient's blood through a dialysis machine containing synthetic filters and a dialysate, a substance used to balance the electrolyte concentration in the blood. The machine can be regulated to remove or retain certain substances as needed for the individual patient. This type of dialysis requires that the patient's circulatory system be accessed as often as 3 times a week for 3 to 4 hours at a time. Therefore, most patients receive a surgical fistula, or graft, between an artery and a vein to make entry with a needle during the procedure easier for the patient. The fistula is often placed in one of the arms, and this arm should not be used for taking blood pressures or for blood draws.

Patients receiving peritoneal dialysis often perform the procedure at home. An appropriately balanced dialysate is administered through a catheter into the abdominal cavity, allowed to remain in the abdominal cavity for a specified time, and then drained into a collecting bag. As the dialysate flows from the peritoneal cavity, it brings with it filtered wastes and excess fluid removed from the patient's blood through the blood vessels in the abdominal cavity. Patients who have had extensive abdominal surgery with disruption of the peritoneal membranes are not good candidates for this type of dialysis. Peritoneal dialysis allows the patient the freedom to move about and continue a more normal lifestyle at home than with hemodialysis, which requires that the patient go to an outpatient facility several times a week. However, an abdominal catheter may result in an altered body image and psychological depression. The surgical opening on the abdomen can also become infected, leading to peritonitis, a serious infection in the abdominal cavity.

Neither type of dialysis is a cure for the underlying renal dysfunction, but both can prolong life almost indefinitely. Chronic renal failure frequently involves other systems as well as the urinary system and requires treatment for that involvement.

 CHECKPOINT QUESTION

1. Which type of dialysis involves the filtering of wastes from the blood directly?

Calculi

Calculi are stone formations that may be found anywhere in the urinary system and may range from granular particles to staghorn structures that fill the renal pelvis. Stones seem most likely to form if the urine is alkaline; the symptoms vary with the size and location of the stone. Hematuria may be present if rough edges of calculi abrade the mucous membrane lining the urinary system. The patient has flank pain if a stone lodges in one of the ureters.

Treatment may not be needed if the stones are small enough to be flushed out with increased fluid intake. Large stones may require surgery or **lithotripsy**, a procedure in which ultrasound is used to crush the stones. In either case, the chemical makeup of the stones is evaluated for the forming components, and the patient's diet may be adjusted to prevent recurrence.

Tumors

The urinary system may be a primary or secondary site for tumors. Tumors are more common in the urinary bladder but may also occur in the kidney. Symptoms vary but usually include hematuria and an unexplained abdominal mass. Treatment is based on the extent and type of tumor and may include surgery, chemotherapy, radiation, or a combination.

 PATIENT EDUCATION

RENAL CALCULI

Clark Watkins, a 45-year-old white man, has severe right flank pain radiating to the suprapubic and inguinal regions of the abdomen. He has a fever of 100.3°F, nausea, and some vomiting. Urinalysis shows gross and microscopic hematuria and calcium crystal casts; it is clear of pyuria and white blood cells.

Dr. Brown performs in-office ultrasonography, and the results suggest renal calculi. He orders an intravenous pyelogram (IVP), which reveals sand-to-gravel calculi.

Your role is to provide patient education. Demonstrate to Mr. Watkins the procedure for filtering his urine and provide him with the strainer so he can bring in the solid material for analysis. Mr. Watkins's diet will be altered in accordance with the composition of the stones. He may be referred to a dietitian or given a diet list after counseling with Dr. Brown. Encourage Mr. Watkins to increase his fluid intake to flush the stones and to walk frequently to assist peristalsis in the ureters and passing the stones. Urge him to drink fruit juices, especially cranberry juice, in addition to water, and discourage caffeine drinks. He may need an antiemetic if nausea and vomiting interfere with fluid intake. Caution him to watch for signs of infection and obstruction, including cloudy urine, which may contain pus, and fever.

 CHECKPOINT QUESTION

2. What are calculi, and when are they more likely to form?

Hydronephrosis

Hydronephrosis is distention of the renal pelvis and calyces resulting from an obstruction in the kidney or ureter that causes a backup of urine. The symptoms include flank pain, hematuria, pyuria, fever, and chills. To restore the flow f urine, the stricture must be corrected, if possible, through **cystoscopy**. If it is not possible to restore the flow of urine to the urinary bladder, it may be necessary to perform a **nephrostomy** (opening the kidney and placement of a catheter in the kidney pelvis) or **ureterostomy** (surgical creation of an opening to the outside of the body from the ureter) (Fig. 34-2).

A

Conventional ileal conduit. The surgeon transplants the ureters to an isolated section of the terminal ileum (ileal conduit), bringing one end to the abdominal wall. The ureter may also be transplanted into the transverse sigmoid colon (colon conduit) or proximal jejunum (jejunal conduit).

Ileal segment

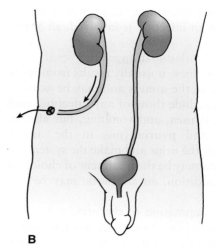

B

Cutaneous ureterostomy. The surgeon brings the detached ureter through the abdominal wall and attaches it to an opening in the skin.

C

Vesicostomy. The surgeon sutures the bladder to the abdominal wall and creates an opening (stoma) through the abdominal and bladder walls for urinary drainage.

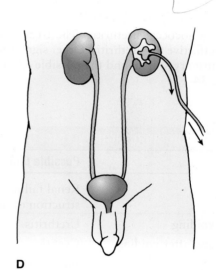

D

Nephrostomy. The surgeon inserts a catheter into the renal pelvis via an incision into the flank or, by percutaneous catheter placement, into the kidney.

Figure 34-2   A ureterostomy. (Reprinted with permission from Smeltzer SC, Bare BG, Hinkle JL, Cheever KH. Brunner & Suddarth's Textbook of Medical-Surgical Nursing. Philadelphia: Lippincott Williams & Wilkins, 2008.)

Urinary System Infections

Glomerulonephritis is inflammation of the glomerulus, or filtering unit, of the kidney. Symptoms range from very mild edema of the extremities, **proteinuria, hematuria**, and oliguria to complete renal failure. It is occasionally seen in children 1 to 4 weeks after a streptococ-cal infection as the large streptococcal antibodies are trapped in the small capillaries of the glomerulus, causing irritation and inflammation. Glomerulonephritis in adults may be chronic, with scarring and hardening of the glomeruli from repeated episodes of acute glomerulonephritis, and may lead to renal failure. Symptoms of the chronic form include proteinuria, casts in the urine (see Chapter 43), and hematuria. Treatment is usually symptomatic, and if an infection is involved, an antibiotic is prescribed.

Pyelonephritis is inflammation of the renal pelvis and the body of the kidney. It usually results from an ascending infection from the ureters and may be acute or chronic. Symptoms include those of any infection, such as chills and fever, nausea, and vomiting, but also include flank pain and **pyuria** (pus in the urine). Medication to acidify the urine and make the system less hospitable to bacteria may be the treatment of choice for pyelonephritis. In addition, an antibiotic may be prescribed.

Cystitis is an inflammation of the urinary bladder. This condition is far more common in women than in men because a woman's urethra is shorter. Symptoms begin with **urinary frequency, dysuria,** and urgency and progress to chills, fever, nausea, vomiting, and flank pain. The causative microorganism is identified with a urine culture, and the treatment usually is an antibiotic once the causative microorganism has been identified.

Urethritis is inflammation of the urethra that may occur before the signs and symptoms of cystitis appear, or it may indicate a sexually transmitted disease, such as gonorrhea or nongonococcal urethritis. The treatment for cystitis is also effective for urethritis. Other signs and symptoms of the urinary system and the possible causes are listed in Table 34-1.

 CHECKPOINT QUESTION

3. Why are women more likely than men to have cystitis?

 PATIENT EDUCATION

URINARY TRACT HEALTH

As the medical assistant, you will teach patients about everyday habits related to good general health. Encourage patients with urinary system symptoms to follow these suggestions to avoid urinary tract infections in the future:

For All Patients

- Drink lots of fluids, which help remove waste products from the fluid compartments. We are all generally advised to drink 8 glasses of water a day so that tissues are well hydrated, feces are soft, and infections in the lower urinary system are relatively unlikely.
- Empty your bladder when you feel the need. Urine held beyond comfort causes bladder stress and irritation. Allowing urine to stagnate in the bladder increases the risk of infection.

TABLE 34-1	Symptoms of Urinary Tract Disorders and Possible Causes
Symptoms	**Possible Causes**
Anuria	Renal failure, acute nephritis, lead or mercury poisoning, complete obstruction of urinary tract
Burning during voiding	Urethritis
Burning during and after voiding	Cystitis
Dysuria	Infection
Enuresis	Normal to age 3 years
Frequency	Infection, diabetes
Hematuria	Diseases of glomeruli, trauma, neoplasm, calculi
Incontinence	Infection, uterine prolapse, nerve damage, neoplasm, senility
Nocturia	Infection, prostatic hypertrophy, abdominal pressure (pregnancy), diabetes
Oliguria	Acute nephritis, dehydration, fever, urinary obstruction, neoplasm
Polyuria	Diabetes mellitus, diabetes insipidus, diuretic use, high fluid intake
Proteinuria	Disease of glomeruli or protein metabolism, infection, nephrotic syndrome
Pyuria	Infection
Renal colic	Calculi
Urgency	Infection, disease of the prostate

- Be aware that cranberry juice and vitamin C help acidify the urine and make the urinary system less attractive to bacteria.

Especially for Women

- Avoid using perfumed products in the perineal area. The female urinary meatus is very short and prone to irritation. Urethral infections quickly become bladder infections with irritation.
- Avoid tight-fitting lower garments, especially nylon underwear. Loose-fitting cotton underwear absorbs moisture and allows for airflow, making both bladder and vaginal infections less likely.
- Wipe carefully from front to back after using the toilet. Wash with soap and water, and rinse well if infections are a recurrent problem.
- If you are prone to urinary tract infections, void immediately after sexual intercourse to flush the area of bacteria that might have intruded into the urethra.
- Avoid tub baths, particularly bubble baths; showers are less likely to contribute to infections.

 W H A T   I F ?

A mother brings her 5-year-old daughter to the office with complaints of burning on urination. What questions do you ask? How do you educate the mother and child?

First, ask if the child urinates when she feels the urge or if she holds her urine. Some young girls are inclined to hold their urine long past the time to void, setting up a perfect situation for bacterial growth. Caution the child to go to the bathroom when the need arises, making sure to use terms she can understand. Next, ask the mother if she uses bubble bath in the child's bath water. Young girls have a very short urethra and are prone to urethritis if they bathe in water with certain types of bubble bath. Finally, explain that the child must learn to wipe from front to back to avoid urinary tract infections.

Common Disorders of the Male Reproductive System

Male patients with disorders of the reproductive system often have signs and symptoms pertaining to the urinary system. If you work in a family practice or internal medicine office, you may care for male patients with repro-

ductive system disorders, or these patients may be referred to urology for specific treatment or surgery. Common disorders are discussed in the following sections.

Benign Prostatic Hyperplasia

As most men reach their middle years, the prostate begins to enlarge, or hypertrophy. Benign prostatic hyperplasia is a noncancerous enlargement of the prostate gland that occurs commonly in men over age 40. Diagnosis is with a digital rectal examination, which should be performed as part of the routine physical examination in men after age 40. Using a gloved hand and water-soluble lubricant, the physician will insert the index finger into the rectum and palpate the prostate for size, shape, and consistency.

As the prostate gland enlarges, it presses on the urethra and urinary bladder, causing urinary symptoms such as frequency and **nocturia**. While this condition is not usually a serious problem, it can be treated medically or surgically by partially or completely removing the prostate gland. The surgical procedure, prostatectomy, can be performed transurethrally or through a surgical opening into the suprapubic area of the lower abdomen. If the prostate is removed transurethrally, the procedure is a transurethral resection of the prostate. Box 34-1 describes the surgical techniques used to treat prostatic hypertrophy in more detail.

BOX 34-1

SURGICAL INTERVENTION FOR PROSTATIC HYPERTROPHY

Transurethral Resection of the Prostate

A cystoscope with an electrocautery wire cutting loop, a resectoscope, is inserted through the urethra and rotated through the prostate to remove pieces of the gland. The pieces are washed out with irrigating fluid introduced through the scope. There is no abdominal incision, making this a relatively safe procedure for the high-risk patient. The whole organ is not usually removed for this surgery; therefore, the obstruction frequently returns. This is not a choice for malignancies.

Suprapubic Prostatectomy

Performed through the abdominal wall and bladder, suprapubic prostatectomy allows the surgeon to peel out the whole organ through a wide surgical field and to check the bladder for involvement. This approach is the choice for large

(continued)

BOX 34-1 *(continued)*

prostate glands or for malignancies. As in all surgeries, there are postoperative risks, particularly for the elderly. These include pain, hemorrhage, urinary leakage, and prolonged convalescence.

Perineal Resection

An incision between the scrotum and the anus is a short, direct route to the prostate without interfering with the bladder and is preferred for some large malignancies. It appears to be relatively nontraumatic for the very old or infirm. Surgeons find that the field offers less room to maneuver than with the suprapubic approach. It is not a good choice for young men because impotence and urinary and fecal incontinence are frequent postoperative complications. The proximity of the anal area also increases the risk of infection.

Retropubic Resection

A low abdominal incision above the pubis but below the bladder avoids trauma to the bladder and thereby allows a shorter convalescence than with the suprapubic approach. It also provides better removal options than the transurethral approach. It is a good choice if pathology is limited to the prostate, with no bladder involvement.

Prostate Cancer

Prostate cancer, like most cancers, is best treated when detected early. In the early stages of the disease, many men are asymptomatic. As a result, male patients over age 40 should be encouraged to have yearly physical examinations that include a digital rectal examination, which often allows the physician to palpate an enlarged gland. If the prostate gland is enlarged, a biopsy of the prostate may be advised to determine the cause of the enlargement.

Another diagnostic test often ordered as part of the routine physical examination is the **prostate-specific antigen**, or PSA, blood test. PSA is normally found in the blood of all men, but its level increases with any inflammation of the prostate, including cancer. While the cause of prostate cancer is not known, it is most common in men over age 50, with 75% of diagnoses in men over age 75. Treatment depends on the extent of the malignancy and the patient's age and general health status. Prostate cancer is often treated by a combination of surgery, chemotherapy, and radiation.

 CHECKPOINT QUESTION

4. Does the patient with benign prostatic hyperplasia have an elevated PSA level? Why or why not?

Testicular Cancer

Although testicular cancer accounts for only about 1% of all malignancies, the metastatic and mortality rates are high. This type of cancer is most often seen in men aged 15 to 34. The cause of testicular cancer is unknown, but predisposing factors may include cryptorchidism, infection, genetic factors, and endocrine abnormalities. The symptoms are gradual and painless and may initially only involve a vague feeling of scrotal heaviness.

Once a diagnosis of testicular cancer has been made, treatment may be orchiectomy, or surgical removal of the testicle. Chemotherapy and radiation may also be used.

Hydrocele

Hydrocele, a collection of fluid in the scrotum and around the testes, may result from trauma or infection or may simply be due to aging. Diagnosis is based on symptoms and inspection. If the condition is extremely uncomfortable, aspiration of the excessive fluid may be required, and if the condition persists, surgical intervention may be the treatment of choice. In most cases, no treatment is necessary, and the fluid is reabsorbed by the body. Hydrocele is common in male infants but generally subsides without treatment.

Cryptorchidism

Normally, the testes descend from the abdominal cavity into the scrotal sac in the male fetus by the eighth month of gestation. In a small percentage of male infants, one or both of the testes fail to descend by the time of delivery (Fig. 34-3). Cryptorchidism refers to either one or both undescended testes. Surgical correction, known as orchiopexy, is usually performed before age 4 years, preferably at 1 or 2 years. If an undescended testis is not

Figure 34-3 Possible locations of undescended testicles.

surgically corrected, it results in sterility of the unde-scended organ and may increase the risk of testicular malignancy later in life.

 CHECKPOINT QUESTION

5. What are the causes of hydrocele?

Inguinal Hernia

After the testes descend in the male fetus and the inguinal canals close, small rings are left open at the anterior base of the abdominal wall as a passage for the spermatic cord. There is no connection between this area and the abdominal contents, but this area remains a possible site for weakness and protrusion of the intestines with age or exertion. The patient with an inguinal hernia is often asymptomatic unless the intestines protrude through the weakened area, which may result in a noticeable bulge and pain. Diagnosis is made in the early stages by having the patient bear down and cough while the physician inserts a finger into a pouch made by the scrotum up into the external and internal inguinal rings. Pressure against the finger indicates weakness of the muscles in this area.

Treatment of an inguinal hernia depends on the patient's physical condition. Surgical correction of a hernia, called a herniorrhaphy, repositions the protruding organ and repairs the opening.

Infections

Infections of the male urinary tract are likely to spread to the reproductive system because they share many of the same organs. The most common infections of the male reproductive system are epididymitis, orchitis, and prostatitis. While not all infections result from a sexually transmitted microorganism, many of the infections of the male reproductive system are caused by sexually transmitted diseases. Refer to Chapter 35 for more information about sexually transmitted diseases that affect both men and women.

Infection in the epididymis usually results from an infected prostate or other inflammation in the urinary tract. Microorganisms that may cause epididymitis include staphylococci, streptococci, *Escherichia coli*, *Chlamydia*, and *Neisseria gonorrhoeae*. Symptoms include a swollen scrotum, pain, tenderness, fever, and malaise. Diagnosis is based on these symptoms and a culture of any drainage from the penis. Treatment includes an antibiotic, bed rest, fluids, and palliative measures for pain.

The microorganisms that cause epididymitis often also cause orchitis, and the treatment is virtually the same. Orchitis may also result in hydrocele, which should be treated if it becomes a severe complication.

Chronic prostatitis is common among the elderly and may be confused with prostatic hypertrophy if repeated infections cause the organs to fibrose. The causative agents are much like those of other infections of the male reproductive system, with the leading cause being *E. coli*. It frequently results from catheterization or cystoscopy. Some pathogens reach the prostate by way of the bloodstream of the lymph system. Signs and symptoms may include inguinal pain, fever, low back and joint pain, burning, dysuria, and urethral discharge. Urine specimens contain blood and pus. Diagnosis is based on signs, symptoms, and urinalysis. Antibiotic treatment is required to treat chronic prostatitis.

 PATIENT EDUCATION

AIDS PREVENTION

When providing instructions about AIDS prevention, explain to your patient that it is safest, of course, to abstain from sex. Encourage your patients to have sex only with a partner who is known not to be infected, who has sex with no one but the patient, and who does not use needles or syringes. Also, advise the patient to use a latex condom if it is not known whether the sexual partner is infected. Generally, instruct patients to:

* Avoid contact with another person's blood, body fluids, semen, and vaginal secretions.
* Avoid sharing needles, syringes, and any objects that come into contact with blood or body fluids.
* Avoid using alcohol and drugs. Use of these substances can hinder clear thinking and lead to unwise decision making.

 CHECKPOINT QUESTION

6. What are some microorganisms responsible for causing infections in the male reproductive system?

Impotence

Impotence, also known as erectile dysfunction, is the inability to achieve or maintain an erection; it may be psychological or organic. **Psychogenic** impotence may be caused by something as simple as exhaustion, anxiety, or depression, and in such cases, it usually disappears with resolution of the underlying cause. Organic impotence may result from disease in almost any other body system, including endocrine imbalance, cardiovascular problems, nervous system impairment, or urinary disease. Organic impotence may also be caused by injury to the pelvic organs or by medication that impairs any of the systems serving the reproductive system.

Diagnosis is based on a detailed medical and sexual history with an analysis of lifestyle and emotional status. Blood studies and measurements of both penile arterial flow and nerve conduction to this area are usually required. Treatment depends on the cause and may include a vacuum tube system that pulls blood into the penis, creating an erection, or vitamin E injections into the penis. Today, many new drugs, such as sildenafil (Viagra) stimulate erections in the impotent male. If none of these are effective, a penile implant can be inserted surgically.

Common Diagnostic and Therapeutic Procedures

Urinalysis

The single most important step in diagnosing urinary diseases is the examination of the patient's urine, or **urinalysis**. Tests should always be performed on a fresh specimen and with the first morning specimen when concentrated urine is needed, such as for pregnancy testing. The urinalysis includes a physical and chemical evaluation, **specific gravity**, and a microscopic examination (see Chapter 43). If an infection is suspected, the physician may also order a urine culture.

The patient may produce the urine specimen by performing a clean-catch midstream procedure after receiving instructions from you on the proper procedure for collecting the specimen. In some cases, the physician may order a urine specimen obtained by **catheterization**, which is the introduction of a sterile flexible tube into the urinary bladder (Fig. 34-4). In the medical office, a straight catheter is used for catheterization and removed once the urine specimen is obtained. Some patients have an indwelling catheter inserted at another facility, such as a hospital. Indwelling catheters are similar to straight

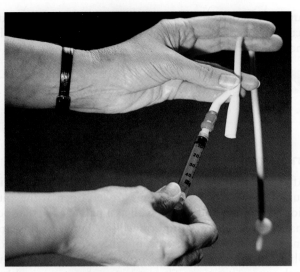

Figure 34-5 Sterile water is inserted into the indicated lumen to inflate the balloon of the indwelling catheter. When the balloon is inflated, the catheter will remain within the bladder.

catheters, but these types are kept in place by a balloon on the end of the catheter inflated after placement in the bladder (Fig. 34-5). Indwelling catheters are not usually inserted in the medical office.

Catheters are sized 8 to 10 fr for children and 14 to 20 fr for adults. Procedures 34-1 and 34-2 describe the procedure for performing a catheterization in females and males, respectively, in the medical office, and Box 34-2 explains some principles of urinary catheterization.

Figure 34-4 Types of catheters. From the top: No. 24 French indwelling catheter; No. 16 French indwelling catheter; No. 16 French straight catheter; coude catheter; and self-contained catheterization collection unit.

LEGAL TIP

CLINICAL TRIALS

Physicians who participate in clinical trials using new drugs or procedures have an ethical and legal obligation to follow specific guidelines, including:

- Notifying the patient that the drug or procedure is experimental and detailing the risks and benefits of the treatment clearly.
- Obtaining an informed, written consent before beginning the drug or performing the procedure.
- Assuring that the drug or procedure is documented appropriately and reported accurately according to the standards for the research being conducted.
- Providing a high standard of care for all patients regardless of whether or not they are participating in a clinical trial.

BOX 34-2

PRINCIPLES OF CATHETERIZATION

Catheterization is usually a last resort for obtaining a urine specimen. Even under the most aseptic conditions, there is a risk of introducing infection into the urinary system. However, some patients require catheterization when there is no other alternative. For example, catheterization is required in the following circumstances:

- It is impossible to obtain a clean-catch midstream specimen for urinalysis.
- The residual urine, or urine left in the bladder after urination, must be measured.
- Medication must be instilled into the bladder to treat an infection.
- The patient has urinary retention or cannot urinate.

Urinary catheter types and sizes vary. They are made of plastic or rubber. If the patient has prostatic hypertrophy, the physician may order a coude catheter (see Fig. 34-4), which is slightly curved and a bit stiffer than the other types so it is easier to advance it beyond the obstructing enlarged prostate gland.

Blood Tests

Serum levels of uric acid, **blood urea nitrogen** (BUN), or creatinine may be indicated for diagnosis of some disease processes of the urinary system. It will likely be your responsibility to draw the patient's blood and process it on site or direct it to the proper testing facility (see Chapter 41).

Cystoscopy or Cystourethroscopy

Cystoscopy is direct visualization of the bladder and urethra with a lighted instrument called a cystoscope (Fig. 34-6). Cystoscopy allows the physician to diagnose many disorders of the lower urinary tract, such as tumors and inflammation. You may be responsible for providing preoperative instructions to the patient as directed by the physician. This procedure is usually done under local anesthesia and may be performed in the urologist's office, but some physicians prefer to have the patient receive a general anesthetic and outpatient hospitalization.

CHECKPOINT QUESTION

7. What is the most common test for disorders of the urinary system performed in the medical office?

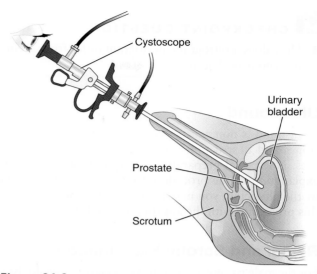

Figure 34-6 The interior of the urinary bladder as seen through a cystoscope. (Modified with permission from Cohen BJ. Medical Terminology: An Illustrated Guide. Philadelphia: Lippincott Williams & Wilkins, 2003.)

Intravenous Pyelogram and Retrograde Pyelogram

An **intravenous pyelogram** (IVP) is radiographic examination of the kidneys and urinary tract using a radiopaque dye injected into the circulatory system. This dye is filtered by the kidneys to serve as a contrast medium and enhance visualization of the renal structures. Although this procedure is not done in the medical office, you will schedule the examination at the appropriate facility and give the patient instructions to be followed before the procedure. Specifically, the patient is required to cleanse the bowels with a laxative the night before the test and to have an enema the morning of the procedure, since feces may prevent adequate visualization of the kidneys. In addition, the patient is asked not to eat or drink anything for at least 8 hours before the dye is injected to increase the blood concentration and visibility of the dye.

You must question the patient carefully about possible iodine allergy, including allergic reactions to seafood, particularly shellfish. Encourage the patient to increase fluid intake after the test to flush out the dye and counteract any dehydration caused by the preliminary cleansing.

A **retrograde pyelogram** is similar to the IVP except that the dye is not injected intravenously but is introduced through a catheter in the ureters through a cystoscope. This test is commonly used when IVP is contraindicated because of poor kidney function. Like IVP, this test is not performed in the medical office, but you may be responsible for making arrangements with the appropriate facility and giving the patient any necessary instructions.

CHECKPOINT QUESTION

8. How does a retrograde pyelogram differ from an intravenous pyelogram?

Ultrasound

Ultrasound is noninvasive use of sound waves to show stones and obstructions in the urinary system and tissues. No special preparation is required other than an explanation of the procedure to the patient. If ordered by the physician, you may be responsible for scheduling this procedure with the appropriate facility.

Rectal and Scrotal Examinations

For the male patient seen in the physician's or urologist's office, you will assist with examination of the reproductive organs by instructing the patient to disrobe from the waist down and providing him with appropriate draping. The physician will inspect and palpate the scrotum for lumps and inguinal hernia. Using a gloved hand and water-soluble lubricant, the physician will perform a digital rectal examination, inserting the index finger into the rectum and palpating the prostate for size, shape, and consistency.

At home, male patients should perform the testicular self-examination because this is the best method for early detection of testicular cancer. The American Cancer Society recommends that all men perform this examination frequently, possibly weekly, and you are responsible for teaching the patient about this disease and the self-examination. You should explain that the best time for the self-examination is after a warm shower or bath, when the scrotal sac is relaxed (Procedure 34-3). If lumps or thickened areas are palpated during the examination, instruct the patient to notify the physician immediately.

CHECKPOINT QUESTION

9. When is the best time to instruct a patient to perform the testicular self-examination?

TRIAGE

While you are working in a medical office, the following three situations occur:

A. Patient A, a 24-year-old patient, has obtained a urine specimen for a work physical.
B. The physician has asked you to teach patient B, a 30-year-old male, to perform the testicular self-examination before discharging him.
C. Patient C is a 67-year-old woman who needs a catheter to relieve bladder distention due to urinary retention.

How do you sort these patients? Who do you see first? Second? Third?

First see patient C, since she has urinary retention and is most likely very uncomfortable. Next, test the urine specimen from patient A. The quality of the urine specimen decreases as the urine specimen sits out, and once it is tested, the results can be given to the physician for diagnosis. Patient B should be addressed last. Patient education should never be rushed, and he should be given an opportunity to ask questions for clarification.

Vasectomy

A popular form of reproductive control is the vasectomy, or surgical removal of all or a segment of the vas deferens to prevent the passage of sperm from the testes. This procedure is frequently performed in the medical office, and you will assist by instructing the patient on preoperative orders as indicated by the physician. Some physicians order light preoperative sedation and may require that the patient have nothing by mouth after midnight on the day of the procedure. On the day of the procedure, you should assist the physician by providing the appropriate surgical tray or instruments and assist the disrobed patient into the lithotomy position with appropriate draping materials to provide privacy. The physician will make two small incisions near the scrotal sac, pull each vas deferens (from the right and left testes) through the incision, clamp each vas deferens proximally and distally, and surgically cut and remove a segment of each. The remaining vas deferens ducts are placed back in the scrotal sac after the clamps are removed, and the site is sutured.

Ejaculation and sexual function are not affected by this procedure. The volume of sperm in the ejaculate is so small that its absence is not noticeable. The sperm produced by the testes after this procedure are absorbed in the testes. Since sterility may not be immediate, the patient should be advised to use another form of birth control, such as a condom, until sperm counts confirm that the ejaculate is free of sperm. You should advise the patient to return to the office for periodic sperm counts until no sperm are found in the ejaculate.

MEDIA MENU

- **Student CD**
  - **CMA/RMA Certification Exam Review**
- **LWW's Medical Assisting Skills DVD**
  - **Procedure 34-1**
- **Premium Online Course**
  http://thePoint.lww.com/Kronenberger3e
- **Internet Resources**

LiveAdvise Online Tutoring & Competency Training
http://thePoint.lww.com/LiveAdvise

Brady Urological Institute, Johns Hopkins Medical Institutions
http://urology.jhu.edu/

Urology Channel
http://www.urologychannel.com/

National Kidney and Urologic Diseases Information Clearinghouse
http://kidney.niddk.nih.gov/kudiseases/pubs/impotence

Urology Notes
http://www.urologyinstitute.com/html/kidney

Prostate Cancer Research Institute
http://www.prostate-cancer.org/

American Cancer Society
http://www.cancer.org/

National Kidney and Urologic Diseases Information Clearinghouse
http://kidney.niddk.nih.gov/kudiseases/pubs/impotence

National Kidney Foundation
http://www.kidney.org

español SPANISH TERMINOLOGY

Orina sin querer?
Do you pass water involuntarily?

Es necesario una muestra de su orina.
Need a urine specimen.

Sera incomodo.
It will be uncomfortable.

Tiene dificultad cuando orina?
Do you have burning when urinating?

Tiene que levantarse por la noche a orinar? Cuantas veces?
Do you have to get up to urinate during the night? How many times?

PROCEDURE 34-1:   Female Urinary Catheterization

Purpose: Using sterile aseptic technique, perform a straight catheterization on a female torso model
Equipment: Sterile straight catheterization tray with 14- or 16-French catheter, sterile gloves, antiseptic solution, sterile specimen cup with lid, lubricant, sterile drape, examination light, anatomically correct female torso model

Steps	Reasons
1. Wash your hands.	Handwashing aids infection control.
2. Identify the patient, explain the procedure, and have the patient disrobe completely from the waist down; provide a gown and adequate draping.	Identifying the patient helps prevent errors in treatment. The privacy of the patient should be maintained at all times.
3. Place the patient in the dorsal recumbent or lithotomy position, draping carefully to prevent unnecessary exposure. Carefully open the tray and place it between the patient's legs. Shine the examination light on the perineum.	The dorsal recumbent or lithotomy position allows the best view of the perineum and urinary meatus. Placing the tray between the legs of the patient allows easy access to the catheter and supplies. Adequate lighting is essential.
4. Remove the sterile glove package and put on the sterile gloves without contaminating them.	
5. Carefully remove the sterile drape and place it under the buttocks of the patient without contaminating your gloves.	If the sterile drape is on top of the tray, it may be carefully lifted out of the tray by the edge with clean hands and carefully placed under the buttocks. This drape is a barrier to protect the examination table from spills.
6. Open the antiseptic swabs and place them upright inside the catheter tray. Open the lubricant and squeeze a generous amount onto the tip of the catheter while it lies in the catheter tray.	The antiseptic swabs should be opened before beginning the actual catheterization. Placing the package upright prevents the antiseptic from spilling. Lubricant applied to the catheter allows for easier insertion.
7. Remove the sterile urine specimen cup and lid and place them to the side of the tray without contaminating your gloves.	Urinary catheterization is a sterile procedure.
8. Using your nondominant hand, carefully expose the urinary meatus by spreading the labia. This hand is now contaminated and must not be moved out of position until the catheter is in the bladder.	
9. Cleanse the urinary meatus using the antiseptic swabs by wiping from top to bottom on each side and down the middle of the exposed urinary meatus. Use a separate swab for each side and the middle.	Continue to hold the labia apart with the nondominant hand.

Step 9. Expose the urinary meatus and cleanse from top to bottom.

(continued)

PROCEDURE 34-1:   **Female Urinary Catheterization** *(continued)*

Steps	Reasons
10. Using your sterile dominant hand, pick up the catheter and carefully insert the lubricated tip into the urinary meatus approximately 3 inches. The other end of the catheter should be left in the tray, which will collect the urine that drains from the bladder.	The adult female urethra is approximately 2 to 3 inches long. Once urine begins flowing into the catheter tray, the catheter is in far enough.
	Step 10. Insert the catheter approximately 3 inches with the sterile hand, while continuing to hold the labia apart with the nondominant hand.
11. Once the urine begins to flow into the catheter tray, hold the catheter in position with your nondominant hand by releasing the labia and moving your fingers down onto the catheter. Use your dominant hand to direct the flow of urine into the specimen cup if a specimen is needed.	
12. When the urine flow has slowed or stopped OR 1000 mL has been obtained, carefully remove the catheter by pulling it straight out.	No more than 1000 mL of urine should be removed from the bladder, since doing so may cause painful spasms of the bladder. Most patients do not have 1000 mL.
13. Wipe the perineum carefully with the drape that was under the buttocks. Dispose of the urine appropriately and discard the catheter, tray, and supplies in a biohazard container.	Once the catheter is removed, it is not necessary to keep your dominant hand sterile.
14. If a urine specimen was obtained, properly label the specimen container and complete the laboratory requisition. Process the specimen according to the guidelines of the laboratory.	
15. Remove your gloves and wash your hands.	Standard precautions must be followed throughout the procedure.
16. Instruct the patient to dress and give any follow-up information regarding test results as necessary.	
17. Document the procedure in the patient's medical record.	Procedures are considered not to have been done if they are not recorded.

Charting Example:

02/14/2008 9:15 AM Catheterization with a 14-fr straight cath, 300 mL dark amber urine obtained, specimen to Acme lab for C & S

—S. Strobb, CMA

PROCEDURE 34-2: Male Urinary Catheterization

Purpose: Using sterile aseptic technique, perform a straight catheterization on a male torso model
Equipment: Sterile straight catheterization tray with 14- or 16-French catheter, sterile gloves, antiseptic solution, sterile specimen cup with lid, lubricant, sterile drape, examination light, anatomically correct male torso model

Steps	Purpose
1. Wash your hands.	Handwashing aids infection control.
2. Identify the patient, explain the procedure, and have the patient disrobe completely from the waist down while providing a gown and adequate draping.	Identifying the patient helps prevent errors in treatment. The privacy of the patient should be maintained at all times.
3. Place the patient supine, draping carefully to prevent unnecessary exposure. Carefully open the tray and place it to the side of the patient on the examination table or on top of the patient's thighs.	The male urinary meatus is on the glans penis. Placing the tray on top of the patient's legs allows easy access to the catheter and supplies.
4. Remove the sterile glove package and put on the sterile gloves without contaminating them.	
5. Carefully remove the sterile drape and place it under the glans penis.	If the sterile drape is the top item in the tray, it may be carefully lifted out of the tray by the edge with clean hands and placed under the penis. This drape is a barrier to protect the examination table and patient from any spills.
6. Open the antiseptic swabs and place them upright inside the catheter tray. Open the lubricant and squeeze a generous amount onto the tip of the catheter as it lies in the bottom of the catheter tray.	The antiseptic swabs should be opened before beginning the catheterization. Placing the package upright helps prevent the antiseptic from spilling. Lubricant on the catheter allows for easier insertion.
7. Remove the sterile urine specimen cup and lid and place them to the side of the tray without contaminating your gloves.	Urinary catheterization is a sterile procedure.
8. Using your nondominant hand, carefully pick up the penis, exposing the urinary meatus. This hand is now contaminated and must not be moved out of position until the catheter is inserted into the urinary bladder.	
9. Cleanse the urinary meatus using the antiseptic swabs by wiping from top to bottom on each side and down the middle of the exposed urinary meatus. Use a separate swab for each side and the middle.	Continue to hold the penis with the dominant hand

Step 9. Expose the urinary meatus and cleanse from top to bottom.

(continued)

PROCEDURE 34-2:   Male Urinary Catheterization *(continued)*

Steps	Purpose
10. Using your sterile dominant hand, pick up the catheter and carefully insert the lubricated tip into the urinary meatus approximately 4 to 6 inches. The other end of the catheter should be left in the tray, which will collect the urine that drains from the bladder.	The adult male urethra is approximately 4 to 6 inches long. Once urine begins flowing into the catheter tray, the catheter is in far enough.

Step 10. Carefully insert the catheter into the urethra.

Steps	Purpose
11. Once the urine begins to flow, hold the catheter in position with your nondominant hand. Use your dominant hand to direct the flow of urine into the specimen cup if a specimen is needed.	
12. When the urine flow has slowed or stopped OR 1000 mL has been obtained, carefully remove the catheter by pulling it straight out.	No more than 1000 mL of urine should be removed from the bladder, since doing so may cause painful spasms of the bladder.
13. Wipe the glans penis carefully with the drape and dispose of the urine, catheter, tray, and supplies appropriately in a biohazard container.	Once the urinary catheter has been removed, it is not necessary to keep the dominant hand sterile.
14. If a urine specimen was obtained, properly label the container and complete the laboratory requisition. Process the specimen according to the guidelines of the laboratory.	
15. Remove your gloves and wash your hands.	Standard precautions must be followed throughout the procedure.
16. Instruct the patient to dress and give any follow-up information regarding test results as necessary.	
17. Document the procedure in the patient's medical record.	Procedures are considered not to have been done if they are not recorded.

Charting Example:

6/17/2008 3:00 PM Catheterization with 14-French straight cath, 600 mL light amber urine obtained, specimen to Acme lab for C & S

—*J. Jones, CMA*

PROCEDURE 34-3: Instructing a Male Patient on the Testicular Self-Examination

Purpose: Teach a male patient to perform the testicular self-examination
Equipment: A patient instruction sheet if available, testicular examination model or pictures

Steps	Purpose
1. Wash your hands.	Handwashing aids infection control.
2. Identify the patient and explain the procedure.	Identifying the patient prevents errors in treatment.
3. Using the testicular model or pictures, explain the procedure, telling the patient to examine each testicle by gently rolling the testicle between the fingers and the thumb with both hands while checking for lumps or thickenings.	Both hands should be used to check each testicle to ensure complete palpation of all areas. Lumps and thickened areas are not normal and should be reported to the physician.

Step 3. (A) Gently roll the testes in a horizontal plane between the thumb and fingers. (B) Follow the same procedure and palpate upward along the testis.

4. Explain that the epididymis is a structure on top of each testicle and should be palpated to avoid incorrectly identifying it as an abnormal growth or lump.	If the epididymis is not correctly identified, the patient may palpate it during the examination and erroneously believe it is an abnormal growth.

Step 4. Locate the epididymis, a cordlike structure on the top and back of the testicle that stores and transports sperm .

5. Instruct the patient to report any abnormal lumps or thickenings to the physician.

(continued)

PROCEDURE 34-3: **Instructing a Male Patient on the Testicular Self-Examination** *(continued)*

Steps	Purpose
6. Allow the patient to ask questions about the self-examination.	The patient should always be encouraged to ask questions to ensure understanding.
7. Document the procedure in the patient's medical record.	Procedures are considered not to have been done if they are not recorded.

Charting Example:

12/13/2008 10:15 AM Pt. given verbal and written instructions on the testicular self-examination; verbal ized understanding

—*C. Brook, CMA*

Chapter Summary

- The urinary system performs many vital functions to maintain the internal environment of the body. Patients may require an examination of the urinary system for:
  - Signs and symptoms that indicate disorders of the urinary system, especially infection of the urinary bladder and urethra.
  - Evaluation during a complete physical examination even if no symptoms are present.
  - Examination of the male reproductive system, which shares the same organs as the male urinary system, for any disorders of the male reproductive system.
- Your role in working with patients with urologic disorders may include:
  - Assisting the physician as necessary during the physical examination.
  - Preparing the patient for urologic procedures.
  - Performing urologic procedures such as urinary catheterization.
  - Providing patient education as directed by the physician.

Warm Ups   for Critical Thinking

1. Differentiate between peritoneal dialysis and hemodialysis. Why are some patients poor candidates for peritoneal dialysis? What can you ask the patient to determine whether or not the peritoneal catheter is functioning or infected?

2. Research the newest pharmacologic agents used to treat impotence and explain the method of action, usual dosages, and side effects.

3. A male patient in your office has just been diagnosed with a low sperm count, and the physician has recommended that he switch from briefs to boxer shorts. How do you think this will affect his sperm count, and why?

4. Create a patient education brochure explaining the procedure for performing the testicular self-examination.

5. Identify the resources in your community for patients diagnosed with renal failure.

6. Elderly patients who experience incontinence may be too embarrassed to discuss this condition with anyone. What interpersonal skills can you use to obtain this information from the patient?

1. The type of dialysis that involves the direct filtering of wastes from the blood is hemodialysis.

2. Calculi are stony formations that are most likely to form when the urine is alkaline.

3. In women, the urethra is short, allowing more bacteria to reach the bladder. Also, the urethra is within the labia, which can harbor other microorganisms.

4. The patient with benign prostatic hyperplasia probably has an elevated PSA because this substance is elevated when the prostate gland is inflamed for any reason.

5. A collection of fluid in the scrotum and around the testes, also known as hydrocele, may result from trauma or infection or may simply be due to aging.

6. Microorganisms that may cause infections in the male reproductive system include staphylococci, streptococci, *Escherichia coli*, *Chlamydia*, and *Neisseria gonorrhoeae*.

7. The urinalysis is the test most commonly performed in the medical office to diagnose disorders of the urinary system.

8. With a retrograde pyelogram, dye is introduced through a catheter inserted into the urinary bladder and ureters, not injected intravenously, as with the IVP.

9. Male patients should be instructed to examine the testicles after a warm shower or bath, when the scrotal sac is relaxed.

CHAPTER
35

Obstetrics and Gynecology

Outline

Gynecologic Disorders
Dysfunctional Uterine Bleeding
Premenstrual Syndrome
Endometriosis
Uterine Prolapse and
    Displacement
Leiomyomas
Ovarian Cysts
Gynecologic Cancers
Infertility
Sexually Transmitted Diseases
**Common Diagnostic and
    Therapeutic Procedures**
The Gynecologic Examination
Colposcopy

Hysterosalpingography
Dilation and Curettage
Obstetric Care
Diagnosis of Pregnancy
First Prenatal Visit
Subsequent Prenatal Visits
Onset of Labor
Postpartum Care
Obstetric Disorders
Ectopic Pregnancy
Hyperemesis Gravidarum
Abortion
Preeclampsia and Eclampsia
Placenta Previa and Abruptio
    Placentae

**Common Obstetric Tests and
    Procedures**
Pregnancy Tests
Alpha-Fetoprotein
Fetal Ultrasonography
Contraction Stress Test and
    Nonstress Test
Contraception
Menopause

Learning Objectives

Upon successfully completing this chapter, you will be able to:

1. Spell and define key terms

2. List and describe common gynecologic and obstetric disorders

3. Identify your role in the care of gynecologic and obstetric patients

4. Describe the components of prenatal and postpartum patient care

5. Explain the diagnostic and therapeutic procedures associated with the female reproductive system

6. Identify the various methods of contraception

7. Describe menopause

1. Instruct the patient on the breast self-examination (Procedure 35-1)

2. Assist with the pelvic examination and Pap smear (Procedure 35-2)

3. Assist with colposcopy and cervical biopsy (Procedure 35-3)

CAAHEP

- Practice standard precautions
- Prepare patient for and assist with routine and specialty examinations
- Prepare patient for and assist with procedures, treatments, and minor office surgeries
- Document appropriately
- Instruct individuals according to their needs

ABHES

- Prepare patients for procedures
- Assist physician with examinations and treatments
- Perform selected tests that assist with diagnosis and treatment
- Document accurately

abortion	cystocele	labor	oligomenorrhea
amenorrhea	dysmenorrhea	laparoscopy	parity
amniocentesis	dyspareunia	lightening	pessary
Braxton-Hicks contractions	Goodell's sign	lochia	polymenorrhea
Chadwick's sign	gravid	menarche	primigravida
colpocleisis	gravida	menorrhagia	primipara
colporrhaphy	gravidity	menses	proteinuria
colposcopy	hirsutism	metrorrhagia	puerperium
culdocentesis	human chorionic gonadotropin (HCG)	multipara	rectocele
curettage	hysterosalpingogram	nulligravida	salpingo-oophorectomy
		nullipara	

The female reproductive system is responsible for the development and maintenance of primary and secondary sexual characteristics and for sexual reproduction. Gynecology and obstetrics are the two medical specialties concerned with female sexual and reproductive functions. Gynecology is a specialty of medicine that deals with development and disorders of the female reproductive system, including the internal and external organs. Obstetrics is the branch of medicine that cares for female patients through pregnancy, childbirth, and the postpartum period. The organs of the female internal reproductive system are shown in Figure 35-1.

Puberty is the onset of production of cyclical hormones that cause secondary sexual characteristics, including **menses**, or menstruation. The age at which a girl begins menses is **menarche**. The menstrual cycle, which is about 28 days, comprises a series of complex events in the internal organs controlled by hormones secreted by the anterior pituitary gland and the ovaries (Fig. 35-2). Always remind and encourage patients, especially adolescents, to record

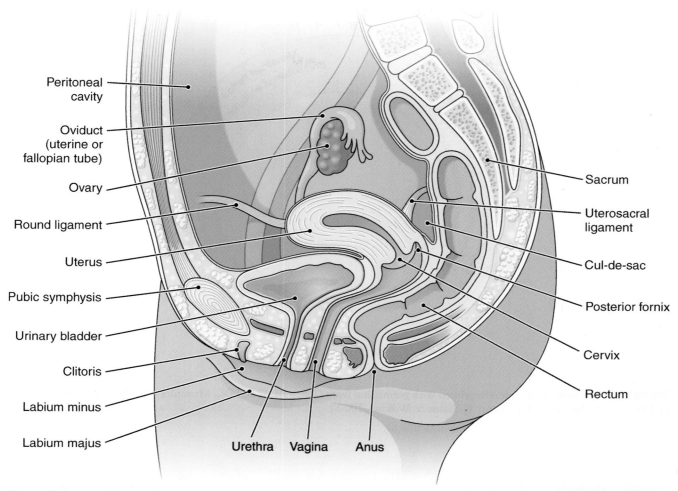

Figure 35-1 Female reproductive system. (Reprinted with permission from Cohen BJ. Memmler's The Human Body in Health and Disease. Philadelphia: Lippincott Williams & Wilkins, 2005.)

and track the menstrual cycle, since the regularity of the cycle is often critical to the physician's assessment of the patient's gynecologic health. In addition, the first day of the last menstrual period (LMP) is necessary for calculating an approximate due date in the pregnant patient. This chapter discusses some of the common disorders of the female reproductive system and caring for the obstetric patient in the medical office before and after delivery.

Gynecologic Disorders

Dysfunctional Uterine Bleeding

Dysfunctional uterine bleeding is abnormal or irregular uterine bleeding, including heavy, irregular, or light bleeding caused by an endocrine imbalance. Abnormal uterine bleeding includes the following:

- **Menorrhagia:** excessive bleeding during menses
- **Metrorrhagia:** irregular bleeding at times other than menses
- **Polymenorrhea:** abnormally frequent menses

- Postmenopausal bleeding: bleeding after menopause that is not associated with tumor, inflammation, or pregnancy

Diagnosis of dysfunctional uterine bleeding consists of ruling out other causes, such as hormonal imbalance, tumor, or another condition of the endometrial lining of the uterus. Treatment includes hormone therapy and oral contraceptives or **curettage** (scraping) of the uterine cavity, depending on the cause. Hysterectomy, surgical removal of the uterus, may be the treatment of choice for patients who do not respond to conservative therapy, who are at increased risk for adenocarcinoma, and who do not desire pregnancy.

Premenstrual Syndrome

Characterized by a wide variety of physical, psychological, and behavioral signs and symptoms, premenstrual syndrome (PMS) occurs on a regular, cyclic basis (Box 35-1). For diagnostic purposes, the patient must have a

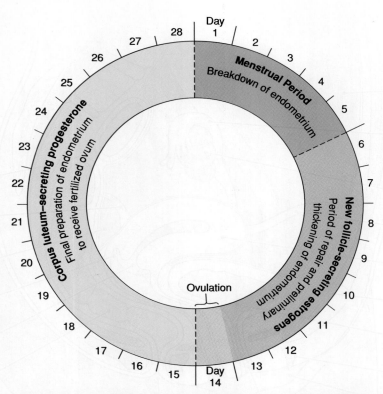

Figure 35-2 The menstrual cycle. (Reprinted with permission from Cohen BJ, Wood DL. Memmler's The Human Body in Health and Disease. Philadelphia: Lippincott Williams & Wilkins, 2000.)

BOX 35-1

PREMENSTRUAL SYNDROME (PMS)

The hormonal flux associated with the menstrual cycle may affect body systems other than the reproductive system in some women. The cascade of events results in the following series of symptoms:

- Acne
- Breast swelling and tenderness
- Feeling tired
- Difficulty sleeping
- Upset stomach, bloating, constipation, or diarrhea
- Headache or backache
- Appetite changes or cravings
- Trouble concentrating or remembering
- Tension, irritability, mood swings, or crying spells
- Anxiety or depression

Although no treatment works the same on all women, the following are some common treatments for PMS that the physician may suggest:

- Take a multivitamin every day that includes 400 micrograms of folic acid.
- Include a calcium supplement with vitamin D to keep bones strong.
- Exercise regularly.
- Eat healthy foods, including fruits, vegetables, and whole grains.
- Avoid salt, sugary foods, caffeine, and alcohol.
- Get enough sleep.
- Find healthy ways to cope with stress.
- Don't smoke.

Over-the-counter medications such as ibuprofen, aspirin, or naproxen sodium may be ordered by the physician for the pain associated with PMS. Severe cases may require the physician to prescribe drugs to prevent ovulation such as birth control pills.

From the Office on Women's Health in the Department of Health and Human Services, 2007, www.womenshealth.gov.

complex of signs and symptoms associated with PMS that occur during the 7 to 10 days before menses. These signs and symptoms must be severe enough to interfere with interpersonal relationships and routine activities. PMS usually diminishes a few hours after the onset of menses, and the cause is idiopathic (unknown). Diagnosis is based on the physician's assessment of the history and physical examination. Patients should chart their symptoms for several months on a calendar that includes the menstrual cycle.

You can have a dramatic influence on the patient's ability to cope with PMS by providing emotional support, teaching the patient about it, and encouraging regular exercise, which may help minimize it. In addition, certain dietary restrictions, such as eliminating caffeine, salt, and animal fats, can decrease the severity of PMS. Patients also should be encouraged to get adequate rest and avoid unnecessary stress.

PATIENT EDUCATION

PREMENSTRUAL DYSPHORIC DISORDER

While many women have symptoms of premenstrual syndrome, a few women have a more severe form of PMS known as premenstrual dysphoric disorder, or PMDD. Diagnosis of PMDD is made when five or more of the following symptoms are present a week before the menstrual cycle begins:

- Feelings of sadness or despair including possible suicidal thoughts
- Feelings of tension or anxiety
- Panic attacks
- Mood swings, crying
- Lasting irritability or anger that affects other people
- Disinterest in daily activities and relationships
- Trouble thinking or focusing
- Tiredness or low energy
- Food cravings or binge eating
- Difficulty sleeping
- Feeling out of control
- Physical symptoms such as bloating, breast tenderness, headaches, and joint or muscle pain

In addition to individual counseling and stress management, the physician may order antidepressants called serotonin reuptake inhibitors (SSRIs), which have been shown to help some women.

Source: Office on Women's Health in the Department of Health and Human Services.

 CHECKPOINT QUESTION

1. What is the difference between menorrhagia and metrorrhagia?

Endometriosis

Endometriosis is a condition of unknown cause in which endometrial tissue grows outside the uterine cavity. Endometrial tissue may be found in the fallopian tubes, the ovaries, the uterosacral ligaments, and in rare cases, in other parts of the abdominal cavity. The patient, who is often of reproductive age, complains of infertility, **dysmenorrhea**, pelvic pain, and **dyspareunia**. The patient's symptoms and physical findings may indicate endometriosis, but the diagnosis and the severity must be confirmed by direct visualization, usually by way of a **laparoscopy** (Fig. 35-3).

Treatment of endometriosis may relieve the pelvic pain, but some treatments reduce fertility. The type of therapy depends on the age of the patient, the severity of the symptoms, and the patient's desire for future pregnancy. Hormone and drug therapy to suppress the growth of the tissue and laparoscopic excision of the tissue using laser or cautery may be used to treat en-

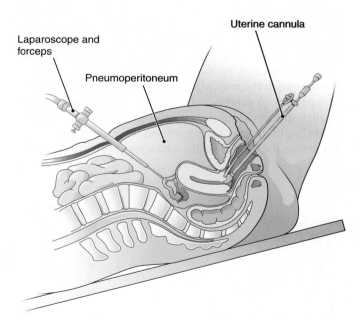

Figure 35-3 Laparoscopy. The laparoscope is inserted through a small incision in the abdomen. A forceps is inserted through the scope to grasp the fallopian tube. To improve the view, a uterine cannula is inserted into the vagina to push the uterus upward. Insufflation of gas creates an air pocket, and the pelvis is raised, which forces the intestines higher into the abdomen. (Reprinted with permission from Cohen BJ. Medical Terminology: An Illustrated Guide. Philadelphia: Lippincott Williams & Wilkins, 2003.)

dometriosis. For patients with severe symptoms, the treatment of choice may be a hysterectomy with possible bilateral **salpingo-oophorectomy**, or surgical removal of the fallopian tubes and ovaries.

Uterine Prolapse and Displacement

Prolapse of the uterus is an abnormal condition in which the uterus droops or protrudes down into the vagina. Often, the condition is accompanied by **cystocele, rectocele**, or both. Cystocele is herniation of the urinary bladder into the vagina, and rectocele is herniation of the rectum into the vagina. The degree of prolapse is usually described as mild, moderate, or severe, or grade I, II, or III. A commonly used method classifies the prolapse in degrees:

- First-degree prolapse occurs when the uterus has descended to the level of the vaginal orifice.
- Second-degree prolapse occurs when the uterine cervix protrudes through the vaginal orifice.
- Third-degree prolapse occurs when the entire cervix and uterus protrude beyond the vaginal orifice.

Diagnosis of uterine prolapse is made during a pelvic examination, at which time the degree of prolapse can be determined. While many women do not have symptoms, others complain of pelvic pressure, dyspareunia, urinary problems, or constipation. Surgical treatment may include vaginal hysterectomy, **colporrhaphy** (suture of the vagina), or **colpocleisis** (surgery to occlude the vagina). Medical management for patients who are elderly or a poor risk for surgery includes hormone therapy to strengthen the muscular floor of the pelvis and the use of a **pessary**. A pessary is a device that is inserted into the vagina and fits around the cervix to support the uterus. You should instruct the patient on the proper procedure for caring for the device by removing it according to the

physician's orders and washing it with soap and warm water before reinserting it into the vagina.

The uterus is normally tilted slightly forward over the bladder with the cervix at a right angle to the direction of the vagina. The uterus is movable, and stress on the supporting ligaments occasionally tilts it from its natural position. This is called uterine displacement (Fig. 35-4). The symptoms of uterine displacement may include pressure in the rectal area or against the bladder that is not usually severe, just troublesome to the patient. Treatment follows the same protocol as required for uterine prolapse. In some instances, the uterus may simply be stitched back into its original position in a hysteropexy.

Leiomyomas

Leiomyomas are benign tumors of the uterus, including fibroid tumors, myomas, and fibromyomas. These tumors may be in any of the uterine tissue layers—endometrium, myometrium, or perimetrium—and they vary greatly in size. Most patients are asymptomatic, but large tumors tend to distort the uterus and are relatively likely to be symptomatic. Symptoms may include abnormal bleeding, pelvic pressure and discomfort, constipation, urinary frequency, and infertility.

A presumptive diagnosis is based on the patient's symptoms and physician's assessment, which initially includes bimanual examination and sounding of the uterus. Sounding of the uterus requires the physician to do a pelvic examination and possibly the insertion of a uterine sound (a long slender instrument; refer to Chapter 21) into the uterine cavity. Obstruction or resistance may be due to the tumor pressing into the uterine cavity. Most physicians request an ultrasound of the uterus to confirm the presence of these tumors.

Treatment of leiomyoma depends on the size of the tumor or tumors. Small asymptomatic tumors are mon-

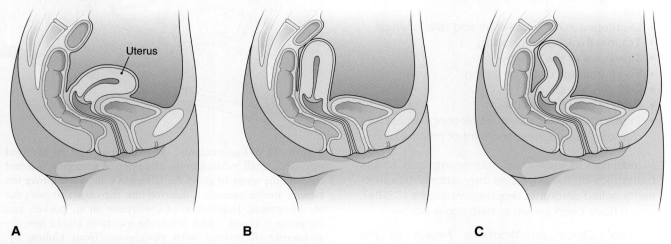

Figure 35-4 Retrodisplacements of the uterus. (**A**) The normal position of the uterus as detected on palpation. (**B**) In retroversion, the uterus turns posteriorly as a whole. (**C**) In retroflexion, the fundus bends posteriorly above the cervical end.

itored to detect excessive growth. Depending on the patient's age and desire for pregnancy, myomectomy or hysterectomy may be indicated.

 CHECKPOINT QUESTION

2. What are some symptoms of endometriosis?

Ovarian Cysts

Numerous types of ovarian cysts, including functional cysts and polycystic ovaries, are benign. Functional ovarian cysts, which are fairly common, include the follicular cyst. This is a fluid-filled sac that causes few if any problems. The patient is most often asymptomatic unless the cyst is large or ruptures. Functional cysts are usually detected during surgery, and treatment is simply puncture or excision.

In contrast, polycystic ovary syndrome (Stein-Leventhal syndrome) is a more troublesome and complex disorder. It affects both ovaries and is most often found in adolescent girls and young women, who have numerous symptoms of an endocrine imbalance. The signs include anovulation, irregular menses or **amenorrhea** (no menses), and **hirsutism**, an abnormal or excessive growth of hair. Diagnosis is based on pelvic examination, ultrasonography, laparoscopy, or exploratory laparotomy. Treatment is difficult and depends on the signs and symptoms and the patient's desire for future pregnancy. Management of this disorder includes hormone therapy or oral contraceptives.

Gynecologic Cancers

The malignant tumors affecting the female reproductive system and their characteristics, diagnosis, and treatment are outlined in Table 35-1. For patient education,

TABLE 35-1	Cancers of the Female Reproductive System			
Cancer	**Warning Signs**	**Risk Factors**	**Early Detection**	**Treatment**
Breast	Breast changes: lumps, pain, thickening, swelling, retraction, dimpling	Over age 40, history of breast cancer, early menarche, nulliparity, first birth at late age	Monthly self-examination, mammogram by age 40 and yearly after 40; yearly clinical breast exam; monthly self-breast exam	Lumpectomy, mastectomy, radiation, chemotherapy
Cervical	Often asymptomatic; irregular bleeding, abnormal vaginal discharge	Intercourse at early age, multiple sex partners, cigarette smoking, history of STDs such as HPV	Annual Pap smear	Cryotherapy; electrocoagulation; surgery; radiation; chemotherapy; new vaccine is available to prevent certain types of HPV that may cause cervical cancer
Endometrial	Irregular bleeding outside menses; unusual vaginal discharge; excessive bleeding during menses; postmenopausal bleeding	Obesity; early menarche; multiple sex partners; late menopause; history of infertility; family history	Endometrial biopsy at menopause for high-risk women	Progesterone therapy; surgery; radiation; chemotherapy
Ovarian	Often asymptomatic; abdominal enlargement; vague digestive disorders, discomfort; gas distention	Risk increases with age (esp. > 60 years), nulliparity, history of breast cancer	Periodic complete pelvic examination	Surgery; radiation; chemotherapy

you should know the recommendations regarding the frequency of pelvic and breast examinations and Pap smears. You should obtain current brochures and literature on various types of cancers from either the American Cancer Society or the American College of Obstetrics and Gynecology and have them readily available to patients.

Cervical and breast cancers have an excellent prognosis when detected and treated early, but left untreated or diagnosed in later stages, these cancers are deadly. Instruct and encourage all female patients to perform a breast self-examination every month (Procedure 35-1). Patients should also be encouraged to have a complete physical that includes a breast examination by the physician and a pelvic examination and Papanicolaou (Pap) test, which is a screening test for early detection of cancer of the cervix. The American College of Obstetricians and Gynecologists (ACOG) recommends that the first Pap test and pelvic exam be performed about 3 years after the first sexual intercourse or by age 21, whichever comes first, and annually until age 30 years. Women over age 30 who have had three negative Pap tests can be screened every 2 to 3 years or annually as recommended by the physician.

Initially, the abnormal growth of cancerous cells in the cervix is asymptomatic, which further necessitates early detection during the physical examination and Pap smear. The Pap test is a grading of any abnormal tissue scraped from the cervix using a classification system such as the one described in Table 35-2. Some laboratories use another classification, the Bethesda system, to provide a more descriptive narrative of the abnormal cells. Cervical cells in the Bethesda system are categorized as normal, atypical squamous cells (ASC), squamous intraepithelial lesions (SIL), atypical glandular cells, or cancer. In addition, the squamous intraepithelial lesions may be noted as high grade (HSIL) or low grade (LSIL). Regardless of the method used by the laboratory to classify the Pap test results, not all abnormal results indicate cancer. However, since this is a deadly

TABLE 35-2	Classification of Papanicolaou Tests
Class	**Characteristics**
I	Normal test, no atypical cells
II	Atypical cells but no evidence of malignancy
III	Atypical cells possible but not conclusive for malignancy
IV	Cells strongly suggest malignancy
V	Strong evidence of malignancy

disease, it must be ruled out using further diagnostic studies such as **colposcopy**, a magnified examination of the cervical tissue with a special instrument called a colposcope. Other reasons for an abnormal Pap result include inflammation of the cervix and some sexually transmitted diseases such as human papilloma virus (HPV) infection.

Infertility

Female infertility is more difficult to diagnose than male infertility. Most testing begins by eliminating the male as the infertile party and then focuses on the female partner. Testing is usually not started until after 1 year of unprotected intercourse without conception.

The causes of infertility may include uterine or cervical abnormalities, tubal occlusion or scarring, a hormonal imbalance, or psychological factors. Diagnosis requires a complete history and physical examination. An endometrial biopsy may diagnose anovulation; progesterone blood levels may indicate hormonal deficiencies; or hysterosalpingography may indicate tubal occlusion or uterine abnormalities. Treatment necessitates identifying and correcting the problem. Procedures such as in vitro fertilization may also be recommended, again, depending upon the nature of the problem.

 CHECKPOINT QUESTION

3. What two factors greatly affect the prognosis of all cancers?

Sexually Transmitted Diseases

Many of the diseases transmitted through sexual contact have serious consequences and may affect men or women. The most deadly of these is acquired immunodeficiency syndrome (AIDS), although other sexually transmitted diseases (STDs) also continue to be a problem. Since STDs are easily transmitted, all STDs must be reported to the local health department by the medical office. This may be your responsibility, or the physician may be required to report the disease according to local policy or the policy of the medical office. In some areas, you may have to file a form or written report; others have a phone reporting system. You need to be familiar with your office policy and procedure manual regarding this requirement and the local laws on reporting. The patient should be encouraged to notify sexual partners so that they may also receive treatment for the appropriate STD.

AIDS

AIDS is an infectious disease that overwhelms the body's immune system. The pathogen that causes AIDS is the human immunodeficiency virus (HIV), which destroys T-helper cells, lowering the body's ability to fight infection. Transmission of HIV most often occurs through an exchange of blood or body fluids, including a sexual act with an HIV-positive partner. A person who is HIV positive may go through the following stages as the infection progresses to AIDS:

1. Acute infectious state with generally mild flulike symptoms
2. Latent period without symptoms but still infectious
3. Weight loss, lymphadenopathy, fever, diarrhea, anorexia, fatigue, and skin rashes
4. Onset of immunodeficiency disorders, such as Kaposi's sarcoma and *Pneumocystis carinii* pneumonia

Although new treatments prolong the HIV-positive individual's life, there currently is no cure; however, research to find more effective treatments and a possible cure is ongoing.

Syphilis

After AIDS, syphilis is the most serious STD. The cause of syphilis is a microorganism known as *Treponema pallidum,* a spirochete. The first sign is a chancre or ulcerated lesion at the primary site of infection on the genitalia. This chancre appears several days to several weeks after infection, heals very quickly, and may not be noticed. Although the chancre heals quickly, the spirochete spreads quickly through the bloodstream and becomes systemic, with far-reaching consequences. The second phase is identified by a rash that may appear anywhere on the body. The patient continues to be infectious at this stage, but treatment with penicillin will stop the progression of the disease to the next, or tertiary, phase. If left untreated, the rash will disappear, and the syphilis may lie dormant for years. At some point, however, the patient will experience cardiovascular damage, central nervous system involvement, and death.

Infants born with syphilis caused by transplacental infection are commonly mentally retarded, deaf, blind, or deformed. Many babies spontaneously abort or are delivered stillborn.

Chlamydia

Chlamydia infections cause urethritis in men, cervicitis in women, and lymphogranuloma venereum in both, all caused by the organism *Chlamydia trachomatis.* Chlamydia is the most common STD in the United States. Female patients may be asymptomatic or may have vague flulike symptoms that are difficult to diagnose without specific reason to suspect infection. In severe cases, there may be extensive lymph gland involvement known as lymphogranuloma venereum.

Chlamydia is one of the leading causes of pelvic inflammatory disease, causing tubal scarring and eventual infertility in women. Infants born to mothers with chlamydial infections may have conjunctivitis and pneumonia. The fetus may spontaneously abort, deliver prematurely, or be stillborn.

Diagnosis is made by a swab culture of the site sent to the laboratory for identification of the microorganism. The disease is treated with an antibiotic such as doxycycline, tetracycline, or sulfamethoxazole until the patient tests negative for the presence of the pathogen.

Condylomata Acuminata

Condylomata acuminata is a viral infection of the genital area causing the growth of soft, papillary warts that appear in a wide variety of places, including the vulva, vagina, cervix, and perineum. The cause is the human papilloma virus, or HPV. The genital warts usually appear about 3 months after exposure. Biopsy of the condyloma is appropriate to rule out the slight possibility of a malignancy. Although HPV is difficult to eradicate, cryotherapy (freezing the involved area) or laser ablation (burning with laser) has moderate success.

HPV has been implicated as a risk for cervical cancer in some women, but currently, there is a vaccine to protect against four types of HPV that are responsible for 70% of cervical cancers and 90% of genital warts (Centers for Disease Control and Prevention). The Advisory Committee on Immunization Practices (ACIP) recommends this vaccine for girls over the age of 9; however, there are no current federal laws requiring administration of this vaccine.

 CHECKPOINT QUESTION

4. Which sexually transmitted disease may cause conjunctivitis and pneumonia in newborns born to infected mothers?

Gonorrhea

Gonorrhea is the second most common STD and is caused by a gram-negative diplococcus, *Neisseria gonorrhoeae.* The symptoms appear in the genitalia 2 to 8 days after exposure. In some female patients, the Bartholin and Skene glands fill with pus, and the infection may spread to the cervix. However, female patients may be asymptomatic and unaware of the disease. The disease may lead to salpingitis with scarring and adhesions or pelvic inflammatory disease. Infants born to mothers infected with gonorrhea may develop purulent conjunctivitis with corneal ulcerations that result in blindness. All infants are now treated prophylactically in the newborn nursery.

Diagnosis is based on the symptoms and through a culture of the drainage if present. Once diagnosed, gonorrhea may be treated with penicillin, although penicillin-resistant strains are now appearing.

Herpes Genitalis

Herpes genitalis is caused by the herpes simplex virus 2 (HSV2) and is characterized by painful vesicular lesions in the vaginal, vulvar, or anorectal area. This genital infection usually appears within 3 to 7 days after exposure. The infected patient may present with painful vesicles in the genital region that rupture and leave equally painful ulcers that eventually heal in about 10 days. In addition, the patient may have swollen and tender lymph nodes and flulike symptoms. After the lesion heals, the patient may be in remission for years, or the symptoms may recur with each stressful situation. Patients with herpes genitalis should be advised to avoid sexual contact during episodes of vesiculation because the exudate is highly contagious. Although there is no cure, the condition is somewhat controlled with an antiviral agent such as acyclovir.

Infants born vaginally to mothers with active lesions may develop the disease within a few weeks of birth. The virus spreads rapidly to the organs of the infant and up to 90% of infected infants die.

Vulvovaginitis, Salpingitis, and Pelvic Inflammatory Disease

Although vulvovaginitis, salpingitis, and pelvic inflammatory disease can be caused by any type of microorganism, these disorders are commonly caused by sexually transmitted infections. Vulvovaginitis is an inflammation of the vulva and vagina and is one of the common complaints of female patients. Symptoms often include pruritus, burning of the vulva or the vagina (or both), and increased vaginal discharge. On examination, the vulva and vagina are reddened. The type of discharge often indicates the cause of the disorder, and effective treatment depends on the cause. The causative agent is confirmed by a microscopic examination of a vaginal smear or by culture of the vaginal discharge and may include the following microorganisms:

- *Trichomonas vaginalis*: Known as trich, this protozoan causes an STD. The signs are a thin, frothy, greenish or gray vaginal discharge with an odor. Signs and symptoms include dysuria with urinary frequency and intense pruritus. Treatment is oral metronidazole for both partners.
- *Candida albicans*: Also known as monilia, this fungus grows best in the presence of glucose. The signs include a thick, curd-like discharge with white patches on the vaginal walls, usually with no odor. Intense itching is

usual. The pathogen is found in the intestines and is most likely to affect the patient during the secretory phase of the menstrual cycle. It is very common during pregnancy and in patients receiving antibiotic therapy. Treatment requires nystatin vaginal suppositories, which may be purchased without a prescription.
- *Gardnerella vaginitis*: This gram-negative bacillus causes a gray discharge with a foul odor. It is treated with metronidazole.

Salpingitis is a bacterial infection of the fallopian tubes that is most often transmitted by sexual intercourse. Young sexually active women, women with multiple sexual partners, and women with intrauterine devices are at increased risk for salpingitis. Numerous microorganisms may cause salpingitis, but the most common microbes include *N. gonorrhoeae*, *C. trachomatis*, genital mycoplasma, and normal flora bacteria. Salpingitis is sometimes called pelvic inflammatory disease when the surrounding structures, including the pelvic peritoneum, uterus, ovaries, and surrounding tissues, are inflamed. Signs and symptoms include varying degrees of abdominal pain and tenderness with or without fever and leukocytosis, an abnormal increase in the white blood cell count.

Cultures for gonorrhea and tests for chlamydia are essential for antibiotic therapy. **Culdocentesis** may be necessary to obtain purulent drainage and determine the exact cause of the infection. Laparoscopy may be performed to determine the extent of the infection. Treatment for mild infections includes antibiotic and analgesic therapy, bed rest, and removal of the source of infection. In patients with pyosalpinx (pus in the fallopian tubes), tubal obstruction, abscess, serious inflammation, and edema, treatment may be a hysterectomy with bilateral salpingectomy-oophorectomy or an incision and drainage.

 CHECKPOINT QUESTION

5. Which sexually transmitted disease is associated with female reproductive cancer?

Common Diagnostic and Therapeutic Procedures

The Gynecologic Examination

As part of the gynecologic examination, the physician examines the patient's breasts, performs a pelvic examination, and obtains a Pap smear. Because of the risk of contracting infection from body fluids, especially blood, you and the physician must observe standard precautions, wearing protective barriers such as gloves as appropriate during the examination. When scheduling the appointment, instruct the patient not to douche, use vaginal medication, or have sexual intercourse for 24 hours before the examination. If a Pap smear will be performed, the appointment should be scheduled about 1 week after the end of menses. When the patient arrives for the scheduled appointment, spend time with the patient to establish rapport, especially with new patients and patients with special needs, such as the young, elderly, and disabled. A procedure that is rushed or seems hurried to the patient may diminish the professional image of the office and the patient's attitude toward the physician and staff.

The physician usually begins the examination by examining the breast and surrounding tissue, including the axillae and chest tissue up to the clavicle. This tissue is inspected for dimpling or size disparity and palpated for lumps or thickenings. Next, the physician examines the external and internal female genitalia to identify or diagnose any abnormal conditions (Procedure 35-2). Although the dorsal lithotomy position provides the best visibility for the physician, this position may be difficult for elderly or some disabled persons. Elevating the head of the table to 30 degrees may be easier for the patient while allowing the physician to do a thorough examination. The elevation of the table does not seem to have any disadvantages, and often the patient finds this position more comfortable, but consult with the physician if the lithotomy position is not possible. If elevating the head of the examination table is not appropriate, an alternative position, such as Sim's, may be necessary.

After visually inspecting the external genitalia, the physician examines the internal female structures. To begin, a vaginal speculum is inserted into the vagina. The vaginal speculum may come in a variety of sizes and is made of either stainless steel (Fig. 35-5) or plastic (Fig. 35-6). Selecting an appropriately sized vaginal speculum is important to maintain the patient's comfort and to facilitate the examination. Although the patient's age and size are the primary factors, the largest speculum that is comfortable for the patient provides the best visibility. Two sizes may be set out to give the physician a choice.

Figure 35-6 A variety of plastic, disposable vaginal specula. (From Weber J, Kelley J. Health Assessment in Nursing. 2nd ed. Philadelphia: Lippincott Williams & Wilkins, 2003.)

Vaginal specula come in pediatric, small, medium, and large sizes, and a variety of sizes should be available in each examination room.

In addition to having the correct size vaginal speculum available for the physician, you should make sure the speculum is warmed for patient comfort. Warm the speculum by running it under warm water (Fig. 35-7) or by storing it on an electric heating pad set on a low setting. Some examination tables are equipped with a special warming drawer for the vaginal specula that heats them automatically as long as the examination table is plugged

Figure 35-5 A stainless steel vaginal speculum. (LifeART image copyright © 2008 Lippincott Williams & Wilkins. All rights reserved.)

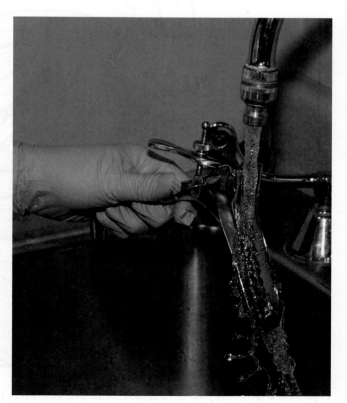

Figure 35-7 Warm the vaginal speculum with warm water.

into an electrical outlet. Some physicians prefer that lubricant not be used on the speculum before insertion since it may interfere with obtaining the cells during the Pap smear. The water used to warm the speculum may serve as a lubricant for easier insertion. Always follow the instructions given by your physician to prepare the patient and the equipment and supplies for this examination.

Once the cervical cells are obtained, the physician will remove the vaginal speculum and perform a bimanual examination using gloved hands. During this part of the examination, the physician may want lubricant applied to gloved fingers for easier insertion into the vaginal and rectum. Specifically, the physician will insert fingers into the vagina and the rectum to feel for the position and size of internal organs (Fig. 35-8). Your role during this part of the examination includes assisting the physician as necessary and supporting the patient. When this part of the examination is finished, you should assist the patient to a sitting position, prepare any specimens obtained for transport to the laboratory, and instruct the patient on the procedure for obtaining the results. You should also reinforce any instructions given by the physician before discharging the patient.

WHAT IF?

The first Pap smear or gynecologic examination for young women may cause great anxiety. What if an 18-year-old woman is to have her first Pap smear today? How should you handle the situation?

Bring the patient into the room and encourage her to talk about her feelings. Do not have her change into an examining gown until she has had an opportunity to speak with the physician or practitioner about the procedure. The physician may require the presence of another health care worker, like the medical assistant, during the examination; however, some physicians feel comfortable performing the examination without assistance. If you remain in the room, you will have an opportunity to provide reassurance and information. Male physicians should have a female health care worker in the room during the examination as a legal precaution.

Figure 35-8 The bimanual examination. (LifeART image copyright © 2008 Lippincott Williams & Wilkins. All rights reserved.)

Colposcopy

Colposcopy is visual examination of the vaginal and cervical surfaces using a stereoscopic microscope called a colposcope. It is often performed to evaluate patients with atypical Pap smear results to locate the origin of abnormal cells; to select areas for cervical, endocervical, or endometrial biopsy; to assess cervical lesions; or for follow-up in patients with a history of cervical dysplasia or cervical cancer.

If a biopsy is to be done, be sure that written consent has been obtained. When possible, label specimen containers and complete laboratory request forms before the procedure. Have the completed forms and labeled containers ready in the examination room for use after the specimen is obtained. Although there is usually very little or no bleeding from the biopsy, chemical cautery using silver nitrate or Monsel solution should be available to control bleeding as necessary. The patient preparation for colposcopy with cervical biopsy is similar to that required for the pelvic examination (Procedure 35-3).

 CHECKPOINT QUESTION

6. What procedures are normally included in the complete gynecologic examination?

Hysterosalpingography

Hysterosalpingography is a diagnostic procedure in which the uterus and uterine tubes are radiographed after injection of a contrast medium. The radiograph is called a **hysterosalpingogram**. This test is often performed to determine the configuration of the uterus and the patency of the fallopian tubes for patients with infertility. Although this test is not usually performed in the physician's office, you may be responsible for scheduling the procedure and explaining to the patient any preparations including where to go and when the procedure will be performed.

Dilation and Curettage

Dilation and curettage (D & C) may be performed to remove uterine tissue for diagnostic testing, to remove endometrial tissue, to prevent or treat menorrhagia, or to remove retained products of conception after a spontaneous **abortion** or miscarriage. During the procedure, the cervical canal is widened with a uterine sound, and the lining of the uterus is scraped with a curet (see Chapter 21 for a picture of a curet). This procedure usually requires anesthesia and may be performed as an inpatient or outpatient procedure. The patient must sign a preoperative consent form, and you may be asked to give any preoperative instructions as directed by the physician. Preoperative instructions may include advising the patient of the need for a perineal pad, not a tampon, to be worn postoperatively and information regarding the signs of infection, hemorrhage, or other follow-up care according to the specifications of the physician.

 CHECKPOINT QUESTION

7. Why would a hysterosalpingography be necessary?

Obstetric Care

Unlike other physicians, obstetricians are frequently called to the hospital to deliver infants during regular office hours. In the absence of the physician, you must use good judgment when pregnant patients come into the office for a scheduled appointment or call with questions and concerns. For instance, you may have to determine whether a situation can wait for the physician's return, whether another physician should be consulted, whether the patient should go to the hospital, or whether, with the physician's permission, you should advise the patient how to manage the problem. Protocols listed in the policy and procedure manual for actions to be taken in specific situations help ensure that, in the physician's absence, safe procedures are followed for your patients and help protect you and your physician from errors in treatment.

Diagnosis of Pregnancy

Many patients suspect that they are **gravid**, or pregnant, because they have signs; however, early signs of pregnancy may indicate other disorders and therefore are considered presumptive until a conclusive diagnostic procedure is done. Presumptive signs include amenorrhea, nausea, vomiting, breast enlargement and tenderness, fatigue, and urinary frequency. Probable signs include **human chorionic gonadotropin (HCG)** in the maternal urine or blood, changes in the uterus and cervix, **Braxton-Hicks contractions**, and enlargement of the uterus (Table 35-3). Braxton-Hicks contractions are irregular uterine contractions that occur fairly frequently but do not affect the cervix like the contractions of active labor. These contractions are normal, and although the patient may or may not be aware, the physician can feel the contractions during a bimanual examination or while palpating the abdomen. The diagnosis of pregnancy is confirmed by the physician or the image of a fetus on ultrasonography.

Cervical changes that occur during pregnancy include softening of the cervix, known as **Goodell's sign**; increased vascularity of the cervix and vagina causing a bluish-violet color (**Chadwick's sign**); and formation of a mucous plug. The mucous plug forms in the cervical os

TABLE 35-3	Signs and Symptoms of Pregnancy	
Presumptive Signs	**Probable Signs**	**Conclusive Signs**
Cessation of menses	HCG in urine, blood	Fetal heart tone
Nausea and vomiting	Braxton-Hicks contractions	Fetal movement detected by
Breast tenderness	Enlargement of abdomen	examiner
Breast enlargement	Uterine changes	Visualization of the fetus
Patient feels quickening or	Goodell's sign	
fetal movement	Chadwick's sign	
Fatigue		
Urinary frequency		

(opening) and protects the developing fetus and the amniotic sac from the external environment. With the onset of **labor**, the mucous plug is expelled with a small amount of blood and is often referred to as the bloody show.

 CHECKPOINT QUESTION

8. Why are presumptive signs and symptoms of pregnancy not considered to be conclusive?

 TRIAGE

While you are working in a gynecology medical office, the following three situations arise:

A. Patient A calls wanting information about the vaginal ring contraception.
B. Patient B is pregnant, and this is the first prenatal visit.
C. Patient C has been seen by the physician and needs to have a hysterosalpingography scheduled at the outpatient ambulatory center.

How do you sort these situations? What do you do first? Second? Third?

First, have the receptionist take a message from patient A and call her back later. This is clearly not an emergency, and you can call her back at a more convenient time. Next you should discharge patient C, letting her know that you will schedule the outpatient procedure later today and call her with the details tomorrow. Finally, call patient B to the examination room and take a thorough medical history and vital signs. Since patient B is new, she may require additional time and reassurance. She may also have questions and concerns about her pregnancy, and you do not want to be rushed during the patient education part of this initial visit.

 PATIENT EDUCATION

FOLIC ACID BEFORE AND DURING PREGNANCY

Women who are planning to get pregnant and those who are pregnant should take folic acid, a B vitamin to prevent neural tube defects. Although medical experts do not know how folic acid works, it is needed to make healthy new cells, like the ones that make up a baby's brain and spine. Taking folic acid every day, starting before and during pregnancy, can reduce the risk for these serious birth defects by 50% to 70%. Every woman who could possibly get pregnant should take 400 micrograms (400 mcg or 0.4 mg) of folic acid daily in a vitamin or in foods that have been enriched with folic acid. Many foods, including cereals, are enriched with folic acid. Encourage patients to check the label since some cereals provide 100% of the daily amount required.

First Prenatal Visit

A pregnant patient's initial prenatal visit is extensive and critical to the ongoing assessment of the pregnancy. The first examination is done to establish a detailed baseline of the patient's physical condition and includes a confirmation of pregnancy, a complete history and physical, determination of the estimated date of delivery, assessment of gestational age, identification of risk factors, and patient education. To elicit complete and accurate information, the health history interview should be conducted in a private room where there will be no interruptions. This is a complete physical examination with a pelvic examination, screening for *N. gonorrhoeae*, chlamydial infection, cervical cancer, syphilis, and tuberculosis. The first prenatal visit also includes the following:

• Blood work: The Venereal Disease Research Laboratory, rapid plasma reagin, or other test for syphilis;

complete blood count with hematocrit, hemoglobin, and white blood cell count with differential; and blood type with Rh factor. Blood for a rubella titer is also collected to determine maternal immunity to German measles, a disease that can result in serious birth defects if contracted during pregnancy.

- Tuberculosis screening: Tine test or purified protein derivative injection.
- Urinalysis: Glucose, albumin, and acetone testing.

The physical and pelvic examination will include laboratory tests such as the Pap smear, urine pregnancy test, clinical pelvimetry, and laboratory blood tests. Also, the estimated date of delivery will be calculated. This is a prediction of the due date, assuming the pregnancy progresses normally (Box 35-2). Normal gestation is 37 to 40 weeks. Infants born before the 37th

week are considered to be premature. Those born after the 41st week are postmature.

Patients should be instructed to notify the physician if any of the following occurs:

- Vaginal bleeding or spotting
- Persistent vomiting
- Fever or chills
- Dysuria
- Abdominal or uterine cramping
- Leaking amniotic fluid
- Alteration in fetal movement
- Dizziness or blurred vision
- Other problems

In addition, advise the pregnant patient to avoid taking any medications or drugs, even over-the-counter preparations, without consulting the physician. Many factors, including medications, nicotine, and alcohol can put the developing fetus at risk. Depending on maternal exposure to the substance and the stage of fetal development, development may be so altered as to cause deformities or damage to other internal organs and may threaten the life of the fetus.

Parity Versus Gravidity

You and the physician will obtain a thorough and detailed history of the patient, including information about previous pregnancies to help predict the outcome of this one. The term **parity** refers to the number of live births, and **gravidity** refers to any pregnancy, regardless of its length and outcome. The pregnant, or gravid, woman is a **gravida**, usually with an indicator of the number. A woman who has never been pregnant is a **nulligravida**, while the woman who is pregnant for the first time is a **primigravida**. The number of live births is also given a prefix indicator, such as **nullipara** (has never borne a living child), **primipara** (first living child), and **multipara** (many live births).

These numbers are listed for the physician's review as gr (or simply g), p, pret (preterm or premature), and ab (abortion, spontaneous or induced). For example, a woman who is pregnant for the third time, has lost no pregnancies, and carried her previous pregnancies to term is listed as gr iii, pret 0, ab 0, p ii. (Arabic numbers are also acceptable.) A woman who is pregnant for the fifth time and who has delivered one set of twins and two single infants, has had no premature infants, and has lost one pregnancy spontaneously would be listed as gr v, pret 0, ab i, p iv.

Subsequent Prenatal Visits

If the pregnancy is progressing as expected and without complications (Fig. 35-9), then the patient is scheduled for office visits monthly at 4, 8, 12, 16, 20, 24, and 28

BOX 35-2

DETERMINING THE ESTIMATED DATE OF CONFINEMENT OR EXPECTED DATE OF DELIVERY

The Estimated Date of Confinement (EDC) is also called the expected date of delivery (EDD). Because of the negative connotations of the word *confinement* and because women are no longer confined during pregnancy or the postpartum period, terminology for the due date is changing to reflect current maternity trends. Many methods are used for determining this projected date. Nagele's rule requires an arithmetic calculation using the following formula:

The first day of the last menstrual period (LMP)
$$- 3 \text{ months} + 7 \text{ days} + 1 \text{ year}$$

Example: LMP = May 3, 2007

LMP =	5	3	2007
	−3	+7	+1
Due date =	2	10	2008

A simpler method is adding 9 months and 7 days to the first day of the LMP. Try that method with the example.

The third common method is to use a gestational wheel. Using the inner wheel, line up the first day of the LMP on the outer wheel with the appropriate arrow and read around the wheel to the indicated milestones in the pregnancy. Many wheels indicate the date of conception and times recommended for blood work and other testing, and all show the date that delivery is expected.

FETAL DEVELOPMENT*

1st Lunar Month (4 weeks)

The embryo is 4 to 5 mm in length.
Trophoblasts embed in decidua.
Chorionic villi form.
Foundations for nervous system,
  genitourinary system, skin,
  bones, and lungs are formed.
Buds of arms and legs begin to form.
Rudiments of eyes, ears, and nose appear.

2nd Lunar Month (8 weeks)

The fetus is 27 to 31 mm in length
  and weighs 2 to 4 g
Fetus is markedly bent.
Head is disproportionately large as
  a result of brain development.
Sex differentation begins.
Centers of bone begin to ossify.

3rd Lunar Month (3 months)

The fetus' average length is 6 to 9
  cm, and weight is 45 g.
Fingers and toes are distinct.
Placenta is complete.
Fetal circulation is complete.

4th Lunar Month (4 months)

The fetus is 12 cm in length and
  weighs 110 g.
Sex is differentiated.
Rudimentary kidneys secrete urine.
Heartbeat is present.
Nasal septum and palate close.

5th Lunar Month (5 months)

The fetus is 19 cm in length and
  weighs approximately 300 g.
Lanugo covers entire body.
Fetal movements are felt by mother.
Heart sounds are perceptible by
  auscultation.

6th Lunar Month (6 months)

The fetus is about 23 cm in length
  and weighs 630 g.
Skin appears wrinkled.
Vernix caseosa appears.
Eyebrows and fingernails develop.

7th Lunar Month (7 months)

The fetus is about 27 cm in length
  and weighs about 1100 g.
Skin is red.
Pupillary membrane disappears
  from eyes.
The fetus has an excellent chance
  of survival.

8th Lunar Month (8 months)

The fetus is 28 to 30 cm in length
  and weighs 1.8 kg.
Fetus is viable.
Eyelids open.
Fingerprints are set.
Vigorous fetal movement occurs.

9th Lunar Month (9 months)

The fetus' average length is 32 cm;
  weight is about 2500 g.
Face and body have a loose
  wrinkled appearance because
  of subcutaneous fat deposit.
Lanugo disappears.
Amniotic fluid decreases.

10th Lunar Month

The average fetus is 36 cm in length
  and weighs 3000 to 3600 g.
Skin is smooth.
Eyes are uniformly slate colored.
Bones of skull are ossified and
  nearly together at sutures.

* All lengths given are crown to rump.

Figure 35-9 Fetal development.

weeks of gestation. The patient is usually seen every 2 weeks during the last 2 months and once a week after the 36th week of gestation. This schedule may be altered according to the patient's condition. Table 35-4 outlines the specific examination and procedures to be performed during subsequent prenatal visits. The height of the fundus (Fig. 35-10) is also palpated at each visit to assess fetal growth. Typically, the top of the uterus, the fundus, can be palpated at or slightly above the level of the maternal umbilicus when the fetus is at 5 months gestation. During the third trimester, the abdomen will be palpated to determine fetal presentation and position, which are important details for a normal vaginal delivery.

The fetal heart tones (FHT) will also be recorded at the subsequent prenatal visits. Around the 10th week of gestation, the fetal heart rate can be heard with the aid

Figure 35-10 Height of the fundus at corresponding gestational dates varies greatly from patient to patient. Those shown are most common. A convenient rule of thumb is that at 5 months of gestation, the fundus is usually at or slightly above the umbilicus. (Reprinted with permission from Weber J. Health Assessment in Nursing. Philadelphia: Lippincott Williams & Wilkins, 2003.)

of a Doppler device (Fig. 35-11), and after the 20th week, a fetoscope can be used. The fetoscope is a special nonelectronic stethoscope (Fig. 35-12). The fetal heart tones should fall within a range of 120 to 160 beats per minute.

 CHECKPOINT QUESTION

9. The pregnant patient should be advised to contact the physician when what problems occur?

TABLE 35-4	Schedule of Prenatal Visits
Month	**Frequency**
1–6	Monthly
7–8	Every 2 weeks
9	Weekly
Included in Visit:	**When Done:**
Weight	Each visit
Blood Pressure	Each visit
Fundal height	Each visit
Fetal heart rate	Each visit
Check of edema	Each visit
Pelvic examination	Middle of ninth month, weekly as indicated
Inquiry about symptoms, signs, problems	Each visit
Prenatal education	Each visit
Nutrition and appetite	Each visit
Urinalysis for glucose, albumin	Each visit
Hematocrit, hemoglobin	32–34 weeks (more often for anemia)
Urine culture	Per signs, symptoms
Rh titer	Initially
AFP	15–20 weeks
Blood glucose	24–28 weeks
Ultrasonography	For fetal age, best 8–16 weeks

From Reeder SJ, Martin LL, Koniak D. Maternity Nursing. 17th ed. Philadelphia: Lippincott Williams & Wilkins, 1992:403.

Figure 35-11 An electronic Doppler used to assess fetal heart tones before the 20th gestational week.

Figure 35-12 A fetoscope. (From Nursing Procedures. 4th ed. Ambler, PA: Lippincott Williams & Wilkins, 2004.)

LEGAL TIP

FETAL PROTECTION

Many medications that might be considered beneficial to the pregnant female may be dangerous to the developing fetus. It is important, therefore, for the professional medical assistant to carefully question female patients who might be pregnant or who are known to be pregnant about any medications including drugs purchased over the counter. This information should be passed along to the physician. The Food and Drug Administration (FDA) has developed a method to classify drugs that are dangerous to the fetus. These categories are listed on package inserts that accompany prescription drugs and in various drug reference books such as the *Physician's Desk Reference*. The categories and a description of dangerous effects on the fetus are listed as follows:

- Category A: Research indicates that there is probably no risk at any point in the pregnancy.
- Category B: Animal research indicates no fetal risk, but human studies are not complete.
- Category C: Research on animals shows this drug to be a danger. Human studies are inconclusive, or no studies are available.
- Category D: There is clear precedence for risk, but the drug may be used if there is no substitution.
- Category X: There is clear evidence of risk, and the drug should not be used by pregnant women.

Onset of Labor

Labor is the physiologic process leading to expelling the fetus from the uterus. About 4 weeks before the onset of labor, **lightening** indicates that the fetus has descended further into the pelvis, and the patient may appear to be carrying the baby lower in the abdomen. The actual onset of labor is characterized by regular uterine contractions that become more intense and more frequent with time. True labor is distinguished from false labor by its effect (dilation and effacement) on the cervix and the increased frequency and intensity of contractions. Another indication of true labor is bloody show, the expulsion of the mucous plug from the cervical os. The patient may call to say her water broke, which indicates rupture of the amniotic sac, another indication of impending labor and delivery.

Whatever signs or symptoms of labor occur, you should know how to advise the patient. The physician makes the decision to send the patient to the hospital, to come to the medical office, or to stay home and wait. You relay the information from the patient to the physician. The office's policy and procedure manual should include specific instructions regarding how the physician wants pregnant patients managed if the physician is not immediately available.

The onset of labor should be discussed with the patient so she knows what to expect and how to manage the situation. Always have the patient's medical record available when talking with the patient or the physician. It is critical to the decision-making process to know the patient's estimated date of delivery and physical condition. Many patients today are choosing options for delivery other than a standard hospital delivery with the physician present. Options include midwife assistance, a birthing center, water birth, and home delivery. The patient must be informed about the advantages and risks of all of these and, together with the physician, make a decision that takes into account the well-being of the mother and the newborn.

Cesarean Section

Sometimes a normal vaginal delivery is not possible or advisable, such as in the following situations:

- Cephalopelvic disproportion: the baby's head is too large for the birth canal
- Placenta previa
- Poor presentation other than an occipital presentation, such as transverse (the baby lying across the cervix) or breech (a buttocks first presentation)
- Failure to progress: inefficient labor or the cervix will not dilate
- Infant or maternal distress

In these situations, the infant is delivered by cesarean section. An incision is made through the abdominal wall into the uterus, and the infant is removed. It was once believed that women who had delivered by cesarean section should not be allowed to deliver vaginally because it was feared that the uterine scar might rupture. Current surgical techniques have lessened that fear, and many women now deliver vaginally after a cesarean delivery.

Postpartum Care

The postpartum period, the **puerperium**, runs from childbirth until involution, when the reproductive structures return to normal. It may take as long as 6 weeks. Once the patient is discharged from the hospital, her care will be managed at the medical office. Hospital reports received in the medical office for the patient's record usually contain certain acronyms and abbreviations related to labor and delivery and the postpartum period. Box 35-3 explains these special terms.

The time for the first postpartum visit depends on the type of delivery and the patient's condition when discharged from the hospital. The needs of postpartum patients today may be greater than in the past because the length of stay in the hospital is typically shorter, with some patients discharged within 24 hours after delivery. Usually the patient is scheduled for the postnatal visit within 4 to 6 weeks of delivery if there were no complications.

At the postpartum visit, the physician performs a complete gynecologic and breast examination. Allow plenty of time for counseling the patient regarding her new role as a parent. Many patients have questions and concerns regarding breastfeeding, birth control, menstruation, and parenting. Before the examination, obtain the patient's weight and vital signs and samples for urinalysis and possibly hematocrit and hemoglobin. During the examination, the physician assesses any uterine discharge. **Lochia**, a discharge from the uterus after delivery, progresses through the following stages:

- Lochia rubra: Blood-tinged discharge within 6 days of delivery
- Lochia serosa: Thin, brownish discharge lasting about 3 to 4 days after the lochia rubra
- Lochia alba: White postpartum discharge that has no evidence of blood and may last up to week 6

The amount of lochia should diminish considerably during the puerperium. The patient should be instructed to notify the physician if there is any abnormality of the lochial progression.

 CHECKPOINT QUESTION

10. What is lochia? Name and describe the three types.

BOX 35-3

ACRONYMS AND ABBREVIATIONS USED IN LABOR AND DELIVERY AND THE POSTPARTUM PERIOD

Following is a brief list of terms frequently used in the medical record.

AROM	Artificial rupture of membranes
AVD	Assisted vaginal delivery
CPD	Cephalopelvic disproportion
L & D	Labor and delivery
NSVD	Normal spontaneous vaginal delivery
PROM	Premature rupture of membranes
SROM	Spontaneous rupture of membranes
VBAC	Vaginal birth after cesarean

Terms for presentations

LOA	Left occiput anterior
LOP	Left occiput posterior
ROA	Right occiput anterior
ROP	Right occiput posterior

Fetal descriptors

AGA	Appropriate for gestational age
LBW	Low birth weight
LGA	Large for gestational age
SGA	Small for gestational age

 PATIENT EDUCATION

KEGEL EXERCISES

The patient's age, gravidity, and past childbearing take their toll on the muscles of the perineum. Kegel exercises can increase the tone of this area. Stronger perineal support helps eliminate stress incontinence and supports the vaginal walls to avoid uterine prolapse.

These exercises should be performed three times every day for 5 minutes each time. In addition, the exercises should be done in three positions: lying down, sitting, and standing. Explain to the patient that she can do Kegel exercises at any time, such as when standing in the grocery line, waiting at a stop light, or sitting in class. Essentially, the exercises involve tightening the pelvic muscles as if stopping the flow of urine. Advise the patient not to tighten the stomach, legs, or other muscles. Also, most patients do not feel bladder control results for 3 to 6 weeks.

Obstetric Disorders

Ectopic Pregnancy

Gestation in which a fertilized ovum implants somewhere other than in the uterine cavity is an ectopic pregnancy. Usually an ectopic pregnancy occurs in the fallopian tube, and when it does, it may be called a tubal pregnancy. Other sites of implantation include the abdomen, the ovaries, and the cervical os. The patient may have signs of early pregnancy, including breast enlargement or tenderness, nausea, and absent or delayed menses. Pelvic pain, syncope, abdominal symptoms, painful sexual intercourse, and irregular menstrual bleeding begin fairly early in the pregnancy. If an ectopic pregnancy is not diagnosed early, there is the potential for rupture of the fallopian tube, which causes hemorrhage into the abdominal cavity and the possibility of shock and death. Diagnostic procedures include urine or serum human chorionic gonadotropin pregnancy test, ultrasound to determine the location of the pregnancy, laparoscopy to visualize the enlarged tube, and perhaps culdocentesis to confirm abdominal bleeding. Treatment is surgical excision of the ectopic pregnancy through either a laparoscopy or laparotomy.

Hyperemesis Gravidarum

Nausea and vomiting, commonly called morning sickness, are expected during early pregnancy and usually can be treated with small frequent meals, adequate hydration, and reassurance. However, if the vomiting becomes unrelenting and leads to dehydration, electrolyte imbalance, and weight loss, the diagnosis is hyperemesis gravidarum. Occasionally the patient must be hospitalized. At early prenatal visits, you may have to discern between morning sickness and the more serious hyperemesis gravidarum by obtaining a complete description of the nausea and vomiting. Of course, the physician makes the diagnosis and orders appropriate treatment, including antiemetics or intravenous fluids if necessary.

Abortion

One of the common disorders of pregnancy is first-trimester spontaneous abortion, also called an early pregnancy loss or miscarriage. With early diagnosis of pregnancy, it is now known whether the spontaneous abortion occurs more often than previously thought. An induced abortion is intentional, while a spontaneous abortion occurs because of fetal or maternal conditions without any outside interference in the pregnancy.

A spontaneous abortion is defined as the loss of pregnancy before the fetus is viable. You need to be familiar with the early signs and symptoms of an impending spontaneous abortion to advise a patient who calls until the physician can be contacted. The first symptom is usually vaginal bleeding, followed by uterine cramps and low back pain. Without telling the patient that she may be in danger of spontaneously aborting her pregnancy (this is diagnosing), you may instruct the patient to come to the medical office, go to the emergency room, or remain at home on bed rest until the physician returns the call, depending on the office policy and procedure.

 CHECKPOINT QUESTION

11. Where is the most common site of implantation for an ectopic pregnancy?

Preeclampsia and Eclampsia

Hypertension that is directly related to the pregnancy is termed pregnancy-induced hypertension (PIH). The two types of PIH are preeclampsia and eclampsia. Preeclampsia is characterized by **proteinuria**, edema of the lower extremities, and hypertension after the 20th week of gestation. As the condition progresses, the patient may complain of blurred vision, headaches, edema, and vomiting. Medical management includes restricted activities, increased bed rest, sexual abstinence, antihypertensive therapy, and well-balanced meals with an increase in protein and a decrease in sodium. Close monitoring of the patient is important, and it requires scheduling the patient for more frequent office visits. The risk of developing eclampsia increases as the pregnancy advances.

Eclampsia is almost always preceded by preeclampsia but has a sudden onset. In eclampsia, the clinical signs of preeclampsia are still present but become more extreme. Eclampsia is always characterized by seizures that may be followed by coma, hypertensive crisis, and shock. The progression of preeclampsia to eclampsia constitutes a medical emergency. Management of eclampsia includes stabilizing the patient and may require induced delivery of the baby, regardless of gestational age.

Placenta Previa and Abruptio Placentae

Placenta previa is a condition in which the placenta is implanted either partially or completely over the internal cervical os, making delivery of the fetus before the placenta difficult. During the second or third trimester of pregnancy, the patient may have painless vaginal bleeding, which may be minimal, such as spotting, or profuse. Placenta previa is easily diagnosed by prenatal ultrasound. Medical management includes bed rest and drug therapy if the patient is preterm. If the patient is near term and if the bleeding is severe and poses a danger to the mother or fetus, then delivery of the baby is essential, usually by cesarean.

The premature separation or detachment of the placenta from the uterus is abruptio placentae. Depending on the severity of the separation, symptoms include pain, uterine tenderness, bleeding, signs of impending shock, and fetal distress or death. If abruptio placentae is confirmed, the baby is usually delivered by cesarean section.

 CHECKPOINT QUESTION

12. What is placenta previa, and how is it managed in a preterm patient?

Common Obstetric Tests and Procedures

Pregnancy Tests

Many over-the-counter pregnancy tests check for HCG in the urine. Chapter 44 has more information about urine pregnancy tests.

Alpha-Fetoprotein

Levels of alpha-fetoprotein (AFP) are obtained from maternal serum to screen the fetus for defects in the neural tube, a part of the fetus that develops into the brain and spinal cord. The test is performed at 16 to 18 weeks of gestation and is used for screening purposes. Elevated AFP levels may indicate nervous system deformities, including spina bifida, but falsely elevated tests can be caused by more than one fetus or incorrect gestational dates. AFP results that are below the normal range may indicate Down syndrome in the developing fetus. Abnormal results indicate the need for further studies, including **amniocentesis** and fetal ultrasound.

Amniocentesis is insertion of a needle through the abdomen and into the gravid uterus to remove fluid from the amniotic sac. This fluid is analyzed for a variety of nervous system disorders. It can also be used to diagnose genetic problems, estimate gestational age, or assess lung maturity of the fetus. It may be performed in the office, and if so, you are responsible for preparing the patient, assisting the physician, preparing the specimen for transportation to the laboratory, and giving the patient any postprocedural instructions from the physician.

Fetal Ultrasonography

An ultrasound of the fetus is performed using high-frequency sound waves to create an image of internal structures. Fetal ultrasound is performed to assess the size, gestational age, position, and number of fetuses as well as fetal structures and development. Some abnormal maternal and fetal conditions, such as ectopic pregnancy, placenta previa, neural tube defects, and cardiac defects may be diagnosed by ultrasound. The gender of the fetus may also be determined, although this is not typically a justification for performing an ultrasound. Although some obstetric offices have a sonographer on staff, fetal ultrasounds may have to be scheduled in an outpatient facility.

Contraction Stress Test and Nonstress Test

A contraction stress test (CST) is performed in the third trimester to determine how the fetus will tolerate uterine contractions. Uterine contractions may be induced by the woman stimulating her nipples, known as the nipple-stimulating CST, or the contractions can be induced by the administration of oxytocin, called an oxytocin-stimulated CST. In both tests, the fetal heart tones and movement are monitored in relation to the uterine contractions. Although the contractions are meant to be temporary, the CST is usually performed in the hospital in case continued contractions and delivery occur.

The nonstress test (NST) is a noninvasive obstetric procedure used to evaluate the fetal heart tones and movement in relation to spontaneous uterine contractions. The NST may be safely performed in the medical office, whereas the CST is usually performed in the hospital setting.

 CHECKPOINT QUESTION

13. In what instances might a fetal ultrasonography be ordered by the physician?

Contraception

Numerous methods of contraception (birth control) are available (Table 35-5). The decision to practice contraception and the selection of an appropriate method involves many factors, including the patient's religious, cultural, and personal beliefs. In addition, the health history, financial situation, and motivation of the patient may be important considerations for the patient, the spouse or partner, and the physician. To reinforce the physician's advice and instructions, you should understand the various methods, including the indications, risk factors, cost, and effectiveness. Both you and the physician should be prepared to educate and advise the patient regarding the choice of contraception.

Menopause

Menopause, also called the climacteric period, is the stage of life during which ovulation ceases because of decreasing ovarian function. This period, characterized by the cessation of the menstrual cycle, usually occurs

TABLE 35-5	Main Methods of Contraception		
Method	**Description**	**Advantages**	**Disadvantages**
Surgical			
Vasectomy, tubal	Tubes carrying gametes cut	Nearly 100% effective; no chemical or mechanical	Not easily reversible; rare surgical complications
Hormonal			
Pill	Oral estrogen or progesterone to prevent ovulation	Highly effective; requires no last-minute preparation	Alters physiology; serious side effects possible
Injection	Inject synthetic progesterone every 3 months to prevent ovulation	Highly effective; lasts 3–4 months	Alters physiology; possible side effects are menstrual irregularity and amenorrhea; expensive
Patch	Patch with progesterone, estrogen worn on skin 3 out of 4 weeks to prevent ovulation	Use is simple; does not require pill or injection	Should be replaced same day of week; pregnancy can occur if patch off for more than 24 hr or left on more than 1 week
Ring	Small, flexible ring in vagina releases synthetic progesterone, estrogen to prevent pregnancy for 1 month	Does not require pill, injection; does not interfere with sexual intercourse	Side effects may include bleeding between periods, breast tenderness, other symptoms associated with hormone therapy
IUD	T-shaped plastic device with copper or progesterone	Spontaneous sexual intercourse	Heavy or long menstrual periods; cramping during and after insertion; periodic check for placement by feeling for string
Barrier			
Male condom	Sheath fits over erect penis, contains ejaculate	Easily available; does not affect physiology; protects from STDs	Must be applied before intercourse; may slip or tear
Female condom	Sheath that fits into vagina, held in place with rings	Easily available; protects from STDs	More expensive than male condom; must be inserted before intercourse
Diaphragm, spermicide	Rubber cap fits over cervix; prevents entrance of sperm	Does not affect physiology; some protection from STDs	Must be inserted before intercourse; requires fitting by physician
Other			
Spermicide	Chemical to kill sperm; best used with a barrier method	Easily available; does not affect physiology; some protection from STDs	Local irritation; must be used just before intercourse
Fertility awareness	Abstinence while fertile per menstrual history, basal temperature, quality of cervical mucus	Does not affect physiology; accepted by certain religions	High failure rate; requires careful record keeping
Emergency contraception	Morning-after pill reduces risk of pregnancy up to 120 hours after unprotected sex	May prevent pregnancy after unprotected sexual intercourse	Nausea, vomiting; no protection from STDs; may not prevent ectopic pregnancy; the closer to ovulation, the greater chance of pregnancy

Adapted from Cohen BJ. Memmler's The Human Body in Health and Disease. 10th ed. Baltimore: Lippincott Williams & Wilkins, 2005.

around 45 to 50 years of age. Changes in the menstrual cycle in early menopause include **oligomenorrhea**, amenorrhea, dysfunctional uterine bleeding, and hot flashes, flushing, or perspiration.

The use of supplemental estrogen, or hormonal replacement therapy (HRT), was prescribed a few years ago to relieve menopausal symptoms such as hot flashes and depression and was believed to also protect against cardiovascular and skeletal disorders. However, in 2002, a research study was published that revealed elevated health risks for women who took hormone replacement therapy. As a result, fewer women today are taking HRT, and most physicians only recommend these medications for women with severe symptoms of menopause. For women with only minor menopausal symptoms, weight-bearing exercises, a healthy diet, and vitamin and mineral supplements have eased the transition through the menopausal stage without the use of hormone replacement medications. In either case, women in this stage of life should continue to have regular pelvic examinations, Pap smears, breast examinations, and mammograms and should speak with the physician about any questions or concerns.

SPANISH TERMINOLOGY

Cuando fue el primer día de su ultimo periodo menstrual?
When was the first day of your last menstrual period?

Usa usted un dispositivo anticonceptivo?
Do you use a contraceptive device?

Cuando se le hizo la ultima mamografía?
When was your last mammogram?

Ha tenido usted la menopausia?
Have you gone through menopause?

MEDIA MENU

- **Student CD**
  - **Case Study**
    Interactive Case Study 4: Patient Interviewing, Education and Confidentiality, and Specimen Handling
  - **CMA/RMA Certification Exam Review**
- **Premium Online Course**
  http://thePoint.lww.com/Kronenberger3e
- **Internet Resources**

LiveAdvise Online Tutoring & Competency Training
http://thePoint.lww.com/LiveAdvise

American College of Obstetricians and Gynecologists
http://www.acog.org

National Center for HIV, STD, and TB Prevention
http://www.cdc.gov/nchstp/dstd/disease_info.htm

American Social Health Association
http://www.ashastd.org/stdfaqs

American Fertility Association
http://www.theafa.org/

American Cancer Society
http://www.cancer.org

National Women's Health Information Center
http://www.womenshealth.gov

PROCEDURE 35-1: Instructing the Patient on the Breast Self-Examination

Purpose: Properly instruct the female patient on the procedure for performing a breast self-examination
Equipment: Patient education instruction sheet if available; breast examination model if available

Steps	Purpose
1. Wash your hands.	Handwashing aids infection control.
2. Explain the purpose and frequency of examining the breasts.	The purpose is to check for lumps, dimples, and thickened areas that can indicate malignancy and allow for early diagnosis and treatment. The patient should be encouraged to examine her breasts at the same time each month, about a week after the menstrual cycle.
3. Describe the three positions necessary for the patient to examine the breasts: in front of a mirror, in the shower, and lying down.	Inspecting and palpating the breasts in a variety of positions allows for a thorough examination of all breast tissue.
4. Explain that she should disrobe and inspect the breasts in front of a mirror with her hands on her hips and with her arms raised above her head. Advise the patient to look for any changes in contour, swelling, dimpling of the skin, or changes in the nipple.	Regular inspection shows what is normal and gives the patient confidence for the examination.
	Step 4. (A) Inspect both breasts in front of a mirror with the hands on the hips. (B) Inspect both breasts with the arms raised over the head. (Reprinted with permission from Pillitteri A. Maternal and Child Health Nursing. Philadelphia: Lippincott Williams & Wilkins, 2007.)
5. In the shower, the patient should feel each breast with her hands over wet skin, using the flat part of the first three fingers. Instruct her to use her right hand to lightly press over all areas of her left breast and her left hand to examine her right breast, checking for any lumps, hard knots, or thickenings.	Palpating the breasts in the shower allows the hands to glide more easily over wet skin.

(continued)

PROCEDURE 35-1: **Instructing the Patient on the Breast Self-Examination** *(continued)*

Steps	Purpose
  Step 5. Examine the breasts in the shower. (Reprinted with permission from Pillitteri A. Maternal and Child Health Nursing. Philadelphia: Lippincott Williams & Wilkins, 2007.)	
6. After showering, the patient should lie down and examine her right breast after placing a pillow or folded towel under her right shoulder and placing her right hand behind her head. With her left hand, she should use the flat part of the fingers to palpate the breast tissue, using small circular motions beginning at the outermost top of her right breast and working clockwise around the breast. **Step 6.** **(A)** While lying down, palpate each breast carefully. (Reprinted with permission from Pillitteri A. Maternal and Child Health Nursing. Philadelphia: Lippincott Williams & Wilkins, 2007.) **(B)** Palpate the breast using the flat part of fingers in a circular motion. (Reprinted with permission from Weber J, Kelley J. Health Assessment in Nursing. Philadelphia: Lippincott Williams & Wilkins, 2003.)	Placing a pillow or folded towel under the right shoulder distributes the breast tissue more evenly on the chest.

(continued)

PROCEDURE 35-1: **Instructing the Patient on the Breast Self-Examination** *(continued)*

Steps	Purpose
7. Encourage the patient to palpate the breast carefully by moving her fingers in toward the nipple, while palpating every part of the breast, including the nipple.	Breast tissue extends from the clavicle to the end of the rib cage and from the sternum to underneath the axilla.
8. Repeat the procedure for the left breast, placing a pillow or folded towel under the left shoulder and the left hand behind the head.	
9. Gently squeeze each nipple between the thumb and index finger. Report any discharge to the physician.	

Step 9. Squeeze each nipple gently. (Reprinted with permission from Pillitteri A. Maternal and Child Health Nursing. Philadelphia: Lippincott Williams & Wilkins, 2007.)

Steps	Purpose
10. Explain to the patient that she should promptly report any abnormalities to the physician.	
11. Document the patient education.	Procedures are considered not to have been done if they are not recorded.

Charting Example:

4/12/2008 2:15 PM Pt. given written and verbal instructions on performing the monthly breast self-examination. She verbalized understanding. Advised to contact the office for any problems or abnormalities

—E. Smith, RMA

PROCEDURE 35-2: Assisting With the Pelvic Examination and Pap Smear

Purpose: Prepare the examination room and the female patient for a pelvic examination and Pap smear and assist the physician as needed

Equipment: Gown and drape; appropriate size vaginal speculum; cotton-tipped applicators; water-soluble lubricant; examination gloves; examination light; tissues; materials for Pap smear: cervical spatula and/or brush, glass slides and fixative solution OR container with liquid medium to preserve the cells, laboratory request form, identification labels, and other materials that may be required by laboratory; biohazard container

Steps	Purpose
1. Wash your hands.	Handwashing aids infection control.
2. Assemble the equipment and supplies.	The vaginal speculum can be warmed under warm running water (see Fig 35-7), on a heating pad set on warm, or in a warming drawer found on some examination tables. Lubricant must not be used on the vaginal speculum before insertion because this will cause inaccurate Pap smear results.
3. If slides are used, label each slide with the date and type of specimen on the frosted end with a pencil. For liquid medium, label the outside of the container.	Each slide should be labeled C for cervical, V for vaginal, or E for endocervical, depending on where the physician obtains the cells for examination. This is not necessary when liquid medium is used.
4. Greet and identify the patient. Explain the procedure.	Identifying the patient prevents errors. Explaining the procedure may reduce anxiety.
5. Ask the patient to empty her bladder and, if necessary, collect a urine specimen.	An empty bladder will make the examination more comfortable.
6. Provide the patient with a gown and drape and ask her to disrobe from the waist down.	If the patient is also having a breast examination, she should be instructed to disrobe completely and put the gown on with the opening in the front. This allows easier access for the breast examination. Allow the patient privacy for changing into the examination gown. **Step 6.** Give the patient a gown and drape while explaining what to remove and how to put the gown on.
7. Position the patient in the dorsal lithotomy position with her buttocks at the bottom edge of the table.	Because this position is embarrassing and may stress the legs and back, assist the patient into this position only when the physician is ready to do the examination.
8. Adjust the drape to cover the patient's abdomen and knees, exposing the genitalia, and adjust the light over the genitalia for maximum visibility.	Good visibility is essential for a thorough examination.
9. Assist the physician with the examination by handing instruments and supplies as needed.	Anticipating the physician's needs during the procedure promotes a more thorough and efficient examination

(continued)

PROCEDURE 35-2: **Assisting With the Pelvic Examination and Pap Smear** *(continued)*

Steps	Purpose
10. After applying examination gloves, hold the microscope slides or container of liquid medium while the physician obtains the specimen. **Step 10.** Hold the slide by the frosted end to receive the smears.	
11. If glass slides are used, spray or cover each slide with fixative solution by holding the slide 4 to 6 inches from the can and spraying lightly once across the slide or dropping the fixative onto the slide.	Spraying the fixative solution too close to the slide will distort the cells or blow them off the slide. The fixative is necessary to preserve the cervical scrapings for cytology analysis. The cells are put into the liquid medium, and no fixative is necessary.
12. When the physician removes the vaginal speculum, have a basin or other container ready to receive it. **Step 12.** Receive the used instruments in a basin or other container to transfer to the soaking solution for sanitizing.	
13. Apply lubricant across the physician's two fingers without touching the end of the lubricant container to the physician's gloves. **Step 13.** Apply about 1 to 2 inches of water-soluble lubricant to the physician's gloved fingers.	Water-soluble lubricant helps make the manual examination more comfortable.

(continued)

PROCEDURE 35-2: **Assisting With the Pelvic Examination and Pap Smear** *(continued)*

Steps	Purpose
14. Encourage the patient to relax during the bimanual examination as needed.	The patient may be more relaxed during the examination if you are supportive.

Step 14. Technique for bimanual examination of the pelvic organs in women. (Reprinted with permission from Smeltzer SC, Bare BG. Textbook of Medical-Surgical Nursing. Philadelphia: Lippincott Williams & Wilkins, 2008.)

Steps	Purpose
15. After the examination, help the patient slide up to the top of the examination table and remove both feet at the same time from the stirrups.	Injury can be prevented if the patient moves up the table before removing feet from the stirrups. Removing both feet at the same time puts less strain on the patient.
16. Offer the patient tissues to remove excess lubricant, and help her sit if necessary, watching for signs of vertigo.	Excess lubricant can be uncomfortable. Some patients, especially the elderly, may be dizzy on sitting up.
17. Ask the patient to get dressed and assist as needed. Provide for privacy as the patient dresses.	
18. Reinforce any physician instructions regarding follow-up appointments and advise the patient on the procedure for obtaining the laboratory findings from the Pap smear.	For quality management, let the patient know when to schedule follow-up appointments and when and how laboratory findings will be obtained.
19. Properly care for or dispose of equipment and clean the examination room. Wash your hands.	
20. Document your responsibilities during the procedure, such as routing the specimen, patient education, and so on.	Procedures are considered not to have been done if they are not recorded

Charting Example:

2/27/2008 3:00 PM Pap and pelvic today per Dr. Todd. Thin Prep sent to Acme lab for cytology. Pt. given written and oral instructions on obtaining results

—B. Lewis, CMA

PROCEDURE 35-3: Assisting With the Colposcopy and Cervical Biopsy

Purpose: Prepare the examination room and the female patient for a colposcopy with cervical biopsy
Equipment: Gown and drape, vaginal speculum, colposcope, specimen container with preservative (10% formalin), sterile gloves in appropriate size, sterile cotton-tipped applicators, sterile normal saline solution, sterile 3% acetic acid, sterile povidone-iodine (Betadine), silver nitrate sticks or ferric subsulfate (Monsel solution), sterile biopsy forceps or punch biopsy instrument, sterile uterine curet, sterile uterine dressing forceps, sterile 4 × 4 gauze, sterile towel, sterile endocervical curet, sterile uterine tenaculum, sanitary napkin, examination gloves, examination light, tissues, biohazard container

Steps	Purpose
1. Wash your hands.	Handwashing aids infection control.
2. Verify that the patient has signed the consent form.	Colposcopy with biopsy is an invasive procedure that requires written consent.
3. Assemble the equipment and supplies.	
4. Check the light on the colposcope.	Properly functioning equipment is crucial to the quality of the examination.
5. Set up the sterile field without contaminating it.	A biopsy is an invasive procedure requiring surgical asepsis.
6. Pour sterile normal saline and acetic acid into their sterile containers. Cover the field with a sterile drape.	Items that can be placed on the sterile field include the sterile cotton-tipped applicators and sterile containers for the solutions. Covering the sterile field maintains sterility as you prepare the patient.
7. Greet and identify the patient. Explain the procedure.	Identifying the patient prevents errors. Explaining the procedure may ease anxiety.
8. When the physician is ready to proceed, assist the patient into the dorsal lithotomy position. If you are to assist the physician from the sterile field, put on sterile gloves after positioning the patient.	Correct positioning is essential for a clear view of the cervix.
9. Hand the physician the applicator immersed in normal saline, followed by the applicator immersed in acetic acid.	Acetic acid swabbed on the area improves visualization and aids in identifying suspicious tissue.

Step 9. Hand the physician an applicator that has been immersed in normal saline.

Steps	Purpose
10. Hand the physician the applicator with the antiseptic solution (Betadine).	The area to be sampled for biopsy must be swabbed with an antiseptic solution to reduce microorganisms and pathogens in the area.

(continued)

PROCEDURE 35-3: **Assisting With the Colposcopy and Cervical Biopsy** *(continued)*

Steps	Purpose
11. If you did not apply sterile gloves to assist the physician, apply clean examination gloves and receive the biopsy specimen into the container of 10% formalin preservative.	Because the specimen may be hazardous, standard precautions must be observed.
12. Provide the physician with Monsel solution or silver nitrate sticks to stop any bleeding if necessary.	If bleeding occurs, a coagulant, such as Monsel solution or silver nitrate, may have to be applied.
13. When the physician is finished with the procedure, appropriately assist the patient from the stirrups and to a sitting position. Explain to the patient that a small amount of bleeding may occur. Have a sanitary napkin available.	Bleeding with a cervical biopsy is usually minimal, and a small sanitary pad should be sufficient.
14. Label the specimen container with the patient's name and date and prepare the laboratory request.	The specimen must be properly identified, and the laboratory request must be complete.

Step 14. Always label the specimen container before sending it to the lab.

Steps	Purpose
15. Ask the patient to get dressed and assist as needed. Provide for privacy as the patient dresses.	
16. Reinforce any physician instructions regarding follow-up appointments, and tell the patient how to obtain the biopsy findings.	For quality management, let the patient know when to schedule follow-up appointments and when and how laboratory findings will be provided.
17. Properly care for or dispose of equipment and clean the examination room. Wash your hands.	
18. Document your responsibilities during the procedure, such as routing the specimen, patient education, and so on.	Procedures are considered not to have been done if they are not recorded.

Charting Example:

10/15/2008 10:45 AM Colposcopy performed per Dr. Lyttle; cervical biopsy obtained and sent to Acme lab for cytology. Minimal bleeding post procedure; pt. given sanitary pad, oral and written instructions on postprocedure care. Verbalized understanding

—J. Pratt, CMA

- Assisting in obstetrics and gynecology is a challenging and fascinating area of medicine. This chapter:
  - Describes the examination of the female reproductive system
  - Explains your role in assisting the patient and the physician in the examination of the female reproductive system
  - Describes a variety of disorders related to the female reproductive system
  - Discusses normal physiologic functions such as menarche and menopause
  - Addresses the care of the pregnant patient including disorders or conditions sometimes seen in pregnancy

- As a professional medical assistant, you will be responsible for:
  - Providing reassurance and emotional support to the gynecologic patient
  - Assisting the physician during the gynecologic exam if needed
  - Processing any specimens for the laboratory using standard precautions
  - Maintaining the examination room, equipment, and supplies

Warm Ups · for Critical Thinking

1. A multiparous patient who is married and has a history of cigarette smoking desires a highly effective method of contraception. What are her best choices for contraception? Explain which choice is best and why.

2. Your patient has both genital herpes and condylomata acuminata. She wants to know whether these disorders are contagious and how they can be cured. How do you respond to these questions?

3. Research the effects of maternal exposure to alcohol, tobacco, and nicotine and prepare a poster describing your findings that could be used to educate pregnant women and those considering pregnancy.

4. In addition to the contraceptives listed in this chapter, list the contraceptives available today, including the advantages and risks associated with each.

5. Using a drug reference book, research some of the newer drugs on the market to treat and/or prevent osteoporosis that may occur after menopause. What are the side effects of these medications?

6. Prepare a patient education poster for your medical office about breast cancer awareness.

Answers · to Checkpoint Questions

1. Menorrhagia is excessive bleeding during menses, and metrorrhagia is irregular bleeding at times other than menses.

2. The symptoms of endometriosis include infertility, dysmenorrhea, pelvic pain, and dyspareunia. The cause is unknown.

3. The prognosis of all cancers is much better with early diagnosis and treatment.

4. Mothers infected with chlamydia may infect the newborn and cause conjunctivitis and pneumonia in the baby. In addition, infected mothers have an increased risk for spontaneous abortion, premature delivery, or stillbirth.

5. Genital warts have been implicated as a risk factor for cervical cancer.

6. The complete gynecologic examination includes a breast examination and a pelvic examination with a Pap smear.

7. A hysterosalpingography would be performed to determine the patency of the fallopian tubes in a patient with infertility.

8. The presumptive signs and symptoms of pregnancy are not conclusive because they may indicate other conditions in the female reproductive system.

9. The pregnant patient should notify the physician if she has vaginal bleeding or spotting, persistent

vomiting, fever or chills, dysuria, abdominal or uterine cramping, leaking amniotic fluid, altered fetal movement, dizziness, or blurred vision.

10. Lochia, a discharge from the uterus after delivery, progresses through several types: lochia rubra (blood tinged), lochia serosa (thin, brownish), and lochia alba (white).

11. The most common site of implantation for an ectopic pregnancy is in the fallopian tube.

12. Placenta previa is a condition in which the placenta is implanted either partly or completely over the cervical os. In a preterm patient, the condition is managed with bed rest and drug therapy.

13. The fetal ultrasound is often performed to assess the size, gestational age, and position of the fetus and the presence of more than one fetus.

Outline

Common Disorders of the Endocrine System
Disorders of the Thyroid
Disorders of the Pancreas

Disorders of the Adrenal Glands
Disorders of the Pituitary Gland

Common Diagnostic and Therapeutic Procedures

Learning Objectives

Upon successfully completing this chapter, you will be able to:

1. Spell and define key terms

2. Identify abnormal conditions of the thyroid, pancreas, adrenal, and pituitary glands

3. Describe the tests commonly used to diagnose disorders of these endocrine system glands

4. Explain your role in working with patients with endocrine systems disorders

Performance Objectives

Upon successfully completing this chapter, you will be able to:

1. Manage a patient with a diabetic emergency (Procedure 36-1)

CAAHEP

- Practice standard precautions
- Prepare patient for and assist with routine and specialty examinations
- Prepare patient for and assist with procedures, treatments, and minor office surgeries
- Document appropriately
- Instruct individuals according to their needs

ABHES

- Prepare patients for procedures
- Assist physician with examinations and treatments
- Document accurately

Key Terms

acromegaly	glycosuria	hypoglycemia	polydipsia
Addison's disease	goiter	insulin-dependent diabetes mellitus	polyphagia
Cushing's syndrome	Graves' disease	ketoacidosis	polyuria
diabetes insipidus	Hashimoto's thyroiditis	ketones	pruritus
dwarfism	hormones	non–insulin-dependent diabetes mellitus	radioimmunoassay
endocrinologist	hyperglycemia		thyrotoxicosis
exophthalmia	hyperplasia		
gigantism			

Common Disorders of the Endocrine System

Together with the nervous system, the endocrine system regulates most body functions (Fig. 36-1). Although the control exerted by the nervous system is immediate and usually elicits a short-term response, the endocrine system regulates chemical metabolism for a longer acting, more widespread response. **Hormones** are the chemical regulators, or messengers, of the endocrine glands. Some hormones stimulate system-wide metabolic processes, while others target specific tissues or organs (Table 36-1).

The endocrine glands differ from the body's other glands, such as sweat glands, because they are ductless. Endocrine glands secrete hormones directly into the bloodstream for transmission rather than having direct access to target tissues. The body regulates the release of hormones through negative feedback, which "tells" the appropriate gland how much hormone to release based on the need for increased or decreased secretion. Some endocrine glands release hormones to maintain a specific range in the blood (thyroid hormones), while others have cyclic or rhythmic fluctuations (estrogen or progesterone).

Although you may see patients with endocrine system disorders in any medical practice specialty, physicians who specialize in the treatment of these disorders specifically are known as **endocrinologists**. Many disorders of the endocrine system result from an oversecretion or undersecretion of hormones. This chapter will focus on some common disorders of the endocrine system.

Disorders of the Thyroid

Hyperthyroidism

The most common form of hyperthyroidism, **Graves' disease**, results from the hypersecretion of thyroid hormones. This condition, also known as **thyrotoxicosis** (Box 36-1), causes an increase in metabolism. In addition to elevated blood levels of thyroid hormones (T_3 and T_4), the patient may have an enlarged thyroid gland

Figure 36-1   The main hormone-secreting glands of the endocrine system.

known as a **goiter** (Fig. 36-2) and unusual protrusion of the eyeballs known as **exophthalmia** (Fig. 36-3). Additional signs and symptoms of Graves' disease include:

- Increased heart rate
- Increased body temperature
- Excessive sweating
- Inability to sleep
- Increased appetite
- Weight loss
- Excitability and nervousness

The treatment for hyperthyroidism includes destruction of part or all of the thyroid gland through the use of radioactive iodine or surgery.

Hypothyroidism

Hypothyroidism results from an undersecretion of thyroid hormones, which may be congenital or acquired. Infants with congenital hypothyroidism are usually diagnosed at birth and treated with appropriate thyroid hormones. However, if a diagnosis is not made in the infant, irreversible mental retardation will occur. In adults, hypothyroidism may occur because of surgical removal of thyroid tissue, radioactivity destruction of the gland, the use of antithyroid medications, or a deficiency of iodine in the diet. One form of hypothyroidism, **Hashimoto's thyroiditis**, is actually a disease of the immune system in which the tissue of the thyroid gland is replaced with fibrous tissue. Treatment of hypothyroidism, regardless of the cause, is replacement of thyroid hormones, which must be taken by the patient for the remainder of his or her life. Your role will include being supportive of the patient to ensure compliance with all physician orders.

☑ CHECKPOINT QUESTION

1. Why does the patient with hyperthyroidism have an increased appetite with weight loss?

Disorders of the Pancreas
Diabetes Mellitus

Dysfunction of the islets of Langerhans cells within the pancreas results in diabetes mellitus, a disorder affecting carbohydrate metabolism. Although the exact cause of diabetes mellitus is not known, the result is a decrease in the production and secretion of insulin from the pancreas. Because insulin is necessary to carry glucose into the cells of the body, a decrease in insulin results in **hyperglycemia** (an elevated blood glucose), which ultimately results in **glycosuria** (glucose in the urine).

Type 1 Diabetes Mellitus

Type 1 diabetes mellitus is sometimes referred to as **insulin-dependent diabetes mellitus** and occurs most often in children and young adults (Fig. 36-4). Usually, the symptoms of type 1 diabetes mellitus are abrupt and include the following:

- **Polydipsia** (increased thirst)
- **Polyuria** (excessive urination)
- **Polyphagia** (abnormal hunger)
- Weight loss

TABLE 36-1	The Major Endocrine Glands and Their Hormones	
Gland	**Hormone**	**Principal Functions**
Anterior pituitary	GH (growth hormone)	Promotes growth of all body tissues
	TSH (thyroid-stimulating hormone)	Stimulates the thyroid gland to produce thyroid hormones
	ACTH (adrenocorticotropic hormone)	Stimulates adrenal cortex to produce cortical hormones
	FSH (follicle-stimulating hormone)	Stimulates growth and hormone activity of ovarian follicles; stimulates growth of testes
	LH (luteinizing hormone)	Causes development of corpus luteum in ruptured ovarian follicle in females; stimulates secretion of testosterone in males
Posterior pituitary	ADH (antidiuretic hormone; vasopressin)	Promotes reabsorption of water in kidney tubules
	Oxytocin	Causes contraction of uterus; causes ejection of milk from mammary glands.
Thyroid	Thyroid hormone (thyroxine and triiodothyronine)	Increase metabolic rate; required for normal growth
	Calcitonin	Decreases calcium level in blood
Adrenal medulla	Epinephrine and norepinephrine	Increase blood pressure and heart rate
Adrenal cortex	Cortisol (95% of glucocorticoids)	Aids in metabolism of carbohydrates, proteins, fats; active during stress
	Aldosterone (95% of mineralocorticoids)	Aids in regulating electrolytes and water balance
Pancreatic islets	Insulin	Aids transport of glucose into cells; required for cellular metabolism of foods, especially glucose; decreases blood glucose levels
	Glucagon	Stimulates liver to release glucose, increasing blood glucose levels
Testes	Testosterone	Stimulates growth and development of male sexual organs
Ovaries	Estrogen	Stimulate growth of primary female sexual organs and development of secondary sexual characteristics

Type 2 Diabetes Mellitus

Type 2 diabetes mellitus may be referred to as **non–insulin-dependent diabetes mellitus**; however, many patients with this condition do require insulin to control elevated blood glucose levels. This type of diabetes mellitus occurs most often in adults over the age of 40 years and has a gradual onset. Although insulin is produced by the pancreas, it cannot exert its effect on cells because of a deficiency of insulin receptors on cell membranes. Risk factors for developing type 2 diabetes are obesity and a family history.

The patient with type 2 diabetes will have symptoms of hyperglycemia similar to patients with type 1 diabetes including polydipsia and polyuria. However, patients with type 2 diabetes mellitus will also have **pruritus** (severe itching) and neuropathy (disorders of the nervous system). Usually, the physician will recommend that the patient lose weight and eat a well-balanced diet, which may help to control the elevated blood glucose levels and reduce the need for parenteral insulin. Oral medications that enable insulin to react with the remaining cell membrane receptors are used as necessary; however, elevated

BOX 36-1

THYROID STORM

A severe form of thyrotoxicosis is thyroid storm, or crisis, which may result in coma and death. Although very few patients suffer from thyroid storm today, symptoms include:

- Very high fever
- Dehydration
- Tachycardia
- Shortness of breath
- Productive cough
- Chest pain
- Agitation
- Mental confusion

Patients diagnosed with thyroid storm require immediate medical intervention to reduce the body temperature and replace fluids and electrolytes.

Figure 36-3 Exophthalmia. (From Goodheart HP. Goodheart's Photoguide of Common Skin Disorders. 2nd ed. Philadelphia: Lippincott Williams & Wilkins, 2003.)

PATIENT EDUCATION

GESTATIONAL DIABETES MELLITUS

Another type of diabetes mellitus occurs only during pregnancy and is known as gestational diabetes mellitus. Although the pregnant patient may have all the signs and symptoms of type 1 or 2 diabetes mellitus, this condition disappears after the patient delivers the baby. It is important that the patient's urine be checked at every medical office visit for the presence of glucose; a blood specimen for glucose should be taken between 24 and 28 weeks of gestation. Early diagnosis of this condition is important to reduce complications such as fetal abnormalities and death.

blood glucose that does not respond to diet control and oral medications must be treated with insulin, which is injected subcutaneously. Long-term complications from uncontrolled hyperglycemia include vascular changes that affect many body systems (Box 36-2).

Diabetic Emergencies

When glucose cannot be used for energy by the cells, the body turns to fats and proteins, which are converted to

Toxic goiter (Graves' disease)

Figure 36-2 An enlarged thyroid gland or goiter. (Asset provided by Anatomical Chart Co.)

Figure 36-4 A young child with diabetes mellitus.

BOX 36-2

DIABETIC RETINOPATHY

Diabetic retinopathy is seen in patients with a history of diabetes mellitus and is caused by small hemorrhages from the capillaries supplying blood to the eye. After the capillaries rupture, scarring occurs that decreases the amount of oxygen to the eye. Over time, this scarring and decrease in oxygen results in permanent damage, causing a decrease in vision and eventual blindness. Controlling blood glucose levels can help control this devastating disease, which is currently the leading cause of blindness in the United States.

ketones by the liver. These ketones accumulate in the blood because the cells cannot use them rapidly. As these acids build up, they lower the pH of the blood, a condition known as **ketoacidosis**. The treatment is immediate intervention with parenterally administered insulin. Left untreated, ketoacidosis will progress to diabetic coma and death. Symptoms of diabetic coma include:

- Flushed, dry skin
- A fruity (acetone) smell on the breath
- Thirst
- Deep respirations
- Rapid, weak pulse
- Abdominal pain
- Elevated blood glucose

Occasionally, a patient with diabetes mellitus has too much insulin in the blood, resulting in **hypoglycemia**, or a decreased blood glucose level. This can result when the patient skips a meal or increases physical activity without adjusting the insulin dose. The result can produce a condition known as insulin shock and includes the following symptoms:

- Pale, moist skin
- Shallow respirations
- Rapid, bounding pulse
- Subnormal blood glucose levels

Procedure 36-1 describes the management of a patient having a diabetic emergency such as hyperglycemia and ketoacidosis or insulin shock.

CHECKPOINT QUESTION

2. What is the difference between type 1 and type 2 diabetes mellitus?

PATIENT EDUCATION

CONTROLLING DIABETES MELLITUS

Use every opportunity to educate diabetic patients about the importance of regulating blood glucose and eating sensibly. Also explain that, although these measures can control diabetes, the long-term effects of hyperglycemia can result in vascular changes that may cause blindness and kidney damage. Specifically, instruct patients how to:

- Maintain good personal hygiene to reduce secondary infections
- Manage their dietary intake of calories and carbohydrates
- Care for their feet properly because peripheral circulation may be poor
- Check blood glucose levels frequently and keep a log of the results
- Dispose of insulin syringes correctly
- Be aware of the signs and symptoms of diabetic ketoacidosis and insulin shock

WHAT IF?

What if your elderly adult patient is having difficulty seeing the numbers on the insulin syringe?

Although many elderly patients have visual difficulties that occur naturally with age, the diabetic patient may have increased visual difficulties from the vascular changes in the eyes that result from the diabetes. Although you should always discuss these problems with the physician before advising the patient, there are visual aids that the patient can get from the pharmacist that fit onto the side of the syringe and magnify the image, making the numbers for "units of insulin" larger in appearance and easier to see. Perhaps a friend, neighbor, or other family member can assist the patient with filling the syringes. In some cases, the physician may want a visiting nurse to come to the patient's house during the week to prefill the syringes for the patient. Whatever the solution, always ask elderly patients about their medications and any difficulties they may be having with administering those medications, and work with the physician to come up with the best plan for the patient.

Disorders of the Adrenal Glands

Addison's disease

Hypoadrenocorticalism, or **Addison's disease**, results from a deficiency of hormone secretion (mineralocorticoids and glucocorticoids) from the adrenal cortex. A decrease in these hormones causes an imbalance of electrolytes, specifically a loss of sodium and an increase in potassium. Other symptoms include weakness, lethargy, weight loss, hypotension, anemia, and a poor tolerance to stress.

The adrenal insufficiency of this disease results in an increase in the release of adrenocorticotropic hormone (ACTH) from the anterior pituitary gland. As this hormone becomes elevated in the blood, the patient will have hyperpigmentation of the skin (Fig. 36-5). Treatment includes the oral replacement of the mineralocorticoid and glucocorticoid hormones.

WHAT IF?

What if your patient asks you if he/she should purchase and wear a medic alert bracelet?

Many of the diseases of the endocrine system are chronic and require monitoring and appropriate administration of hormones for the remainder of the patient's life. Unfortunately, if these patients become unresponsive or unable to verbalize their condition in an emergency, the appropriate treatment may be overlooked and have serious consequences for the patient. Always encourage any patient with a chronic disease to wear a medic alert necklace or bracelet to avoid a delay in treatment should an emergency arise.

Figure 36-5 Hyperpigmentation seen in Addison's disease. (From Goodheart HP. Goodheart's Photoguide of Common Skin Disorders. 2nd ed. Philadelphia: Lippincott Williams & Wilkins, 2003.)

Cushing's Syndrome

Hyperadrenocorticalism, also known as **Cushing's syndrome**, may be caused by **hyperplasia** of the adrenal cortex or a tumor, resulting in an increased production of ACTH from the pituitary. Excessive cortisol promotes fat deposits in the trunk of the body, with the extremities remaining thin. Osteoporosis is accelerated, whereas the skin is fragile and heals slowly after injuries. The face is characteristically round (Fig. 36-6).

Cushing's syndrome may also be present in patients who are taking corticosteroids for medical reasons. Patients who may be prescribed corticosteroids include transplantation recipients and those with severe asthma or rheumatoid arthritis. Treatment for hyperadrenocorticalism requires removal of the cause of the hypersecretion, which could be either a pituitary or an adrenal tumor.

 CHECKPOINT QUESTION

3. Which disorder of the adrenal gland results in elevated cortisol levels?

Disorders of the Pituitary Gland

Gigantism and Acromegaly

The pituitary gland, also known as the hypophysis, is the master gland responsible for controlling many aspects of the endocrine system. Hyperpituitarism is marked by an excess production of human growth hormone (HGH) secreted from the anterior lobe of the pituitary gland. Normally, HGH is secreted only up to the time of maturity when the epiphyseal lines on the long bones seal; however, hyperpituitarism during childhood or adolescence will result in an increase in bone length and a final height of 7 or 8 feet. This con-

Figure 36-6 The round face of Cushing's syndrome. (From Weber J, Kelley J. Health Assessment in Nursing. 2nd ed. Philadelphia: Lippincott Williams & Wilkins, 2003.)

dition is called **gigantism** and is noted by an excessive size and stature.

If hyperfunction of the anterior pituitary occurs near the end of puberty or during adulthood after epiphyseal closure, bone length does not change, but bone width increases, resulting in a condition known as **acromegaly** (Fig. 36-7). The patient with this disorder will have physical features such as a prominent jaw, an enlarged nose, and unusual thickening of the hands, feet, and skin. Unusual hyperactivity of the pituitary gland is associated with a tumor of the gland. Treatment of acromegaly requires surgical removal of the tumor or its destruction by radiation.

Dwarfism

Hypopituitarism is a deficiency of the anterior pituitary hormones, which may be caused by injury, atrophy of the gland, or certain types of tumors. If this condition occurs early in life, growth will be retarded, and **dwarfism** will result. A person with dwarfism is extremely short but has normal body proportions. Children who are diagnosed with this disorder can be given growth hormone (GH) to stimulate growth.

Adult hypopituitarism may be classified according to whether the various anterior pituitary hormones are selectively or completely deficient. If all the hormones are deficient, the condition is called panhypopituitarism, and if only certain hormones are deficient, the condition is named for the specific deficiency.

 CHECKPOINT QUESTION

4. How are hypopituitarism and hyperpituitarism different?

Figure 36-7 Acromegaly. (From Willis MC. Medical Terminology: A Programmed Learning Approach to the Language of Health Care. Baltimore: Lippincott Williams & Wilkins, 2002.)

Diabetes Insipidus

Diabetes insipidus results from a deficiency of antidiuretic hormone (ADH) secreted by the posterior pituitary gland. A deficiency in this hormone causes the renal tubules in the kidneys to reabsorb water and salts, resulting in polyuria with an increased urine output between 5 to 10 liters a day. Other clinical symptoms include polydipsia as the body tries to compensate for the dehydration caused by the increased urine production. Although the cause may be unknown, damage to the posterior pituitary gland from trauma or a pituitary tumor may result in this condition. Treatment involves correction of the causative factor if known and the administration of synthetic ADH by tablets, injection, or nasal spray.

Common Diagnostic and Therapeutic Procedures

A variety of laboratory tests and diagnostic procedures may be ordered by the physician to assist in the correct identification of endocrine disorders. Your assistance with performing or scheduling these laboratory or other diagnostic procedures is important so that treatment may be initiated as quickly as possible. In most cases, testing of blood and urine can be used to measure the various hormone levels. Although the procedures for collecting these specimens are discussed in the clinical laboratory section of this text, you should be familiar with the procedures for collecting the specimen in addition to the procedure for processing the specimen appropriately. In some situations, you may have to schedule the patient for specimen collection at an outside laboratory facility.

Some examples of commonly performed tests for diabetes mellitus include the fasting glucose test and the glucose tolerance test (GTT), both using blood samples to check the levels of glucose. Although the urine glucose test is not used to diagnose or monitor diabetes mellitus, it is commonly part of the reagent strips used to check a variety of substances in the urine when performing a urinalysis (see Chapter 43, Urinalysis, for additional information). The glycohemoglobin, or hemoglobin A1C, blood test may be ordered by the physician to determine how well the blood glucose has been controlled in a patient with type 2 or type 2 diabetes mellitus during the previous 2 to 3 months. Ideally, a hemoglobin A1C level of 7% or lower is generally a good sign that the average blood glucose levels have been 170 mg/dL or less over the past 6 to 12 weeks. Table 36-2 describes the hemoglobin A1C levels and the corresponding mean glucose levels, and Table 36-3 describes other blood tests used to diagnose disorders of the endocrine system.

Thyroid functions tests measure the levels of thyroxine (T_4), triiodothyronine (T_3), and thyroid-stimulating hormone in the blood. In addition, the physician may

TABLE 36-2	Correlation of Hemoglobin A1C Values and Mean Blood Glucose Levels
Hemoglobin A1C (%)	Mean Blood Glucose Levels (mg/dL)
6	135
7	170
8	205
9	240
10	275
11	310
12	345

order diagnostic imaging procedures to diagnose abnormalities with the thyroid gland. Specifically, a thyroid scan and the radioactive iodine uptake are ordered to diagnose thyroid disorders. During a thyroid scan, a radioactive compound is administered and localizes in the thyroid gland. The gland is then visualized with a scanner device to detect tumors or nodules. The radioactive iodine uptake procedure determines the amount of thyroid function by having the patient take an oral dose of radioactive iodine and measuring the absorption of this iodine in the thyroid gland.

Another test for endocrine disorders is the **radioimmunoassay (RAI)**, which measures hormone levels in blood by introducing radioactive substances into the body. The test is based on the ability of antibodies to bind specifically to radioactively labeled hormone molecules and to nonradioactive molecules. Computed tomography (CT) scans, magnetic resonance imaging (MRI), and ultrasonography are also used in the diagnosis of pathologic conditions of the endocrine system. Although you will not be performing the imaging procedures used in diagnosing endocrine system disorders, your role will include scheduling the patient for these procedures as ordered by the physician.

 CHECKPOINT QUESTION

5. What is the purpose of the hemoglobin A1C blood test?

 TRIAGE

While you are working in a medical office, the following three situations occur at the same time:

A. Patient A is a 62-year-old man who is waiting for you to obtain a blood specimen that the physician has ordered for T_3 and T_4.

B. Patient B is a new patient who has just been taken back to an examination room and needs to have vital signs taken.

C. Someone from the laboratory is on the phone with the results for a diabetic patient who had a hemoglobin A1C drawn yesterday.

How do you sort these patients? What do you do first? Second? Third?

First, have someone take the message from the laboratory personnel. Anyone from the clinical staff can take these results. Patient B should have his vital signs taken and recorded. After checking for completion of the necessary new patient paperwork, you should notify the physician that he is ready to be seen. While the physician is examining patient B, you should perform a venipuncture on patient A. Unless the physician has indicated a need to speak with patient A, he can be discharged after the blood specimen is taken.

TABLE 36-3	Laboratory Tests for Endocrine System Disorders
Endocrine Gland	Blood Test
Thyroid	Thyroxine (T4)
	Triiodothyronine (T3)
Anterior pituitary	TSH (thyroid-stimulating hormone)
	GH (growth hormone)
	FSH (follicle-stimulating hormone)
	LH (luteinizing hormone)
Pancreas	Glucose
	Hemoglobin A1C
Adrenal cortex	Corticoids

español
SPANISH TERMINOLOGY

Tiene usted sed excesiva?
Do you have excessive thirst?
Necesito una muestra de su orina.
I need a urine specimen.
Como es su apetito?
How is your appetite?
Necesito tomarle una muestra de la sangre.
I need to take a blood sample.

MEDIA MENU

- Student CD
  - CMA/RMA Certification Exam Review
- Premium Online Course
  http://thePoint.lww.com/Kronenberger3e
- Internet Resources

  LiveAdvise Online Tutoring & Competency Training
  http://thePoint.lww.com/LiveAdvise

  The Hormone Foundation
  www.hormone.org

National Graves' Disease Foundation
www.ngdf.org

American Diabetes Association
www.diabetes.org

American Dietetic Association
www.eatright.org

The Thyroid Foundation of America
www.allthyroid.org

PROCEDURE 36-1:   Manage a Patient With a Diabetic Emergency

Purpose: Respond to a patient who comes into the office with signs and symptoms consistent with a diabetic emergency, either hyperglycemia or hypoglycemia

Equipment: Gloves, blood glucose monitor and strips, fruit juice or oral glucose tablets

Steps	Reasons
1. Wash your hands.	Handwashing aids infection control.
2. Recognize the signs and symptoms of hyperglycemia and hypoglycemia. *Hyperglycemia:* • Flushed, dry skin • A sweet, fruity smell on the breath • Thirst • Deep respirations • Rapid, weak pulse • Abdominal pain *Hypoglycemia:* • Pale, moist skin • Shallow, fast respirations • Rapid, bounding pulse • Weakness • Shakiness	
3. Identify the patient and escort him/her into the examination room. 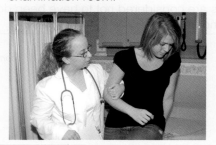 **Step 3.** Assist the patient to the examination room.	This prevents error in treatment, helps gain the patient's compliance, and eases anxiety.

(continued)

PROCEDURE 36-1:   Manage a Patient With a Diabetic Emergency (continued)

4. Determine whether the patient has been previously diagnosed with diabetes mellitus.

You may ask a patient if he or she is a diabetic; however, if the patient is confused, they may say "no" when they are in fact diabetic. You may also check the medical record or look for a medic alert bracelet or necklace.

Step 3. Determine if the patient is a known diabetic.

5. Ask the patient if he or she has eaten today or taken any medication.

The signs and symptoms of hyperglycemia and hypoglycemia may be difficult to distinguish. A patient who has eaten but has not taken insulin may be hyperglycemic. A patient who has not eaten but has taken insulin may be hypoglycemic.

6. Notify the physician about the patient and perform a capillary stick for a blood glucose measure as directed.

A patient experiencing hyperglycemia will have a blood glucose between 250 and 800 mg/dL. A patient experiencing hypoglycemia will have a blood glucose of less than 70 mg/dL.

Step 6. Perform a finger stick as directed by the physician.

7. Notify the physician with the results of the blood glucose and treat the patient as ordered by the physician.
   A. Administer insulin subcutaneously to a patient with hyperglycemia.
   B. Administer a quick-acting sugar, such as an oral glucose tablet or fruit juice, for a patient with hypoglycemia.

It is important to act quickly while remaining calm when treating a patient having a diabetic emergency.

8. Be prepared to notify EMS as directed by the physician if the symptoms do not improve or worsen.

9. Document any observations and treatments given.

Procedures are considered not to have been done if they are not recorded.

(continued)

PROCEDURE 36-1:   **Manage a Patient With a Diabetic Emergency** *(continued)*

Charting Example:

10/14/2008 11:00 AM Pt. presented to office with complaint of weakness since last evening that has gotten worse this morning. Awake and answers questions appropriately, but seems lethargic. BP 110/62 (R) sitting, pulse 122. Skin pale, skin cool, moist. Denies being diabetic, but wearing a medic alert bracelet indicating that he is diabetic. Dr. Smith notified
—J. Jones, CMA
10/14/2008 11:05 AM Blood glucose 65 mg/dL. Pt. given 8 oz. orange juice orally and a glucose tablet as ordered
—J. Jones, CMA
10/14/2008 11:10 AM Pt. states he "feels better" but continues to look pale, pulse 110, BP 120/72. Given another 8 oz. orange juice as ordered
—J. Jones, CMA

Chapter Summary

- The endocrine system controls many bodily processes indirectly through chemical messengers called hormones.
- Hormones are secreted directly into the blood stream.
- Disorders of the endocrine system include alterations in hormone secretion, and either too much hormone is secreted (hypersecretion or excess) or not enough hormone is secreted (hyposecretion or deficiency).
- Disorders of the thyroid gland include Graves' disease and Hashimoto's thyroiditis.

- Diabetes mellitus is a disorder of the pancreas involving the production of insulin and its ability to take glucose into the cells of the body.
- Depending on when the anterior pituitary gland secretes too much growth hormone, the patient may have gigantism or acromegaly.
- Your role in working with patients with endocrine system disorders includes emotional support to ensure compliance with treatments that are often required for the life of the patient.

1. A 40-year-old female patient is seen in the office with a complaint of weight gain and hair loss. After the physical examination, she asks you why the physician felt the front of her neck. How would you respond? What gland is located there?

2. Your 56-year-old diabetic patient cannot understand why his blood glucose levels are above 200 mg/dL, and he tells you that he "does not eat candy or sweets." Upon furthering questioning, you find out his diet consists of pasta and diet soda. What education does this patient need, if any? Create a brochure that would help this patient understand diabetes mellitus using language a patient would understand.

3. Research the transphenoidal hypophysectomy surgical procedure used to remove pituitary gland tumors. How is this procedure performed? What hormone replacement medications will the patient have to take postoperatively?

4. Your patient is concerned about the thyroid function tests that the physician has ordered and asks you to explain what these tests involve. What could you say to this patient? Would you tell the patient that this test would determine the presence of a thyroid tumor? Why or why not?

5. Create a brochure for the newly diagnosed diabetic patient explaining the hemoglobin A1C test.

Answers   to Checkpoint Questions

1. A patient with hyperthyroidism will have an increased appetite with weight loss due to the increased metabolism from elevated thyroid hormones in the blood.

2. Type 1 diabetes mellitus has a rapid onset in young children and adolescents, while type 2 diabetes mellitus has a gradual onset, affecting adults over the age of 40. Type 1 patients always require parenteral insulin, whereas type 2 patients may control their condition by losing weight and eating a balanced diet.

3. Hyperadrenocorticalism, or Cushing's syndrome, results from an elevated level of cortisol secreted from the adrenal gland.

4. Hypopituitarism is an undersecretion of the anterior pituitary hormones, whereas hyperpituitarism is marked by an excess secretion of growth hormone.

5. The purpose of the hemoglobin A1C is to determine the average blood sugar, or glucose, in a diabetic patient over the previous 2 to 3 months. This will allow the physician to determine compliance with controlling the blood glucose with diet and insulin.

Outline

The Pediatric Practice
Safety
Types of Pediatric Office Visits
Child Development
Psychological Aspects of Care
Physiologic Aspects of Care
Role of the Parent
**The Pediatric Physical
  Examination**
The Pediatric History
Obtaining and Recording
  Measurements and Vital
  Signs

Administering Medications
Oral Medications
Injections
Collecting a Urine Specimen
Understanding Child Abuse
**Pediatric Illnesses and
  Disorders**
Impetigo
Meningitis
Encephalitis
Tetanus

Cerebral Palsy
Croup
Epiglottis
Cystic Fibrosis
Asthma
Otitis Media
Tonsillitis
Obesity
Attention Deficit Hyperactivity
  Disorder

Learning Objectives

*Upon successfully completing this chapter, you
will be able to:*

1. Spell and define key terms

2. List safety precautions for the pediatric office

3. Explain the difference between a well-child and a sick-child visit

4. List types and schedule of immunizations

5. Describe the types of feelings a child might have during an office visit

6. List and explain how to record the anthropometric measurements obtained in a pediatric visit

7. Identify two injection sites to use on an infant and two used on a child

8. Describe the role of the parent during the office visit

9. List the names, symptoms, and treatments for common pediatric illnesses

Performance Objectives

*Upon successfully completing this chapter, you
will be able to:*

1. Obtain an infant's length and weight (Procedure 37-1)

2. Obtain the head and chest circumference (Procedure 37-2)

3. Apply a urinary collection device (Procedure 37-3)

CAAHEP

- Practice standard precautions
- Prepare patient for and assist with routine and specialty examinations
- Prepare patient for and assist with procedures, treatments, and minor office surgeries
- Document appropriately

ABHES

- Prepare patients for procedures
- Assist physician with examinations and treatments
- Document accurately

Key Terms

aspiration
autonomous
congenital anomaly

immunization
neonatologist
pediatrician

pediatrics
psychosocial
restrain

sick-child visit
well-child visit

The Pediatric Practice

Medical assistants who work in an office where infants and children are seen must understand that the needs of children and adolescents are often different from those of adult patients. Pediatrics is the medical specialty devoted to the care of infants, children, and adolescents. This care includes diagnosis and treatment of childhood diseases, prevention of accidents and trauma, and monitoring the physical and **psychosocial**, or mental and emotional, development of the child. These patients are not simply small adults; however, they may contract some of the illnesses that are seen in adult patients. Pediatric patients are also susceptible to a unique array of illnesses and problems not present in adults. Some young patients have **congenital anomalies** that are life threatening or debilitating. Because children have immature nervous systems, faster metabolism, and accelerated growth patterns, they are subject to complications that may not occur in adult patients.

A **pediatrician** is a physician who is specially trained to care for both the well child and diseases of infants, children, and adolescents. While most traditional pediatricians treat all children up through the teen years, pediatric specialists include **neonatologists**, physicians who treat only newborns, and physicians who specialize in the treatment of adolescents. In addition, the medical assistant working in the family practice will see patients of all ages, including children.

Safety

A pediatric office decorated and furnished in a manner appropriate to children's physical and psychosocial needs creates an unthreatening and possibly even inviting environment. Child-size furniture helps these patients feel comfortable and welcome. Popular toys evoke happy associations. Safe toys allow for hands-on activity while the child is waiting to see the physician. Popular storybooks and magazines give parents an opportunity to read quietly to a child who may not feel well enough to play. Some offices provide waiting rooms that are designed to separate sick and well children to prevent the transmission of communicable diseases between patients.

Safety should be a prime concern for choosing toys and equipment for a pediatric office. Waiting room toys should be examined frequently and replaced when damaged or soiled. All toys should be washable and should be cleaned according to office policy to reduce the risk of disease transmission. Try to see the office from a child's viewpoint. If necessary, get down to a child's level to discover dangers, such as sharp table corners and exposed electrical outlets, that an adult standing to observe and evaluate the environment might overlook.

The examination room should also be designed for children's safety. Keep all medical equipment out of a child's reach, and never leave a young child alone in the examining room. Follow these tips to ensure your patient's safety:

- Place infant scales on a sturdy table, and never leave an infant alone on a scale.
- Store any disinfectants away from patient care areas.
- Store and dispose of all sharps in proper containers.
- Practice stringent handwashing and standard precautions with every patient. Many childhood diseases are highly contagious and can be transmitted by poor medical asepsis.

 CHECKPOINT QUESTION

1. What are three safety precautions that should be used in a pediatric office?

Types of Pediatric Office Visits

The Well-Child Office Visit

Well-child visits are regularly scheduled office visits whose goal is to maintain the child's optimum health. Although these visits are typically scheduled to correspond with the immunization schedule (Figs. 37-1 and 37-2), the first newborn visit is often required within 1 week after birth. At this visit, you may be required to obtain a blood specimen from the newborn patient to check for the absence of the enzyme phenylalanine hydroxylase, also known as a PKU test. This test must be performed between 1 and 7 days after birth since an absence of this enzyme may result in mental retardation if not treated by 3 to 4 weeks of age. Treatment of the newborn with this deficiency includes a diet low in phenylalanine.

In addition to including a complete examination and an evaluation of the child's neurologic and psychosocial development, any other concerns on the part of the caregiver are also addressed at these visits. The neurologic examination consists of the physician checking for the presence or absence of various reflexes. Table 37-1 describes various infant reflexes and the normal responses typically assessed at the well-child infant visit. In addition to the reflexes, the physician observes for development appropriate for the age of the infant or child. The child is observed or the caregiver is questioned about areas such as social development, fine motor development, gross motor development, language, and nutrition using a guide such as the Denver II (Fig. 37-3).

The well-child visit also provides an opportunity to administer **immunizations** to protect children from diseases that in the past caused early death or long-term health problems. Immunizations produce immunity by slowly introducing an altered form of the disease-producing bacteria or virus into the body, which stimulates the body to produce antibodies to protect against the specific disease. Immunization schedules are developed by the American Academy of Pediatrics (AAP) and the Centers for Disease Control and Prevention, and they change periodically as new vaccines become available. These schedules include one for children ages 0 to 6 years and another for children ages 7 to 18 years (see Figs. 37-1 and 37-2). You should post these schedules prominently in the office and replace as necessary with the latest information. All children must be current with their immunizations before they are permitted to attend public school.

Vaccine manufacturers have established protocols that must be followed to ensure full immunity to the specific diseases. If you are responsible for administering vaccines, you must read all package inserts and become familiar with the correct administration and possible adverse effects before administering the medication. In addition, you must give the parent or caregiver of the child the written vaccine information statement (VIS) about each vaccine you are administering detailing the benefits and risks that may be associated with each vaccine (Fig. 37-4). In some cases, it may be necessary to obtain written consent before administering the vaccine. The VIS for individual vaccines describes the disease and provides information specific to the immunization, such as recommended ages and adverse reactions. The most current vaccine schedules and information sheets can be found on the Centers for Disease Control and Prevention website.

The Sick-Child Office Visit

A **sick-child visit** occurs whenever an infant or child requires medical treatment for signs or symptoms of illness or injury. The goal of these visits is diagnosis and treatment of the child's immediate illness or injury. After examining the child, the physician may pursue diagnostic tests and treatments including radiography, laboratory tests, medication, or simply the reassurance that the illness will run a predictable and manageable course. Table 37-2 lists three common childhood illnesses and their causes, signs and symptoms, and treatments.

DEPARTMENT OF HEALTH AND HUMAN SERVICES • CENTERS FOR DISEASE CONTROL AND PREVENTION

Recommended Immunization Schedule for Persons Aged 0–6 Years—UNITED STATES • 2007

Vaccine▼ Age►	Birth	1 month	2 months	4 months	6 months	12 months	15 months	18 months	19–23 months	2–3 years	4–6 years	
Hepatitis B[1]	HepB	HepB		see footnote 1		HepB				HepB Series		Range of recommended ages
Rotavirus[2]			Rota	Rota	Rota							
Diphtheria, Tetanus, Pertussis[3]			DTaP	DTaP	DTaP		DTaP				DTaP	
Haemophilus influenzae type b[4]			Hib	Hib	Hib[4]	Hib		Hib				
Pneumococcal[5]			PCV	PCV	PCV	PCV				PCV / PPV		Catch-up immunization
Inactivated Poliovirus			IPV	IPV		IPV					IPV	
Influenza[6]						Influenza (Yearly)						
Measles, Mumps, Rubella[7]						MMR					MMR	Certain high-risk groups
Varicella[8]						Varicella					Varicella	
Hepatitis A[9]						HepA (2 doses)				HepA Series		
Meningococcal[10]										MPSV4		

This schedule indicates the recommended ages for routine administration of currently licensed childhood vaccines, as of December 1, 2006, for children aged 0–6 years. Additional information is available at http://www.cdc.gov/nip/recs/child-schedule.htm. Any dose not administered at the recommended age should be administered at any subsequent visit, when indicated and feasible. Additional vaccines may be licensed and recommended during the year. Licensed combination vaccines may be used whenever any components of the combination are indicated and other components of the vaccine are not contraindicated and if approved by the Food and Drug Administration for that dose of the series. Providers should consult the respective Advisory Committee on Immunization Practices statement for detailed recommendations. Clinically significant adverse events that follow immunization should be reported to the Vaccine Adverse Event Reporting System (VAERS). Guidance about how to obtain and complete a VAERS form is available at http://www.vaers.hhs.gov or by telephone, 800-822-7967.

1. Hepatitis B vaccine (HepB). *(Minimum age: birth)*
At birth:
- Administer monovalent HepB to all newborns before hospital discharge.
- If mother is hepatitis surface antigen (HBsAg)-positive, administer HepB and 0.5 mL of hepatitis B immune globulin (HBIG) within 12 hours of birth.
- If mother's HBsAg status is unknown, administer HepB within 12 hours of birth. Determine the HBsAg status as soon as possible and if HBsAg-positive, administer HBIG (no later than age 1 week).
- If mother is HBsAg-negative, the birth dose can only be delayed with physician's order and mother's negative HBsAg laboratory report documented in the infant's medical record.

After the birth dose:
- The HepB series should be completed with either monovalent HepB or a combination vaccine containing HepB. The second dose should be administered at age 1–2 months. The final dose should be administered at age ≥24 weeks. Infants born to HBsAg-positive mothers should be tested for HBsAg and antibody to HBsAg after completion of ≥3 doses of a licensed HepB series, at age 9–18 months (generally at the next well-child visit).

4-month dose:
- It is permissible to administer 4 doses of HepB when combination vaccines are administered after the birth dose. If monovalent HepB is used for doses after the birth dose, a dose at age 4 months is not needed.

2. Rotavirus vaccine (Rota). *(Minimum age: 6 weeks)*
- Administer the first dose at age 6–12 weeks. Do not start the series later than age 12 weeks.
- Administer the final dose in the series by age 32 weeks. Do not administer a dose later than age 32 weeks.
- Data on safety and efficacy outside of these age ranges are insufficient.

3. Diphtheria and tetanus toxoids and acellular pertussis vaccine (DTaP). *(Minimum age: 6 weeks)*
- The fourth dose of DTaP may be administered as early as age 12 months, provided 6 months have elapsed since the third dose.
- Administer the final dose in the series at age 4–6 years.

4. Haemophilus influenzae type b conjugate vaccine (Hib).
(Minimum age: 6 weeks)
- If PRP-OMP (PedvaxHIB® or ComVax® [Merck]) is administered at ages 2 and 4 months, a dose at age 6 months is not required.
- TriHiBit® (DTaP/Hib) combination products should not be used for primary immunization but can be used as boosters following any Hib vaccine in children aged ≥12 months.

5. Pneumococcal vaccine. *(Minimum age: 6 weeks for pneumococcal conjugate vaccine [PCV]; 2 years for pneumococcal polysaccharide vaccine [PPV])*
- Administer PCV at ages 24–59 months in certain high-risk groups. Administer PPV to children aged ≥2 years in certain high-risk groups. See *MMWR* 2000;49(No. RR-9):1–35.

6. Influenza vaccine. *(Minimum age: 6 months for trivalent inactivated influenza vaccine [TIV]; 5 years for live, attenuated influenza vaccine [LAIV])*
- All children aged 6–59 months and close contacts of all children aged 0–59 months are recommended to receive influenza vaccine.
- Influenza vaccine is recommended annually for children aged ≥59 months with certain risk factors, health-care workers, and other persons (including household members) in close contact with persons in groups at high risk. See *MMWR* 2006;55(No. RR-10):1–41.
- For healthy persons aged 5–49 years, LAIV may be used as an alternative to TIV.
- Children receiving TIV should receive 0.25 mL if aged 6–35 months or 0.5 mL if aged ≥3 years.
- Children aged <9 years who are receiving influenza vaccine for the first time should receive 2 doses (separated by ≥4 weeks for TIV and ≥6 weeks for LAIV).

7. Measles, mumps, and rubella vaccine (MMR). *(Minimum age: 12 months)*
- Administer the second dose of MMR at age 4–6 years. MMR may be administered before age 4–6 years, provided ≥4 weeks have elapsed since the first dose and both doses are administered at age ≥12 months.

8. Varicella vaccine. *(Minimum age: 12 months)*
- Administer the second dose of varicella vaccine at age 4–6 years. Varicella vaccine may be administered before age 4–6 years, provided that ≥3 months have elapsed since the first dose and both doses are administered at age ≥12 months. If second dose was administered ≥28 days following the first dose, the second dose does not need to be repeated.

9. Hepatitis A vaccine (HepA). *(Minimum age: 12 months)*
- HepA is recommended for all children aged 1 year (i.e., aged 12–23 months). The 2 doses in the series should be administered at least 6 months apart.
- Children not fully vaccinated by age 2 years can be vaccinated at subsequent visits.
- HepA is recommended for certain other groups of children, including in areas where vaccination programs target older children. See *MMWR* 2006;55(No. RR-7):1–23.

10. Meningococcal polysaccharide vaccine (MPSV4). *(Minimum age: 2 years)*
- Administer MPSV4 to children aged 2–10 years with terminal complement deficiencies or anatomic or functional asplenia and certain other high-risk groups. See *MMWR* 2005;54(No. RR-7):1–21.

The Recommended Immunization Schedules for Persons Aged 0–18 Years are approved by the Advisory Committee on Immunization Practices (http://www.cdc.gov/nip/acip), the American Academy of Pediatrics (http://www.aap.org), and the American Academy of Family Physicians (http://www.aafp.org).

SAFER • HEALTHIER • PEOPLE™

CS103164

Figure 37-1 An immunization schedule, 2007, 0–6 years.

DEPARTMENT OF HEALTH AND HUMAN SERVICES • CENTERS FOR DISEASE CONTROL AND PREVENTION

Recommended Immunization Schedule for Persons Aged 7–18 Years—UNITED STATES • 2007

Vaccine ▼　　　　　　　　Age ▶	7–10 years	11–12 YEARS	13–14 years	15 years	16–18 years
Tetanus, Diphtheria, Pertussis[1]	*see footnote 1*	Tdap	Tdap		
Human Papillomavirus[2]	*see footnote 2*	HPV (3 doses)	HPV Series		
Meningococcal[3]	MPSV4	MCV4	MCV4[3] MCV4		
Pneumococcal[4]		PPV			
Influenza[5]		Influenza (Yearly)			
Hepatitis A[6]		HepA Series			
Hepatitis B[7]		HepB Series			
Inactivated Poliovirus[8]		IPV Series			
Measles, Mumps, Rubella[9]		MMR Series			
Varicella[10]		Varicella Series			

Range of recommended ages

Catch-up immunization

Certain high-risk groups

This schedule indicates the recommended ages for routine administration of currently licensed childhood vaccines, as of December 1, 2006, for children aged 7–18 years. Additional information is available at http://www.cdc.gov/nip/recs/child-schedule.htm. Any dose not administered at the recommended age should be administered at any subsequent visit, when indicated and feasible. Additional vaccines may be licensed and recommended during the year. Licensed combination vaccines may be used whenever any components of the combination are indicated and other components

of the vaccine are not contraindicated and if approved by the Food and Drug Administration for that dose of the series. Providers should consult the respective Advisory Committee on Immunization Practices statement for detailed recommendations. Clinically significant adverse events that follow immunization should be reported to the Vaccine Adverse Event Reporting System (VAERS). Guidance about how to obtain and complete a VAERS form is available at http://www.vaers.hhs.gov or by telephone, 800-822-7967.

1. Tetanus and diphtheria toxoids and acellular pertussis vaccine (Tdap).
(Minimum age: 10 years for BOOSTRIX® and 11 years for ADACEL™)
- Administer at age 11–12 years for those who have completed the recommended childhood DTP/DTaP vaccination series and have not received a tetanus and diphtheria toxoids vaccine (Td) booster dose.
- Adolescents aged 13–18 years who missed the 11–12 year Td/Tdap booster dose should also receive a single dose of Tdap if they have completed the recommended childhood DTP/DTaP vaccination series.

2. Human papillomavirus vaccine (HPV). *(Minimum age: 9 years)*
- Administer the first dose of the HPV vaccine series to females at age 11–12 years.
- Administer the second dose 2 months after the first dose and the third dose 6 months after the first dose.
- Administer the HPV vaccine series to females at age 13–18 years if not previously vaccinated.

3. Meningococcal vaccine. *(Minimum age: 11 years for meningococcal conjugate vaccine [MCV4]; 2 years for meningococcal polysaccharide vaccine [MPSV4])*
- Administer MCV4 at age 11–12 years and to previously unvaccinated adolescents at high school entry (at approximately age 15 years).
- Administer MCV4 to previously unvaccinated college freshmen living in dormitories; MPSV4 is an acceptable alternative.
- Vaccination against invasive meningococcal disease is recommended for children and adolescents aged ≥2 years with terminal complement deficiencies or anatomic or functional asplenia and certain other high-risk groups. See *MMWR* 2005;54(No. RR-7):1–21. Use MPSV4 for children aged 2–10 years and MCV4 or MPSV4 for older children.

4. Pneumococcal polysaccharide vaccine (PPV). *(Minimum age: 2 years)*
- Administer for certain high-risk groups. See *MMWR* 1997;46(No. RR-8):1–24, and *MMWR* 2000;49(No. RR-9):1–35.

5. Influenza vaccine. *(Minimum age: 6 months for trivalent inactivated influenza vaccine [TIV]; 5 years for live, attenuated influenza vaccine [LAIV])*
- Influenza vaccine is recommended annually for persons with certain risk factors, health-care workers, and other persons (including household members) in close contact with persons in groups at high risk. See *MMWR* 2006;55 (No. RR-10):1–41.
- For healthy persons aged 5–49 years, LAIV may be used as an alternative to TIV.
- Children aged <9 years who are receiving influenza vaccine for the first time should receive 2 doses (separated by ≥4 weeks for TIV and ≥6 weeks for LAIV).

6. Hepatitis A vaccine (HepA). *(Minimum age: 12 months)*
- The 2 doses in the series should be administered at least 6 months apart.
- HepA is recommended for certain other groups of children, including in areas where vaccination programs target older children. See *MMWR* 2006;55 (No. RR-7):1–23.

7. Hepatitis B vaccine (HepB). *(Minimum age: birth)*
- Administer the 3-dose series to those who were not previously vaccinated.
- A 2-dose series of Recombivax HB® is licensed for children aged 11–15 years.

8. Inactivated poliovirus vaccine (IPV). *(Minimum age: 6 weeks)*
- For children who received an all-IPV or all-oral poliovirus (OPV) series, a fourth dose is not necessary if the third dose was administered at age ≥4 years.
- If both OPV and IPV were administered as part of a series, a total of 4 doses should be administered, regardless of the child's current age.

9. Measles, mumps, and rubella vaccine (MMR). *(Minimum age: 12 months)*
- If not previously vaccinated, administer 2 doses of MMR during any visit, with ≥4 weeks between the doses.

10. Varicella vaccine. *(Minimum age: 12 months)*
- Administer 2 doses of varicella vaccine to persons without evidence of immunity.
- Administer 2 doses of varicella vaccine to persons aged <13 years at least 3 months apart. Do not repeat the second dose, if administered ≥28 days after the first dose.
- Administer 2 doses of varicella vaccine to persons aged ≥13 years at least 4 weeks apart.

The Recommended Immunization Schedules for Persons Aged 0–18 Years are approved by the Advisory Committee on Immunization Practices (http://www.cdc.gov/nip/acip), the American Academy of Pediatrics (http://www.aap.org), and the American Academy of Family Physicians (http://www.aafp.org).

SAFER • HEALTHIER • PEOPLE™

CS10013

Figure 37-2　An immunization schedule 2007, 7–18 years.

Catch-up Immunization Schedule
for Persons Aged 4 Months–18 Years Who Start Late or Who Are More Than 1 Month Behind

UNITED STATES • 2007

The table below provides catch-up schedules and minimum intervals between doses for children whose vaccinations have been delayed. A vaccine series does not need to be restarted, regardless of the time that has elapsed between doses. Use the section appropriate for the child's age.

CATCH-UP SCHEDULE FOR PERSONS AGED 4 MONTHS–6 YEARS

Vaccine	Minimum Age for Dose 1	Minimum Interval Between Doses			
		Dose 1 to Dose 2	Dose 2 to Dose 3	Dose 3 to Dose 4	Dose 4 to Dose 5
Hepatitis B[1]	Birth	4 weeks	8 weeks (and 16 weeks after first dose)		
Rotavirus[2]	6 wks	4 weeks	4 weeks		
Diphtheria, Tetanus, Pertussis[3]	6 wks	4 weeks	4 weeks	6 months	6 months[3]
Haemophilus influenzae type b[4]	6 wks	**4 weeks** if first dose administered at age <12 months / **8 weeks (as final dose)** if first dose administered at age 12-14 months / **No further doses needed** if first dose administered at age ≥15 months	**4 weeks**[4] if current age <12 months / **8 weeks (as final dose)**[4] if current age ≥12 months and second dose administered at age <15 months / **No further doses needed** if previous dose administered at age ≥15 months	**8 weeks (as final dose)** This dose only necessary for children aged 12 months–5 years who received 3 doses before age 12 months	
Pneumococcal[5]	6 wks	**4 weeks** if first dose administered at age <12 months and current age <24 months / **8 weeks (as final dose)** if first dose administered at age ≥12 months or current age 24–59 months / **No further doses needed** for healthy children if first dose administered at age ≥24 months	**4 weeks** if current age <12 months / **8 weeks (as final dose)** if current age ≥12 months / **No further doses needed** for healthy children if previous dose administered at age ≥24 months	**8 weeks (as final dose)** This dose only necessary for children aged 12 months–5 years who received 3 doses before age 12 months	
Inactivated Poliovirus[6]	6 wks	4 weeks	4 weeks	4 weeks[6]	
Measles, Mumps, Rubella[7]	12 mos	4 weeks			
Varicella[8]	12 mos	3 months			
Hepatitis A[9]	12 mos	6 months			

CATCH-UP SCHEDULE FOR PERSONS AGED 7–18 YEARS

Vaccine	Minimum Age for Dose 1	Dose 1 to Dose 2	Dose 2 to Dose 3	Dose 3 to Dose 4	
Tetanus, Diphtheria/ Tetanus, Diphtheria, Pertussis[10]	7 yrs[10]	4 weeks	**8 weeks** if first dose administered at age <12 months / **6 months** if first dose administered at age ≥12 months	**6 months** if first dose administered at age <12 months	
Human Papillomavirus[11]	9 yrs	4 weeks	12 weeks		
Hepatitis A[9]	12 mos	6 months			
Hepatitis B[1]	Birth	4 weeks	8 weeks (and 16 weeks after first dose)		
Inactivated Poliovirus[6]	6 wks	4 weeks	4 weeks	4 weeks[6]	
Measles, Mumps, Rubella[7]	12 mos	4 weeks			
Varicella[8]	12 mos	**4 weeks** if first dose administered at age ≥13 years / **3 months** if first dose administered at age <13 years			

1. Hepatitis B vaccine (HepB). *(Minimum age: birth)*
- Administer the 3-dose series to those who were not previously vaccinated.
- A 2-dose series of Recombivax HB® is licensed for children aged 11–15 years.

2. Rotavirus vaccine (Rota). *(Minimum age: 6 weeks)*
- Do not start the series later than age 12 weeks.
- Administer the final dose in the series by age 32 weeks. Do not administer a dose later than age 32 weeks.
- Data on safety and efficacy outside of these age ranges are insufficient.

3. Diphtheria and tetanus toxoids and acellular pertussis vaccine (DTaP). *(Minimum age: 6 weeks)*
- The fifth dose is not necessary if the fourth dose was administered at age ≥4 years.
- DTaP is not indicated for persons aged ≥7 years.

4. *Haemophilus influenzae* type b conjugate vaccine (Hib). *(Minimum age: 6 weeks)*
- Vaccine is not generally recommended for children aged ≥5 years.
- If current age <12 months and the first 2 doses were PRP-OMP (PedvaxHIB® or ComVax® [Merck]), the third (and final) dose should be administered at age 12–15 months and at least 8 weeks after the second dose.
- If first dose was administered at age 7–11 months, administer 2 doses separated by 4 weeks plus a booster at age 12–15 months.

5. Pneumococcal conjugate vaccine (PCV). *(Minimum age: 6 weeks)*
- Vaccine is not generally recommended for children aged ≥5 years.

6. Inactivated poliovirus vaccine (IPV). *(Minimum age: 6 weeks)*
- For children who received an all-IPV or all-oral poliovirus (OPV) series, a fourth dose is not necessary if third dose was administered at age ≥4 years.
- If both OPV and IPV were administered as part of a series, a total of 4 doses should be administered, regardless of the child's current age.

7. Measles, mumps, and rubella vaccine (MMR). *(Minimum age: 12 months)*
- The second dose of MMR is recommended routinely at age 4–6 years but may be administered earlier if desired.
- If not previously vaccinated, administer 2 doses of MMR during any visit with ≥4 weeks between the doses.

8. Varicella vaccine. *(Minimum age: 12 months)*
- The second dose of varicella vaccine is recommended routinely at age 4–6 years but may be administered earlier if desired.
- Do not repeat the second dose in persons aged <13 years if administered ≥28 days after the first dose.

9. Hepatitis A vaccine (HepA). *(Minimum age: 12 months)*
- HepA is recommended for certain groups of children, including in areas where vaccination programs target older children. See *MMWR* 2006;55(No. RR-7):1–23.

10. Tetanus and diphtheria toxoids vaccine (Td) and tetanus and diphtheria toxoids and acellular pertussis vaccine (Tdap). *(Minimum ages: 7 years for Td, 10 years for BOOSTRIX®, and 11 years for ADACEL™)*
- Tdap should be substituted for a single dose of Td in the primary catch-up series or as a booster if age appropriate; use Td for other doses.
- A 5-year interval from the last Td dose is encouraged when Tdap is used as a booster dose. A booster (fourth) dose is needed if any of the previous doses were administered at age <12 months. Refer to ACIP recommendations for further information. See *MMWR* 2006;55(No. RR-3).

11. Human papillomavirus vaccine (HPV). *(Minimum age: 9 years)*
- Administer the HPV vaccine series to females at age 13–18 years if not previously vaccinated.

Information about reporting reactions after immunization is available online at http://www.vaers.hhs.gov or by telephone via the 24-hour national toll-free information line 800-822-7967. Suspected cases of vaccine-preventable diseases should be reported to the state or local health department. Additional information, including precautions and contraindications for immunization, is available from the National Center for Immunization and Respiratory Diseases at http://www.cdc.gov/nip/default.htm or telephone, 800-CDC-INFO (800-232-4636).

DEPARTMENT OF HEALTH AND HUMAN SERVICES • **CENTERS FOR DISEASE CONTROL AND PREVENTION** • **SAFER • HEALTHIER • PEOPLE**

CS103164

Figure 37-2 *(continued)*

TABLE 37-1	Infant Reflexes and Responses
Reflex	**Response**
Sucking or rooting	Stroking the cheek causes the infant to turn toward the stroke with its mouth open to suck. This reflex subsides by 3–6 months.
Moro or startle	A loud noise or sudden change in position causes the infant to look startled; the back arches, the arms and legs fly out and then quickly come back close to the body, and the infant cries. The Moro reflex results in the thumbs and forefingers forming a C while the other fingers spread open (in the startled reflex, the fingers remain clenched). Both reflexes disappear by 6 months.
Grasp	Stroking the infant's palm causes the fingers to grasp; stroking the plantar surface causes the toes to flex to grasp. The palmar grasp disappears by 3 months. The plantar grasp disappears by 9–12 months.
Tonic neck or fencing	With the infant supine, the physician turns the head to either side. The arm and leg on the side the infant is facing will flex, and the limbs on the opposite side will extend. This reflex disappears by 3–4 months.
Placing or stepping	The physician holds the infant upright at the edge of the examining table with the heel just below the edge. When the tops of the feet touch the table edge, the infant will place each foot up on the table and make walking movements. This reflex disappears by 6 weeks.
Babinski	When the plantar surface of the foot is stroked, the toes flare outward. This reflex disappears by 12 months.

CHECKPOINT QUESTION

2. What is the difference between well-child and sick-child visits?

Child Development

Psychological Aspects of Care

Understanding a child's psychological needs and development helps you provide safe and effective care. During an office visit, the patient may have the same feelings as adults: fear and powerlessness. However, depending on the child's age and ability to understand, the behaviors associated with these feelings are different from those of the adult patient. Specifically, children may have these feelings:

- Fear that something painful and frightening will be done
- Anxiety about repetition of a previous bad experience
- Guilt and feelings of being punished for being bad or misbehaving
- Powerlessness and loss of physical autonomy
- Curiosity about new surroundings and experiences

Some children verbalize these feelings, while others can express them only by crying and resisting the approach of the medical staff. As a professional medical assistant, you can reassure patients and family members by demonstrating your understanding of the child's feelings and displaying a kind and gentle manner. Include the child in the explanation of procedures on an age-appropriate level. Children who are encouraged to "help" during the examination or procedure (such as holding the adhesive bandage before receiving an injection) may also feel part of the examination and may be more cooperative.

Physiologic Aspects of Care

To anticipate age-appropriate behavior and to provide proper psychological support and physical care, you must have a broad knowledge of child growth and development patterns. Never expect a child to react or respond beyond his or her developmental age. For example, a 2-year-old child is naturally reluctant to be examined and may resist your advances. Many 4- or 5-year-old children are curious and willing to cooperate if you turn the examination into a game. Children older than 4 years should understand the need to comply, but this age group may still have to be restrained during some procedures, such as injections. A normal child's growth and development of mind, body, and personality follow an orderly progression. Table 37-3 describes the stages of growth and development and lists special considerations for the medical assistant.

The nervous system is complete but immature at birth. During regular visits to the pediatrician, the infant is tested for infantile automatisms—reflexes found in the newborn that disappear later in childhood (Fig. 37-5).

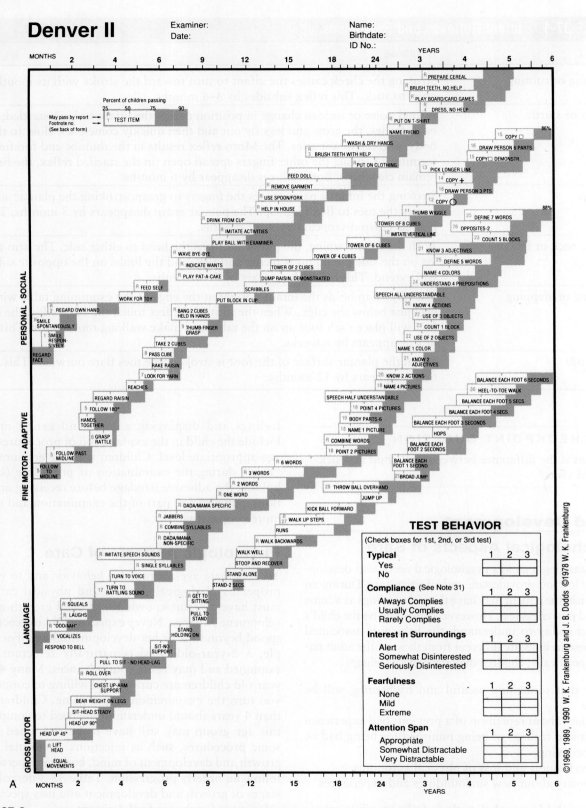

Figure 37-3 (A) The Denver Developmental Screening Test II. (B) Instructions for the test. Test kits, test forms, and reference manuals, which must be used to ensure accuracy, may be ordered from Denver Developmental Materials Incorporated, P.O. Box 6919, Denver CO 80206-0919.

DIRECTIONS FOR ADMINISTRATION

1. Try to get child to smile by smiling, talking or waving. Do not touch him/her.
2. Child must stare at hand several seconds.
3. Parent may help guide toothbrush and put toothpaste on brush.
4. Child does not have to be able to tie shoes or button/zip in the back.
5. Move yarn slowly in an arc from one side to the other, about 8″ above child's face.
6. Pass if child grasps rattle when it is touched to the backs or tips of fingers.
7. Pass if child tries to see where yarn went. Yarn should be dropped quickly from sight from tester's hand without arm movement.
8. Child must transfer cube from hand to hand without help of body, mouth, or table.
9. Pass if child picks up raisin with any part of thumb and finger.
10. Line can vary only 30 degrees or less from tester's line. V
11. Make a fist with thumb pointing upward and wiggle only the thumb. Pass if child imitates and does not move any fingers other than the thumb.

12. Pass any enclosed form. Fail continuous round motions.
13. Which line is longer? (Not bigger.) Turn paper upside down and repeat. (pass 3 of 3 or 5 of 6)
14. Pass any lines crossing near midpoint.
15. Have child copy first. If failed, demonstrate.

When giving items 12, 14, and 15, do not name the forms. Do not demonstrate 12 and 14.

16. When scoring, each pair (2 arms, 2 legs, etc.) counts as one part.
17. Place one cube in cup and shake gently near child's ear, but out of sight. Repeat for other ear.
18. Point to picture and have child name it. (No credit is given for sounds only.)
    If less than 4 pictures are named correctly, have child point to picture as each is named by tester.

19. Using doll, tell child: Show me the nose, eyes, ears, mouth, hands, feet, tummy, hair. Pass 6 of 8.
20. Using pictures, ask child: Which one flies?... says meow?... talks?... barks?... gallops? Pass 2 of 5, 4 of 5.
21. Ask child: What do you do when you are cold?... tired?... hungry? Pass 2 of 3, 3 of 3.
22. Ask child: What do you do with a cup? What is a chair used for? What is a pencil used for?
    Action words must be included in answers.
23. Pass if child correctly places <u>and</u> says how many blocks are on paper. (1, 5)
24. Tell child: Put block **on** table; **under** table; **in front of** me, **behind** me. Pass 4 of 4.
    (Do not help child by pointing, moving head or eyes.)
25. Ask child: What is a ball?... lake?... desk?... house?... banana?... curtain?... fence?... ceiling? Pass if defined in terms of use, shape, what it is made of, or general category (such as banana is fruit, not just yellow). Pass 5 of 8, 7 of 8.
26. Ask child: If a horse is big, a mouse is __? If fire is hot, ice is __? If the sun shines during the day, the moon shines during the __? Pass 2 of 3.
27. Child may use wall or rail only, not person. May not crawl.
28. Child must throw ball overhand 3 feet to within arm's reach of tester.
29. Child must perform standing broad jump over width of test sheet (8½ inches).
30. Tell child to walk forward, ⬭⬯⬭⬯➤ heel within 1 inch of toe. Tester may demonstrate.
    Child must walk 4 consecutive steps.
31. In the second year, half of normal children are noncompliant.

B **OBSERVATIONS:**

Figure 37-3 *(continued)*

Figure 37-4 Provide VIS to caregiver before administering any vaccines.

Examples include the stepping reflex, the Moro (or startle) reflex, and the rooting reflex. The absence of infantile automatisms or continuation of these reflexes beyond infancy suggests central nervous system dysfunction and requires further testing. One of the most popular tools for evaluating specific gross and fine motor coordination is the Denver Developmental Screening Test (DDST) II (see Fig. 37-3). The DDST II evaluates children from the most basic reflexes to complex interpersonal reactions. If you perform the assessment, you should be trained in proper testing to evoke the most diagnostic response. The indicators are registered in a vertical line drawn at the child's age. Children should register within the normal range for their age. The DDST does not measure intelligence levels.

Role of the Parent

Parents are a source of support and comfort to a child. Their presence minimizes stress in unfamiliar surroundings. Encourage parents to remain with young children and to assist in care when appropriate. For instance, ask the parent to stand beside the child as you weigh him or her. Many children are more compliant if much of the

preliminary workup is performed while the parent **restrains**, or holds, the child (Fig. 37-6).

As a child develops and becomes more **autonomous**, or independent, a parent's immediate presence may be less meaningful as long as the child knows that the parent is close by. Many adolescent patients prefer to be alone with the physician to demonstrate their independence and to discuss matters that they may not be comfortable talking about with the parent present. Depending on the maturity of the adolescent, ask the patient, not the parent, if the parent should be present during the examination.

 CHECKPOINT QUESTION

3. What kinds of feelings might a pediatric patient experience during an office visit?

 LEGAL TIP

MAKE SURE YOUR INTERVIEW QUESTIONS ARE APPROPRIATE

Some states require obtaining parental permission before treating a minor patient. The exceptions to this rule may include:

- Pregnancy or prenatal care
- Sexually transmitted disease
- Rape
- Life-threatening injury

Emancipated minors (children under age 18 years who support themselves financially), minors enlisted in the armed services, and married minors may obtain treatment without parental consent. You are responsible for knowing your state's laws regarding the treatment of minors. Refer to Chapter 2 for more information related to legal and ethical implications.

TABLE **37-2**	**Common Childhood Illnesses**		
Illness	**Signs and Symptoms**	**Cause**	**Treatment**
Common cold	Congestion, cough, malaise, sore throat, fever	Virus	Increase PO fluids, rest, cold mist humidifier, medications if ordered by the MD
Gastroenteritis	Vomiting, diarrhea, fever	Virus OR bacteria	Increase PO fluids, medications if ordered by the MD
Otitis media	Earache (may accompany or follow a cold), reduced hearing, fever, tugging at the affected ear in infants	Virus OR bacteria	Increased PO fluids, medications if ordered by the MD

TABLE 37-3	Pediatric Growth and Developmental Stages			
Age	Growth	Stage	Development	Medical Assistant Considerations
Infancy (0–1 yr)	Triples birth weight; increases physical control of body; may walk by 1st birthday	Trust	Newborn can see, hear, smell, feel pain, and communicate. Protective mechanisms include blink reflex, pulling in for warmth, and pulling away from pain or restraint. Development cephalic to caudal: head control; then full-body control (e.g., rolling over, crawling, walking); then motor development (e.g., picking up small objects). Fastest period of growth and development, from total dependence to walking and talking.	Involve parent; keep parent in child's view; approach child slowly; use soft, soothing voice; speak reassuringly. Advise parents to call about fever over 100.5°F rectally, diarrhea, vomiting, failure to nurse or take a bottle. Encourage appropriate use of car seat as required by law in most states.
Toddler (1–3 yr)	Growth rate slows; body proportions change; language skills begin	Autonomy	Growth levels off but exploration and social development continue. Negativism precedes autonomy. The child will begin to seek relationships and is acutely aware of strangers.	Use all skills above; explain procedures so child can understand; expect resistance; use firm, direct approach; ignore negative behavior; restrain to maintain child's safety; allow child to hold security object. Warn parents of increased potential for accidents. Continue to encourage use of car seat and proper restraint in motor vehicle.
Preschool (3–6 yr)	Language and self-control develop; motor skills increase	Initiative	Socialization continues, with fairly clearly marked stages of social development in next 10 years. Many early-stage problems resolve. Except for usual communicable diseases, generally a time of good health. Diseases such as leukemia, Hodgkin's disease, and various sarcomata may present, but these years are usually spent establishing relationships with peers, exercising autonomy, and completing growth process.	Use all skills above. Encourage child to speak feelings; explain why procedure is being done; have child help as much as possible (e.g., hold equipment). Advise parents to be alert for risks of accidents and trauma with riding toys such as tricycles and bicycles. Encourage the use of helmet. *Children over 40 lb or 4 years can use booster seat until age 8 or 4 ft 9 in tall. Check your state laws.*

(continued)

				Medical Assistant
Age	**Growth**	**Stage**	**Development**	**Considerations**
School age (6–12 yr)	Social skills develop; peer group becomes important; self-concept develops	Industry		Involve child in decision making; involve child in care (e.g., collecting specimens, choosing which procedure is done first; encourage and support questions). Children may indicate what hurts and how they feel, so include child when asking questions. *Encourage use of booster seat to age 8 and seat belt thereafter according to state law.*
Adolescent (12–18 yr)	Emotional changes; identity, place in world being defined	Identity		Discuss procedures so adolescent can understand; adolescents may resist authority figures; be sure patient education includes smoking, alcohol, and perhaps birth control and STDs. At physician's discretion, this information may be discussed without parent. As children in this age group begin to drive, encourage use of seat belts for self and passengers.

TABLE 37-3   Pediatric Growth and Developmental Stages *(continued)*

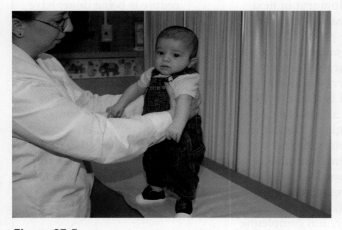

Figure 37-5   The presence or absence of reflexes is determined during the pediatric examination.

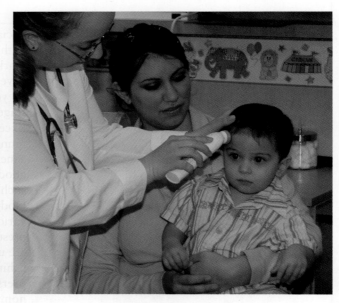

Figure 37-6   Much of the examination can be performed while the caregiver holds the baby.

The Pediatric Physical Examination

Typically, you prepare the pediatric patient for examination, and you may also assist with the examination by restraining the child. Often, you are responsible for documenting much of the history and the chief complaint and for collecting specimens for diagnostic testing. When approaching the patient, you should have a calm and cheerful manner and use a firm but gentle touch to increase the patient's feeling of security. Involve the parents as much as possible during the examination and keep them in the infant or child's view to reduce anxiety for both the patient and the parent.

During the examination, the physician will systematically review the body systems of the patient. The general appearance of the infant or child is assessed; the heart and lungs are auscultated; the eyes, ears, nose, and throat are inspected; and developmental issues appropriate for the age of the child are discussed with the parent or caregiver. The child who is preschool age or older will have vision and hearing tested. Your role includes obtaining relevant data from the parent, obtaining anthropometric measurements, and performing hearing and vision screening tests as appropriate. Of course, you will be responsible for recording this information in the patient's medical record.

The Pediatric History

A child's medical history differs greatly from an adult patient's history. During the early years, it is important to know the prenatal history, including details of the mother's pregnancy, labor, and delivery. The length of the pregnancy, any maternal illnesses or complications, neonatal complications, and risk factors must be recorded as predictors of the infant's health and development. Most newborn charts contain a copy of the delivery record or birth summary outlining the delivery with the Apgar score and progress notes from the newborn nursery (Box 37-1). As the child grows, the history expands to include childhood illnesses, developmental milestones, immunizations, and nutritional status.

Obtaining and Recording Measurements and Vital Signs

Before the physical examination is conducted, you should obtain some or all of the following measurements: height or length, head and chest circumference, weight, temperature, and the pulse and respiratory rate. The blood pressure may or may not be required, depending on the child's age and the preference of the examiner. The measurements and schedule for obtaining them should be detailed in the office policy and procedure manual.

BOX 37-1

THE APGAR SCORE

Named for pediatrician Virginia Apgar, the Apgar score is a method for describing the general health of newborns at 1 minute and 5 minutes after delivery. Signs assessed include:

- Heart rate
- Respiratory effort
- Muscle tone
- Response to a suction catheter in the nostril
- Color

A perfect score for each sign is 2; a total absence of any sign is 0. A perfect score of 10 indicates the following:

- Heart rate is greater than 100 beats per minute.
- Respirations are eupneic, or the baby is crying.
- Muscle tone is good, and the baby is active.
- Baby coughs or sneezes in response to suction catheter.
- Skin is completely pink, with no acrocyanosis.

Most babies have 1-minute scores of 7 to 9 because many have a bit of acrocyanosis until respiration is fully established. Babies with 1-minute scores below 4 usually require medical assistance, particularly respiratory intervention with oxygen.

The Apgar score is not considered an indicator of future intelligence or health problems. Rather, it is used by the obstetrician, pediatrician, and delivery room personnel to assess newborns who may require closer observation or intervention.

For a well-child visit, you typically measure the child's height or length, head and chest circumference, and weight. These measurements show the child's growth and development patterns and are good indicators of health status. Weight is the most frequently obtained measurement in pediatrics; it is often needed by the physician to assess nutritional status and determine medication dosages. Head and chest measurements may alert the physician to cardiac or intracranial abnormalities. Procedures 37-1 and 37-2 describe the steps for obtaining the weight, length, and head and chest circumference.

After obtaining these measurements, you may be required to graph the weight, height or length, and head circumference on a separate growth chart that is placed into the patient's medical record (Fig. 37-7). These charts are designed to show the child's growth patterns using data obtained at each well-child visit. Once the

Figure 37-7 Growth charts. (A) For girls, birth to 36 months for length, weight, and head circumference. (B) For boys, 2 to 20 years for height and weight.

2 to 20 years: Boys
Stature-for-age and Weight-for-age percentiles

NAME _____

RECORD # _____

Published May 30, 2000 (modified 11/21/00).
SOURCE: Developed by the National Center for Health Statistics in collaboration with
the National Center for Chronic Disease Prevention and Health Promotion (2000).
http://www.cdc.gov/growthcharts

CDC
SAFER • HEALTHIER • PEOPLE™

B

Figure 37-7   *(continued)*

measurements are plotted, the child's percentile can be determined. The percentile is used to compare the patient's growth with those of children of the same age. The head circumference is not included on growth charts for children older than 36 months, and chest circumference is usually not graphed.

 CHECKPOINT QUESTION

4. Why is it important to track a child's anthropometric measurements?

Pediatric Vital Signs

Temperature

A child's temperature may be measured by the axillary, oral, rectal, tympanic, or temporal artery method. If the child is compliant, the axillary route is satisfactory, but the tympanic and temporal artery methods have gained popularity because they are rapid, reliable, and most readily accepted at all ages (see Fig. 37-6). Oral measurement may be used with an older child but should not be used if the child is congested, coughing, vomiting, or uncooperative. The rectal route should not be used for newborns and small infants or if the child has diarrhea.

Pulse and Respirations

The pulse rate reflects the heart rate and usually is easily measured. Pulse rate can be affected by activity, body temperature, emotion, and illness. The pulse of children under 2 years of age should be assessed apically. To do this, place the stethoscope on the chest between the sternum and left nipple. Count the rate for 1 full minute. For children older than 2 years, take the radial pulse. Expect the child's heart rate to be considerably higher than an adult's rate. A newborn may have a pulse rate of 100 to 180 beats per minute, and with fever, a rate of 200 beats per minute or more is not unusual. As the child matures, the rate will slow. By age 2, a child's rate may range from 70 to 100 beats per minute. By puberty, the rate is comparable to that of an adult. Table 37-4 details normal pulse rates for children.

Measure respiratory rate by observing the rise and fall of the child's chest. It is not necessary to disguise the

TABLE 37-5	Normal Respiratory Rates for Children
Age	**Rate/Minute**
Newborn	30–35
1–2 yr	25–30
4–6 yr	23–25
8 yr and older	16–20

fact that you are counting respirations as with adults. Because infants breathe using the abdominal muscles more than the chest, observe abdominal movements and count for 1 full minute. For children over age 2 years, use the same method as adults: count the respiratory rate for 30 seconds and multiply by two. Expect a newborn's respiratory rate to be as high as 35 per minute (Table 37-5). Like the pulse rate, the respiratory rate will slow as the child matures. At age 2 years, it will be about 25, and by puberty, it will be comparable to an adult's rate.

Blood Pressure

Blood pressure measurements are not required for most pediatric patients but may be appropriate at times. Blood pressure is the most difficult measurement to obtain in an infant or child because it is so difficult to prevent movement. Infants and children have smaller extremities than adults and require a smaller cuff. Because of their soft, nonresistant vessels and smaller bodies, children have lower blood pressure than adults. You may have problems determining the diastolic pressure in some children using a standard sphygmomanometer. In children less than 1 year of age, expect a blood pressure of about 90/50. The blood pressure will gradually rise as the child matures. By age 10, a child's blood pressure will be in the low normal range of 110/60 (Table 37-6). Blood pressure checks become routine when children are about school age.

 CHECKPOINT QUESTION

5. How does a child's pulse and respiratory rate differ from an adult's?

TABLE 37-4	Normal Pulse Rates for Children	
Age		**Rate/Minute**
Newborn		100–180
3 mo–2 yr		80–150
2–10 yr		65–130
10 yr and older		60–100

TABLE 37-6	Normal Blood Pressure for Children	
Age	**Systolic**	**Diastolic**
Newborn	<90	<70
1–5 yr	<110	<70
10 yr and older	<120	<84

Blood pressure measured in millimeters of mercury.

WHAT IF?

What if you have an uncooperative infant or child?

During the examination and certain procedures, you may need to help restrain the child. Restraining is sometimes necessary to protect the child from injury and to help the physician complete the examination in a timely manner. Many children understandably resist the examination or procedure because they are frightened and do not want to be touched. Calm and gentle restraint is in the best interest of everyone involved.

Mummy restraint. Place the child diagonally on a small receiving blanket. **(A)** Wrap the right corner across the torso, covering the right arm and shoulder. Pull it snugly under the child's left arm and tuck it under the child's body. **(B)** Pull the left corner across the child's left arm and shoulder and tuck it snugly under the torso at the back so that the child's weight secures the end. **(C)** Wrap the end of the blanket up around the child.

Administering Medications

Administering medications to children challenges you and the parents who are responsible for home administration. Medication dosages for children are calculated by weight or by body surface area. However, because children vary in weight, age, and fat-to-muscle ratio, they metabolize and absorb medication at varying rates. As a result, the physician prescribes medication according to how much the child weighs, and you must give only the amount prescribed. To prevent errors, always check drug dosage calculations for an infant or child with another staff member. The formulas for calculating pediatric dosages are described in Chapter 24. Before administering any medication, you should know the safe

amount, correct administration procedure, intended actions, and side effects. In most pediatric practices, the physician uses only 50 or so medications that are suitable for children, making it relatively easy for you to learn all that is necessary about each medication. As for any medication, the seven "rights" of drug administration remain the same: the *right patient, right drug, right dose, right route, right time, right method,* and *right documentation.*

Oral Medications

Use caution when administering oral medications to a child to prevent **aspiration.** Hold infants in a semi-reclining position, not lying down. Place the medication in the mouth beside the tongue. Depending on the child's age, use a medication spoon, syringe, dropper, or medicine cup. Many children will suck medication from a syringe easily and safely. Administer small amounts of medication, allowing the child time to swallow. Always explain to children who are old enough to understand why medications are important, and then proceed in a swift and safe manner to give the medication.

Injections

Medications are given to infants and children by injection when there is no choice. Children commonly fear injections more than any other medical procedure. You should approach the child in a calm and firm manner, but never lie to the child or say that the injection will not hurt. Although it is important for the child to know that an injection is about to be given, you can prevent some anxiety by not letting the child see the syringe. Offer the child an age-appropriate explanation, and then quickly give the medication. After administering any medication, praise and comfort the child.

Most children's injections are given in the vastus lateralis, at least until age 2 years (Fig. 37-8). The dorsogluteal site is not used for children under age 2 years because the muscles have not developed well. Chapter 24 lists the steps in administering an intramuscular injection.

 CHECKPOINT QUESTION

6. How is medication dosage calculated for children?

Collecting a Urine Specimen

Because infants and small children cannot void into a specimen container on command, if a urine specimen is needed, you must use a collection device. Procedure 37-3 describes the procedure for applying a urinary collection device. Once applied, the device should be left in place

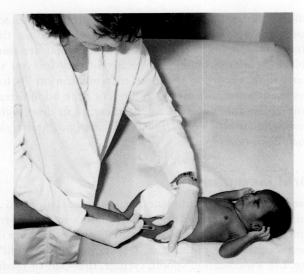

Figure 37-8 The vastus lateralis is the site of choice for infant injections.

until the infant urinates. The infant may wear a diaper over the collection device until the specimen is obtained.

Understanding Child Abuse

A child's social and physical well-being may be compromised by physical or emotional abuse or neglect or by sexual abuse. Abuse is thought to be the second most common cause of death in children under age 5 years. Although many children are permanently disabled or seriously injured as a result of physical abuse, many more carry emotional scars that will never heal. Medical assistants should be aware of the signs of abuse—either obvious indications or subtle warnings—that must be pursued for the child's safety.

These are the obvious indications of child abuse:

- Reports of physical or sexual abuse by the child
- Previous reports of abuse in the family with current indicators
- Conflicting stories about the "accident" or injury from the parents and the child
- Injuries inconsistent with the history
- Injuries blamed on siblings or someone other than the parent
- Repeated emergency room visits for injuries
- Fractures, burns, or skeletal injuries of a suspicious nature

These indications of child abuse are hidden or not apparent:

- Dislocations
- Nervous system trauma, particularly shaken baby syndrome
- Internal injuries, particularly to the abdominal area

These are behavioral indications of child abuse:

- Too-willing compliance, overeagerness to please
- Passive avoidance, such as refusing to make eye contact, shrinking from contact
- Extremely aggressive, demanding, rage-filled behavior
- Role reversal, parenting the parent
- Developmental delay (the child may be using energy needed for maturation to defend against abuse)

These are the warning signs of child abuse:

- Malnutrition
- Poor growth pattern
- Poor hygiene
- Gross dental disorders
- Unattended medical needs

If you suspect a child is being abused, approach the child and the parent in a calm and supportive manner. Discuss any suspicions about the cause of a child's injuries privately with the physician right away. State laws vary regarding the procedure for reporting abuse; local regulations should be outlined in the policies and procedures manual. As a medical assistant, you have an ethical and moral responsibility to report suspected cases of abuse or neglect.

LEGAL TIP

REPORTING SUSPECTED CHILD ABUSE

The Federal Child Abuse Prevention and Treatment Act mandates that threats to a child's physical and mental welfare be reported by anyone having contact with children in a professional or employment setting (e.g., teachers, physicians, nurses, medical assistants, day care workers). Health care workers, teachers, social workers, and others who work with children are protected against liability if they report their suspicions in good faith.

Pediatric Illnesses and Disorders

Because children do not have a well-developed immune system, they are particularly susceptible to viruses and bacterial infections. As a result, sick-child visits occur frequently during early childhood. Some infants and small children have febrile seizures during illness because of the child's immature nervous system. This does not mean that the child will be prone to seizures as he or she matures. Parents should be instructed how to obtain a child's temperature and be encouraged to call the office for any evidence of a fever. All parents should be advised never to give aspirin to young children with viral fever, since aspirin has been associated with Reye's syndrome. This syndrome causes encephalopathy and fatty infiltration of the internal organs and may cause either mental retardation or death. Check with the physician about the type of medication to use before suggesting any antipyretic, including over-the-counter medications.

WHAT IF?

What if a child's mother complains that her baby vomits everything he eats?

If the vomiting is projectile, the child may have pyloric stenosis, a disorder usually seen in infants several days to several months old. Diagnosis is usually made by parental history, physical examination, and radiography. The physician often can palpate an olive-shaped lump in the right upper quadrant of the abdomen while the child is supine. Surgery (pyloroplasty) is the treatment. Although pyloric stenosis is not an emergency, surgery is usually scheduled promptly to prevent dehydration. Inform the parents about the disorder and reassure them as needed.

Vomiting may also be caused by gastroenteritis, or an infection of the stomach and intestines caused by a bacterium or virus. These infants may also have diarrhea. Regardless of the cause, infants may dehydrate very quickly and should be seen by the physician without delay.

Impetigo

A common skin disorder in children is impetigo, a contagious bacterial infection that may be caused by either the *Staphylococcus* or *Streptococcus* bacteria. The lesions commonly occur on the face, neck, and other exposed areas of the body (Fig. 37-9). Patches of exudative vesicles produce honey-colored crusts. These vesicles leave red areas when the crusts are removed.

The treatment for impetigo is washing the area two to three times a day and applying a topical antibiotic. An oral antibiotic may be prescribed for severe cases. Discourage scratching and advise parents to keep separate and wash frequently any towels, washcloths, and bed linens to prevent the spread of the disease.

Meningitis

Inflammation of the meninges covering the spinal cord and the brain, termed meningitis, can result from either a bacterial or a viral infection. Viral meningitis is usually not life threatening and is short lived, but bacterial meningitis is often severe and may be fatal. The infectious process is usually precipitated by an upper respiratory, sinus, or ear infection, and since these infections commonly occur in children under age 5 years, they are the most likely age group to develop this disease. Meningitis can also result from head trauma in which an open area allows the microorganisms to enter the nervous system. Older adolescents living in college dormitories or residence halls are also at high risk for meningitis and should be immunized before leaving for college.

The signs and symptoms of meningitis include nausea, vomiting, fever, headaches, and a stiff neck. A rash with small, reddish-purple dots may appear on the body. As the patient becomes sicker, he or she may become comatose and develop seizures. To diagnose meningitis, the physician usually orders a complete blood count, and if the white blood cell count is elevated, a lumbar puncture is performed to withdraw cerebrospinal fluid for analysis. The treatment of meningitis is based on the microorganism. Viral meningitis is treated with oral fluids and bed rest, and bacterial meningitis is treated with an antibiotic and generally hospitalization.

CHECKPOINT QUESTION

7. How does treatment of viral meningitis differ from that of bacterial meningitis?

Encephalitis

Encephalitis is inflammation of the brain that frequently results from a viral infection following chickenpox, measles, or mumps. A strain of the virus is transmitted by mosquitoes. This type is primarily seen on the East and Gulf coasts. Symptoms of all forms include drowsiness, headache, and fever in the early stages; however, seizures and coma may occur in the later stages. Diagnosis is by a lumbar puncture and analysis of the cerebrospinal fluid. Treatment requires hospitalization for intravenous therapy and supportive care, but the

Figure 37-9 Impetigo lesions are commonly found on the face and neck.

prognosis is usually good if the diagnosis is made early and treatment begins quickly.

Tetanus

Tetanus, commonly called lockjaw, is an infection of nervous tissue caused by the tetanus bacillus, *Clostridium tetani*, which lives in the intestinal tract of animals and is excreted in their feces. The organisms are found in almost all soil. The bacilli enter the body through a puncture wound or open area in the skin. Wounds caused by farm equipment in which manure is present are especially susceptible to tetanus. All deep, dirty wounds should be treated as high risk for tetanus. You should always ask about previous tetanus immunization in patients with accidental laceration or puncture wounds.

 CHECKPOINT QUESTION

8. What is the best way to prevent tetanus?

Cerebral Palsy

Cerebral palsy is a term for a group of neuromuscular disorders that result from central nervous system damage sustained during the prenatal, neonatal, or postnatal period of development. Although cerebral palsy is not progressive, the damage may become more obvious as developmental delays are discovered. Impairment may range from slight motor dysfunction to catastrophic physical and mental disabilities. Prognosis varies with the site of the damage and its severity. Treatment is supportive and rehabilitative. There is no cure.

Croup

Laryngotracheobronchitis, also known as croup, is a disease primarily seen in children 3 months to 3 years of age. This disease is caused by a viral infection of the larynx resulting in swelling and narrowing of the airway. This results in dyspnea (difficulty breathing) characterized by stridor (high-pitched crowing wheeze) on inspiration and a sharp barking cough. Treatment may include hospitalization, cool mist vaporizer, and medication to decrease the swelling.

Epiglottitis

Swelling of the epiglottis may resemble croup, but it is usually more serious and may be life threatening if it progresses to complete obstruction of the airway. It occurs most frequently in children aged 2 to 6 years, although it can be seen in all age groups. It is caused by a bacterial infection, usually *Haemophilus influenzae*. A child diagnosed with epiglottitis in the medical office must be transported immediately to the hospital, since the first priority is maintaining and possibly establishing an airway. As with any medical emergency in the office, you must be prepared to assist the physician as needed while contacting the emergency medical services for transport. In addition, the parents of the sick child will need support and guidance during this emotional time.

Cystic Fibrosis

Cystic fibrosis is an inherited disease that affects the exocrine glands of the body, changing their secretions and making the mucus extremely thick and sticky. Although it affects several areas of the body, the most serious complications of cystic fibrosis are usually respiratory. Children with this disease are prone to repeated respiratory infections because of the difficulty in clearing the mucus from their airways. Treatment of cystic fibrosis includes medication to reduce the thickness of secretions and frequent breathing treatments to maintain open airways. Many new treatments are being developed, and much exciting research into prevention and cure is under way.

 CHECKPOINT QUESTION

9. Why is epiglottitis considered a medical emergency?

Asthma

As discussed in Chapter 30, asthma is a reversible inflammatory process of the bronchi and bronchioles. When a patient with asthma has dyspnea, it is due to bronchospasm and constriction of the smooth muscle lining the airways. Patients have an increase in mucus production with a productive cough. It becomes difficult for the patient to move air into and out of the lungs. In children, asthma attacks may be triggered by exposure to an allergen in the environment such as mold or dust, an inhaled irritant such as cigarette smoke, or upper respiratory infection. Many children who develop asthma outgrow it by adulthood.

The treatment for asthma includes the administration of bronchodilators through an inhaler, which may not be appropriate for a small child or infant, or through a nebulizer machine (see Chapter 30 for more information about nebulized breathing treatments). An infant or small child will not be able to hold the mouthpiece tightly between the lips during the treatment; however, masks are available (Fig. 37-10). As with adult patients taking bronchodilators, the pulse rate should be monitored before, during, and after the treatment.

Otitis Media

Otitis media, an inflammation or infection of the middle ear, is frequently caused by an upper respiratory infection (URI) in infants and children. This disorder is par-

Figure 37-10 Breathing treatments may be administered through a mask.

ticularly common in infants and children because of the relatively horizontal position of the eustachian tube between the nasopharynx and middle ear (see Chapter 29). Symptoms include severe pain, fever of varying degrees, and mild to moderate hearing loss. Infants may be fussy and tug at their ears. Any elevation in a child's temperature should be a warning to check for otitis media.

Diagnosis is usually made by inspecting the tympanic membrane with an otoscope, which reveals a reddened, bulging tympanic membrane. If the suspected pathogen is bacterial, an antibiotic may be prescribed. With the exception of aspirin, analgesics are often recommended for the relief of the pain. If nasal congestion is present, a decongestant may reduce some of the swelling. In severe chronic cases, surgery may be performed to relieve pressure, and tubes may be inserted through the tympanic membrane to equalize the pressure.

PATIENT EDUCATION
MIDDLE EAR INFECTIONS

Explain to the child's parents that children have short, straight eustachian tubes. Upper respiratory infections, particularly with coughing, may force microorganisms into the middle ear spaces. As the infection grows, the eustachian tubes swell and eventually close. Exudate from the mucous membrane continues to be produced, causing fluid to build with resulting pressure and pain.

While the infecting microorganism can be bacterial or viral, bacterial otitis media may be caused by putting the child to bed with a bottle of milk, juice, or formula. The drink and bacteria from the mouth set up a medium for growth within the eustachian tube. Provide patient education to caregivers whenever possible.

TRIAGE

While working in a family practice office, you have to complete the following three tasks:

A. Patient A is a 2-month-old child who has just been placed in examination room 1. You are to take the vital signs and measurements, including length, weight, and head circumference.
B. Patient B is a 14-month-old child who was seen today and diagnosed with otitis media. The physician has asked you to give the parent a prescription for an antibiotic and schedule a referral with an ear, nose, and throat physician for possible myringectomy and tubes.
C. A mother is on the phone and is concerned because patient C, her newborn, is vomiting.

How do you sort these tasks? What do you do first? Second? Third?

First, speak to the mother of patient C. This infant will dehydrate very quickly, and the situation must be assessed promptly and efficiently. Give advice about increasing fluids or giving pediatric electrolyte solutions *only* after assessing the situation, consulting with the physician, and receiving instructions from the physician to pass along to the mother. Next, deal with patient B by giving the parent the prescription and clarifying any other orders from the physician. The information regarding the referral can be given to the parent to make the arrangements, or you may make the appointment later in the day, when time permits. Of course, the required paperwork for the referral must be faxed to the referral physician, and this may be delegated to an administrative assistant according to the office policy and procedure manual.

See patient A after patient B is discharged. When obtaining a history for a well-child checkup, you want to give the parent your undivided attention and take extra time to establish rapport with the parent and the infant.

Tonsillitis

Pharyngitis, or a sore throat, may be caused by inflammation of the tissues of the throat and/or the tonsils (see Chapter 29). Inspection of the throat may reveal the tissue to be red and swollen, possibly with pustules on the tonsils or in the throat. When a diagnosis of tonsillitis is made, you may be asked to take a sample for a throat culture to rule out *Streptococcus* bacteria as the causative pathogen. (Chapter 44 describes the steps for obtaining a throat culture.) If the throat culture is positive for *Streptococcus*, an antibiotic will be ordered. If the throat culture is negative but the infection appears bacterial, an antibiotic may still be prescribed. Chronic tonsillitis may be treated by surgical removal of the tonsils—a tonsillectomy—by a surgeon who specializes in disorders of the ears, nose, and throat.

 CHECKPOINT QUESTION

10. Why is otitis media more common in children than adults?

Obesity

According to the American Academy of Pediatrics (AAP), obesity in children has become an epidemic. The importance of assessing the weight and length of infants and children and plotting this information on the appropriate growth chart is essential in assisting the physician in early recognition; however, prevention of obesity is even more important in preventing long-term complications, such as heart disease and diabetes. You must ask parents or caregivers during each visit to the office about the eating patterns, nutrition status, and activity levels of the child and offer education and support when necessary or as indicated by the physician. Since children develop eating habits early in life and take these habits into adulthood, you should teach parents about eating in moderation and increasing physical activity as a means to reduce the weight of an overweight child or prevent abnormal gains in weight. If the physician prescribes a specific diet or reduces caloric intake, you should offer support and guidance to the caregiver as needed.

Attention Deficit Hyperactivity Disorder

Attention deficit hyperactivity disorder (ADHD) is a condition of the brain affecting boys more frequently than girls and causing difficulty in controlling behavior. The problematic behavior in children with ADHD includes the following signs of inattention in the school-age child:

- Daydreaming or difficulty paying attention
- Easy distraction
- Inability to complete tasks
- Forgetfulness
- Reluctance to perform tasks that require mental effort
- Low grades in school

The hyperactivity is often seen thus:

- Excessive talking
- Inability to sit quietly for any length of time
- Breaking rules regarding running or jumping

In addition to inattention and hyperactivity, children with ADHD are often impulsive and behave irrationally to others, even after being repeatedly warned about a specific behavior, dangerous or not. These children have difficulty taking turns and may be disruptive, shouting out answers before being called on in the classroom.

The diagnosis for a child with ADHD is often based on a thorough history of the child's behaviors, including reports from teachers or other professionals who work with the child. The AAP publishes guidelines for diagnosing ADHD in children aged 6 to 12 years. There is no one test for diagnosing this disorder; instead, the diagnosis is based on certain behaviors in several settings (i.e., school and home). Once the physician has made the diagnosis, an individual treatment plan is devised; it may include behavior therapy, psychological counseling for the child and the family, education about ADHD, coordination of the treatment plan with the family and involved teachers, and stimulant medications.

 MEDIA MENU

- **Student CD**
  - **CMA/RMA Certification Exam Review**
- **LWW's Medical Assisting Skills DVD**
  - **Procedure 37-1**
- **Premium Online Course**
  http://thePoint.lww.com/Kronenberger3e
- **Internet Resources**
  LiveAdvise Online Tutoring & Competency Training
  http://thePoint.lww.com/LiveAdvise

español
SPANISH TERMINOLOGY

Ha tenido la criatura alguna enfermedad o lesiónes?
  Has the child had any illnesses or injuries?
Necesitamos una muestra de su orina.
  We need a urine specimen.
Que vacunas se han dado a la criatura?
  Which immunizations has the child received?
Tose el niño por la noche?
  Does the child cough at night?
Con que frecuencia evacua la criatura?
  How often does the child have a bowel movement?

PROCEDURE 37-1:   Obtaining an Infant's Length and Weight

Purpose: Accurately determine the length and weight of an infant
Equipment: Examination table with clean paper, tape measure, infant scale, protective paper for the scale, appropriate growth chart

Steps	Reasons
1. Wash your hands.	Handwashing aids infection control.
2. Explain the procedure to the parent and ask him or her to remove the infant's clothing except for the diaper.	
3. Place the child on a firm examination table covered with clean table paper. If using a measuring board, cover the board with clean paper.	Measurements may not be correct if the surface is not firm. Clean paper prevents cross-infection.
4. Fully extend the child's body by holding the head in the midline. Grasp the knees and press flat onto the table gently but firmly. Make a mark on the table paper with your pen at the top of the head and at the heel of the feet.	Most infants assume a flexed position, requiring you to extend the legs for accurate measurement. If you need assistance, ask the parent or a co-worker to hold the child in position. A foot board against the soles will give the most accurate measurement. **Step 4.** Straighten the leg of the infant.
5. Measure between the marks in either inches or centimeters, according to the preference of the physician.	
6. Record the child's length on the growth chart and in the patient's chart.	Procedures are considered not to have been done if they are not recorded. To plot the measurement on the growth chart, find the child's measurement in inches or centimeters and move in that line across to the age column. Make a mark where the two values intersect. **Step 6.** Make a mark where the child's length and age intersect.

PROCEDURE 37-1: Obtaining an Infant's Length and Weight (continued)

Steps	Reasons
7. Either carry the infant or have the parent carry the infant to the scales.	
8. Place protective paper on the scale and balance the scale.	Protective paper prevents transmission of microorganisms. The balance beam must be centered before each use.
9. Remove the diaper just before laying the infant on the scale.	For the most accurate weight, infants should be weighed without any clothing. However, cool air against the infant's skin may cause voiding. Some offices permit the infant to be weighed in the diaper as long as it is dry and clean.
10. Place the child gently on the scale. Keep one of your hands over or near the child on the scale at all times.	

A

B

Step 10. (A) Infants are weighed lying down.
(B) Infants who can sit may be weighed while sitting if this is less frightening for them.

Steps	Reasons
11. Quickly but carefully move the counterweights to balance the apparatus exactly.	This will ensure accurate measurement.
12. Pick up the infant and instruct the parent to replace diaper if removed for the weight.	
13. Record the weight on the growth chart and in the patient's chart.	Procedures are considered not to have been done if they are not recorded. To plot the measurement on the growth chart, find the child's measurement in pounds or kilograms, and then move in that line across to the age column. Make a mark where the two values intersect.

Charting Example

02/08/2008 10:00 AM 12-month-old, length 30 inches, wt. 22 lb. 6 oz.

—J. DeBard, CMA

PROCEDURE 37-2: Obtaining the Head and Chest Circumference

Purpose: Accurately determine the head and chest circumference of an infant
Equipment: Paper or cloth measuring tape, growth chart

Steps	Reasons
1. Wash your hands.	Handwashing aids infection control.
2. Place the infant supine on the examination table or ask the parent to hold the child.	
3. Measure around the head above the eyebrow and posteriorly at the largest part of the occiput. For an accurate reading, measure the largest circumference.	 **Step 3.** Measure around the head above the eye brow and posteriorly at the largest part of the occiput.
4. Record the child's head circumference on the growth chart and in the patient's chart.	Procedures are considered not to have been done if they are not recorded. To plot the measurement on the growth chart, find the child's measurement in inches or centimeters, and then move in that line across to the age column. Make a mark where the two values intersect. **Step 4.** Make a mark where the child's head circumference in inches or centimeters and age intersect.
5. With the clothing removed from the chest, measure around the chest at the nipple line, keeping the measuring tape at the same level anterior and posterior.	The tape should be at the same level to ensure the most accurate reading.

(continued)

PROCEDURE 37-2: Obtaining the Head and Chest Circumference *(continued)*

Steps	Reasons
	Step 5. Measure around the chest at the nipple line, keeping the measuring tape at the same level anteriorly and posteriorly.
6. Record the child's chest circumference on the growth chart and in the patient chart.	Procedures are considered not to have been done if they are not recorded. To plot the measurement on the growth chart, find the child's measurement in inches or centimeters, and then move in that line across to the age column. Make a mark where the two values intersect.

Note: If the head and chest growth are within normal limits, this measurement is not usually required after 12 months.

Charting Example

10/15/2008 9:45 AM Wt. 14 lb. Length 24 in., Head 15 in., Chest 17 in.

—B. Brady, CMA

PROCEDURE 37-3: Applying a Urinary Collection Device

Purpose: Correctly apply a urinary collection device to a child
Equipment: Gloves, personal antiseptic wipes, pediatric urine collection bag, completed laboratory request slip, biohazard transport container

Steps	Reasons
1. Wash your hands.	Handwashing aids infection control.
2. Explain the procedure to the caregivers.	
3. Place the child supine. Ask for help from the parents as needed.	The child may be more cooperative if a parent helps.
4. After putting on gloves, clean the genitalia with the antiseptic wipes: A. For girls: Cleanse front to back with separate wipes for each downward stroke on the outer labia. The last clean wipe should be used between the inner labia. B. For boys: Retract the foreskin if the baby has not been circumcised. Cleanse the meatus in an ever-widening circle. Discard the wipe and repeat the procedure. Return the foreskin to its proper position.	For girls, cleansing front to back will remove debris from the area and avoid introducing bacteria into the urethra. For boys, cleansing outward will avoid introducing bacteria into the urethra. Returning the foreskin to the correct position will prevent constriction of the penis.

(continued)

PROCEDURE 37-3: Applying a Urinary Collection Device (continued)

Steps	Reasons
5. Holding the collection device, remove the upper portion of the paper backing and press it around the mons pubis. Remove the second section and press it against the perineum. Loosely attach the diaper.	The collection device must be securely attached to ensure collection of the next voiding. Reattaching the diaper will avoid soiling if the child has a stool.

Step 5. The collection device fits over the genitalia.

6. Give the baby fluids unless contraindicated, and check the diaper frequently.	
7. When the child has voided, remove the device, clean the skin of residual adhesive, and diaper.	Adhesive left on the skin may be irritating.
8. Prepare the specimen for transport to the laboratory or process it according to the office policy and procedure manual.	
9. Remove your gloves and wash your hands.	Standard precautions must be followed when handling body fluids.
10. Record the procedure.	Procedures are considered not to have been done if they are not recorded.

Charting Example

> 08/16/2008 11:45 AM Urine collection device applied; approximately 50 mL clear amber urine obtained after 20 minutes. Specimen sent to Acme Laboratory for urinalysis
>
> —S. Schein, CMA

Working with children offers many rewards; however, the special developmental needs and unique physiology of children make these patients challenging and must always be taken into consideration. This chapter focuses on:

- The skills necessary to assist with a well-child visit including obtaining and recording normal growth information. It is important to record this information carefully to assist the physician in detecting problems as early as possible.
- Caring for the child who comes to the office for a sick-child visit. This includes maintaining the reception area by separating sick and well children if possible and disinfecting any toys to avoid cross-contamination in other children.
- Common diseases that may be seen in childhood including ear infections, upper respiratory infections, and gastrointestinal problems. Although these diseases are common, they are not pleasant for the child or the caregiver. You will have a role in reassuring

anxious parents while caring for their sick children competently and professionally.

- Education of the pediatric patient caregiver including vaccine information. Parents should always be encouraged to ask questions and should expect to get honest and clear answers.
- Legal and ethical issues related to immunizations, child abuse, and neglect. You must always be alert for signs of neglect and/or abuse and be ready to report your suspicions to the physician.
- Your role in preventing disease in the pediatric patient and assisting with pediatric procedures. In addition to caring for children, you must also provide patient education to caregivers and older children to prevent the spread of disease. Also, your expertise in working with pediatric patients will be appreciated by the physician and the other staff who may find it necessary to have you assist with a variety of pediatric procedures.

Warm Ups   for Critical Thinking

1. During years of practice, Dr. Hernandez has found that many new parents are unfamiliar with basic child care needs. He decides to publish a short booklet for his new parents describing various aspects of child care. The booklet should be informative and professional and show genuine concern for children. Using your creativity and your knowledge of child care, develop a sample booklet for Dr. Hernandez's patients after choosing two of the following topics:
   - General safety tips
   - Types of office visits
   - Immunizations (what they are, why they are important, at what ages they are given, side effects and adverse effects)
   - What a parent can expect during an office visit
   - Brief explanation of child development
   - Tips for administering oral medications to children

2. You obtained the weight on Lillian Parks, a 7-month-old girl. She weighs 16½ pounds according to your balanced pediatric scales. What percentile is this patient according to the growth chart? How would you explain a percentile to the mother of the infant?

3. The father of a toddler is insistent that you give the child an immunization in the arm rather than the thigh. How would you handle this situation?

4. Research one of the following conditions that may be found in pediatric patients and prepare a poster detailing the causes, signs and symptoms, and treatment. Include information for the caregivers or school personnel who may have questions about these conditions:
   - Strep throat
   - Pediculosis
   - Conjunctivitis

5. Compare the developmental skills of a 3-year-old and 5-year-old child. What are the similarities? What are the differences?

1. The following are safety precautions to consider for a pediatric practice:
   - Keep all medical equipment out of a child's reach.
   - Never leave a child alone in the examining room.
   - Place infant scales on a sturdy table and never leave a child alone on a scale.
   - Store disinfectants away from patient care areas.
   - Dispose of all sharps in proper containers.
   - Practice stringent handwashing and standard precautions with every patient.

2. Well-child visits are scheduled at regular intervals and are designed to maintain the child's optimum health. Sick-child visits are scheduled as needed with the goal of diagnosing and treating a child's immediate illness or injury.

3. A child may feel fear, anxiety, guilt, powerlessness, or curiosity during an office visit.

4. A child's anthropometric measurements show the growth and are good indicators of the health status.

5. A child's pulse and respiratory rates are higher than an adult's.

6. Medication dosage in children is calculated by weight or by body surface area.

7. For viral meningitis, fluids and bed rest are encouraged. For bacterial meningitis, an antibiotic is prescribed, and hospitalization may be required.

8. The best way to prevent tetanus is through immunization.

9. Epiglottitis is a medical emergency because the small airways of the infant or child can become occluded or blocked as the epiglottis swells, causing respiratory arrest.

10. Otitis media is common in infants and children because of the horizontal position of the eustachian tube. Microorganisms travel easily from the mouth, throat, and nasal passages to the middle ear.

Outline

Concepts of Aging
Reinforcing Medical
Compliance in the Elderly
Reinforcing Mental Health in
the Elderly
Coping With Aging
  Alcoholism
  Suicide

Long-Term Care
Elder Abuse
Medications and the Elderly
Systemic Changes in the
Elderly
Diseases of the Elderly
  Parkinson's Disease
  Alzheimer's Disease

Maintaining Optimum Health
Exercise
Diet
Safety

Learning
Objectives

Upon successfully completing this chapter, you will be able to:

1. Spell and define key terms

2. Explain how aging affects thought processes

3. Describe methods to increase compliance with health maintenance programs among the elderly

4. Discuss communication problems that may occur with the elderly and list steps to maintain open communication

5. Recognize and describe the coping mechanisms used by the elderly to deal with multiple losses

6. Name the risk factors and signs of elder abuse

7. Explain the types of long-term care facilities available

8. Describe the effects of aging on the way the body processes medication

9. Discuss the responsibility of medical assistants with regard to teaching elderly patients

10. List and describe physical changes and diseases common to the aging process

Key Terms

activities of daily living (ADL)
biotransform
bradykinesia
cataracts
cerebrovascular accident (CVA)

compliance
degenerative joint disease (DJD)
dementia
dysphagia
gerontologist
glaucoma

Kegel exercises
keratosis (senile)
kyphosis (dowager's hump)
lentigines
osteoporosis
potentiation

presbycusis
presbyopia
senility
syncope
transient ischemic attack (TIA)
vertigo

Concepts of Aging

As the elderly population has increased, established concepts about aging have also changed. The greeting card image of a cozy, gray-haired grandmother in her rocking chair is being replaced by a trim, active woman rushing out the door with a briefcase or tennis racket under her arm. **Gerontologists**, specialists in aging, describe many of the elderly today as healthy enough to maintain homes well into their 80s and 90s. The branch of medicine that deals with the elderly population is geriatrics, and while some physicians today are treating only geriatric patients, any physician in family practice or internal medicine will take care of the elderly. Other specialties, such as ophthalmology, also treat many geriatric patients daily. Box 38-1 outlines some myths and stereotypes about the elderly. How many are far from typical of this age group today?

Stereotyping the elderly is a subtle and usually unconscious way to disassociate ourselves from the prospect of growing old. Although other cultures respect their elderly for their wealth of wisdom and experience, the American media perpetuate myths and stereotypical reactions by implying that graying hair and wrinkles in the skin are repulsive and should be avoided at all costs.

Those costs include billions of dollars spent on delaying the physical signs of aging. Consider how the following situations take on new meaning when applied to different age groups.

- You are running late again. Dashing out of the door, you remember that you left the keys to the car on the kitchen table—again.
- You stride purposefully from the bedroom into the kitchen with a specific goal in mind, only to reach the kitchen without any idea why you were in such a hurry to get there.

We have all done these things and will no doubt do them again. However, if these things are done by an elderly person, they are considered to be a sign of approaching **senility** or **dementia**. While some memory loss and difficulty with thought processes are inevitable as a result of aging, memory loss in the elderly is often the result of various disease processes and medications. The next section describes some techniques that you can use to enhance **compliance** with patients who have difficulty with thought processes, whether the cause is natural aging or a specific disease or medication regimen.

BOX 38-1

MYTHS AND STEREOTYPES ABOUT THE ELDERLY

Myths

- Old people are weak and sick.
- Old people can no longer learn.
- Old people have no more contributions to make.
- Old people are boring.
- Old people are a drag on the economy.
- Old people are always lonely.
- Old people cannot live alone.
- Old people cannot be trusted to make rational decisions.
- Old people have lost all interest in life.

Stereotypes

- Old people have sensory losses.
- Old people have erratic sleep patterns and nap a lot.
- Old people do everything slower.
- Old people have lost stature and slump a lot.
- Old people cannot remember what happened this morning but can recall everything that happened 40 years ago.

Reinforcing Medical Compliance in the Elderly

Working with elderly patients who may have problems with memory loss or thought processes is extremely important to ensure that they take their medications as prescribed and follow the physician's instructions precisely. A patient who has good rapport with the office staff is likely to be truthful about the need for memory aids, and compliance may be increased. A patient who has difficulties with memory may benefit from the following approaches:

- Write out instructions in easy-to-understand terms.
- Use large print.
- Have the patient repeat instructions to you for reinforcement.
- Ask the patient to show you how he or she will perform a procedure before leaving the office.
- Give the patient a copy of a large appointment calendar and list the times and days for treatments and medications, which should be crossed off as completed.

Many chronic illnesses that affect the elderly require medication or treatment for the remainder of the pa-

tient's life. In these situations, the patient may not notice much improvement, making compliance over a long period problematic. You should reinforce the fact that, although the patient may not return to his or her former health status, the prescribed treatment will maintain health at a manageable level. A patient's diabetes or heart disease will not be cured, but treatment will help the patient maintain a reasonable standard of health and independence.

It is important that, each time a patient visits the medical office, you ask for a complete account of all medications being taken, including prescribed and over-the-counter medications, herbal supplements, and vitamins. To maintain a complete and accurate list of these medications, you may have patients bring all medications to the office at each visit and ask the patient to state how often each is taken (Fig. 38-1). If you ask, "Mrs. Jones, are you still taking your heart medicine?" she may answer yes whether or not she is actually taking the medication as prescribed. In addition to difficulty with thought processes and occasional forgetfulness, some patients simply grow tired of the constraints that illness and medications impose on their lives, and some must make the financial choice between medication and food on the table. Assisting the patient to find ways to fit health requirements into a fairly normal lifestyle or coordinating with community resources to relieve financial constraints will help to ensure that treatment plans are followed and that the patient achieves the best level of health possible.

 CHECKPOINT QUESTION

1. What are some reasons a patient may not comply with a prescribed treatment plan?

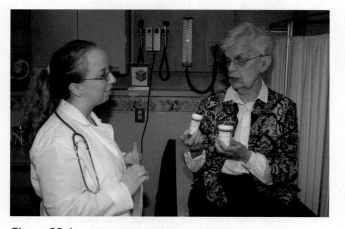

Figure 38-1   Ask patients about medications at every visit.

Reinforcing Mental Health in the Elderly

With the recognized correlation between physical and mental health, we must be acutely aware of the patient's mental status in patients who have acute or chronic physical problems. Some elderly patients are adapting to new roles of dependency after a lifetime of social interaction, career objectives, and family development. Some have been relieved of social responsibility whether they welcome it or not, and if they are ill, they must take on a dependent role. Adjusting to pain or disability is often easier than adjusting to loss of social interaction or dependency.

Paradoxically, if you open yourself to patients, including the elderly, and you are accessible and caring, you are likely to be the object of anger simply because you are seen as a safe outlet for venting frustrations. A suffering patient is less likely to release pent-up rage at someone who may respond with hostility or corresponding anger; consequently, the patient may hold these feelings in, and the problem is compounded. Making yourself available to field these emotions can be as therapeutic as any treatment administered to this patient. To do this effectively:

1. Maintain open communication, freely discussing hopes and fears realistically, listening attentively, and offering advice without diagnosing or offering false hope.
2. By listening and being supportive to the patient and family members, help the patient to cope with and express feelings of guilt for being ill, anger at self and others nearby, and the loss of health and independence.
3. Work toward maintaining the patient's positive self-image by reinforcing the positive qualities of the patient's physical health or personal situation as appropriate.
4. Assist family members to maintain a positive support system by listening to concerns and possibly serving as a liaison for outside social services or resources if available.
5. Without being discouraging or offering false hope, prepare the patient for the possibility that a return to the previous state of health may not be feasible.
6. Direct the patient and family to specific support groups, such as the American Heart Association, the American Cancer Society, or another group specific to the patient's problem, to assist them with acquiring information about the patient's condition.

CHECKPOINT QUESTION

2. How can you help promote good mental health in your elderly patients?

P A T I E N T   E D U C A T I O N

HERBAL SUPPLEMENTS

The herb ginkgo, also known as ginkgo biloba, maidenhair tree, kew tree, fossil tree, ginkyo, and yinhsing, is advertised in the United States as a natural way to improve memory and concentration. It is for this reason that the elderly have been targeted for the purchase of this product. After all, it can be purchased over the counter at many pharmacies and health food stores, and so many patients do not consider it a medication. However, it is extremely important that you obtain a thorough history from your patients each time they visit the office and specifically ask about any over-the-counter medications, including herbs and vitamin supplements. This drug may improve memory in some patients, but it causes an increase in clotting time in anyone who takes it and should not be used by patients with bleeding or clotting disorders. Any patient being scheduled for a surgical procedure must also be asked about the use of herbs. Patients who are taking the following medications should avoid taking ginkgo:

- Warfarin (Coumadin)
- Aspirin
- Nonsteroidal anti-inflammatory drugs (NSAIDs), such as ibuprofen, naproxen, and indomethacin

The physician should be informed of any patient taking this herbal supplement because reactions with other medications in addition to those listed could have serious consequences.

P A T I E N T   E D U C A T I O N

TIPS FOR IMPROVING MEMORY IN THE ELDERLY

Many research studies have been done regarding improving the forgetfulness that sometimes results from aging and that is not associated with an organic brain disorder such as Alzheimer's disease or cerebrovascular disease. The factors that seem to play an important role in maintaining and improving memory include many of the same factors necessary for general good health:

- Regular physical exercise
- Maintaining a healthy body weight

(continued)

- Eating a healthy diet that includes a variety of foods (grains, fruits, vegetables, etc.) and is low in fats

In addition, eating breakfast and regularly exercising the brain with puzzles, word searches, and other activities that require thinking skills may also affect cognitive function.

Coping With Aging

Although most elderly people are generally healthy and satisfied with their lives, those who live in long-term care facilities or whose health and economic situation are unstable have every right to feel overwhelming stress and grief. Stress will compromise the immune system, raise the blood pressure and blood sugar level, and strain the heart and lungs—all at a time when the patient needs all available resources to fight a debilitating disease process. You can help patients to cope with stress by listening to their fears and concerns, respecting their right to have these feelings, and helping them to reduce the stressors in their lives. Keep in mind that the coping mechanisms (e.g., denial, projection, repression) used to protect ourselves from stress may become more pronounced with age.

The ability of patients to cope with their losses is in direct relation to the importance of the losses and their own personal habits for coping with loss in the past. Be aware of a patient's loss of specific senses, abilities, or important things in life, such as sight, hearing, movement, perception, health, employment, home, and spouse. Also, be alert to the loss of nonspecific things, such as life purpose, goals, a sense of achievement, self-worth, recognition, and security. Some elderly patients react to these losses by disengaging emotionally and relinquishing all decision making to family members. This may compound their grieving and lead to a sense of hopelessness and resignation. To prevent this reaction, involve elderly patients, like all patients, as much as possible by allowing them to have a voice in decisions that will affect their care. The elderly who are encouraged to make decisions and take responsibility for themselves are happier, more sociable, and live longer than those who are not.

Alcoholism

Some elderly, like adults coping with other losses, turn to alcohol as a way to escape dealing with the various losses associated with aging. Because alcohol slows brain activity and impairs mental processes, coordination, and judgment, a patient who comes to the office under the influence of alcohol may be mistaken for having dementia (mental deterioration), a transient ischemic attack (TIA), or central nervous system impairment.

Also, many medications taken by the elderly affect the central nervous system and react badly with alcohol, compounding the problem. For example, alcohol increases the effect of opioids, barbiturates, and depressants of all types, and caretakers may not recognize this reason for the **potentiation**.

Identifying an elderly patient who is using or abusing alcohol may require the entire office to work as a team with the patient's family or caregiver to seek causes of various symptoms, such as impaired judgment or coordination. As often as necessary, you should reinforce with elderly patients and their caregivers the effects of alcohol on mental processes and undesirable interactions with medications. In addition, the patient and responsible caregivers may require a referral to a mental health professional or other community resource to deal effectively with alcohol abuse. You may be required to make this referral as ordered by the physician.

Suicide

When ill health, multiple losses, and deep depression become too much for the patient to bear, suicide may seem preferable to life. Unlike suicide among younger people, suicide among the elderly is likely to be well planned and successful. Most elderly suicides are white men over age 65, especially those who have recently lost a spouse to death or divorce. These suicides are not usually a cry for help but a genuine effort to end life. Watch for these signs of intent:

- Deepening confusion and scattered attention
- Increasing anger, hostility, or isolation
- Increase in alcoholism or requests for opioids or sedatives
- Marked loss of interest in matters of health
- Secretive behavior
- Sharp mood swings from deep depression to euphoria
- Giving away favored objects

Always take seriously a patient who expresses an intent to commit suicide, and communicate this to the physician. You should work with the health care team to restore mental health as aggressively as to restore physical health.

 CHECKPOINT QUESTION

3. What are some signs of suicidal intent?

Long-Term Care

Although many elderly are able to live in their own homes, some enter long-term care facilities if they cannot return to health and independence. There are three main types of long-term care:

- *Group homes* or *assisted living facilities* are for the elderly who are able to tend to their own **activities of daily living (ADL)** (e.g., bathing, dressing, eating) but who need companionship and light supervision for safety.
- *Long-term care facilities* are for those who need help with most areas of personal care and moderate medical supervision. Many of these patients are ambulatory but have a chronic disease that makes living at home alone impossible.
- *Skilled nursing facilities* are for those who are gravely or terminally ill and need constant supervision. If the illness is acute and short term, the patient may return to an intermediate stage of care after recovery and possibly to full independence.

Expect some elderly patients to react to a move to long-term care with sorrow and a deep sense of loss. The patient may show the signs and symptoms of grief: poor appetite, headaches, insomnia, deep depression, and vague aches and pains. Report all signs and symptoms to the physician. Many physicians continue to care for patients residing in long-term care facilities. You may be responsible for blocking time in the daily schedule for the physician to visit these patients, and you may receive phone calls at the medical office from facilities regarding changes in patient's care and physical condition.

 CHECKPOINT QUESTION

4. How are long-term facilities and skilled nursing facilities different?

 LEGAL TIP

ADVANCE DIRECTIVES

An advance directive is a legal document outlining the wishes of an adult should he/she become mentally incompetent or otherwise unable to communicate decisions about end-of-life care. Although physicians as medical professionals are dedicated to sustaining life, a patient's autonomy must be respected at all times, including decisions to avoid or terminate life-sustaining procedures or equipment. As unpleasant as the prospect of death may be, documenting and communicating the wishes of the patient to the physician will assist with avoiding any confusion about the wishes of the patient should a life-threatening situation arise. Also, if the patient has an advanced directive on file somewhere other than the medical office, this should be noted in the patient's medical record.

 WHAT IF?

What if a patient's relative asks you about options for home care for an elderly parent?

Explain that many options allow patients to remain in their home. One option is the use of home health aides. Some insurance plans pay for this service. Home health aides do light housecleaning and cooking and promote patient safety. A second option is a community resource center. Some communities have senior citizen programs that provide transportation for shopping, doctor appointments, and entertainment. These programs get the older patient out of the house, preventing boredom and enhancing self-esteem. A third option is day care for the elderly. These programs keep the patient safe, entertained, and cared for during the day. The advantages of day care are that it relieves the caregiver of the need to place a parent in a long-term care facility, keeps the patient safe during the day, and allows the relative the freedom to continue employment or attend to personal needs. Community programs for senior citizens are good sources of information for caregivers or for relatives searching for respite or permanent care.

Elder Abuse

Although elder abuse is not as widely publicized as child abuse, it is thought to be almost as prevalent. The following are common risk factors for elder abuse:

- Multiple chronic illnesses that stress the family's physical, emotional, and financial resources
- Senile dementia that precludes reasoning or interaction
- Bladder or bowel incontinence
- Age-related sleep disturbances that interfere with the caretaker's rest
- Dependence on the caretaker for ADL

Elder abuse and neglect may take several forms, but family members (adult children and spouses) are the typical perpetrators.

- Passive neglect may result from the caretaker's ignorance regarding the patient's physiologic and psychological needs.
- Active neglect may take many forms, including overmedicating to render the patient passive and easier to care for or depriving the victim of adequate nutrition to decrease physical resources.

Figure 38-2 You should always be alert to signs of elder abuse. (From Weber J, Kelley J. Health Assessment in Nursing. 2nd ed. Philadelphia: Lippincott Williams & Wilkins, 2003.)

- Psychological abuse may include threatening imprisonment in the home, perhaps locking in a room, or physical abuse, withholding food or medication, or physical isolation.
- Financial abuse may involve only small amounts of money or entire substantial estates. The patient's financial resources may be embezzled, squandered, or frankly stolen, leaving the victim destitute.
- Physical abuse may be as simple as pinches and slaps or may be life threatening, sexual, or so well concealed that even perceptive health care providers do not suspect it (Fig. 38-2).

Some elderly patients fear reprisal or abandonment by their caregivers, just as children do, and are reluctant to complain of any improprieties. Separate the caregiver from the patient for the examination if possible, and treat the patient with the utmost compassion and care. Document all findings with full descriptions. It may be necessary to photograph the suspected injuries.

LEGAL TIP
ELDER ABUSE

If you suspect abuse or neglect, you are responsible ethically and legally for bringing it to the attention of the physician, who should assess the situation and, if it is confirmed, notify the proper authorities. Most states require that health care professionals report all suspected cases of elder abuse to the department of social services, just as is required for suspected child abuse. The entire medical staff may be held responsible if the abuse is not reported immediately. The following signs may indicate elder abuse:

- Wound of suspicious origin in various stages of healing

- Signs of restraints having been used, such as wrist or ankle abrasions or bruising
- Neglected large, deep pressure ulcers
- Poor hygiene or poor nutrition with little or no effort at correction
- Dehydration not caused by a disease process
- Untreated injury or medical condition
- Excessive and unwanted agitation or apathetic resignation

 CHECKPOINT QUESTION

5. What are the types of elder abuse?

Medications and the Elderly

The need to teach some elderly patients about self-medication is a challenge that will become increasingly common as the general population ages. At the same time that elderly patients need more medications for various disorders, the body is coping with the stress of illness, disease, or injury along with slowing of many bodily functions. The gastrointestinal system is no longer moving medications along as efficiently because peristalsis has slowed. The circulatory system is not absorbing the dissolved medication from the intestines or the injection site and delivering it to the target tissue as quickly. The liver does not **biotransform** (convert) the medication as quickly, so that it remains in the body longer than might be desirable and possibly adds to cumulative effect. Finally, the kidneys are receiving less blood, so that less medication is filtered and removed from the body. All of these decreases in body systems can result in possible toxic effects of medications in the elderly.

Your responsibility is to elicit information from the patient about all medications they are taking, including prescribed and over-the-counter medications and herbal or vitamin supplements. Follow these guidelines to help ensure that your elderly patient adheres to the prescribed medication regimen:

1. Explain all side effects, precautions, interactions, and expected actions in a manner the patient can understand.
2. Explain the proper dosage and how to measure it. For patients with failing eyesight, mark plastic measuring cups with indelible ink at the correct level so they can easily see it.
3. Write out a schedule and suggest methods to help the patient remember. Suggestions may include a daily dose pack available at pharmacies, an egg carton with hours for taking the medications marked on the

cups, and a calendar marked with the medications and hours, to be checked off after taking the medication.

4. Tell the patient to take the most important medication first and space out the other medications according to the physician's order. Medications that are ordered to be taken once a day may not have to be taken in the morning.

5. Encourage the patient not to rush when taking medications. The patient should be sitting or standing, not reclining. One pill should be taken at a time with lots of water. If the medication is difficult to swallow, have the patient try putting the pill on the back of the tongue and drinking water with a straw.

6. A patient who has difficulty reading or has failing eyesight can ask the pharmacist for large print on the label (Fig. 38-3). This makes medication errors less likely. Childproof containers are not necessary if there are no children in the home, and the patient may find them difficult to open.

7. Explain that the medication must be taken until it is gone (if this is the case). No medication should be taken by other family members or saved for another illness.

8. Encourage patients to take an active role in therapy. Teach them to apply ointments or transdermal patches or to give themselves injections. A patient who feels in charge is more likely to complete a course of medication or to remain on the medication for the long term than one who feels passive.

CHECKPOINT QUESTION

6. How can you help your elderly patients follow the medication regimen prescribed by the physician?

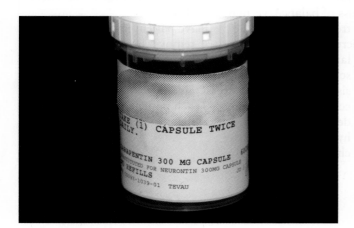

Figure 38-3 Large print on a medication label.

Systemic Changes in the Elderly

Although longevity is considered largely hereditary, environmental factors play a significant part in how long and how well we will live. An obese, physically inactive smoker is much less likely to be in good health than a nonsmoker whose diet is well balanced and who exercises. In addition, certain occupational hazards, such as black lung disease from coal mining, may shorten a life that should have lasted for decades longer.

The aging changes are thought to be programmed into our cells along with our genetic material. Some experts suggest that when cells reach a specific reproduction level, they either do not replace themselves or replicate more slowly or ineffectively. These changes manifest themselves at varying rates for all persons but follow a recognized order as outlined in Table 38-1.

WHAT IF?

You are organizing your charts at the beginning of the day and you notice that one of your patients, an 88-year-old man, has HOH (hard of hearing) stamped inside his chart. How can you best communicate with him?

When speaking to an elderly patient who is hearing impaired, it is important not to shout. Instead, get closer to the patient, face the patient directly, and speak slowly and distinctly. Try to give written instructions whenever possible, and encourage the patient to ask questions for clarification. Avoid speaking to the hard-of-hearing patient with your back to the light, since this may cast shadows and prevent the patient from being able to lip read.

Diseases of the Elderly

The degenerative conditions noted in Table 38-1 are typically part of the aging process. Many of these changes cause problems that must be managed by the health care team; others are mere inconveniences for the patient. Diseases related to aging are described in the preceding chapters on specialties. The following sections describe two conditions commonly associated with aging that may appear in the middle years as well.

Parkinson's Disease

Parkinson's disease is a slow, progressive neurologic disorder affecting specific cells of the brain that produce the

TABLE 38-1	Effects of Aging on Body Systems		
System	**Physiologic Effects**	**Signs and Symptoms**	**Suggestions**
Integumentary system	Loss of subcutaneous fat Loss of pigment Loss of elasticity Receding capillaries Slower reproduction of hair, skin cells Diminished oil, sweat production Erratic pigment, cell production	Wrinkling, sagging, decreased ability to maintain hydration, reduced protection against temperature change Less protection against sun damage, paler skin, graying hair Increased skin dryness, risk of trauma Sallow skin, thickened nails Balding; thin, fine hair; slower healing Dry, fragile skin; intolerance to heat Senile **lentigines, keratoses**	Encourage drinking plenty of fluids, dressing appropriately for weather. Encourage use of sunscreen with appropriate UV protection. Suggest good lubricating lotion and bathing less often; caution patient to guard against injuries. Suggest ways to avoid overheating. Teach patient to conduct skin checks and to notify physician of concerns.
Musculoskeletal system	Loss of muscle strength, size Loss of bone density, typical loss of height with osteoporosis Degenerative joint cartilage	Loss of strength, flexibility, endurance Vertebral compression with diminished height, **kyphosis; osteoporosis** with frequent fractures Less clear margins with spurs of bone that restrict movement, **degenerative joint disease,** arthritis	Suggest frequent exercise appropriate to age and ability. Explain weight-bearing exercise. Encourage home safety check to avoid falls. Physician may recommend calcium supplement, dietary consultation, estrogen replacement. Physician may limit phosphorus intake.
Nervous system	Slow nerve conduction Reduced cerebral circulation Referred circulatory problems	Slow reaction time, slow learning, slow perception of pain with resulting increase in injuries Loss of balance, **vertigo,** frequent falls Increase in cardiovascular diseases (atherosclerosis, arteriosclerosis) reflected as **cerebrovascular accident (CVA),** cerebral hypoxia, **transient ischemic attack (TIA)**	Allow extra time as needed and teach about hazards of delayed reaction times. Aim teaching at comprehension level. Encourage home safety checks. Have patient install bath rails, remove throw rugs, conduct home safety check. Encourage use of walking aid. Teach patient and family about danger signs for CVA, TIA.

(continued)

TABLE 38-1	Effects of Aging on Body Systems (continued)		
System	**Physiologic Effects**	**Signs and Symptoms**	**Suggestions**
Cardiovascular system	Atherosclerosis, arteriosclerosis, narrowing of blood vessels Slow response to demands for increased output Diminished function	Loss of peripheral circulation, fatty plaques with risk of MI, CVA, cold extremities, slow healing time, hypertension Complaints of fatigue on exertion Pulmonary involvement with edema, dyspnea	Encourage exercise; balanced, low-fat, low-salt diet; dressing appropriately for weather; home safety check. Help patient pace exercise and exertion. Explain about low-salt diets and orthopneic positions. Explain about smoking hazards, emphysema. Encourage moderate exercise.
Respiratory system	Stiffening costal cartilage Decreased gas exchange General loss of muscle mass	Decreased expansion, contraction; barrel chest; decreased lung capacity Fatigue, breathlessness on exertion; impaired healing due to insufficient oxygen, **syncope** Difficulty coughing deeply, may lead to pneumonia	Encourage exercise as appropriate and use of walking aid. Caution about upper respiratory infection; encourage home safety check. Encourage drinking adequate fluids to liquefy respiratory secretions.
Gastrointestinal system	Drying of secretions, including saliva Decreased enzyme activity Slower peristalsis Loss of teeth	Dry mouth, **dysphagia** Incomplete digestion, poor conversion of nutrients with malnourishment Constipation, flatulence, indigestion Poor chewing, choking on large pieces, loss of appetite, poor nutrition	Teach oral hygiene, adequate fluid intake. Encourage small, frequent well-balanced meals. Refer to a dentist; teach good oral hygiene. Suggest dietary counseling.
Urinary system	Decreased bladder capacity Decreased bladder muscle tone Fewer functioning nephrons	Urinary frequency Urinary retention with urinary tract infection or incontinence Less blood flowing through kidneys to be cleaned of wastes, creating possibly lethal levels of medications or normal body wastes	Encourage patient to respond to initial urge to void. Suggest exercises for strengthening pelvic floor. Urge patient to empty bladder completely when voiding. Suggest increase in fluid intake to maintain hydration.

(continued)

TABLE 38-1	Effects of Aging on Body Systems *(continued)*		
System	**Physiologic Effects**	**Signs and Symptoms**	**Suggestions**
Endocrine system	Decreased enzyme activity	Menopause, glucose intolerance with NIDDM, slower metabolism	Physician will supplement as needed.
Immune system	Diminished production of T cells, B cells Diminished ability of body to distinguish self from foreign substances Diminished other defenses (e.g., GI enzymes)	Loss of resistance to illness Increase in autoimmune illnesses Overload on compromised immune systems	Encourage age-appropriate immunization. Explain symptoms of autoimmunity. Encourage age-appropriate immunizations, guarding against communicable diseases.
Eyes	Less time spent in deep sleep Diminished lens accommodation Lens cloud Loss of ciliary function	Less restful sleep, more frequent naps **Presbyopia** **Cataracts** (lens opacity) that dim vision as less light reaches the retina **Glaucoma** (increased intraocular pressure), intolerance to light or glare, poor night vision	Encourage rest periods as needed. Obtain referral to ophthalmologist. Recommend adequate lighting, large-print books, brochures, pamphlets. Obtain referral to ophthalmologist. Recommend adequate lighting. Obtain referral to ophthalmologist. Recommend adequate lighting, avoidance of night driving.
Ears	Loss of auditory hair cells (organ of Corti) Ossicle becomes fixed	Hearing loss in upper frequencies, problems distinguishing sibilants **Presbycusis**	Obtain referral to otologist. Speak clearly, facing patient, in area with few distractions. Obtain referral to otologist. Speak clearly, facing patient, in area with few distractions.
Other senses	Diminished sense of smell Diminished sense of taste	Loss of appetite, poor nutrition Loss of appetite, poor nutrition, perhaps increased use of salt, other seasonings	Suggest dietary consultation. Suggest dietary consultation. Encourage use of seasonings other than salt.
Female reproductive system	Decreased egg production system Decreased estrogen production Poor perineal muscle tone	Menopause Hot flashes; thinner, drier vaginal walls with itching, painful intercourse; osteoporosis Rectocele, cystocele, stress incontinence	Physician may prescribe supplemental estrogen. Suggest **Kegel exercises** to strengthen pelvic floor.

(continued)

TABLE 38-1	Effects of Aging on Body Systems *(continued)*		
System	**Physiologic Effects**	**Signs and Symptoms**	**Suggestions**
Male reproductive system	Smaller penis, testicles Atherosclerosis, arteriosclerosis Benign prostatic hypertrophy (BPH)	Loss of libido Impotence Urgency, frequency, nocturia, retention	Physician may refer patient for counseling. Explain good nutrition to avoid atherosclerosis. Encourage patient to have yearly checks for BPH.

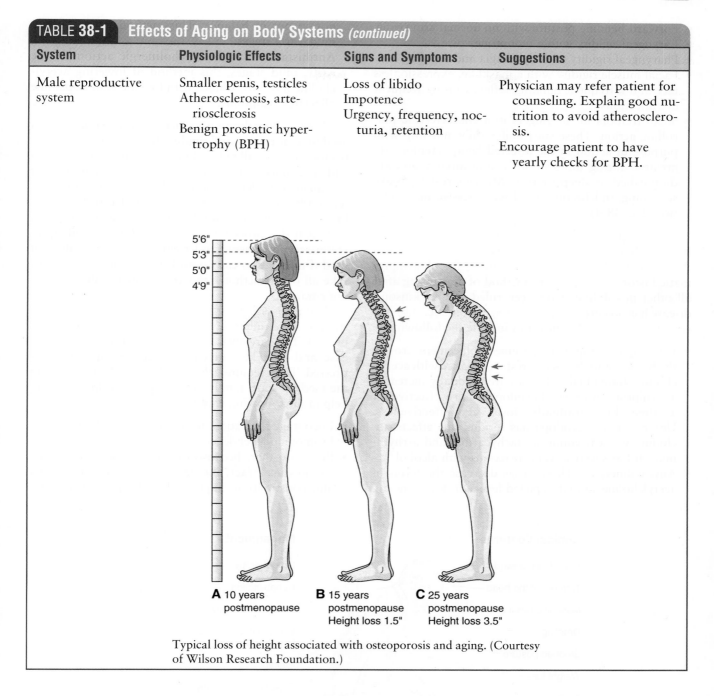

A 10 years postmenopause

B 15 years postmenopause Height loss 1.5"

C 25 years postmenopause Height loss 3.5"

Typical loss of height associated with osteoporosis and aging. (Courtesy of Wilson Research Foundation.)

neurotransmitter dopamine. The initial symptoms frequently include muscle rigidity, involuntary tremors, and difficulty walking. Parkinson's disease affects men more than women and is estimated to affect in some form approximately 1 in 100 persons over age 60. This disease may progress for 10 years or more before resulting in complete debilitation or death.

Normally, dopamine and acetylcholine, another neurotransmitter, are in balance and produce smooth, controlled muscle movement. With lower levels of dopamine, acetylcholine is not counterbalanced. This leads to involuntary movements of muscles and inability to control these movements. While the causes of Parkinson's disease are unknown, researchers are working to determine whether there is a genetic component. Some evidence suggests that certain toxins may cause the disease. These toxins may be environmental or related to certain medications. The following are the signs and symptoms of Parkinson's disease:

- Muscle rigidity
- **Bradykinesia** (abnormally slow voluntary movements)
- Difficulty walking, with a shuffling, mincing gait

- Forward-bending posture with no normal arm swing
- Laryngeal rigidity with a monotone voice
- Pharyngeal rigidity with dysphagia and drooling
- Facial muscle rigidity with a masklike, expressionless face and infrequent blinking reflex, causing frequent eye infections
- Small tremors in the fingers in a characteristic pill-rolling action. These start unilaterally and stop with purposeful action in the affected hand. Tremors are greatest during times of stress and anxiety and are diminished at sleep or rest. Muscles resist passive stretching and become rigid with passive manipulation (Fig. 38-4).

The diagnosis of Parkinson's disease is usually made by excluding other causes; however, testing may show decreased levels of dopamine in the urine. A symptomatic history is the primary method of diagnosing after all other possibilities have been ruled out. Parkinson's disease has no cure. Treatment is symptomatic, supportive, and palliative. Medications include the following:

- Levodopa (L-dopa). Dopamine replacement crosses the blood–brain barrier to restore balance with acetylcholine. Individualized doses are gradually increased as symptoms progress. Levodopa is fairly effective for a time but gradually loses its effectiveness. Unfortunately, levodopa has serious side effects, including nausea, vomiting, tachycardia, and arrhythmias. It has severe adverse reactions with alcohol.
- Anticholinergics. These drugs decrease the levels of acetylcholine so that depleted levels of dopamine are not so out of balance. This method works best in mild, early stages.
- Antihistamines with anticholinergic action. In the early, mild stages, this method of lowering acetylcholine levels to balance with low levels of dopamine alleviates symptoms.

A procedure known as deep-brain stimulation is used to treat tremor and rigidity. In this procedure, electrodes are surgically placed in certain areas of the brain and are connected by wires to an impulse generator that is implanted under the skin of the chest. This transmitter sends electrical impulses to the electrodes in the brain, blocking the impulses that cause the tremors. Although this procedure is effective for controlling involuntary movements and tremors, it is generally not used if medication can control the patient's symptoms. Like all other methods, this treatment is palliative and not curative.

Parkinson's patients retain their mental and cognitive functions unless an organic brain disturbance is also present. They are aware of the outward signs of the disease and may be embarrassed and emotionally depressed. They require great psychological support from the medical staff, family, and support groups. You can help in the following ways:

- Encourage the patient to participate in all ADL.
- Promote independence.
- Be aware that, because rigidity extends to the gastrointestinal tract, the patient may have dysphagia and constipation. Suggest that the patient increase

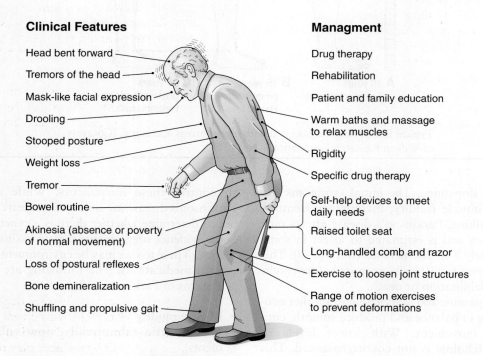

Clinical Features

- Head bent forward
- Tremors of the head
- Mask-like facial expression
- Drooling
- Stooped posture
- Weight loss
- Tremor
- Bowel routine
- Akinesia (absence or poverty of normal movement)
- Loss of postural reflexes
- Bone demineralization
- Shuffling and propulsive gait

Managment

- Drug therapy
- Rehabilitation
- Patient and family education
- Warm baths and massage to relax muscles
- Rigidity
- Specific drug therapy
- Self-help devices to meet daily needs
- Raised toilet seat
- Long-handled comb and razor
- Exercise to loosen joint structures
- Range of motion exercises to prevent deformations

Figure 38-4   The Parkinson's patient.

fluid intake, eat a balanced diet, and increase fiber intake.

- Tell the patient that a decreased cough reflex can lead to choking. Suggest that the patient take small bites and chew each mouthful of food carefully before attempting to swallow.
- Encourage the patient to use eating aids such as a no-spill cup, plate with high sides, and special utensils. High toilet seats and handrails in the bath also help increase the patient's independence and safety.
- Listen to the patient. Intelligence is still intact and needs to be stimulated.
- Educate the patient about safety factors. The forward-bending posture and altered gait frequently lead to falls. Encourage these patients to hold on to handrails and pick up feet carefully to avoid falling. Also, the home should be free from rugs and loose cords that may cause accidental tripping.
- Enlist the help of support groups. Include the caregiver and urge respite care when exhaustion and stress become overwhelming.

 CHECKPOINT QUESTION

7. How can you assist a patient with Parkinson's disease?

Alzheimer's Disease

Roughly half of the cases of dementia in the elderly are due to Alzheimer's disease. The symptoms of Alzheimer's disease may be similar to those caused by TIA, cerebral tumor, and dementia other than Alzheimer's. Unfortunately, the cause of Alzheimer's is not known.

The symptoms of Alzheimer's disease may begin as early as age 40, with a gradual loss of memory and slight personality changes. The changes may occur over as long as 15 years and are frequently so gradual that diagnosis is difficult and may be made only by ruling out all other possibilities. Autopsy reveals organic brain changes, including a loss of neurons and neurotransmitters. Plaques or deposits may be present as a residue of the neural cell deterioration.

Alzheimer's disease has seven recognized stages. The progression from one stage to the next may be gradual. Some stages may last for years, but a patient may pass through other stages so quickly that the progression goes unnoticed. Expect varying levels of response from patients in these different levels (Table 38-2). When caring for Alzheimer's patients, you must remember that anger and hostility are symptoms of the disease and should not to be taken personally. Be sure to do the following:

- Respond with the utmost patience and compassion.
- Speak calmly and without condescension.

TABLE 38-2	Levels of Alzheimer's Disease
Level	**Description**
I, II	Presenile dementia may end here, with no further progression. Brain changes insignificant; only remarkable symptom may be forgetfulness. ADL done with reasonable ease.
III	Patient losing ability to remember facts, faces, and names but still aware enough to recognize problem and becomes increasingly frustrated and angry. Most ADL still performed reasonably well.
IV	Late confusional or mild Alzheimer's. Patient beginning to misplace things, has increasing difficulty remembering, and neglects ADL. Most patients aware of a problem but deny any concern.
V	Early dementia or moderate Alzheimer's. Patient must have custodial care, has severe memory lapses, disorientation, anger, and great frustration.
VI	Middle dementia or moderately severe Alzheimer's with severe memory loss, no self-care at any level, disoriented most of the time with immense anger, hostility, and combativeness. Fear of water.
VII	Late dementia. Patient requires full-time care and is rarely seen in the office. Unless home care is an option, physician will probably visit long-term care facility. Patient rarely speaks, almost never intelligibly; incontinent; may require tube feeding.

- Never argue with the patient, even if the patient blames you unfairly for something the patient forgot.
- Do not expect the patient to remember you from previous visits. Reintroduce yourself.
- Explain even common procedures as if the patient has never had them explained.
- Approach the patient quietly and professionally in an unthreatening manner, and remind the patient who you are and what you must do.
- Speak in short, simple, direct sentences, and explain only one action at a time.
- Keep a list of support contacts for family members to call.

Home care agencies usually offer respite care, which can be vitally important for caregivers, who need to maintain their own mental and physical health. An exhausted, distraught family member may not be thinking clearly. The most therapeutic action may be for you to assist the family with proper contacts to help make caring for a family member with this devastating disease less traumatic.

TRIAGE BOX

While you are working in a medical office, the following three patients are waiting to be seen:

A. Patient A is a 76-year-old woman who is active but underweight, with a history of osteoporosis. She is here for a physical examination, and the doctor has just instructed you to obtain some blood work for laboratory analysis.

B. Patient B is an 87-year-old man brought in by his daughter, who takes care of him in her home since his stroke 3 years ago. His wife is deceased, and his daughter is concerned because his memory seems to be failing him.

C. Patient C is a 90-year-old man residing in an assisted-living facility with his wife, who is 88. They were brought to the office today because the husband is due for a blood pressure check and possible medication adjustment. They are alert and sharp mentally, although both move more slowly than usual and the wife requires a walker.

How would you sort these patients? Who do you see first? Second? Third?

When working with elderly patients, it is important to remember not to rush them or appear inattentive. Since patient B is having new symptoms and may require a longer time with the physician, you should check him in first and get vital signs and any appropriate medical information from both the patient and his daughter. The husband and wife should be seen next, since all that is required is a brief chief complaint and obtaining vital signs. When both the husband and wife are comfortable and safely seated, you may leave them alone until the doctor is available to see them. Patient A should be seen last because obtaining blood from the elderly requires special attention to detail and patience. Once the blood sample is obtained, patient A may be discharged after checking the medical record to assure that no physician orders have been missed.

Maintaining Optimum Health

No one realistically expects to have the same strength and agility at age 70 as at age 20. With attention to exercise and good nutrition, however, it is possible to maintain a good level of fitness that adds to quality of life.

Exercise

Exercise plays a vital role in maintaining overall physical and mental health (Table 38-3). Older patients should begin an exercise program only after a thorough physical examination and should follow the physician's recommendation. Provide the following guidelines for elderly patients who are starting an exercise program with the physician's approval:

1. Before exercise, always warm up cold muscles for at least 10 minutes. Slow and rhythmic movements, such as walking, raise the heart rate and increase metabolism. Then do slow, easy stretching to lengthen sluggish muscles.

2. Begin by exercising for brief periods. Exercise only 5 to 10 minutes a day the first week, then progress to 10 to 15 minutes a day the next week. Gradually work up to about 30 to 45 minutes of a pleasantly challenging strength and cardiovascular endurance activity after about a month. This routine reduces the chance of injury and is likely to be an attainable goal.

3. Stop if you feel pain, shortness of breath, or dizziness. Never try to work through pain.

4. Breathe deeply and evenly. If you cannot carry on a conversation, slow down. Never hold your breath while you exercise.

5. Rest when you get tired. Do not try to exercise to the point of exhaustion.

TABLE 38-3	Benefits of Exercise
System	**Benefits**
Cardiovascular	Increases endurance Lowers cholesterol to avoid atherosclerosis Maintains vascular elasticity to delay arteriosclerosis
Musculoskeletal	Increases bone mass to reduce osteoporosis Decreases fat–muscle ratio and increases metabolism Retains strength and flexibility to ensure mobility, improve posture
Nervous	Improves mental health by reducing stress, fatigue, tension, boredom Maintains or restores balance to reduce risk of falls
Endocrine	May decrease need for insulin or oral hypoglycemic medication in diabetes

6. Keep a record of your progress. It is motivational to watch your performance improve.
7. Exercise with a friend, with a group, or to music that you enjoy (Fig. 38-5).
8. Make exercise a part of your daily routine, but do not make it a chore. Do something vigorous every day and take pride in it.

 CHECKPOINT QUESTION

8. What are the physical signs that indicate a patient should stop exercising?

Diet

Many elderly patients have difficulty maintaining good nutrition. Reduced activity means a corresponding decrease in hunger. Decaying teeth or poorly fitting dentures cause pain, making it hard to chew. Saliva production decreases, making it harder to swallow. The senses of smell and taste diminish, interfering with the cephalic phase of digestion. Many elderly patients eat alone or are not able to enjoy the socializing that adds immeasurably to the pleasure of eating.

A balanced diet is vital to good health at any age. Although activity levels, and hence calorie requirements, are lower among the elderly, vitamin and mineral requirements do not decrease with age. Efforts must be made to increase the nutritional level of the elderly. Smaller, more frequent meals may be easier to digest than infrequent large meals. Water should be encour-

aged to maintain hydration and to aid digestion and elimination.

Talk to patients or their families about valuable social services that may deliver nutritious meals to the home daily or 5 days a week. These programs may ensure that at least one well-balanced meal a day is available. Most services prepare meals to meet special dietary needs, such as low sodium or low fat. The program volunteer is alert to the needs of the patient and will report to a coordinator if the patient does not answer the door or seems ill or confused. These resources will help to reassure the family that the patient's nutritional and social needs are being met.

 PATIENT EDUCATION

LIQUID DIETARY SUPPLEMENTS

There are many liquid dietary supplements available on the market today, and some are specifically marketed for the elderly. When interviewing the elderly, always assess their nutritional status by asking about the frequency of meals and types of food eaten and obtaining a weight at each visit. Let the physician know if you notice a trend in weight loss or other signs of poor nutrition. With permission of the physician, encourage your patient with nutritional problems to get a liquid supplement in his or her favorite flavor; most come in vanilla, chocolate, and strawberry. Advise your patient that these supplements should not replace a meal, but rather provide extra nutrition between meals.

Safety

Alert the patient and caregivers to hazards in the home of an elderly patient and offer the following suggestions:

- Remove any scatter rugs, especially on highly polished floors.
- Never allow electrical cords to cross passageways.
- Remove or reduce clutter as much as possible.
- Strengthen handrails on stairs and install them in tubs and near the commode.
- Install a telephone by the bedside and near a favorite chair.
- Install and carefully maintain smoke alarms and carbon monoxide detectors throughout the house.
- Establish a system in which someone calls and checks on the patient every day.

Many communities have programs in which volunteers call the sick or elderly daily to check on their needs and offer a few minutes of conversation. If the patient

Figure 38-5 Participating in group exercise helps to maintain overall physical and mental health.

fails to answer, someone goes to the home to check on the patient. This service ensures that the patient is never without contact for long. Lifeline, an emergency service, is another option that increases the feeling of safety for patients who live alone.

CHECKPOINT QUESTION

9. What are some reasons an elderly patient may have poor nutritional status?

---

español SPANISH TERMINOLOGY

Asi se toma este medicamento.
This is how you take this medication.

Tiene usted dolor junto con la rigidez?
Do you have pain with the stiffness?

La auxiliar sanitaria le ayudara con su cuidado personal.
The home health aide will help with your personal care.

Ha notado usted algún cambio en su habilidad de recordar cosas?
Have you noticed a change in your memory?

MEDIA MENU

- **Student CD**
  - **Case Studies**
    Interactive Case Study 2: Vital Signs, Patient Education, and Refusal of Treatment
  - **CMA/RMA Certification Exam Review**
- **Premium Online Course**
  http://thePoint.lww.com/Kronenberger3e
- **Internet Resources**

  LiveAdvise Online Tutoring & Competency Training
  http://thePoint.lww.com/LiveAdvise

  The Center for Social Gerontology
  http://www.tcsg.org

  American Association of Retired Persons
  http://www.aarp.org

  National Center on Elder Abuse
  http://elderabusecenter.org

  National Institute on Aging
  http://www.nia.nih.gov/

  Centers for Medicare and Medicaid Services
  http://www.cms.hhs.gov

Chapter Summary

Regardless of the type of specialty you work in, you will encounter the elderly patient. Some important things to remember about the elderly include:

- Avoid stereotyping the elderly into passive, dependent roles.
- Be alert to the normal physiologic changes of aging and adjust your communication techniques accordingly.

- Not all elderly patients are affected by diseases such as dementia, Alzheimer's disease, or Parkinson's disease.
- Having patients who are diagnosed with Parkinson's or Alzheimer's disease will require you to understand the disease process and develop excellent interpersonal skills.
- Use patient education opportunities to discuss issues of safety whenever possible.

1. Mrs. Moss, aged 78, lives with her son and daughter-in-law and their two school-age children. She has dysphagia and a poor appetite. Identify ways in which Mrs. Moss can improve or maintain her nutritional status while participating in the family meals.

2. Mr. Brown is 90, and his wife is 86. They live alone, and Mrs. Brown is the primary caregiver. During the physical examination, Mr. Brown is found to have several large decubital ulcers. Summarize the various types of elder abuse or neglect. What is likely the problem in this case? Explain how you would handle this situation.

3. The pharmacist calls you at the office and says he has an elderly patient waiting to have a prescription for a high blood pressure medication filled. This prescription was filled just 2 weeks ago, but the patient says he is "all out of my medicine." What do you advise the pharmacist to do?

4. Your 68-year-old male patient tells you that he is thinking about joining the senior citizens exercise group at the local community college. He appears to be healthy and is not currently on any medications. How would you respond?

5. The daughter of an elderly woman comes to the office with her 76-year-old mother who lives alone. Would it be permissible to have the daughter present during the interview and physical exam? What about confidentiality?

1. Elderly patients may not comply with treatment plans because of memory loss from normal aging or because they are growing tired of the constraints imposed on their life by illness. Some patients may have financial difficulties that force them to choose between medication and other essential needs, such as food.

2. You can help your elderly patients maintain good mental health by encouraging open communication, helping them deal with their feelings, promoting a positive self-image, helping family members to be supportive, and suggesting support groups as needed.

3. The signs of suicidal intent include deepening confusion, increasing anger, increased alcohol or drug use, lack of interest in health, secretive behavior, sharp mood swings, and giving away personal possessions.

4. Long-term care facilities are for individuals who need help with personal care and some medical supervision. Skilled nursing facilities are for gravely or terminally ill individuals who need constant supervision.

5. Elder abuse may be passive or active neglect, or it can be psychological, financial, or physical.

6. To help your elderly patient follow the prescribed medication regimen, provide a full explanation of the medication in a way that the patient understands; explain the proper dosage and techniques for measuring; develop a written schedule for taking the medication; instruct the patient to take the most important medication first; tell the patient not to rush when taking the medication; have the patient ask the pharmacist for large print on the label; explain the appropriate use of the medication; and encourage patients to take an active role in their therapy.

7. To assist a patient with Parkinson's disease, encourage activity and independence, promote good nutrition and hydration, caution the patient about the potential for choking, educate the patient about safety, use therapeutic communication skills, and enlist the help of support groups for the patient and his or her caregivers.

8. Elderly patients who are exercising should be warned to stop if they experience pain, shortness of breath, or dizziness.

9. The nutritional status of some elderly patients may be decreased due to decaying teeth or poorly fitting dentures, decreased saliva production, diminished taste and smell, and lack of socialization from having to eat alone.

CLINICAL DUTIES RELATED TO MEDICAL SPECIALTIES
(Chapters 27–38)

1. The busy family practice office where you work employs three medical assistants, two physicians, and one nurse practitioner. This morning, you are covering for one of the medical assistants who called off work due to illness. The 24-year-old patient in the first examination room needs a pre-employment physical, and the physician has asked you to get a pulmonary function test and check his visual acuity. A 6-month-old baby girl in another examination room is due to have her scheduled immunizations. The local outpatient radiology center has just left a message with you that another patient's lower GI performed yesterday is negative according to the radiologist and a formal report will be faxed to the office later today.

   A. What immunizations are typically scheduled at the 6-month well-baby visit? (knowledge)
   B. How would you explain the pulmonary function test to a patient who has never had this test? (comprehension)
   C. What approach would you use to prioritize the tasks in this scenario? (application)
   D. Why would a visual acuity test be included in the pre-employment physical examination? (analysis)
   E. Would lower GI results that were positive for a tumor change the way you would proceed with managing these tasks? (synthesis)
   F. Would it be better if the 6-month-old child were rescheduled to come back at a later date for immunizations when the office is less busy and all the employees are present? (evaluation)

2. Today, the physician you work for has scheduled a medical sales representative to explain a newly purchased ECG machine to the clinical staff during lunch. The sales rep has arrived early and is waiting in the reception area for you to escort him to the staff lounge. The patient in examination room A is a new 46-year-old patient who has the following vital signs: T 98.8°F (O), P 76, R 16, BP 180/98 (R) sitting. An established patient in examination room B is 82 years old and appears exceptionally frail today. Her vital signs are T 100.4°F (O), P 110, irregular R 28. Her BP is inaudible today but has typically been around 104/66 at the past several office visits. She complains of abdominal discomfort and generalized weakness. Earlier this morning, the only tray for removal of an ingrown toenail was used, and the instruments need to be prepared for another ingrown toenail removal scheduled for later this afternoon.

   A. What are considered normal vital signs for an adult? (knowledge)
   B. Explain the steps for preparing the ingrown toenail removal surgical tray before it can be used this afternoon. (comprehension)
   C. Can you think of another way to assess the blood pressure of the 82-year-old patient whose BP is inaudible today? (application)
   D. Why do you think the physician has asked the sales representative to explain the new ECG machine to the clinical staff since everyone at the office already knows how to perform an ECG? (analysis)
   E. What would happen if the 46-year-old patient indicated to you that he suddenly had chest discomfort? (synthesis)
   F. Can you anticipate what tests, procedures, or treatments the physician might order for the patients in this scenario? (evaluation)

3. Because flu season is quickly approaching, the physicians in your office have agreed to provide immunizations to adults at a reduced cost. These patients do not need to see the physician. Looking at today's schedule, you note that there are 35 patients scheduled for flu shots, two minor office surgical procedures, and a full schedule of established patients to be seen for a variety of medical issues. The first patient to be seen by the physician is a developmentally disabled adult who has Down syndrome and asthma and is being seen today for a routine check on his breathing status and preventative asthma medications.

   A. What causes asthma? (knowledge)
   B. Can you explain why the patients coming into the office for flu shots do not need to see the physician? (comprehension)
   C. How would the developmentally disabled patient benefit from getting a flu shot if ordered by the physician? (application)
   D. What is the motive of the physicians in offering the flu immunization at a reduced cost? (analysis)
   E. Can you think of a way to administer the many flu shots in your office without causing the rest of the patient schedule to get behind? (synthesis)
   F. What additional information would you need to

know about the developmentally disabled adult before you obtained the vital signs and chief complaint? (evaluation)

4. A newly diagnosed diabetic patient has come into the office today for a follow-up visit. Although he says he feels fine, you notice that his face is flushed and his breath is "fruity." Another patient complains of a sore throat and headache and has the following vital signs: T 104.2°F (O), P 124, R 32, BP 130/84 (R) sitting. The physician has made a diagnosis of strep throat and has ordered you to give an intramuscular injection of penicillin. In the third examination room, a mother is with her 10-year-old daughter who was sent home from school today with pediculosis.

A. How would you explain the fruity odor of the diabetic patient's breath? (knowledge)
B. Can you explain why the patient with strep throat has a temperature of 104.28F? (comprehension)
C. Based on what you know about pediculosis, what precautions would you take when interacting with this patient? (application)
D. Why do you think the physician has ordered an intramuscular injection of penicillin for the patient with strep throat? (analysis)
E. What would happen if you gave the injection and then realized that the patient is allergic to penicillin? How could you prevent this from happening? (synthesis)
F. How would you prioritize the tasks in this scenario? (evaluation)

5. Although one of the physicians in the group practice where you work is out of the office at a conference, the other two physicians are busy and have asked you to fill in for another medical assistant who is on vacation. This morning, there are two female physical examinations scheduled, a suspicious skin lesion to be removed on one patient, and several patients to be seen for general illness complaints. The scheduler has just informed you that a patient is coming into the office to have a laceration to his right index finger examined by the physician and a new mother is bringing in her 3-month-old baby who is fussy and pulling at both ears.

A. What equipment and supplies are necessary for the female examinations? (knowledge)
B. How would you interpret a "suspicious" skin lesion? (comprehension)
C. What questions should you be prepared to ask the patient coming into the office with the lacerated finger? (application)
D. What inference can you make about the fussy baby who is pulling at both ears? (analysis)
E. What would happen if the patient to have the skin lesion removed refused to sign the consent form? (synthesis)
F. Based on what you know about tetanus, how would you explain the physician ordering a tetanus injection for the patient with the lacerated finger? (evaluation)

PART

IV

The Clinical Laboratory

Fundamentals of Laboratory Procedures

Introduction to the Clinical Laboratory

Outline

Types of Laboratories
Reference Laboratory
Hospital Laboratory
Physician Office Laboratory
Laboratory Departments
Hematology
Coagulation
Clinical Chemistry
Toxicology

Urinalysis
Immunohematology
Immunology
Microbiology
Anatomic and Surgical
Pathology
Laboratory Personnel
**Physician Office Laboratory
Testing**

Laboratory Request Forms
Laboratory Test Panels
Laboratory Equipment
Cell Counter
Microscope
Chemistry Analyzer
Centrifuge
Incubator
Refrigerators and Freezers

Learning Objectives

Upon successfully completing this chapter, you will be able to:

1. Spell and define key terms

2. List reasons for laboratory testing

3. Outline the medical assistant's responsibility in the clinical laboratory

4. Name the kinds of laboratories where medical assistants work and the functions of each

5. Name the types of departments found in most large laboratories and give their purposes

6. List the types of personnel in laboratories and describe their jobs

7. Explain how to use a package insert to determine the procedure for a laboratory test

8. List the equipment found in most small laboratories and give the purpose of each

9. List and describe the parts of a microscope

Performance Objectives

Upon successfully completing this chapter, you will be able to:

1. Care for the microscope (Procedure 39-1)

CAAHEP

- Perform handwashing
- Practice standard precautions
- Perform routine maintenance of clinical equipment
- Care of the microscope
- Document appropriately

ABHES

- Operate and maintain facilities and equipment safely
- Practice standard precautions
- Document accurately
- Care of the microscope

Key Terms

aliquots	coagulation	immunology	quality control (QC)
anticoagulant	cytogenetics	microbiology	specimens
clinical chemistry	cytology	normal values	toxicology
Clinical Laboratory Improvement Amendments (CLIA)	hematology	panels	urinalysis
	histology	quality assurance (QA)	
	immunohematology		

The medical laboratory provides the physician with powerful diagnostic tools. Laboratory staff analyze blood, urine, and other body samples to facilitate identification of diseases and disorders. Results of laboratory testing are compared with normal or reference values (acceptable ranges for a healthy population) to determine the relative health of body systems or organs. Blood levels of various medications are determined to adjust dosages to therapeutic levels. Bacteria, viruses, parasites, and other microorganisms are identified to begin the treatment process. (See Appendix I for a list of commonly performed laboratory tests and their **normal values**.)

Laboratory testing is most commonly used for the following:

- Detecting and diagnosing disease
- Following the progress of a disease and its response to treatment
- Meeting legal requirements (e.g., drug testing, a marriage license)
- Monitoring a patient's medication and treatment
- Determining the levels of essential substances in the body
- Identifying the cause of an infection

- Determining a baseline value
- Preventing disease

As a medical assistant, you have an important role in laboratory analysis even when testing is performed at sites other than the medical office. In general, you may be responsible for the following:

- Informing patients of the proper procedure or preparation for obtaining laboratory **specimens** (samples, such as blood or urine, used to evaluate a patient's condition)
- Obtaining a quality specimen
- Arranging for appropriate transport if the specimen is to be analyzed at another site
- Performing common laboratory tests in the physician's office or clinic in compliance with the **Clinical Laboratory Improvement Amendments (CLIA)**, which are federal quality standards for all laboratory testing to ensure the accuracy, reliability, and timeliness of patient test results regardless of where the test was performed
- Documenting and maintaining a **quality assurance (QA)** program designed to ensure thorough patient care and a **quality control (QC)** protocol designed to

monitor and evaluate testing procedures, supplies, and equipment to ensure accuracy in laboratory performance

• Maintaining laboratory instruments and equipment to manufacturers' standards

Medical assistants also may control purchase of laboratory supplies and selection of reagents, which are substances used to produce a reaction in tests. In addition, you may be in charge of biohazard safety and waste disposal for the workplace. This chapter outlines the basic information you will need to ensure the quality of the laboratory testing in your facility.

PATIENT EDUCATION
SPECIMEN COLLECTION

Before collecting a specimen, instruct the patient on the proper preparation for testing. For instance, does the test require that the patient fast or follow a specific dietary regimen? Does the test require stopping any medications or modifying dose patterns? Is the timing of collection imperative, or will a random sample be sufficient? Failure to inform the patient properly before testing may result in erroneous (invalid) test results, which can cause a delay in treatment or incorrect diagnosis.

At the time of specimen collection, tell the patient:

• The name of the test (e.g., blood cell count)
• The type of specimen required (e.g., blood, stool, urine)

Be sure to tell the patient approximately how long it will take for the results to be available and how and by whom the patient will be contacted regarding the results.

Patient education requirements for drawing an HIV test vary from state to state, although most require pretest and posttest counseling. Most states do not allow HIV test results to be given over the telephone.

Types of Laboratories

Three types of laboratories significant to the medical assistant are reference, hospital, and physician office laboratories (POLs). Hospital and reference laboratories may perform hundreds of specialized tests and may process thousands of specimens per day. In contrast, POLs perform only a few types of tests on a limited number of patients.

Reference Laboratory

A reference or referral laboratory is a large facility in which thousands of tests of various types are performed each day. A reference laboratory's direct patient contact is limited to its own satellite specimen procurement stations. It also receives specimens from physicians' offices, hospitals, and clinics across the region it serves. The specimens are delivered by special courier, US mail, or other ground or air transportation delivery service. Specimens sent to reference laboratories must be packaged to withstand rough handling, pressure changes, and temperature extremes during shipment. Packaging includes placement in a special leak-proof secondary transport container (Fig. 39-1) that meets federal regulations for transportation of biohazardous materials.

Tests are performed in batch test runs, and results and reports are managed by information systems. Reference laboratories usually are not responsible for re-

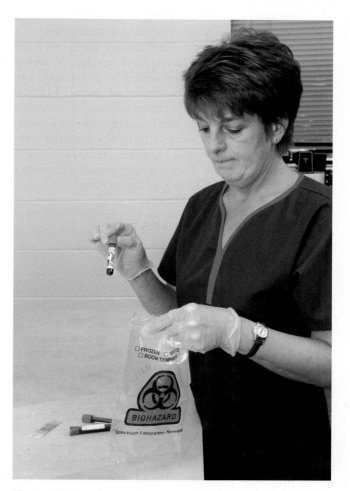

Figure 39-1 Transport containers are constructed to maintain the integrity of the specimen and to protect those who are responsible for the care and handling of possibly hazardous bodily fluids and substances.

porting test results to patients. Test results generally are returned to the referring physician, who relays the results to the patient.

Employees of reference laboratories have specific job descriptions. Specimen processors receive the specimens and log patient data and specimen information into the laboratory information system, which assigns each specimen an accession (testing identification) number. Processors also centrifuge, separate, and prepare **aliquots** (portions of specimens used for testing) if indicated and send them to the correct departments for analysis.

Testing is performed by medical technologists, medical laboratory technicians, or laboratory assistants, depending on the complexity of the procedure. Most testing is performed in large batches on automated instruments. Testing personnel are responsible for QC procedures, such as checking instruments, performing daily maintenance, and running and evaluating quality control specimens. Testing duties include loading specimens and reagents into the instruments to perform test runs and managing test results by accepting or rejecting, recording, and reporting results of QC and patient specimens.

Customer services personnel answer questions from the sites submitting specimens, track specimens, report results, add or delete tests requested by physicians, and troubleshoot problems primarily by telephone. Medical assistants may work in specimen-processing or client services. They may also be employed in testing, provided that they meet the Clinical Laboratory Improvement Amendments of 1988 (CLIA 1988) federal requirements, which include documented testing experience and supervision by a CLIA-qualified person.

 CHECKPOINT QUESTION

1. What are the requirements for medical assistants to be employed in laboratory testing?

Hospital Laboratory

The hospital laboratory serves inpatients (patients who stay overnight or longer) and outpatients (patients who come for services and leave the same day).

The hospital laboratory staff includes phlebotomists to collect and sometimes process blood specimens, laboratory assistants to collect and process specimens and perform limited testing, and medical laboratory technicians and medical technologists to perform most of the testing. Laboratories also have receptionists or secretaries who process outpatients and manage the large volume of requisitions, test results, and other information and paperwork generated daily. Medical assistants work as laboratory secretaries, receptionists, phlebotomists, or laboratory assistants.

Hospital test menus are restricted to the most commonly requested tests and tests for which results are needed immediately. Less commonly ordered tests are sent to reference laboratories. Whether the test is performed on site or sent to a reference laboratory, results generally are available within 24 to 48 hours. Results for some of the less common or more sophisticated tests may take a week or longer.

Physician Office Laboratory

The most common type of laboratory is the physician office laboratory (POL), which may vary greatly in size and diversity. POLs generally perform a limited number of waived (or low-complexity) to moderate-complexity tests (discussed in Chapter 40). Samples for less common or high-complexity tests may be obtained here but are sent to hospital or reference laboratories for testing.

The most common tests in this type of laboratory are urinalysis, blood cell counts, hemoglobin and hematocrit, and blood glucose levels. In POLs, pregnancy tests and quick screening tests for diseases such as mononucleosis and strep throat are also available. Like hospital and reference laboratories, POLs use forms that list normal ranges for various tests (Fig. 39-2).

A POL may have medical assistants who, in addition to other tasks, perform laboratory duties, such as collecting samples, performing tests, managing QC, maintaining instruments, keeping accurate records, and reporting results. Medical assistants may perform all of these tasks only if a physician monitors QC and abnormal results. The chapters in this unit will introduce you to the skills and knowledge necessary to operate a POL.

 CHECKPOINT QUESTION

2. What is a reference laboratory, and how does it differ from a POL? Name and describe the kinds of positions that a medical assistant may hold in a reference laboratory.

 LEGAL TIP

TEST RESULTS

While working in a laboratory, you will have access to the results of many confidential blood tests, such as tests for HIV, drugs, pregnancy, and sexually transmitted diseases. You have an ethical responsibility not to communicate any results to unauthorized persons. Only patients and their physicians are entitled to the results. The only exception is the provision in state laws requiring the reporting of certain test results for public safety.

Time Order Received:		Doctor:
Time Collected:	**Third Street** **PHYSICIAN'S OFFICE, INC.** **123 Main Street** **Baltimore, MD 21201**	Date:
Time Reported:		

LABORATORY

| Patient Name | Chart No. |

URINALYSIS

PHYSICAL

Color _____

Clarity_____

CHEMICAL

Leuk. Esterase _____

Nitrite _____

Urobilinogen _____

Protein _____

pH _____

Specific Gravity _____

Blood _____

Bilirubin _____

Ketones _____

Glucose _____

PREGNANCY

Urine HCG _____

Serum HCG _____

PROTHROMBIN TIME

Seconds _____

INR _____

SEDIMENTATION RATE

_____ Males 0-10

_____ Females 0-20

GLUCOSE

_____ 80-110 mg/dl

MONO

_____ NEG

STREP SCREEN

_____ NEG

PROVIDER PERFORMED MICROSCOPY

URINE MICROSCOPIC

Epis _____

WBCs_____

RBCs _____

Bacteria _____

Mucus _____

Amorphous _____

Other _____

KOH

_____

_____

WET PREP

_____

_____

_____

_____

Performed by: _____

Figure 39-2 Laboratory result form. Normal values are provided for the various tests.

Laboratory Departments

Most large laboratories are divided into departments. This is because the term laboratory includes several specialties that require varying equipment and techniques. Small laboratories, such as POLs, may have only one department. Even so, understanding the basic divisions of laboratory testing may make it easier to understand the nature of the tests and the information they provide. Following is a list of common laboratory departments, possible subdivisions, and the kinds of testing performed in each.

Hematology

The **hematology** department performs tests on blood and blood-forming tissues. The various types of cells in

the blood and the amount or number of each type of cell is determined. Common tests include complete blood count, white blood cell (WBC) count, red blood cell (RBC) count, platelet count, hemoglobin, hematocrit, WBC differential, erythrocyte sedimentation rate, and reticulocyte count.

Coagulation

Often a part of the hematology department, **coagulation** testing entails evaluating how well the body's blood clotting process is performing. The most common tests are prothrombin time and activated partial thromboplastin time. These tests are used to monitor levels of **anticoagulant** drugs, such as heparin and Coumadin, during medication therapy. An anticoagulant is anything that prevents or delays blood clotting.

Clinical Chemistry

The **clinical chemistry** department measures chemical substances in blood or serum. These substances may include hormones, enzymes, electrolytes, gases, medicines and drugs, sugars, proteins, fats, and waste products. The most common tests in small laboratories are glucose, cholesterol, blood urea nitrogen, and electrolytes.

Toxicology

Toxicology is often a separate department in the chemistry laboratory. Toxicology testing entails measuring blood levels of both therapeutic drugs and drugs of abuse.

Urinalysis

The **urinalysis** department may stand alone or be a part of one of the other laboratory sections. The most common urinalysis assay is the complete urinalysis (UA), an evaluation of the physical, chemical, and microscopic properties of urine. CLIA approves medical assistants to perform the physical and chemical evaluations of urine. With additional training and documentation, medical assistants may perform urine microscopic analysis under the supervision of a physician or medical technologist. Urine pregnancy tests also may be performed in this department.

Immunohematology

Commonly called the blood bank, this department is found only in hospitals and blood donor centers. The **immunohematology** department performs blood typing and compatibility testing of patient's blood with blood products for transfusion purposes. Blood products prepared, stored, and dispensed include whole blood, packed red cells, platelets, fresh-frozen plasma, cryoprecipitate (substances that settle out of blood after freezing), and Rh immune globulin, such as RhoGAM. Other services may include autologous donation (donation of blood by prospective patients for their own use), tissue typing for transplantation purposes, and paternity testing.

Immunology

Testing in the **immunology** department is based on the reactions of antibodies formed against certain diseases in the presence of proteins called antigens. Increased need for testing to evaluate the body's cellular immune response has resulted from treating autoimmune diseases and AIDS. Rapid tests for Group A *Streptococcus* and infectious

mononucleosis join more highly specialized flow cytometry procedures in the immunology department.

Microbiology

The **microbiology** department identifies the various microorganisms that cause disease. Through sensitivity testing, this department identifies which antibiotics will successfully treat pathogens grown from patients' specimens. Microbiology may include one or more of the following:

- Bacteriology, the study of bacteria
- Virology, the study of viruses
- Mycology, the study of fungi and yeasts
- Parasitology, the study of parasitic protozoa and worms

Anatomic and Surgical Pathology

The anatomic and surgical pathology department studies tissue and body fluid specimens from aspirations, autopsies, biopsies, organ removal, and other procedures to identify or evaluate the effects of cancer and other diseases. The following are common subdivisions of pathology, which may be individual departments in larger institutions.

Histology

Histology is the study of the microscopic structure of tissue. In histology, samples of tissue are prepared, stained, and evaluated under a microscope to determine whether disease is present. Types of histology specimens include tissue obtained through biopsy and surgical frozen sections that must be evaluated immediately to determine whether further surgery is needed.

Cytology and Cytogenetics

Cytology is the study of the microscopic structure of cells. In cytology, the individual cells in body fluids and other specimens are evaluated microscopically for the presence of disease, such as cancer. The most common cytology test is the Papanicolaou (PAP) test, in which vaginal secretions containing cells brushed or scraped from the cervix are evaluated. **Cytogenetics** is a type of cytology in which the genetic structure of the cells obtained from tissue, blood, or body fluids, such as amniotic fluid, are examined or tested for chromosome deficiencies related to genetic disease.

CHECKPOINT QUESTION

3. What departments may be found in a large laboratory? Summarize the testing done in each.

Laboratory Personnel

Within the various departments of reference and hospital laboratories, specially trained professionals oversee laboratory operations or perform testing required by physicians. Each professional position requires a particular level of education and training and has specific responsibilities (Box 39-1).

BOX 39-1

LABORATORY PERSONNEL

- Pathologist. A physician who studies disease processes. Commonly, a pathologist oversees the technical aspects of a laboratory.
- Chief technologist or laboratory manager. A supervisor who manages the day-to-day operations of a laboratory, including staffing, test menu and pricing, purchasing, and QC.
- Medical technologist or clinical laboratory scientist. A graduate of a Bachelor's (4-year) degree program (or equivalent) in medical laboratory science, who has been certified by a national certification agency. Laboratory technologists perform all levels of testing and are approved by CLIA to supervise laboratory departments.
- Medical laboratory technician or clinical laboratory technician. A graduate of an Associate (2-year) degree program (or equivalent) in medical laboratory science who is nationally certified. Laboratory technicians perform specimen testing within limits defined by CLIA.
- Laboratory assistant. A person with a high school diploma or equivalent who is a graduate of a vocational or on-the-job laboratory assistant training program. Laboratory assistants collect and process specimens and can perform waived and certain moderately complex testing if CLIA qualified.
- Phlebotomist. A professional trained to draw blood and to process blood and other samples. A phlebotomist may be a laboratory assistant, medical assistant, or person trained specifically in phlebotomy. A nationally certified phlebotomist has a high school diploma or equivalent and either is a graduate of an approved training program or has a minimum of 1 year of full-time work in phlebotomy.
- Histologist. A technician trained to process and evaluate tissue samples, such as biopsy or surgical samples.
- Cytologist. A professional trained to examine cells under the microscope and to look for ab-

normal changes; PAP smears are generally examined by cytologists.
- Specimen processor or accessioner. A professional trained to accept shipments of specimens and to centrifuge, separate, or otherwise process the samples to prepare them for testing. In addition, this position usually includes numbering and labeling the specimens and entering specimen information into a computer.

Physician Office Laboratory Testing

Many tests can be performed in an office laboratory that meets the standards set forth in the Clinical Laboratory Improvement Amendments and in modifications of the original amendment (discussed in Chapter 42). Most tests performed in the POL fall into one of two general categories: tests performed on a semiautomated machine and tests conducted with a self-contained kit. Tests in these categories vary among manufacturers.

The best source of information for safe and accurate testing is the package insert shipped inside the test kit or the instrument reagents and QC instructions specific for various office test instruments. Box 39-2 outlines the type of information contained in test package inserts.

BOX 39-2

UNDERSTANDING KIT PACKAGE INSERTS

Test package inserts provide the following basic pieces of information:

- Procedure. Explains the test method in numbered steps, usually with illustrations.
- Test principles. Outlines the test.
- Specimen required. Tells whether the test is done on blood, urine, or other body fluids and what collection method is acceptable. Indicates if the specimen may be stored for later testing and, if so, under what conditions.
- Reagents needed (or included). Lists the reagents in the kit and any other reagents or materials necessary to perform the test.
- Quality control. States recommendations for testing procedures to ensure that test results are accurate.
- Expected values. Lists normal values for comparison to results obtained.
- Interferences. Explains any factors that may alter test results or compromise test accuracy.

For many kit tests, the package insert is the only information provided to guide the performance of the test and to evaluate the results. The package insert information should be combined with routine laboratory practice in a written procedure for each test performed in the laboratory. The Commission on Office Laboratory Accreditation (discussed in Chapter 40) provides step-by-step instructions for writing a clinical procedure that meets CLIA standards.

Understanding key information needed for test performance and QC makes package inserts a simple and integral part of office laboratory testing. Ask your laboratory procedures instructor for examples of package inserts from rapid test kits for practice in obtaining this information.

Laboratory Request Forms

Laboratories provide and utilize request forms appropriate to their individual operations (Fig. 39-3). All forms should be convenient to use, with clear instructions for complete patient and physician identification to avoid errors. Most request forms cover a variety of tests, so that a single form can be used for tests in hematology, chemistry, immunology, and so on. Some forms serve as both a request and report form, listing expected values by test. Many requisitions now contain bar codes that allow fast, accurate processing and reduce specimen identification errors. Most hospitals use computer-generated forms that also contain specimen labels. Box 39-3 lists the information required on all laboratory request forms.

Laboratory Test Panels

To effectively evaluate disease processes or organ systems, laboratory tests are organized into standard groups or **panels**. The Centers for Medicare and Medicaid Services (CMS) mandate the use of panels defined by the American Medical Association (AMA) for national standardization of nomenclature and testing. The tests included in the Comprehensive Metabolic, Basic Metabolic, Electrolyte, Hepatic Function, and Lipid Panels are defined in Table 39-1.

LEGAL TIP

ORDERS FOR LABORATORY TESTS

- A written request authorized by a practitioner licensed to order laboratory tests is required before a medical assistant can proceed with collection of a specimen for any laboratory procedure.

- In the communication of a laboratory order, the licensed provider (not a delegated representative) must obtain the patient's informed consent to undergo the procedure prior to referring the patient to the laboratory for testing.
- A licensed provider must be one of three people: the physician, the physician's assistant, or the nurse practitioner (not an RN, BSN, or MSN).
- This ordering process is both an ethical and a legal requirement in all 50 states.
- Depending on institutional policy, phoned orders from the licensed provider may be accepted only if their authenticity is later documented in the patient's record by the practitioner responsible for the verbal order.
- A licensed provider may write one single order for laboratory testing to be repeated at the ordered time interval lasting up to 6 months. This is called a Standing Order and must be renewed by the licensed provider every 6 months.

Laboratory Equipment

Laboratory equipment and supplies for performing physician office tests come in a variety of types and sizes. It is not necessary to become familiar with every possible type of laboratory equipment. However, a few basic pieces are common to most small laboratories. These include the following:

- Automated cell counter
- Microscope
- Chemistry analyzer
- Centrifuge
- Incubator
- Refrigerator or freezer

Cell Counter

A cell counter is an automated analyzer used to count and size blood cells. The simplest cell counter counts only red and white blood cells and performs hemoglobin and hematocrit testing. Specimens are inserted individually, and results may be printed or read from a screen (see Chapter 42).

Cell counters also include more complex analyzers that accept hundreds of specimens and perform 12 to 15 tests, calculations, and cell differentials on each specimen. Medical assistants test specimens using a cell counter if they have received documented training in its use from a CLIA-qualified person.

THIRD SHEET PHYSICIANS OFFICE ☐ A ☐ B ☐ C ☐ D

VISIT NUMBER			DATE OF SERVICE		
MRN #			DR. NAME	
CPI #			DR #	
PATIENT NAME			US PROVIDER NAME	
DATE OF BIRTH		SUB PROVIDER NO.	BILLING AREA	

DATE OF INJURY _____ LOCATION _____ SPECIAL FSC _____

INJURY TYPE: ☐ ACCIDENTAL ☐ CAR ☐ WORKER'S COMP

EMPLOYER'S NAME & ADDRESS

PRE-AUTH. #/CAROLINA ACCESS #

REF PHYS
UPIN # _____ DOCTORS NAME _____
ADDRESS _____
CITY _____ STATE _____
TELEPHONE NO. ( )
ONSET DATE _____

I authorize any holder of medical or other information about me to release to my healthcare provider, third party processor, the Health Care Financing Administration or its intermediaries or carriers any information needed for this health care encounter or a related claim. I permit a copy of this authorization to be used in place of the original, and request payment of authorized insurance benefits be made on my behalf to the WFU Physicians. I understand I am responsible for payment of these charges. I am also responsible for payment if my insurance carrier decides this is a non-covered service or requires prior authorization which I did not obtain.

X _____
   SIGNATURE   DATE

IF ACCIDENTAL, * DATE OF ONSET   OTHER DIAGNOSIS

Code	Diagnosis	Code	Diagnosis	Code	Diagnosis	Code	Diagnosis
789.00	Abdominal Plan	700	Corns and Calluses	684	Impetigo	601.01	Prostatitis, Chronic
706.1	Acne	733.6	Costochrondritis	487.1	Influenza	569.3	Rectal Bleeding
314.00	ADD - w/o hyperactivity	595.0	Cystitis, Acute	780.52	Insomnia	714.0	Rheumatoid Arthritis
314.01	ADD - w/hyperactivity	331.0	Dementia, NOS	564.1	Irritable Bowel	477.9	Rhinitis, Allergic
309.0	Adjust React. Breif Depression	311	Depressive Disorder	702.0	Keratosis, Actinic	472.0	Rhinitis - Chronic
995.2	Adverse Drug Reaction	691.8	Dermatitis, Atopic	702.19	Keratosis, Seborrheic	460	Rhinitis - Purulent
331.0	Alzheimer's Disease	691.0	Dermatitis, diaper	386.35	Labyrinthitis	133.0	Scabies
626.0	Ameorrhea	692.6	Dermatitis, Poison Ivy*		Laceration, Uncomp. (Specify Site)*	706.2	Sebaceous Cyst.
280.0	Anemia, Fe defic., Blood loss	692.9	Dermatitis & Eczema			345.10	Seizure Gen. Convul. Epileptic
280.1	Anemia, Fe defic., Dietary Def.	250.01	Diabetes Mellitus, Insulin dep.	464.0	Laryngitis, Acute	461. __	Sinusitis, Acute (Specify sinus)
281.0	Anemia, pernicious	250.00	Diab. Mellitus, Non-insulin dep.	132. __	Lice (Specify Site)		
300.02	Anxiety Disorder, Generalized	780.4	Dizziness/Vertigo, Light-headedness			473. __	Sinusitis, Chronic (Specify sinus)
308.0	Anxiety Reaction to Stress		Drug Dependence (Specify Drug)	214.1	Lipoma, skin		
414.00	A.S.H.D.			785.6	Lymph Nodes, Enlargement	701. __	Skin Tags (Specify Sites)
493.00	Asthma, childhood	995.2	Drug Reaction, Adverse	627.2	Menopausal Symptoms		
493.00	Asthma, extrinsic	625.3	Dysmenorrhea	626.1	Menstruation, Infrequent	845.00	Sprain, Ankle*
493.10	Asthma, intrinsic	536.8	Dyspepsia	626.2	Menstrucation, Excess or Freq.	847.2	Sprain, Lumbar*
427.31	Atrial Fibrillation	788.1	Dysuria	424.0	Mitral Valve Prolapse		Sprain/Strain (Specify Site, Lig.)*
724.2	Back Pain, Low	692.9	Eczema and Dermatitis	075	Mononucleosis	034.0	Strep Throat
596.0	Bladder Neck Obstruction	345.10	Epilepsy, General Convulsive		Nevus/Mole (Specify Site)	438.	Stroke, s/p, specific
	Boil & Carbuncle (Specify Site)	784.7	Epistaxis				
		381.81	Eustachian Tube Dysfunction	278.00	Obesity, NOS		
610.0	Breast, fibrocycstic	780.7	Fatigue	715. __	Osteoarthritis (Specify Site)		Tendonitis (Specify Site)
611.72	Breast, Mass	610.1	Fibrocystic Breast Disease				
466.0	Bronchitis, Acute	729.1	Fibromyalgia	380.22	Otitis Externa, Acute	110.5	Tinea Corporis
491.20	Bronchitis, Chronic	729.0	Fibrositis	382.00	O.M., Acute Suppurative	V15.82	Tobacco Use
727.3	Bursitis	535.00	Gastritis, Acute Non-alcoholic	381.10	O.M., Chronic Serous	703.0	Toenail, Ingrown
3544.0	Carpal Tunnel Syndrome	008.8	Gastroenteritis, Viral	719. __	Pain In Joint (Specify Joint)	463	Tonsillitis, Acute
	Cellulitis (Specify Site)	530.81	GERD			465.9	Upper Respiratory Infection
		274.0	Gout, arthropathy	729.5	Pain in Limb	099.40	Urethritis, non-GC
380.4	Cerumen in Ear	309.0	Grief Reaction	723.1	Pain, Neck	788.41	Urinary Frequency
616.0	Cervicitis	346.00	Headache, Migraine, Classical	785.1	Palpitations	599.0	UTI, Site Not Specified
786.51	Chest Pain	346.10	Headache, Migraine Common	300.01	Panic Attack	623.8	Vaginal Bleeding
052.9	Chicken Pox, no complications	784.0	Headache, Muscle Tension	795.0	Pap Smear, Abnormal	627.3	Vaginitis, Post Menopausal Atrophic
078.11	Condyloma Acumination	599.7	Hematuria	533.30	Peptic Ulcer, acute, no compl.	112.1	Vulvo Vaginitis, Monilial
428.0	Congestive Heart Failure	455.44	Hemorrhoids, Ext. Thrombosed	533.70	Peptic Ulcer, chronic, no compl.	131.01	Vulvo Vaginitis, Trichomonal
372.03	Conjunctivitis	455.5	Hemorrhoids, Ext. c-Comp.	462	Pharyngitis	616.10	Vulvo Vaginitis, Other
564.0	Constipation	455.2	Hemorrhoids, Int. c-Complication	614.0	PID, Acute	078.19	Warts, Plantar
V25.01	Contraception, Birth Control Pills	054.10	Herpes, Genital	614.1	PID, Chronic	078.10	Warts, Viral
V25.02	Contraception, Other	553.3	Hiatal Hernia	486	Pneumonia	783.1	Weight Gain, Abnormal
	Contusion (Specify Site)*	272.0	Hypercholesterolemia	V22.0	pregnancy, Normal, G1	783.2	Weight Loss, Abnormal
		272.2	Hyperlipidemia	V22.1	Pregnancy, Normal, not G1	V70.0	Well Adult Physical
491.20	C.O.P.D. w/o Acute Exacerbation	401.1	Hypertensionn, Benign Essential	625.4	Premenstrual Tension Syn.	V72.3	Well Woman Gyne.
491.21	C.O.P.D. w/Acute Exacerbation	402.10	Hypertensive H.D. w/o CHF	600	Prostate, Hyperpl.		
918.1	Corneal Abrasion*	244.9	Hypothyrodism, Acquired	601.0	Prostatitis, Acute		

Figure 39-3 Laboratory requisition. (Courtesy of Quest Diagnostics, 2007.)

BOX 39-3

LABORATORY REQUEST FORMS: COMMONLY REQUIRED INFORMATION

- Patient's database. This includes name, address, social security number, and the medical office identification number to avoid errors with identical names. Other identifying information may be included.
- Patient's birth date and gender. Many test results vary with age and sex.
- Date and time of collection. Often test results are affected by the passage of time or the time of day the specimen was collected.
- Physician's name and address or identification number. Results may have to be reported immediately; this information also avoids errors in reporting.

- Checklist of the test or tests to be performed. These may be grouped under one heading as a panel, such as a renal panel or liver panel, which includes more than one test to determine the state of health of one organ, or a general health profile, such as a complete blood count.

Other required information may include the source of the specimen, such as culture swabs for microbiology tests; medications the patient is taking that may alter certain test results (e.g., anticoagulants affecting prothrombin time); directions for reporting (e.g., an immediate need should be marked STAT); and total volume of a 24-hour urine specimen.

TABLE 39-1 Test Panels Defined by the AMA and Mandated by CMS

Comprehensive Metabolic	Basic Metabolic	Electrolyte	Hepatic Function	Lipid
Glucose	Glucose	Sodium	Albumin	Cholesterol
Calcium	Calcium	Potassium	Total protein	Triglycerides
Sodium	Sodium	Chloride	Alkaline phosphatase (ALP)	HDL
Potassium	Potassium	CO2	Alanine aminotransferase (ALT; SGPT)	LDL
Chloride	Chloride		Aspartate aminotransferase (AST; SGOT)	
CO2	CO2			Total bilirubin
BUN	BUN			Direct bilirubin
Creatinine	Creatinine			
Albumin				
Total protein				
Alkaline phosphatase (ALP)				
Alanine aminotransferase (ALT; SGPT)				
Aspartate aminotransferase (AST; SGOT)				
Total bilirubin				

CHECKPOINT QUESTION

4. Why are package inserts crucial for safe and accurate testing?

Microscope

The microscope is used to identify and count cells and microorganisms in blood and other body specimens. Learning how to use a microscope properly requires time and repeated practice. The compound microscope is the type most commonly used in the medical office. The compound microscope is a two-lens system in which ocular and objective lenses together provide the total magnification. A light source illuminates the objects as they are magnified. Figure 39-4 shows a microscope and its various parts.

The *frame*, which consists of the arm and base, is the basic structural component of the microscope. The oculars at the top of the instrument are for the user's eyes. Each is marked with its magnification, usually ×10. Binocular microscopes (two eyepieces) minimize eyestrain and have adjustments to allow for variations in spacing between the user's eyes.

To bring the object to be viewed into focus, the *coarse adjustment knob* is used with the lower powered objective to focus on the object; the *fine adjustment knob* is used with the higher powered objective or the oil immersion lens for the greatest definition. Always focus in two steps. First look at the slide and objective from the side (not through the ocular or oculars), bringing the slide very close to the lens. Then look through the ocular or oculars as you move the slide farther from the lens to bring it into focus. This procedure will prevent damage to the lens from contact with the slide.

The *nosepiece* houses three or four objective lenses and rotates to bring the objective into working position. Pressure to the objectives should never be used to rotate lenses. Only the grip should be used to make this adjustment. The magnification power is marked on each objective. The shorter, or low-power, objective magnifies ×10. The higher power magnifies ×40 for closer observation. With the use of oil, the third objective, called the oil immersion lens, magnifies ×100. Some microscopes have a fourth objective with a ×4 lens to scan larger specimens. To determine the total magnification of a specimen, multiply the magnification of the working objective by the magnification of the ocular lens (×10):

- Low power: 10 × 10 = 100
- High power: 40 × 10 = 400
- Oil immersion: 100 × 10 = 1000

The *stage* is the flat surface that holds the slide for viewing. An opening in the solid surface allows illumination of the slide from below. Many stages have clips to hold the slide in place and to allow manual movement of the slide as needed. Some stages mechanically adjust the position vertically or horizontally by moving adjustment knobs, also called X- and Y-axis knobs.

The *condenser* concentrates the light rays to focus on the slide. The condenser is adjustable. In the lower position, the light focus is reduced; in the higher position, it is increased.

The *diaphragm*, in the condenser, consists of interlocking plates that adjust into a variable-sized opening, or iris, to regulate the amount of light from the source in conjunction with the condenser. The more highly magnified the slide must be, the greater the need for light.

The *light source* is housed in the base.

Microscopes are delicate, expensive instruments. To ensure that the microscope used in your clinical laboratory is kept in good working order, you must handle it properly (Box 39-4) and maintain it according to the manufacturer's standards (Procedure 39-1). Be sure to place it in a low-traffic area and away from any source of vibration, such as a centrifuge. It should always be covered when not in use.

 CHECKPOINT QUESTION

5. How do the three objective lenses of the microscope differ?

Figure 39-4 Basic components of the standard light microscope. (Courtesy of Nikon, Melville, NY.)

Eyepiece
Body tube
Nosepiece
Objective lens
Stage
Diaphragm
Condenser
Light source
Arm
Coarse adjustment knob
Fine adjustment knob
Base

Chemistry Analyzer

Like cell counters, traditional chemistry analyzers vary from simple instruments that perform one or a few tests and require manual operation to complex analyzers that

BOX 39-4

PROPER HANDLING OF A MICROSCOPE

- Always lift your microscope with one hand holding the "arm" and the other hand under the base; avoid bumping or jarring the scope. This delicate instrument can easily go out of alignment if it is handled roughly. You will only be able to carry one microscope or lamp at a time, if you are to avoid the possibility of damage.
- Use your microscope on a sturdy, solid surface and away from the edge. Vibrations can also cause the microscope to go out of alignment.
- Never touch the lenses of the eyepieces and objectives with your finger. Keep all glass and optical lenses clean. Use lens paper dipped in a lens cleaning solution to gently wipe dust and oils off the eyepieces, objectives, condenser, and illumination glass. (Never use a paper towel, tissue, or Kleenex to wipe a lens—the fibers in them will scratch the lenses.)
- Keep the stage and the other metal parts free of excess oil. An alcohol wipe is best but is not recommended for use on the lenses.
- To keep your microscope in top condition for years, our manufacturer recommends that you have the microscope professionally serviced once a year.
- When you are finished using your microscope, rotate the nosepiece so that it is on the low-power objective, roll the nosepiece so that it is all the way down to the stage, and then replace the dust cover.
- Always keep the dust cover on your scope when it is not in use.

to the strip with an automated pipette. Other analyzers use wet reagent systems with special reagent packs required for each type of test. These machines can usually be interfaced with an office computer to allow for storage and retrieval of results. Whatever the analyzer, the operator must follow the specific manufacturer's instructions for proper care and use.

Centrifuge

A centrifuge swings its contents in a circle to separate liquids into their component parts. A whole blood specimen, when centrifuged, is separated into a bottom layer of heavy red blood cells, a thin middle layer of platelets and white blood cells called the buffy coat (Fig. 39-5), and a top liquid layer that is the lightest of the components. The top layer is serum if the specimen was allowed to clot before centrifuging or plasma if the specimen was anticoagulated and not allowed to clot.

Tubes must always be balanced in the centrifuge. If an uneven number of tubes is to be spun, a tube with water must counterbalance the odd tube. Try to place tubes with approximately the same level of liquid in opposing spaces. All tubes must be securely capped. Never start centrifugation until the lid is locked (most will not start until the lid is securely locked). Never open the centrifuge until all motion has stopped, and never stop the spin with your hand. Follow the manufacturer's recommendations for cleaning, oiling, and maintaining the centrifuge. As with all equipment, read the instructions before operation.

perform 30 or more tests per sample and are operated by computer.

Advances in laboratory instrumentation have led to the development of portable and even hand-held devices for point-of-care testing. These devices are especially suited to POL testing because they are simple to operate, require only small amounts of sample for testing and provide results in minutes. The machine computes the result and displays it on a screen and/or provides a printout of results.

For high-volume testing and to perform a large variety of tests, a number of bench-top chemistry analyzers are suitable for POL testing. Several use dry reagent technology, in which all reagents are impregnated into a special strip or card. The strip or card is inserted into the machine, and a drop of whole blood or serum is applied

Figure 39-5 Centrifuged blood specimen. (Reprinted with permission from McCall R. Phlebotomy Essentials. Baltimore: Lippincott Williams & Wilkins, 2003.)

A special type of centrifuge called a microhematocrit centrifuge is used to perform hematocrit testing, further discussed in Chapter 42.

 CHECKPOINT QUESTION

6. How does the centrifuge work, and what is its purpose?

Incubator

Microbiology specimens require a suitable environment to thrive and reproduce.

Culture media inoculated with specimens are stored in an incubator for approximately 24 hours to allow microbes to reproduce to a large enough quantity to be identified. The incubator is set at about body temperature (99°F or 37°C), and a daily log is maintained to record the incubator temperature.

Refrigerators and Freezers

Laboratory refrigerators and freezers are similar to those used in the home, but their uses are very different. They are used to store reagents, kits, and specimens. The temperature is critical and must be measured and recorded daily. The refrigerator should be able to maintain a constant temperature of 4 to 8°C to remain in service. Food should never be stored in these refrigerators because of the possibility of biohazard contamination. These also vary in size and can be purchased according to office needs and space.

 MEDIA MENU

- Student CD
  - CMA/RMA Certification Exam Review
- LWW's Medical Assisting Skills DVD
  - Procedure 39-1
- Pemium Online Course
  http://thePoint.lww.com/Kronenberger3e
- Internet Resources

  LiveAdvise Online Tutoring & Competency Training
  http://thePoint.lww.com/LiveAdvise

  Commission on Office Laboratory Accreditation
  www.cola.org

  Centers for Medicare and Medicaid Services
  http://www.cms.hhs.gov/

PROCEDURE 39-1:   Caring for a Microscope

Purpose: To protect the integrity and function of the microscope
Equipment: Lens paper, lens cleaner, gauze, mild soap solution, microscope, hand disinfectant, surface disinfectant

Steps	Reasons
1. Wash your hands.	Handwashing aids infection control.
2. Assemble the equipment.	
3. If you need to move the microscope, carry it in both hands, one holding the base and the other holding the arm. (See Box 39-4.)	Jarring or dropping the microscope will damage the optics.
4. Clean the optical areas following these steps: A. Place a drop or two of lens cleaner on a piece of lens paper. B. Wipe each eyepiece thoroughly with the lens paper. Do not touch the optical areas with your fingers.	Do not use tissue or gauze because either may scratch the lenses. Direct contact will transfer oils from your skin to the optical surfaces.

(continued)

PROCEDURE 39-1:　Caring for a Microscope *(continued)*

Steps	Reasons

C.　Wipe each objective lens, starting with the lowest power and continuing to the highest power (usually an oil immersion lens). If the lens paper appears to have dirt or oil on it, use a clean section of the lens paper or a new piece of lens paper with cleaner.

Step 4B. Wipe each eyepiece with lens paper and lens cleaner.
Wiping in this manner ensures that you progress from the cleanest area to the least clean area (oil immersion lens).

D.　Using a new piece of dry lens paper, wipe each eyepiece and objective lens so that no cleaner remains.

E.　With a new piece of lens paper moistened with lens cleaner, clean the condenser and illuminator optics.

Step 4C. Wipe each objective lens with lens paper and lens cleaner. Clean oil objective last so you won't carry its oil to the other objective lenses.
Removing the cleaner completely prevents distortion by residue.

5.　Clean the areas other than the optics:
A.　Moisten gauze with mild soap solution or use an alcohol wipe and wipe all areas other than the optics, including the stage, base, and adjustment knobs.
B.　Moisten another gauze with water and rinse the washed areas.

Step 4E. Clean and dry the condenser and illuminator optics.

This removes oil and dirt from mechanical and structural surfaces.

(continued)

PROCEDURE 39-1: Caring for a Microscope *(continued)*

Steps	Reasons
6. To store the cleaned microscope, ensure that the light source is turned off. Rotate the nosepiece so that the low-power objective is pointed down toward the stage. Cover the microscope with the plastic dust cover that came with it or a small trash bag.	This protects the mechanism and surfaces between uses.
7. Document microscope cleaning on the microscope maintenance log sheet.	Documentation of instrument service history is required for all laboratory equipment.

Step 7. Sample instrument log sheet.

Note: To maintain precision focusing, the microscope should be used in a low-traffic area and away from any source of vibration, such as a centrifuge.

Note: Follow the manufacturer's recommendations for changing the light bulb and servicing the microscope.

Charting Example:

8/26/2008 11:30 AM Microscope cleaned according to manufacturer's recommendations

—D. Howell, CMA

Chapter Summary

- Laboratory staff analyze blood, urine, and other body samples to facilitate identification of diseases and disorders.
- The most common tests in a POL are urinalysis, blood cell counts, hemoglobin and hematocrit, and blood glucose levels.

- The test kit or reagent package insert is the key tool for accurate testing and QC instructions.
- Laboratory test panels defined by the AMA and mandated by CMS provide national standardization of nomenclature and testing to evaluate disease processes and organ systems.

1. Review Box 39-2 on understanding package inserts. Ask your instructor for a copy of a package insert from a test kit you will be using in class. Locate each bulleted item listed in the box and find the corresponding information on your sample package insert.

2. Review the section of this chapter describing reference laboratories. The physician requests a laboratory test that is unfamiliar to you. You do not find the test listed in the reference laboratory's test catalogue. How would you get the appropriate patient preparation and specimen collection, processing, and transport instructions for the requested test?

Answers to Checkpoint Questions

1. Medical assistants may be employed in testing, provided they meet the Clinical Laboratory Improvement Amendments of 1988 (CLIA 1988) federal requirements, which include documented testing experience and supervision by a CLIA-qualified person.

2. A reference laboratory is a large facility that serves a particular region, performing thousands of specialized tests daily. In contrast, the POL performs only a few kinds of common tests and refers other specimens to a reference laboratory for testing. Medical assistants working in reference laboratories may be employed as specimen processors, sorting specimens and entering data into computers. They may also work as customer service personnel, answering telephones, tracking specimens, and reporting results to the centers from which the specimens were collected.

3. A large laboratory may have the following departments:

   - Hematology, testing for abnormalities of blood and blood-forming tissues
   - Coagulation, measuring the blood's ability to clot
   - Clinical chemistry, measuring substances in blood
   - Toxicology, measuring drug levels in blood
   - Urinalysis, evaluating physical, chemical, and microscopic properties of urine
   - Immunohematology, performing blood typing and compatibility testing for transfusion
   - Immunology, evaluating antigen–antibody reactions
   - Microbiology, identifying pathogens and effective antibiotic treatment
   - Anatomic and surgical pathology, studying tissue and body fluid specimens to identify or evaluate the effects of disease

4. Because tests vary among manufacturers, the package insert is the best source of information on performing the test and evaluating the results.

5. The low-power objective lens magnifies objects ×10 and is used for scanning. The high-power objective lens magnifies objects ×40 and is used for close observation. The oil immersion lens magnifies objects ×100 for close visualization.

6. A centrifuge swings its contents in a circle to separate liquids into their component parts. Various tests require different components of the specimen.

CHAPTER 40

CLIA Compliance and Laboratory Safety

Outline

Clinical Laboratory Improvement Amendments
Laws Governing the Clinical Laboratory
Levels of Testing
Laboratory Standards
Laboratory Quality Assurance
Patient Test Management

Quality Control
Proficiency Testing
Reagent Management
Instrument Calibration and Maintenance

Laboratory Safety
Occupational Safety and Health Administration (OSHA)
Safety Guidelines
Incident Reports

Learning Objectives

Upon successfully completing this chapter, you will be able to:

1. Spell and define the key terms

2. Explain the significance of the Clinical Laboratory Improvement Amendments and how to follow their regulations to ensure quality control

3. Using CLIA guidelines, identify laboratory tests that are and are not within the scope of practice for a medical assistant

4. Define panic values and document the proper notification to the health care professional

5. Identify results that require follow-up and document action in chart

6. Identify how to handle all test results whether normal or abnormal and document on a flow sheet

7. Identify and use quality control methods

8. Define OSHA and state its purpose

9. List the laboratory safety guidelines

Performance Objectives

Upon successfully completing this chapter, you will be able to:

1. Screen and follow-up test results and document laboratory results appropriately (Procedure 40-1)

2. Use methods of quality control (Procedure 40-2)

3. Perform routine maintenance of clinical equipment (Procedure 40-3)

CAAHEP

- Screen and follow-up test results
- Document appropriately
- Perform routine maintenance of clinical equipment
- Use methods of quality control

ABHES

- Use quality control
- Screen and follow-up patient test results
- Document accurately
- Maintain licenses and accreditation
- Perform routine maintenance of clinical equipment safely
- OSHA compliance rules and regulations

Key Terms

aerosol
calibration
Chemical Hygiene Plan (CHP)
Clinical and Laboratory Standards Institute (CLSI)

Clinical Laboratory Improvement Amendments (CLIA)
flow sheet
laboratory procedure manual

material safety data sheet (MSDS)
normal values
Occupational Safety and Health Administration (OSHA)

panic values
quality assurance (QA)
quality control (QC)
reportable range
shifts
trends

Clinical Laboratory Improvement Amendments

Laws Governing the Clinical Laboratory

With the goals of standardizing laboratory testing and enforcing quality protocols, Congress originally passed the **Clinical Laboratory Improvement Amendments (CLIA)** in 1988 to establish regulations governing any facility that performs testing for the diagnosis, prevention, or treatment of human disease or for assessment of patients' health status. While final modification of the amendments was made on January 24, 2003, with an effective date of April 24, 2003, the amendments maintain their original name, CLIA `88.

Standards were developed to cover all laboratories from large regional laboratories to the smallest physician office laboratory (POL). The Centers for Medicare and Medicaid Services (CMS) regulate all laboratory testing (except research) performed on humans in the United States through CLIA. The Division of Laboratory Services of the Survey and Certification Group in the Center for Medicaid and State Operations is responsible for implementing the CLIA program.

CLIA regulations set standards for the following:

- Laboratory operations
- Application and user fees
- Procedures for enforcement of the amendment
- Approval of programs for accreditation

Levels of Testing

CLIA regulations established the three levels of testing discussed next based on the complexity of the testing method.

Waived Tests

Waived tests are low-complexity tests that require minimal judgment or interpretation. They include many tests simple enough for the patient to perform at home (e.g., dipstick urinalysis and glucose monitoring). If these are the only types of tests performed on site, the laboratory can apply for a certificate of waiver (CLIA Waiver Registration), but it still must follow all manufacturers' recommendations for each piece of equipment or product used for testing.

The following are a few of the tests listed in the waived category:

- Urine dipstick or reagent tablets
- Fecal occult blood packets

- Ovulation testing in packets with color comparison charts
- Urine pregnancy testing kits using color comparison charts
- Nonautomated erythrocyte sedimentation rate tests
- Nonautomated copper sulfate testing for hemoglobin
- Centrifuged microhematocrits
- Low-complexity blood glucose determination testing
- Hemoglobin by single analyte instruments with self-contained reagent and specimen interaction and direct measurement and readout

Many additional tests, including rapid strep kits, have waived methodologies available, but the Food and Drug Administration (FDA) has not provided waived status to every manufacturer. The most up-to-date listing of available waived tests can be found on the CMS website.

Moderate-Complexity Tests

Most of the testing performed in large, established laboratories has moderate complexity. The following are some moderate-complexity tests commonly performed in POLs with moderate-complexity certification:

- Urine and throat cultures
- Automated testing for cholesterol, high-density lipoproteins, and triglycerides
- Gram staining
- Microscopic urinalysis
- Automated hematology procedures with or without a differential requiring no operator intervention during the analytic process and no interpretation of a histogram
- Manual white blood cell count differentials without identification of atypical cells
- Automated coagulation procedures that do not require intervention during analysis
- Automated chemistry procedures that do not require intervention during analysis
- Automated urinalyses that do not require intervention during analysis

A subcategory of moderate-complexity testing called provider-performed microscopy (PPM) requires POLs to have a special registration certificate. PPM can be performed only by a physician or dentist or by a nurse midwife, nurse practitioner, or physician assistant under the direct supervision of a physician. PPM tests include the following:

- All direct wet-mount preparations to be tested for bacteria, fungi, parasites, and human cellular elements
- All potassium hydroxide preparations
- Pinworm examinations
- Fern tests
- Postcoital direct qualitative examinations of vaginal or cervical mucus

- Urine sediment examinations
- Nasal smear examinations for granulocytes
- Fecal leukocyte examinations
- Qualitative semen analysis (limited to the presence or absence of sperm and detection of motility)

High-Complexity Tests

High-complexity tests, which are rarely performed in medical offices, include the following:

- Advanced cell studies (cytogenetics)
- Cytology (e.g., Pap tests)
- Histocompatibility
- Histopathology
- Manual cell counts

If the level of testing to be performed is in question, it must be considered high complexity until its level can be designated by CMS. CMS publishes a list of all tests in the moderate-complexity category. States may establish stricter rules than those set by the governing body, but they may not adopt less strict rules.

Laboratory personnel must also meet the educational levels set forth by CLIA. These guidelines and their updates can be found in the *Federal Register*. The *Federal Register* is the official daily publication for rules, proposed rules, and notices of federal agencies and organizations, as well as executive orders and other presidential documents. You can access the *Federal Register* through this website: http://www.gpoaccess.gov/fr/index.html. CLIA considers any facility to be a laboratory if it performs tests on human specimens for the purpose of providing information for the diagnosis, prevention, or treatment of any disease or impairment of a human being or the assessment of the health of a human being. Laboratories must meet federal requirements. CLIA applies even if you only perform one or a few basic tests and even if you are not charging for testing. Your laboratory must have a CLIA certificate to meet federal requirements. The application for a CLIA certificate (Form CMS116) is available via the following website: http://www.cms.hhs.gov/cmsforms/downloads/cms116.pdf. The CLIA application collects information about your laboratory's operation that is necessary to calculate fees to be assessed and to fulfill the requirements of CLIA. Waived tests are not exempt from CLIA. Laboratories performing only tests categorized as waived must apply for a CLIA certificate of waiver.

As a source of CLIA '88 compliance support for POLs, the Commission on Office Laboratory Accreditation (COLA) was established. COLA was subsequently granted deemed status under CLIA. The Joint Commission on Accreditation of Healthcare Organizations (JCAHO) also recognized COLA's laboratory accreditation program and granted it deemed status under JCAHO standards. COLA works to support the health care industry by providing knowledge and resources for maintaining quality laboratory operations.

CHECKPOINT QUESTION

1. List the three levels of laboratory testing defined by CLIA. Which level of testing is approved for performance by medical assistants?

Laboratory Standards

Laboratories that perform moderate- or high-complexity testing may be inspected in an unannounced visit every year by representatives from CMS or the Centers for Disease Control and Prevention (CDC) under the direction of the Department of Health and Human Services. They must meet all standards set by CLIA. Penalties for failure to comply include fines and testing restrictions.

Laboratory Quality Assurance

Quality assurance (QA) is a plan for ensuring the quality of all areas of the laboratory's technical and support functions. Quality assurance should monitor the following laboratory functions:

- Patient preparation
- Specimen collection, processing, preservation, and transportation
- Test analysis, reporting and interpretation

The laboratory must have a written QA policy that is communicated to all of the laboratory staff. This document should contain methods for monitoring and assessment of all phases of the total laboratory process. The purpose of the QA policy is to prevent problems before they occur. Since all the problems that could happen cannot be anticipated, the QA plan should be continually reviewed and annually updated. When an there is an error or problem, corrective action must begin and be documented. Outcomes of correcting the problem should lead to new QA policies to prevent recurrence. When the lab is inspected, the inspector will expect to see a well-written QA policy that monitors all phases of the laboratory process, is actively reviewed, and shows evidence of corrective action when a problem is discovered and evaluation of that remedial action for effectiveness.

The laboratory's policy and procedure manual should cover recommendations for continuing education for the laboratory personnel and evaluation methods for ensuring that workers are competent. The qualifications and responsibilities of all laboratory workers are specified by CLIA, with education and training requirements for all levels of personnel. Employers must ascertain the educational background of employees,

provide opportunities for continuing education, and conduct or provide for proficiency testing. This information must be documented and available for inspection by CLIA representatives.

The following are standard issues that should be covered in the POL Quality Assurance Plan:

- Patient test management
- Quality control
- Proficiency testing
- Reagent management
- Instrument calibration and maintenance

CHECKPOINT QUESTION

2. What is the purpose of a laboratory quality assurance policy?

Patient Test Management

A written system must be in place to ensure that the specimens are properly maintained and identified and that the results are accurately recorded and reported. Policies must be written for standards of patient care and employee conduct. Each test performed will be evaluated for safety, reliability, and diagnostic indication for its performance.

Policy and procedure manuals will clearly outline patient preparation, specimen handling, how tests are to be performed, alternatives to the usual testing methods for specific situations, and what to do in the event of questionable testing results.

CLIA Standards for Laboratory Procedure Manuals

The laboratory procedure manual is the primary reference in operating the POL. CLIA regulations require each laboratory to have its own procedure manual describing how to perform every test in the laboratory. The physician laboratory director is required to review and sign the procedure manual. If a change in procedure is made, it must be approved, signed, and dated by the director. This eliminates the need for an annual review of the manual. If there is a change in directors, the new director must review and sign the manual. All procedures must be dated when they are put into use and when they are discontinued. Written procedures must be kept on file for 2 years after they are discontinued.

Laboratories performing moderate-complexity testing, such as using cell counters for complete blood counts, must have procedures for performing these tests and reporting the patient results, calibrating the instrument, quality control, and resolving problems. Some suggestions for developing a procedure manual are listed in Box 40-1.

BOX 40-1

SUGGESTED SHORTCUTS FOR DEVELOPING A LABORATORY PROCEDURE MANUAL

- Use test package inserts and operator's manuals as the primary reference.
- Use a standard format so all procedures contain the essential elements.
- Keep a computer file and a hard copy of your manual.
- Use a binder with tabs and sheet protectors so that it is easy to update the manual as changes occur.
- You may use package inserts in your manual if you supplement them with instructions for reporting patient results, protocols for reporting panic values, actions if the test becomes inoperable, and criteria and procedures for referring the specimens to another laboratory including specimen submission and handling.

When using package inserts, the physician laboratory director must review and approve any modifications in the procedure.

CHECKPOINT QUESTION

3. What does a laboratory procedure manual contain, and why is it necessary?

ETHICAL TIP

Laboratory Code of Ethics

I. Duty to the Patient

Laboratory professionals are accountable for the quality of the laboratory services they provide. This includes maintaining individual competence in judgment and performance and striving to safeguard the patient from incompetent or illegal practice by others.

Laboratory professionals exercise sound judgment in establishing, performing, and evaluating laboratory testing.

Laboratory professionals maintain confidentiality of patient information and test results. They safeguard the dignity and privacy of patients and provide accurate information to other health care professionals about the patient services they have provided.

II. Duty to Colleagues and the Profession

Laboratory professionals strive to maintain a reputation of honesty, integrity, and reliability.

Laboratory professionals actively strive to establish cooperative and respectful working relationships with other health care professionals with the primary objective of ensuring a high standard of care for the patients they serve.

III. Duty to Society

Laboratory professionals have the responsibility to contribute to the general well-being of the community.

Laboratory professionals comply with laws and regulations pertaining to the practice of laboratory medicine and seek with conscience to change those that do not meet high standards of care and practice.

Source: The American Society for Clinical Laboratory Science: http://www.utmem.edu/ascls/Region3/Ethics.html.

Screen and Follow-Up Test Results

The Medical Assistant's responsibilities do not stop with being familiar with the laboratory tests performed in a specific office laboratory. Key information needed to screen and follow-up any report will be documented on the report (Procedure 40-1).

The **normal values** (normal range or reference interval) for the test or tests included in the report will be listed. They are the test results usually seen in a healthy population. The best normal value source for the POL is the manufacturer's package insert for the test being reported. Reference laboratories have a more detailed process for establishing normal ranges. Manufacturer's data and reference books are sources for target ranges. The reference lab itself, however, must perform extensive testing to prove that the normal range it prints on its reports is true for the population it tests. When screening a laboratory report, start by noting test results that fall outside the listed normal values.

Panic values are also known as alert values or critical limits. Critical limits define the boundaries of the life-threatening values of laboratory test results. See Box 40-2 for results considered to be panic values in some offices. Urgent clinician notification of critical results is a responsibility of the laboratory. Documentation of the proper notification of such test results to the health care professional responsible for the patient is essential. Each medical office should establish a list of panic values agreed upon by the physician(s) in

BOX 40.2

EXAMPLE CRITICAL VALUES FOR SOME COMMON LABORATORY TESTS

Analyte (Lab Test)	Critical Values Low	High
Serum glucose	<40 or 45 mg/dL	>500 mg/dL
Serum sodium	<120 mEq/L	>160 mEq/L
Serum potassium	<2.5 mEq/L	>6.0 mEq/L
Serum calcium (total)	<7.0 mg/dL	>13.0 mg/dL
White blood cell count	$<2 \times 10^{-9}$/L	$>50 \times 10^{-9}$/L
Platelet count	$<20 \times 10^{-9}$/L	$>1,000 \times 10^{-9}$/L
Prothrombin time	Not applicable	International normalized ratio (INR) >5
Partial thromboplastin time	Not applicable	>100 seconds

that office. In addition, an office protocol for alerting the physician and documenting this communication should be defined.

In addition to responding to panic values, the medical assistant must obtain from the physician an understanding of abnormal test results that require follow-up, what that follow-up should entail, and a format for documenting that action in the patient's chart. A standard protocol for managing abnormal results will ensure that the physician is alerted to all the conditions that require action or intervention. Each office will have its own procedure for handling all test results, whether normal or abnormal. Steps in this procedure should include:

- Receiving and processing incoming laboratory reports.
- Review of reports for results requiring priority action.
- Paper flow for priority and routine results.

 CHECKPOINT QUESTION

4. What are the two essential steps in following up on a panic value?

Each state has laws for reporting communicable diseases. The Department of Public Health for your state requires health care providers to notify them of the occurrence of a reportable disease. Check with your state for a list of all conditions that should be reported to your city/county health department. There will be requirements that some conditions be reported within 24 hours of suspected or confirmed diagnosis by the most rapid means available and that others be reported within 3 days of suspected or confirmed diagnosis. Check your office policy manual or with your practice manager for the assignment of reporting responsibilities in your office.

For the tests performed in the POL, the medical assistant must know how to reference the **reportable range**

of each assay reported from that laboratory. The reportable range is the very lowest and highest value the manufacturer has documented the test can determine. Manufacturers provide these ranges in their package inserts and instrument manuals. If a test result reads 12 on the laboratory instrument, but the manufacturer documents the reportable range to be 40 to 500, the medical assistant must report the test result as less than 40 instead of reporting the instrument reading of 12.

Using Flow Sheets to Improve Patient Care

A **flow sheet** is a form that gathers all the important data regarding a patient's condition. The flow sheet stays in the patient's chart and serves as a reminder of care and a record of whether care expectations have been met. Each time the patient makes an office visit, no matter the chief complaint, the doctor will look at the flow sheet and address the patient's condition that warrants the flow sheet in addition to the sore throat or whatever the reason for the patient visit. Each time a lab report or test result monitored on the flow sheet comes back to the chart, the data is logged in its spot on the flow sheet. This allows the patient's critical indicator(s) to be monitored at a glance, as in Figure 40-1.

Medical assistants (MA) play a key role in maintenance of patient flow sheets and in bringing trends to the attention of the physician. Flow sheets only serve their purpose if they are used consistently. Since MAs have their hands on patients' charts for multiple tasks (i.e., documenting phone messages and prescription refills) there are multiple opportunities to keep the charts current. If the office maintains a patient registry (i.e., a list of patients who are being tracked with a certain flow sheet), this can be managed on schedule because you will know exactly which charts to pull. And since the information you will need to review will now be organized into a single page, the task is manageable. With the

DIABETES CARE FLOW SHEET

Name: RUTH PERKINS

Date of birth: 11-17-27

HGB A1C   5.4-8.0   4-6 months

Date:	12-04-99	5-7-00						
Result:	9.7	9.1						
Date:		10-2-00						
Result:		10.3						

BP   130/80

Date:								
Result:	157/92	149/85						
Date:	1-19-00							
Result:	162/88	180/92						

BUN   7-18 mg/dL   annually

Date:								
Result:	24							

Creatinine   0.5-1.2 mg/dL   annually

Date:								
Result:	1.3							

LIPIDS   annually

Date:								
Result:	279							
Trig:	198							
HDL:	32							
LDL:	220							

Figure 40-1 Diabetes care flow sheet.

physician's approval you can then send reminder postcards to patients who are due for testing.

Quality Control

A comprehensive **quality control (QC)** program monitors each phase of the laboratory process, including specimen collection, specimen processing, testing, and reporting results. The programs also monitor reagents, instruments, and personnel in addition to actual test performance. Each laboratory must have its own written policies and procedures that include instructions to ensure that all QC standards for monitoring the accuracy and quality of each test are in place for all levels of testing the laboratory conducts. The protocols ensure reliable findings and identification and elimination of errors. Control sample manufacturers provide specimens comparable to human specimens with known reference ranges. Testing control samples at the same time the patient specimen is tested or when a new reagent kit is received ensures that all components are performing as required. Reagent and instru-

ment manufacturers document frequencies for performing QC on their products. The performance of these controls must be recorded in the QC log.

To record compliance with CLIA measures, a record must be kept of each control sample result. The log must show the date and time of the test, the control or standard results expected, what results were obtained, the action taken for correction, if any, and the initials of the person performing the test. Documentation must be consistent, and the records must be retained for at least 2 years. Computer software programs are also available for maintaining this data.

The **Clinical and Laboratory Standards Institute (CLSI)** establishes rules to ensure the safety, standards, and integrity of all testing performed on human specimens. Figure 40-2 is an example of a form containing information recommended by CLSI on which control sample testing can be recorded. If controls do not fall in the range given in the manufacturer's package insert, testing cannot be conducted. The cause must be discovered and corrected before reporting any patient results. Start by

QUALITATIVE QC LOG SHEET FOR _____ RECORD LOT NUMBER IF DIFFERENT FROM LAST LOT NUMBER.								
TEST DATE	KIT LOT	POSITIVE CONTROL LOT #	NEGATIVE CONTROL LOT #	POSITIVE CONTROL RESULT	NEGATIVE CONTROL RESULT	OK TO USE?	IF NO, CORRECTIVE ACTION	INITIALS

Figure 40-2 Quality control log sheet.

checking the reagents and controls for expiration dates, accurate reconstitution, and expiration dates once reconstituted. Next check to see that the testing instrument is clean and functioning properly. If all of this has been done, reconstitute or open a new control sample or reagent and begin the process again.

 CHECKPOINT QUESTION

5. List seven areas monitored by a comprehensive quality control program.

Methods of Quality Control

Quality control for qualitative tests (tests with a positive or negative result) requires different methods than quality control for quantitative tests (tests with a measure result).

QC for Qualitative Methods

To satisfy CLIA requirements for quality control, the actual testing personnel must run, review for acceptability, and document the results produced by positive and negative controls at a frequency established by the reagent manufacturer. Corrective action must be taken and documented for unacceptable QC results. Controls can be internal to the testing device or external. Laboratories must follow a manufacturer's quality control instructions. Failure to follow the instructions results in a use that extends beyond the scope of a test system's FDA-approved indications and results in the test not being CLIA-waived and not approved for the medical assistant to perform.

QC for Quantitative Methods

The basic tool for manually recording quantitative quality control is the Levey-Jennings QC Chart (Fig. 40-3). Using the chart builds a picture of how your test is performing over time. Monitoring the charts for **shifts** and **trends** will warn you that a test may not be performing optimally. A laboratory test is exhibiting a shift when QC results make an obvious change in performance levels. A laboratory test is exhibiting a trend when results

Figure 40-3 Levey-Jennings Chart.

progressively increase or decrease over time. See examples of shifts and trends in Figure 40-4. Being alerts for shifts or trends will allow you to investigate a potential reagent problem and prevent having controls fail, causing repeat testing and delayed reporting of patient results. Procedure 40-2 describes how to perform quality control monitoring using a QC chart.

 CHECKPOINT QUESTION

6. How does a QC shift differ from a trend?

Proficiency Testing

Proficiency testing facilitates external evaluation of the laboratory. To continue testing and maintain Medicare el-

igibility, all laboratories, even those conducting only waived tests, must participate in three proficiency tests a year and must be available for at least one on-site inspection. Three times a year, the laboratory is shipped specimens prepared by an approved agency. These specimens must be tested by the same procedures used for patients' evaluation and the results mailed to the proficiency testing agency. The proficiency testing agency evaluates the results and provides feedback on performance.

Reagent Management

Reagents are chemicals used to produce a reaction. In the case of the lab tests you perform, the reaction will provide a measurement or test result. All reagents have a manufacturer's lot number and expiration date. These

Figure 40-4 QC charts representing a shift and a trend.

must be recorded on the QC log sheet when quality control is validated. The date the package is opened and the initials of the person who opened the package should be documented on each package. If the reagent consistently performs inappropriately, the lot number will help the manufacturer identify defects. All supplies and equipment, reagents, and testing components must be labeled with identification, storage requirements, date of preparation or when opened, and expiration date.

CLIA requires each laboratory to have a procedure to test new reagents (or kit lots) for acceptability before using them to perform patient's tests. Specifically, new reagent lots must be compared to previously used reagent lots to ensure comparability between the newly received lots and lots that have already been in use. Documentation of this verification process is required. An example of this is mon-

itoring and documenting fecal occult blood test kits (see Chapter 44) and developer lot numbers for this purpose. Use of a reagent kit component is restricted to the kit in which it was originally contained, unless otherwise specified by the manufacturer. It is unacceptable to use fecal occult blood test cards and developer from different lots together for patient testing unless this practice has been approved by the manufacturer of the reagents.

Instrument Calibration and Maintenance

Laboratory equipment is sensitive and requires strict compliance with operation and maintenance standards. Manufacturers provide maintenance schedules and methods for evaluating performance. Maintenance of equipment and supplies must be documented in the QC log book; this includes maintenance either by an employee or by a manufacturer's representative. Any corrective action required for equipment or supply malfunction must be documented. Figures 40-5 and 40-6 show sample CLSI forms on which this information can be recorded.

Instruments are designed to produce results within a documented reportable range. If the QC results are not within the stated reference range, the instrument's **calibration** (standardization) should be checked by the manufacturer's instructions, and patient and QC specimens should be retested. If the calibration is correct and the results of QC specimens run in the same manner as the pa-

tients' specimens are within the stated reference range, the patients' results are correct. The flow chart in Figure 40-7 shows how you can evaluate test results for errors.

The laboratory's procedure manual must state the manufacturer's recommendation for the performance of calibration procedures, and supporting documentation must show that controls are performed as directed. Some procedures may require that controls be performed at each testing. Documentation must show the action taken to verify results, what was done when a problem arose, what the solution to the problem was, when the testing equipment was serviced and by whom, and what was done. Procedure 40-3 describes

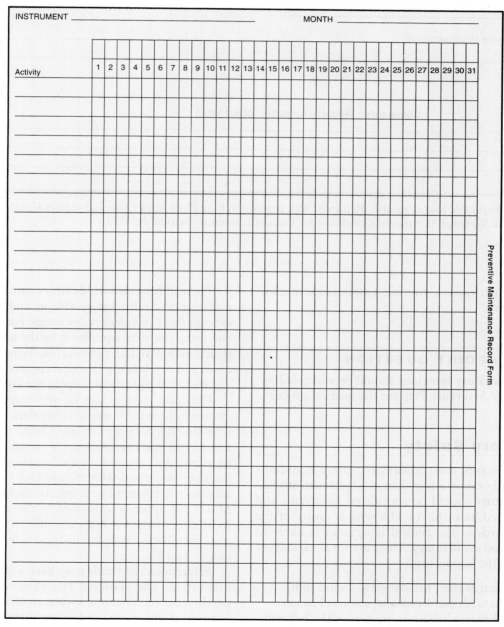

Figure 40-5 Preventative maintenance record form. (Reprinted with permission from Physician's Office Laboratory Guidelines and Procedure Manual. 3rd ed. Wayne, PA: National Committee for Clinical Laboratory Standards, 1995.)

Instrument History Record				Instrument: _____

Instrument History Record

Model No.: _____

Date Purchased: _____

Manufacturer: _____

_____

Telephone: _____

Dealer: _____

_____

Telephone: _____

Warranty: _____

_____

Technical Service Representative: _____

Telephone: _____

Instrument: _____

Serial No.: _____

Cost: _____

State: _____ Zip: _____

Contact
Person: _____

State: _____ Zip: _____

Contact
Person: _____

Expiration Date: _____

Service Record

Date   **Comments** Who was contacted, action taken

_____

_____

_____

Figure 40-6 Instrument history record. (Reprinted with permission from Physician's Office Laboratory Guidelines and Procedure Manual. 3rd ed. Wayne, PA: National Committee for Clinical Laboratory Standards, 1995.)

the steps for performing routine maintenance of clinical equipment.

 CHECKPOINT QUESTION

7. Which laboratory functions should be addressed in the Quality Assurance Plan for the medical office?

Laboratory Safety

Medical assistants must always be safety conscious when using laboratory equipment. All specimens studied in the laboratory should be considered hazardous and must be treated as such. An MA who is aware of the types of hazards in the clinical laboratory is likely to work safely and avoid injury. There are three basic types of hazards in the laboratory:

- Physical hazards (fire, broken glass, liquid spills)
- Chemical hazards (acids, alkalis, chemical fumes)
- Biological hazards (diseases such as HIV, hepatitis, and tuberculosis)

Physical hazards include fires caused by an electrical malfunction. Staff must be able to find and operate fire extinguishers and identify fire escape routes. Maintaining and using electrical equipment by the manufacturer's instructions will reduce fire hazards. Avoid using extension cords and overloading electrical circuits. Before servicing any electrical equipment, unplug the instrument.

Chemical hazards can be minimized by labeling all chemicals with the **material safety data sheet (MSDS)** information. MSDS are obtained from the manufacturer and provide the manufacturer's instructions for storage, handling, and disposal of the chemical. They describe the risks associated with the product and indicate steps necessary to prevent exposure. An up-to-date volume of MSDS for all chemicals used in the laboratory is the focal part of the facility's chemical hygiene plan. The plan should also include chemical safety protocols specific to that facility.

Hazardous chemicals may have additional labels of precaution. The National Fire Protection Association developed a classification system to identify areas where hazardous chemicals and other materials are stored. This system uses a diamond-shaped symbol, divided into

Figure 40-7 Flow chart for the evaluation of test results result for random error: a simple strategy for determining whether an individual test result is reasonable and correlates with other results. Y, yes; N, no. A and B (far left) show interconnection between evaluation of repeat testing and a where decision-making strategy should resume. For example, if an impossible value is obtained and repeat analysis does not show the same value, the uppermost horizontal line of chart says that testing procedure should return to symbol A, where the steps are begun again with examine result. (Adapted from Cembrowksi GS. Use of patient data for quality control. Clin Lab Med 6:715, 1986).

four quadrants, to represent different types of hazards (Fig. 40-8). The blue section indicates health hazards; the red section indicates fire hazards; and the yellow section indicates reactive hazards. The white section is left blank unless there is a specific hazard such as an oxi-dizer, water reactive, or radiation hazard. There will be a number from 0 (no hazard) to 4 (serious hazard) in each colored section. Hazardous materials classification posters that explain the significance of each diamond should be prominently displayed in all laboratory areas.

Identification of Health Hazard Color Code: **BLUE**		Identification of Flammability Color Code: **RED**		Identification of Reactivity (Stability) Color Code: **YELLOW**	
	Type of possible injury		Susceptibility of materials to burning		Susceptibility to release of energy
SIGNAL		SIGNAL		SIGNAL	
4	Materials that on very short exposure could cause death or major residual injury even though prompt medical treatment was given.	4	Materials that will rapidly or completely vaporize at atmospheric pressure and normal ambient temperature, or that are readily dispersed in air and that will burn readily.	4	Materials that in themselves are readily capable of detonation or of explosive decomposition or reaction at normal temperatures and pressures.
3	Materials that on short exposure could cause serious temporary or residual injury even though prompt medical treatment was given.	3	Liquids and solids that can be ignited under almost all ambient temperature conditions.	3	Materials that in themselves are capable of detonation or explosive reaction but require a strong initiating source or that must be heated under confinement before initiation or that react explosively with water.
2	Materials that on intense or continued exposure could cause temporary incapacitation or possible residual injury unless prompt medical treatment is given.	2	Materials that must be moderately heated or exposed to relatively high ambient temperatures before ignition can occur.	2	Materials that in themselves are normally unstable and readily undergo violent chemical change but do not detonate. Also materials that may react violently with water or that may form potentially explosive mixtures with water.
1	Materials that on exposure would cause irritation but only minor residual injury even if no treatment is given.	1	Materials that must be preheated before ignition can occur.	1	Materials that in themselves are normally stable, but that can become unstable at elevated temperatures and pressures or that may react with water with some release of energy, but not violently.
0	Materials that on exposure under fire conditions would offer no hazard beyond that of ordinary combustible material.	0	Materials that will not burn.	0	Materials that in themselves are normally stable, even under fire exposure conditions, and that are not reactive with water.

Figure 40-8 Hazardous materials rating system. (Reprinted with permission from McCall R. Phlebotomy Essentials. Baltimore: Lippincott Williams & Wilkins, 2007.)

WHAT IF?

What if you stick yourself with a contaminated needle?

- Cleanse the wound thoroughly with soap and water or substance for tissue cleaning.
- Report incident to the practice manager or appropriate person for documentation.
- Complete the required institutional incident report form.
- Ask the practice manager any questions about follow-up on the patient source of contamination.

  It is recommended that you:

- Seek care from the nearest emergency room or health care facility.
- Have blood drawn as soon as possible for HBsAg, antibody to hepatitis B surface antigen (anti-HBs), hepatitis C antibody, and anti-HIVe.

The primary purpose of the initial visit is to document the incident and offer prophylactic therapy for HIV exposure. If health care providers at the facility have questions about appropriate care, they can call the national HIV Post-Exposure Prophylaxis Hot-Line for Clinicians at 1-888-HIV-4911, which is open 24 hours per day.

Biological hazards refer to specimens capable of transmitting disease. Personal protective equipment (PPE) used according to Occupational Safety and Health Administration (OSHA) requirements and strict compliance with handwashing protocols are the best tools for preventing exposure. Methods for handling each of these hazards must be outlined in detail in your facility's policy and procedure manual. Each member of the staff must be familiar with safety protocols to ensure that risks are kept to a minimum.

CHECKPOINT QUESTION

8. What are the major pieces of information provided on a material safety data sheet?

Occupational Safety and Health Administration

The **Occupational Safety and Health Administration (OSHA)** is a federal agency in the US Department of Labor that monitors and protects the health and safety of workers. OSHA standards are federal regulations that protect workers by eliminating or minimizing chemical,

physical, and biological hazards and preventing accidents. OSHA standards supersede all other regulatory agency requirements. Two OSHA standards of particular importance to medical laboratories are the Occupational Exposure to Blood-borne Pathogens Standard and the Hazardous Communication (HazCom) Standard, or the "right to know law."

Prevention of disease transmission in a medical facility is often called infection control or biohazard risk management. The OSHA Blood-borne Pathogens Standard (review the use of standard precautions in Chapter 2) requires all medical employers to provide training for their employees in techniques that will protect them from occupational exposure to infectious agents, including blood-borne pathogens. Safety manuals must be available or incorporated into the policy and procedure manual to guide employees in correct procedures and emergency protocols.

In addition, OSHA standards require that all workers who are at risk for exposure to potentially hazardous material wear PPE supplied by the employer and readily available for use. PPE includes the following:

- Gloves
- Gown
- Apron
- Face shield
- Goggles
- Glasses with side shields
- Mask
- Lab coat

All PPE must be appropriate to the level of exposure. Workers who are sensitive to allergens such as latex must be supplied with latex-free equipment. Box 40-3 provides a review of the symptoms of latex allergies and evaluation criteria to determine their level of severity. A medical assistant performing phlebotomy or assisting with collection of most tissue samples is safe with glove protection. Situations that may result in splashes, splatters, or spreading of an **aerosol** (particles suspended in gas or air), however, require full coverage, including a face shield and footwear.

According to OSHA requirements, employers are required to provide free immunization against hepatitis B virus and other blood-borne pathogens if vaccines are available to employees within 10 days of being assigned to duties with possible exposure to blood-borne pathogens. Patient care and laboratory test duties carry the risk of exposure to blood-borne pathogens. Exposure can occur if the skin is pierced or if any body fluid splashes into the eyes, nose, mouth, other opening, or abrasion.

The OSHA HazCom Standard requires all hazardous materials to be labeled by their manufacturers. Hazardous chemicals must be labeled with a warning, such as "danger"; a statement of the hazard, such as

BOX 40-3

THREE MAJOR TYPES OF LATEX REACTIONS

1. Irritant dermatitis—Skin irritation not an allergic response. Some causes include inadequate drying after handwashing, aggressive scrubbing technique or detergents, abrasive effect of glove powder, climatic irritation (cold climates can cause dry, chapped skin, and hot weather can cause excessive sweating), and emotional stress. Irritant hand dermatitis can cause breaks in the skin, which can allow easier entry of the sensitizing latex protein or glove chemicals, and in turn lead to latex allergy.

2. Delayed cutaneous hypersensitivity (type IV allergy)—A contact (hand) dermatitis generally due to the chemicals used in latex glove production. It is mediated via T cells. The skin reaction is seen 6–48 hours after contact. The reaction is local and limited to the skin that has contacted the glove. Those with type IV allergy are at increased risk of developing type I allergy. One route of sensitization is latex proteins more easily entering the body if the skin barrier is broken.

3. Immediate reaction (type I allergy)—Systemic allergic reactions caused by circulating IgE antibodies to the proteins in natural latex. Symptoms include hives, rhinitis, conjunctivitis, asthma due to bronchoconstriction, and, in severe cases, anaphylaxis and hypotension. Symptoms occur within about 30 minutes of exposure to latex. Several routes of exposure that can lead to type I sensitivity are cutaneous, mucosal, parenteral, and aerosol (from inhaling latex glove powder).

BOX 40-4

MATERIAL SAFETY DATA SHEET

An MSDS is required for each of the hazardous materials at a particular site. In the laboratory, these can include disinfectants, cleaning compounds, laboratory chemicals, and some office supplies (e.g., toners, printing compounds). All of these must be labeled as hazardous, with the contents listed on the label. Protocols for each hazardous agent used on site must be listed on the MSDS with the following information:

- Product name and identification. Include all names (trade and generic) by which it may be known.
- Hazardous components. List all hazardous components if the agent contains more than one.
- Health hazard data. Note the risks to those using the agent.
- Fire and explosive data. If this is a volatile agent, note what precautions are necessary to prevent an accident.
- Spill and disposal procedures. Note how to handle spills and disposal to avoid danger.
- Recommendations for personal protection equipment. Note whether gloves, gown, face shield, or other equipment should be worn during use of this agent.
- Handling, storage, and transportation precautions. List any special precautions that must be observed.

"flammable"; precautions to avoid exposure; and first aid measures for exposure incidents. In addition, manufacturers must supply an MSDS for their products. Employers are responsible for obtaining or developing a protocol for each hazardous agent used on site. This protocol should include an MSDS supplied by the manufacturer for each substance used in the medical office. The extensive information on the MSDS includes items such as storage guidelines, flammability, and exposure precautions. These sheets should be maintained in an office binder near the site of use and should be reviewed routinely by all office staff (Box 40-4).

OSHA specifically mandates that a **Chemical Hygiene Plan (CHP)** be written by office management and made available to employees exposed to chemical hazards. A chemical hygiene plan is a part of the HazCom standard and must address the following concerns:

1. Standard Operating Procedures to be used when working with hazardous chemicals
2. Criteria to be used to determine and implement control measures to reduce exposure to hazardous chemicals
3. Measures to be taken to ensure that fume hoods and other protective equipment are functioning properly
4. The employee information and training program
5. Particular operations or procedures that are hazardous enough that prior approval will be required before employees carry them out
6. A medical examination and consultation policy
7. Designation of a Chemical Hygiene Officer
8. Additional provisions for work with "select carcinogens," reproductive toxins, and substances with "high acute toxicity"

CHECKPOINT QUESTION

9. What are three types of hazards found in the laboratory? Give suggestions for preventing exposure to them.

Safety Guidelines

The following guidelines are some of the most important safety factors required in all laboratories. Follow them carefully to protect yourself, your co-workers, and your patients.

1. Never eat, drink, or smoke in the laboratory area.
2. Never touch your face, mouth, or eyes with your gloves or with items such as a pen or pencil used in the laboratory.
3. Do not apply makeup or lipstick or insert contact lenses in the laboratory.
4. Wear gloves and appropriate protective barriers whenever contact with blood, body fluids, secretions, excretions, broken skin, or mucous membranes is possible. If a splatter, splash, spill, or exposure to aerosols is possible, wear appropriate PPE.
5. Label all specimen containers with biohazard labels.
6. Store all chemicals according to the manufacturer's recommendations. Discard any container with an illegible label. Never store chemicals in unlabeled containers.
7. Wash hands frequently for infection control. Always wash hands before and after gloving and before leaving the work site.
8. Clean reusable glassware and other containers with recommended disinfectant or soap and dry thoroughly before reuse. Wear gloves to prevent cuts.
9. Avoid inhaling the fumes of any chemicals found in the laboratory or wearing contact lenses when working with these types of chemicals. Use of chemicals with hazardous fumes should be limited to facilities equipped with a fume hood.
10. Know the location and operation of all safety equipment, such as fire extinguishers, eyewashes (Fig. 40-9), and safety showers. Keep fire extinguishers close at hand because many chemicals are flammable.
11. Use safe practices when operating laboratory equipment. Read the manuals and know how to operate the equipment. Avoid contact with damaged electrical equipment.
12. Disinfect all laboratory surfaces concurrently and at the end of the day with a 10% bleach solution or appropriate disinfectant. Never allow clutter to accumulate.
13. Dispose of needles and broken glass in sharps containers. Use biohazard containers for any other contaminated articles.
14. Use mechanical pipetters, but never the mouth, to apply suction to the pipette.
15. Use the proper procedure for removing chemical or biological spills. If the spill is chemical, follow the manufacturer's directions; commercial kits are available for such cleanups. If the spill is biological:
    - Put on gloves and other protective equipment as indicated by the size of the spill.
    - Cover the area with absorbent material, such as paper towels, to soak up the spill; discard in a biohazard container.
    - Flood the area with disinfecting solution, such as a 10% bleach solution, and allow it to sit for 10 to 15 minutes.
    - Wipe up the solution with disposable material.
    - Dispose of all waste in a biohazard container.
    - With gloves on, remove eyewear and discard or disinfect per office policy. Remove remaining protective items and place in biohazard container or the biohazard laundry bag (for reusable linen).
    - Remove and dispose of gloves. Wash your hands.

Figure 40-9 Eyewash basin. (**A**) Press the lever at the right of the basin. (**B**) The stream of water forces the caps from the nozzles. Lower your face and eyes into the stream and continue to wash the area until the eyes are clear.

16. Avoid spills:
    - Pour carefully (palm the label).
    - Pour at eye level if possible or practical; never pour close to the face.
    - Tightly cap all containers immediately after use.
17. Use a splatter guard or splash shield whenever there is any risk of splatter or exposure to aerosols. Spills, splatters, and exposure to aerosols commonly occur in the following circumstances:
    - Taking the stopper off a blood collection tube
    - Transferring blood from a collection syringe to a specimen receptacle
    - Conducting centrifugation
    - Preparing a smear
    - Flaming the inoculation loop
18. When removing a stopper, hold the opening away, use gauze around the cap, and twist gently. Avoid glove contact with the specimen.
19. Immediately report to your supervisor any work-related injury or biohazard exposure.
20. Follow all guidelines for standard precautions and the requirements of the various types of transmission-based precautions as described in Chapter 2.
21. When opening a tube or container, hold the mouth away from you to avoid aerosols, splashes, and spills.

 CHECKPOINT QUESTION

10. How would you clean up a biological spill?

Incident Reports

When there is an occurrence in the medical setting for which liability could be considered, an incident report should be completed. An incident report is indicated if a patient, employee, or visitor is injured, if an employee is stuck with a contaminated needle, in case of medication error, or if blood is drawn from the wrong patient. The incident report should be completed by the staff member involved in the incident or closest to the patient or visitor involved in the incident.

Information necessary on an incident report includes the injured person's name, address, telephone number, and date of birth; the date and time; name and address of the facility where the incident occurred; and a brief description of the incident, including any diagnostic procedures or treatments performed. Witnesses to the incident should be listed with names, addresses, and phone numbers for insurance investigation if necessary. In addition to the signature of the person completing the form, a supervisor or doctor should review and sign the form in accordance with the office incident report policy.

 WHAT IF?

What if your laboratory is not in compliance with OSHA's safety regulations?

In such a situation, your health and that of your colleagues is in jeopardy. OSHA developed the guidelines to protect you from serious injury or death. OSHA can impose significant fines for noncompliance. Continued noncompliance may result in loss of the laboratory's license. In some situations, the physician may not be allowed to file for Medicare compensation. Other situations may incur large fines. To bring the laboratory back into compliance, any citations must be addressed and corrected. OSHA inspectors will revisit the site and reconsider licensure.

PROCEDURE 40-1: Screen and Follow-Up Laboratory Test Results and Document Appropriately

Purpose: To alert physician to a patient's critical lab results as soon as possible and document appropriately

Equipment: Patient laboratory results, Critical Values List for office, patient's chart, telephone (as needed)

Steps	Reasons
1. Review laboratory reports received from reference laboratory.	Laboratory reports may contain results that require immediate intervention for patient safety.
2. Note which reports may be placed directly on the patient's chart for the physician's routine review and which require immediate notification due to critical results.	
3. Notify the physician of the result. Take any immediate instructions from the physician.	Lab results requiring immediate follow-up should be reported to the physician by the most direct method. The physician will want to contact the patient for immediate action.
4. Follow instructions and document notification and follow-up.	Relaying instructions to the patient is the first priority. Documenting physician notification and, if directed, patient notification verifies that the process was completed.
5. Chart remaining reports appropriately.	All laboratory results should be routed according to laboratory policy for timely follow-up with the patient.

Charting Example:

02/12/2007 10:00 AM Panic level glucose of 597 mg/dL reported to Dr. Peters. Dr. will follow-up with
patient
M. Miller, CMA

PROCEDURE 40-2: Quality Control Monitoring Using a QC Chart

Purpose: To determine the acceptability of quality control results in compliance with CLIA standards
Equipment: Instrument test results and quality control charts

Steps	Reasons
1. Assemble the charts and data.	
2. On the QC chart (see Fig. 40-3), plot the control results obtained for the test run.	Levey-Jennings charts list the acceptable control results and provide an ongoing report of test performance.
3. Evaluate chart for acceptability of results.	
4. If results are within accepted limits, report patient results.	For waived testing, CLIA requires that quality control procedures be performed in compliance with the manufacturer's instructions.
5. If results are not within accepted limits, do not report patient results. Troubleshoot the test. Repeat testing on the patient and control specimens.	If control results are not acceptable, the patient results are not valid.
6. If results are within accepted limits, report patient results. Document corrective action and acceptable control results.	For waived testing, CLIA requires that quality control procedures be performed in compliance with the manufacturer's instructions.
7. If results are not within accepted limits, notify the physician of test malfunction. Arrange to have patient specimen referred for testing or store the pecimen appropriately until repairs can be made.	The specimen may deteriorate if left at room temperature for too long.
8. Troubleshoot within manufacturer's guidelines for operator troubleshooting. Document this in the maintenance log. If this is not successful, arrange repairs for the instrument. Document any manufacturer-supplied repairs in the maintenance log.	CLIA requires that all maintenance on an instrument be documented in the maintenance log.
9. Keep physician informed of testing status.	The physician needs to know the status of test availability.
10. Before returning the instrument to service, validate calibration and quality control. Document appropriately.	For waived testing, CLIA requires that quality control procedures be performed in compliance with the manufacturer's instructions.

Charting Example:

02/12/2008 10:00 AM QC results plotted and within acceptable limits
CDH, CMA

PROCEDURE 40-3: Perform Routine Maintenance of Laboratory Equipment (Glucose Meter Example)

Purpose: To meet CLIA standards for quality performance by maintaining clinical equipment according to manufacturer's instructions

Equipment: Laboratory instrument to be maintained, instrument manual from manufacturer, instrument maintenance log, maintenance supplies as indicated in the instrument manual, personal protective equipment, hand sanitizer, surface sanitizer, contaminated waste container

Steps	Reasons
1. Wash your hands. Put on gloves.	The meter is used for patient testing. In maintaining it, you will be exposed to remaining specimen residue.
2. Read or review the maintenance section of the instrument manual.	CLIA requires that maintenance be performed as according to manufacturer recommendations.
3. Follow the manufacturer's step-by-step instructions for maintaining the instrument.	Following the manufacturer's instructions ensures optimum instrument performance.
4. Turn on the instrument and ensure that it is calibrated.	Calibration of the instrument is essential for accurate test results.
5. Perform the test on the quality control material. Record results. Determine whether QC is within control limits. If yes, proceed with patient testing. If no, take corrective action and recheck controls. Document corrective action. Proceed with patient testing when acceptable QC results are obtained.	For waived testing, CLIA requires that quality control procedures be performed in compliance with the manufacturer's instructions.
6. Document maintenance procedures performed in instrument maintenance log.	Maintenance is not considered performed unless procedures are documented.
7. Properly care for or dispose of equipment and supplies.	
8. Clean the work area. Remove personal protective equipment and wash your hands.	Attention to infection control is important when working the parts of an instrument that analyzes patient specimens.

Charting Example: Glucose Meter Maintenance Log Entry

02/12/2008 10:00 AM *Routine maintenance performed on glucose meter per manufacturer's instructions. Meter was then calibrated and quality control material was tested with acceptable results*
DHW, CMA

MEDIA MENU

- **Student CD**
  - **CMA/RMA Certification Exam Review**
- **LWW's Medical Assisting Skills DVD**
  - **Procedure 40-3**
- **Premium Online Course**
  http://thePoint.lww.com/Kronenberger3e
- **Internet Resources**

LiveAdvise Online Tutoring & Competency Training
http://thePoint.lww.com/LiveAdvise

Commission on Office Laboratory Accreditation
www.cola.org

Centers for Medicare and Medicaid Services
www.cms.hhs.gov/

Clinical and Laboratory Standards Institute
www.clsi.org/

Occupational Safety and Health Administration
www.osha.gov/

Federal Register
www.gpoaccess.gov/fr/index.html

CLIA website to access certificate application
http://www.cms.hhs.gov/cmsforms/downloads/cms116.pdf

español
SPANISH TERMINOLOGY

Buenos Días. Este es _____ de la oficina del doctor _____. (For a female, change "este" to "esta" and for a woman doctor, use "de la doctora.")

Hello. This is _____*name*_____ from doctor _____*name*_____'s office.

Necesito hablar con _____?

May I speak with _____*name*_____?

_____, el doctor _____ me pidió llamarle con las resultas de su examen.

_____*name*_____, Dr. _____*name*_____ asked me to call you about your test results.

Su _____ fue demasiado alto (o bajo).

Your _____*test name*_____ was too high (or too low)."

El médico quiere que usted siga estas instrucciones.

The doctor wants you to follow these instructions.

Usted puede llamar la oficina mañana para arreglar una cita para la semana próxima.

You need to call the office tomorrow to schedule a follow-up appointment next week.

Entiende usted lo que le pido hacer?

Do you understand what I am asking you to do?

- As the CLIA list of waived tests continues to grow, medical assistants can provide numerous laboratory findings to aid diagnosis.
- By maintaining an up-to-date working knowledge of the CLIA standards, medical assistants can validate and document the quality and dependability of the results they report.

- Maintaining awareness of the types of hazards in the clinical laboratory allows the medical assistant to perform these critical tasks safely.

Warm Ups for Critical Thinking

1. List all items that must be documented in the laboratory. Design a form to meet these requirements. Who should complete the form? Where should it be kept? Explain your responses.

2. Working with another student, develop a plan of corrective action to use in case your controls do not come into range.

3. Review the laboratory safety rules and create a poster summarizing these rules for display in the laboratory.

Answers to Checkpoint Questions

1. The three levels of laboratory testing defined by CLIA are waived, moderate complexity, and high complexity. Medical assistants may perform any CLIA-waived test.

2. The purpose of the QA policy is to prevent problems before they occur.

3. The laboratory procedure manual is the primary reference in operating the POL. CLIA regulations require each laboratory to have its own procedure manual describing how to perform every test in the laboratory.

4. Urgent clinician notification of critical results is a responsibility of the laboratory. Documentation of the proper notification of such test results to the health care professional responsible for the patient is essential.

5. A comprehensive quality control program monitors each phase of the laboratory process, including specimen collection, specimen processing, testing, and reporting results. The programs also monitor reagents, instruments, and personnel in addition to actual test performance.

6. A QC is considered to shift when the results make an obvious change in performance levels. QC re-

sults are in a trend when they progressively increase or decrease over time.

7. The Quality Assurance Plan for the medical office should include monitors for the quality of patient preparation; specimen collection, processing, preservation, and transportation; and test analysis, reporting, and interpretation.

8. The major information provided on a material safety data sheet includes flammability, precautions to avoid exposure, first aid measures for exposure incidents, storage guidelines, and methods for safe disposal.

9. The three basic types of hazards are physical (e.g., fire, broken glass, and liquid spills), chemical (e.g., acids, alkalis, and chemical fumes), and biological (e.g., diseases such as HIV, hepatitis, and tuberculosis).

10. To clean up a biological spill, first put on gloves. Cover the area with disposable material, such as paper towels; discard these in an appropriate container. Next, flood the area with disinfecting solution and allow it to sit for 10 to 15 minutes. Wipe up the spill. Dispose of all waste in a biohazard container.

41 Phlebotomy

Outline

General Phlebotomy Equipment
Blood Drawing Station
Gloves
Antiseptics
Spill Kit Supplies and Instructions
Gauze Pads
Bandages
Sharps Containers
Venipuncture Equipment
Tourniquets
Needles
Blood Collection Systems

Capillary Puncture (Microcollection) Equipment
Puncture Devices
Microhematocrit Tubes
Microcollection Containers
Filter Paper Test Requisitions
Warming Devices
Phlebotomy Quality Control
Patient Preparation
Performing a Venipuncture With a Multisample Needle or a Winged Infusion Set

Selection of the Venipuncture Site
Special Concerns Using the Winged Infusion Set
Venipuncture Using the Evacuated Tube
Complications of Venipuncture
Performing a Capillary Puncture
Selection of the Capillary Puncture Site
Complications of Capillary Puncture

Learning Objectives

Upon successfully completing this chapter, you will be able to:

1. Define and spell the key terms

2. Identify equipment and supplies used to obtain a routine venous specimen and a routine capillary skin puncture

3. List the major anticoagulants, their color codes, and the suggested order in which they are filled from a venipuncture

4. Describe the location and selection of the blood collection sites for capillaries and veins

5. Explain the importance of correct patient identification and complete specimen and requisition labeling

6. Describe the steps in preparation of the puncture site for venipuncture and skin puncture

7. Describe care for a puncture site after blood has been drawn

8. List precautions to be observed when drawing blood

Performance Objectives

Upon successfully completing this chapter, you will be able to:

1. Obtain a blood specimen by evacuated tube or winged infusion set (Procedure 41-1)

2. Obtain a blood specimen by capillary puncture (Procedure 41-2)

CAAHEP

- Perform venipuncture
- Perform capillary puncture
- Dispose of biohazardous materials
- Practice standard precautions
- Document appropriately
- Use quality control

ABHES

- Personal protective equipment
- Venipuncture specimen collection
- Finger puncture specimen collection
- OSHA compliance rules and regulations
- Apply principles of aseptic technique and infection control
- Use quality control
- Dispose of biohazardous materials
- Practice standard precautions

Key Terms

antecubital space	evacuated tube	hemolysis	palpate
anticoagulant	gauge	luer adapter	prophylaxis
antiseptic	gel separator	multisample needle	sharps container
barrier precautions	hematoma	order of draw	syncope
bevel	hemoconcentration		

Successfully obtaining blood specimens requires knowledge, skill, practice, and empathy for all patients. A comfortable routine that complies with facility policy is established by each phlebotomist. Blood is collected by several methods, including arterial puncture, skin puncture, and venipuncture. The quality of a laboratory test result is only as good as the quality of the specimen collected for testing. The quality of the specimen starts with the phlebotomist's attention to several factors:

- Accurate patient identification
- Patient compliance with preparation requirements
- Timing of collections
- Collection techniques
- Accurate specimen labeling
- Provision of any special handling techniques to ensure integrity of the specimen
- Timely specimen transportation to the laboratory

This chapter describes blood collection equipment and supplies for safe venipuncture and skin puncture. While collection of arterial specimens is another common specimen type, it is limited to the evaluation of respiratory function and not performed by medical assistants. You must perform blood collection in the safest manner possible. Blood is a biohazardous material, so it should be handled with standard precautions and appropriate **barrier precautions**, which are physical products or equipment used specifically for the purpose of protecting the patient and the health care worker from exposure to potentially infectious material.

Needlestick injuries contribute to the overall burden of health care worker injuries. Estimates indicate that 600,000 to 800,000 such injuries occur annually, and about half go unreported. Needlestick injuries may expose workers to blood-borne pathogens, such as human immunodeficiency virus (HIV), hepatitis B virus, and/or hepatitis C virus. A health care worker's risk of infection depends on the pathogen, the severity of the needlestick injury, and the use of vaccination before the exposure and **prophylaxis** (protective treatment for the prevention of disease once exposure has occurred) after it. Become familiar now with the instructions for immediate action from the Centers for Disease Control and Prevention (CDC) in case of a needlestick injury (Box 41-1).

BOX 41-1

IMMEDIATE ACTION AFTER NEEDLESTICK INJURY

If you are exposed to the blood or other body fluid of a patient by needlestick or other means during the course of your work, immediately follow these steps:

- Wash needlesticks and cuts with soap and water.
- Flush splashes to the nose, mouth, or skin with water.
- Irrigate eyes with clean water, saline, or sterile irrigant.
- Report the incident to your supervisor.
- Initiate written documentation of the incident as directed by facility procedure.
- Immediately seek medical treatment.

Courtesy of the Centers for Disease Control and Prevention.

General Phlebotomy Equipment

Blood Drawing Station

A blood drawing station is equipped for performing phlebotomy procedures on outpatients or patients in medical offices sent by their physicians for laboratory testing (Fig. 41-1). The station should be out of the regular office traffic pattern for safety. The station should include a table close at hand for supplies and a chair or bed for the patient. The table should be at a convenient height for working with enough space to hold numerous supplies. Phlebotomy chairs are available from several manufacturers. The chair should be comfortable and have adjustable armrests to allow proper positioning of

Figure 41-1 A well-stocked blood drawing station.

either arm. The surface of the armrest should be disinfected by wiping with a solution such as 10% bleach. A safety device locks the armrest in place in front of the patient to prevent falling from the chair if fainting occurs. A bed or reclining chair should be available for patients with a history of fainting and to perform heel sticks or other procedures on infants and small children.

Gloves

Guidelines from the CDC and the Occupational Safety and Health Administration (OSHA) require that gloves be worn during phlebotomy procedures. A new pair of gloves must be used for each patient and removed when the procedure is finished. Nonsterile, disposable latex, nitrile, vinyl, or polyethylene gloves are acceptable.

Standard precautions require handwashing after glove removal. Good glove fit enhances safe manipulation. Gloves that are dusted with powder can be a source of contamination for some tests, especially those collected by capillary puncture. Gloves are not required to be sterile. They should fit snuggly to enhance manual dexterity.

Some users have allergic responses to glove powder. Powder in latex gloves can also facilitate suspension of latex particles in the air, posing danger to those with latex allergy. Gloves are available powder free and/or latex free. Best practice for the medical assistant is to ask the patient whether he or she has a latex allergy before starting the phlebotomy procedure. The phlebotomist can avoid gloves, tourniquets, and bandages containing latex before exposing the patient.

Antiseptics

Antiseptics inhibit the growth of bacteria. They are safe for use on human skin and are used to clean the skin before skin puncture or venipuncture. The most commonly used antiseptic for routine blood collection is 70% isopropyl alcohol. Other antiseptics used for blood collection are povidone iodine, 0.5% chlorhexidine gluconate, and benzalkonium chloride. These other alternatives are required when collecting blood specimens for tests that may be compromised if contaminated with alcohol. These tests are identified in the specimen collection procedure or manual.

Spill Kit Supplies and Instructions

The supplies available in a biohazard spill kit should include but are not limited to the following:

- A copy of the biohazardous spill cleanup instructions
- Nitrile disposable gloves
- Laboratory coat
- Absorbent material, such as absorbent paper towels or granular absorbent material

- All-purpose disinfectant, such as normal household bleach (diluted 1:10) or an iodophor
- Bucket for diluting disinfectant (can be used to store the kit contents when not in use)
- Dustpan, broom, hand broom (for picking up broken glass and other contaminated sharps)
- Sharps containers
- Biohazard waste bags

All reusable items should be autoclavable or compatible with the disinfectant used. Most of the listed items and other biohazard spill control items are sold in biohazardous spill control kits.

When cleaning blood spills, you should wear disposable gloves of sufficient sturdiness so they will not tear while you clean. If the gloves develop holes, tears, or splits, remove them, wash hands immediately, and put on fresh gloves. Disposable gloves must never be washed or reused.

Spills of blood and blood-contaminated fluids should be properly cleaned using either a chemical germicide approved for use as a hospital disinfectant and tuberculocidal at recommended dilution or a solution of 5.25% sodium hypochlorite (household bleach) diluted 1:10 with water. Steps for cleaning a biological spill are outlined in Chapter 40.

Gauze Pads

Clean 2 × 2 gauze pads are used to hold pressure on the venipuncture site following removal of the needle. Clean 2 × 2 gauze pads folded in fourths are used to hold pressure over the puncture site when secured by a bandage. Cotton or rayon balls may be used but are not recommended because of their tendency to stick to the site and cause bleeding when removed.

Bandages

An adhesive bandage (e.g., Band-Aid) is used to cover the site once the bleeding has stopped. If a patient is allergic to adhesive bandages, use paper, cloth, or knitted tape over a folded gauze square. Do not use a bandage on infants under 2 years of age because of the danger of aspiration and suffocation. Latex-free bandages are available in case of latex allergy.

Sharps Containers

Regardless of safety features, immediately dispose of used needles, lancets, and other sharp objects in a puncture-resistant, leak-proof disposable container called a **sharps container**. These containers are marked as biohazard and are red or bright orange for easy identification. Needles should never be cut, bent, or broken before disposal.

 CHECKPOINT QUESTION

1. What phlebotomy equipment might cause allergic reactions from the patient?

Venipuncture Equipment

Venipuncture procedures require the use of the following special equipment.

Tourniquets

The tourniquet constricts the flow of venous blood in the arm and makes the veins more prominent so that they are easier to find and penetrate with a needle. The tourniquet is a soft, pliable rubber strip, usually 1 inch wide and 15 to 18 inches long. It can easily be released with one hand, does not cut into the patient's arm, and is inexpensive enough that a new tourniquet can be used for each patient. The maximum time limit for leaving the tourniquet in place is 1 minute. Extending the time limit can alter test results by causing **hemoconcentration** (decrease of the fluid content of blood) and **hemolysis** (rupturing of red blood cells, causing release of intracellular contents into the plasma). If the tourniquet is released prior to completion of the venipuncture procedure, reapplication should be delayed for at least 2 minutes.

The decrease of fluid in hemoconcentrated blood results in an increase of cellular components in that blood. Normal concentration of cellular components is approximately 46%. Hemoconcentration causes too many cells to be present for the amount of serum or plasma. When the phlebotomist is inattentive to good techniques in performing phlebotomy, the resulting hemoconcentration of the specimen produces inaccurate test results. This false elevation results in inaccurate laboratory measurement of iron, calcium, and some enzymes.

To avoid hemoconcentration, the phlebotomist should:

1. Ensure that the tourniquet is not on too tight or left on too long.
2. Instruct the patient to avoid pumping his or her hand and to just make a fist
3. Avoid probing with the needle ("fishing" for a vein)
4. Avoid sclerosed or occluded veins

By taking similar precautions, the phlebotomist will also avoid hemolysis. Hemolysis contamination is not always visible. Alterations of patient test results occur long before hemolysis reaches the level of a visible color change of plasma or serum from slightly yellow to pink or red. When cells are hemolyzed, they are not recognized as red blood cells by hematology cell counters, resulting in falsely decreased results in cell counts and hemoglobin determinations. When the red cells rupture, all of their intracellular contents are released into the serum or plasma. Fluid inside the cell contains components different from regular plasma. An example is the electrolyte, potassium. The fluid inside the cell has a much higher concentration of potassium than the plasma. Even hemolysis not perceived visibly can cause clinically significant increases in the patient's potassium measurement.

As an additional precaution, the phlebotomist can avoid hemolysis by using a needle with a large enough diameter that it does not cause rupture of RBCs as they pass through the needle into the collection tube. Selecting the appropriately sized needle is discussed in the next section.

Needles

Due to the frequency of phlebotomist exposure to communicable disease by needlestick, OSHA requires needles to have safety features to minimize accidental needlesticks. Manufacturers provide needles with various features to facilitate this requirement. Users can select products that both meet requirements and provide ease of use.

Sterile, disposable, single-use only needles are used for venipuncture. They are silicon coated, which enables them to penetrate the skin smoothly. The end of the needle that pierces the vein is cut on a slant or **bevel**. The bevel allows the needle to penetrate the vein easily and prevents coring (removal of a portion of skin or vein). The long, cylindrical portion of the needle is called the

shaft, and the end that connects to the blood-drawing apparatus is called the hub.

The **gauge** of a needle indicates the size of the lumen (bore size or opening) of the needle. The larger the gauge number is, the smaller the diameter of the needle (e.g., 20 gauge is larger than 25 gauge). Selection of the gauge is based on the size and condition of the patient's vein. A 21- or 22-gauge needle is used for most routine blood collection. Never use a needle smaller than 23-gauge to collect blood because the lumen is too small and will rupture blood cells, causing hemolysis of the specimen.

✔ CHECKPOINT QUESTION

2. What is the benefit of using a new tourniquet for each patient?

Blood Collection Systems

The primary blood collection system most commonly used today for venipuncture is the vacuum or **evacuated tube** system. A less common collection method incorporates the use of the syringe method and is useful in certain types of difficult venipunctures.

Evacuated Tube System

The evacuated tube system consists of a tube holder (adapter) (Fig. 41-2) and a needle designed specifically

Figure 41-2 Traditional components of the evacuated tube system. (Reprinted with permission from McCall R. Phlebotomy Essentials. Baltimore: Lippincott Williams & Wilkins, 2007.)

for use with the evacuated tube. This is a closed system allowing the patient's blood to flow from the vein through the needle and into the collection tube without exposure to the air. This system facilitates collecting multiple tubes with a single venipuncture. Evacuated tube systems are composed of three components: a **multisample needle** (allows collection of multiple tubes of blood during one venipuncture), a plastic needle holder that holds the collection tubes, and various collection tubes. Multisample needles with safety features are shown in Figure 41-3. Figure 41-4 is a traditional needle and tube holder. A safety needle-retracting device in the needle holder allows the safety to be provided as part of the needle holder rather than as a part of the needle itself (Fig. 41-5).

With beveled points on both ends, multisample needles are threaded in the middle to screw into the needle holder. One end of the needle is longer and is exposed for piercing the patient's skin and entering the vein. The shorter end penetrates the rubber stopper of the collection tube and, with its retractable rubber sleeve, prevents leakage of blood during tube changes. The sleeve is pushed back when it goes into the stopper, allowing blood to flow into the tube, and re-covers the end of the needle when the tube is removed.

The holder, sometimes called an adapter, has an indentation about half an inch from the hub (see Fig. 41-5). This indentation marks the point where the short, sleeved end of the needle starts to enter the rubber stopper of the tube. The open end of the holder accepts the

Figure 41-4 Traditional needle and tube holder. (Reprinted with permission from McCall R. Phlebotomy Essentials. Baltimore: Lippincott Williams & Wilkins, 2003.)

blood collection tube. There are flanges (extensions) on the sides of the rim of the holder to aid in tube placement and removal. Holder safety features may include a shield that covers the needle or a device that retracts the needle into the holder after it is withdrawn from the vein (see Fig. 41-3).

Evacuated tubes contain a vacuum with a rubber stopper sealing the tube. These tubes are made of glass or plastic and range in size from 2 to 15 mL. Tube size is selected according to the patient's age, amount of blood needed, and the size and condition of the patient's vein. The tubes are sterile to prevent contamination of the specimen and the patient.

Because of the vacuum inside the tube, evacuated tubes fill with blood automatically. The vacuum is premeasured by the manufacturer to draw the precise amount of blood into the tube. The tube fills until the vacuum is exhausted, so that a tube that has lost all or part of its vacuum will not fill completely, if at all.

Tube Additives

Different laboratory tests require different types of blood specimens. For tests requiring serum samples; the blood is drawn into a tube that allows clotting. The clotting process takes 30 to 60 minutes at 22 to 25°C. The specimen should be allowed to complete the clotting process prior to being centrifuged for separation of the serum from the clot; this is required to attain the optimum specimen. Other tests require whole blood or plasma, and these samples are drawn into a tube that

Figure 41-3 BD Eclipse multisample safety needle attached to traditional tube holder. (Courtesy of Becton-Dickinson, Franklin Lakes, NJ.)

Figure 41-5 Safety tube holder. (**A**) Venipuncture Needle-Pro with needle-sheathing device. (**B**) Vanish point tube syringe with needle-retracting device. (Retractable Technologies, Little Elm, TX.)

contains an **anticoagulant** additive because it prevents clotting.

An additive is any substance (other than the tube coating) that is placed in a tube. Additives have specific functions. Following is a list of the most common additives and their functions:

- Anticoagulants prevent the blood from coagulating or clotting.
- Clot activators enhance coagulation.
- Thixotropic **gel separator**, an inert substance, forms a physical barrier between the cellular portion of a specimen and the serum or plasma portion after the specimen has been centrifuged. This protects the serum from interaction with the red cells or fibrin that would alter test results.

The evacuated tube system uses color-coded stoppers as a means of identifying the additive contained in each type of tube (Table 41-1). It is necessary to use the correct anticoagulant because improper anticoagulant use can alter test results. It is also necessary to fill the tube until the vacuum is exhausted. Under-filled tubes will alter patient test results due to overdilution of the specimen by the tube additive.

 CHECKPOINT QUESTION

3. In what ways is plasma different from serum?

Order of Draw

A designated **order of draw** is recommended to avoid contamination of nonadditive tubes by additive tubes, cross-contamination between different types of additive tubes, contamination with tissue thromboplastin, and microbial contamination.

The Clinical and Laboratory Standards Institute (CLSI), formerly the National Committee for Clinical Laboratory Standards (NCCLS), is an organization of representatives from the health care community, industry, and government who use consensus to develop voluntary guidelines and standards for the laboratory. CLSI recommends one order of draw for both collection of evacuated tubes and filling evacuated tubes from a syringe (Table 41-2). Recommended protocols from various manufacturers and the CLSI, as well as policies of individual laboratories, may slightly differ. The protocol for your facility should be the order you use.

If you make a mistake in the order of draw, record the actual order of draw on the request form or in the computer so that it is visible in the laboratory testing area. Findings are reviewed for evidence of contamination before they are reported. If interference is suspected, the laboratory can suggest recollection of the specimen to validate the original test results.

 CHECKPOINT QUESTION

4. What is the proper order of draw when using the evacuated tube system? Why is this important?

Syringe System

As discussed previously, evacuated tubes remove the blood from the vein because they contain a vacuum. A syringe is helpful with fragile veins because the vacuum can be applied slowly and gently, rather than all at once as with vacuum tubes. Syringes are made of disposable plastic and vary in volume from 1 to 50 mL. Choose the smallest syringe volume that will accommodate the total amount of blood necessary for the tests the physician has requested.

TABLE 41.1   Evacuated Tube System: Color Coding

BD Vacutainer® Venous Blood Collection
Tube Guide

For a full line of BD Vacutainer® Specimen Collection Products, visit www.bd.com/vacutainer.

BD Helping all people live healthy lives

BD Vacutainer Tubes with BD Hemogard Closure	BD Vacutainer Tubes with Conventional Stopper	Additive	Inversions at Blood Collection*	Laboratory Use	Your Lab's Draw Volume/Remarks
Gold	Red/Black	• Clot activator and gel for serum separation	5	For serum determinations in chemistry. May be used for routine blood donor screening and diagnostic testing of serum for infectious disease.** Tube inversions ensure mixing of clot activator with blood. Blood clotting time: 30 minutes.	
Light Green	Green/Gray	• Lithium heparin and gel for plasma separation	8	BD Vacutainer® PST™ Tube for plasma determinations in chemistry. Tube inversions prevent clotting.	
Red	Red	• None (glass) • Clot activator (plastic)	0 5	For serum determinations in chemistry. May be used for routine blood donor screening and diagnostic testing of serum for infectious disease.** Tube inversions ensure mixing of clot activator with blood. Blood clotting time: 60 minutes.	
Orange	Gray/Yellow	• Thrombin	8	For stat serum determinations in chemistry. Tube inversions ensure complete clotting, which usually occurs in less than 5 minutes.	
Royal Blue		• Clot activator (plastic serum) • K₂EDTA (plastic)	8 8	For trace-element, toxicology, and nutritional-chemistry determinations. Special stopper formulation provides low levels of trace elements (see package insert).	
Green		• Sodium heparin • Lithium heparin	8 8	For plasma determinations in chemistry. Tube inversions prevent clotting.	
Gray		• Potassium oxalate/sodium fluoride • Sodium fluoride/Na₂EDTA • Sodium fluoride (serum tube)	8 8 8	For glucose determinations. Oxalate and EDTA anticoagulants will give plasma samples. Sodium fluoride is the antiglycolytic agent. Tube inversions ensure proper mixing of additive and blood.	
Tan		• K₂EDTA (plastic)	8	For lead determinations. This tube is certified to contain less than .01 μg/mL(ppm) lead. Tube inversions prevent clotting.	
Yellow		• Sodium polyanethol sulfonate (SPS) • Acid citrate dextrose additives (ACD): **Solution A -** 22.0 g/L trisodium citrate, 8.0 g/L citric acid,	8 8	SPS for blood culture specimen collections in microbiology. Tube inversions prevent clotting. ACD for use in blood bank studies, HLA phenotyping, and DNA and paternity testing.	

Tube	Additive	Inversions	Use
	24.5 g/L dextrose **Solution B -** 13.2 g/L trisodium citrate, 4.8 g/L citric acid, 14.7 g/L dextrose	8	
Lavender	• Liquid K_3EDTA (glass) • Spray-coated K_2EDTA (plastic)	8 8	K_2EDTA and K_3EDTA for whole blood hematology determinations. K_2EDTA may be used for routine immunohematology testing and blood donor screening.*** Tube inversions prevent clotting.
White	• K_2EDTA with gel	8	For use in molecular diagnostic test methods (such as but not limited to polymerase chain reaction [PCR] and/or branched DNA [bDNA] amplification techniques).
Pink (New)	• Spray-coated K_2EDTA	8	For whole blood hematology determinations. May be used for routine immunohematology testing and blood donor screening.*** Designed with special cross-match label for patient information required by the AABB. Tube inversions prevent clotting.
Light Blue (Clear)	• Buffered sodium citrate 0.105 M (≈3.2%) glass 0.109 M (≈3.2%) plastic • Citrate, theophylline, adenosine, dipyridamole (CTAD)	3-4 3-4	For coagulation determinations. CTAD for selected platelet function assays and routine coagulation determination. Tube inversions prevent clotting.
Clear (New / Red/Gray)	• None (plastic)	0	For use as a discard tube or secondary specimen collection tube.

Partial-draw Tubes (2 mL and 3 mL: 13 x 75 mm)   **Small-volume Pediatric Tubes** (2 mL: 10.25 x 47 mm, 3 mL: 10.25 x 64 mm)

Tube	Additive	Inversions	Use
Red	• None	0	For serum determinations in chemistry. May be used for routine blood donor screening, immunohematology testing,*** and diagnostic testing of serum for infectious disease.** Tube inversions ensure mixing of clot activator with blood. Blood clotting time: 60 minutes.
Green	• Sodium heparin • Lithium heparin	8 8	For plasma determinations in chemistry. Tube inversions prevent clotting.
Lavender	• Spray-coated K_2EDTA (plastic)	8 8	For whole blood hematology determinations. May be used for routine immunohematology testing and blood donor screening.*** Tube inversions prevent clotting.
Light Blue	• 0.105 M sodium citrate (≈3.2%)	3-4	For coagulation determinations. Tube inversions prevent clotting.

* Invert gently, do not shake
** The performance characteristics of these tubes have not been established for infectious disease testing in general; therefore, users must validate the use of these tubes for their specific assay-instrument/reagent system combinations and specimen storage conditions.
*** The performance characteristics of these tubes have not been established for immunohematology testing in general; therefore, users must validate the use of these tubes for their specific assay-instrument/reagent system combinations and specimen storage conditions.

BD Diagnostics
Preanalytical Systems
1 Becton Drive
Franklin Lakes, NJ 07417 USA

BD Global Technical Services: 1.800.631.0174
vacutainer_techservices@bd.com
BD Customer Service: 1.888.237.2762
www.bd.com/vacutainer

BD, BD Logo and all other trademarks are property of Becton, Dickinson and Company. © 2006 BD

Printed in USA   07/06   VS5229-8

Courtesy and © Becton, Dickinson and Company.

TABLE **41-2**	CLSI Order of Draw and Rationale for Collection Order	
Order of Draw	**Tube Stopper Color**	**Rationale for Collection Order**
Blood cultures (sterile collections)	Yellow, culture bottles (SPS) (or sterile media containers)	Minimizes chance of microbial contamination.
Plain (nonadditive) tubes	Red	Prevents contamination by additives in other tubes.
Coagulation tubes	Light blue	Second or third position in order of draw; prevents tissue thromboplastin contamination. Must be the first additive tube in the order because all other additive tubes affect coagulation tests.
Serum separator gel tubes (SSTs)	Red and gray rubber; gold plastic	Prevents contamination by additives in in other tubes. Comes after coagulation tests because silica particles activate clotting and affect coagulation tests. Carryover of silica into subsequent tubes can be overridden by the anticoagulant in them.
Plasma separator gel tubes (PSTs)	Green and gray rubber; light green plastic	Contains heparin, which affects coagulation tests and interferes in collection of serum specimens. Causes the least interference in tests other than coagulation tests.
Heparin tubes	Green	Same as PST.
Ethylenediaminetetraacetic acid (EDTA) tubes	Lavender	Causes more carryover problems than any other additive. Elevates sodium and potassium levels. Chelates and decreases calcium and iron levels. Elevates prothrombin time and partial thromboplastin time results.
Oxalate/fluoride tubes	Gray	Sodium fluoride and potassium oxalate elevate sodium and potassium levels, respectively. Comes after hematology tubes because oxalate damages cell membranes and causes abnormal red blood cell morphology.

Pulling on the plunger of the syringe creates a vacuum in the barrel. The plunger often sticks and is hard to pull. A technique called "breathing the syringe" makes the plunger easier to move. To do this, before beginning the procedure, pull back the plunger to about halfway up the barrel, and then push it back. This makes the plunger move more smoothly and reduces the tendency to jerk when it is first pulled after insertion into the vein. The vacuum created by pulling on the plunger while a needle is in a patient's vein fills the syringe with blood. Pulling the plunger slowly and resting between pulls allows the vein time to refill with blood.

Using a syringe for blood collection requires transfer of blood to a collection tube. Various brands of devices ensure safety during the transfer of blood from a syringe into an evacuated tube. When performing this transfer, force on the syringe plunger is not required because the vacuum in the tube will draw the specimen from the syringe. Blood specimens collected by syringe must be transferred to evacuated tubes following proper order of draw.

Winged Infusion Set

The butterfly collection system, or winged infusion set, has a stainless steel beveled needle with attached winged-shaped plastic extensions connected to a 6- to 12-inch length of tubing. It is preferred in geriatric and pediatric phlebotomy because the tubing length allows more flexibility for patients who cannot keep still and those whose limbs may be not be able to extend adequately enough to accommodate the needle holder and stationary needle. The most common butterfly needle sizes are 21- to 25-gauge and half an inch to three-quarters of an inch long. The butterflies come with attachments to be used with syringes and a special multisample **luer adapter** (a device for connecting a syringe or evacuated holder to the needle) that allows them to be used in an evacuated tube system (Fig. 41-6). Figure 41-7 demonstrates the use of the butterfly system.

Examine the needle gauge of the winged infusion set prior to using it for phlebotomy. Blood specimens for laboratory testing should be drawn with 22-guage needles or larger (smaller gauge number). Infusion sets commonly stocked in patient care facilities have gauges of 23 to 25. During withdrawal of the specimen into the collection device, the red blood cells endure tremendous pressure. The combination of the pull of the vacuum with the small bore of the needle can result in more pressure than the cell structure can withstand, causing red blood cells to rupture. As described earlier in this chapter, hemolysis is the result of rupturing red blood cells

Figure 41-6 Winged infusion sets. Left: Attached to a syringe. Right: Attached to evacuated tube holder by means of a Luer adapter. (Reprinted with permission from McCall R. Phlebotomy Essentials. Baltimore: Lippincott Williams & Wilkins, 2003.)

releasing their contents into the plasma. Hemolysis contamination of the plasma can result in significant inaccuracies in test results.

 CHECKPOINT QUESTION

5. Why is it important that the gauge of the phlebotomy needle be 22 or less (larger opening)?

 LEGAL TIP

ASSESS THE RISK OF PHLEBOTOMY LIABILITY

To reduce a laboratory's exposure to phlebotomy liability, address the following issues in your policy manual, your new employee training program, and in your employee competency assessments.

- Put the proper information on every tube of blood, including the time and date of collection and the phlebotomist's initials.
- Note that phlebotomy textbooks set a range between 15 and 30 degrees for the angle of needle insertion.
- Require adherence to facility protocol regardless of an employee's experience.
- Perform regular competency evaluations on all phlebotomy staff members.
- In vein selection, the vein of choice is the medial vein, which typically lies in a depression in the center of the antecubital area. It is the vein of choice because it is usually larger, more stationary, closer to the surface of the skin, and more isolated from other underlying structures than the other veins.
- The error considered most critical for a health care facility is misidentifying a patient. Avoiding this risk requires strict adherence to the facility's patient identification policy.

Capillary Puncture (Microcollection) Equipment

Capillary puncture or skin puncture requires penetration of the capillary bed in the dermis of the skin with a puncture device. The small specimen volumes required by point-of-care instruments allow more laboratory tests to be collected by skin puncture. The equipment used to collect the specimen depends on the patient's age and condition and on the test being performed.

Figure 41-7 Procedure for using butterfly in a hand vein. (**A**) Hand with tourniquet in place reveals prominent vein. (**B**) With the skin pulled taut over the knuckles, the needle is inserted into the vein until there is a flash of blood in the tubing. (**C**) Using the nondominant hand, a wing of the butterfly is held against the patient's hand to steady the needle while the blood collecting tube is pushed onto the blood collecting needle. (**D**) Once the proper tubes have been drawn, gauze is placed over the vein, and the needle is removed. (Reprinted with permission from McCall R. Phlebotomy Essentials. Baltimore: Lippincott Williams & Wilkins, 2003.)

Puncture Devices

A sterile disposable puncture device is used to pierce the skin to obtain drops of blood for testing. These devices are designed to control depth of puncture and have a spring-loaded point or blade to reduce accidental sharps injuries. Manufacturers offer puncture devices in a range of lengths and depths to facilitate varying puncture situations and sample requirements. Figure 41-8 shows several types of puncture devices used for microcollection.

Microhematocrit Tubes

Microhematocrit tubes are narrow-bore glass or plastic disposable capillary tubes used for hematocrit determinations. They fill by capillary action and hold 50 to 75 μL of blood. Capillary action is a scientific principal that explains how the blood can flow upwards. Microhematocrit tubes for sampling specimens directly from a

lavender-top tube are plain; those used for collecting hematocrit specimens directly from a capillary puncture are coated with ammonium heparin. Plain tubes have a blue band on one end of the capillary tube, and ammonium heparin–coated tubes have a red band. A plastic or clay sealant is used to close one end of the tube (Fig. 41-9).

Microcollection Containers

Microcontainers consist of small, nonsterile plastic tubes with color-coded stoppers that indicate the presence or absence of an additive. The color coding is identical to evacuation tubes used in venipuncture, but the microcontainer contains no vacuum to remove the blood from the patient. Microcontainers are used for measuring, stoppering, centrifuging, and storing blood, all in one container. Samples for light-sensitive

Figure 41-8 Several types of finger and heel puncture lancets. (**A**) Vacutainer Genie Lancets. (Courtesy of Becton-Dickinson, Franklin Lakes, NJ.) (**B**) Tenderlett toddler, junior, and adult lancet devices. (Courtesy of ITC, Edison, NJ.) (**C**) Tenderfoot toddler, newborn, preemie, and micro-preemie heel incision devices. (Courtesy of ITC, Edison, NJ.)

analytes, such as bilirubin, are collected in an amber-colored plastic tube that protects the blood from the light exposure, which would damage the substance to be measured.

Filter Paper Test Requisitions

Microcollection may also be accomplished using filter paper attached to a test requisition. Filter paper is a special paper product made to be thick and absorbent. It is used to collect blood specimens to test newborns for genetic defects, such as hypothyroidism and phenylketonuria. The filter paper is printed with circles that must be filled with blood. Figure 41-10 is an example of how the requisition and attached filter paper could look. The lateral surface of the newborn's heel is punctured, and

the blood droplet is absorbed into individual circles on a filter paper card. A large drop of blood must be applied from one side of the paper, and the blood must soak through to the other side. The specimen should air dry in a horizontal position and not be stacked with other collection requisitions.

Warming Devices

Important especially for heel sticks, warmers increase blood flow before the skin is punctured. Heel-warming devices (Fig. 41-11) provide a temperature not exceeding 42°C. Alternatively, a diaper or towel may be wet with warm tap water and used to wrap the hand or foot before skin puncture. Do not use water that is so hot that it might burn the patient.

Phlebotomy Quality Control

Many factors must be addressed to ensure specimen quality. Phlebotomy errors may cause serious harm to patients. Quality control consists of methods practiced in every capillary puncture or venipuncture to optimize the quality of each specimen. The list includes:

• Patient identification
• Patient preparation

Figure 41-9 Microcollection tubes and clay sealant.

Figure 41-10 Newborn screening specimen forms. (**A**) Initial specimen form. (**B**) Second specimen form. (Courtesy of Daniel Gray, State of New Mexico Scientific Laboratory, Albuquerque, NM.)

Figure 41-11 Infant heel warmer. (Reprinted with permission from McCall R. Phlebotomy Essentials. Baltimore: Lippincott Williams & Wilkins, 2007.)

- Communicating with the patient
  - Diet
  - Medications
  - Lifestyle habits
- Specimen collection
  - Selection of the venipuncture or capillary puncture site
  - Type of collection and amount of specimen to be collected
  - Need for special timing for collection
  - Types and amounts of preservatives and anticoagulants
  - Patient posture
  - Duration of tourniquet use
  - Actual time of specimen collection
  - Choosing the correct equipment
  - Order of draw
  - Need for special handling between time of collection and time received by the laboratory (e.g., refrigeration, protection from light)
- Specimen labeling
- Specimen processing and storage

- Time
- Temperature
- Needed clinical data when indicated
- Specimen-interfering substances

Quality control begins with a thorough specimen collection manual that specifies the instructions for collecting every type of specimen. The phlebotomist must meet the written standards at all times. The supervisor observes phlebotomists at work to verify compliance with facility protocol. In the absence of a phlebotomy supervisor, co-workers can observe each other to validate compliance.

Patient Preparation

Gaining the patient's trust and confidence and putting the patient at ease will help divert attention from any discomfort associated with the procedure. To accomplish this, use good interpersonal skills, introduce yourself, explain the procedure in simple terms, and communicate effectively with the patient.

Many patients know from experience where it is easiest to find an accessible vein. In conjunction with your knowledge and skill, choosing the best site will make the procedure less traumatic. Talk quietly with the patient and progress through the procedure with confidence.

After identifying the patient and explaining the procedure, verify that the patient has followed any dietary instructions or restrictions ordered by the physician or required by the test requested. If the patient indicates that fasting instructions or dietary restrictions were not followed, notify the physician for a decision whether or not to proceed with the venipuncture. If you are unable to reach the physician or instructed to proceed in obtaining the specimen, write "nonfasting" on both the test requisition and the specimen label.

Fasting

Fasting, the most common dietary restriction, requires the patient to refrain from eating for a certain period, usually from midnight until specimen collection the following morning. Fasting does not require the patient to refrain from drinking water; in fact, adequate hydration is necessary to ensure that veins are palpable and accessible for venipuncture. Dehydration from abstaining from all fluids can falsely elevate some test results, making them appear abnormal when they really are not.

NPO

NPO orders require that the patient have absolutely nothing by mouth for a certain period. This type of order is usually used if the patient is scheduled for surgery or other anesthesia procedures or for some radiology procedures. The purpose of an NPO order is to minimize secretions by reducing the body's fluid level.

Always believe patients who say they faint during venipuncture. Have these patients lie down during the procedure. This reduces the chance of **syncope** (fainting), and if the patient does faint, he or she will not fall. If the patient is sitting and feels faint or mentions feeling weak, have the patient lower his of her head and take deep breaths. Call for assistance without leaving the patient unattended.

One of the most important steps in specimen collection is identification of the patient. Ask the patient to state his or her name, date of birth, or any other information to verify identity. After you collect the blood specimen, label the sample with the patient's first and last names, an assigned identification number if available, the date and time, and your initials to verify who drew the sample. Specimens should be labeled before the patient exits the facility using the collection protocol for that facility.

PATIENT EDUCATION

INSTRUCTING PATIENTS ON DIETARY RESTRICTIONS

Fasting and NPO are two common dietary restrictions. Because most patients will not understand the differences between these requirements, you must provide clear explanations. Instruct patients to follow the correct protocol for dietary restrictions to ensure accurate test results and procedure outcomes.

CHECKPOINT QUESTION

6. How do the patient instructions for fasting differ from having nothing by mouth?

Performing a Venipuncture With a Multisample Needle or a Winged Infusion Set

The forearm veins in the **antecubital space** (the inside of the elbow) are commonly used for venipuncture. The three main veins in this area are the cephalic, median cubital, and basilic (Fig. 41-12). The commonly used vein for venipuncture is the median cubital vein.

Selection of the Venipuncture Site

Begin the procedure by washing your hands and putting on gloves. Equipment and supplies should be assembled near the phlebotomy chair. The tourniquet should be placed 3 to 4 inches above the planned venipuncture site and secured with a half-bow knot. Apply the tourniquet tightly enough to slow venous blood flow without affecting arterial blood flow. The half-bow makes it easy to remove the tourniquet with one hand. Rapid removal is important in collection procedures and emergencies. Leaving the tourniquet in place for longer than 1 minute will change the blood components as a result of hemoconcentration. Velcro closure, rubber tubing, or a blood pressure cuff may also be used as a tourniquet.

Ask the patient to make a fist so that the veins in the arm become more prominent. Do not allow the patient to open and close the fist because it will cause hemocon-

centration (pooling of blood components) and lead to erroneous test results.

Although some veins are visible, the best choice for venipuncture is found by touch. Use the tip of the index finger to **palpate** (evaluate by feeling) veins to determine their suitability. Palpating helps locate veins and determine their size, depth, and direction. Do not slap the arm when trying to locate a vein because this can cause bruising. If no suitable antecubital vein can be found, release the tourniquet and repeat the procedure to this point on the other arm.

If no suitable antecubital vein is found in either arm, check hand veins and finally wrist veins. Massaging the arm from wrist to elbow increases blood flow and makes veins more palpable. Warming the site with a warm towel can produce the same effect. Geriatric patients may require the phlebotomist to use a smaller (flatter) angle when inserting the needle. Their veins may be more shallow due to decreased muscle mass. Holding the skin near the site extra tight will prevent veins from "rolling."

Figure 41-12 (**A**) Principal veins of the arm, including major antecubital veins subject to venipuncture. (**B**) Forearm, wrist, and hand veins subject to venipuncture. (Reprinted with permission from McCall R. Phlebotomy Essentials. Baltimore: Lippincott Williams & Wilkins, 2003.)

Contraindications for using a specific site for venipuncture are:

- Burns or scars
- Areas with a hematoma or bruising
- Thrombosed veins (lack resilience, feel like rope cord and roll easily)
- Edema (swollen area due to excess tissue fluid)
- Partial or radical mastectomy on one or both sides
- Intravenous (IV) lines in both arms

The complete procedure for performing a venipuncture is outlined in Procedure 41-1. Always use aseptic techniques to prevent infection of the venipuncture site. For example:

- Do not touch the site after cleaning.
- Do not remove the needle cap until right before venipuncture.
- Do not open bandages ahead of time.

Special Concerns Using the Winged Infusion Set

To attach the winged infusion set, thread or attach the end of the winged infusion set to the tube holder. To avoid specimen contamination by transferring additives with the winged infusion system, hold the collection tube horizontally or slightly lowered. To enhance the use of the winged infusion set, use the smallest evacuated collection tube. This puts less pressure on small, fragile veins.

A drawback in using the winged infusion system is that, in some sets, the bevel cut is more blunt than the multisample needle, resulting in more painful punctures. Because the needle part of the system is much shorter than the multisample needle, it cannot reach deeper veins.

Several studies have shown that winged sets cause increased numbers of needlesticks to phlebotomists. After withdrawing the needle from the patient, it tends to hang loose on the end of the tubing, offering less control than the multisample needle. Phlebotomists should use extra caution and activate the safety device as quickly as possible.

Due to their limitations, winged sets should be used only for small, fragile veins in pediatrics and geriatrics.

Venipuncture Using the Evacuated Tube

When blood does not immediately flow into the tube, you may have to change the position of the needle. Figure 41-13 shows proper and improper needle positions. Make a slight (less than one-quarter) turn because the bevel of the needle may be against the wall of the vein. If the needle has not penetrated the vein, slowly advance it farther into the vein. If the needle has penetrated too far into the vein, pull it back a little. The tube may not have sufficient vacuum; try another tube before withdrawing the needle.

Comply with your facility's protocol for the allowed number of attempts to obtain a specimen. A common number of attempts is two. If a blood specimen cannot be obtained by that number of attempts, have another person attempt the draw or do a microcollection (skin puncture) if possible. Box 41-2 lists some common errors in venipuncture that you need to guard against.

Complications of Venipuncture

The most common complication of venipuncture is **hematoma** formation caused by blood leaking into the tissues during or after venipuncture. Hematomas are painful, cause unsightly bruising, and can cause compression injuries to nerves. Box 41-3 describes situations that may trigger hematoma formation. If a hematoma begins to form during the venipuncture, release the tourniquet immediately, withdraw the needle, and hold pressure on the site for at least 2 minutes. Cold compresses reduce pain and swelling.

Accidental puncture of an artery is recognized by the blood's bright red color and the pulsing of the specimen into the tube. In this case, it is important to hold pressure over the site for a full 5 minutes after the needle is removed. Permanent nerve damage may result from poor site selection, movement of the patient during needle insertion, inserting the needle too deeply or quickly, or excessive blind probing.

Performing a Capillary Puncture

Adult skin punctures are performed when no veins are accessible, to save veins for procedures such as chemotherapy, and for point-of-care testing. Technology now allows some tests to be performed on very small blood samples. However, some results are more accurate on venipuncture specimens than on capillary specimens. The phlebotomist must be aware of these tests in choosing the appropriate procedure for the patient. Tests that cannot be performed on skin puncture specimens include erythrocyte sedimentation rate methods, coagulation studies on plasma, cultures, and tests that require large blood volumes.

The skin puncture is the preferred method to obtain blood from infants and children. Venipuncture on infants and children can damage veins and surrounding tissues. Restraining the infant or child can cause injury.

Selection of the Capillary Puncture Site

The location of the puncture must be carefully considered in addition to the patient's age, accessibility of ac-

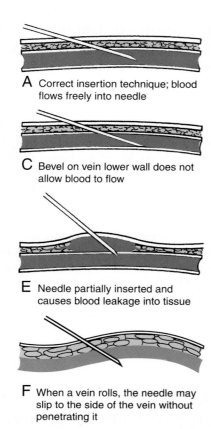

A Correct insertion technique; blood flows freely into needle

B Bevel on vein upper wall does not allow blood to flow

C Bevel on vein lower wall does not allow blood to flow

D Needle inserted too far

E Needle partially inserted and causes blood leakage into tissue

G Collapsed

F When a vein rolls, the needle may slip to the side of the vein without penetrating it

Figure 41-13 Proper and improper needle positioning. **(A)** Needle correctly positioned in a vein; blood flows freely into the needle. **(B)** Bevel on the upper wall of the vein prevents blood flow. **(C)** Bevel on the lower wall of the vein prevents blood flow. **(D)** Needle inserted too deep runs through the vein. **(E)** Partially inserted needle causes blood to leak into tissue. **(F)** Needle slipped beside the vein, not into it; this occurs when a vein rolls to the side. **(G)** Collapsed vein prevents blood flow. (Reprinted with permission from McCall R. Phlebotomy Essentials. Baltimore: Lippincott Williams & Wilkins, 2007.)

BOX 41-2

SOURCES OF ERROR IN VENIPUNCTURE

Errors in Venipuncture Preparation

- Improper patient identification
- Failure to check patient adherence to dietary restrictions
- Failure to calm patient prior to blood collection
- Use of improper equipment and supplies
- Inappropriate method of blood collection
- Failure to dry the site completely after cleansing with alcohol

Errors in Venipuncture Procedure

- Inserting needle bevel side down
- Use of needle that is too small, causing hemolysis of specimen
- Venipuncture in an unacceptable area
- Prolonged tourniquet application
- Wrong order of tube draw

- Failure to mix blood collected in additive-containing tubes immediately
- Pulling back on syringe plunger too forcefully
- Failure to release tourniquet prior to needle withdrawal

Errors After Venipuncture Completion

- Failure to apply pressure immediately to venipuncture site
- Vigorous shaking of anticoagulated blood specimens
- Forcing blood through a syringe needle into tube
- Mislabeling of tubes
- Failure to label appropriate specimens with infectious disease precaution
- Failure to put date, time, and initials on requisition
- Slow transport of specimens to laboratory

Reprinted with permission from McCall R. Phlebotomy Essentials. Baltimore: Lippincott Williams & Wilkins, 2003.

BOX 41-3

SITUATIONS THAT MAY TRIGGER HEMATOMA FORMATION

1. The vein is fragile or too small for the needle.
2. The needle penetrates all the way through the vein.
3. The needle is only partly inserted into the vein.
4. Excessive or blind probing is used to find the vein.
5. The needle is removed while the tourniquet is still on.
6. Pressure is not adequately applied after venipuncture.

Complications of Capillary Puncture

Obtaining a specimen without clots is a challenge in microcollection. The capillary puncture activates the body's clotting system to stop the bleeding as soon as the skin is punctured. If an anticoagulated specimen is required, it should be drawn first to get an adequate volume before the blood begins to clot. Any other additive specimens are collected next, and clotted specimens are collected last. If the blood has begun to produce microscopic clots while you are filling the last tube, this is not a problem because clotting is required in this tube.

Avoid excessive squeezing of the fingertip or heel because the red blood cells will rupture and contaminate the specimen. If excessive squeezing is required because of inadequate blood flow, discontinue the puncture. Choose another site and warm the site prior to the puncture. Box 41-4 lists common sources of errors in microcollection that should be avoided.

ceptable sites, and the tests ordered. Skin puncture in adults and older children most often involves one of the fingers. Recommended sites are the fleshy pad of the third or fourth finger of the patient's nondominant hand only. For finger puncture sites, it is best to have the hand below the heart.

For infant heel punctures in children under 1 year of age, the CLSI (described earlier in this chapter) set the standard of a maximum of 2 mm for heel punctures to avoid hitting bone. Because the thickness of the tissue on the side of an infant's heel can be as little as 2.0 mm and as little as 1.0 mm at the positive curvature of the heel, heel punctures on infants must never be performed on the back of the heel. If performed on the side of the heel, they must be no deeper than 2.0 mm. Contraindications for using a specific site for capillary puncture are:

- Bruised, infected, swollen, or traumatized sites on fingers or heels
- Thumb, because the skin is often too thick
- Second finger, because it is much more sensitive than other fingers
- Fifth finger, because the flesh may be so thin that the bone could be pierced

If the patient has cold hands, warm them by holding them under warm running water or by vigorously rubbing them. The complete procedure for performing a skin puncture is outlined in Procedure 41-2.

BOX 41-4

SOURCES OF ERROR IN SKIN PUNCTURE

- Misidentification of patient
- Puncturing wrong area of infant heel
- Puncturing bone in infant heel
- Puncturing fingers of infants
- Puncturing wrong area of adult finger
- Contaminating specimen with alcohol or Betadine
- Failure to discard first blood drop
- Excessive massaging of puncture site
- Collecting air bubbles in pH or blood gas specimen
- Hemolyzing specimen
- Failure to seal specimens adequately
- Failure to chill specimens requiring refrigeration
- Erroneous specimen labeling
- Failure to document skin puncture collection on the requisition or in the computer
- Failure to warm site
- Delaying specimen transport
- Bruising site as a result of excessive squeezing

WHAT IF?

What if your patient feels faint while you are drawing blood?

1. Remove the tourniquet and withdraw the needle as quickly as possible.
2. Talk to the patient to divert attention from the procedure and to help keep him or her alert.
3. Have the patient lower his or her head and breathe deeply while you physically support the patient to prevent injury in case of collapse.
4. Loosen a tight collar or tie if possible.
5. Apply a cold compress or washcloth to the forehead and back of the patient's neck.
6. Call for the physician if the patient does not respond.

Modified with permission from McCall R. Phlebotomy Essentials. Baltimore: Lippincott Williams & Wilkins, 2003.

MEDIA MENU

- Student CD
  - **Video Procedures**
  Procedure 41-1 and 41-2 video clips
  - **CMA/RMA Certification Exam Review**
- Premium Online Course
  http://thePoint.lww.com/Kronenberger3e
- Internet Resources

LiveAdvise Online Tutoring & Competency Training
http://thePoint.lww.com/LiveAdvise

The Internet Pathology Laboratory for Medical Education, Florida State University College of Medicine
http://library.med.utah.edu/WebPath/TUTORIAL/PHLEB/PHLEB.html

Phlebotomy Pages
www.phlebotomypages.com/

Austin Community College—Phlebotomy Quizzes
www2.austin.cc.tx.us/kotrla/phlebquiz.htm

Centers for Disease Control and Prevention—Phlebotomy Information
www.cdc.gov/ncbddd/hemochromatosis/training/pdf/phlebotomy_info.pdf

---

PROCEDURE 41-1: Obtaining a Blood Specimen by Evacuated Tube or Winged Infusion Set

Purpose: To obtain blood for diagnostic purposes and/or monitoring of prescribed treatment
Equipment: Multisample needle and adaptor or winged infusion set, evacuated tubes, tourniquet, sterile gauze pads, bandages, sharps container, 70% alcohol pad, permanent marker or pen, appropriate personal protective equipment (e.g., gloves, impervious gown, face shield)

Steps	Reasons
1. Check the requisition slip to determine the tests ordered and specimen requirements.	This ensures proper specimen collection.
2. Wash your hands.	Handwashing aids infection control.
3. Assemble the equipment. Check the expiration date on the tubes.	Assembling the equipment ensures that everything you need is available. Discard expired supplies.
4. Greet and identify the patient. Explain the procedure. Ask for and answer any questions.	Identifying the patient maintains sample integrity. Explaining the procedure helps ease anxiety and ensure compliance.

(continued)

PROCEDURE 41-1: **Obtaining a Blood Specimen by Evacuated Tube or Winged Infusion Set** *(continued)*

Steps	Reasons
5. If a fasting specimen is required, ask the patient for the last time he or she ate or drank anything other than water.	For fasting specimens, the patient should not have eaten within at least 8 hours.
6. Put on nonsterile latex or vinyl gloves. Use other personal protective equipment as defined by facility policy.	Standard precautions protect the phlebotomist and the patient.
7. *For evacuated tube collection*: Break the seal of the needle cover and thread the sleeved needle into the adaptor, using the needle cover as a wrench. *For winged infusion set collection*: Extend the tubing. Thread the sleeved needle into the adaptor. *For both methods*: Tap the tubes that contain additives to ensure that the additive is dislodged from the stopper and wall of the tube. Insert the tube into the adaptor until the needle slightly enters the stopper. Do not push the top of the tube stopper beyond the indentation mark. If the tube retracts slightly, leave it in the retracted position.	This ensures proper needle placement and tube positioning and prevents loss of vacuum in the evacuated tubes.
8. Instruct the patient to sit with a well-supported arm.	Veins in the antecubital fossa are most easily located when the arm is straight.
9. Apply the tourniquet around the patient's arm 3–4 inches above the elbow.	The tourniquet makes the veins more prominent.

A. Apply the tourniquet snuggly, but not too tightly. .

Step 9. Apply the tourniquet 3–4 inches above the elbow.

Step 9A. Apply the tourniquet snuggly, but not tightly.

(continued)

PROCEDURE 41-1: **Obtaining a Blood Specimen by Evacuated Tube or Winged Infusion Set** *(continued)*

Steps	Reasons
B. Secure the tourniquet by using the half-bow knot.	
	Step 9B. Secure the tourniquet by using a half-box knot.
C. Make sure the tails of the tourniquet extend upward to avoid contaminating the venipuncture site.	
D. Ask the patient to make a fist and hold it but not to pump the fist.	**Step 9C.** The tourniquet should extend upwards. Making a fist raises the vessels out of the underlying tissues and muscles.
10. Select a vein by palpating. Use your gloved index finger to trace the path of the vein and judge its depth.	The index finger is the most sensitive for palpating.
	Step 10. Trace the path of the vein.
11. Release the tourniquet after palpating the vein if it has been left on for more than 1 minute. Have the patient release the fist.	The tourniquet should not be left on for more than 1 minute at a time during the procedure.

(continued)

PROCEDURE 41-1: Obtaining a Blood Specimen by Evacuated Tube or Winged Infusion Set *(continued)*

Steps	Reasons
12. Cleanse the venipuncture site with an alcohol pad, starting in the center of the puncture site and working outward in a circular motion. Allow the site to dry, or dry the site with sterile gauze. Do not touch the area after cleansing.	The circular motion helps avoid recontamination of the area. Puncturing a wet area stings and can cause hemolysis of the sample.
13. If blood being drawn for culture will be used in diagnosing a septic condition, make sure the specimen is sterile. To do this, apply alcohol to the area for 2 full minutes. Then apply a 2% iodine solution in ever-widening circles. Never move the wipes back over areas that have been cleaned; use a new wipe for each sweep across the area.	Ensuring sterility of the specimen will add in accurate identification of the pathogen, if present.
14. Reapply the tourniquet if it was removed after palpation. Ask the patient to make a fist.	Tourniquet time greater than 1 minute may alter test results.
15. Remove the needle cover. Hold the needle assembly in your dominant hand, with your thumb on top of the adaptor and your fingers under it. Grasp the patient's arm with the other hand, using your thumb to draw the skin taut over the site. This anchors the vein about 1–2 inches below the puncture site and helps keep it in place during needle insertion.	Anchoring the vein allows easier needle penetration and less pain.
16. With the bevel up, line up the needle with the vein approximately one-quarter to half an inch below the site where the vein is to be entered. At a 15- to 30-degree angle, rapidly and smoothly insert the needle through the skin. Use a lesser angle for winged infusion set collections. Place two fingers on the flanges of the adapter, and with the thumb, push the tube onto the needle inside the adapter. Allow the tube to fill to capacity. Release the tourniquet and allow the patient to release the fist. When blood flow ceases, remove the tube from the adapter by gripping the tube with your non-dominant hand and place your thumb against the flange during removal. Twist and gently pull out the tube. Steady the needle in the vein. Avoid pulling up or pressing down on the needle while it is in the vein. Insert any other necessary tubes into adapter and allow each to fill to capacity.	The sharpest point of the needle is inserted first. Proper tube filling ensures correct ratio of blood to additive. Removal of the tourniquet releases pressure on the vein and helps prevent blood from seeping into adjacent tissues and causing a hematoma.

(continued)

| **PROCEDURE 41-1:** | **Obtaining a Blood Specimen by Evacuated Tube or Winged Infusion Set** (continued) |

Steps | **Reasons**

Step 16. Insert the needle at a 15–30° angle.

17. With the tourniquet released, remove the tube from the adapter before removing the needle from the arm. | Removing the last tube from the adapter before removing the needle from the vein prevents excess blood from dripping from the tip of the needle onto the patient. Pressure decreases the amount of blood escaping into the tissues.

18. Place a sterile gauze pad over the puncture site at the time of needle withdrawal. Do not apply any pressure to the site until the needle is completely removed. | Removing the last tube from the adapter before removing the needle from the vein prevents any excess blood from dripping from the tip of the needle onto the patient. Pressure decreases the amount of blood escaping into the tissues.

Step 18. Place a gauze pad over site.

19. After the needle is removed, immediately activate the safety device and apply pressure, or have the patient apply direct pressure for 3–5 minutes. Do not bend the arm at the elbow. | Bending the arm increases the chance of blood seeping into the subcutaneous tissues. Unfolding the bent arm disturbs the clot forming at the puncture site and causes bleeding.

Step 19. Apply pressure for 3–5 minutes.

20. If the vacuum tubes contain an anticoagulant, they must be mixed immediately by gently inverting the tube 8–10 times. Do not shake the tube. | Mixing anticoagulated tubes prevents clotting of blood.

(continued)

PROCEDURE 41-1: **Obtaining a Blood Specimen by Evacuated Tube or Winged Infusion Set** *(continued)*

Steps	Reasons
21. Label the tubes with patient information as defined in facility protocol.	Proper labeling of blood specimens maintains accurate sample identification.
22. Check the puncture site for bleeding. Apply a dressing, a clean 2 × 2 gauze pad folded in quarters, and hold in place using an adhesive bandage or 3-inch strip of tape.	
23. Thank the patient. Instruct the patient to leave the bandage in place for at least 15 minutes and not to carry a heavy object (such as a purse) or lift heavy objects with that arm for 1 hour.	Courtesy helps the patient have a positive attitude about the procedure and the physician's office.
24. Properly care for or dispose of all equipment and supplies. Clean the work area. Remove personal protective equipment and wash your hands.	Standard precautions must be followed throughout the procedure to prevent the spread of microorganisms.

Step 24. Properly dispose of sharps.

25. Test, transfer, or store the blood specimen according to the medical office policy.	
26. Record the procedure.	Procedures are considered not to have been performed if they are not recorded.

Charting Example:

05/31/2008 10:00 AM OP venipuncture for platelet count, dx code ###.## per Dr. Jacobs

—J. Simpson, RMA

PROCEDURE 41-2: ## Obtaining a Blood Specimen by Capillary Puncture

Purpose: To obtain blood for diagnostic purposes and/or monitoring of prescribed treatment

Equipment: Skin puncture device, 70% alcohol pads, 2 × 2 gauze pads, microcollection tubes or containers, heel-warming device if needed, small bandages (Band-Aids), pen or permanent marker and personal protective equipment (e.g., gloves, impervious gown, face shield).

Steps	Reasons
1. Check the requisition slip to determine the tests ordered and specimen requirements.	This ensures proper specimen collection.
2. Wash your hands.	Handwashing aids infection control.
3. Assemble the equipment.	Having the equipment ready will speed collection so the puncture site does not clot off before the entire specimen has been collected.
4. Greet and identify the patient. Explain the procedure. Ask for and answer any questions.	Identifying the patient maintains sample integrity. Explaining the procedure helps ease anxiety and ensure compliance.
5. Put on gloves.	Standard precautions protect both the phlebotomist and the patient.
6. Select the puncture site (the lateral portion of the tip of the middle or ring finger of the non-dominant hand or lateral curved surface of the heel of an infant). The puncture should be made in the fleshy central portion of the second or third finger, slightly to the side of center and perpendicular to the grooves of the fingerprint.	The ring and middle fingers are less calloused than the forefinger. The lateral part of the tip is the least sensitive part of the finger. A puncture made across the fingerprints will produce a large, round drop of blood. In an infant skin puncture, the area and the depth designated reduces the risk of puncturing the bone.

Site

This

Not this

Step 6. Recommend site and direction of finger puncture. (Reprinted with permission from McCall R. Phlebotomy Essentials. Baltimore: Lippincott Williams and Wilkins, 2003).

Perform heel puncture only on the plantar surface of the heel, medial to an imaginary line extending from the middle of the great toe to the heel and lateral to an imaginary line drawn from between the fourth and fifth toes to the heel. Use the appropriate puncture device for the site selected.

(continued)

PROCEDURE 41-2: Obtaining a Blood Specimen by Capillary Puncture (continued)

Steps	Reasons

Step 6. Acceptable areas for heel punctures on newborns. (Reprinted with permission from McCall R. Phlebotomy Essentials. Baltimore: Lippincott Williams and Wilkins, 2003).

Steps	Reasons
7. Make sure the site chosen is warm and not cyanotic or edematous. Gently massage the finger from the base to the tip, or massage the infant's heel.	Massaging the area increases the blood flow. Good circulation at the chosen site yields a better blood sample for analysis.
8. Grasp the finger firmly between your non-dominant index finger and thumb, or grasp the infant's heel firmly with your index finger wrapped around the foot and your thumb wrapped around the ankle.	The area must be dry to eliminate alcohol residue, which can cause the patient discomfort and interfere with test results.

Cleanse the selected area with 70% isopropyl alcohol and allow to air dry.

Step 8. Grasp the finger firmly.

Step 8. Cleanse the site with alcohol and allow to air dry.

Steps	Reasons
9. Hold the patient's finger or heel firmly and make a swift, firm puncture. Perform the puncture perpendicular to the whorls of the fingerprint or footprint. Dispose of the used puncture device in a sharps container.	Maintaining your hold at the site prevents the patient from contaminating the cleansed puncture area and allows you to have control of the puncture site.

(continued)

PROCEDURE 41-2: Obtaining a Blood Specimen by Capillary Puncture *(continued)*

Steps	Reasons
	  Step 9. Hold the patient's finger or heel firmly and make a swift, firm puncture.
10. Obtain the first drop of blood and wipe it away with dry gauze. Apply pressure toward the site but do not milk the site.	The first discarded drop may be contaminated with tissue fluid or alcohol residue.
	Step 10. (A) Obtain the first drop of blood. **(B)** Wipe it away.
11. Collect the specimen in the chosen container or slide. Touch only the tip of the collection device to the drop of blood. Blood flow is encouraged if the puncture site is held downward and gentle pressure is applied near the site. Cap microcollection tubes with the caps provided and mix the additives by gently tilting or inverting the tubes 8–10 times.	Milking the site will dilute the specimen with tissue fluid. Scraping the collection device on the skin activates platelets and may cause hemolysis. Mixing the specimens prevents clotting. Touching the tube to the site may cause contamination.

(continued)

PROCEDURE 41-2: Obtaining a Blood Specimen by Capillary Puncture *(continued)*

Steps	Reasons

Step 11. Apply pressure with clean gauze.

12. When collection is complete, apply clean gauze to the site with pressure. Hold pressure or have the patient hold pressure until bleeding stops. Label the containers with the proper information. Do not apply a dressing to a skin puncture of an infant under 2 years of age. Never release a patient until the bleeding has stopped.	Proper labeling of blood specimens maintains accurate sample identification. Younger children may develop a skin irritation from the adhesive bandage. Also, a young child may put the bandage in the mouth and choke.
13. Thank the patient. Instruct the patient to leave the bandage in place for at least 15 minutes.	Courtesy helps the patient have a positive attitude about the procedure and the physician's office.
14. Properly care for or dispose of equipment and supplies. Clean the work area. Remove gloves and wash your hands.	Standard precautions protect the phlebotomist and the patient.
15. Test, transfer, or store the specimen according to the medical office policy.	
16. Record the procedure.	Procedures are considered not to have been done if they are not recorded.

Note: Several precautions should be observed to produce the most accurate specimen. The greatest concern with microcollection specimens is hemolysis, the rupture of erythrocytes with the release of hemoglobin. Do not squeeze or milk the heel or finger to increase blood flow. Never scrape the microcollection device on the skin. Allow the container to touch only the drop of blood. Also, be careful to avoid additional sources of errors, which are listed in Box 41-4.

Charting Example:

07/12/2008 9:00 AM OP fingerstick for prothrombin time dx ###.## per Dr. Robins
—S. Smith, CMA

- Maintain your professional attitude and be sympathetic to the fears and anxieties of the patient in all areas of patient care. For many patients, venipuncture is particularly frightening. Demonstrate compassion and understanding to allay their fears. Your skill and knowledge, coupled with a caring approach, will help ensure that the patient's experience in phlebotomy is not unpleasant.

- Selection of the proper equipment and blood collection system provide the safest and most gentle stick for the patient and also provide the highest quality specimens.

- The quality of the test result is only as good as the quality of the specimen. Several essential steps ensure successful blood collection. These steps include accurate patient identification, verification of proper dietary restrictions prior to testing, good venipuncture site selection, and obtaining and handling the specimen so that minimal damage is done to the cells and the specimen is thoroughly mixed with the tube additives as soon as possible. Medical assistants are responsible for collecting specimens properly and testing them accurately.

- The office laboratory provides a challenge and opportunity to work with the physician in improving and promoting the health of the patient.

Warm Ups   for Critical Thinking

1. What effects do hemoconcentration and hemolysis of the specimen have in test results?

2. Your patient complains of serious pain when you insert the needle into the vein. Explain the steps to improve the patient's comfort.

3. How can you help ease patient anxiety about venipuncture? List the steps to take.

4. Your patient asks you how long you have been drawing blood and whether you are "good"? How do you respond? Justify your response.

5. Describe the steps you would take if you started a venipuncture and got no specimen in the tube. Explain how each step could result in a successful blood collection.

Answers   to Checkpoint Questions

1. Patients and phlebotomists may have allergic reactions to latex products and glove powder. The reactions to latex can be severe.

2. Discarding tourniquets after one use is a good infection control practice. Reusing a blood-flecked tourniquet is not in agreement with any infection control policy and also reduces the patient's confidence in you as a phlebotomist.

3. Plasma is the liquid portion of the specimen in an anticoagulated specimen. Serum is the liquid portion of the specimen from a clotted specimen. Serum does not contain blood coagulation components because they were exhausted to produce the clot.

4. When using the evacuated tube system, the proper order of draw is blood culture tubes, plain red, light blue, red/gray and gold, green, lavender, and gray. It is important to follow the correct order of draw to avoid specimen cross-contamination with additives.

5. The red blood cells move from the collection site, through the needle, and into the tube. Needle gauges of 23 and smaller cause damage to the red blood cells that contaminates the specimen. The gauge number gets larger as the needle get smaller.

6. The term NPO means "nothing by mouth." The purpose is to empty the gastric system and minimize secretions. The term fasting means nothing by mouth except water. In addition to the great difference in the patient's comfort, the water keeps the patient more hydrated, making veins more supple.

CHAPTER

42

Hematology

Outline

Formation of Blood Cells
Pathophysiology and
   Hematologic Testing
Complete Blood Count
  White Blood Cell Count and
   Differential
  Red Blood Cell Count

Hemoglobin
Hematocrit
Erythrocyte Indices
Platelet Count
Erythrocyte Sedimentation
  Rate

Coagulation (Hemostasis)
  Tests
Prothrombin Time
Partial Thromboplastin Time

Learning Objectives

Upon successfully completing this chapter, you will be able to:

1. Spell and define the key terms

2. List the parameters measured in the complete blood count and their normal ranges

3. State the conditions associated with selected abnormal complete blood count findings

4. Explain the functions of the three types of blood cells

5. Describe the purpose of testing for the erythrocyte sedimentation rate

6. List the leukocytes seen normally in the blood and their functions

7. Explain the hemostatic mechanism of the body

8. List and describe the tests that measure the body's ability to form a fibrin clot

9. Explain how to determine the prothrombin time and partial thromboplastin time

Performance Objectives

Upon successfully completing this chapter, you will be able to:

1. Make a peripheral blood smear (Procedure 42-1)

2. Stain a peripheral blood smear (Procedure 42-2)

3. Perform a hemoglobin determination (Procedure 42-3)

4. Perform a microhematocrit determination (Procedure 42-4)

5. Determine a Westergren erythrocyte sedimentation rate (Procedure 42-5)

CAAHEP

- Perform handwashing
- Dispose of biohazardous materials
- Practice standard precautions
- Perform hematology testing
- Screen and follow-up test results
- Use methods of quality control
- Document appropriately

ABHES

- Apply principles of aseptic techniques and infection control
- Collect and process specimens
- Perform selected CLIA-waived tests that assist with diagnosis and treatment
- Dispose of biohazardous waste
- Practice standard precautions
- Perform hematology testing
- Document appropriately
- Use methods of quality control
- Specimen collection
- OSHA compliance rules and regulations

Key Terms

anisocytosis	erythrocyte sedimen- tation rate	hematopoiesis	morphology
basophil		hemoglobin	neutrophil
complete blood count	erythropoietin	hemostasis	poikilocytosis
eosinophil	folate	leukocytes	sickle cell anemia
erythrocytes	granulocytes	lymphocyte	thrombocytes
erythrocyte indices	hematocrit	monocyte	thromboplastin

The hematology laboratory analyzes the blood cells, their quantities, and their characteristics for diagnosis and management of many conditions. Anemias, leukemias, and infections are some of the more common disorders detected and managed by hematologic testing. In addition, hematology includes the study of **hemostasis**, or the ability of the patient's blood to form and dissolve a clot. Thus, the hematology laboratory is helpful in evaluating individuals who have difficulty forming a clot and those who form clots spontaneously within their blood vessels.

Formation of Blood Cells

Blood is made up of fluid (plasma) and three general types of cells, **erythrocytes** (red blood cells or RBCs), **leukocytes** (white blood cells or WBCs), and **thrombocytes** (platelets) (Fig. 42-1). Blood cells are formed in the bone marrow. The long bones, skull, pelvis, and sternum manufacture most of these cells. Other blood cell–making sites are the liver and spleen. The yolk sac of the developing fetus also produces blood cells. (The yolk sac is the structure that nourishes the embryo until the seventh week, when the placenta takes over.) **Hematopoiesis** (blood cell production) starts with very young, immature cells within the bone marrow that eventually divide and differentiate (acquire distinct or individual characteristics and mature) (Fig42-2). These cells become erythrocytes, leukocytes, and thrombocytes according to the body's needs. Each type of cell has a particular function, discussed later in this chapter. Hematopoiesis is influenced by hormones and requires adequate nutrients, such as iron, to produce functional cells. Once these cells have reached maturity, they are released from the bone marrow and travel into the bloodstream.

Figure 42-1 (**A**) A blood smear. (**B**) RBCs (large, round cells) and platelets (stained purple). (**C**) Segmented neutrophil. (**D**) Neutrophil band. (**E**) Lymphocyte. (**F**) Monocyte. (**G**) Eosinophil. (**H**) Basophil.

 CHECKPOINT QUESTION

1. What is hematopoiesis, and how is it influenced?

Pathophysiology and Hematologic Testing

Although hematologic testing is often used to diagnose and manage disease of the blood cells and coagulation proteins, it is also useful in the study of other diseases, such as metabolic, nutritional, immunologic, and neoplastic disorders. Common hematologic tests include the **complete blood count** (CBC), erythrocyte sedimentation rate (ESR or sed rate), and coagulation tests. Clinical Laboratory Improvement Amendment (CLIA) regulations limit the types of hematology testing medical assistants can perform. The list of tests medical assistants can perform, updated regularly by the Centers

for Medicare and Medicaid Services (CMS), includes the following:

- Erythrocyte sedimentation rate (not automated)
- Hematocrit (all spun microhematocrit procedures)
- Hemoglobin (selected methods)
- Prothrombin time (selected methods)

Complete Blood Count

The complete blood count (CBC), or hemogram, is one of the most frequently ordered tests in the laboratory (Box 42-1). It consists of a number of parameters, including the following:

- WBC count and differential
- RBC count
- Hemoglobin (Hgb) determination
- Hematocrit (Hct) determination

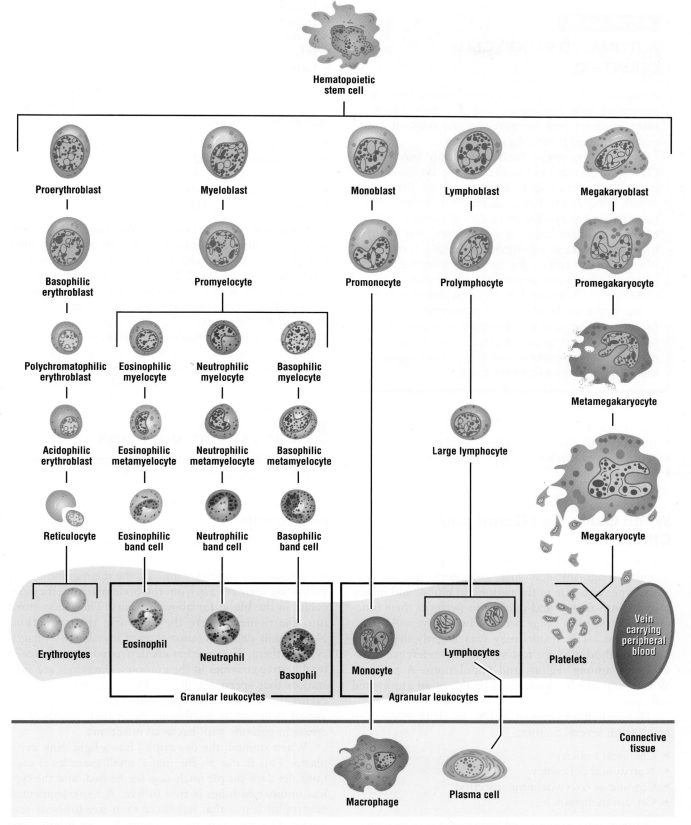

Figure 42-2 Maturation of blood cell lines. (From Eroschenko V. di Fiore's Atlas of Histology, With Functional Correlations. 9th ed. Baltimore: Lippincott Williams & Wilkins, 2000.)

BOX 42-1

AUTOMATED BLOOD CELL COUNTERS

A number of biotechnology companies have instruments that can count and size blood cells. Although each has its own specific method, the main operating principles are similar.

A portion of whole blood (anticoagulated with EDTA) is taken in and diluted. These dilutions are moved into counting chambers, where they are drawn through tiny holes (apertures). As the cells pass through the holes, an electrical current, a light beam, or a laser beam is interrupted. The instrument registers the interruption as a cell. It can tell the size of the cell by the length of time the beam is interrupted or the amount of light scatter.

These instruments have become so sophisticated that a white blood cell differential now can be reported accurately. Hemoglobin is also measured, along with other parameters, such as mean corpuscular hemoglobin, adding to the diagnostic value of the complete blood count.

- Mean cell volume (MCV)
- Mean corpuscular hemoglobin (MCH)
- Mean corpuscular hemoglobin concentration (MCHC)
- Platelet count

White Blood Cell Count and Differential

WBCs (leukocytes) provide the main line of defense against foreign invaders such as bacteria and viruses. Some types circulate in the peripheral blood, and others migrate into tissues and cavities to perform their functions. The normal range for a WBC count is 4300 to 10,800/mm^3. Test results may vary slightly depending on the method used for testing. Normal reference intervals vary among regions and populations. A patient's WBC count can be determined by use of an automated cell counter.

Diminished numbers of leukocytes (leukopenia) can result from several factors:

- Chemical toxicity
- Nutritional deficiency
- Chronic or overwhelming infection
- Certain malignancies

Patients with pronounced leukopenia may be vulnerable to infections. Leukocytosis (increased numbers of WBCs) can stem from many sources:

- Infection
- Inflammatory condition
- Certain drugs
- Injury to tissue
- Certain malignancies

The WBC differential determines the amounts of various WBC types in the peripheral blood. These types include the following:

- Neutrophils (Fig. 42-1, C and D)
- Lymphocytes (Fig. 42-1E)
- Monocytes (Fig. 42-1F)
- Eosinophils (Fig. 42-1G)
- Basophils (Fig. 42-1H)

Because all of these types of leukocytes are colorless, a drop of blood is smeared on a glass slide and then stained so that they can be seen with a microscope (Procedures 42-1 and 42-2). Once the peripheral blood is stained, 100 WBCs are counted, tallied according to type, and reported as percentages. This count is known as the WBC differential. These cell types fall into three general categories: **granulocytes** (subdivided into neutrophils, eosinophils, and basophils; so named because of granules in their cytoplasm that have distinctive staining characteristics), **lymphocytes**, and **monocytes**. Each of the three has a distinct purpose in fighting infection.

 CHECKPOINT QUESTION

2. What is leukopenia, and what are four conditions that may cause it?

Neutrophils

Neutrophils—also called polymorphonuclear neutrophils, polys, segmented neutrophils, or segs—are the most abundant leukocyte and are the main granulocyte. Following their release from the bone marrow, they circulate in the blood for about 7 hours. They then move into the tissues, where they perform their function. Neutrophils defend against foreign invaders by phagocytizing them. The invaders are destroyed inside the cells by digestive enzymes in the granules. (Enzymes are substances that speed reactions.) These digestive enzymes eventually kill the neutrophil too. The normal percentage of neutrophils is 50% to 70%; their numbers increase in patients with bacterial infections.

When stained, the neutrophil has a light pink cytoplasm. This is due to the many small granules it contains. Its dark purple nucleus is segmented, and the typical number of lobes is two to five. A hypersegmented neutrophil is one that has more than five lobes or segments. This can indicate a vitamin B$_{12}$, or **folate**, deficiency. (Folate, a salt of folic acid, is an essential nutrient.) A band (or stab) is a younger, less mature version of the neutrophil. The band's appearance is the same as that of the more mature counterpart, but its nucleus is not segmented. The percentage of bands is 0% to 5%. Higher percentages of bands may indicate any of a variety of acute conditions that necessitate immediate attention. In combination with leukocytosis, this is called a left shift.

PATIENT EDUCATION

DIETARY FOLATE

Folate plays an active part in normal RBC maturation. When it is decreased in the body, anemia develops. The body acquires folate via the food chain. Some natural sources of folate are:

- Leafy green vegetables, such as spinach or turnip greens
- Citrus fruits and juices
- Dried beans and peas

Folate may also be taken as a dietary supplement. In addition to anemia, more subtle signs may indicate a folate deficiency:

- Diarrhea
- Sore tongue
- Heart palpitations
- Behavioral disorders

CHECKPOINT QUESTION

3. What is the function of neutrophils?

Lymphocytes

Lymphocytes (lymphs) are the second most numerous WBC. The main function of lymphocytes is to recognize that a particular cell or particle is foreign to the body and to make antibodies specific to its destruction. The antibodies coat this foreign mass, resulting in one of two possible outcomes: the phagocytic system is activated to destroy the pathogen, or the complement system (a series of chemicals in the blood) is activated to destroy the cellular invaders by puncturing holes in their membranes. The normal percentage of lymphocytes is 20% to 35%. Higher numbers, especially of atypical ones, can signal a viral infection such as infectious mononucleosis. The life span of the lymphocyte is generally 3 to 4 days, longer than that of the neutrophil. However, some have much longer lives, spanning into years or even decades.

The lymphocyte is the smallest of the leukocytes. When stained, it has a small, round, dark purple nucleus. The surrounding cytoplasm is scant and sky blue. Atypical lymphs are larger, with more cytoplasm that is either darker or lighter.

Monocytes

Monocytes (or monos) are the third most abundant leukocyte. Like neutrophils, monocytes phagocytize foreign material. They also aid the lymphocyte in providing the humoral response (destruction of foreign particles by antibodies). Monocytes stay in the bloodstream for about 3 days and then move into tissues.

The shape of the monocyte nucleus varies but tends to be indented or horseshoe-shaped. It is much larger than the lymphocyte and closer in size to the neutrophil. When stained, the monocyte's cytoplasm is gray-blue and has a ground-glass appearance. The normal percentage of monocytes is 3% to 8%. Monocytosis (increase in monocytes) occurs with inflammatory responses and certain bacterial infections, such as syphilis and tuberculosis. Monocytopenia may occur after administration of certain drugs or after an overwhelming infection.

Eosinophils

Eosinophils (or eos) are fourth in abundance. Their function is not completely understood. The normal percentage of eosinophils is 0% to 6%. They are higher during allergic reactions and some infections, especially parasitic. The typical number of nuclear lobes in granulocytes is two to five. The eosinophil has a bilobed nucleus with large red granules in the cytoplasm.

Basophils

Basophils (or basos) are the least numerous WBC, accounting for fewer than 1% of circulating WBCs. The nucleus is either bilobed or trilobed, and on staining, very large dark blue–purple granules are seen in the cytoplasm. Basophils appear to be a factor in allergic asthma, in contact allergies, and in hypothyroidism and chronic myeloid leukemia.

CHECKPOINT QUESTION

4. Elevated eosinophils and basophils are both seen with what condition?

Red Blood Cell Count

RBCs (erythrocytes) transport gases (mainly oxygen and carbon dioxide) between the lungs and the tissues. Their special structure, a biconcave disk containing hemoglobin, lets them readily exchange gases in the tissues and lung fields. As blood moves through the capillary bed of the lungs, RBCs release carbon dioxide that was picked up at the tissues and then bind oxygen. As the blood leaves the lungs and circulates to the organs, oxygen is released from the RBCs into the tissues. At the same time, carbon dioxide (the byproduct of metabolism) diffuses into the blood and is brought back to the lungs to be exhaled.

RBCs are made in the bone marrow along with all other blood cells. Their production is influenced by the hormone **erythropoietin**, which is released from the kidneys. When the kidney detects decreased oxygen concentration in circulating blood, increased levels of this hormone migrate from the kidney to the marrow to increase RBC production (erythropoiesis), which corrects the anemia by releasing more RBCs into the circulation to carry more oxygen. Other factors can also influence the quality and quantity of erythropoiesis. For example, vitamin B_{12} and folic acid are required for the cells to mature properly. The globin molecule needs iron to make functional hemoglobin. Initially, erythrocytes have a nucleus, but as they mature, the nucleus is pushed out, and the color of their cytoplasm changes from blue to red. The mature RBC is a pale red biconcave disk that can squeeze through very small capillaries. The average RBC lives about 120 days.

Hematology analyzers provide measurements of RBCs and associated parameters (Fig. 42-3) provide a useful guide for detecting anemia, which can be caused by decreased erythrocyte production (as in iron deficiency) (Fig. 42-4), increased RBC destxruction (as in hemolytic anemia), or blood loss. The normal range of RBCs for men is 4.6 to 6.2 million/mm^3, and for women, it is 4.2 to 5.4 million/mm^3.

Figure 42-4 Blood smear from a patient with iron deficiency anemia showing RBCs that are hypochromic and microcytic. (From Rubin R, Strayer D. Rubin's Pathology. 4th ed. Baltimore: Lippincott Williams & Wilkins, 2005.)

A WBC differential of the peripheral blood includes a report on RBC **morphology** or appearance. This report contains comments on the variation in size (**anisocytosis**) and shape (**poikilocytosis**) of the RBCs. Table 42-1 describes some common erythrocyte abnormalities and their associated conditions.

PATIENT EDUCATION

IRON DEFICIENCY ANEMIA

Patients who have iron deficiency anemia should be taught proper dietary management.

They should be instructed to eat foods high in iron, such as liver, oysters, kidney beans, lean meats, turnips, egg yolks, whole-wheat bread, carrots, raisins, and dark greens. A vitamin supplement with iron can be added to the diet. Patients should be warned that iron supplements can cause constipation and dark stools.

Hemoglobin

Hemoglobin is the functioning unit of the red blood cell. Each hemoglobin molecule contains four protein chains called globins. Alpha and beta are the most common types of globin chains, with some gamma chains (fetal) in newborns. Defects in the globin chains result in abnormal hemoglobins, such as S (sickle) found in persons having **sickle cell anemia** or carrying the sickle trait. In the folds of each globin is a heme unit that contains one iron molecule; the iron can reversibly bind gases such as oxygen and carbon dioxide. The iron also gives RBCs

Figure 42-3 Coulter Ac-T diff2 Hematology Analyzer. (Courtesy of Beckman-Coulter, Fullerton, CA.)

TABLE 42-1	Erythrocyte Abnormalities	
Abnormality	**Associated Conditions**
Hypochromasia—diminished hemoglobin in RBCs; appear paler with more area of central pallor	Anemias (especially iron deficiency), thalassemia (a hemolytic anemia)
Hyperchromasia—increased hemoglobin in RBCs; appear to have less or no area of central pallor	Megaloblastic anemia (characterized by large, dysfunctional RBCs), hereditary spherocytosis (condition in which nearly all the RBCs are spherocytes)
Polychromasia—some RBCs have a blue color	Hemolysis, acute blood loss
Microcytosis—RBCs are smaller than usual	Iron deficiency anemia, thalassemia
Macrocytosis—RBCs are larger than normal	Vitamin B12 and folate deficiencies, megaloblastic anemias
Elliptocytes/ovalocytes—RBCs are distinctly oval in shape	Hereditary elliptocytosis, iron deficiency anemia, myelofibrosis (disorder in which bone marrow tissue develops in abnormal sites), sickle cell anemia (hereditary anemia characterized by the presence of sickle-shaped RBCs)
Target cells—RBCs resemble a target with light and dark rings	Liver impairment, anemias (especially thalassemia), hemoglobin C disease (genetic blood disorder)
Schistocytes—RBCs are fragmented	Hemolysis, burns, intravascular coagulation (clot formation within the vessels)
Spherocytes—RBCs show no area of central pallor	Hereditary spherocytosis, hemolytic anemias, burns
Burr cells—RBCs have small, regular spicules (sharp points)	Artifact as blood dries, hyperosmolarity (a condition of increased numbers of dissolved substances in the plasma)

their distinctive red color. There are millions of hemoglobin molecules in each RBC. The normal range for hemoglobin is 13 to 18 g/dL (or g/100 mL) in men and 12 to 16 g/dL in women. Anemia is detected with a hemoglobin measurement, which is a direct indicator of the body's ability to oxygenate tissues (Procedure 42-3). There are also point-of-care methods approved for use by medical assistants. An example is the HemoCue System Hemoglobin Plasma/Low Hemoglobin Analyzer.

Hematocrit

The **hematocrit** is the percentage of RBCs in whole blood. For example, a hematocrit of 40% indicates that 40% of the total blood volume consists of RBCs. The remaining 60% is plasma, WBCs, and platelets.

To measure the hematocrit, the blood is centrifuged to pack the RBCs, and the percentage is determined. Automated instruments do not measure the hematocrit but rather calculate it from the RBC count and mean cell volume (MCV). The purpose of measuring the hematocrit is to detect anemia. The normal range is 45% to 52% in men and 37% to 48% in women (Procedure 42-4).

 CHECKPOINT QUESTION

5. A patient has a hematocrit of 20%. What does this percentage signify?

Erythrocyte Indices

Three measurements are included in the **erythrocyte indices**: mean cell volume (MCV), mean cell hemoglobin (MCH), and mean cell hemoglobin concentration (MCHC). These measurements indicate the size of the RBC and how much hemoglobin the RBC holds. Erythrocyte indices are significant in diagnosing and treating the anemias.

Mean Cell Volume

Because RBCs vary in size, MCV measures the average size of RBCs. For example, a patient with an MCV of 85 femtoliters (fL; unit of measure signifying one quadrillionth of a liter) may have RBCs that range in size from 75 to 95 fL but that average 85 fL. The MCV can be an indicator of anemias such as those caused by the nutritional deficiencies that affect RBC production. The normal range for MCV is 80 to 95 fL.

Microcytosis (MCV below 80 fL) is most commonly caused by iron deficiency. This finding, coupled with RBC count, hemoglobin, and hematocrit, will indicate anemia and may lead to a diagnosis of iron deficiency anemia. Likewise, macrocytosis (MCV above 95 fL) may be caused by a deficiency of vitamin B_{12} or folic acid. These abnormalities can also result in anemia. Liver disorders sometimes raise the MCV.

Mean Cell Hemoglobin and Mean Cell Hemoglobin Concentration

MCH and MCHC indicate relative hemoglobin concentration in the blood. Both the MCH and MCHC are calculated. RBCs with inadequate amounts of hemoglobin are termed hypochromic. The MCH is derived from the ratio of hemoglobin to the number of RBCs in the specimen. The normal range for MCH is 27 to 31 picograms. An increase may be seen in macrocytic anemias, and a decrease is consistent with microcytic, hypochromic anemias.

The MCHC is derived from the ratio of hemoglobin to hematocrit. The normal range for MCHC is 32 to 36 g/dL. The MCHC is reduced in true hypochromic anemia and may be increased when spherocytes (RBCs with high hemoglobin content) are present.

Platelet Count

Platelets (thrombocytes), like other blood cells, are made in the bone marrow. However, they are not actually cells but cell fragments that adhere to damaged endothelium. Platelets are essential to hemostasis because they not only aid in sealing wounds and stopping bleeding until a clot can form but also help initiate the clotting factors to form the more stable fibrin clot.

The normal range for platelets is 200,000 to 400,000/mm³. Thrombocytopenia (decreased platelets) can be caused by a variety of conditions and may be associated with increased bleeding. The bleeding is usually from many small capillaries. The risk of bleeding increases as the platelet count decreases. Treatment requires a specific diagnosis of the cause of the thrombocytopenia, which may be anemia, infectious disease, drug, acute leukemia, radiation treatment, or chemotherapy. Thrombocytosis (increased platelets) is most often benign. It can be seen after splenectomy or during inflammatory disease. Marked thrombocytosis (< 1 million/mm³) may be associated with an increased clotting tendency or severe bleeding if the platelet function is impaired.

Platelets are much smaller than RBCs. They stain a light purplish-blue, have an irregular shape, and contain visible granules but no nucleus.

Erythrocyte Sedimentation Rate

The erythrocyte sedimentation rate (ESR) measures the rate in millimeters per hour at which RBCs settle out in a tube. Performing the test includes placing anticoagulated blood in a calibrated column and allowing it to settle undisturbed for 1 hour. At the end of the hour, the distance the RBCs have fallen is measured. Although there are several methods for determining the ESR, such as the Wintrobe and the Westergren methods, the principle remains the same. The Westergren method is most commonly used in POLs. This method has the safety feature of a closed system that reduces the medical assistant's exposure to the patient's blood. Procedure 42-5 describes the steps and Figure 42-5 outlines the steps for the Westergren method.

Always verify the following conditions to ensure accurate ESR results:

- Test should be started within 2 hours of specimen collection.
- Test should be conducted at room temperature.
- The blood column must contain no bubbles.
- The tube must remain completely vertical during testing.
- The sedimentation rack must be placed on a counter with no vibrations. (Do not place near a centrifuge.)
- The sedimentation rack must be away from all drafts and direct sunlight.
- Test results should be read at exactly 60 minutes.

Figure 42-5 Westergren Dispette System for ESR determination. *Left:* EDTA-anticoagulated whole blood is poured into a vial containing 3.8% sodium citrate. *Center:* Dispette is placed in vial using a twisting motion until blood reaches bottom of safety autozeroing plug. *Right:* Vial and Dispette are placed upright in a special rack for 60 minutes before reading the ESR. (Courtesy of Ulster Scientific, Highland, NY.)

The normal range for men is 0 to 10 mm/hr, and for women, it is 0 to 20 mm/hr. Elevations in ESR values are not specific for any disorder but indicate either inflammation or any other condition that causes increased or altered proteins in the blood (e.g., rheumatoid arthritis). The more rapidly the RBCs fall in the column, the greater the degree of inflammation. Physicians use this as a guideline when monitoring the course of inflammation in rheumatoid arthritis. The ESR can also be elevated with infection and pregnancy.

Coagulation (Hemostasis) Tests

Coagulation tests measure the ability of whole blood to form a clot. Coagulation proteins in the blood act in sequential order when stimulated by cell membrane disruptions (cuts, tears, or other injuries) to form a clot. This clot stabilizes the platelet plug, which is the first link in the chain of events that occur on injury. Both the platelet plug and the fibrin clot are needed for continued hemostasis. When vascular damage occurs, the following sequence of events occurs:

1. *Vasoconstriction.* The vein constricts to reduce blood loss.
2. *Platelet plug formation.* The platelets adhere to the wound and form a plug, temporarily slowing or stopping the blood flow.
3. *Fibrin clot formation.* When activated, the clotting factors form an insoluble clot at the wound site. (The two most common tests for determining how well a fibrin clot can form are prothrombin time and partial thromboplastin time, discussed in the next sections).
4. *Clot lysis and vascular repair.* Another set of proteins slowly dissolves the fibrin clot as the surrounding endothelial tissue of the blood vessel wall replicates to repair the damage.

Prothrombin Time

The prothrombin time (PT) is a test in which calcium and **thromboplastin** (a complex substance that starts the clotting process) are added to the patient's plasma and the clotting time is observed. The normal range is 12 to 15 seconds, but each laboratory establishes its own range. Among the factors that may prolong a patient's PT are liver disease, vitamin K deficiency, and warfarin (Coumadin; oral anticoagulant) therapy.

The PT is the primary monitor of Coumadin anticoagulant therapy. The PT is reported along with its corresponding international normalized ratio (INR) to standardize results. The INR is a mathematical calculation that compares the patient's PT to a reference standard. Several point-of-care instruments allow medical assistants to determine prothrombin time and INR in the office.

 CHECKPOINT QUESTION

6. What is the function of thromboplastin?

 WHAT IF?

Your patient is taking Coumadin and does not return for scheduled prothrombin tests? What should you do?

Let the physician know. The physician will determine whether a refill prescription should be called in to the pharmacy. Document all phone conversations with the patient, including the date, time, and message. Also document the patient's responses, quoting him or her whenever possible. The patient should be informed of the dangers of self-dosing Coumadin, such as excessive bleeding with overdose or clotting with underdose. Make sure the patient understands the purpose of the medication and why blood tests are so important. Determine why the patient is not coming in for blood work; the reason may be as simple as transportation. Many communities have visiting nurse associations or hospital outreach programs whose staff members will draw blood for patients in the home.

Partial Thromboplastin Time

The partial thromboplastin time (PTT) is a two-stage test in which first partially activated thromboplastin is incubated with the patient's plasma and then calcium is added. The clotting time is then determined. The normal range is 32 to 51 seconds, but each laboratory establishes its own range, so there may be a slight variation. PTT may be prolonged in certain factor deficiencies, especially those that cause hemophilia. Heparin (anticoagulant) therapy also prolongs the PTT. Thus, it is used to monitor dosages.

 CHECKPOINT QUESTION

7. What are the two most common tests used to determine how well a fibrin clot will form?

MEDIA MENU

- **Student CD**
  - **Case Studies**
    Clinical Interactive Case Study 1: Triage in an Emergency Situation, Communication and Documentation
  - **Animations**
    Hemostasis
  - **CMA/RMA Certification Exam Review**
- **LWW's Medical Assisting Skills DVD**
  - **Procedure 42-4**
- **Premium Online Course**
  http://thePoint.lww.com/Kronenberger3e

- **Internet Resources**
  LiveAdvise Online Tutoring & Competency Training
  http://thePoint.lww.com/LiveAdvise

  American Society of Hematology
  http://www.hematology.org/

  Lab Tests Online
  http://www.labtestsonline.org/understanding/analytes/esr/test.html

  The Medical Biochemistry Page
  http://web.indstate.edu/thcme/mwking/blood-coagulation.html#top

  University of Minnesota Hematography
  http://www1.umn.edu/hema/

PROCEDURE 42-1:   Making a Peripheral Blood Smear

Purpose: To prepare a blood sample for microscopic examination
Equipment: Clean glass slides with frosted ends, pencil, well-mixed whole blood specimen, transfer pipette, hand disinfectant, surface disinfectant, gloves, biohazard container

Steps	Purpose
1. Wash your hands.	Handwashing aids infection control.
2. Assemble the equipment.	
3. Greet and identify the patient. Explain the procedure. Ask for and answer any questions.	
4. Put on gloves.	
5. Obtain an EDTA (lavender-top tube) blood specimen from the patient, following the steps for venipuncture described in Chapter 41.	
6. Place a drop of blood 1 cm from the frosted end of the slide.	

Step 6. Drop of blood on slide with spreader placed in front. (Reprinted with permission from McCall R. Phlebotomy Essentials. Baltimore: Lippincott Williams & Wilkins, 2003.)

(continued)

PROCEDURE 42-1:   **Making a Peripheral Blood Smear** *(continued)*

Steps	Purpose
7. Place the slide on a flat surface. With the thumb and forefinger of the dominant hand, hold the second (spreader) slide against the surface of the first at a 30° angle. Draw the spreader slide back against the drop of blood until contact is established. (Note: The angle of the spreader slide may have to be greater than 30° for large or thin drops of blood and less than 30° for small or thick drops.) Allow the blood to spread under the edge, and then push the spreader slide at a moderate speed toward the other end of the slide, keeping contact between the two slides at all times.	A flat surface allows for smooth movements. A 30° angle allows the blood to be spread in a thin film for viewing.

Step 7. Spreader slide with drop of blood spreading to its edges. (Reprinted with permission from McCall R. Phlebotomy Essentials. Baltimore: Lippincott Williams & Wilkins, 2003.)

Steps	Purpose
8. Label the slide on the frosted area.	The slide must be labeled with the patient's name or identification number; the frosted end will retain the markings.
9. Allow the slide to air dry.	

Step 9. A properly prepared smear will yield a slide that is easy to read. (Reprinted with permission from McCall R. Phlebotomy Essentials. Baltimore: Lippincott Williams & Wilkins, 2003.)

Steps	Purpose
10. Properly care for or dispose of equipment and supplies. Clean the work area. Remove gloves and wash your hands.	

Note: Too much blood will make the smear invalid.

PROCEDURE 42-2:   Staining a Peripheral Blood Smear

Purpose: To aid in identifying the types of blood cells in a patient sample for diagnosis and treatment of infectious processes and blood dyscrasias

Equipment: Staining rack, Wright's stain materials, prepared slide, tweezers, hand disinfectant, surface disinfectant, gloves, impervious gown and face shield

Steps	Purpose
1. Wash your hands.	Handwashing aids infection control.
2. Assemble the equipment.	
3. Put on gloves, impervious gown, and face shield.	
4. Obtain a recently made dried blood smear. Verify that the slide is labeled with identification of the appropriate patient.	A smear that is more than 2 hours old may have deteriorated.
5. Place the slide on a stain rack blood side up. Place staining solution(s) onto slide according to manufacturer's instructions.	This provides a stable surface for staining. Wright's stain contains alcohol to fix blood to the slide and to stain the cells according to their characteristics. **Step 5.** Place slide on stain rack and stain onto slide.
6. Holding the slide with tweezers, gently rinse the slide with water. Wipe off the back of the slide with gauze. Stand the slide upright and allow it to dry.	This rinses and removes the excess stain for viewing under a microscope. **Step 6.** Rinse slide, and then wipe it with gauze.
7. Properly care for or dispose of equipment and supplies. Clean the work area. Remove gloves, gown, and face shield and wash your hands.	

Note: Some manufacturers provide a simple one-step method that consists of dipping the smear in a staining solution and then rinsing. Directions provided by the manufacturer vary with the specific test.

PROCEDURE 42-3:　Performing a Hemoglobin Determination

Purpose: To determine the oxygen-carrying capacity of the blood in a patient sample for diagnosis and treatment of anemia

Equipment: Hemoglobinometer, applicator sticks, whole blood, hand disinfectant, surface disinfectant, gloves, biohazard container

Steps	Purpose
1. Wash your hands.	Handwashing aids infection control.
2. Assemble the necessary equipment.	
3. Put on gloves.	
4. Obtain a blood specimen from the patient by capillary puncture following the procedures in Chapter 41. An EDTA (lavender-top tube) blood specimen from the patient is also acceptable.	EDTA is the anticoagulant required for hematology testing.
5. Place well-mixed whole blood into the hemoglobinometer chamber as described by the manufacturer.	This prepares the sample for the hemoglobin determination.
6. Slide the chamber into the hemoglobinometer.	The chamber must be in the receiving slot for the reading.
7. Record the hemoglobin level from the digital readout.	
8. Clean the work area with surface disinfectant. Dispose of equipment and supplies appropriately. Remove gloves and wash your hands.	

Note: This procedure may vary with the instrument. Some manufacturers offer a digital readout that is less subjective and is therefore considered more accurate and easier to use.

Charting Example:

12/02/2008 10:30 AM Cap puncture L ring finger. Hgb 9.5. Dx code ###.## per Dr. Royal. Dr. Royal notified of results

—R. Smith, CMA

PROCEDURE 42-4: Performing a Microhematocrit Determination

Purpose: To determine the quantity of erythrocytes in a centrifuged blood specimen for diagnosis and treatment of anemia

Equipment: Microcollection tubes, sealing clay, microhematocrit centrifuge, microhematocrit reading device, hand disinfectant, surface disinfectant, gloves, biohazard container, sharps container

Steps	Purpose
1. Wash your hands.	Handwashing aids infection control.
2. Assemble the equipment.	
3. Put on gloves.	

4. Draw blood into the capillary tube by one of two methods:
  A. Directly from a capillary puncture (see Chapter 41) in which the tip of the capillary tube is touched to the blood at the wound and allowed to fill to three-quarters or the indicated mark.
  B. From a well-mixed EDTA tube of whole blood; again, the tip is touched to the blood and allowed to fill three-quarters of the tube.
	Whole blood from a capillary puncture has not clotted and is acceptable. If blood from a tube is not well mixed, the reading is likely to be inaccurate.

5. Place the forefinger over the top of the tube, wipe excess blood off the sides, and push the bottom into the sealing clay.	Holding the finger over the tip stops blood from dripping out the bottom. The clay seals one end of the tube to contain it during centrifugation.
6. Draw a second specimen in the same manner.	A second tube is necessary for duplicate testing as a quality control measure.
7. Place the tubes, clay-sealed end out, in the radial grooves of the microhematocrit centrifuge opposite each other. Put the lid on the grooved area and tighten by turning the knob clockwise. Close the centrifuge lid. Spin for 5 minutes or as directed by the centrifuge manufacturer.	Specimens should always be placed opposite each other to balance the centrifuge. Read the manufacturer's directions for the specific centrifuge used in your facility; 5 minutes is normal.
8. Remove the tubes from the centrifuge and read the results; instructions are printed on the device. Results should be within 5% of each other. Take the average and report as a percentage.	Results with greater than 5% variation have been found to offer unreliable results.

Step 8. Results from the centrifuge reading device.

(continued)

PROCEDURE 42-4:   Performing a Microhematocrit Determination *(continued)*

Steps	Purpose

Step 8. Centrifuged tube reader.

9. Dispose of the microhematocrit tubes in a biohazard container. Properly care for or dispose of other equipment and supplies. Clean the work area. Remove gloves and wash your hands.

Note: Some microhematocrit centrifuges have the scale printed in the machine at the radial grooves.

Charting Example:

03/28/2008 4:20 PM Capillary puncture, left ring finger. Hct: 42%. Dx code XXX.XX per Dr. Erikson.
Dr. notified of results

—M. Mays, CMA

PROCEDURE 42-5:   Westergren Erythrocyte Sedimentation Rate

Purpose: To determine the rate at which erythrocytes separate from plasma and settle in a tube for diagnosis of nonspecific inflammatory processes

Equipment: Hand disinfectant, gloves, EDTA blood sample less than 2 hours old, ESR kit, sedimentation rack, pipette, timer, surface disinfectant, biohazard disposal container, sharps container, impervious gown, face shield

Steps	Purpose
1. Wash your hands.	Handwashing aids infection control.
2. Assemble the necessary equipment.	
3. Put on gloves, impervious gown, and face shield.	
4. Verify that the patient information on the specimen tube is that of the appropriate patient. Gently mix EDTA lavender-stoppered anticoagulation tube for 2 minutes.	The blood must not be allowed to clot; it must be drawn into an anticoagulation tube.
5. Using a vial from the ESR kit and a pipette, fill vial to the indicated mark. Replace stopper and invert vial several times to mix (see Fig. 42-5).	

(continued)

PROCEDURE 42-5: Westergren Erythrocyte Sedimentation Rate (continued)

Steps	Purpose
6. Using an ESR calibrated pipette from the kit, insert the pipette through the tube's stopper with a twist and push down slowly but firmly until the pipette meets the bottom of the vial (see Fig. 42-5). The pipette will autozero with the excess flowing into the holding area. If the blood column does not reach the autozero point, discard used materials and start again at Step 4.	Presence of the full calibrated volume is necessary for an accurate test result. Bubbles and incorrect filling will alter the test results.
7. Place the tube in a holder that will keep the tube vertical (see Fig. 42-5).	Any deviation from being absolutely vertical will produce inaccurate test results.
8. Wait exactly 1 hour; use a timer for accuracy. Keep the tube straight upright and undisturbed during the hour.	
9. Record the level of the top of the RBCs after 1 hour. Normal results for men are 0–10 mL/hr; for women, normal results are 0–15 mL/hr.	Never use a shorter time and multiply the reading; less time will give inaccurate results.
10. Properly care for or dispose of equipment and supplies. Clean the work area. Remove gloves, gown, and face shield. Wash your hands.	

Charting Example:

02/21/2008 12:30 PM ESR performed D code XXX.XX per Dr. North's order. Westergren ESR test
results 12 mL/hr. Dr. North notified

—B. White, CMA

Chapter Summary

- The hematology laboratory analyzes the blood cells, their quantities, and their characteristics for diagnosis and management of many conditions.
- Several hematology screening tests are CLIA waived and can be performed by the medical assistant in a typical physician office setting.

- Coagulation testing aids in determining the ability of a patient to maintain hemostasis.

1. A patient was taking a medication that caused him to become neutropenic. To what might he be susceptible?

2. A patient lives at a very high elevation, where there is less oxygen than at sea level. Would you expect her hemoglobin to be greater than, less than, or the same as if she lived at sea level?

3. On microscopic review, a patient's RBCs are described as macrocytic. What impact would that characteristic have on the patient's MCV?

4. A patient with rheumatoid arthritis has an ESR of 77 mm/hr when she has her blood tested at the doctor's office; 2 weeks later, she returns, and now the rate is 31 mm/hr. With her condition in mind, would you expect that she is improving or not?

5. A patient has a platelet count of 75,000/mm^3. How would that impact the patient's coagulation studies?

Answers to Checkpoint Questions

1. Hematopoiesis is the medical term for blood cell production. It is influenced by hormones and depends on adequate nutrients such as iron.

2. Leukopenia is a diminished number of leukocytes. It can be caused by chemical toxicity, nutritional deficiency, overwhelming or chronic infection, or certain malignancies.

3. Neutrophils defend against foreign invaders by phagocytosis.

4. Elevated eosinophils and basophils are both seen with allergic reactions.

5. A hematocrit of 20% indicates that 20% of the total blood volume consists of RBCs.

6. Thromboplastin initiates the clotting process.

7. The two most common tests for determining how well a fibrin clot can form are prothrombin time and partial thromboplastin time.

CHAPTER 43

Urinalysis

Outline

Specimen Collection Methods
Random Specimen
First Morning Void
Postprandial Specimen
Clean-Catch Midstream Urine
  Specimen
24-Hour Collection
Bladder Catheterization
Suprapubic Aspiration
Drug Testing
Physical Properties of Urine
Color

Clarity
Specific Gravity
Chemical Properties of Urine
pH
Glucose
Ketones
Proteins
Blood
Bilirubin
Urobilinogen
Nitrite
Leukocyte Esterase

Confirmatory Testing
Copper Reduction Test
Nitroprusside Test
Precipitation Test
Diazo Test
Urine Sediment
Structures Found in Urine
  Sediment

Learning Objectives

Upon successfully completing this chapter, you will be able to:

1. Spell and define the key terms

2. Describe the methods of urine collection

3. List and explain the physical and chemical properties of urine

4. List confirmatory tests available and describe their use

5. List and describe the components that can be found in urine sediment and describe their relationships to chemical findings

Performance Objectives

Upon successfully completing this chapter, you will be able to:

1. Explain to a patient how and/or assist a patient to obtain a clean-catch midstream urine specimen (Procedure 43-1)

2. Explain the method of obtaining a 24-hour urine collection (Procedure 43-2)

3. Determine color and clarity of urine (Procedure 43-3)

4. Accurately interpret chemical reagent strip reactions (Procedure 43-4)

5. Prepare urine sediment for microscopic examination (Procedure 43-5)

CAAHEP

- Obtaining a clean-catch midstream urine specimen
- Determining color and clarity of urine
- Chemical reagent strip analysis
- Preparing urine sediment
- Obtaining a 24-hour urine specimen

ABHES

- Obtaining a clean-catch midstream urine specimen
- Obtaining a 24-hour urine specimen
- Determining color and clarity of urine
- Chemical reagent strip analysis
- Preparing urine sediment

Key Terms

bilirubinuria	ketones	quantitative	supernatant
diurnal variation	leukocyte esterase	sediment	threshold
glycosuria	nitrite	specific gravity	urobilinogen
hemoglobinuria	proteinuria	sulfosalicylic acid	

A urinalysis is a physical and chemical examination of urine to assess renal function and other possible problems. Because so many urinalyses are done in the office laboratory, proficiency in this skill is essential for the medical assistant. As indicated by clinical symptoms or physical and chemical findings in the urine, a microscopic examination may be added. CLIA (Clinical Laboratory Improvement Amendments) regulations limit the types of testing medical assistants can perform. The list of tests medical assistants can perform, which is updated regularly by the Centers for Medicare and Medicaid Services (CMS), does not include the urinalysis microscopic procedure. The medical assistant may prepare urine sediment for microscopic examination (see Procedure 43-5). The microscopic examination may be performed by the physician under the CLIA category Physician-Performed Microscopy. Insight into many systemic diseases or conditions can be gained from urinalysis. Diabetes mellitus, shock, malnutrition, preeclampsia, and blood transfusion reactions are several of the disorders that can be diagnosed or assessed by an examination of the urine. As with all body fluids, urine must be handled using OSHA-mandated personal protective equipment and safety guidelines.

Specimen Collection Methods

Proper collection of a urine specimen varies with the test to be performed. Unless otherwise specified by the physician, a freshly voided specimen is all that is necessary.

This is called a random urine. The patient voids the urine into a clean, dry container. To diagnose a urinary tract infection (UTI), the specimen is collected either as a clean-catch midstream or by catheter and submitted to the laboratory in a sterile container with a lid (Fig. 43-1). Detecting the microorganism causing disease may require that a culture be performed. A culture is a laboratory test in which microorganisms are grown in a nutrient medium to be identified and tested for antibiotic susceptibility. All cultures require the specimen not be contaminated during the preliminary testing process. Proper patient instruction in the clean-catch procedure avoids contamination with microorganisms from the perineal area, which would produce misleading results in urine culture or microscopic analysis.

Once the urine is collected, many of its elements deteriorate within 1 hour. If testing cannot be performed within this time, the specimen is refrigerated at 4° to 8°C for up to 4 hours. Multiplication of microorganisms in an unrefrigerated specimen changes the pH from acidic to alkaline. Glucose in the urine may be used as a nutrient by the microorganisms, resulting in a false-negative or lowered glucose result.

The timing of collection is sometimes an important consideration. First morning urine specimens are the most concentrated and are useful for many tests that are more easily determined with concentrated components (e.g., pregnancy testing); 2-hour postprandial (after a meal) specimens are used for glucose testing.

Figure 43-1 Sterile specimen cup with lid

Random Specimen

When a random specimen is indicated, the patient voids the urine into a clean, dry container. Label all specimens directly on the container and not on the lid. The lid may become separated from the specimen. Check the office policy manual for minimum label requirements. Always check with female patients and note on the test requisition if the patient is on her menstrual period because the specimen may be contaminated with blood. These precautions are necessary for all types of urine collections.

First Morning Void

It is easiest to identify urine abnormalities in a more concentrated urine specimen. Urine formed over a 6- to 8-hour period provides the preferred concentration. This is called a first morning specimen or an early morning void. It may be necessary to clarify this term for the patient with alternative sleep patterns.

Postprandial Specimen

A postprandial urine specimen is one that is collected exactly 2 hours after the patient consumes a meal. The patient should be instructed to empty the bladder prior to eating the meal. This will ensure that the collected urine is entirely postprandial.

Clean-Catch Midstream Urine Specimen

A clean-catch midstream urine is the most commonly ordered random specimen. It is useful when the physician suspects an infection because any microorganisms present after this collection will be from the urinary tract and not contaminated by an area, such as the perineal area. This specimen can be used for a culture if nothing has been allowed to contaminate the urine, such as a pipette or reagent strip. Collection is done after the urinary meatus and surrounding skin have been cleansed. The urine is voided into a sterile container.

Clean-Catch

Most patients are not familiar with aseptic technique. Procedure 43-1 outlines the specific patient education instructions for both males and females. Disabled or elderly patients may require assistance with the procedure.

Midstream

Midstream specimen collection avoids contaminants from the urethra or the urinary meatus and ensures that the specimen represents bladder contents. Instruct the patient to begin the void directly into the toilet. The patient stops the flow and voids the middle third of urine into the collection container. Once the patient has collected about 25 mL of urine, the bladder may be emptied into the toilet.

24-Hour Collection

Because some substances such as proteins are excreted with **diurnal variation** (variation during a 24-hour period), a 24-hour collection is a better indicator of values than a random specimen. To obtain this kind of specimen, the patient collects all voided urine within a 24-hour period (Procedure 43-2). Providing an information sheet with written instructions for collecting a 24-hour urine specimen helps ensure the patient's compliance.

Other Specified Number of Hours

There may be circumstances that prompt the physician to order a specimen over a time frame that is less than 24 hours. Such collections may be requested as 2-hour, 6-hour, or 12-hour specimens. The basic protocol described in Procedure 43-2 applies with modifications made in timing.

1. Void into the toilet, and note this time and date as the beginning.
2. After the first voiding, collect each void, and add it to the urine container for the number of hours indicated by the physician.
3. At precisely the number of hours indicated by the physician after beginning the collection, empty the bladder even if there is no urge to void, and add this final volume of urine to the container.
4. Note on the label the ending time and date.

Bladder Catheterization

Another method for aseptic urine collection is catheterization. A thin sterile tube (catheter) is inserted into the bladder through the urethra. This procedure usually is performed by a physician or a nurse. Some medical assistants may be trained by their physicians to perform catheterizations. Bladder catheterization is recommended when the patient cannot give a urine specimen in a sterile manner using the clean-catch method.

Suprapubic Aspiration

Suprapubic aspiration is the least common method of urine collection. A needle is inserted into the bladder through the skin of the abdominal wall above the symphysis pubis, and urine is withdrawn (aspirated). This method is not common and is performed by a physician. The medical assistant may be asked to assist with the procedure.

 CHECKPOINT QUESTION

1. What is the time frame for testing urine that is not refrigerated? Why is this important?

Drug Testing

Each urine specimen submitted for drug testing must be analyzed using an initial test approved for commercial use by the Food and Drug Administration. Several techniques are available to screen for the five drug classes. Two tests are required to prove a positive drug result. The initial test eliminates negative urine specimens from further testing. A negative specimen either contains no drug or has a concentration less than a specified cutoff level. Gas chromatography/mass spectrometry (GC/MS) technology is used for confirmation testing.

Chain of Custody

The term chain of custody indicates the ability to guarantee the identity and integrity of a specimen from collection through all steps of transport and processing to the reporting of the test results. The chain-of-custody process is used to maintain and document the history of the specimen and ensures that the sample has been in possession of, or secured by, a responsible person at all times. It should eliminate doubt about sample identification or that the sample has been tampered with. The chain-of-custody document should include the name or initials of the individual collecting the specimen, each person who subsequently had custody of it, and the date the specimen was collected or transferred. A secure chain of custody leads to the production of a legally defensible test report.

Patient Preparation

To perform a chain-of-custody specimen collection, you must first see a photo ID issued by the patient's employer or the federal, state, or local government (e.g., a driver's license). You may not accept faxes or photo-

copies of identification. Positive identification by an employer representative (not a co-worker or another employee being tested) is also acceptable. If the patient cannot produce positive identification, you do not continue with the specimen collection procedure.

Explain the basic collection procedure to the patient. Direct the patient to remove outer clothing (e.g., jacket, coat, hat) that could conceal substances that could be used to tamper with a specimen. These garments and any briefcase, purse, or other personal belongings must remain with you or in a mutually agreeable location. The patient must empty his or her pockets and display the items in them to ensure that nothing is present that could be used to adulterate the specimen. After ensuring that nothing is present that can be used in that manner, the patient may return the items to his or her pockets.

Instruct the patient to wash and dry his or her hands and not to wash his or her hands again until after delivering the specimen to you. You must eliminate the patient's access to water or other materials that could be used to adulterate the specimen.

Allow the patient to select an individually wrapped or sealed collection container from collection kit materials. The container must be unwrapped and seal broken with both the collector and the patient present. Do not break the seal on the actual specimen bottle at this time. The patient cannot take anything from the collection kit into the room used for urination except the collection container.

Direct the patient to go into the room used for urination, to provide a specimen of at least 45 mL, to not flush the toilet, and to return to you with the specimen as soon as he or she has completed the void. Complete the specimen handling and chain-of-custody form documentation according to the testing laboratory's instructions.

 LEGAL TIP

SPECIMEN COLLECTION FOR DRUG SCREENING

The Mandatory Guidelines for Federal Workplace Testing Programs establish scientific and technical guidelines, including specimen collection for Federal Workplace drug testing programs. Executive Order 12564 (Drug-Free Federal Workplace, 1986) and the Mandatory Guidelines apply to programs established by Executive agencies of the Federal Government. The Urine Specimen Collection Handbook for the new Federal Custody and Control Form provides guidance for collecting urine specimens in accordance with the Mandatory Guidelines.

(continued)

- A collector performs the essential steps in conducting a urine specimen collection for drug testing.
- The collection site may be a permanent or temporary facility located either at the work site or at a remote site. The Drug and Alcohol Testing Industry Association provides a searchable database of certified specimen collectors.
- Once a site has been selected, the collector must ensure that the appropriate supplies are available to conduct proper collections.
- The donor must be positively identified as the individual selected for testing.
- All urine specimens must be collected while maintaining chain of custody. Chain of custody is the term used to describe the process of documenting the handling of a specimen from the time a donor gives the specimen to the collector, during the testing at the laboratory, and until the results are reported by the laboratory. For specimens collected under Federal regulations, a newly approved Office of Management and Budget (OMB) Custody and Control Form (CCF) must be used to document the collection of a specimen at the collection site.
- A donor may be unable to provide a urine specimen upon arrival at the collection site because he or she either urinated recently or has a "shy bladder." Generally the term "shy bladder" refers to a person's inability to produce a urine sample on demand. If this is the case, those following the Federal guidelines should see Chapter 7 of the Urine Specimen Collection Handbook for the new Federal Custody and Control Form (available online at http://workplace.samhsa.gov/DrugTesting/Specimen Collection/UrnSpcmnHndbk.html#Ch7.)
- A direct observed collection (i.e., the collector or agency-designated representative accompanies the donor into the stall/toilet area and observes the act of urination) may occur only under very specific circumstances.

Source: United States Department of Health and Human Services, Substance Abuse and Mental Health Services Administration, Division of Workplace Programs; website: http://workplace.samhsa.gov/DrugTesting/DTesting.aspx.

Physical Properties of Urine

The physical properties include the urine's color, appearance (such as clarity or turbidity), specific gravity, and odor. While the odor may not be included in the urinalysis report, odors can alert the experienced medical assistant to specific conditions. A diabetic patient's urine may smell sweet, and bacteria may give urine a foul odor. Color and clarity are assessed visually and are subjective, which means the individual performing the testing will determine whether these properties can be considered within the normal range (Table 43-1).

Color

Urine color can be affected by many things, including diet, drugs, diseases, and the concentration of the urine. The normal color of urine is a pale straw color to dark yellow. The yellow color is due to the pigment urochrome. Pale urine is typically very dilute and is seen after high fluid intake and after diuretic therapy. Likewise, deep, dark yellow can signify highly concentrated urine, such as when fluids are withheld or the patient is dehydrated. It also may mean that the patient recently took a multiple vitamin pill.

WHAT IF?

A patient asks you what drugs can be detected in the urine? What do you say?

Many employers are requiring routine urine drug testing for their employees. Urine tests are preferred to blood tests because they are less expensive and are noninvasive. The following drugs can be detected in the urine: amphetamines, barbiturates, benzodiazepines, cocaine, marijuana, opioids, PCP, and methadone. If you must obtain urine specimens for drug testing, it is essential that you ensure security of the urine and confidentiality of the results.

Clarity

Normal, freshly voided urine is usually clear (transparent). Haziness or turbidity (cloudiness) indicates the presence of particulate matter. Some alkaline urine may appear turbid because of a high concentration of phos-

TABLE 43-1	Expected Ranges for Urine Physical Properties
Property	**Expected Range**
Color	Pale yellow to amber
Clarity	Clear
Odor	Slightly aromatic but not fruity, no ammonia
Specific gravity	1.001–1.035

phates. Some acidic urine may become turbid (cloudy) on standing as a result of precipitation of urates (nitrogenous compounds resulting from the body's metabolism of protein). Turbidity caused by either of these is considered normal. Red or white blood cells, bacteria, or mucus can also cause turbidity.

Laboratories vary in terminology used to express clarity or turbidity of urine. Common terminology dictates that when a small amount of turbidity is present, so that black lines on white paper can be seen through the specimen, it is hazy. As turbidity increases and these black lines can no longer be seen, it is called cloudy (Procedure 43-3). The three terms most commonly used to describe clarity are clear, hazy, and cloudy. Table 43-2 summarizes the common causes of variations in the color and clarity of urine.

Specific Gravity

The **specific gravity** reflects the concentration of a urine specimen. The weight of the urine is compared to the weight of water. Normal urine is slightly heavier than water. If you were to compare the weight of distilled water to itself, the specific gravity of the water would be 1.000. Urine, which contains cells and elements such as sodium, potassium, and chloride, is heavier than water. Specific gravity for a normal urine specimen is 1.001 to 1.035.

Urine with low specific gravity is dilute. As stated previously, this may result from a high fluid intake. Abnormal conditions that produce dilute urine are diabetes insipidus and kidney infection or inflammation. Urine with high specific gravity is concentrated. A patient who is dehydrated, perhaps from sweating, vomiting, or diarrhea, may produce a concentrated specimen because the body is trying to conserve water. High specific gravity can occur in diabetes mellitus.

Specific gravity can be determined by a variety of methods. The specific gravity pad on the reagent strip takes a drop of urine, and the color change is compared to a chart to determine the value. This allows specific gravity to be determined in combination with the other chemical assays on the reagent strip and is the most common and efficient method of measurement. An older tool for measuring specific gravity is the refractometer or total solids meter, which requires a drop of urine and is read using a scale that measures the amount of light bent by the particles in urine. The oldest tool is the urinometer, a floating measuring instrument that requires 10 mL or more of urine. The urinometer offers a good visual image of specific gravity (Fig. 43-2) but is obsolete for today's laboratory because of the large volume of urine required and the potential for mercury contamination should the urinometer be broken.

　CHECKPOINT QUESTION

2. What are the three physical properties of urine, and which two are assessed visually?

Chemical Properties of Urine

Urine contains chemicals produced in the body and ingested from the environment. The reagent strip produces 10 chemical measurements. If more **quantitative** (measurement of a specific amount or quantity) information is needed (e.g., protein), the test is performed in the chemistry laboratory (see Chapter 45). Table 43-3 gives the expected value for each chemical property. Detecting and measuring chemical properties can facilitate the diagnosis of many conditions. Included in the discussion of each urine chemistry are the disease processes that might be indicated by abnormal readings.

TABLE **43-2** Common Causes of Variations in the Color and Clarity of Urine	
Color and Clarity	**Possible Causes**
Yellow-brown or green brown	Bile in urine (as in jaundice)
Dark yellow or orange	Concentrated urine, low fluid intake, dehydration, inability of kidney to dilute urine, fluorescein (intravenous dye), multivitamins, excessive carotene
Bright orange-red	Pyridium (urinary tract analgesic)
Red or reddish-brown	Hemoglobin pigments, pyrvinium pamoate (Povan) for intestinal worms, sulfonamides (sulfa-based antibiotics)
Green or blue	Artificial color in food or drugs
Blackish, grayish, smoky	Hemoglobin or remnants of old red blood cells (indicating bleeding in upper urinary tract), chyle, prostatic fluid, yeasts
Cloudy	Phosphate precipitation (normal after sitting for a long time), urates (compound of uric acid), leukocytes, pus, blood, epithelial cells, fat droplets, strict vegetarian diet

Figure 43-2 Determining specific gravity of urine using a urinometer.

Several manufacturers produce reagent strips that can be dipped into urine. These strips have chemicals embedded in pads that react with the chemicals in the urine. A reagent pad will change color as the chemical reaction takes place. All reagent pad colors are compared with a color chart to interpret the reactions at the specific time indicated for each reaction (Procedure 43-4). This color measurement may be performed visually or with a semi-automated strip-reading instrument (Fig. 43-3).

pH

The kidneys excrete acids produced during normal metabolic processes. Hydrogen ions and ammonia are excreted as well. Ammonia is produced by decomposition of nitrogen. The kidneys regulate the acid-base balance of the body by reabsorbing water, sodium, chloride, potassium, bicarbonate, glucose, calcium, and amino acids. Because the body produces more acids than bases, urine is usually acidic.

Expected values for urine pH can range from 5.0 (acidic) to 8.0 (slightly basic). The typical value for freshly voided urine is slightly acidic at 6.0. While acidic

Figure 43-3 Bayer Clinitek Dipstick Reader

urine is normal, it also occurs with a high-protein diet and uncontrolled diabetes. Alkaline urine (above 7.0) can occur after meals and with a vegetarian diet, certain renal diseases, and urinary tract infection.

Glucose

Glucose is filtered and reabsorbed in the kidneys. If plasma renal **threshold** levels exceed 180 g/dL, not all of the glucose will be reabsorbed, and detectable amounts of it will be present in the urine. This can vary and requires measuring the actual blood level for a diagnostic assessment. The amount of glucose in urine corresponds to plasma levels; normal urine does not contain glucose. Glucose-negative urine corresponds to a plasma level of less than 180 mg/dL. In a hyperglycemic state, such as diabetes mellitus, **glycosuria** (glucose in urine) can occur if plasma levels are greater than 180 mg/dL (Box 43-1).

Ketones

Ketones are a group of chemicals produced during fat metabolism. In normal circumstances, energy is derived pri-

TABLE **43-3**	Expected Range of Chemical Properties
Property	**Expected Range**
Glucose	Negative
Bilirubin	Negative
Ketones	Negative
Blood	Negative
pH	5.0–8.0
Protein	Negative to trace
Urobilinogen	0.1–1.0 mg/dL
Nitrite	Negative
Leukocyte esterase	Negative

BOX 43-1

RENAL THRESHOLD AND GLYCOSURIA

Glucose is resorbed in the proximal convoluted tubule. When blood glucose levels exceed 180 mg/dL, depending on the individual, not all of the glucose can be reabsorbed into the bloodstream. Rarely does a healthy person's blood glucose level exceed this threshold value. Diabetics, however, may pass some glucose in their urine because of the high level in their blood. A frequently used term, spilling sugar, means that not all of the sugar is reabsorbed and some is excreted in the urine.

marily from carbohydrate metabolism. In conditions of insufficient carbohydrates, as in starvation, low-carbohydrate diet, and inadequately managed diabetes, fats are used by the body for energy, and ketones are produced.

In normal urine, ketones are typically too low to be measurable. A positive ketone test indicates that the body is burning more fat than normal.

Proteins

Small quantities of proteins are found in normal urine. Proteinuria (increased amounts of protein in the urine) is an important indicator of renal disease. Other events that can cause protein in urine include strenuous physical exercise, pregnancy, infection, hematuria (blood in urine), pyuria (white cells in urine), and multiple myeloma. Microscopic examination of the urine can help determine whether the proteinuria is caused by bacteria, casts, or cellular elements.

Blood

Small numbers of red blood cells are occasionally observed in urine. Intact capillaries in the glomerulus usually do not allow the passage of cells into the Bowman's capsule. Hematuria not due to contamination from menstrual flow indicates bleeding in the urinary tract that may result from renal disorders, certain neoplasms, urinary tract infection, or trauma to the urinary tract.

The reagent strip reacts to hemoglobin, which is the primary constituent of red cells. **Hemoglobinuria** may occur with transfusion reaction, chemical toxicity, or burn. The strip also reacts to myoglobin, a protein found in muscles. Myoglobin may be released into the bloodstream from a crushing injury or other trauma and may then be excreted in the urine.

Bilirubin

Bilirubin is formed during breakdown of hemoglobin. It is processed in the liver before being excreted into the intestines. Urine contains very low levels of bilirubin, reflecting the usual low serum levels. **Bilirubinuria** (bilirubin in the urine) can occur with certain liver diseases (e.g., hepatitis), biliary tract obstruction, and hemolytic states, such as transfusion reactions.

The reagent strip is designed to react to bilirubin; however, dark yellow urine can make it difficult to read the reaction because bilirubin is also a yellow pigment.

Important Note: Bilirubin is a highly unstable substance and will break down with exposure to light. Specimens must be shielded from light and processed as soon as possible to avoid deterioration of the specimen.

Urobilinogen

When bilirubin is secreted into the intestines in the bile, bacterial action converts it to **urobilinogen**. Some of this is reabsorbed into the bloodstream and excreted by the kidneys. The remaining urobilinogen leaves the body in the feces.

Small amounts of urobilinogen are normally found in urine, usually 0.1 to 1.0 mg/dL. As with bilirubin, increased levels of urobilinogen can be found with conditions that have a high rate of red cell destruction. Also, bowel obstructions cause the feces to remain in the intestines for longer periods, resulting in greater reabsorption of urobilinogen along with the rest of the fluid portion. Urobilinogen levels rise both in urine and in serum when this occurs. Liver impairment can also lead to increased levels of urobilinogen because some of the urobilinogen that is reabsorbed from the intestinal tract is processed by the liver and excreted in the feces.

 CHECKPOINT QUESTION

3. What does a positive bilirubin test indicate?

Nitrite

Some types of bacteria that infect the urinary tract have an enzyme that can reduce nitrate to **nitrite**. This factor is used to assess the presence of bacteria in urine. If these types of bacteria are present, nitrates will be converted to nitrites, and the resulting pink color development can be observed on the reagent pad. A positive nitrite test result indicates bacteriuria, which occurs with urinary tract infections. A negative nitrite test result does not indicate the absence of bacteriuria since all types of bacteria do not reduce nitrate to nitrite.

Leukocyte Esterase

Leukocytes in the urine indicate a urinary tract infection. Phagocytic white cells, such as neutrophils, are called to the kidney to fight the infection. These leukocytes contain an enzyme called esterase. This is detected with the **leukocyte esterase** reaction on the reagent strip. Normal urine may contain a few white cells but not in sufficient numbers to produce a positive leukocyte esterase test.

 CHECKPOINT QUESTION

4. Which two indicators on a dipstick suggest a urinary tract infection?

Confirmatory Testing

Confirmation of positive reagent strip reactions (e.g., bilirubin, protein) are sometimes part of laboratory protocol as defined by the facility where the test is performed. Box 43-2 lists several types of confirmation tests. Check your laboratory procedure manual for the confirmation testing used in your laboratory.

BOX 43-2

URINE CONFIRMATORY TESTING

Reagent strip tests are screening tests. Confirmation with a more sensitive and/or specific method may be requested to follow-up some positive results. Your laboratory will have a specific procedure outlining the performance of confirmation tests.

Analyte	Common Confirmatory Test
Protein	Sulfosalicylic acid test
Ketones	Acetest
Bilirubin	Ictotest
Glucose	Clinitest

Copper Reduction Test

The copper reduction method (Clinitest) (Fig. 43-4) has been used for many years to detect reducing sugars in urine. This test is used to detect any reducing sugar (sugar that gives up electrons easily in chemical reactions), such as glucose, galactose, lactose, or fructose. Its use is significant in children aged 2 years or less to screen for galactosuria. (Galactosuria, or an increased level of galactose in the blood and urine, is a condition in newborns lacking an enzyme that metabolizes galactose.) Other sugars and ascorbic acid (vitamin C) can react with the reagent and cause inaccuracies in the test result. The reagent strips are specific for glucose and are preferred for their accuracy; however, the Clinitest tablets may be used as confirmation for chemical reagent strips. Note, the reaction produces heat, so always use a glass tube.

Nitroprusside Test

A nitroprusside reaction is used to detect ketone. (Nitroprusside is a nitrogen cyanic compound that reacts with ketones to produce a purple reaction.) This is the method used on both reagent strips and tablet tests. Many laboratories choose to confirm results with the nitroprusside tablet (Acetest). The lactose present in the tablet method serves to enhance the color reaction with that method.

Precipitation Test

Turbidity or precipitation tests confirm a protein on the reagent strip. The most common confirmation test is observing the amount of cloudiness when equal amounts of urine and **sulfosalicylic acid** are mixed. The urine used must be centrifuged to remove all particulate matter before adding the acid.

If the amount of protein is negligible and produces a negative reagent strip reaction, there should be no cloudiness when the sulfosalicylic acid is added to the urine. When the concentration of urine protein reaches approximately 20 mg/dL, turbidity will result as sulfosalicylic acid combines with the urine. As protein levels increase, so will the degree of turbidity during the reaction with the acid.

Diazo Test

Many laboratories confirm a positive strip result using a diazo tablet method (Ictotest) (Fig. 43-5). The diazo tablet procedure is good for confirmation because it is more sensitive than the strip procedure. The tablet method can detect as little as 0.05 to 0.1 mg/dL of bilirubin in a urine sample.

Urine Sediment

The microscopic examination of urine can corroborate the findings of the urinalysis and may produce additional data with diagnostic value. Cells and other structures are noted and counted during a microscopic exam-

5-Drop Method Standard Procedure

DIRECTIONS FOR TESTING:

1. Collect urine in clean container. With dropper in upright position, place **5 drops** of urine in test tube. Rinse dropper with water and add 10 drops of water to test tube.

2. Drop one tablet into test tube. Watch while complete boiling reaction takes place. Do not shake test tube during boiling, or for the following 15 seconds after boiling has stopped.

3. At the end of this 15-second waiting period, shake test tube gently to mix contents. Compare color of liquid to Color Chart below. Ignore sediment that may form in the bottom of the test tube. Ignore changes after the 15-second waiting period.

4. Write down the percent (%) result which appears on the color block that most closely matches the color of the liquid.

NEGATIVE	1/4%	1/2%	3/4%	1%	2% or more

Figure 43-4 Clinitest for reducing sugars. Clinitest package insert. (Courtesy of Bayer Corporation, Elkhart, IN.)

Figure 43-5 The diazo tablet test for bilirubin. Ictotest package insert. (Courtesy of Bayer Corporation, Elkhart, IN.)

ination. Microscopic examination of urine is not a CLIA-waived procedure. Urine **sediment** is prepared by centrifuging urine and saving the button of cells and other particulate matter that collects in the bottom of the tube. This button is resuspended in the residual **supernatant** (urine above the sediment when the tube of urine is centrifuged), and a drop of this suspension is placed on a slide and viewed with a microscope. Making a sediment button concentrates all of the structures in the urine so that it is unlikely that any components will be missed (Procedure 43-5).

A slide system used in conjunction with a unique centrifuge tube is available to examine sediments. This provides some standardization of the procedure so that the numbers in the findings have meaning with regard to abnormal results. Glass slides, with or without coverslips, may still be used by some laboratories.

Structures Found in Urine Sediment

The following structures may appear in the urine: red blood cells, white blood cells, bacteria, epithelial cells, crystals, casts, and others. Correlations with chemical properties of the urine are described as appropriate.

Red Blood Cells

The presence of red cells in urine, as stated previously, can occur with a number of conditions, including renal damage. When sediment contains red cells, the reagent strip should be positive for blood. Protein may also be positive if hemolysis is occurring. A positive reagent strip test for blood with no red cells seen microscopically may occur with various kinds of hemolysis, such as with transfusion reactions and sickle cell crisis (see Chapter 42). As stated earlier, myoglobin will cause a positive reaction.

White Blood Cells

Leukocytes in the sediment indicate a urinary tract infection. The leukocyte esterase test on the chemical strip

will be positive when white cells are present in significant numbers. The protein test may be positive if some of the white blood cells lyse (break apart) or if the infection is damaging the renal tubules, as in glomerulonephritis.

Bacteria

Bacteria are always present on the skin but not usually in the bladder. Urine normally does not contain bacteria if a clean-catch specimen is collected properly. The presence of significant amounts (more than a trace) of bacteria in a urine specimen is considered an indication of a urinary tract infection. A positive nitrite result may be obtained when bacteria are seen.

Epithelial Cells

Epithelial cells cover the skin and organs and line pathways, such as the digestive and urinary tracts. Their shapes vary according to their location of origin. Epithelial cells normally slough off and are found in the urine, but increased amounts can indicate an irritation, such as inflammation somewhere in the urinary system. The three types of epithelial cells in the urine are squamous, transitional, and renal. Squamous epithelial cells cover external skin surfaces and are considered a normal finding in urine, since urine comes in contact with skin during urination. Transitional epithelial cells line the bladder and are seen with infections of the lower urinary tract, such as cystitis. Renal epithelial cells line the nephrons and are seen with infections and inflammations of the upper urinary tract.

There is no chemical test for epithelial cells. However, if renal epithelial cells are seen in urinary sediment, damage to the renal tubules is likely, and the protein test may be positive.

 CHECKPOINT QUESTION

5. List the three types of epithelial cells found in urine. Note the most common condition in which each type is found.

Crystals

Crystals are made up of a chemical substance in the urine in sufficient quantities to form a solid three-dimensional structure that can be seen microscopically. The three most common crystals found in urine sediment—calcium oxalate, uric acid (both of which occur in urine with a pH < 7.0), and triple phosphate (found in urine with a pH > 7.0)—are not independently pathologic. However, uric acid crystals can be seen with fever, leukemia, or gout. Crystals can contribute to the formation of stones in the urinary tract.

Casts

Cast formation occurs in the tubules of the nephron. When protein is present in sufficient quantities, it will cement together whatever solutes or cells are in the tubule as well; this is called a cast. Most casts eventually break free and flow into the urine. The type of cast can indicate certain pathologies. For instance, in pyelonephritis, white cells that are present to combat the infection become trapped in the protein network and form white cell casts. Casts are counted using low-power magnification with reduced light and are reported as a number per low-power field.

 CHECKPOINT QUESTION

6. What are three of the most common crystals found in urine?

Other Structures

Other structures can be found in urine sediment. Yeast in the urine can result from vaginal contamination of the specimen or may be the causative agent of a urinary tract infection, especially in a diabetic patient. The parasite *Trichomonas vaginalis* is a contaminant from the genital tract of an infected person. Mucus may be present if there is an inflammation in the urinary tract. Mucus threads are usually reported in quantities, such as few, moderate, or many. Spermatozoa may be found when there has been a recent emission.

 PATIENT EDUCATION

Instructions for 24-Hour Urine Collection

The following instructions can be given to patients to ensure proper collection:

Instructions to Patients

- Instructions must be followed exactly. Your test results are based on the total amount of urine excreted by your body over a 24-hour period. Not following instructions will result in inaccurate results reported to your physician.
- Some tests have dietary and/or drug restrictions. Check with your physician or the laboratory before starting the collection. Drink the amount of fluid you normally would during the 24-hour collection period.
- The physician or laboratory will give you a special container to collect the urine. A preservative may be in the container. Do not throw away the preservative. Preservatives may be caustic or toxic. Do not void directly into the container. Be very careful not to spill the preservative on you or anything else.* Refrigerate the container during collection. The urine must be kept cold.

Day 1

- Empty your bladder into the toilet. Record this specific date and time on your 24-hour urine container.
- Collect all specimens during the day, evening, and night for the entire 24-hour period. Add all of the specimens to the container. Gently shake the container after each urine specimen is added. Keep the urine container refrigerated during the collection period and until you take it to the physician or laboratory for testing.

Day 2

- Exactly 24 hours later, completely empty your bladder and add this specimen to the container. This last specimen completes your 24-hour collection. Record the ending date and time on the container. Replace the cap and tighten firmly. Refrigerate the specimen until you can turn it in. Take the specimen to the physician or laboratory as soon as possible.
- If you were on a special diet for this test, you may resume your normal diet after the specimen is collected.

* If you do spill the preservative, immediately wash with large amounts of water. You will have to get a new container from your physician or laboratory to collect the specimen.

 MEDIA MENU

- **Student CD**
  - **Video Procedures**
    Procedure 43-4 video clip
  - **CMA/RMA Certification Exam Review**
- **LWW's Medical Assisting Skills DVD**
  - **Procedures 43-1, 43-3, 43-4, 43-5**
- **Premium Online Course**
  http://thePoint.lww.com/Kronenberger3e
- **Internet Resources**

  LiveAdvise Online Tutoring & Competency Training
  http://thePoint.lww.com/LiveAdvise

  National Institutes of Health—Urinalysis
  http://www.nlm.nih.gov/medlineplus/ency/article/003579.htm

  Lab Tests Online
  http://www.labtestsonline.org/understanding/analytes/urinalysis/test.html

  Medical Technology
  http://www.irvingcrowley.com/cls/urin.htm

PROCEDURE 43-1: Obtaining a Clean-Catch Midstream Urine Specimen

Purpose: To minimize contamination of a voided urine specimen
Equipment: Sterile urine container labeled with patient's name, cleansing towelettes (two for males, three for females), gloves if you are to assist patient, hand sanitizer

Steps	Reasons
1. Wash your hands. If you are to assist the patient, put on gloves.	Handwashing aids infection control.
2. Assemble the equipment.	
3. Identify the patient and explain the procedure. Ask for and answer any questions.	
4. If the patient is to perform the procedure, provide the necessary supplies.	
5. Have the patient perform the procedure. A. Instruct the male patient:	
i. If uncircumcised, expose the glans penis by retracting the foreskin, then clean the meatus with an antiseptic wipe. The glans should be cleaned in a circular motion away from the meatus. A new wipe should be used for each cleaning sweep.	The antiseptic solution removes bacteria from the urinary meatus and the surrounding skin. Wiping away from the meatus will remove bacteria from the area; wiping toward the meatus or returning to the area with a used wipe will reintroduce bacteria to the site.
ii. Keeping the foreskin retracted, initially void a few seconds into the toilet or urinal.	Organisms in the lower urethra and at the meatus will be washed away.
iii. Bring the sterile container into the urine stream and collect a sufficient amount (about 30–60 mL). Instruct the patient to avoid touching the inside of the container with the penis.	Collecting the middle of the stream ensures the least contamination with skin bacteria. Touching the inside with the penis may contaminate the specimen.
iv. Finish voiding into the toilet or urinal.	Prostatic fluid may be expressed at the end of the stream and may contaminate the specimen.
B. Instruct the female patient:	
i. Kneel or squat over a bedpan or toilet bowl. Spread the labia minora widely to expose the meatus. Using an antiseptic wipe, cleanse on either side of the meatus, and then cleanse the meatus itself. Use a wipe only once in a sweep from the anterior to the posterior surfaces, and then discard it.	The antiseptic solution removes bacteria from the urinary meatus. Bringing a wipe back to the surface already cleaned will recontaminate the area. The antiseptic solution is washed away before the specimen is collected at midstream.
ii. Keeping the labia separated, initially void a few seconds into the toilet.	Organisms remaining in the meatus will be washed away.
iii. Bring the sterile container into the urine stream and collect a sufficient amount (about 30–60 mL).	
iv. Finish voiding into the toilet or bedpan.	
6. Cap the filled container and place it in a designated area.	
7. Transport the specimen in a biohazard container for testing.	

(continued)

PROCEDURE 43-1:   Obtaining a Clean-Catch Midstream Urine Specimen (continued)

Steps	Reasons
8. Properly care for or dispose of equipment and supplies. Clean the work area. Remove gloves and wash your hands.	

Charting Example:

05/31/2008 1:30 PM Pt instructed in midstream collection of urine with antiseptic wipe. U/A: Color, straw;
clarity, clear; specific gravity, 1.020; dipstick negative; pH 7.0

S. Miller, CMA

PROCEDURE 43-2:   Obtaining a 24-Hour Urine Specimen

Purpose: To determine the quantity and proportion of substances in a 24-hour urine sample
Equipment: Patient's labeled 24-hour urine container (some patients require more than one container), preservatives required for the specific test, chemical hazard labels, graduated cylinder that holds at least 1 L, serologic or volumetric pipettes, clean random urine container, fresh 10% bleach solution, gloves, impervious gown, face shield, hand disinfectant, surface disinfectant

Steps	Reasons
1. Wash your hands.	Handwashing aids infection control.
2. Assemble the equipment.	
3. Identify the type of 24-hour urine collection requested and check for any special requirements, such as any acid or preservative that should be added. Label the container appropriately.	Proper identification avoids errors. Special additives protect the integrity of the specimen. **Step 3.** Tweny-four–hour urine containers containing hazardous chemicals should be labeled appropriately.
4. Put on gloves, impervious gown, and face shield.	
5. Add to the 24-hour urine container the correct amount of acid or preservative using a serologic or volumetric pipette. Some reference laboratories provide these specimen containers to clients with the preservative already added.	This prevents altered findings due to incorrect preparation.
6. Use the provided label or make a label with spaces for the patient's name, beginning time and date, and ending time and date so that the patient can fill in the appropriate information.	This ensures that the patient documents the testing times.

(continued)

PROCEDURE 43-2:   Obtaining a 24-Hour Urine Specimen *(continued)*

Steps	Reasons
7. Instruct the patient to collect a 24-hour urine sample as follows: A. Void into the toilet, and note this time and date as the beginning. B. After the first voiding, collect each void and add it to the urine container for the next 24 hours. C. Precisely 24 hours after beginning collection, empty the bladder even if there is no urge to void and add this final volume of urine to the container. D. Note on the label the ending time and date.	
8. Explain to the patient that, depending on the test requested, the 24-hour urine may have to be refrigerated the entire time. Instruct the patient to return the specimen to you as soon as possible after collection is complete.	Proper care of the specimen prevents degradation of the urine components, which may alter findings.
9. Record in the patient's chart that supplies and instructions were given to collect a 24-hour urine specimen and the test that was requested.	This documents patient education and instructions.
10. When you receive the specimen, verify beginning and ending times and dates before the patient leaves. Check for any acids or preservatives to be added before the specimen goes to the testing laboratory.	This protects the integrity of the specimen.
11. Wearing gloves, impervious gown, and face shield, pour the urine into a cylinder to record the volume. Pour an aliquot of the urine into a clean container to be sent to the laboratory. (Label the specimen with the patient's identification.) Record the volume of the urine collection and the amount of any acid or preservative added on the sample container and on the laboratory requisition. If permitted, you may dispose of the remainder of the urine. Note that some reference labs will accept the entire 24-hour specimen and make this measurement at the laboratory. **Step 11.** CMA pouring 24-hour urine into a graduated cylinder to measure the specimen's total volume.	
12. Record the volume on the patient's test requisition and chart.	

(continued)

PROCEDURE 43-2: **Obtaining a 24-Hour Urine Specimen**
(continued)

Steps	Reasons
13. Clean the cylinder with fresh 10% bleach solution and then rinse with water. Let it air dry. If you are using a disposable container, be sure to dispose of it in the proper biohazard container.	
14. Clean the work area and dispose of waste properly. Remove personal protective equipment and wash your hands.	

Note: Some containers come with the preservative already added. In either case, be sure the patient is instructed not to discard preservative and not to allow it to be handled.

Warning! Use caution when handling acids and other hazardous materials. Be familiar with the material safety data sheets for each chemical in your site.

Note: Depending on the type of office and laboratory, you may not need the aliquot.

Charting Example:

3/8/2008 9:30 AM Pt instructed to collect urine for 24 hours and verbalized understanding. Pt was given
container and written instructions to begin collecting at 8:00 AM on 3/9 and to end on 3/10 at 8:00 AM
Will bring specimen in on 3/10
M. Smith, CMA

3/10/2008 10:10 AM Pt returned with 24-hour specimen collection. Total volume is 1850 mL. Labeled 50-
mL aliquot to reference laboratory
M. Smith, CMA

PROCEDURE 43-3:   Determining Color and Clarity of Urine

Purpose: To determine the visible characteristics of a urine specimen
Equipment: Gloves, impervious gown, 10% bleach solution, patient's labeled urine specimen, clear tube, usually a centrifuge, white paper scored with black lines, hand disinfectant, surface disinfectant

Steps	Reasons
1. Wash your hands.	Handwashing aids infection control.
2. Assemble the equipment.	
3. Put on personal protective equipment.	
4. Verify that the name on the specimen container and the name on the report form are the same.	This prevents reporting errors.
5. Pour about 10 mL of urine into the tube. If the specimen volume is less that 10 mL, note this on the test result form.	This provides an adequate quantity for testing and allows for visual assessment of the urine.
6. In bright light against a white background, examine the color. The most common colors are straw (very pale yellow), yellow, dark yellow, and amber (brown-yellow).	The intensity of the yellow color, which is due to urochrome, depends on urine concentration. (Table 43-2 has information about other urine colors.)
7. Determine clarity. Hold the tube in front of the white paper scored with black lines. If you see the lines clearly (not obscured), record as clear. If you see the lines but they are not well delineated, record as hazy. If you cannot see the lines at all, record as cloudy.	The lines help discern clarity by providing contrast.
8. Properly care for or dispose of equipment and supplies. Clean the work area using a surface disinfectant. Remove personal protective equipment. Wash your hands.	

Note: Rapid determination of color and clarity is necessary because some urine turns cloudy if left standing. Bilirubin, which may be found in urine in certain conditions, breaks down when exposed to light. Protect the specimen from light if urinalysis is ordered but testing is delayed. If further testing is to be done but is delayed for more than an hour, refrigerate the specimen to avoid alteration of chemistry.

Charting Example:

05/31/2008 2:45 PM Random urine collected. Yellow/clear
H. Henderson, CMA

PROCEDURE 43-4: Chemical Reagent Strip Analysis

Purpose: To determine the level of constituents in a patient's urine to aid in the diagnosis of urinary or metabolic disorders

Equipment: Patient's labeled urine specimen, chemical strip (such as Multistix or Chemstrip), manufacturer's color comparison chart, stopwatch or timer, personal protective equipment, hand disinfectant, surface disinfectant

Steps	Reasons
1. Wash your hands.	Handwashing aids infection control.
2. Assemble the equipment.	
3. Put on personal protective equipment.	
4. Verify that the name on the specimen container and the name on the report form are the same.	This prevents reporting errors.
5. Mix the patient's urine by gently swirling the covered container.	
6. Remove the reagent strip from its container and replace the lid to prevent deterioration of strips by humidity.	
7. Immerse the reagent strip in the urine completely, and then immediately remove it, sliding the edge of the strip along the lip of the container to remove excess urine. Pooling of excess urine on the dipstick causes cross-contamination among the reactions, possibly obscuring accurate color detection.	Immersing the reagent strip resuspends particulate matter in urine. Immediate removal of the strip prevents colors from leaching during prolonged exposure to urine.
8. Start your stopwatch or timer immediately.	Reactions must be read at specific intervals as directed on the package insert and on the color comparison chart.
9. Compare the reagent pads to the color chart, determining results at the intervals stated by the manufacturer. Example: Glucose is read at 30 seconds. To determine results, examine that pad 30 seconds after dipping and compare with color chart for glucose.	This adheres to strict time-sensitive testing protocol.

(continued)

PROCEDURE 43-4:   Chemical Reagent Strip Analysis (continued)

Steps	Reasons

2161

Multistix® 10 SG

Reagent Strips for Urinalysis
For In Vitro Diagnostic Use

COLOR CHART

Bayer

READ PRODUCT INSERT BEFORE USE.
IMPORTANT: Do not expose to direct sunlight.
Do not use after 12/99.

TESTS AND READING TIME

LEUKOCYTES 2 minutes	NEGATIVE		TRACE	SMALL +	MODERATE ++	LARGE +++
NITRITE 60 seconds	NEGATIVE		POSITIVE	POSITIVE	(Any degree of uniform pink color is positive)	
UROBILINOGEN 60 seconds	NORMAL 0.2	NORMAL 1	mg/dL 2	4	8	(1 mg = approx. 1EU)
PROTEIN 60 seconds	NEGATIVE	TRACE	mg/dL 30 +	100 ++	300 +++	2000 or more ++++
pH 60 seconds	5.0	6.0	6.5	7.0	7.5	8.0	8.5
BLOOD 60 seconds	NEGATIVE	NON-HEMOLYZED TRACE	NON-HEMOLYZED MODERATE	HEMOLYZED TRACE	SMALL +	MODERATE ++	LARGE +++
SPECIFIC GRAVITY 45 seconds	1.000	1.005	1.010	1.015	1.020	1.025	1.030
KETONE 40 seconds	NEGATIVE	mg/dL	TRACE 5	SMALL 15	MODERATE 40	LARGE 80	LARGE 160
BILIRUBIN 30 seconds	NEGATIVE		SMALL +	MODERATE ++	LARGE +++	
GLUCOSE 30 seconds	NEGATIVE	g/dL (%) mg/dL	1/10 (tr.) 100	1/4 250	1/2 500	1 1000	2 or more 2000 or more

©1997 Bayer Corporation, Diagnostics Division, Tarrytown, NY 10591   Rev. 12/97 0401123

Step 9. Multistix package insert. (Courtesy of Bayer Corporation, Elkhart, IN.)

10. Read all reactions at the times indicated and record the results.

11. Discard the reagent strips in the proper receptacle. Discard urine unless more testing is required.

12. Clean the work area with surface disinfectant. Remove personal protective equipment. Wash your hands.

Warning: Do not remove the desiccant packet in the strip container; it ensures that minimal moisture affects the strips. The desiccant is toxic and should be discarded appropriately after all of the strips have been used.
Note: The manufacturer's color comparison chart is assigned a lot number that must match the lot number of the strips used for testing. Record this in the quality assurance (QA/QC) log. False-positive and false-negative results are possible. Review the manufacturer's package insert accompanying the strips to learn about factors that may give false results and how to avoid them. Aspirin may cause false-positive ketones. Document any medications the patient is taking. If the patient is taking pyridium, do not use a reagent strip for testing because the medication will interfere with the color. Outdated materials give inaccurate results. If the expiration date has passed, discard the materials.

PROCEDURE 43-5: **Preparing Urine Sediment**

Purpose: To aid in the determination and identification of formed elements and solid particles in a urine specimen

Equipment: Patient's labeled urine specimen, urine centrifuge tubes, transfer pipette, centrifuge (1500–2000 rpm), gloves, impervious gown, face shield, hand disinfectant, surface disinfectant

Steps	Reasons
1. Wash your hands.	Handwashing aids infection control.
2. Assemble the equipment.	
3. Put on personal protective equipment.	
4. Verify that the name on the specimen container and the name on the report form are the same.	This prevents reporting errors.
5. Swirl specimen to mix. Pour 10 mL of well-mixed urine into a labeled centrifuge tube or standard system tube. Cap the tube with a plastic cap or parafilm.	Capping the tube prevents a biohazardous aerosol when the centrifuge is running.
6. Centrifuge the sample at 1500 rpm for 5 minutes.	Centrifugation ensures that cellular and particulate matter is pulled to the bottom of the tube.
7. When the centrifuge has stopped, remove the tubes. Make sure no tests are to be performed first on the supernatant. Remove the caps and pour off the supernatant, leaving 0.5–1.0 mL of it. Suspend the sediment again by aspirating up and down with a transfer pipette, or follow the manufacturer's directions for a standardized system.	The concentrated urine is now prepared for microscopic examination.
8. Properly care for and dispose of equipment and supplies. Clean the work area with surface disinfectant. Remove personal protective equipment. Wash your hands.	

Note: If the urine is to be tested by chemical reagent strip, perform the dip test before spinning the urine. Preparing a urine specimen of less than 3 mL for sediment is not recommended because that is not enough urine to create a true sediment. However, some patients cannot provide a large amount of urine. In such cases, document the volume on the chart under sediment to ensure proper interpretation of results. Centrifuge maintenance requires periodic checks to ensure that the speed and timing are correct. Document this information on the maintenance log.

- Urine tests help the physician determine or rule out abnormalities to make a correct diagnosis.
- The medical assistant ensures a properly collected clean-catch midstream specimen by thoroughly instructing the patient in the collection procedure.
- Another important factor the medical assistant can influence is the elapsed time from collection to examination in the laboratory.
- Changes over time after collection include (1) decreased clarity due to crystallization of solutes, (2) ris-

ing pH, (3) loss of ketone bodies, (4) loss of bilirubin, (5) dissolution of cells and casts, and (6) overgrowth of contaminating microorganisms. Urinalysis may not reflect the findings of absolutely fresh urine if the sample is more than 1 hour old.
- Proper performance of the urinalysis, including confirmation tests as indicated, is an important function of the medical assistant.

Warm Ups   for Critical Thinking

1. Most laboratories pour off a portion of a urine specimen to test rather than dipping the chemical reagent strip directly into the urine container. Why?

2. You report a positive dipstick result for blood to the physician. The physician asks you to prepare the urine sediment for microscopic examination and

comes to the lab to review the slide. Microscopic examination does not reveal any RBCs in the specimen. What is the explanation for the dipstick test result? Can it be accurate?

3. What is the preferred specimen for urinalysis? Why is this preferred, and how should it be collected?

Answers   to Checkpoint Questions

1. Urine should be tested within 1 hour of collection. (If testing cannot be performed within 1 hour, refrigerate the specimen at 4° to 8°C until testing can be performed.) If the urine is not properly refrigerated, the specimen can deteriorate.

2. The three reported physical properties of urine are color, clarity and specific gravity.

3. A positive bilirubin test can indicate problems such as liver disease, hepatitis, and bile duct destruction.

4. Positive nitrates and leukocytes on a dipstick would suggest a urinary tract infection.

5. The three types of epithelial cells in the urine are squamous, transitional, and renal. Squamous epithelial cells are a normal finding. Transitional epithelial cells are seen with infections of the lower urinary tract, such as cystitis. Renal epithelial cells line the nephrons and are seen with infections and inflammations of the upper urinary tract.

6. Three of the most common crystals found in urine are calcium oxalate, uric acid, and triple phosphate.

Microbiology and Immunology

Outline

Microbiological Life Forms
Bacteria
Rickettsias and Chlamydiae
Fungi
Viruses
Protozoa
Metazoa
Specimen Collection and Handling
Types of Specimens
Types of Culture Media
Transporting the Specimen

Microscopic Examination of Microorganisms
Smears and Slides
Identification by Staining
Inoculation
Sensitivity Testing
Antigens and Antibodies
Immunology Testing Principles
Reagent and Kit Storage and Handling

Immunology Tests
Infectious Mononucleosis
Pregnancy Test
Group A Streptococcus
Immunohematology
ABO Group
Rh Type

Learning Objectives

Upon successfully completing this chapter, you will be able to:

1. Spell and define the key terms

2. List and describe primary microorganisms

3. Describe how bacteria are named

4. Identify various bacterial illustrations

5. Describe the classifications of rickettsiae, chlamydiae, fungi, protozoa, and metazoa

6. Describe the medical assistant's responsibilities in microbiological testing

7. List the most common types of microbiological specimens collected in the physician's office laboratory

8. State the factors necessary for microbial growth

9. Describe the different types of media used for microbial testing

10. List the steps used in caring for media plates

11. List each step in Gram staining and state the purpose of each step

12. State the purpose of sensitivity testing and give the meaning of sensitive and resistant results

13. Describe the antigen-antibody reaction

14. Explain the storage and handling of test kits

15. List and describe immunology tests most commonly encountered through the medical office

Upon successfully completing this chapter, you will be able to:

1. Collect throat specimens (Procedure 44-1)
2. Collect nasopharyngeal specimens (Procedure 44-2)
3. Collect wound specimens (Procedure 44-3)
4. Collect sputum specimens (Procedure 44-4)
5. Collect stool specimens (Procedure 44-5)
6. Collect blood specimens for culture (Procedure 44-6)
7. Collect genital specimens (Procedure 44-7)
8. Test stool specimen for occult blood (Procedure 44-8)
9. Prepare a smear for microscopic evaluation (Procedure 44-9)
10. Perform a Gram stain (Procedure 44-10)
11. Inoculate a culture (Procedure 44-11)
12. Perform mononucleosis testing (Procedure 44-12)
13. Perform HCG pregnancy testing (Procedure 44-13)
14. Perform rapid group A strep testing (Procedure 44-14)

Competencies

CAAHEP

- Perform handwashing
- Dispose of biohazardous materials
- Use quality control
- Practice standard precautions
- Prepare patients for procedures
- Obtain specimens for microbiological testing
- Instruct patients in the collection of fecal specimens
- Perform microbiology testing
- Perform immunologic testing
- Document accurately

ABHES

- Practice OSHA compliance rules and regulations
- Practice standard precautions
- Collect and process specimens
- Instruct patients in the collection of fecal specimens
- Obtain throat specimen for microbiological testing
- Perform selected tests that assist with diagnosis and treatment
- Perform wound collection procedure for microbiological testing
- Prepare patients for procedures
- Perform microbiology testing
- Perform immunologic testing
- Dispose of biohazardous materials

Key Terms

aerobes	bacteriology	normal flora	sensitivity testing
anaerobes	cocci	nosocomial infection	specificity
antibody	media	parasitology	virology
antigen	morphology	pathogens	
bacilli (singular, bacillus)	mycology	sensitivity	

Microbiology means the study of small life, too small to be seen without a microscope. **Pathogens**, microorganisms likely to cause disease, are those that thrive at temperatures between 96°F and 101°F in a fairly neutral environment. Many **normal flora** (bacteria that are not pathogens) live and thrive on the human body without causing disease. As a medical assistant, to protect yourself, the physician, patients, and all co-workers from **nosocomial infections** (infections acquired in a medical setting), you need to be aware of the organisms present around us and their potential for causing disease.

Bacteria require the following five elements for survival: nutrients, warmth, moisture, darkness, and oxygen (**aerobes**) or lack of oxygen (**anaerobes**). The human body provides all five elements. These same five elements are simulated in the microbiology laboratory with the use of culture media, incubators, and techniques to control the specimen's exposure to oxygen.

Medical microbiology is performed using cultures and smears of patients' specimens referred to the laboratory. The specimens may be taken from wounds or other areas, such as the throat, vagina, urethra, or skin, by using a swab, a stick topped with cotton or other absorbent manmade fiber. Specimens may be drawn from the body by surgical puncture or by venipuncture. Specimens are also excreted from the body as sputum, stool, or urine.

As a medical assistant, you will frequently collect specimens or assist the physician with the collection. You may collect specimens from wounds or from the throat, but the physician usually collects specimens from the eye, ear, rectum, or reproductive organs. In all instances, you must practice aseptic technique to ensure the integrity of the specimen. (see Chapter 17). In addition, standard precautions are necessary to protect all health care workers and patients.

Microbiological Life Forms

Bacteria

Bacteriology is the study of bacteria. Organisms have both a genus and species name. The genus is always spelled with a capital letter, and the species begins with a lowercase letter (e.g., *Staphylococcus aureus*). In print, the name is in italics or underlined.

Several groups of bacteria, including the spore-forming bacteria, are significant in medical microbiology. Bacteria are unicellular (one-celled) simple organisms, each with its own characteristics. Bacteria do not require a host for their life stages as long as they have the five survival requirements. The organisms can be identified by their distinct shapes, or morphology (Table 44-1); chemical tests; and other means, such as motility tests.

Cocci (spherical bacteria) are responsible for many diseases. Some species of staphylococci are found on all

TABLE 44-1	Categorizing Bacteria
Morphology	**Types**
Round (spherical)	Cocci
Grape-like clusters	Staphylococci
Chain formations	Streptococci
Paired	Diplococci
Rod-shaped	Bacilli
Somewhat oval	Coccobacilli
End-to-end chains	Streptobacilli
Spiral	Spirochetes
Flexible (usually with flagella, whip-like extremities that aid movement)	Spirilla
Rigid, curved rods (comma-shaped)	Vibrios

surfaces of the skin and many mucous membranes. They are generally not pathogenic unless they reach an area that is usually sterile, where they may cause abscess formation or another form of infection. Species of streptococci may cause sore throat, scarlet fever, rheumatic fever, many pneumonias, and various skin infections. Diplococci (cocci in pairs) cause bacterial meningitis, gonorrhea, and some of the pneumonias. Figure 44-1 shows the **morphology** (structural characteristics) of various cocci.

Bacilli (bacteria with a rod shape) are usually aerobic (requiring oxygen to live). They are longer than they are wide. There are approximately six variations in the bacillus shape: cigar, curved, oval, rod, staff, and tapered rod. Most bacteria are bacillus-shaped and often found in soil. Diseases caused by bacilli include tetanus, botulism, gas gangrene, tuberculosis, pertussis, salmonellosis, certain pneumonias, and otitis media.

Spirochetes are long, spiral, flexible organisms; spiral bacteria are classified as spirilla if they are rigid rather than flexible. Spirochetes are responsible for syphilis and Lyme disease. Vibrios are very motile comma-shaped bacteria. They cause cholera.

PATIENT EDUCATION

LYME DISEASE

The deer tick is an arthropod capable of transmitting *Borrelia burgdorferi*, the spirochete responsible for Lyme disease (Fig. 44-2). When the infected deer tick bites a human, the spirochete enters the body and can produce mild to severe symptoms, including a rash, joint aches, fever, general body

Arrangement	Description	Appearance	Example	Disease
Diplococci	Cocci in pairs		*Neisseria gonorrhoeae*	Gonorrhea
Streptococci	Cocci in chains		*Streptococcus pyogenes*	Strep throat
Staphylococci	Cocci in clusters		*Staphylococcus aureus*	Boils
Tetrad	A packet of 4 cocci		*Micrococcus luteus*	Rarely pathogenic
Octad	A packet of 8 cocci		*Sarcina ventriculi*	Rarely pathogenic

Figure 44-1 Morphologic arrangements of cocci. (From Engelkirk P. Burton's Microbiology for the Health Professions. 8th ed. Baltimore: Lippincott Williams & Wilkins, 2007.)

aches, and alterations in neurologic and cardiac function.

Lyme disease, which has been documented in 47 states, can be prevented with proper education. Instruct patients to avoid tick habitats, to apply insect repellent, and to wear shoes and light-colored clothing when working outside in wooded areas. Clothing should be checked for ticks and washed in hot water with strong soap. Stress the importance of looking for ticks and removing them properly when they are found.

Figure 44-3 shows the various forms of bacteria.

 CHECKPOINT QUESTION

1. What are the two basic morphologic forms of bacteria?

Rickettsias and Chlamydiae

Specialized forms of bacteria that fit in a category of their own are the rickettsias and chlamydiae. They are smaller than bacteria but larger than viruses. Because they require a living host for replication and survival, they are referred to as obligate intracellular parasites. Rickettsias cause Rocky Mountain spotted fever. The chlamydiae cause lymphogranuloma venereum, a prevalent sexually transmitted disease.

Figure 44-2 Lyme disease organism, the *Borrelia burgdorferi* spirochete. (Asset provided by Anatomical Chart Co.)

Figure 44-3 Various forms of bacteria including single cocci, diplococci, single bacilli, diplobacilli, spirochetes, and other bacterial forms. (From Engelkirk P. Burton's Microbiology for the Health Professions. 8th ed. Baltimore: Lippincott Williams & Wilkins, 2007.)

Figure 44-4 Tissue section taken from an individual with coccidioidomycosis. (From McClatchey KD. Clinical Laboratory Medicine. 2nd ed. Philadelphia: Lippincott Williams & Wilkins, 2002.)

Fungi

Mycology is the study of fungi. Infectious fungi are small organisms like bacteria with the potential to produce disease in susceptible hosts. Some fungi are microscopic, but many can be seen without the aid of a microscope. Fungi resemble plants, whereas bacteria appear to resemble one-celled animals. Fungi may be in the form of yeasts or molds in the human body. They are opportunistic, usually becoming pathogenic when the host's normal flora can no longer counterbalance the colony's growth.

Fungal diseases, called mycoses or mycotic infections, include the following.

Molds

- Aspergillus. Often affects the ear but may affect any organ or surface; may be fatal if widespread.
- Blastomycosis. Usually asymptomatic but may cause skin ulcers or bone lesions and may spread to the viscera.
- Coccidioidomycosis. May cause acute flulike respiratory symptoms or may become chronic and infect almost any body part (Fig. 44-4).
- Histoplasmosis. Spreads through contaminated soil; usually asymptomatic but may lead to pneumonia (Figs. 44-5 and 44-6).
- Tinea. Cutaneous mycoses (e.g., tinea pedis [athlete's foot], tinea corporis [ringworm of the body], tinea capitis [ringworm of the scalp], and tinea unguium [nail fungus]).

WHAT IF?

What if your patient asks you how to prevent cutaneous mycoses, such as tinea pedis?

Explain to your patient that tinea pedis is a common fungal infection. Then offer the following suggestions, which can aid prevention:

- Practice good basic hygiene.
- Thoroughly dry between the toes.
- Do not share footwear.
- Use antifungal powder between the toes and in shoes.
- Wear foot protection when using public showers.

Yeasts

- Candidiasis causes thrush (skin and mouth), vaginitis, and endocarditis. It may be spread by contact (Fig. 44-7).

Viruses

Virology is the study of viruses, the smallest microorganisms. Viruses cause influenza, infectious hepatitis, rabies, polio, and acquired immunodeficiency syndrome (AIDS). They are so small that they can be seen only with an electron microscope, not the usual bright-field microscope found in the medical office. They require a living host for survival and replication and are referred to as obligate intracellular parasites. Because viruses are not susceptible to antibiotics, most are extremely difficult to treat. Antiviral therapies are being developed for many of the

Figure 44-6 Microscopic appearance of the mold phase of Histoplasma capsulatum. (From McClatchey KD. Clinical Laboratory Medicine. 2nd ed. Philadelphia: Lippincott Williams & Wilkins, 2002.)

viruses, and researchers continue to work on cures for many viral diseases, such as AIDS and herpes.

Protozoa

Single-celled parasitic animals that may be diagnosed in the **parasitology** laboratory are the protozoa. These microorganisms and the conditions they cause include the following:

- Entamoeba: diarrhea, dysentery, and liver and lung disorders
- Giardia: giardiasis, diarrhea, and malabsorption of nutrients
- Trichomonas: trichomoniasis, vaginitis, and urinary tract infection
- Plasmodium: malaria
- Toxoplasma: toxoplasmosis and fetal abnormalities

Figure 44-5 Photomicrographs illustrate the fungus *Histoplasma capsulatum* grown at 25°C (top) and at 37°C (bottom). (From Engelkirk P. Burton's Microbiology for the Health Professions. 8th ed. Baltimore: Lippincott Williams & Wilkins, 2007.)

Figure 44-7 *Candida albicans* (original magnification ×3600). (From McClatchey KD. Clinical Laboratory Medicine. 2nd ed. Philadelphia: Lippincott Williams & Wilkins, 2002.)

Metazoa

Metazoa include helminths, nematodes, and arthropods. The helminth family includes roundworms, flatworms, and flukes. Most survive almost anywhere in the human body or may migrate through the body until they find a place to settle. Helminths can cause schistosomiasis, liver fluke infestations, and beef or pork tapeworm infestation. The nematodes cause roundworm infestations, gastrointestinal obstruction, bronchial damage, pinworm infestation, and trichinosis. Arthropods include mites, lice, ticks, and fleas along with bees, spiders, wasps, mosquitoes, and scorpions. All may cause injury by their bites or stings, and several are also capable of transmitting disease by their bite or sting.

Specimen Collection and Handling

Laboratory tests are most often performed on specimens that are easily obtained from the body, such as blood, urine, feces, sputum, and other body secretions and fluids. The specimen gives the physician a view of the condition of the system from which the specimen was obtained. For instance, a urine culture will indicate the infectious process at work within the urinary system; a sputum culture will grow the organism responsible for the patient's respiratory signs and symptoms.

As a medical assistant, you may be responsible for collecting most of the specimens in the medical office. To ensure that the office or reference laboratory receives a sample that will indicate the disease process for which the specimen was collected, you must collect the specimen from the appropriate site using the proper method. You also must handle the specimen so that it will yield accurate findings (Box 44-1).

Types of Specimens

Microbiology entails extensive work with cultures of the referred biological specimen. Cultures are media that will support the growth of microorganisms. The organisms are encouraged to replicate under controlled conditions for the purpose of diagnosing disease. Protocols for patient instruction, collection, and assisting physician collection of specimens for microbiology testing are outlined in Procedures 44-1 through 44-7.

Types of Culture Media

Media (liquid, solid, or semisolid preparations) support the growth of microorganisms for identification. The microorganism will multiply for diagnosis of disease when it is provided an environment for optimal growth.

Various types of **media** are prepared with a mixture of substances that nourish pathogens. All of the sus-

---

BOX 44-1

GUIDELINES FOR SPECIMEN COLLECTION AND HANDLING

- Follow standard precautions for specimen collection as outlined by the Centers for Disease Control and Prevention.
- Review the requirements for collecting and handling the specimen, including the equipment, the type of specimen to be collected (e.g., exudate, blood, mucus), the amount required for laboratory analysis, and the procedure to be followed for handling and storage.
- Assemble the equipment and supplies. Use only the appropriate specimen container as specified by the medical office or laboratory.
- Ensure that the specimen container is sterile to prevent contamination of the specimen by organisms not present at the collection site.
- Examine each container before use to make sure that it is not damaged, the medium is intact and moist, and it is well within the expiration date.
- Label each tube or specimen container with the patient's name and/or identification number, the date, the name or initials of the person collecting the specimen, the source or site of the specimen, and any other information required by the laboratory. Use an indelible pen or permanent marker. Make sure you print legibly, document accurately, and include all pertinent information.

---

pected microorganism's requirements for growth must be present. The medium provides nutrients, moisture, and the proper pH. Specimens submitted for laboratory study are most frequently cultured on blood agar, a solid medium prepared by adding 5% sheep's blood to agar, a firm, jello-like, transparent and colorless substance made from seaweed. The agar congeals the blood and forms a firm surface to support the growth of microorganisms. The firm surface makes it easy to observe the culture growth. The blood adds the nourishment required for replication of the microorganisms. A Petri plate is a glass or plastic dish used to hold a solid culture medium, such as blood agar. The plate is fitted with a cover to maintain the integrity of the specimen. Petri plates are clear and allow visual examination of a culture as it grows (Fig. 44-8).

The temperature and darkness are maintained by an incubator (Fig. 44-9). The presence or absence of oxygen is provided by the type of incubator (oxygen for aerobes and carbon dioxide for anaerobes). Media designed for anaerobic bacteria (bacteria that live without oxygen)

Figure 44-8 Solid media are supplied on Petri plates wrapped in a plastic sleeve. Petri plates are always stored medium side up.

may contain a tablet that generates carbon dioxide and eliminates oxygen in the closed environment of the medium container. Figure 44-10 displays one type of anaerobic culture set-up.

Caring for the Media

Commercially prepared culture media in disposable plastic Petri plates are available for use in medical offices. The plates are supplied in a plastic sleeve and must be stored in the refrigerator with the side containing the medium on top (see Fig. 44-9). The plates should be stored in the plastic wrapper to keep the medium moist.

Figure 44-9 Standard laboratory incubator. (Courtesy of So-Low Environmental Equipment, Cincinnati, OH.)

Figure 44-10 The Bio-Bag anaerobic culture set. It includes a plate of CDC-anaerobic blood agar in an oxygen-impermeable bag. The system contains its own gas-generating kit and cold catalyst. (Courtesy of Becton Dickinson, Franklin Lakes, NJ.)

Petri plates stored with the medium down may form condensation on the lids that will drip onto the surface, making it too moist for an accurate culture. Check the expiration date and the condition of the medium surface before using the plates. Discard any plates that are past the expiration date or any medium that has dried or cracked. When the shipment arrives, date each sleeve.

Rotate the media in the refrigerator so that the oldest is in front and used first, based on the date it expires, not the date it was received. Note, the temperature of the refrigerator should be checked and recorded daily. Be sure not to overfill the refrigerator or allow media to be placed against the back wall or sides. This will raise the temperature.

Agar must be refrigerated until needed and then warmed to room temperature before use. A cold plate or tube will kill many microorganisms, most of which require a warmer temperature for growth. Most physician offices are equipped with an incubator set at about 99°F (37°C), or just about body temperature. Check and record the incubator temperature daily.

 CHECKPOINT QUESTION

2. Why is it important to store the Petri plates with the medium side uppermost?

Transporting the Specimen

Care must be taken to transport or process the specimen as soon as possible so the organisms do not die. The sooner the specimen is processed, the sooner the pathogen can be identified and treatment can begin. Some microorganisms, such as *N. gonorrhoeae*, are very fragile and must be cultured under controlled conditions as quickly as possible.

Specimens to be processed in outside or regional laboratories must be placed in transport medium, such as Culturette (Marion Scientific) (Fig. 44-11) or Precision Culture CATS (Precision Dynamics). All directions appropriate for the specimen are stated on the package. Most transport systems are designed to be self-contained and include a plastic tube with a sterile swab and transport medium appropriate for the type of specimen (Fig. 44-12). Most are stored at room temperature.

Special care must be taken in filling out all identification slips and information.

Properly prepared transport media may be mailed or routed by a courier. The outside laboratory may provide a mailing or shipping container, either cardboard or plastic foam, to protect the specimen during transport. A label indicating the presence of a biohazardous biological specimen is attached to the outside of the container. In many instances, specimens are collected and transported on days that ensure their arrival during the business week to avoid having them remain in transit until the start of a new week. Delays in testing may cause some of the microorganisms to die or to overproliferate, possibly compromising the results of the test.

For the most reliable results, laboratory tests should be performed on fresh specimens within 1 hour after collection. When this is not possible, the specimen must be stored properly to preserve the physical and chemical properties necessary for accurate diagnosis. Specimens should never be subjected to extreme temperature changes. Table 44-2 lists general guidelines for handling and storing specimens commonly collected in the medical office.

Actual testing of the stool specimen for the presence of occult blood is performed via the guaiac method as described in Procedure 44-8. Box 44-2 provides tips for collecting special types of stool specimens.

Figure 44-12 Preparing transport media for use.

PATIENT EDUCATION

PATIENT PREPARATION FOR FECAL OCCULT BLOOD TESTING

Guaiac Methods Only

- A high-residue diet starting 2 days prior to and continuing through testing. Note: CHECK YOUR TEST METHOD. There are new testing methods available that do not require diet restrictions.

Diet May Include:

- Meats: small amounts of well-cooked chicken, turkey, and tuna.
- Vegetables: large amounts of raw and cooked vegetables including lettuce, corm, spinach, carrots and celery. Note vegetables that should be avoided listed below.
- Fruits: large amounts of fruits, especially prunes and apples.
- Cereals: bran and bran-containing cereals.
- Moderate amounts of peanuts and popcorn daily.
- Drink large amounts of fluids.

To Be Avoided:

- Meat: diet should not include and red or rare meat
- Vegetables: some have a chemical reaction that interferes with the test: turnips, cauliflower, red radishes, broccoli, cantaloupe, horseradish, parsnips

Other Factors Requiring Instructions:

- Medications: For 7 days prior to and during the testing, do not take aspirin or other NSAIDs (anti-

Figure 44-11 Transport media.

inflammatory medicines) or iron supplements. For 2 days prior to and during testing, do not use rectal medications, tonics or vitamin preparations containing vitamin C (ascorbic acid) in excess of 250 mg/day).
- Bleeding hemorrhoids: Do not test.
- Menses: Do not test during menses or for 3 days after menses.

Microscopic Examination of Microorganisms

Smears and Slides

Specimens grown on a culture may be spread onto a glass slide for morphologic inspection under a microscope as described in Procedure 44-9. Sometimes a special treatment with stain or fixative will be applied to aid in identification. Some pathogens are more easily identified if they are allowed to move freely in a wet mount. For more information about wet mounts, see Box 44-3. These are best viewed immediately, but at the latest, they should be viewed within 30 minutes of collection. To preserve the specimen for longer term evaluation, the procedure described in Procedure 44-9 should be used.

Identification by Staining

Staining the microorganisms may help the physician narrow the field of possible pathogens and initiate treat-

---

BOX 44-2

SPECIAL STOOL SPECIMENS

Follow these tips when collecting stool specimens to test for pinworms or parasites or to obtain a swab for culture. Remember to follow standard precautions.

- *Pinworms:* Schedule the appointment early in the morning, preferably before a bowel movement or bath. Pinworms tend to leave the rectum and lay eggs around the anus during the night. Press clear adhesive tape against the anal area. Remove it quickly and place it sticky side down on a glass slide for the physician to inspect.
- *Parasites:* Caution the patient not to use a laxative or enema before the test to avoid destroying the evidence of parasites. If the stool contains blood or mucus, include as much as possible in the specimen container because these substances are most likely to contain the suspected organism.
- *Stool culture:* A sterile cotton-tipped swab is passed into the rectal canal beyond the sphincter and rotated carefully. Place it in the appropriate culture container or process as directed for smear preparation.

TABLE 44-2	Handling and Storing Commonly Collected Specimens	
	Handling	**Storage**
Urine	Clean-catch midstream with care to avoid contaminating the inside of the container; must not stand more than 1 hour after collection.	Refrigerate if cannot be tested within 1 hour; add preservative at direction of laboratory; preservatives not usually used for urine culture.
Blood	Handle carefully, as hemolysis may destroy microorganisms; collect in anticoagulant tube at room temperature; specimen must remain free of contaminants; see laboratory manual for proper anticoagulant.	For most specimens, refrigerate at 4°C (39°F) to slow changes in physical and chemical composition.
Stool	Collect in clean container. To test for ova and parasites, keep warm.	Deliver to laboratory immediately. If delayed, mix with preservative provided or recommended by laboratory, or use transport medium.
Microbiology specimens	Do not contaminate swab or inside of specimen container by touching either to surface other than site of collection. Protect anaerobic specimens from exposure to air.	Transport specimen as soon as possible. If delayed, refrigerate at 4°C (39°F) to maintain integrity

Observe standard precautions while handling any of these specimens.

BOX 44-3

PREPARING A WET MOUNT SLIDE

To prepare a wet mount, follow these steps:

1. Place a drop of the specimen on a glass slide with sterile saline or 10% potassium hydroxide (KOH).
2. Place a coverslip over the specimen to reduce evaporation.
3. To decrease evaporation, coat the rim of the coverslip with petrolatum.
4. Inspect the slide by microscope using the high-power objective lens with diminished light.

Wet mount slide preparation. **(A)** A drop of fluid containing the organism is placed on a glass slide. **(B)** The specimen is covered with a coverslip ringed with petroleum jelly.

ment before a culture has been incubated. Most bacteria are colorless and hard to see or identify without special treatment such as staining. The primary stain used in the microbiology lab is the Gram stain. In the Gram stain process, certain bacteria (cocci and bacilli), which are stained with crystal violet and safranin, retain crystal violet dye. These bacteria can be seen with the use of a bright-field microscope. Bacteria that retain the purple color are said to be Gram positive. Those that do not retain the crystal violet will stain red with the safranin stain, also called the counterstain. These are said to be Gram negative (Fig. 44-13). Procedure 44-10 details the steps for Gram staining a smear. The Gram stain is read with the use of a bright-field microscope. CLIA regulations allow the medical assistant to prepare the Gram stain to be read and reported by the physician.

Inoculation

Microbiological inoculation is the introduction of a microorganism into culture medium and placement in an environment that will support growth of pathogens. To ensure that the specimen is placed on or in the culture medium in the proper manner to encourage maximal growth, you will inoculate it with the specimen swab or remove a portion of the specimen with a sterile inoculating loop. Procedure 44-11 describes the steps for culture inoculation.

 CHECKPOINT QUESTION

3. Why are bacteria stained?

Sensitivity Testing

To determine the antibiotic that will most effectively treat the pathogen isolated from the patient's culture, the pathogen is inoculated to large agar plate. Paper disks impregnated with antibiotics are applied to the culture plate with the organism, and the prepared plate is incubated for 24 hours. When the plate is observed for growth, the antibiotic disks that exhibit a margin with no bacterial growth indicate that the pathogen is sensi-

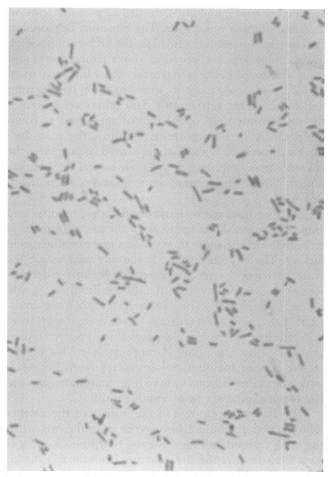

Figure 44-13 Gram-negative bacteria. (From Sweet RL, Gibbs RS. Atlas of Infectious Diseases of the Female Genital Tract. Philadelphia: Lippincott Williams & Wilkins, 2005.)

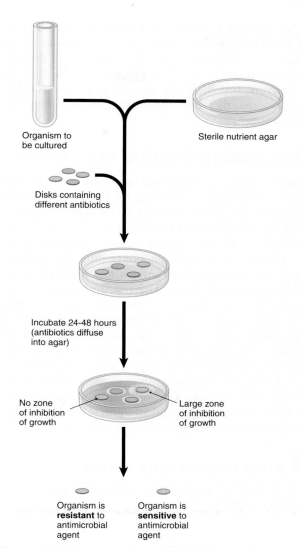

Figure 44-14 Manual disk antibiotic susceptibility testing.

tive or susceptible to this medication. If there is no zone around the disk, the organism is said to be resistant to that antibiotic. If there is a small zone, it may be reported as intermediate. The antibiotic of choice will be the one with the largest zone of inhibition (no growth). Multiple antibiotics can be tested on one plate. Figure 44-14 shows a plate testing one antibiotic with a significant zone indicating resistance. This is the manual technique for **sensitivity testing.** Automated instruments perform this testing in large laboratories.

 CHECKPOINT QUESTION

4. What is the purpose of sensitivity testing?

Antigens and Antibodies

Antigens are substances recognized as foreign to the body that cause the body to initiate a defense response, including the production of antibodies. Pathogenic mi-

crobes are among the substances recognized by the body as antigens. **Antibodies** are proteins produced by the body in response to a specific antigen that bind to that specific antigen. Antibodies float freely in the bloodstream and are found in serum. Each antibody combines with (in most instances) only one antigen; this is called **specificity.** It allows laboratory personnel to test the exact substance desired without interference from any other substance in serum.

Because an antibody has a particularly strong attraction for its antigen, little antigen need be present in a sample for the antibody to find it; this is referred to as **sensitivity.** A test is very sensitive if it can determine the presence of a substance even if only a small amount is present. Tests using antigen antibody reactions are very specific and very sensitive. These tests can detect small amounts of a substance and pick it out of a solution, such as serum, that contains millions of other substances.

An antibody is named by using its specific antigen's name and adding the prefix anti-. In the blood for instance, if the antigen on the RBC's name is A, then the antibody's name is anti-A. If the antigen is B, then the antibody is anti-B. If the antigen is a bacteria, like *Streptococcus*, then the antibody's name is antistreptococcal antigen.

Immunology Testing Principles

In immunology, the substance to be tested is identified or the amount present (quantity) is measured using the binding of a specific antibody to its specific antigen. Either the antigen is detected by use of a solution containing the antibody (antisera) or the antibody is detected by using a solution containing the antigen. Usually the binding of an antigen and antibody is not visible to the naked eye. The reaction has to be enhanced. These immunoassays use highly sensitive antibodies that are specific for the antigen being tested. Test kits include reagents to extract the antigen from the specimen. The protein fragments in the extraction react with reagents in the test strip or cartridge. If the extracted specimen contains the antigen, a color change (usually blue or red) will indicate a positive result. Accuracy of testing is dependent upon following the specific manufacturer's instructions (Box 44-4).

 CHECKPOINT QUESTION

5. How does an immunoassay indicate the presence of the test substance?

Reagent and Kit Storage and Handling

Immunoassay reagents are manufactured as kits. These kits contain all of the reagents and often supplies, such as pipettes, tubes, and cups, needed to perform tests on a certain number of samples. The kits must be stored at the temperature recommended on the kit box or package insert. Some kits are stored at room temperature, and some are stored in the refrigerator; other kits have to be divided, with some reagents stored at room temperature and others in the refrigerator. Still others are stored in the refrigerator until opened and then stored at room temperature. It is important to follow the manufacturer's directions. If the kits are stored improperly, the reagents may deteriorate, and false results may be obtained. Tips for performing immunoassays are noted in Box 44-4.

Each kit package is marked with a lot number and expiration date. All reagents with the same lot number were made at the same time in the same manufacturing facility. The expiration date is the day past which the reagents are no longer guaranteed to perform correctly. Reagents from kits with different lot numbers should not be used together. The manufacturer will not guarantee that they will work correctly when components from different lots are mixed. Reagents should never be used past their expiration date. A more complete list of corrective actions for immunology assays is in Box 44-5, which describes actions to take if an immunoassay control is not producing an acceptable result.

The date of opening and the initials of the worker who opened it should also be written on the box when the kit is opened and used for the first time. Some kits have a new expiration date starting from the day the kit is opened. Always read the package insert for details about storing and handling the reagents and supplies.

There may be specific specimen collection guidelines indicated on each kit. Be sure to read and follow the manufacturer's instructions

---

BOX 44-4

TIPS FOR PERFORMING IMMUNOASSAYS

1. Follow the times exactly.
2. Add reagents in correct order.
3. Use reagents only with other reagents from the same kit.
4. Use the exact amount of reagents stated in directions.
5. Ensure that reagents and samples are at room temperature.
6. Ensure that reagents have not expired.

BOX 44-5

IMMUNOASSAY TROUBLESHOOTING TIPS

If an immunoassay control is not producing an acceptable result, try the following:

1. Reread the procedure to be sure a step was not omitted.
2. Check the labels of reagents to be sure the correct reagents were added in the correct order.
3. Visually check reagents for signs of contamination, such as cloudiness or color change.
4. Repeat the test with a new bottle of control.
5. Repeat the test with a new kit or reagent.
6. Call the manufacturer for assistance.

CHECKPOINT QUESTION

6. Why is it important to store reagent kits at specified temperatures?

Immunology Tests

There are many immunoassay test kits available today, and the number is growing. This is an area of CLIA-waived testing that is making an increasing number of diagnostic test results available in the physician's office. The three most common immunoassays will be discussed here.

Infectious Mononucleosis

Infectious mononucleosis is caused by the Epstein-Barr virus. The symptoms are fever, sore throat, and swollen lymph glands. Because these symptoms are common to several illnesses, the immunoassay test is useful for a differential diagnosis (Procedure 44-12). False-negative results can occur early in the disease before antibodies are produced.

Pregnancy Test

The test for pregnancy (Procedure 44-13) is based on the detection of the hormone human chorionic gonadotropin (HCG). Today's tests are sensitive enough to determine pregnancy before the first missed menses. A pregnancy test is frequently used to rule out pregnancy before a medical procedure that might harm the fetus (Fig. 44-15). A urine specimen that is too dilute can give a false-negative reaction. The first morning urine specimen is the most likely to contain HCG if the patient is pregnant. Certain tumors (testicular and some fibroids) produce HCG and can cause a false-positive result.

Figure 44-16 Rapid Strep Test Kit.

Group A Streptococcus

Group A streptococcus (*Streptococcus pyogenes*) is one of the most common bacterial causes of sore throat and upper respiratory tract infections. Because of the need for rapid diagnosis to begin appropriate treatment, many immunoassay kits are available to test quickly for group A beta-hemolytic streptococcus or *Streptococcus pyogenes* (Fig. 44-16). If the test result is positive, treatment can begin at once.

Group A strep infection can be diagnosed by bacterial culture or immunoassay for the antigenic presence of the bacteria (Fig. 44-17). (See Procedure 44-14.) If improper technique is used in collecting the throat swab or an inadequate specimen is obtained, a false-negative result can occur. Culture testing is considered more sensitive and should be used to confirm negative immunoassay test results.

Figure 44-15 Pregnancy test kit.

Figure 44-17 Positive and negative rapid strep test results.

CHECKPOINT QUESTION

7. What are the benefits and drawbacks of using immunoassay testing versus cultures for group A streptococcus?

Immunohematology

ABO Group

Each person belongs to one of four blood groups: A, B, O, or AB. Approximately 45% of the population are O, 40% are A, 11% are B, and 4% are AB. Serum contains antibodies to the ABO antigens that a person lacks. These antibodies occur naturally. Shortly after birth, these antibodies are found in serum, even though the person has never received blood.

- A person in the A group has the A antigen.
- A person in the B group has the B antigen.
- A person in the AB group has both the A and B antigen.
- A person in the O group lacks both antigens.
- A person in the A group lacks the B antigen and has an antibody to B (anti-B) in serum.
- Someone who is B lacks the A antigen and has anti-A in serum.
- A person who is O has both anti-A and anti-B in serum.
- A person who belongs to the AB group has neither antibody in serum.

The lack of either A or B antigens on O cells makes this group the universal donor. This means type O blood may be given to patients no matter what their ABO group.

Rh Type

The presence of the D antigen is termed Rh positive. The absence of the D antigen is termed Rh negative. Antibodies to D do not occur naturally. A person lacking the D antigen must be exposed to the D antigen of foreign RBCs to produce antibodies. This can happen if an Rh-negative (D-negative) patient is transfused with Rh-positive (D-positive) blood. This can also happen if an Rh-negative mother is exposed to the Rh-positive cells of her baby before or during childbirth. Rh-nega-

 WHAT IF?

What if a patient asks you about the criteria for donating blood?

The American Red Cross bases criteria for donating blood on recommendations from government agencies and the Centers for Disease Control and Prevention and findings of research projects. In addition, each state has its own laws regulating blood donors. Generally, blood donors must meet the following criteria:

- Age 16 years or older (donors who are 16 years of age require a parent's permission; donors who are 65 years of age or older require a physician's consent)
- Weight of 110 lb or more
- Hemoglobin at least 12.5 g/dL (women) or 13.5 g/dL (men)
- Pulse of 50 to 110 beats per minute
- Blood pressure lower than 180/100

The donor also must provide a brief history. The entire procedure lasts approximately an hour; the actual blood donation time is about 10 minutes. Blood can be donated every 56 days. Only 1 unit (pint) will be taken at a time. All blood will be tested by the American Red Cross for HIV, hepatitis, and syphilis.

tive mothers can be prevented from producing antibodies to the Rh (D) antigen by injection of immune-D serum, or RhoGAM. This injection prevents the production of antibodies that might cause hemolytic disease of the next baby (erythroblastosis fetalis) by destroying its RBCs.

ABO and Rh testing are not CLIA-waived procedures and may only be performed by those who meet CLIA qualifications for moderate-complexity testing.

PATIENT EDUCATION

EXPECTANT MOTHERS AND RHOGAM

If you are employed in an obstetrician's office, you will have the opportunity to teach many expectant mothers who are Rh negative about the purpose of RhoGAM. Here are some pointers:

- Explain what it means to be Rh negative in terms appropriate to the patient's level of understanding.
- Point out that if the Rh factor of the baby's father is either positive or unknown, the baby could be born with Rh-positive blood. Also note that if the Rh factor of the baby's father is negative, there should be no problem.
- Explain that, if the baby's Rh-positive blood comes in contact with the mother's Rh-negative blood, the mother will make antibodies against the baby's blood. In future pregnancies, her antibodies will fight with the fetal blood (if Rh positive), causing severe hemolytic anemia in the fetus.
- Tell the patient that RhoGAM is an immune globulin that prohibits the production of Rh-positive antibodies in the mother. It is given during and after labor and requires that a consent form be signed.
- After a miscarriage or abortion, the Rh-negative mother must receive RhoGAM unless it is documented that the baby's father was Rh negative.

MEDIA MENU

- **Student CD**
  - **Animations**
    Acute Inflammation; Immune Response
  - **CMA/RMA Certification Exam Review**
- **LWW's Medical Assisting Skills DVD**
  - **Procedures 44-1, 44-8, 44-9, 44-10, 44-13, 44-14**
- **Premium Online Course**
  http://thePoint.lww.com/Kronenberger3e
- **Internet Resources**

LiveAdvise Online Tutoring & Competency Training
http://thePoint.lww.com/LiveAdvise

MedlinePlus Health Information from the National Library of Medicine
http://medlineplus.gov/

Microbiology Microbes Bacteria Information and Links
http://www.microbes.info/

American College of Allergy, Asthma and Immunology (ACAAI)
http://www.acaai.org/

PROCEDURE 44-1 — Collect a Throat Specimen

Purpose: Obtain a throat specimen for rapid strep testing or culture
Equipment: Tongue blade, light source, sterile specimen container and swab, personal protective equipment, hand sanitizer, surface sanitizer, biohazard transport bag (if to be sent to the laboratory for analysis)

Steps	Reasons
1. Wash your hands.	Handwashing aids infection control.
2. Assemble the equipment and supplies.	
3. Put on personal protective equipment.	Following standard precautions prevents the transmission of infectious microorganisms.
4. Greet and identify the patient. Explain the procedure.	Identifying the patient prevents errors in treatment.
5. Have the patient sit with a light source directed in the throat.	Enhancing visualization of specimen site improves accuracy of sampling.
6. Carefully remove the sterile swab from the container. If performing both the rapid strep and culture or confirming negative results with a culture, swab with two swabs held together.	Swabbing with two swabs at once eliminates the discomfort to the patient of having to perform the procedure twice.

Step 6. Carefully remove the sterile swab from the container.

Steps	Reasons
7. Have the patient say "Ah" as you press down on the midpoint of the tongue with the tongue depressor.	Saying "Ah" raises the uvula to avoid contaminating the specimen and decreases the gag reflex. If the tongue depressor is placed too far forward, it will not be effective; if it is placed too far back, the patient will gag unnecessarily.
8. Swab the mucous membranes, especially the tonsillar area, the crypts, and the posterior pharynx in a "figure 8" motion. Turn the swab to expose all of its surfaces to the membranes. Avoid touching tongue, teeth, sides of mouth, and uvula.	Pathogens must be collected with a twisting motion for maximum collection. Touching the areas noted to avoid will contaminate the specimen with normal flora and inhibit testing accuracy.

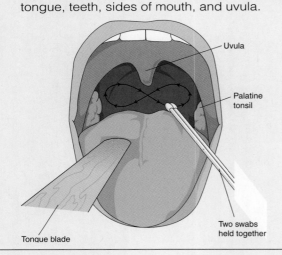

Uvula

Palatine tonsil

Two swabs held together

Tongue blade

Step 8. Technique for obtaining a throat sample

(continued)

| PROCEDURE 44-1: | **Collect a Throat Specimen** *(continued)* |

Steps	Reasons
	Step 8. Avoid touching areas that will contaminate the specimen.
9. Maintain the tongue depressor position while withdrawing the swab from the patient's mouth.	Keeping the tongue down prevents contaminating the swab with normal flora.
	Step 9. Withdraw the swab with the tongue depressor still in position.
10. Follow the instructions on the specimen container for transferring the swab or processing the specimen in the office using a commercial kit. Label the specimen with the patient's name, the date and time of collection, and the origin of the material.	Improper handling of the specimen will compromise test results. Improper labeling will result in test delay and require the patient to have the procedure repeated.
11. Properly dispose of the equipment and supplies in a biohazard waste container. Remove personal protective equipment and wash your hands.	This prevents the spread of microorganisms.
12. Route the specimen or store it appropriately until routing can be completed.	Delay in transport to the testing site or improper storage will compromise test results.
13. Document the procedure.	Procedures that not documented are considered to have not been performed.
14. Sanitize the work area.	Sanitation aids in infection control.
	Step 14. Sanitize the work area.

Charting Example:

*11/20/2008 10:30 AM Throat specimen obtained, Dx code **###.##** per Dr. Lewis. Rapid strep test negative, specimen to reference lab for C&S*

M. Mohr, CMA

PROCEDURE 44-2:   Collecting a Nasopharyngeal Specimen

Purpose: This test is used to evaluate nasopharyngeal secretions for the presence of pathogenic organisms
Equipment: Penlight, tongue blade, sterile flexible wire swab, transport media, personal protective equipment, hand sanitizer, surface sanitizer, biohazard transport bag (if to be sent to the laboratory for analysis)

Steps	Reasons
1. Wash your hands.	Handwashing aids infection control.
2. Assemble the equipment and supplies.	
3. Put on personal protective equipment.	Following standard precautions prevents the transmission of infectious microorganisms.
4. Greet and identify the patient. Explain the procedure.	Identifying the patient prevents errors in treatment.
5. Position the patient with his head tilted back.	
6. Using a penlight and a tongue blade, inspect the nasopharyngeal area.	Enhancing visualization of specimen site improves accuracy of sampling.
7. Gently pass the swab through the nostril and into the nasopharynx, keeping the swab near the septum and floor of the nose. Rotate the swab quickly, and then remove it and place it in the transport media. Do not let the swab touch the sides of the patient's nostril or his tongue to prevent specimen contamination.	

Step 7. Gently swab through the nostril.

Steps	Reasons
8. Label the specimen with the patient's name, the date and time of collection, and the origin of specimen.	Improper labeling will result in test delay and require the patient to have the procedure repeated.
9. Properly dispose of the equipment and supplies in a biohazard waste container. Remove personal protective equipment and wash your hands.	This prevents the spread of microorganisms.
10. Route the specimen or store it appropriately until routing can be completed.	Delay in transport to the testing site or improper storage will compromise test results.
11. Document the procedure.	Procedures not documented are not performed.
12. Sanitize the work area.	Sanitation aids in infection control.

Charting Example:

11/20/2008 10:30 AM Nasopharyngeal specimen obtained, Dx code ###.## per Dr. Lewis. Specimen to reference lab for C&S
M. Mohr, CMA

PROCEDURE 44-3: Collecting a Wound Specimen

Purpose: This test is used to evaluate wound exudate for the presence of pathogenic organisms
Equipment: Sterile swab, transport media, personal protective equipment, hand sanitizer, surface sanitizer, biohazard transport bag (if to be sent to the laboratory for analysis)

Steps	Reasons
1. Wash your hands.	Handwashing aids infection control.
2. Assemble the equipment and supplies.	
3. Put on personal protective equipment.	Following standard precautions prevents the transmission of infectious microorganisms.
4. Greet and identify the patient. Explain the procedure.	Identifying the patient prevents errors in treatment.
5. If dressing is present, remove it and dispose of it in biohazard container. Assess the wound by observing color, odor, and amount of exudate. Remove contaminated gloves and put on clean gloves.	Thorough visualization of specimen site improves accuracy of sampling.
6. Use the sterile swab to sample the exudate. Saturate swab with exudate, avoiding the skin edge around the wound. **Step 6.** Saturate swab with exudate.	
7. Avoid skin edge around wound.	Normal skin flora may contaminate specimen and compromise viability of pathogens in specimen.
8. Place swab back into container and crush the ampule of transport medium. **Step 8. (A)** Place swab in culturette tube. **(B)** Crush the ampule of media at the bottom of the tube.	Fastidious bacteria may require transport medium environment to maintain viability.
9. Label the specimen with the patient's name, the date and time of collection, and the origin of specimen.	Improper labeling will result in test delay and require the patient to have the procedure repeated.
10. Route the specimen or store it appropriately until routing can be completed.	Delay in transport to the testing site or improper storage will compromise test results.
11. Clean the wound and apply a sterile dressing using sterile technique.	
12. Properly dispose of the equipment and supplies in a biohazard waste container. Remove personal protective equipment and wash your hands.	This prevents the spread of microorganisms.

(continued)

PROCEDURE 44-3: Collecting a Wound Specimen (continued)

Steps	Reasons
13. Document the procedure.	Procedures not documented are not performed.
14. Sanitize the work area.	Sanitation aids in infection control.

Charting Example:

> *11/20/2008 10:30 AM Wound specimen obtained from right heel, Dx code* **###.##** *per Dr. Lewis.*
>
> *Specimen to reference lab for C&S*
>
> M. Mohr, CMA

PROCEDURE 44-4: Collecting a Sputum Specimen

Purpose: This test is used to evaluate sputum for the presence of disease
Equipment: Sterile specimen container, personal protective equipment, hand sanitizer, surface sanitizer, biohazard transport bag.

Steps	Reasons
1. Wash your hands.	Handwashing aids infection control.
2. Assemble the equipment and supplies.	
3. Put on personal protective equipment.	Following standard precautions prevents the transmission of infectious microorganisms.
4. Greet and identify the patient. Explain the procedure.	Identifying the patient prevents errors in treatment. Explanations will help gain compliance and ease anxiety.
5. Provide patient with a cup of water and instruct the patient to rinse mouth with water.	Rinsing the mouth reduces contamination of sputum specimen with normal mouth flora.
6. Ask the patient to cough deeply, using the abdominal muscles as well as the accessory muscles to bring secretions from the lungs and not just the upper airways.	The desired specimen should contain pathogens and epithelial cells from the lining of the lower respiratory tract.
7. Ask the patient to expectorate directly into the specimen container without touching the inside and without getting sputum on the outsides of the container. About 5–10 mL is sufficient for most sputum studies.	Touching the inside of the container will contaminate the container and specimen. Sputum on the outside of the container may be hazardous.
8. Handle the specimen container according to standard precautions. Cap the container immediately and put it into the biohazard bag for transport to the laboratory. Fill out a laboratory requisition slip to accompany the specimen.	The specimen is a biohazard, and capping the container immediately eliminates the danger of spreading microorganisms. A laboratory requisition will tell the laboratory personnel the type of specimen and the specific tests ordered.
9. Label the specimen with the patient's name, the date and time of collection, and the origin of specimen.	Improper labeling will result in test delay and require the patient to have the procedure repeated.

(continued)

PROCEDURE 44-4: Collecting a Sputum Specimen *(continued)*

Steps	Reasons
10. Route the specimen to the laboratory.	Delay in transport to the testing site will compromise test results. The pathogens may either proliferate, causing overgrowth, or die, causing a false-negative result.
11. Properly dispose of the equipment and supplies in a biohazard waste container. Remove personal protective equipment and wash your hands.	This prevents the spread of microorganisms.
12. Document the procedure.	Procedures not documented are not performed.
13. Sanitize the work area.	Sanitation aids in infection control.

Charting Example:

11/20/2008 10:30 AM Moderate amount of thick, yellow sputum, Dx code ###.## per Dr. Lewis.
Specimen to reference lab for C&S
M. Mohr, CMA

PROCEDURE 44-5: Collecting a Stool Specimen

Purpose: This test is used to evaluate stool for pathogens and/or blood

Equipment: Specimen container dependent on test ordered (sterile container or Para-Pak Collection System for C&S or ova and parasites; test kit or slide for occult blood testing; see laboratory procedure manual), tongue blade or wooden spatula, personal protective equipment, hand sanitizer, surface sanitizer, biohazard transport bag

Para-Pak stool collection containers.

Steps	Reasons
1. Wash your hands.	Handwashing aids infection control.
2. Assemble the equipment and supplies.	
3. Greet and identify the patient. Explain the procedure. Explain any dietary, medication, or other restrictions necessary for the collection. (These restrictions and instructions for the patient are detailed earlier in this chapter in the Patient Education box titled Patient Preparation for Fecal Occult Blood Testing.) Instruct patient to defecate into a disposable plastic container or onto plastic wrap placed over the toilet bowl.	Identifying the patient prevents errors in treatment. Explanations will help gain compliance and ease anxiety. Noncompliance with preparation for specimen collection may cause false-positive results and unnecessary follow-up testing.

(continued)

PROCEDURE 44-5: Collecting a Stool Specimen (continued)

Steps	Reasons
4. When obtaining a stool specimen for C&S or ova and parasites, the patient should collect a small amount of the first and last portion of the stool after the bowel movement with the wooden spatula or tongue blade and place it in the specimen container without contaminating the outside of the container. Fill Para-Pak until fluid reaches "fill" line, and recap the container.	Touching the inside of the container will contaminate the container and specimen. Stool on the outside of the container may be hazardous. The specimen is a biohazard, and capping the container immediately eliminates the danger of spreading microorganisms.
5. Upon receipt of the specimen, the MA should put on gloves and place the specimen into the bio hazard bag for transport to the reference laboratory. Fill out a laboratory requisition slip to accompany the specimen.	A laboratory requisition will tell the laboratory personnel the type of specimen and the specific tests ordered.
6. Label the specimen with the patient's name, the date and time of collection, and the origin of specimen.	Improper labeling will result in test delay and require the patient to have the procedure repeated.
7. Transport the specimen to the laboratory or store the specimen as directed. Refer to laboratory procedure manual since some samples require refrigeration; others are kept at room temperature, and some must be placed in an incubator at a laboratory as soon as possible after collecting.	Improper storage and/or delay in transport to the testing site will compromise test results.
8. Properly dispose of the equipment and supplies in a biohazard waste container. Remove personal protective equipment and wash your hands.	This prevents the spread of microorganisms.
9. Document the procedure including patient instructions.	Procedures not documented are not performed.
10. Sanitize the work area.	Sanitation aids in infection control.

Charting Example:

11/20/2008 10:30 AM Patient instructed on preparation for and collection of stool for occult blood. Patient demonstrated understanding and will return specimen to lab upon completion. Dx code ###.## per Dr. Lewis
M. Mohr, CMA

11/21/2008 8:00 AM Patient delivered stool specimen to the laboratory
M. Mohr, CMA

PROCEDURE 44-6: Collecting Blood for Culture

Purpose: This test is used to evaluate blood for pathogens

Equipment: Specimen container depends on testing site (yellow-top sodium polyanethol sulfonate vacutainer tubes or aerobic and anaerobic blood culture bottles), blood culture skin prep packs (or 70% isopropyl alcohol wipes and povidone-iodine solution swabs or towelettes), venipuncture supplies (see Chapter 41), personal protective equipment, hand sanitizer, surface sanitizer

Steps	Reasons
1. Wash your hands.	Handwashing aids infection control.
2. Assemble the equipment and supplies, checking expiration dates.	Expired collection or culture supplies must be discarded.
3. Put on personal protective equipment.	Following standard precautions prevents the transmission of infectious microorganisms.
4. Greet and identify the patient. Explain the procedure. Verify that the patient has not initiated antibiotic therapy. If therapy has started, document antibiotic, strength, dose, duration, and time of last dose.	Identifying the patient prevents errors in treatment. Antibiotic therapy can cause false-negative test results.
5. Using skin preparation kits or supplies, apply alcohol to venipuncture site and allow to air dry. Apply povidone-iodine prep in progressively increasing concentric circles without wiping back over skin that is already prepped. Let stand for at least 1 minute and allow the site to air dry. Do not touch skin following preparation. **Step 5.** Swab the antecubital space of the arm using a povidone-iodine swab, cleaning in progressively increasing circles.	The povidone-iodine reduces false-positive culture results from skin contaminants. Touching the site following preparation may reintroduce contaminants.
6. Wipe bottle stoppers with povidone-iodine solution.	Bottle tops require decontamination to prevent specimen contamination.
7. Perform venipuncture as described in Procedure 41-1.	
8. Fill bottles or tube according to specific laboratory procedure. Invert each 8–10 times as soon as collected. If using culture bottles, fill the aerobic bottle first.	Inversion mixes blood with media. Collecting the aerobic bottle first removes any residual air in the needle to avoid contaminating the anaerobic bottle.
9. Complete venipuncture. Use an isopropyl alcohol wipe to remove residual povidone-iodine from skin. Label the specimen with the patient's name, the date and time of collection, and the origin of specimen.	Leaving iodine solution on skin can cause irritation.
10. Remove gloves and wash hands. In preparation for the second collection 30 minutes after the first, put on new gloves and repeat Steps 5–9 at a second venipuncture site.	A minimum of 30 mL of blood should be collected between the two venipunctures. Using two collection sites increases success of isolating pathogen if present.

(continued)

PROCEDURE 44-6: Collecting Blood for Culture *(continued)*

Steps	Reasons
11. Label the specimens with the patient's name and the date and time of collection.	Improper labeling will result in specimen rejection by the testing laboratory.
12. Properly dispose of the equipment and supplies in a biohazard waste container. Remove personal protective equipment and wash your hands.	This prevents the spread of microorganisms.
13. Document the procedure.	Procedures not documented are not performed.
14. Sanitize the work area.	Sanitation aids in infection control.

Charting Example:

11/20/2008 10:30 AM *Blood culture specimens collected from antecubital area of left and right arms,*

Dx code **###.##** *per Dr. Lewis*

M. Mohr, CMA.

PROCEDURE 44-7: Collecting Genital Specimens for Culture

Purpose: This test is used to evaluate for pathogens
Equipment: Specimen container depends on testing requested (bacterial, viral, and *Chlamydia* specimens require different media), personal protective equipment, hand sanitizer, surface sanitizer

Steps	Reasons
1. Wash your hands.	Handwashing aids infection control.
2. Assemble the equipment and supplies, checking expiration dates.	Expired collection or culture supplies must be discarded.
3. Put on personal protective equipment.	Following standard precautions prevents the transmission of infectious microorganisms.
4. Your role will be to assist the physician in the collection and handling of these specimens. Be sure to verbally verify patient identification.	Identifying the patient prevents errors in treatment.
5. Accept specimens from the physician, securing them in the appropriate medium follow the instructions for that particular medium.	Isolating the pathogen is dependent upon providing the appropriate environment for transport and culture. **Step 5.** Physician places swab into culturette tube in medical assistant's gloved hand.
6. Label the specimen with the patient's name, the date and time of collection, and the origin of specimen.	Improper labeling will result in specimen rejection by the testing laboratory.
7. Repeat Steps 5 and 6 for each specimen.	

(continued)

PROCEDURE 44-7:   Collecting Genital Specimens for Culture
(continued)

Steps	Reasons
8. Store specimens per procedure instructions until transport. Transport to testing facility as soon as possible.	Improper storage and/or delay in transport to the testing site will compromise test results.
9. Properly dispose of the equipment and supplies in a biohazard waste container. Remove personal protective equipment and wash your hands.	This prevents the spread of microorganisms.
10. Document the procedure.	Procedures not documented are not performed.
11. Sanitize the work area.	Sanitation aids in infection control.

Charting Example:

*11/20/2008 10:30 AM Vaginal specimens collected for C&S, herpes, and Chlamydia and referred to reference lab, Dx code **###.##** per Dr. Lewis*

M. Mohr, CMA

PROCEDURE 44-8:   Testing Stool Specimen for Occult Blood: Guaiac Method

Purpose: Test stool for occult blood in a sample obtained by the patient using a test kit and brought or mailed into the office

Equipment: Gloves, patient's labeled specimen pack, developer or reagent drops, personal protective equipment, hand sanitizer, surface sanitizer, contaminated waste container

Steps	Reasons
1. Wash your hands and put on clean examination gloves.	Handwashing aids infection control. Follow standard precautions when handling stool specimens.
2. Assemble the supplies and verify the patient identification on the patient's prepared test pack. Check the expiration date on the developing solution.	Proper identification prevents errors. Solution that has expired may yield inaccurate results.
	Step 2. Assemble the supplies and check expiration dates.
3. Open the test window on the back of the pack and apply one drop of the developer or testing reagent to each window according to manufacturer's directions. Read the color change within the specified time, usually 60 seconds.	Following the manufacturer's instructions ensures accurate results.

(continued)

PROCEDURE 44-8: **Testing Stool Specimen for Occult Blood: Guaiac Method** *(continued)*

Steps	Reasons
4. Apply one drop of developer as directed on the control monitor section or window of the pack. Note whether the quality control results are positive or negative as appropriate. If results are acceptable, patient results may be reported. If results are not acceptable, notify the physician.	Patient test results cannot be reported if quality control results are not acceptable.
5. Properly dispose of the test pack and gloves. Wash your hands.	Follow standard precautions throughout the procedure.
6. Record the procedure.	Procedures not documented are not performed.
7. Sanitize the work area.	Sanitation aids in infection control.

Charting Example:

> 3/28/2008 3:00 PM Occult blood slides ×3 returned to office via mail; testing performed Dx ###.## per
>
> Dr. Franklin; findings positive. Dr. Franklin notified
>
> J. Smith, RMA

PROCEDURE 44-9: **Preparing a Smear for Microscopic Evaluation**

Purpose: To aid in the identification of microorganisms in a specimen
Equipment: Specimen, Bunsen burner, slide forceps, slide, sterile swab or inoculating loop, pencil or diamond-tipped pen, personal protective equipment, hand sanitizer, surface sanitizer, contaminated waste container

Steps	Reasons
1. Wash your hands.	Handwashing aids infection control.
2. Assemble the equipment.	
3. Label the slide with the patient's name and the date on the frosted edge with a pencil.	Labeling will ensure proper identification. Pencil markings will not rinse off during staining.
4. Put on personal protective equipment.	Always comply with standard precautions.
5. Hold the edges of the slide between the thumb and index finger. Starting at the right side of the slide and using a rolling motion of the swab, gently and evenly spread the material from the specimen over the slide. The material should thinly fill the center of the slide within half an inch of each end.	Spread the material thinly to avoid obscuring the slide with too much material. Rolling ensures that as much of the specimen as possible is deposited on the slide. Sweeping the loop accomplishes the same purpose. Confining the specimen to the area within half an inch of the edges avoids contaminating the gloves.

Step 5. The material should thinly fill the center of the slide.

(continued)

PROCEDURE 44-9:   Preparing a Smear for Microscopic Evaluation *(continued)*

Steps	Reasons
6. Do not rub the material vigorously over the slide.	Doing so may destroy fragile microorganisms.
7. Dispose of the contaminated swab or disposable inoculating loop in a biohazard container.	The swab and the loop contain body fluid and are biohazardous.
8. Allow the smear to air dry in a flat position for at least half an hour. Do not blow on the slide or wave it about in the air. Heat should not be applied until the specimen has been allowed to dry. Some specimens (e.g., Pap smear) require a fixative spray.	The cells will dry slowly at room temperature. If you blow on the slide, you may contaminate the specimen with bacteria from your mouth. Fixative may be sprayed from 4–6 inches to protect the cells from contaminants or to keep them from becoming dislodged. Heat at this point may destroy the microorganisms.
9. Hold the dried smear slide with the slide forceps. Pass the slide quickly through the flame of a lighter or safety match three or four times. The slide has been fixed properly when the back of the slide feels slightly uncomfortably warm to the back of the gloved hand. It should not feel hot. CAUTION: Any excess heat will distort and probably destroy the specimen material on the slide.	Passing the slide through the heat kills the microorganisms and attaches them firmly to the slide so they do not wash off during staining and are not dislodged during viewing. Excessive heat may distort the specimen cells.
10. Properly dispose of the equipment and supplies in a biohazard waste container. Remove personal protective equipment and wash your hands.	This prevents the spread of microorganisms.
11. Document the procedure.	Procedures not documented are not performed.
12. Sanitize the work area.	Sanitation aids in infection control.

Charting Example:

07/23/08 10:00 AM Specimen taken from nostril and prepared as a direct smear Dx. **###.##** *per*
Dr. York
B. White, RMA

PROCEDURE 44-10: Performing a Gram Stain

Purpose: To aid in the identification of pathogens in a specimen
Equipment: Crystal violet stain, staining rack, Gram iodine solution, wash bottle with distilled water, alcohol-acetone solution, counterstain (e.g., safranin), absorbent (bibulous) paper pad, specimen smear on glass slide labeled with a pencil or diamond-tipped pen (as prepared in Procedure 44-9), Bunsen burner, slide forceps, stopwatch or timer, personal protective equipment, hand sanitizer, surface sanitizer, contaminated waste container

Steps	Reasons
1. Wash your hands.	Handwashing aids infection control.
2. Assemble the equipment.	
3. Make sure the specimen is heat-fixed to the labeled slide and the slide is room temperature (see Procedure 44-9).	
4. Put on personal protective equipment.	
5. Place the slide on the staining rack with the smear side up.	The staining rack collects the dye as it runs off the slide for disposal.
6. Flood the smear with crystal violet. Time for 60 seconds. **Step 6.** Flood the smear with crystal violet.	
7. Hold the slide with slide forceps. A. Tilt the slide to an angle of about 45° to drain the excess dye. B. Rinse the slide with distilled water for about 5 seconds and drain off excess water.	Washing the slide stops the staining process.
8. Replace the slide on the slide rack. Flood the slide with Gram iodine solution for 60 seconds.	The iodine acts as a mordant and fixes, or binds, the crystal violet to the Gram-positive bacteria. The stain will be permanent in the receptive Gram-positive cells after it is fixed with the iodine solution.
9. Using the forceps, tilt the slide at a 45° angle to drain iodine solution. With the slide tilted, rinse the slide with distilled water from the wash bottle for about 5 to 10 seconds. Slowly and gently wash with the alcohol-acetone solution until no more stain runs off.	The alcohol-acetone removes the crystal violet stain from the Gram-negative bacteria. The Gram-positive bacteria retain the purple dye. If the process is carried on too long or too vigorously, dye may leach out of the Gram-positive bacteria and lead to incorrect findings.
10. Immediately rinse the slide with distilled water for 5 seconds and return the slide to the rack.	Rinsing stops the decolorizing.
11. Flood with safranin or suitable counterstain for 60 seconds.	The Gram-negative bacteria stain pink or red with the counterstain.
12. Drain the excess counterstain from the slide by tilting it at a 45° angle. Rinse the slide with distilled water for 5 seconds to remove the counterstain. Gently blot the smear dry with bibulous paper. Take	Moisture or excess solution may obscure the slide and hinder identification.

(continued)

PROCEDURE 44-10: Performing a Gram Stain *(continued)*

Steps	Reasons
care not to disturb the smeared specimen. Wipe the back of the slide clear of any solution. It may be placed between the pages of a bibulous paper pad and gently pressed to remove excess moisture.	
	Step 12. Gently blot smear dry with bibulous paper.
13. Properly dispose of the equipment and supplies in a biohazard waste container. Remove personal protective equipment and wash your hands.	This prevents the spread of microorganisms.
14. Document the procedure.	Procedures not documented are not performed.
15. Sanitize the work area.	Sanitation aids in infection control.

Note special precautions: Results may be misinterpreted if a reagent is defective or near expiration or if the timing is not as directed. The bacteria may overstain, or color may leach from the cells if care is not taken to observe the time limits. The results will not be accurate if the specimen was not heated properly (killing the bacteria) or was not incubated long enough or if the general technique was not performed correctly. Prepared smears of known Gram-positive and Gram-negative organisms are processed with the patient's specimen for quality control.

Charting Example:

07/23/08 10:10 AM Slide of patient's specimen Gram stained and submitted to Dr. York to review.
Dx. ###.##
<div align="right">*B. White, RMA*</div>

PROCEDURE 44-11: Inoculating a Culture

Purpose: To introduce a portion of a specimen into the culture medium for growth and replication of microorganisms and to produce isolated colonies

Equipment: Specimen on a swab or loop, china marker or permanent laboratory marker, sterile or disposable loop, Bunsen burner, labeled Petri dish of culture medium (the patient's name should be on the side of the plate containing the medium because it is always placed upward to prevent condensation from dripping onto the culture), personal protective equipment, hand sanitizer, surface sanitizer, contaminated waste container.

Steps	Reasons
1. Wash your hands.	Handwashing aids infection control.
2. Assemble the equipment.	
3. Put on personal protective equipment.	
4. Label the medium side of the plate with the patient's name, identification number, source of specimen, time collected, time inoculated, your initials, and date.	Because culture incubation may take 24–72 hours, dating ensures that the plate is read at the proper time. Labeling the medium side will prevent misplacing culture. **Step 4.** Correctly labeled specimen plate.
5. Remove the Petri plate from the cover (the Petri plate is always stored with the cover down), and place the cover on the work surface with the opening up. Do not open the cover unnecessarily.	Each time the cover is removed, there is a chance of contamination. Having the cover's opening upward avoids contamination from the work surface.
6. Using a rolling and sliding motion, streak the specimen swab across half of the plate, starting at the top and working to the center. Dispose of the swab in a biohazard container. The specimen will spread in gradually thinning colonies of bacteria.	 **Step 6.** Use a rolling and sliding motion to apply specimen to plate.
7. Use a disposable loop.	
8. Turn the plate a quarter turn from its previous position. Pass the loop a few times in the original inoculum, and then across the medium approximately a quarter of the surface of the plate. Do	The loop draws into the clean surface a bit of the specimen that was streaked in the first part of the procedure.

(continued)

PROCEDURE 44-11:   Inoculating a Culture *(continued)*

Steps	Reasons
not enter the originally streaked area after the first few sweeps.	
	Step 8. Streak lightly from the original inoculum across the next quarter of the plate.
9. Turn the plate another quarter turn so that now it is 180° to the original smear. Working in the previous manner, draw the loop at right angles through the most recently streaked area. Again, do not enter the originally streaked area after the first few sweeps. **Step 9.** Streak the third quadrant of the plate.	The loop pulls out gradually thinning bits of the specimen to isolate colonies. Large groups of colonies close together are more difficult to identify than isolated colonies. Pale yellow colonies of *Staphylococcus aureus.* Colonies demonstrate growth of the microbe on a properly streaked plate.
FOR QUANTITATIVE CULTURES: A. Streak the plate with the specimen from side to side across the middle.	
	Step 9A. Streak the plate from one side to the other in a straight line across the middle.
B. Streak the entire plate back and forth across the initial inoculate. This allows bacteria to grow in a way that colonies can be counted.	
	Step 9B. Streak the entire plate from side to side over the original inoculum.
10. Properly dispose of the equipment and supplies i n a biohazard waste container. Remove personal protective equipment and wash your hands.	This prevents the spread of microorganisms.
11. Document the procedure.	Procedures not documented are not performed.
12. Sanitize the work area.	Sanitation aids in infection control.

(continued)

PROCEDURE 44-11: Inoculating a Culture *(continued)*

Charting Example:

7/14/08 9:15 AM Swab specimen taken of (L) heel wound, transferred to culture medium for incubation.
To be read 7/16/08. Dx ###.## per Dr. Brehmer. Pt instructed on wound care and infection control;
verbalized understanding of instructions
G. Gray, RMA

PROCEDURE 44-12: Mononucleosis Testing

Purpose: To determine the presence or absence of infectious mononucleosis
Equipment: Patient's labeled specimen (whole blood, plasma, or serum, depending on the kit), CLIA-waived mononucleosis kit (slide or test strip), stopwatch or timer, personal protective equipment, hand sanitizer, surface sanitizer, contaminated waste container

Steps	Reasons
1. Wash your hands.	Handwashing aids infection control.
2. Verify that the names on the specimen container and the laboratory form are the same.	
3. Assemble the equipment and ensure that the materials in the kit and the patient specimen are at room temperature.	
4. Label the test pack or test strip (depending on type of kit) with the patient's name, positive control, and negative control. Use one test pack or strip per patient and control.	This ensures accurate testing.
5. Aspirate the patient's specimen using the transfer pipette and place volume indicated in kit package insert on the sample well of the test pack or dip test strip labeled with the patient's name.	
6. Sample the positive and negative controls as directed in Step 5.	This satisfies quality assurance and quality control standards.
7. Set timer for incubation period indicated in package insert.	
8. Read reaction results at the end of incubation period.	Waiting the appropriate amount of time ensures that testing is complete.
9. Verify the results of the controls before documenting the patient's results. Log controls and patient information on the worksheet.	This satisfies quality assurance and quality control standards
10. Properly dispose of the equipment and supplies in a biohazard waste container.	
11. Remove personal protective equipment and wash your hands.	This prevents the spread of microorganisms.
12. Document the procedure.	Procedures not documented are not performed.
13. Sanitize the work area.	Sanitation aids in infection control.

Note: Kits vary with the manufacturer; read instructions carefully before beginning. Controls for test kits may be performed at different intervals depending on laboratory protocol. Follow procedures to ensure quality.

Charting Example:

04/23/2008 10:00 AM Mono test performed, Dx ###.## per Dr. Scott. Results negative
S. Miller, CMA

PROCEDURE 44-13:   HCG Pregnancy Test

Purpose: To detect the production of HCG to determine pregnancy
Equipment: Patient's labeled specimen (plasma, serum, or urine depending on the kit), HCG pregnancy kit (test pack and transfer pipettes or test strip; kit contents will vary by manufacturer), HCG positive and negative control (different controls may be needed when testing urine), timer, personal protective equipment, hand sanitizer, surface sanitizer, contaminated waste container

Steps	Reasons
1. Wash your hands.	Handwashing aids infection control.
2. Assemble the equipment. 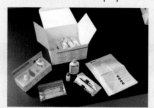	**Step 2.** Assembled equipment from an HCG test kit.
3. Verify that the names on the specimen container and the laboratory form are the same.	
4. Label the test pack or strip (depending on type of kit) with the patient's name, positive control, and negative control. Use one test pack or strip per patient and control.	
5. Note in the patient's information and in the control log whether you are using urine, plasma, or serum. Be sure that the kit and controls are at room temperature.	
6. Aspirate the patient's specimen using the transfer pipette and place volume indicated in kit package insert on the sample well of the test pack or dip test strip labeled with the patient's name.	
7. Sample the positive and negative controls as directed in Step 6.	This satisfies quality assurance and quality control standards.
8. Set timer for incubation period indicated in package insert.	
9. Read reaction results at the end of incubation period.	Waiting the appropriate amount of time ensures that testing is complete.
10. Verify the results of the controls before documenting the patient's results. Log controls and patient information on the worksheet.	This satisfies quality assurance and QC standards
11. Properly dispose of the equipment and supplies in a biohazard waste container.	
12. Remove personal protective equipment and wash your hands.	This prevents the spread of microorganisms.
13. Document the procedure.	Procedures not documented are not performed.
14. Sanitize the work area.	Sanitation aids in infection control.

(continued)

PROCEDURE 44-13: HCG Pregnancy Test *(continued)*

Note: Kits vary with the manufacturer; read instructions carefully before beginning. Controls for test kits may be performed at different intervals depending on laboratory protocol. Perform at least the minimum controls required in the product information to ensure quality. Your office protocol may require more frequent quality control testing.

Charting Example:

12/14/2008 9:30 AM HCG test performed on urine, dx ###.## per Dr. Schanzer. Positive result reported to doctor

J. Simpson, CMA

PROCEDURE 44-14: Rapid Group A Strep Testing

Procedure Note: To validate negative rapid group A strep results, set up a culture on beta-strep agar with the addition of a bacitracin disk to the first quadrant. Check the plate after 24 hours for presence of beta-hemolytic colonies. If beta-hemolytic colonies are present, the patient is positive for group A strep. A culture is more sensitive than a rapid immunoassay test. The culture procedure is not CLIA waived and cannot be performed by medical assistants. This additional step will require that a second swab be collected or that the agar plate be inoculated before the swab is used for the rapid test.

Purpose: To determine the presence of *Streptococcus pyogenes* in the specimen

Equipment: Patient's labeled throat specimen, group A strep kit (controls may be included, depending on the kit), timer, personal protective equipment, hand sanitizer, surface sanitizer, contaminated waste container

Rapid strep kit.

Steps	Reasons
1. Wash your hands.	Handwashing aids in infection control.
2. Verify that the names on the specimen container and the laboratory form are the same.	
3. Label one extraction tube with the patient's name, one for the positive control, and one for the negative control. 	**Step 3.** Label extraction tubes for patient and each control.
4. Follow the directions for the kit. Add the appropriate reagents and drops to each of the extraction tubes. Avoid splashing, and use the correct number of drops.	Following the manufacturer's instructions exactly will ensure that you adhere to the appropriate testing guidelines.

(continued)

PROCEDURE 44-14: Rapid Group A Strep Testing *(continued)*

Steps	Reasons
5. Insert the patient's swab into the labeled extraction tube.	**Step 5.** Insert patient's swab into labeled extraction tube.
6. Add the appropriate controls to each of the labeled extraction tubes.	This begins the chemical reaction and provides the proper dilution factor for proper control results.
7. Set the timer for the appropriate time to ensure accuracy.	
8. Add the appropriate reagent and drops to each of the extraction tubes.	
9. Use the swab to mix the reagents. Then press out any excess fluid on the swab against the inside of the tube.	This maximizes the volume of the extraction solution for testing.
10. Add three drops from the well-mixed extraction tube to the sample window of the strep A test unit or dip the test stick labeled with the patient's name. Do the same for each control.	
11. Set the timer for the time indicated in the kit package insert.	
12. A positive result appears as a line in the result window within 5 minutes. The strep A test unit or strip has an internal control; if a line appears in the control window, the test is valid.	**Step 12.** Picture of positive and negative control strips or packs.
13. Read a negative result at exactly 5 minutes to avoid a false negative.	
14. Verify results of the controls before recording or reporting test results. Log the controls and the patient's information on the worksheet.	This satisfies quality assurance and quality control standards
15. Properly dispose of the equipment and supplies in a biohazard waste container.	
16. Remove personal protective equipment and wash your hands.	This prevents the spread of microorganisms.
17. Document the procedure.	Procedures not documented are not performed.
18. Sanitize the work area.	Sanitation aids in infection control.

(continued)

PROCEDURE 44-14: Rapid Group A Strep Testing *(continued)*

Note: Kits vary with the manufacturer; read instructions carefully before beginning. Controls for test kits may be performed at different intervals depending on laboratory protocol. Follow procedures to ensure quality.

Charting Example:

05/22/2007 11:15 AM Group A rapid strep test performed, dx code ###.##, per Dr. Harrison. Positive result reported to physician
B. White, CMA

- The key of microbiology is starting with a good specimen, a specimen with nothing but the microorganisms from that patient.
- Recovering the organism from the culture so that it can be identified and an effective antibiotic chosen requires maintaining the environment required for survival.

- Immunoassay is based on the reaction of an antigen with its antibody.
- Increasing numbers of CLIA-waived immunoassays are available, offering expanded test menus for POLs.

Warm Ups for Critical Thinking

1. You are asked to give a brief talk to a group of elementary school children on microbiological life forms. Develop an age-appropriate discussion of this topic. How would you make it possible for the children to correlate the presence of microbes with the need to wash their hands?

2. Write a policy that explains how to care for media and how to transport specimens.

3. Create a patient education brochure for streptococcal pharyngitis infections. Include information about what it is, how it is transmitted, signs and symptoms, and the testing procedure.

4. In performing an immunoassay, your controls do not give acceptable results. How would you resolve this problem and provide results for the patient?

Answers to Checkpoint Questions

1. The two basic morphologic forms of bacteria are cocci and bacilli.

2. If Petri plates are stored with the medium downward, condensation may form on the lids and drip onto the surface, making it too moist for an accurate culture.

3. Staining bacteria helps the physician narrow the field of possible pathogens and begin treatment before a culture has been incubated. Most bacteria are colorless and hard to see or identify without special treatment such as staining.

4. Sensitivity testing is done to determine which antibiotic inhibits bacterial growth.

5. Immunoassays indicate the presence of the test substance by producing a color change.

6. Improper storage of the kit may result in deterioration of the reagents and, hence, false test results.

7. Immunoassays are easier to perform and provide results more quickly, but cultures are more sensitive.

Outline

Renal Function
Electrolytes
Nonprotein Nitrogenous
Compounds
Liver Function
Bilirubin
Enzymes
Thyroid Function
Thyroid-Stimulating Hormone
Cardiac Function
Creatine Kinase-MB

Troponin
Pancreatic Function
Pancreatic Enzymes
Pancreatic Hormones
Glucose
Fasting Glucose
Random Glucose
Two-Hour Postprandial
Glucose

Oral Glucose Tolerance Test
Glucose Tolerance Testing in
Obstetric Patients
Hemoglobin A1C
Lipids and Lipoproteins
Cholesterol
Low-Density Lipoprotein
High-Density Lipoprotein
Triglycerides

Learning Objectives

Upon successfully completing this chapter, you will be able to:

1. Spell and define the key terms

2. List the common electrolytes and explain the relationship of electrolytes to acid-base balance

3. Describe the nonprotein nitrogenous compounds and name conditions with abnormal values

4. List and describe the substances commonly tested in liver function assessment

5. Explain thyroid function and the hormone that regulates the thyroid gland

6. Describe how an assessment for a myocardial infarction is made with laboratory tests

7. Describe how pancreatitis is diagnosed with laboratory tests

8. Describe glucose use and regulation and the purpose of the various glucose tests

9. Describe the function of cholesterol and other lipids and their correlation to heart disease

Performance Objectives

Upon successfully completing this chapter, you will be able to:

1. Perform blood glucose testing (Procedure 45-1)

2. Perform blood cholesterol testing (Procedure 45-2)

3. Perform routine maintenance of a glucose meter (Procedure 45-3)

CAAHEP

- Perform chemistry testing
- Perform maintenance of clinical equipment

ABHES

- Perform CLIA-waived tests that assist with diagnosis and treatment
- Perform chemistry testing
- Perform routine maintenance of clinical equipment safely

Key Terms

amylase	cations	extracellular	ions
anions	creatinine	fast	lipase
bicarbonate	electrolytes	intracellular	lipoproteins

Clinical chemistry entails testing for many of the chemical components found in serum, plasma, whole blood, and other body fluids (fluids that accumulate in the body's compartments). The chemical components can be electrically charged atoms called ions (K^+, Na^+, Cl^-), metabolic byproducts (urea, creatinine), proteins (albumin, globulin), or hormones (e.g., testosterone and thyroid-stimulating hormone [TSH]). Quantifying the amount of these chemicals can help the physician:

- Assess organ function (e.g., bilirubin level is an indicator of liver function)
- Gain a better understanding of the patient's overall health status (e.g., glucose and cholesterol levels can aid in assessing a patient's health)

Only a few specific chemistry tests may be performed in the physician office laboratory, but it is important for you to understand the purpose of chemistry tests because they comprise a significant percentage of laboratory testing in general. Specimen collection, reporting, and follow-up of patient care will be your responsibility. This information is often vitally important to the treatment and recovery of the patient.

Much chemical analysis is performed in reference laboratories on automated systems that mechanically sample, dilute, or add reagents (chemicals) to the patient's blood for quantifying components. Automation has allowed more rapid analyses, reduced operator error, and helped control the cost of testing by reducing human intervention. The normal ranges included in this text may vary among laboratories because of the use of different substrates, temperatures, and instruments.

Many chemistry tests are grouped according to body system. These are called panels or profiles and are described in Chapter 39.

CHECKPOINT QUESTION

1. How does the physician use chemistry test results?

Renal Function

The kidneys rid the body of waste products and help maintain fluid balance and acid-base balance. When the kidneys begin to fail, waste products, such as urea, ammonia, and creatinine, build up in the blood. The patient becomes edematous, and the delicate acid-base balance is upset. Abnormal increases or decreases in the substances that affect acid-base balance compromise health and may cause death. To assess renal function, the physician may order tests for serum measurements of electrolytes, blood urea nitrogen (BUN), creatinine, and other components. These tests, combined with information from urinalysis, can significantly aid in renal assessment.

Electrolytes

Electrolytes are **ions** (chemicals that carry an electrical charge) in blood and body fluids. They may be positively charged (**cations**) or negatively charged (**anions**).

Electrolytes conduct electrical impulses across cell membranes to maintain fluid and acid-base balance, aid in the functioning of nerve cells and muscle tissue, and are activators in the blood coagulation process.

Electrolytes include sodium, potassium, chloride, **bicarbonate** (dissolved carbon dioxide), calcium, magnesium, and phosphorus. The renal system helps regulate electrolytes and fluid and acid-base balance. In the presence of an electrolyte imbalance, electric impulses are not transmitted properly, resulting in fluid and acid-base imbalances and impaired functioning of nervous and muscle tissue.

Sodium

Sodium (chemical symbol: Na) is the major cation of the **extracellular** fluid (the fluid outside the cell). Normal serum levels range from 135 to 145 mmol/L. The sodium level depends on intake and output of water and the kidney's ability to regulate the sodium level. See Table 45-1 for sodium reference ranges.

Hyponatremia (sodium level below 135 mmol/L), one of the most common electrolyte imbalances, can result from many factors, including gastrointestinal losses (vomiting, diarrhea), burn, cardiac or renal failure, and hepatic cirrhosis. Symptoms of hyponatremia range in severity with the value. Symptoms of a slightly decreased sodium level are generally gastrointestinal and as the level continues to drop, symptoms proceed to neurologic malfunctions, including seizures.

Hypernatremia (sodium level above 145 mEq/L) results from excess water loss or decreased water intake caused by increased urination, profuse sweating, diarrhea, severe burns, diabetes insipidus, and other pathologies. Typically, the kidneys help the body adjust to this more saline (salty) environment by not excreting as much water. In this way, sodium is diluted to an acceptable level. Because treatment of hypernatremia involves water retention, it must be done gradually to avoid cerebral edema in the patient.

Potassium

Potassium (chemical symbol: K) is the major cation of the **intracellular** fluid (fluid within the cell). Potassium concentration is 20 times greater inside the cell than outside, so serum levels are much lower than those of sodium: 3.4 to 5.0 mmol/L (Table 45-2). Potassium's major function in the body is with contraction of skeletal and cardiac muscles.

Hypokalemia (potassium level below 3.4 mmol/L) may occur with gastrointestinal or urinary losses. Symptoms of hypokalemia range from weakness, fatigue, and constipation with slightly decreased levels to muscle weakness and difficulty breathing in very decreased values.

Hyperkalemia (potassium level above 5.0 mmol/L) commonly occurs secondary to another disorder (e.g., renal deficiency or diabetes mellitus). Artifactual (caused by outside interference) hyperkalemia resulting from red blood cell lysis, as with a traumatic venipuncture or the tourniquet left on the arm too long or applied too tightly, may result in reporting a falsely elevated potassium result. The medical assistant must take special care in collecting and processing blood specimens for potassium analysis. Hyperkalemia can result in muscle weakness, numbness, mental confusion, and cardiac arrhythmias.

Chloride

Chloride (chemical symbol: Cl) is the major anion of the extracellular fluid. The normal range for chloride is 98 to 107 mmol/L. Hypochloremia is a condition in which the serum chloride level is below 98 mmol/L. In hyperchloremia, the serum chloride level is above 107 mmol/L. Chloride is closely associated with acid-base balance and is adversely affected in such conditions as diabetic ketoacidosis and metabolic acidosis (a condition of increased metabolic acids).

Bicarbonate

Bicarbonate (chemical symbol: HCO_3) is formed when carbon dioxide dissolves in the bloodstream, forming another negatively charged ion in the extracellular fluid. Bicarbonate is the major factor in acid-base balance; increased levels result in alkalosis (the body pH is too basic), and decreased levels may result in acidosis (the body pH is too acidic). Normal venous carbon dioxide levels are 22 to 29 mmol/L.

TABLE **45-1**	Reference Ranges for Sodium
Measure	**Range**
Serum, plasma	135–145 mmol/L
24-hour urine	40–220 mmol/day, varies with diet
Spinal fluid	138–150 mml/L

TABLE **45-2**	Reference Ranges for Potassium
Measure	**Range**
Plasma, serum	3.4–5.0 mmol/L
24-hour urine	25–125 mmol/day

The acid-base system is extremely sensitive and cannot tolerate large pH fluctuations. The body's normal pH range is 7.35 to 7.45, very slightly basic (neutral = 7.0). The renal and respiratory systems work to regulate acid-base balance. Bicarbonate is breathed out in the form of carbon dioxide and is also excreted through the kidneys. Measurement of carbon dioxide is considered more useful for pH balance assessment than for measuring renal function, but it also aids in the overall assessment of renal function.

Magnesium

Magnesium (chemical symbol: Mg) is a cation found in intracellular fluid. Normal magnesium levels range from 1.2 to 2.1 mEq/L. Magnesium has many significant roles in the body, especially in cardiovascular, metabolic, and neuromuscular function. Clinical use of serum magnesium levels is increasing as more information about magnesium is discovered.

Hypomagnesemia (magnesium level below 1.2 mEq/L) may result from shifts in body fluids and other electrolytes and is usually seen in patients experiencing a long-term severe illness. Gastrointestinal disorders can decrease magnesium absorption in the intestine resulting in excess magnesium loss in the feces. Disruptions in absorption, such as prolonged vomiting, diarrhea, or laxative abuse, may lead to hypomagnesemia. Renal disorders that cause excess magnesium loss in the urine and several endocrine disorders result in decreased magnesium levels. Symptoms of magnesium loss usually involve cardiovascular, neuromuscular, psychiatric, and metabolic abnormalities.

Hypermagnesemia (magnesium level above 2.1 mEq/L) is most commonly from impaired excretion caused by kidney failure. Symptoms of mildly increased serum magnesium levels are hypotension, bradycardia, skin flushing, nausea, vomiting, and lethargy. The symptoms grow in severity as the magnesium level increases.

Calcium

Calcium (chemical symbol: Ca) is a cation, with normal serum levels ranging from 8.6 to 10.0 mg/dL. Blood levels are regulated by three hormones: parathyroid hormone, vitamin D, and calcitonin. Most of the body's calcium is in the bone. Hypocalcemia (calcium level significantly below 8.6 mg/dL) may occur due to abnormal vitamin D metabolism, due to hypoparathyroidism, or secondary to hypomagnesemia. Symptoms of hypocalcemia include muscle cramps and cardiac arrhythmia. Hypercalcemia (calcium level above 10.0 mg/dL) is primarily due to hyperparathyroidism and is frequently associated with malignancies. Mild hypercalcemia is usually asymptomatic.

Phosphorus

Phosphorus (chemical symbol: P), the major anion in the intracellular fluid, is the building block for the body's genetic material. Normal phosphorus levels range from 2.7 to 4.5 mg/dL. Eighty percent of the body's phosphorus is in the bone. Hypophosphatemia (phosphorus level below 2.7 mg/dL) can result from a number of factors, including inadequate absorption, gastrointestinal losses, electrolyte shifts, and endocrine disorders. Hyperphosphatemia (phosphorus level above 4.5 mg/dL) may occur with hypocalcemia, hypoparathyroidism, and renal impairment or failure. In patients with renal failure, soft tissue calcification is a long-term effect of hyperphosphatemia.

 CHECKPOINT QUESTION

2. What is hyperkalemia? Name three possible causes.

Nonprotein Nitrogenous Compounds

Three nonprotein nitrogenous compounds that can be increased as a consequence of impaired renal function are urea, creatinine, and uric acid.

Urea

Urea is the major end product of protein and amino acid metabolism. Because urea is formed in the liver and excreted mainly by the kidneys, it can be an indicator for both liver and renal function. Typically urea, measured as BUN, ranges from 7 to 18 mg/dL. Various factors besides renal and liver function, such as dietary intake of protein and state of hydration, affect BUN levels. Azotemia is the clinical term for increased BUN levels. Conditions that affect BUN concentrations are listed in Table 45-3.

Creatinine

Creatinine is a breakdown product of creatine, which aids in delivering energy to cells. Normal range for creatinine is 0.5 to 1.2 mg/dL, with normal ranges varying

TABLE 45-3	Causes of Elevated BUN Concentrations
Prerenal	Congestive heart failure Corticosteroid therapy Dehydration Increased protein catabolism Shock, hemorrhage
Renal	Acute and chronic renal failure Glomerular nephritis
Postrenal	Urinary tract obstruction

slightly among laboratories. Creatinine is more specific than BUN for assessing renal function. Creatinine enters the bloodstream at a rate that maintains its proportion to the patient's muscle mass. Only trace amounts of creatinine are reabsorbed in the renal tubules, whereas urea is reabsorbed to a certain extent. Urinary excretion of this compound equals the amount produced in the body. This is useful in determining the filtering ability of the kidneys.

A test called creatinine clearance is used to evaluate the filtering ability of the kidney. A 24-hour urine sample is collected for a creatinine clearance because excretion of creatinine varies throughout the day. (See Chapter 43 for 24-hour urine collection instructions.) The clearance of something is a measure of the volume of plasma from which that substance (in this case, creatinine) can be removed in a set amount of time (in this case, 24 hours). A key point for the medical assistant to remember is that the test requires a blood specimen to be drawn during the 24-hour collection. That specimen is assayed for creatinine, and those results are used in calculating the actual clearance result. Arranging the logistics of obtaining that specimen from the patient is a part of educating the patient to complete the procedure.

Uric Acid

Uric acid is a metabolic end product of proteins containing purine, so it is highly influenced by diet. For men, the normal range is 3.5 to 7.2 mg/dL, and for women, it is 2.6 to 6.0 mg/dL. Increased amounts of uric acid are more significant than decreased amounts. Hyperuricemia may occur with renal failure, use of diuretics (substances that promote urine formation and excretion), obesity, and atherosclerosis. Diets high in proteins (meat, legumes, and yeast) can cause mild hyperuricemia. The disease gout is characterized by high uric acid accumulation in the joints; the joints become inflamed and painful (Fig. 45-1).

 WHAT IF?

What if a patient is diagnosed with gout and asks you about dietary restrictions?

First and foremost, speak to the physician to determine whether the patient has any other medical conditions that warrant a special diet. Most patients with gout are prescribed a low-purine diet initially. Foods that are high in purine are liver, kidneys, sweetbreads, sardines, anchovies, and meat extracts. Diet and medications can often keep gout under control. Dietary retraining is usually done by the physician or a registered dietitian.

Figure 45-1 Gout of the foot.

Liver Function

The liver is the largest gland of the body and one of the most complex. Among its major functions are the production of bile, metabolism of many compounds used by the body (glucose, fats, proteins, and vitamins), processing of bilirubin, and detoxifying substances in the blood. Alkaline phosphatase (ALP), alanine aminotransferase (ALT), and aspartate aminotransferase (AST) are some of the commonly tested enzymes that help determine liver function, in addition to the measurement of bilirubin, a component of bile.

Bilirubin

Red blood cells live approximately 120 days; the liver and spleen remove worn-out cells from the circulation. The worn-out cells break down, and hemoglobin is released and converted to bilirubin. It travels through the bloodstream until it enters the liver and is excreted into the bile. Bilirubin is yellow-orange; if excess amounts settle into the skin and sclera, it makes the patient appear yellow (jaundiced).

 CHECKPOINT QUESTION

3. Name the nonprotein nitrogenous compounds important for assessing renal function.

Enzymes

An enzyme is a protein produced by living cells that speeds up chemical reactions. The liver has many enzymes. Reference ranges for enzyme tests are the most sensitive to deviation among laboratories. In evaluating patient results, be sure to compare them to the reference ranges for the laboratory that performed the test.

Alkaline Phosphatase (ALP)

ALP is present in the bones, liver, intestines, kidneys, and placenta. Circulating ALP is primarily from the liver and bone. Levels of ALP rise in bone and liver disorders.

Normal values vary with age. High levels of ALP are considered normal during periods of bone growth, such as childhood growth spurts and third-trimester pregnancy. An approximate reference range for ALP is 30 to 95 U/L.

Alanine Aminotransferase (ALT) and Aspartate Aminotransferase (AST)

ALT and AST are enzymes in the liver. AST is present in many other organs as well. Increased levels of ALT and AST occur with liver disorders. Approximate reference ranges for ALT and AST are 6 to 37 U/L and 5 to 30 U/L, respectively.

 CHECKPOINT QUESTION

4. Name four common tests that evaluate liver function.

Thyroid Function

The thyroid gland regulates metabolism by secreting the hormones triiodothyronine and thyroxine. The thyroid gland is controlled by another hormone, thyroid-stimulating hormone (TSH), which is produced in the anterior pituitary gland. Normal thyroid function is dependent on a normally functioning hypothalamus and pituitary gland in addition to a healthy thyroid gland.

Thyroid-Stimulating Hormone

In the absence of disease, when additional thyroid hormones are needed, more TSH is secreted to stimulate the thyroid gland. In the same manner, when lesser amounts of the hormones are required, less TSH is secreted, and the thyroid gland reduces its production. However, many situations can cause an imbalance in this delicate endocrine system. Malfunction of the anterior pituitary gland results in oversecretion or undersecretion of TSH. If the thyroid gland is malfunctioning, it cannot be stimulated regardless of the amount of TSH secreted (Fig. 45-2). TSH levels may be quite high in cases such as this. The TSH reference range is 0.5 to 5.0 μU/mL.

Cardiac Function

When a myocardial infarction occurs, the damaged heart muscle releases into the bloodstream large quantities of specific substances referred to as cardiac markers. A single marker that will quickly and accurately assess cardiac function is not available, so the markers are tested in combination with each other. We will consider the two most common markers: creatine kinase-MB (CKMB) and troponin.

Change in T3 and T4 levels sensed by the pituitary gland

Hypothalamus

Pituitary gland

TSH

Thyroid

Figure 45-2 Thyroid disorders.

Creatine Kinase-MB

Creatine Kinase (CK) is an enzyme found almost exclusively in skeletal muscle and myocardium. CK has three isoenzymes, designated MM (muscle), MB (heart), and BB (brain). CKMB levels, along with total CK, are tested in persons who have chest pain to determine whether they have had a heart attack. Within 2 to 8 hours of a myocardial infarction, CK levels will increase. CK also increases in crushing injuries to muscles, such as those sustained in car accidents. Most of the normal levels of CK consist of the MM fraction. The MB fraction rises with myocardial infarction. A high total CK may indicate damage to either the heart or other muscles, but a high CKMB suggests that the damage was to heart muscle. CKMB results indicate heart involvement when they are ≥ 6% of the total CK result.

Troponin

Troponin is a protein specific to heart muscle, making it a valuable marker in the diagnosis of acute myocardial infarction. Troponin blood levels begin to rise within 4 hours of the onset of myocardial damage and stay elevated for up to 14 days, which means levels can be measured to monitor the effectiveness of thrombolytic therapy in heart attack patients.

Pancreatic Function

The pancreas (Fig. 45-3) is a large gland that functions in both the endocrine and exocrine systems. Amylase and lipase, two of its exocrine system products, are released as excretory enzymes into the intestines to aid in digestion. Insulin and glucagon, hormonal products of its endocrine function, are released into the bloodstream to regulate carbohydrate metabolism.

Pancreatic Enzymes
Amylase and Lipase

Amylase is markedly increased with pancreatitis (inflammation of the pancreas). The salivary glands also produce amylase, which accounts for the elevated levels occurring with inflammatory diseases of the salivary glands, such as mumps. **Lipase** levels also rise with pancreatitis and stay elevated longer than amylase levels.

Pancreatic Hormones
Insulin and Glucagon

Glucose is a primary energy source for the body. When foods are metabolized, nutrients including glucose are released. For glucose to be used for stored energy in the form of glycogen, it must be brought into the cells. Two hormones, insulin and glucagon, regulate this process. Blood glucose levels must be maintained within narrow limits or adverse physical effects may occur. By their ac-

tions, insulin and glucagon keep these levels within the approximate range.

Insulin brings the glucose used for energy into cells for immediate use or for storage. If sufficient energy is available for cell use, the glucose is stored as either glycogen (long chains of glucose) in the liver and muscles or as fat. Insulin is an important hormone; cells starve if insulin is not available or if the cells cannot bring glucose in for energy. By facilitating glucose storage, insulin keeps glucose levels down, thereby maintaining a stable blood level.

The hormone glucagon releases into the bloodstream glucose stored as glycogen, thereby raising glucose levels. Whenever blood glucose levels drop, glucagon acts on glycogen to break it apart so that molecules of glucose are available for cellular use.

 CHECKPOINT QUESTION

5. Which enzyme can assist the physician to diagnose a myocardial infarction within 3 hours of onset? Why?

Glucose

For diagnostic usefulness, the time a blood sample is taken for glucose testing must be related to length of fasting or to the time of the previous meal.

The glucose reflectance photometer (glucose meter) is a quick, accurate, easy in-office procedure to measure a patient's blood glucose level. Glucose meters are sold under several names, including Accu-Chek, Ascensia, and One Touch, among others (Fig. 45-4). The testing principle is application of whole blood to a reagent strip, which is read optically by the instrument after a designated time (Procedure 45-1). The amount of color change correlates with glucose concentration and the value is measured and reported.

Figure 45-3 The pancreas.

Figure 45-4 Various blood glucose monitoring systems.

PATIENT EDUCATION
USING A GLUCOSE METER

Many diabetic patients routinely monitor glucose levels at home. As a medical assistant, you can help reinforce use of this procedure. Help the patient get familiar with the analyzer. Instruct the patient to adhere to the manufacturer's instructions. Here are points to stress:

- Teach patients about the need to test and document glucose levels regularly.
- Instruct the patient in maintaining a quality control record for the instrument using control materials within the expiration date and as directed by the manufacturer.
- Offer instructions in the proper technique for obtaining a blood sample (e.g., cleanse the area well before beginning and do not milk the finger).
- Caution patients against self-regulating with insulin. Have patients call the physician if glucose levels are abnormal.
- Alert patients to the signs and symptoms of high and low glucose levels and the treatments for each.

Most pharmacies and surgical supply stores that sell glucose meters will teach patients how to use them. The strips for glucose meters are expensive and may be covered by certain insurance companies if the physician clearly documents the need.

Fasting Glucose

A fasting blood sugar (FBS) level can be obtained from the patient after an 8- to 12-hour **fast** (nothing other than water is ingested during the fast). Procedure 45-1 describes obtaining an FBS level using a glucose meter. The main purpose of an FBS is to detect either diabetes mellitus or hypoglycemia. The American Diabetes Association's (ADA) cutoff point for normal fasting blood glucose levels is 100 mg/dL. A value of 100 mg/dL or above leads to a diagnosis of impaired fasting glucose, included in the term prediabetes. Prediabetes occurs when a person's glucose levels are higher than normal but not yet high enough for a diagnosis of diabetes. Studies indicate that many people in the prediabetic range go on to develop diabetes within 10 years.

Further testing by a 2-hour postprandial glucose test confirms the diagnosis. Hypoglycemia is a syndrome characterized by FBS levels below 45 mg/dL and a variety of symptoms: sweating, weakness, dizziness, headache, trembling, lethargy, and other nervous manifestations.

Random Glucose

Although a random glucose test is not as diagnostically useful as a fasting test, it is a good screening tool. A random glucose specimen can be drawn anytime during the day. Because glucose fluctuates so much according to diet, activity levels, and insulin levels, references attempting to quote a reference range for a random blood glucose vary from < 130 mg/dL to < 180 mg/dL.

Two-Hour Postprandial Glucose

A 2-hour postprandial (PP) glucose test is used to screen for diabetes and to monitor insulin therapy of diabetic patients. The patient must eat a high-carbohydrate meal after a 10- to 12-hour fast. Patients who may not be compliant are given a glucose solution to drink as a substitute for the meal. Then, 2 hours after the meal, a blood sample is drawn, and glucose is measured. Timing of the specimen collection is extremely important for this test result. "Good control" of diabetes has been defined as a 2-hour PP value of less than 140 mg/dL.

Oral Glucose Tolerance Test

The ADA does not encourage the use of the glucose tolerance test (GTT) to diagnose diabetes. For those situations in which it is still used, the procedure should begin with effective patient preparation. For 3 days prior to the test, the patient should be mobile and eating a normal to high-carbohydrate diet. The patient should fast (consuming only water) for 10 to 16 hours prior to starting the test, and the test should be performed in the morning because of diurnal variations in glucose levels. In preparation for the test and during the test, the patient should not exercise, smoke, or consume anything other than water. The patient is given 75 g of a glucose solution such as glucola; then blood glucose levels are checked at intervals to see how the body metabolizes the glucose. The first step of the GTT is to check the fasting glucose. Blood is obtained 30 minutes and 1 and 2 hours after the glucose has been administered. For a valid evaluation, blood sampling must occur at the precise times. Urine specimens may also be collected during the timed intervals. A serum, plasma or whole blood specimen may be collected, depending on laboratory protocol. If using serum or plasma, the specimen should be centrifuged and separated as soon as possible to prevent metabolism of glucose by red blood cells. Specimens collected in gray stopper tubes containing sodium fluoride are stable for up to 3 days even without centrifugation.

Numerous methods are used to interpret the values obtained from a GTT. The criteria proposed by the National Diabetes Data Group and the World Health Organization and endorsed by the American Diabetes Association recommend a diagnosis of diabetes if the

Figure 45-5 Glucose tolerance test.

fasting glucose level is greater than 110 mg/dL and the 2-hour measurement is equal to or above 155 mg/dL. See Figure 45-5 to see a graph of various glucose tolerance responses.

 CHECKPOINT QUESTION

6. What is hypoglycemia? List its signs and symptoms.

Glucose Tolerance Testing in Obstetric Patients

An increase of glucose intolerance has been frequently noted among pregnant patients in the second and third trimesters. Because gestational diabetes can endanger the fetus, the pregnant patient's glucose level must be monitored. The widely accepted screening method used for this purpose is to administer a 50-g glucose load in drink form and draw blood 1 hour later. If the value exceeds 155 mg/dL, a GTT is indicated for a diagnosis of gestational diabetes. This screen is usually done during the second trimester.

 CHECKPOINT QUESTION

7. Do the terms "fasting" and "NPO" have the same meaning?

Hemoglobin A1C

Although blood glucose levels are used to detect and monitor diabetic patients, the test of choice for long-term blood glucose regulation is hemoglobin A1C. The best health goal for a diabetic patient is to keep nondiabetic blood glucose levels as much as possible. Glucose molecules normally attach to hemoglobin molecules of the RBCs circulating in the blood. RBCs have a life span of about 120 days. The hemoglobin A1C is a test that

measures just the glucose that is attached to hemoglobin molecules. This glucose result gives the physician a picture of the patient's glucose levels over the past 3 months.

Lipids and Lipoproteins

Cholesterol and associated lipids (free fatty acids) and **lipoproteins** (substances composed of lipids and proteins) have long been implicated in heart disease. However, these compounds are important building blocks of our bodies and in proper quantities are vital to health maintenance. They are a component of every cell membrane and of the myelin sheath around the nerves. They also cushion and support organs. Testing for these quantities aids the physician in assessing the risk of heart disease (Fig. 45-6). Figure 45-7 is a diagram of the body's major lipoprotein metabolism pathways.

Cholesterol

Bile acids, partly formed by cholesterol, are produced in the liver, stored in the gallbladder, and released into the intestine as needed for the digestion of fats. Vitamin D is formed from cholesterol at the skin's surface during exposure to sunlight. Various hormones, such as cortisol, testosterone, and estrogen, are also synthesized from cholesterol. Only in proportions not necessary for cell maintenance and other body functions should cholesterol be considered a health hazard. Measurement of cholesterol is done on a 10- to 12-hour fasting blood specimen. The ideal range for cholesterol is less than 200 mg/dL (as recommended by the American Heart Association) (Table 45-4). Anyone with a cholesterol level above 200 mg/dL is considered to be at risk for developing atherosclerosis.

Figure 45-6 The Cholestech analyzer can perform tests for cholesterol, triglyceride, low-density lipoprotein, and high-density lipoprotein. (From Cholestech, Heywood, CA.)

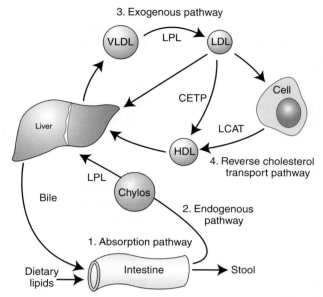

Figure 45-7 Diagram of major lipoprotein metabolism pathways.

Much research has been directed along the lines of increasing HDL because high levels of it correlate with reduction in the risk of heart disease. In contrast, decreased HDL levels correlate with increased risk of heart disease.

Triglycerides

Triglycerides store energy. They are stored in adipose tissue and muscle and released and metabolized between meals according to the body's energy demands. Adipose (fatty) tissue is composed almost entirely of triglycerides. The normal range is less than 150 mg/dL (see Table 45-4). Research identifies triglycerides as a risk factor in heart disease.

A summary of the common chemistry tests is presented in Table 45-5.

 CHECKPOINT QUESTION

8. Which lipoprotein is beneficial? Why?

Low-Density Lipoprotein

Low-density lipoprotein (LDL) is a plasma protein that transports cholesterol from the liver to the walls of large- and medium-sized arteries. Atherosclerotic plaques form, causing the affected vessel to thicken and become more rigid. Circulation to the organs and other areas normally supplied by these arteries is reduced. Atherosclerosis is the major cause of coronary heart disease, angina pectoris, myocardial infarction, and other cardiac disorders. As LDL values rise above the normal range (see Table 45-4), the risk of heart disease increases.

High-Density Lipoprotein

High-density lipoprotein (HDL) is the protein molecule that carries cholesterol from the cell back to the liver to be excreted in bile. Quantities of HDL typically are less than those of LDL (see Table 45-4).

TABLE 45-4	Adult Reference Ranges for Lipids
Analyte	**Reference Range**
Total cholesterol	< 200 mg/dL
HDL cholesterol	> 40 mg/dL
LDL cholesterol	< 130 mg/dL
Triglyceride	< 150 mg/dL

 PATIENT EDUCATION

BAD AND GOOD CHOLESTEROL

There are two main types of cholesterol that affect health:

- "Bad" cholesterol: Low-density lipoproteins, or LDL, are known as bad cholesterol and clog arteries and put patients at risk for heart disease.
- "Good" cholesterol: High-density lipoproteins, or HDL, are known as good cholesterol and help remove bad cholesterol from the body.

Controlling diet and getting plenty of exercise are great ways to help get your bad cholesterol down. Managing cholesterol also includes getting your good cholesterol up. Here is a saying to help remember which is the "bad" or "good" cholesterol: Keep your **L**DL **l**ow and keep your **H**DL **h**igh.

How do you know if your bad cholesterol is high? Many people don't. **People with high LDL cholesterol usually do not have any symptoms.** That is why it is so important for adults to get a cholesterol screening at least every 5 years.

TABLE 45-5	Common Chemistry Panel Tests			
Test	**Body Function**	**Normal Values**	**Causes of Increase**	**Causes of Decrease**
BUN	Metabolic byproduct	7–18 mg/dL	Kidney disease, kidney obstruction, dehydration	Liver failure, malnutrition
Calcium	Structural element for bones, teeth, muscles	8.6–10.0 mg/dL	Hyperparathyroidism, hyperthyroidism, Addison disease, bone cancer, multiple myeloma, other malignancies	Hypoparathyroidism, renal failure
Chloride	Acid-base balance, component of stomach acid	98–107 mmol/L	Dehydration, Cushing syndrome, hyperventilation	Severe vomiting, severe diarrhea, severe burn, pyloric obstruction, heat exhaustion
Cholesterol	Building block for cell membranes, steroid hormones, bile acids	140–200 mg/dL	Atherosclerosis, heart disease, certain liver diseases with obstruction, hypothyroidism	Liver disease, hyperthyroidism, malabsorption syndrome
Creatinine	Metabolic byproduct	Males: 0.6–1.2 mg/dL Females: 0.5–1.1 mg/dL	Kidney disease, muscle disease	Muscular dystrophy
Glucose (fasting)	Energy source	70–110 mg/dL	Diabetes mellitus, Cushing syndrome, liver disease	Excessive insulin, Addison disease, bacterial sepsis, hypothyroidism
Phosphorus	Used in bone, endocrine processes	2.7–4.5 mg/dL	Renal disease, hypoparathyroidism, hypocalcemia, Addison disease	Hyperparathyroidism, bone disease
Potassium	Acid-base balance	3.4–5.0 mmol/L	Kidney disease, cell damage, Addison disease	Diarrhea, starvation, severe vomiting, severe burn, some liver diseases
Sodium	Fluid balance	135–145 mmol/L	Dehydration, Cushing syndrome, diabetes insipidus	Severe burns, diarrhea, vomiting, Addison disease
Triglycerides	Energy source; lipid deposits for stored energy, organ support	67–157 mg/dL	Atherosclerosis, liver disease, poorly controlled diabetes, pancreatitis	Malnutrition
Uric acid	Metabolic byproduct	Men: 3.5–7.2 mg/dL Women: 2.6–6.0 mg/dL	Renal failure, gout, leukemia, eclampsia	Drug therapy to lower uric acid levels

MEDIA MENU

- Student CD
  - **CMA/RMA Certification Exam Review**
- LWW's Medical Assisting Skills DVD
  - **Procedure 45-1**
- Premium Online Course
  http://thePoint.lww.com/Kronenberger3e
- Internet Resources

  LiveAdvise Online Tutoring & Competency Training
  http://thePoint.lww.com/LiveAdvise

  American Diabetes Association
  www.diabetes.org

  American Heart Association
  www.americanheart.org

  World Health Organization
  www.who.int/en/

  National Diabetes Information Clearinghouse
  www.diabetes.niddk.nih.gov

PROCEDURE 45-1:   Perform Blood Glucose Testing

Standard: This task should take about 10 minutes.
Purpose: To determine the level of glucose in the blood for diagnosis and treatment of hypoglycemia and hyperglycemia
Equipment: Glucose meter, glucose reagent strips, control solutions, capillary puncture device, alcohol pad, gauze, paper towel, adhesive bandage, personal protective equipment, hand sanitizer, surface sanitizer, contaminated waste container

Steps	Purpose
1. Wash your hands. Put on gloves.	Handwashing and personal protective equipment aid infection control.
2. Assemble the equipment and supplies.	
3. Review the instrument manual for your glucose meter.	Following the manufacturer's instructions ensures accurate testing.
4. Turn on the instrument and ensure that it is calibrated.	Calibration of the glucose meter is essential for accurate test results.
5. Perform the test on the quality control (QC) material. Record results. Determine whether QC is within control limits. If yes, proceed with patient testing. If no, take corrective action and recheck controls. Document corrective action. Proceed with patient testing when acceptable QC results are obtained.	For waived testing, CLIA requires that quality control procedures be performed in compliance with the manufacturer's instructions.

(continued)

PROCEDURE 45-1: Perform Blood Glucose Testing *(continued)*

Steps	Purpose
6. Remove one reagent strip, lay it on the paper towel, and recap the container.	The paper towel will serve as a disposable work surface and will absorb excess blood added to the strip. The strips are sensitive to humidity and will deteriorate if allowed to absorb moisture.
7. Greet and identify the patient. Explain the procedure. Ask for and answer any questions.	
8. Have the patient wash hands in warm water.	Sugar residues on hands can falsely elevate glucose results if the strip is touched. Washing removes sugar residues from the skin, and the warm water stimulates blood flow.
9. Cleanse the selected puncture site (finger) with alcohol.	Alcohol removes bacteria from the site.
	Step 9. Cleanse the selected puncture site with alcohol.
10. Perform a capillary puncture, following the steps described in Chapter 41. Wipe away the first drop of blood.	The first drop of blood is contaminated with tissue fluid and will produce erroneous test results.
	Step 10. Wipe away the first drop of blood.
11. Turn the patient's hand palm down and gently squeeze the finger to form a large drop of blood.	Gentle squeezing obtains a blood specimen without diluting the sample with tissue fluid.
	Step 11. Turn the patient's hand palm down and gently squeeze the finger to form a large drop of blood.

(continued)

PROCEDURE 45-1:   **Perform Blood Glucose Testing** *(continued)*

Steps	Purpose
12. Bring the reagent strip up to the finger and touch the pad to the blood. Do not touch the finger. Completely cover the pad or fill the testing chamber with blood.	The entire pad must be covered or testing chamber filled for accurate reading. There is no chance of contamination by oils or other residue remaining on the finger if this surface is not touched. **Step 12.** Touch the pad to the blood. Do not touch the finger.
13. Insert reagent strip into analyzer, while applying pressure to the puncture wound with gauze. The meter will continue to incubate the strip and measure the reaction.	This allows time for the reaction. **Step 13.** Apply pressure to puncture wound with gauze.
14. The instrument reads the reaction strip and displays the result in milligrams per deciliter.	The reaction is now complete. The color change is photo-optically measured and reported in milligrams per deciliter. **Step 14.** Record the reading from the instrument display.
15. Apply a small adhesive bandage to the patient's fingertip.	
16. Properly care for or dispose of equipment and supplies.	
17. Clean the work area. Remove personal protective equipment and wash your hands.	

Note: These are generic instructions for using a glucose meter. Refer to the manufacturer's instructions for instructions specific to the particular instrument.

Charting Example:

02/12/2007 10:00 AM. Capillary puncture left middle finger for glucose DX ###.## per Dr. Miller.
Glucose tested with meter. Results: 60 mg/dL. Dr. Peters notified.
—M. Miller, CMA

PROCEDURE 45-2: Perform Blood Cholesterol Testing

Standard: This task should take about 10 minutes.
Purpose: To determine the level of cholesterol in the blood for diagnosis and treatment of lipid disorders

Equipment: Cholesterol meter and supplies or test kit, control solutions, capillary puncture equipment or blood specimen as indicated by manufacturer, personal protective equipment, hand sanitizer, surface sanitizer, contaminated waste container

Steps	Purpose
1. Wash your hands. Put on gloves	Handwashing and personal protective equipment aid infection control.
2. Assemble the equipment and supplies.	
3. Review the instrument manual for your cholesterol meter or kit.	Following the manufacturer's instructions ensures accurate testing.
4. Perform the test on the quality control material. Record results. Determine whether QC is within control limits. If yes, proceed with patient testing. If no, take corrective action and recheck controls. Document corrective action. Proceed with patient testing when acceptable QC results are obtained.	For waived testing, CLIA requires that quality control procedures be performed in compliance with the manufacturer's instructions.
5. Follow manufacturer's instructions in using a patient specimen obtained by capillary puncture or from vacutainer tube.	
6. Follow manufacturer's instructions for applying the sample to the testing device and inserting the device into the analyzer. Record results.	
7. Properly care for or dispose of equipment and supplies.	
8. Clean the work area. Remove personal protective equipment, and wash your hands.	

Note: These are generic instructions for performing cholesterol testing. Refer to the manufacturer's manual or package insert for instructions specific to the particular instrument or test kit.

Charting Example:

02/12/2007 10:00 AM Cholesterol test performed. Dx ###.## per Dr. Peters. Results: 274 mg/dL. Dr.
Peters notified
—M. Miller, CMA

PROCEDURE 45-3: **Perform Routine Maintenance of a Glucose Meter**

Standard: This task should take about 20 minutes.
Purpose: To comply with manufacturers' and CLIA guidelines for maintaining equipment in optimum functional condition
Equipment: Glucose meter, maintenance and testing supplies, manufacturer's manual for glucose analyzer, control solutions, personal protective equipment, hand sanitizer, surface sanitizer, contaminated waste container

Steps	Purpose
1. Wash your hands. Put on gloves	Handwashing and personal protective equipment aid infection control.
2. Assemble the equipment and supplies.	
3. Review the instrument manual for your glucose meter.	Following the manufacturer's instructions for instrument maintenance is a CLIA requirement.
4. Perform the maintenance procedures listed in the manufacturer's instructions. Document the performance of these procedures in the instrument maintenance log.	
5. Perform the test on the quality control material. Record results. Determine whether QC is within control limits. If yes, maintenance was successful and instrument is ready for patient testing. If no, take corrective action and re-check controls. Document corrective action. Instrument is available for patient testing when acceptable QC results are obtained.	For waived testing, CLIA requires that quality control procedures be performed in compliance with the manufacturer's instructions.
6. Properly care for or dispose of equipment and supplies.	
7. Clean the work area. Remove personal protective equipment and wash your hands.	

Note: These are generic instructions for performing maintenance of a glucose analyzer. Refer to the manufacturer's manual for instructions specific to the particular instrument.

Chapter Summary

- Blood chemistry tests measure important substances in the blood. They can help show how well organs like the liver and kidneys are working and can provide useful information about drug side effects.
- Most chemistry testing is referred to reference laboratories that house large automated analyzers that produce these test results at a lower cost than can be achieved in smaller laboratories.
- The key focus for the medical assistant is that, no matter where the tests are performed, the results are only as good as the specimen submitted for testing.
- It is important for the medical assistant to have a basic understanding of the principles involved, proper sampling procedures required, and specific handling requirements necessary for the specimen to arrive at the testing facility with the analyte to be tested intact for measurement.

1. A patient with edema is told by her physician to restrict her salt intake. Why may this help improve her condition?

2. A diabetic patient gave herself too much insulin by mistake. Would you expect her glucose to be very high or very low? Why?

3. A patient's glucose level is repeatedly normal at routine office visits, but she continues to have worsening side effects of hyperglycemia. What test might the physician request that would reflect her glucose levels over a period of weeks?

4. A medical assistant draws a red-top tube for a number of chemistry tests. Unfortunately, the tube is left on the counter for several hours before being centrifuged and refrigerated. Which chemistries may be affected by this? Why?

5. A physician needs to evaluate a patient's kidney function. Which chemistry measurements will the physician request? Which of these measurements is least impacted by the patient's diet?

6. Describe three ways cholesterol is beneficial to the body.

Answers | to Checkpoint Questions

1. Physicians use chemistry test results to assess organ function and to gain a better understanding of the patient's overall health status.

2. Hyperkalemia, or elevated potassium, can occur with cell injuries, renal failure, and artifactual causes.

3. Urea, creatinine, and uric acid are important for assessing renal function.

4. Results of bilirubin, ALP, AST, and ALT levels aid in the evaluation of liver function.

5. CKMB can help diagnose myocardial infarction within 3 hours of onset because CK levels increase within 2 to 8 hours of an infarction.

6. Hypoglycemia is a syndrome characterized by fasting blood sugar levels below 45 mg/dL. Symptoms include sweating, weakness, dizziness, headache, trembling, lethargy, and other nervous manifestations.

7. The term fasting indicates that the patient should have nothing to eat or drink other than water. The patient should be encouraged to drink water while fasting. The term NPO indicates that the patient should have no oral intake at all.

8. High-density lipoprotein is beneficial because it works to eliminate lipids via bile.

UNIT SIX

Power Critical Thinking Exercises

FUNDAMENTALS OF LABORATORY PROCEDURES (CHAPTERS 39–45)

1. An elderly gentleman was seen with the following symptoms: nausea, vomiting, decreased respiration, hypotension, and a pulse rate of 46. Physical exam indicated skin warm to the touch and flushed. Review the laboratory results for this case.

Laboratory Results

Test	Result	Reference Range
Calcium	8.2 mg/dL	8.6–10.0 mg/dL
Magnesium	8.0 mEq/L	1.2–2.1 mEq/L
Sodium	129 mmol/L	135–145 mmol/L
Potassium	5.3 mmol/L	3.4–5.3 mmol/L
Chloride	96 mmol/L	98–106 mmol/L
Bicarbonate	16 mmol/L	22–29 mmol/L

A. Define hypermagnesemia and hypocalcemia; describe the outcomes from each disorder.

B. State the normal ranges for respiration rate, blood pressure, and pulse.

C. What is the most likely cause for this patient's symptoms? What is the most likely cause for the hypermagnesemia? What could be the cause for the hypocalcemia?

2. Matt is the phlebotomist at the clinic today. He has received an order for phlebotomy on Dr. Kay's patient, Emma Schanzer. Mrs. Schanzer, age 87, had a right mastectomy in 1998. In 2001 Mrs. Schanzer suffered a stroke resulting in paralysis of her entire left side. The paralysis prevents her from extending her left arm. Her left hand is frozen turned under that arm.

A. List the following items:

- Common specimen characteristics that cause laboratory test interference

- Basic tools used for phlebotomy

- Common venipuncture sites

B. What phlebotomy considerations are required for postmastectomy patients? What sites should Matt consider for venipuncture on this patient? Why?

C. What choices of venipuncture supplies could Matt make? Why?

D. What specimen interference could be a problem depending on Matt's choice of venipuncture site and venipuncture equipment? Why? If the specimen collection results in this type of interference, what test results would be affected?

3. Cheryl performed a urinalysis on Dr. Hall's patient, Lydia Snelling. She obtained the following results:

Color	Yellow-orange
Clarity	Hazy
Specific Gravity	1.020
pH	6.5

Protein	1+
Glucose	Negative
Ketone	Negative
Bilirubin	3+
Blood	Negative
Urobilinogen	2.0 mg/dL
Nitrites	Negative
Leukocyte esterase	Negative

A. Define urine threshold, and list the causes of variations in the color of urine. Identify at least five diseases that would produce these urinalysis results.

B. List the common urinalysis confirmatory tests, and describe how each is used. Which of the patient's urinalysis results are abnormal?

C. What urine confirmation test(s) may Dr. Hall order on Mrs. Snelling's urine specimen? The results indicate a potential dysfunction with what body organ? What results should Cheryl expect to see in Mrs. Snelling's blood chemistries?

4. Robert entered the laboratory and found a spill on the laboratory counter.

A. Define the following terms:

- Biohazard

- Chemical hazard

- Material Safety Data Sheet

B. Describe the suggested spill clean-up procedures for biohazardous spills and chemical spills.

C. What action(s) should Robert take? Why? Would Robert's action(s) be different if someone told him exactly what the spill was? Why or why not? List the supplies Robert will need depending upon your answers to these questions.

+2sd = 102	x																														
101		x																													
100			x																												
mean = 99				x																											
98					x																										
97																															
−2sd = 96																															
Date	1	2	3	4	5	6	7	8	9	10	11	12	13	14	15	16	17	18	19	20	21	22	23	24	25	26	27	28	29	30	31

5. Stephanie was recording her QC results. She noticed that her Level I control was in range. The accepted range for Level I was (96–102). The following is the graph of her control results over the past 5 days:

A. Define the following terms:

- Quality Control

- Accuracy

- Precision

- Shifts

- Trends

B. Evaluate the QC results posted on the graph. Was Stephanie's Level I control acceptable? Were the results exhibiting a trend or a shift?

C. Determine follow-up actions. Are any corrective actions required to report patient results? Would any troubleshooting be required or useful for this test? If yes, then what actions should Stephanie take?

PART

V

Career
Strategies

Competing in the Job Market

Congratulations! You have reached a pivotal point in your medical assisting career. This unit prepares you to make the transition from student to employee. The first chapter introduces you to the externship program. Your externship is the springboard to starting your career. The remainder of chapter 46 focuses on how to acquire the job that you have worked so hard to prepare for. The last chapter is a mock certification examination. You will now prepare for the next phase in your goal of becoming a medical assistant. You will be prepared to enter this fascinating and exciting career with confidence and professionalism while enjoying the rewards and accepting the challenges that face you. Good luck in your new adventure!

Making the Transition: Student to Employee

Outline

EXTERNSHIPS
 Types of Facilities
 Externship Benefits
 Externship Responsibilities
 Guidelines for a Successful
  Externship
Externship Documentation
Externship Evaluations
Graduate Surveys
Employer Surveys

ESTABLISH THE JOB FOR YOU
 Setting Employment Goals
 Self-Analysis
FINDING THE RIGHT JOB
APPLYING FOR THE JOB
 Answering Newspaper
  Advertisements
 Preparing Your Résumé
 Preparing Your Cover Letter

 Completing an Employment
  Application
THE INTERVIEW
 Preparing for the Interview
 Crucial Interview Questions
 Follow-Up
LEAVING A JOB
BE A LIFELONG LEARNER
Recertification
Professionalism

Upon successfully completing this chapter, you will be able to:

1. Spell and define the key terms
2. Explain the purpose of the externship experience
3. Understand the importance of the evaluation process
4. List your professional responsibilities during externship
5. List personal and professional attributes necessary to ensure a successful externship
6. Determine your best career direction based on your skills and strengths
7. Identify the steps necessary to apply for the right position and be able to accomplish those steps
8. Draft an appropriate cover letter
9. List the steps and guidelines in completing an employment application
10. List guidelines for an effective interview that will lead to employment
11. Identify the steps that you need to take to ensure proper career advancement
12. Explain the process for recertification of a medical assisting credential
13. Describe the importance of membership in a professional organization

Upon successfully completing this chapter, you will be able to:

1. Write a résumé to properly communicate skills and strengths (Procedure 46-1)

ABHES

• Allied health professions and credentialing

externship
networking

portfolio
preceptor

résumé

Graduation from a medical assisting program is an important milestone in your life. It is normal to have conflicting emotions ranging from excitement to anxiety. The purpose of this chapter is to help you make this transition from student to employee. The first part of the chapter discusses externships. An externship is your first opportunity to use your knowledge in a clinical setting. The chapter also discusses the benefits of externship programs, how to get the most out of your externship, and the documentation that accompanies an externship. The later part of the chapter prepares you to begin searching for employment. Résumé preparation is discussed along with successful interviewing techniques. An introduction to key employment laws is also discussed.

Externships

Accredited medical assisting programs are required to provide an **externship** as part of the course requirement. An externship is a training program that gives you the experience of working in a professional medical office under the supervision of a preceptor or supervisor who will help you to apply the theories and procedures you learned during classroom training. This is the opportunity for you to perform and perfect the skills that you have learned during the academic portion of your program.

In an externship, you will discover areas of interest in certain types of practices or health care specialties (Fig. 46-1). Rotating through clinical sites will expose you to different offices you may pursue as possible opportunities for future employment. The length and schedule of your externship will depend on your school's curriculum and the medical site where you will be working, but most externships range from 160 to 240 hours in a semester. You are not paid for this externship experience, but you will receive curriculum credit based on the hours earned.

Figure 46-1 By working side by side with practicing allied health professionals, you will prepare for the real world in your extern site.

Types of Facilities

The health care industry is diversified, with a wide variety of specialty offices and clinics. As a medical assisting student, you will experience an extensive scope of procedures during an externship in a general or family practice clinic or office. Family practices are generally referred to as primary care providers. Patients range in age from newborns to the elderly and typically have a broad range of complaints and illnesses. General practice facilities provide the best exposure to all types of procedures performed by medical assistants.

Your externship may be more limited in specialty practices. For example, staff members in obstetric offices usually do not perform electrocardiograms, and staff members in orthopedic offices wouldn't perform gynecologic examinations. Working in these types of practices, however, will give you experience in special examinations and procedures in areas that you might not observe in a general practice setting. Each specialty has advantages and disadvantages as a site, but all offer invaluable experience that cannot be adequately simulated in the classroom.

Extern Sites

Most schools have extern sites they have used for years. Based on the experience of former students, personnel in these sites know what the student must do to complete the clinical experience. An ideal site should provide a variety of experiences, both in administrative (front office) and clinical (back office) procedures.

A **preceptor** works with externship students the same as the instructor in the classroom. Preceptors typically are graduate medical assistants who have been through a similar externship program.

The school is careful to choose externship sites with preceptors who are willing to work with you and help you feel comfortable in the medical setting. They understand that all of your experience up to this point has been with fellow students in a protected classroom. They understand how nervous you are and will help you to ease the transition from classroom to the medical office. Your clinical sites are usually chosen within easy travel distance.

 CHECKPOINT QUESTION

1. What is the role of the preceptor?

Externship Benefits
Benefits to the Student

Externship is a vital part of medical assisting training. You will develop self-confidence and professionalism during the externship portion of your training. No amount of classroom training can compare with the experience of applying skills and knowledge in a medical facility. An externship also allows you to broaden your knowledge base by learning new and different equipment and techniques. You will adapt your base of knowledge to your environment.

Benefits to the Medical Assisting Program

As you gain experience from the externship, the school also benefits from the affiliation, or connection, with the medical community. Many sites have a long history of training students. Schools rely on good training sites to enhance the medical assisting curriculum. Medical assisting programs also rely on the medical profession to aid in updating and revising the curriculum and course content to ensure that the methods and procedures presented to the students from year to year are current.

The school, the program director, and externship preceptors review students' extern experiences to change the program to reflect the needs of the community and the profession as health care constantly changes, such as with new technology. If students are routinely required to perform a procedure or examination that is not a part of the curriculum, for example, this will usually be considered for an addition to future lectures and laboratory sessions. If the accepted practice of a procedure has changed, changes will be made in the way it is taught to ensure that students are kept abreast of health care advances.

Benefits to the Externship Site

The student and the school are not the only ones to benefit from the externship period. The site also gains information about how well different areas of the facility are functioning. Site personnel may discover through the presence and questions of students that they should review certain policies or add others to help the office run more smoothly. Medical facilities must be updated on a continuing basis. Items may be deleted or added to policy, and procedure manuals or parts may have to be revised to provide clearer instructions.

As a student, you will be looking at the office as a newcomer, with a fresh perspective, and you may have many questions for the staff. As you become more familiar with the office routine, you will be more comfortable asking questions without the fear of appearing inexperienced. These questions may help point out to the office personnel things that should be changed or clarified.

ETHICAL TIP

HIPAA and Students

The HIPAA Privacy Rule does not prohibit students accessing patient medical information as part of their education. The wording of the privacy rules defines "health care operations" in a way that includes training of health care providers and professionals. Students are part of the covered entity's workforce for HIPAA compliance purposes. The rule does require that students receive training about the organization's policies and procedures related to protected health information. This training must be completed within a reasonable period of time after the student begins the externship. Documentation of this training must be kept for 6 years.

Externship Responsibilities

Responsibilities of the Student

You will develop many attributes, or characteristics, of a professional health care worker during the externship program. You should foster characteristics during this time to ensure that you continue to grow professionally and are an asset to the profession.

You must be dependable. Dependability is a good sign of maturity. Students who are not at the site on time, who take excessive numbers of breaks, or who do not follow through on assignments cannot properly provide for the needs of the patients who rely on the medical staff of the facility.

You must act in a professional manner. All concepts of professionalism include a positive, pleasant, confident attitude with a sincere desire to help the physician, the patient, and the staff.

You must be well groomed and meet the program's dress code. If the medical facility requires clothing that differs from your school's requirements, you are usually asked to comply with the site's requirements.

Many programs require you to keep a journal listing the events of each day at the extern site. Students will be expected to assist in the completion of the evaluation form and must therefore keep records of dates and procedures observed and performed. You will also keep a record of the time you spent at the site.

CHECKPOINT QUESTION

2. List three responsibilities that you have during your externship.

Responsibilities of the Medical Assisting Program

The primary responsibility of the program is to arrange for the best possible clinical experience for students. The program usually has a coordinator who matches students to appropriate sites. Once a site has been chosen, you will meet with the externship coordinator to discuss the particulars of the medical facility. An interview is sometimes held to acquaint you with your preceptor before the externship begins.

After your site rotation has begun, the program's externship coordinator will visit or call frequently to follow your progress. If either you or the site has concerns, the coordinator will mediate to eliminate problems or concerns as they arise.

The externship coordinator will make an evaluation, or appraisal, of your progress at the site. These evaluations, which are discussed later, will be used to determine whether you are prepared for the profession or your skills are deficient and need more reinforcement. The school is also responsible for maintaining liability insurance for students during clinical hours. You may pay a small premium when you pay your tuition. Students are required in most instances to provide proof of general immunizations and vaccination for hepatitis B. Some schools may provide the vaccine for students. Most programs require a current physical examination, a serology profile, and a tuberculin skin test before students are admitted to the program or before they make contact with patients.

WHAT IF?

You notice that on several occasions your preceptor does not follow standard precautions. Why is this dangerous? Whom should you tell? Would you tell your instructor at school? Why or why not? How would you discuss this with your preceptor?

Not following standard precautions when handling body fluids may expose you to blood-borne pathogens like HIV and hepatitis. When you see dangerous practices, it is usually best to confront the employee first. As an extern, you may or may not feel comfortable doing that. You will have a faculty member who has been designated as the externship coordinator. This person needs to be notified. He or she will help you decide the best way to handle the situation. If necessary, the office manager or clinical supervisor might address the issue with everyone in an office meeting rather than singling out particular employees.

Responsibilities of the Externship Site

The medical facility is, of course, responsible for providing opportunities for training. The staff will help orient you to the office and its policies. In some sites, students are allowed only to observe certain procedures but are given permission to perform some basic or routine procedures. Even if you are not allowed to perform specific procedures, the opportunity to observe and ask questions will be useful. In this way, you will become as familiar as possible with all clinical areas and functions. In many cases, the site preceptor will plan and oversee your externship experience, verify time sheets and other documentation generated at the extern site, and report to the externship coordinator from your school.

Guidelines for a Successful Externship

Success in your externship is important for you to obtain employment. Your success in your externship is evaluated according to certain standards, or criteria. The person or persons evaluating you during your externship are professional medical personnel who know the standards for the health care field as they relate to medical assisting. These areas include the following:

- Procedural performance
- Preparedness
- Attendance
- Appearance
- Attitude

Procedural Performance

You will be judged on your ability to measure up to the standard of care for an entry-level medical assistant. This means you are expected to perform at the level of a new employee in the field. Your preceptor is there to assist you, not to teach you the basics that you should have learned in the classroom. Come to your externship prepared. Ask questions, when in doubt, before starting any procedure. Ask questions outside the patient's room. Never perform a procedure alone, unless otherwise directed by your instructor.

Preparedness

Preparation is the best insurance for success, regardless of the goal. Personal preparation for the externship helps prevent losing time because of other extracurricular obligations. Make sure in advance that you have prepared:

- Reliable transportation
- Reliable day care services

- Backup systems for a sick child, snow cancellations of school, or early dismissals from school
- Financial coverage and support for any hours that you are unable to work at your usual job because of your extern site hours

Attendance

If you have planned well for transportation, family considerations, and finances, you are more likely to attend all sessions at the clinical sites. You must also be healthy. A good diet, regular exercise, and proper rest help you maintain good health. Careful attention to hygiene and medical asepsis help ensure that you do not bring illnesses home from the clinical sites.

If at any time you will be late or will not be able to attend the site for any reason, you must notify both the externship coordinator and the site preceptor. Never be a no-call or no-show. Almost all sites have an answering service for leaving messages, as do most schools. There is no excuse for not notifying all parties involved if you will be unavoidably late or will not be able to attend the scheduled session.

Office hours vary from site to site; it is always a good practice, however, to arrive a few minutes before the scheduled opening. This allows time to check for telephone messages, arrange the day's appointments, turn on office equipment, and generally get into the routine of the office. Plan your transportation, leaving plenty of time for any problems that may occur. Arriving in a flurry, frustrated by traffic or home problems, with no time to ease into your day causes a high level of tension and anxiety. This makes it more difficult to have the caring and compassionate attitude necessary to deal with the complex problems in the medical office.

Appearance

You have only one opportunity to make a first impression, which is usually based on appearance. Appearance is much more than looks. A beautiful face on a poorly groomed person is not seen as professional and does not inspire trust and confidence in patients or co-workers. The key to a professional appearance is careful preparation and planning.

If you wear a uniform for your externship, it must be freshly laundered and pressed; clean but wrinkled is not acceptable. Plan your wardrobe for ease of care and a professional appearance. Fad or trendy clothing, suggestive clothing, and flashy clothing are not appropriate for clinical sites. All clothing should be in good repair, with no missing buttons, hanging hems, tears, rips, or stains. Duty shoes should be clean, polished frequently, and kept in good condition. Laced shoes look better

with fresh, clean shoelaces. Check nylon hosiery for runs and snags and replace them as needed. You may wear laboratory coats in some programs; uniforms may be worn in others. The clinical preceptor or the externship coordinator will inform you of the dress code in advance.

Professional appearance includes hair and makeup. Your hair should be conservatively styled, and long hair must be kept away from the face. Wash it frequently so that it is fresh and clean. Makeup should be minimal and tastefully applied. Never use perfume or cologne, which may be irritating to co-workers and patients. Keep fingernails short to avoid transferring pathogens or ripping gloves when you perform procedures.

Wear only minimal, tasteful jewelry. Rings can puncture gloves, possibly causing exposure to a pathogen. Therefore, it is a good idea to avoid wearing them in the clinical site.

 CHECKPOINT QUESTION

3. Describe the proper attire for your externship.

Attitude

Attitude is also part of appearance. Most patients and co-workers will see your emotions through facial expressions and body language. A person who looks eager is usually perceived as a good, diligent worker.

Attitude is determined by how well you handle change and direction and how adaptable and flexible you are during difficult assignments.

The medical profession is constantly changing, making it imperative for all professionals to stay flexible. In the classroom, you learn generic methods for treatments and procedures. Because of the constantly changing technology, you may have to adjust to other methods in the field. If you learned a procedure one way in the classroom training but find that it is performed differently in the clinical site, the new method must be accepted and performed as well as possible. Frequently, there is more than one right way to do a procedure, and the classroom method you learned may be just one of the accepted methods. The next physician or clinical site may use yet another equally correct procedural method.

Your attitude determines your altitude. Students who work with a positive attitude during their externship are likely to reach higher levels of the profession than those who see the externship as an imposition or a burden. Box 46-1 offers some additional suggestions.

LEGAL TIP

WHO'S THE BOSS?

In Chapter 2, you learned that a medical assistant practices under the license of a physician. As an extern, you are not an employee of the physician; therefore, the legal doctrine of respondeat superior does not apply. Since you are participating in a college activity, any liability issues are covered by the college's insurance. If you fall on a wet floor, the college is responsible. You should also have malpractice insurance to cover any issues with patient care in the medical site. Most colleges arrange for this malpractice coverage, and fees are included with other tuition expenses. It is important that you identify yourself as a student. You must be wearing a name tag with your student status clearly visible. Patients have the right to know who is participating in their care.

BOX 46-1

STRATEGIES FOR A SUCCESSFUL EXTERNSHIP

Your externship will be successful if you:

- Show enthusiasm and interest in learning.
- Be a team player.
- Offer to assist with as many tasks as possible.
- Ask questions or clarification before doing any procedures or tasks about which you are unsure.
- Immediately admit to any errors or mistakes that you make.
- Accept corrections and suggestions by staff members.
- Anticipate tasks that need to be done, and do them before you are asked.
- Do not make remarks such as: "I can't believe that you don't have that on the computer." "This office is outdated." "Don't you know about these new regulations?"

Externship Documentation

Most programs use a time sheet or record of some sort to document your hours in the externship (Fig. 46-2). The beginning and ending hours of each day are recorded. How breaks are handled depends on the externship coordinator, program requirements, and specific site. Some sites allow half an hour for lunch, and others allow an hour; some close for an hour or more midday, while others are open and staffed from morning until evening. Some programs make students responsible for time sheet signatures; others delegate the responsibility to the site preceptor. However the form is handled, it is used to validate your time in the externship and is a requirement for completion of most programs.

Journals are required by many programs. These provide proof that tasks are performed and learning takes place. The student will list each day's activities, and this is reviewed by the externship coordinator. Checklists serve as further documentation of tasks observed and performed. In many cases, the site supervisor actually assigns a grade to the student using criteria provided by the college. Site evaluations performed by the student are another form of externship documentation and are discussed in the next section.

Every accredited school will use surveys to gather information from students. Sample evaluations are available through AAMA's website. Evaluations are used to improve performance and services offered to students. Most medical assisting programs have advisory boards whose members use the results of such surveys to make necessary changes to existing programs. Your input is vital to this ongoing quest for excellence. Take these evaluations seriously and be honest. Do not take the opportunity to complain about individual problems that may have been encountered. It is more appropriate to address these concerns under comments. For example, if a particular instructor's grading criteria are more strict than others' criteria, your evaluation of that instructor should not be based on the fact that you got a lower grade in his or her class. You should be fair and objective and evaluate the instructor on his or her actual performance in the classroom. Evaluations are not designed to prove popularity but to report strengths and deficiencies in areas that can be improved.

Externship Evaluations

The preceptor or office manager at your site will evaluate you on a completed form that contains detailed areas to be graded; these are equivalent to grades on a test or examination. The externship coordinator is responsible for compiling evaluations and keeping you abreast of your progress. Frequent conferences with your coordinator usually help accomplish this. After your externship is completed, your input in the quality of your experience helps program administrators choose the best extern sites in the future.

Most schools use a site evaluation form to gather impressions of the program's extern sites and the students' overall externship experience (Fig. 46-3). This form helps determine the effectiveness of the site for training and whether any issues should be addressed be-

CLINICAL EXPERIENCE
STUDENT'S TIME REPORT

To obtain proper credit, an account of time and days in attendance must be recorded by each intern student. This report must be verified by the job supervisor and attached to the final 55-day roster. This information is kept strictly confidential.

Student's Name: _____

Program: _____

Minimum Contact Hrs. Required: _____

Course No.: _____

Course Title: _____

Quarter/Year: _____

WEEK OF (DATES)		TIME OF DAY						TOTAL HOURS	SITE SUPERVISOR
	M	T	W	TH	F	S			

TOTAL HOURS FOR QUARTER: _____

I certify that the above time report is a true statement of the hours worked.

I approve this statement of hours in attendance for the quarter covered.

_____   _____
Student's Signature   Date

_____   _____
Externship Coordinator's Signature   Date

Figure 46-2 Sample extern time sheet.

fore assigning other students. Be objective and honest in your evaluation of the site. When completing a site evaluation, consider these questions:

- Was the overall experience positive or negative?
- Were opportunities for learning abundant and freely offered or hard to obtain?
- Were staff personnel open and caring or unwelcoming?
- Was the preceptor available and easily approachable or preoccupied and distant?

If the site is not providing a positive learning experience, the program should discontinue using it.

Graduate Surveys

When you graduate, the college will want to know your opinion of its instruction and services. You will be asked to evaluate your experience at the college in general, your course work, and your extern experience. Take the time to think back over your overall experience at the school. Information provided is tabulated and distributed to those evaluated. This is an integral part of the quality improvement and planning processes of educational institutions. Figure 46-4 illustrates a sample graduate survey.

Employer Surveys

After you have been on a job for awhile, the college will survey your employer to assess his/her satisfaction with your performance, skills, and professionalism. Figure 46-5 is a sample of an employer evaluation. You must always do your best. Your performance is not only a reflection of you but also of your medical assisting program and the college you attended.

CHECKPOINT QUESTION

4. What is the purpose of having students evaluate their externship experience?

Establish the Job for You

Setting Employment Goals

Once your externship is complete, you are one step closer to getting the job that you desire. Before beginning to search for a job, decide what you want and need from a job and make that your goal. People who do not set employment goals too often accept only what is presented to them. They often end up unhappy in their work because they did not choose their job in the first place. The average person approaches the job search with the attitude, "I wonder what is available," rather than, "Here is what I would like to do, and here is the facility where I would like to work." *That* is setting a goal. It is also a positive, proactive approach to the job market rather than a reactive position to what is available. In general, the medical field is looking for proactive people. You will work harder and more enthusiastically if you choose your workplace.

The best way to set a goal and eventually get what you want is to study your strengths and weaknesses and, from that self-knowledge, design the best job for

Figure 46-3 Sample site evaluation form.

Figure 46-4 Sample graduate survey.

EMPLOYER SURVEY

Pittssylvania Community College
Medical Assisting Program

The primary goal of a Medical Assisting Education program is to prepare each graduate to function as a competent Medical Assistant. This survey is designed to help program faculty determine their program's strengths and those areas that need improvement. All data will be kept confidential and will be used for program evaluation purposes only. We request that this survey be completed by the graduate's immediate supervisor.

BACKGROUND INFORMATION:

Name of Graduate (Optional): _____

Certification Status (check all that apply):
☐ CMA   ☐ RMA

Length of employment at time of survey: _____ years and _____ months

Place of employment: _____

Name of evaluator completing this form: _____

INSTRUCTIONS: Consider each item separately and rate each item independently of all others. Circle the rating that indicates the extent to which you agree with each statement. Please do not skip any rating.
5 = Strongly Agree   4 = Generally Agree   3 = Neutral (acceptable)   2 = Generally Disagree   1 = Strongly Disagree

I.   KNOWLEDGE   (Cognitive Learning Domain)

THE GRADUATE:

A.	Has medical assisting knowledge appropriate to his/her level of training.	5	4	3	2	1
B.	Has general medical knowledge appropriate to his/her level of training.	5	4	3	2	1
C.	Is able to collect pertinent data accurately from charts and patients.	5	4	3	2	1
D.	Is able to perform appropriate diagnostic and medical procedures as directed.	5	4	3	2	1
E.	Uses good judgment while functioning in the ambulatory healthcare setting.	5	4	3	2	1

Comments: _____

II.   SKILLS   (Psychomotor Learning Domain)

THE PROGRAM:

A.	Prepared the graduate to perform all clinical skills appropriate to entry level medical assisting.	5	4	3	2	1
B.	Prepared the graduate to perform all administrative skills appropriate to entry level medical assisting.	5	4	3	2	1

Comments: _____

III.   BEHAVIORS   (Affective Learning Domain)

THE GRADUATE:

A.	Communicates effectively in the healthcare setting.	5	4	3	2	1
B.	Conducts himself/herself in an ethical and professional manner.	5	4	3	2	1
C.	Functions effectively as a member of the healthcare team.	5	4	3	2	1
D.	Accepts supervision and works effectively with supervisory personnel.	5	4	3	2	1
E.	Is self-directed and responsible for his/her actions.	5	4	3	2	1
F.	Arrives to work prepared and on time.	5	4	3	2	1
G.	Contributes to a positive environment in the department.	5	4	3	2	1

Comments: _____

IV.   GENERAL INFORMATION   (Circle yes or no)

A.   Do you encourage/motivate employees to take and pass the CMA Certification exam?   Yes   No
B.   Do you encourage/motivate employees to take and pass the RMA Registry exams?   Yes   No
C.   If you answered NO to any of the above questions, please explain why:

Comments: _____

V.   ADDITIONAL COMMENTS

OVERALL RATING:

Please rate and comment on the OVERALL quality of this graduate:
5 = Excellent   4 = Very Good   3 = Good   2 = Fair   1 = Poor

Comments: _____

What qualities or skills did you expect of the graduate upon employment that he/she _did not_ possess?
_____

Please provide comments and suggestions that would help this program to better prepare future graduates.
_____

What are strengths of the graduate(s) of this program?
_____

Name and Title of Evaluator:

(Please Print) _____   Date: _____

Signature: _____

Thank you in advance

February 2006

February 2006

Figure 46-5   Sample employer evaluation.

you. Goal setting means describing the ideal job for you and deciding that this is the job that you will someday have.

On a sheet of paper, describe the best job for you if you had your choice. For example, you might describe these elements:

- Specialty area (e.g., obstetrics, pediatrics, surgery)
- Duties (clinical or administrative)
- Type of employer and supervisor
- Other employees and co-workers
- Type of facility
- Desired atmosphere (casual or formal)
- Ideal hours
- Availability of flextime (a system of scheduling that allows for a personal choice in hours or days worked)

Next, write down where you expect to be in 2 years and in 5 years, in terms of both position and income. Now you are more focused on where you want to work, what you want to do, and the direction you want to be going. The next question is how to get there.

To win the position you want, you have to learn to sell yourself. Generally, employers will not come looking for you; you will have to go to them. They will compare you with all of the other equally well-qualified candidates who are interested in the same position. If 25 people interview for a job, even if you are second best,

you still lose. The one who is best suited for a job does not necessarily get it; instead, frequently the one who performs best in the interview does. Marketing yourself takes real effort.

Self-Analysis

A good presentation of your qualifications begins with self-analysis. You must know what strengths you have to offer a potential employer as well as your weaknesses. Make an honest list of your strengths and weaknesses. Each of your strengths presents an opportunity to sell yourself and your value as an employee. When you are interviewing for a position, concentrate on projecting your strengths to the interviewer.

Just as your strengths give you a special advantage, each weakness is a reason someone may not want to offer you the position. Recognize and work to resolve your weaknesses. Recognizing your weaknesses as a threat to securing the position you want will help you develop strategies to eliminate these problems or turn them into strengths. As long as you are aware of your weaknesses, you are better prepared to handle them.

Once you know the type of job you want and have identified your positive and negative qualities, it is time to begin to look for the right job.

CHECKPOINT QUESTION

5. What is the purpose of self-analysis?

Finding the Right Job

The internet offers employment services that allow you to search for a certain type job in a specific geographic location. Even though searching the internet is easier and less time consuming than the traditional ways of looking for a job, an internet search may not be the best way to find a job. For jobs in your hometown, it is helpful to begin with the newspaper. Keep in mind that many of the most desirable job openings are never advertised; they are posted internally and filled from within. Membership in your professional organization is an excellent way to network.

Many studies show that most positions are never advertised in the media. Open positions that are posted internally are often filled with current employees or by referrals from current employees. Any organization that looks within and obtains a recommendation from a current employee to fill an available position accomplishes two things: (1) it saves the cost of advertising, and (2) the recommendation itself is usually a good one because it comes from someone who presumably knows the demands and special needs of that particular organization.

It is important for someone seeking employment in the medical field to build as many contacts within the field as possible. These contacts help you with **networking**. Networking is using friends, family members, and professional colleagues to advance or obtain information in the workplace. It is impossible to have too many contacts. Everyone with whom you associate should know that you are looking for employment. Friends and acquaintances cannot tell you about a job or recommend you for a job if they do not know that you are searching.

Traditional sources of information for job openings:

- *Local, state, or federal government employment offices.* These agencies are designed to find work for the unemployed. They frequently have listings of positions that are not found anywhere else. Rather than calling the office with inquiries, make an appointment to visit. Register with the service. Get to know the contact person with whom you will be contacting frequently.
- *School placement office.* If your school has a placement office, contact the coordinator or personnel officer and outline what you are looking for and where you want to work. Their job is to assist you in securing the position you want. If you establish a working relationship with a contact person, you will probably have better results.

- *Medical facilities.* Do not wait for an advertisement. Go to the office or facility where you would like to work and leave a résumé—a document summarizing your professional qualifications—and a cover letter explaining how much you want to work there. Find out the name of the office manager or personnel officer and call first for an appointment. This shows better planning and foresight and is more professional than dropping by unannounced.
- *Private agencies.* Many medical facilities solicit privately to avoid being swamped by applications from unqualified applicants. A fee is charged for the service but is usually paid by the employer. Call the agency to make an appointment with a representative who will interview you and tell you what steps to follow.
- *Temporary services.* These agencies fill short-term vacancies for medical offices. If you are new in an area, this is a good way to learn which facilities would be good choices for you. You may be assigned for several days or several weeks. If you work well as a temporary replacement and like the site, leave your résumé and let the appropriate individuals know that you would like to work in this place if an opening occurs. Check with the temporary agency regarding any fees that you may be charged or that the medical office may have to pay if it hires you, often called a finder's fee.

CHECKPOINT QUESTION

6. List four resources that you may use to identify potential job opportunities.

APPLYING FOR THE JOB

Answering Newspaper Advertisements

When responding to a newspaper advertisement, be sure to do exactly what the advertisement asks you to do; one of the qualities that many interviewers look for is the ability to follow directions. At the same time, try to make your response more distinctive (yet still professional) than others they may receive. The medical profession rarely responds well to those who do not fit its image and almost never accepts someone who does not conform at the entry level. Most employers will require you to submit a résumé. A well-prepared résumé and cover letter are essential to job hunting.

Preparing Your Résumé

Many resources can help you write your **résumé**. Start with your school library. Most schools have books on how to create résumés. Numerous websites also offer this information. Caution: Many websites have free information, but some charge fees. Focus on free resources before paying for these services. Many word processing programs have templates for résumés. Put your résumé on a computer disk and be sure to personalize it for the position you are seeking. For example, if you give a career objective, try putting in the title a description of the particular job you are seeking. Keep changing this for every different position so that your résumé is personalized for each interview.

The résumé is a flash picture of yourself; if it is neat and professional, the reviewer will presume that it is a reflection of you. Procedure 46-1 outlines the steps in writing a résumé. Here are some guidelines that will help you create a résumé that will capture the reviewer's interest.

1. Evaluate your skills, goals, and what you have to offer. With this list in hand, you can better concentrate on highlighting your strengths.
2. Confine your résumé to one page, selecting carefully what you want to include. The résumé must state just what the reviewer needs to know and no more.
3. Include the following key information:
   - Name, address, and telephone number: Include these at the top of your résumé (usually centered). (Because you are including your telephone number, you should expect calls from prospective employers. Box 46-2 offers some tips for handling such calls.)
   - Education: Start with the most recent and work backward.
   - Affiliations or volunteer work (if appropriate): If this information shows that you have good orga-

nizational skills or have held an office for the group, you should include it.
   - Experience: This may be listed in either of two standard forms: functional or chronological. A functional résumé focuses on skills and qualifications rather than employment and works well for those who recently graduated or who are re-entering the job market after a period of years (Fig. 46-6). A chronological résumé is useful for those who have an employment history, particularly if the history is relevant to the position being sought. Start with the most recent employment and work backward. Include your title, position, and a few of your key responsibilities (Fig. 46-7). Explain any gaps such as pregnancy, schooling, relocations, and so on.
   - References: You may or may not include your references on a separate sheet. When you have chosen the people you want to use as references, be sure to ask their permission. Start by asking your instructors if you can use them as references. Other medical professionals (physicians or nurses) will also make strong references. Previous employers also make very good references. You should have a minimum of three references. Do not bring a list of more than five people. Prospective employers are not interested in your neighbors, pastor, or relatives as references.
4. Do not include hobbies and personal interests unrelated to work. It is not relevant that you play the guitar, but it would be impressive to know that you volunteer at a free clinic.
5. Use action words (Box 46-3).
6. Center the résumé on white or off-white heavy bond or high rag content paper, 8.5 × 11 inches. (Colors are not acceptable, and cheap paper will not convey the professional impression you hope to make.) Keep a 1-inch margin around the text. Single space within the sections of information, but leave a blank line between the sections.
7. Use regular type. Avoid fonts that are cute or fancy. Use black ink. Do not print your résumé in color.
8. Have someone proofread your work. It is difficult to find your own errors or see areas that are not clearly worded.
9. Mail the résumé in an 8.5 × 11–inch manila envelope. This will present the interviewer with a résumé and cover letter that are smooth, with no fold lines. Many prefer to work with résumés that have not been folded for an envelope.
10. Many employers are now allowing applicants to send their résumés as an e-mail attachment. Use a well-known software to create your résumé, and keep it simple because some formatting may not transmit properly.

BOX 46-2

HANDLING CALLS FROM PROSPECTIVE EMPLOYERS

Here are some tips for handling calls from prospective employers:

- Tell family members or other household members that you are expecting important telephone calls.
- Keep a pen and paper by the telephone.
- Instruct people to take a complete message. Ask them to write down the person's name, phone number, message, and what time the call was received.
- Leave a professional message on your answering machine. Avoid leaving cute or silly messages.

Tina Elmwood C.M.A.
22 Brandy Drive
Dayton, Ohio 00000
444-777-6666

Employment Objective: To use my medical assisting skills in a challenging position. My goal is to work with children. (*Change this sentence to reflect the type of office that you are applying to.*)

Experience:

Externship (160 hours) at Family Practice Associates, Bayview Drive, Dayton, Ohio (*If you have a positive evaluation from your preceptor, bring it with you to the interview. Do not attach it to the resume.*)

Education:

Medical Assisting Program, Diploma. Graduated June 2008. West County Community College, Dayton Ohio (*Bring a copy of your diploma and transcripts to the interview. Do not attach them unless employer has specifically requested them.*)
Dayton High School, Diploma. Graduated June 2006. Dayton, Ohio

Skills:

Clinical and Laboratory skills listed on Role Delineation for Medical Assisting

Administrative skills listed on Role Delineation for Medical Assisting

Comfortable using all types of standard office equipment

Familiar with XYZ software programs (*List software programs that you are comfortable with. If you know what type of software the office uses, list that as well.*)

Certifications:

Certified Medical Assistant, American Association of Medical Assistants (*Bring copy to interview or attach to résumé.*)
Cardiopulmonary Resuscitation, American Heart Association (*Bring copy to interview or attach to résumé.*)

Figure 46-6 Sample functional résumé.

11. Be honest. Do not embellish your résumé or add fictional information. This could get you fired.

 CHECKPOINT QUESTION

7. What is the difference between a functional résumé and a chronological résumé?

Preparing Your Cover Letter

When contacting a prospective employer about a job, you need to send a résumé along with a cover letter. Keep your cover letter brief and meaningful. You want it to be read, and you want the reader to be impressed by what it says. Be sure that you mention the job itself in your letter. You may even consider a statement such as, "This is the type of position I would prefer." If you are applying to a pediatrician's office, you may write, "My goal is to work with children." If you know something favorable about the facility, include that in your letter. If you know anyone who works for the company, mention it. *Do not* mention the person by name unless you have secured his or her permission.

Make sure you address your letter to the right person. Call the personnel department or office manager and ask the name of the person handling the applications. Determine the correct spelling of the name and the preferred honorific, such as Mr., Ms., or Mrs.

The standard form for a cover letter has three brief paragraphs:

- First paragraph: State the position for which you are applying.

Beatrice Meza C.M.A.
123 Main Street
West Harford, CT 00000
888-999-6666

Employment Objective: To use my medical assisting skills in a challenging position. My goal is to work in an obstetrical office. (*Change this sentence to reflect the type of office that you are applying to.*)

Education:

2008–2009 Medical Assisting Program; Mountain Laurel Community College, West Hartford, Connecticut (*Bring a copy of your diploma and transcripts to the interview. Do not attach them unless employer has specifically requested them.*)

Externship:

July 2009–(160 hours) Women's Health Care Center, Hartford, Connecticut (*If you have a positive evaluation from your preceptor, bring it with you to the interview. Do not attach it to the résumé.*)

Work Experience:

July 2008–present Receptionist, Dermatology Consultants, West Hartford, Connecticut. Worked part time while I was in school. Answered and triaged telephone calls. Assisted with various other medical administrative responsibilities. (*If you have a reference letter from this employer, bring it with you to the interview. Be prepared to answer questions about why you are leaving this position.*)
May 2005–July 2008 Cashier/Clerk for SuperMarket Grocers, West Hartford, Connecticut. Worked part time. Responsible for training new employees. Promoted to senior cashier.

Skills:

Clinical and Laboratory skills listed on the Role Delineation for Medical Assisting
Administrative skills listed on the Role Delineation for Medical Assisting
Comfortable using all types of standard office equipment
Familiar with XYZ software programs (*List software programs that you are comfortable with. If you know what type of software the office uses, list that as well.*)

Activities/Honors

Student Government representative
Most Improved Medical Assisting Student in 2008

Figure 46-7 Sample chronological résumé.

BOX 46-3

ACTION WORDS

Achieved	Established	Planned
Assisted	Filed	Prepared
Attained	Generated	Processed
Conducted	Handled	Scheduled
Completed	Implemented	Screened
Composed	Maintained	Selected
Created	Operated	Solved
Developed	Organized	Systemized
Directed	Participated	Wrote
Ensured	Performed	

- Second paragraph: Stress your skills. Do not be redundant, since you will also send a résumé, but mention or highlight specifically the skills needed for this job.
- Third paragraph: Request an interview. Offer to call in a week to set up an interview (then do so). Keep a copy of your letter to refer to when calling.

Use the same good-quality paper for the cover letter that you use for your résumé. Include your name, address, and telephone number at the top of the page, centered or in block form. Single space the letter, and double space between paragraphs. Either block or modified block form is acceptable.

As mentioned earlier, many employers are now accepting résumés via e-mail. Although this may eliminate the need for a cover letter, the information included should still be communicated as an e-mail message. Accuracy is just as important in an electronic communication as in any other form.

Completing an Employment Application

Some sites will have you fill out an employment application while you wait for your interview; others may mail one to you to be filled out and taken to the interview. Although résumés have their place and are indispensable, many facilities rely more on an application form. Many organizations accept online applications. The guidelines for completing an online application are similar to those of manual completion of an application:

1. Read through completely before beginning.
2. Follow the instructions exactly. Prospective employers notice neatness, erasures, evasions, and indecision.
3. Answer every question. If the question does not apply to you, draw a line or write N/A so that the interviewer will know that you did not overlook the question.
4. In the line for wage or salary desired, write "negotiable" or find out before the interview what is usual for the area for this type of position.
5. In spaces requesting your reason for leaving a previous position, try to sound positive. Answers such as "to explore a new career direction" are general enough to fill many needs. If the reason for leaving was relocation, schooling, or pregnancy, say so.
6. Type, or print legibly, being as neat as possible.
7. Use a black or blue pen. Never use a pencil or colored pen (red, green, purple) to complete the application. It does not portray a professional image.
8. You may attach your résumé to the application if you did not mail one already.

The Interview

Interviewing well is a skill that takes effort to develop. As with any skill, if you want to stay proficient and keep your skills in good working order, you have to practice. Ask friends or family members to work with you to develop a relaxed approach to answering the questions most often asked during an interview. Have them try to trip you up or confuse you by throwing in tricky questions. Although the effect will not be the same with a friend or family member as with an interviewer, this practice can make a difference between getting the job and losing the chance. You can also rehearse in front of a mirror.

Usually, the person who interviews best is hired for the position. An excellent interview is absolutely crucial

for obtaining any job. It is highly unlikely that you will get the job you want without doing well in the interview. Remember what the employer is looking for. Every employer is looking for something special from each employee. Medicine has special needs. The employer must believe that you possess a number of skills necessary to do the job:

- *Technical skills.* You must have the necessary proficiency to get the job done.
- *Confidentiality.* In medicine, you are exposed to sensitive information about patients. Is the interviewer convinced that you can be relied on to keep those confidences?
- *Human relations skills.* Will you get along with the others in the workplace?
- *Communication skills.* Do you have the verbal and writing skills that the job demands? Remember the importance of correct English. You will not be hired if your English and grammar are not exemplary.

If you fail to impress the interviewer with your grasp of these skills, you will never be considered for the position. The interviewer knows that whatever you display in the interview will also be displayed to the patients.

WHAT IF?

You become tongue-tied during an interview. What should you do?

It's not unusual to feel nervous during the interview. To stay calm, take a deep breath and count to 3 before answering a question. Doing this also gives you time to think before you speak. Remember: Believe in yourself and your skills. Say to yourself, "I am going to get this job." Rehearse your answers to the common interview questions. Doing this exercise in front of a mirror is beneficial. Visit the websites listed in this chapter. Some of these sites offer virtual interviewing skills and have excellent tips for interviewing. Finally, arrive prepared and relaxed. Avoid excessive caffeine ingestion before the interview. Caffeine will increase your anxiety level.

Preparing for the Interview

Before the day of the interview, find out all you can about the facility. What is its reputation? Does it have a big turnover of employees? Review your textbooks that cover the specialty so that you can ask informed questions about procedures performed at the site. Think of questions to ask and write them down. Anticipate questions that might be asked of you. Find out the name of the interviewer; if it is a difficult name, practice saying it. Go to the site ahead of time to be sure of its location and time the trip so that you will not be late for your appointment. Do this ideally at the same time of day as your appointment to judge traffic delays, parking problems, and so on.

Dress appropriately for the interview. The general rule is to dress one step above what is required for the job. Do not overdress, as if for a party; make sure your outfit is professional. Your personal hygiene must be above reproach. If you normally smoke, avoid smoking before the interview. Those who do not smoke are acutely aware of the odor of smoke on one's clothes and breath. Avoid large jewelry and apply makeup carefully. Avoid perfumes; some people are very sensitive to scents.

Arrive on time or a few minutes early. Go alone; do not take a friend or family member for moral support. When you are introduced to the interviewer, offer your hand for a handshake and sit only when and where you are directed. Do not fidget, swing your foot, play with your hair, or tap your fingers on the chair arm. Make eye contact when the interviewer speaks with you and when you respond to the questions (Fig. 46-8). Sit up straight but relaxed, with your portfolio on your lap. A **portfolio** is a folder containing all of the information you will need to impress the interviewer. If you do not have a special folder or briefcase, a neat, new manila folder will be adequate. This folder or portfolio will contain items crucial to your interview (Box 46-4).

Crucial Interview Questions

Every interviewer must have the answers to three basic questions. When you respond to the interviewer's questions, keep these in mind:

1. Do you have the necessary skills to do the job? (Don't forget to include any foreign language skills; Box 46-5).

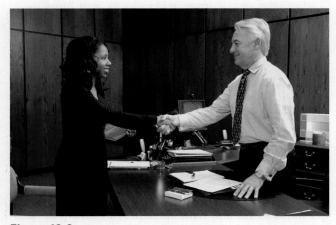

Figure 46-8   Dress and act professionally for the interview.

BOX 46-4

CONTENTS OF A PORTFOLIO

Take these items with you to the interview:

- Two pens
- A notepad
- Your Social Security card
- Verification or at least the dates of immunizations (hepatitis B, TB test)
- Two copies of your résumé
- Two letters of reference
- Typed list of three references including names, phone numbers, and addresses
- Documentation of any special projects
- Copies of awards received

---

2. Do you have the necessary drive, energy, and commitment to get the job done?
3. Will you work well with the rest of the team?

A positive answer to all of these questions is not a guarantee that you will be offered the job, but a negative answer to any one of these will most assuredly mean that you will *not* get the job. Make sure that your comments make a positive impression regarding these

---

BOX 46-5

KNOWLEDGE OF A FOREIGN LANGUAGE

If you are applying for a position that encourages bilingual applicants, be prepared for questions during the interview regarding your ability to speak another language. Know what languages are commonly spoken in your community. Whether it is Spanish, Polish, Italian, or any other language, take the time to become familiar with simple greetings: "Hello." "What is your name?" "Can I help you?" Tell the interviewer that you know a few words but are not fluent. It is not fair to the employer or to the patients to pretend otherwise if you are unable to communicate effectively. Most community colleges offer language courses. A local hospital may offer these courses with a focus on medical terms. Finally, the best way to learn a new language is to use it. If your classmates speak another language, ask them to tutor you. Being bilingual in the medical profession is always an asset.

three questions. In the medical field, the interviewer will need to establish your professionalism and ability to keep confidentiality. The interviewer will also want to know how interested you are in increasing and continuing your education and skills. Be sure that your answers will satisfy the interviewer.

Many interviewers use a prepared list of questions to direct the flow of the interview. Table 46-1 contains some commonly asked interview questions and guidance for responses. Be prepared with answers that will reflect well on your professionalism and qualifications.

When the interviewer finishes asking questions, he or she will usually ask if you have any questions. Refer to your notepad, on which you have listed questions such as these:

- What are the responsibilities of the position offered?
- If it is not personal, why is the current employee leaving?
- What are the opportunities for future advancement?
- How long is the training or probation period?

- How does the facility feel about continuing education? Do they pay membership dues to your professional organization? Is time off offered to employees to upgrade their skills? Does the facility subsidize the expense?
- Is there a job performance or evaluation process?
- What is the benefit package? Is there access to a 401(k) plan or other retirement plan? Health insurance? Life insurance?

Make notes of the answers for future reference. Avoid asking about time off or vacations during the interview. These questions imply that you are more interested in being paid to avoid work than you are in contributing to the work at hand.

Make sure the interviewer knows how important continuing education is to you. Talk about the types of continuing education courses you would like to attend and the subjects you would like to study. Show that you realize that the only constant in medicine is change and that you expect to keep abreast of the information in your area. Thank the interviewer for the opportunity to apply for the position and ask the time frame for a decision. As you leave, offer your hand for a handshake

TABLE 46-1 Interview Questions and Responses	
Common Interview Questions	**Possible Responses and Points to Mention**
1. Tell me about yourself.	"I enjoy working with other people." Stress the good points you wrote on your self-analysis. Keep the comments professional. Do not give long explanations about personal topics. ("I have three brothers." "I like basketball.")
2. What are your strengths?	"My strengths are honesty and dependability." List any clinical or administrative skills that you excel at.
3. What are your weaknesses?	Be honest; everyone has a weakness. "My weakness is phlebotomy skills," and add, "but I have improved my skills by reading magazine articles about blood drawing and by practicing in the school laboratory." Do not say, "I am perfect" or "I have no weaknesses." State one weakness and explain how you are trying to improve it.
4. Why do you want this position?	"I like this office setting." "I always wanted to work for [as an example] a cardiologist." Mention that you are aware of the office's good reputation in the community, and if the location of the office is convenient, say so.
5. What are your goals?	List two or three immediate goals: "My priority is to acquire a medical assisting position that will be challenging and rewarding." Have at least two goals in your mind for where you want to be in 5 years.
6. Why did you leave your last position?	Always place a positive spin on why you left: "Looking for new challenge." Never criticize past employers, their offices, or your co-workers.
7. What salary rate are you looking for?	Know the average pay in your area. Check with your placement office if you are unsure of the typical salaries. Never demand a certain pay rate.

(continued)

TABLE **46-1** Interview Questions and Responses *(continued)*	
Common Interview Questions	**Possible Responses and Points to Mention**
8. How do you handle pressure?	Possible answers can include, "I set priorities" and "I remain calm and well organized." Avoid comments such as "I hate stress" or "I panic when I feel pressured."
9. Do you work better alone or as part of a team?	Stress that you can work as a team member but that you can also function independently.
10. Who was your best supervisor and why?	Possible remarks may include phrases such as "always fair," "supportive," and "encouraging." Avoid comments such as "She gave us long lunch breaks" or "She didn't make us work hard."
11. How do you handle conflict?	Indicate that you begin trying to resolve any problems in a professional manner. Indicate that you are always open to constructive criticism.
12. How would your classmates describe you?	Include remarks such as "good student," "team worker," and "helpful."
13. I noticed your grades in computer class were poor. Why?	Be honest: "It was a tough course" or "Although my grade was poor, I have restudied the course material, and my computer skills have improved." If you have taken any additional studies or tutoring to help in this subject area, mention that. Never say the teacher was unfair, the class was boring, or you didn't care about the class.
14. Describe the term confidentiality and how you would use it in our office.	Review the term. Stress to the interviewer that you know how important patient confidentiality is from a legal and ethical view point.

and ask if you may call again before the decision date to clear up any questions that the interviewer may have during the decision-making process.

Follow-Up

The day of the interview or no later than the day after, write a short thank you note for the opportunity to be interviewed and restate how interested you are in the job (Fig. 46-9). Remind the interviewer that you are available for additional questions. Call several days after the interview. Reintroduce yourself politely and add any new information or ask any questions that might have occurred to you after the interview. Thank the interviewer again for this opportunity.

Think back to your performance in the interview. Determine what skills you still need to develop or enhance in order to improve your interview skills. Remember that experience is the best teacher and each interview helps you continue to improve.

CHECKPOINT QUESTION

8. What are the three basic questions in every interviewer's mind?

September 15, 2008

Dear Dr. Whitten,

I would like to thank you for the opportunity to meet with you today to discuss employment. I enjoyed meeting everyone. Your employees made me feel welcome. After meeting with you and spending some time in your office, I feel that I would be a good addition to your team. Thank you for considering me in filling your CMA position. I look forward to hearing from you.

Sincerely,

Jan Joyce, CMA

Figure 46-9 Sample thank you letter.

Leaving a Job

Should you leave, or should you stay? Almost everyone comes to this question at some point in his or her career. *Should I look for a new place to work and leave this place where I am safe and comfortable? Would another job be better or more satisfying? Would benefits be better?*

An important factor in many relocations is salary. In addition to the financial aspects, however, employees today are looking for other elements that contribute to job satisfaction, such as:

- A sense of achievement
- Recognition
- Opportunity for growth and advancement
- Harmonious peer group relationships
- A good working relationship with supervisors
- Status
- Job security
- Comfortable working conditions
- Fair company policies

If you are no longer happy in your job, the reason probably lies in one or more of these elements. Before you make the decision to change jobs, do some internal soul searching to determine exactly what type of position would make you happy.

If you decide to leave your job, follow these steps:

- Always give adequate notice (minimum 2 weeks, optimal a month).
- Write a resignation letter. Keep the letter positive: "I am leaving this position to explore new opportunities." This is often the last item in your personnel file.
- Be positive during your exit interview. Do not criticize employees or the position.
- Clean and empty your locker, desk, and any other assigned space.
- Return your pager and any other equipment that has been assigned to you.
- Finish all duties and tie up any loose ends.
- Alert your supervisor to any unfinished business.
- Ask for a letter of reference.

Be a Lifelong Learner

You are about to embark on the career you have spent time, money, and energy to prepare for. Even though your formal schooling is coming to an end, you must continue to learn. Be a lifelong learner. In the medical field, changes occur frequently. You must stay abreast of new technologies, procedures, and legal issues. In addition to facility training, inservices, and seminars, you will need to stay current with your CPR certification and recertify your credential.

Recertification

You now face the process of acquiring certification in your field. As discussed in Chapter 1, whether you become a certified medical assistant or a registered medical assistant, you must keep your credential current. Both credentialing bodies require recertification. For AAMA, recertification is mandatory. A CMA wishing to recertify must either retake the examination or complete 60 hours of continuing education units. A CMA who does not recertifiy by the end of the month of his or her birthday 5 years after the last date of certification loses the right to use the credential. RMAs are required to renew their certification each year by renewing their membership in the American Medical Technologists. If their membership lapses for more than 1 calendar year, the RMA must begin the process of becoming certified again. Both groups offer continuing education seminars and products. Information about the specific requirements and issues involving recertification is available on the organizations' websites.

To prepare for the process of recertifying, maintain a file with information about all educational sessions you attend. You should keep a brochure of the event with the following information: the topic, hours of session, learning objectives, and an outline of the program. You should also have proof of your attendance. When the time to apply for recertification comes, you will be prepared to complete the application.

Professionalism

Experts say that professionalism is the one quality all employers seek. An allied health care career holds excitement, variety, and prestige. But with that comes a responsibility to the patients you serve. This requires professionalism and a commitment to excellence. As a member of the health care team, you are expected to conduct yourself professionally. One sign of professionalism and seriousness of purpose is membership in your professional organization. Whether you are a member of AAMA or AMT, the benefits of membership will be invaluable to you and your future. Participation in a professional organization keeps you abreast of changes and issues facing your profession. If you are a student member, continue as an active member. If not, consider joining. Many employers will pay dues and other expenses for professional activities. Information about joining these organizations can be found at their websites.

 CHECKPOINT QUESTION

9. What is the policy of the AAMA regarding recertification of the CMA credential?

MEDIA MENU

- **Student CD**
  - **CMA/RMA Certification Exam Review**
- **Premium Online Course**
  http://thePoint.lww.com/Kronenberger3e
- **Internet Resources**

  LiveAdvise Online Tutoring & Competency Training
  http://thePoint.lww.com/LiveAdvise

  Careerspan.com
  www.careerspan.com

  Resume.com
  www.resume.com

  Resume Writers.com
  www.resumewriters.com

  Seeking Success.com
  www.seekingsuccess.com

  10 Minute Resume
  www.10minuteresume.com

  US Equal Employment Opportunity Commission
  www.eeoc.gov

  American Medical Technologists
  www.amt1.com

  American Association of Medical Assistants
  www.aama-ntl.org

PROCEDURE 46-1: Writing a Résumé

Purpose: To summarize your skills and experience and to make yourself marketable in the medical assisting profession
Equipment: Word processor, paper, personal information

Steps	Reason
1. At the top of the page, center your name, address, and phone numbers.	The reader should be able to get your contact information easily.
2. List your education starting with the most current and working back. List graduation dates and areas of study.	Give the reader only the most vital information.
3. For the chronological format, list your prior related work experience with dates, responsibilities, company, and supervisor's name. The most recent should be first. For the functional format, list skills and qualifications. (Refer to Figs. 46-6 and 46-7 for examples.)	If you have a long work history, include only jobs that used skills needed for the job for which you are applying.

(continued)

PROCEDURE 46-1:　**Writing a Résumé** *(continued)*

Steps	Reason
4. List any volunteer work with dates and places.	This will serve as proof of organizational and team-building skills. It will also show the reader that you are interested in going the extra mile and/or helping others.
5. List skills you possess including those acquired in your program and on your externship.	This will show the prospective employer exactly what skills you possess.
6. List any certifications or awards received.	This proves your competence.
7. List any information relevant to a certain position. For example, list competence in spreadsheet applications for a job in a patient billing department.	Supplying information specific to a certain position proves your competence and shows your attention to detail.
8. After obtaining permission and/or notifying the people, prepare a list of references with their addresses and phone contact information.	It is unprofessional to use someone for a reference without their knowledge and permission.
9. Carefully proofread the résumé for accuracy and typographical errors.	Many employers will automatically reject a résumé with errors.
10. Have someone else proofread the résumé for errors other than content.	Another set of eyes will ensure a perfect document.
11. Print the résumé on high-quality paper.	The appearance and professionalism of your résumé is a direct reflection of you.

Chapter Summary

- Your externship is the transition from classroom to employment. A successful externship helps lead to your ultimate goal—employment.
- During your externship, you will perform in the workplace the skills that you have learned in the classroom and laboratory.
- There are many resources to help you locate job openings. A job should be fulfilling and rewarding in ways beyond just the income. Learn how to promote yourself and earn the position you want.

- A properly written cover letter, résumé, and thank you letter will enhance your chances of getting the job.
- Continuing education, recertification, and membership in a professional organization should be sought as you look to your future as a medical assistant.
- You will work hard, but there are many rewards. Welcome to the world of medical assisting!

1. Search the internet for local job openings for medical assistants. List any available positions and any other resources identified.

2. Read the Classified section of the Sunday newspaper and select a job advertisement that interests you. Write a cover letter and résumé tailored to this position. Assume you have been called for an interview. What questions do you ask the prospective employer? What questions do you expect to be asked? Explain your responses.

3. Obtain two employee application forms from the human resources department of your local hospital. Complete one application form yourself and invite a fellow student to complete the other. Swap applications and evaluate each other's work.

Determine which areas are appropriately addressed and which need further attention.

4. Visit the Equal Employment Opportunity Commission (EEOC) website. What is the purpose of the EEOC? Where is your nearest EEOC district office? Would you talk to your supervisor if you felt that you were discriminated against? Why or why not?

5. Suppose you were just hired into your dream position. On day 2, you overhear your supervisor telling another employee, "Don't report that billing error to Medicare. They won't catch us." What would you do? Whom would you tell, or would you pretend you didn't hear it? Would you report to Medicare? Why or why not?

1. The preceptor acts as the instructor in the clinical site, providing supervision and technical direction to medical assisting students.

2. You must be dependable, professional, and well groomed.

3. The proper attire includes a freshly laundered uniform, clean shoes, neatly groomed hair, limited makeup, and jewelry kept to a minimum.

4. A student evaluation helps determine the effectiveness of the site for training and whether any issues should be addressed before assigning other students.

5. A self-analysis helps you identify your strengths and weaknesses.

6. Sources of job information include government employment offices, your school placement office,

medical facilities, private agencies, and temporary services.

7. A functional résumé stresses skills and qualifications rather than employment history. A chronological résumé lists positions held, starting with the most recent and working backward.

8. The three basic questions in every interviewer's mind are: do you have the skills I need; do you have the drive, energy, and commitment to get the job done; and will you work well with the rest of the team?

9. The recertification of the AAMA's medical assisting credential, CMA, is mandatory. You must recertify every 5 years to remain current.

CHAPTER 47 — Comprehensive Final Examination

Note: This test is based on the information in this textbook only. Students should consult the content outline of the certification examination that they plan to take (CMA or RMA) to determine the possible content of the exam.

1. A medical assistant's training focuses on:

    A. The hospital setting
    B. Outpatient services
    C. Nursing skills
    D. Secretarial skills

2. Maslow's hierarchy of human needs is based on the concept that:

    A. Physiologic needs are the most basic and must be met first
    B. Esteem must always come from people around us
    C. A safe environment is placed above all other needs
    D. People never really reach self-actualization

3. A computer program that tells the computer what to do is the:

    A. Hardware
    B. Peripheral
    C. Software
    D. CPU

4. Which of the following medical specialists cares for people who are recovering from a stroke?

    A. Endocrinologist
    B. Internist
    C. Neurologist
    D. Emergency medicine

5. Gathering information about a patient's present health care needs and abilities in preparation for teaching the patient a new diet is referred to as what?

    A. Implementation
    B. Planning
    C. Assessment
    D. Evaluation

6. A system that selects the order of patients to receive urgent medical treatment is referred to as what?

    A. Triage
    B. Selection
    C. Streamlining
    D. Matrixing

7. Which of the following is NOT required when taking a telephone message?

    A. The caller's name and phone number
    B. Time and date
    C. The name of the person to whom the call is directed
    D. The caller's account number

8. The basic elements of communication include which of the following?

    A. A message to be sent
    B. A person to send the message
    C. A person to receive the message
    D. All of the above

9. Which of the following is NOT an example of nonverbal communication?

    A. Facial expression
    B. Touch
    C. Tone
    D. Posture

10. Patients should be given instructions in writing because:

    A. Most patients cannot read
    B. Most patients do not hear well
    C. Most patients do not really care to hear the details
    D. The human memory does not perform well in stressful situations

11. Why is understanding cultural differences important?

    A. Everyone is unique and their health care needs differ
    B. One should never have predetermined notions
    C. Perceptions may vary among nationalities
    D. All of the above

12. A legally required disclosure is one that:

    A. Is given without the consent of the patient
    B. Is designed to protect the public
    C. Represents an exception to the rights of patients
    D. All of the above

13. A patient's medical record:

    A. Is considered a legal document
    B. Is only to be seen on a need-to-know basis
    C. Is the property of the physician
    D. All of the above

14. Medical ethics require physicians to:

    A. Be of good moral character
    B. Not accept money if they make a mistake
    C. Not charge a finance fee
    D. All of the above

15. A physician who treats a patient without his consent, may be charged with:

    A. Assault
    B. Negligence
    C. Ethical behavior
    D. All of the above

16. Which of the following is considered an ethical issue?

    A. Long waits for patients in physician offices
    B. Certification of physicians
    C. Allocation of scarce resources such as donated organs
    D. An unlicensed nurse

17. A patient who is noncompliant is one who:

    A. Does not pay the bill in a timely fashion
    B. Has a difficult time understanding the physician's directions
    C. Should be given instructions in writing
    D. Does not follow the doctor's orders

18. When a hearing-impaired patient is communicating with the physician:

    A. Instructions should be given to a family member
    B. The office should require that they bring an interpreter
    C. The office is responsible for providing an interpreter
    D. The two of them can write back and forth to each other

19. A physician who dispenses narcotic drugs listed in the schedule of the Controlled Substances Act must keep the narcotic records:

    A. For 4 years
    B. For 6 years

    C. Forever
    D. For 2 years

20. HIPAA is the acronym for which of the following?

    A. Health Insurance Privacy and Accountability Act
    B. Health Insurance Portability and Accounta-bility Act
    C. Healthcare Information Privacy and Accuracy Act
    D. Healthcare Information and Patient Advocacy Act

21. Among other things, HIPAA is concerned with:

    A. Protecting personal health information
    B. Patient safety
    C. Patient advocacy
    D. Patient compliance

22. Which of the following elements is NOT included in a memorandum?

    A. A heading
    B. A subject line
    C. To and from lines
    D. A complimentary close

23. A facsimile transmittal cover page:

    A. Is only necessary if you are sending the fax to someone you don't know
    B. Should include a confidentiality statement
    C. Should not be counted in the total number of pages being sent
    D. Requires postage

24. When sorting mail, you should:

    A. Place the physician's personal mail on top
    B. Dispose of any "junk mail"
    C. Place letters from other physicians in the appropriate chart
    D. Place all mail in the physician's mailbox

25. The minutes of a business meeting include all of the following, except:

    A. Motions passed
    B. Members present
    C. Members absent and the reasons for their absences
    D. A list of reports that were submitted

26. Missed appointments:

    A. Should be documented in two places
    B. Should be rescheduled by either the patient or the office
    C. Give the physician time to get caught up
    D. All of the above

27. In the following list of names, which one comes first in an alphabetical list?

    A. Stephen W. Long
    B. Jacqueline Stephens-Long
    C. Wilma Long-Adams
    D. Yolanda Long-Woodson

28. Your physician-employer is a participating provider with Mrs. Smith's insurance company. The difference in the fee for an office visit and the amount the insurance company "allows" for that service must be:

    A. Billed to the patient
    B. Adjusted off of the patient's account
    C. Collected at the patient's next visit
    D. Sent to a collection agency

29. A physician's fee schedule is determined by using UCRs, which means what?

    A. United compared resources
    B. Universal customary regulation
    C. Resource-based relative value scale
    D. Usual, customary, and reasonable

30. ICD-9 CM is a coding system used to report what?

    A. Services provided by a nurse practitioner
    B. Services provided by a physician
    C. Medical necessity for services and procedures
    D. Procedures performed on the patient

31. CPT-4 Codes include E&M codes, which are used to report what?

    A. Office procedures performed by a provider
    B. Anesthesia and surgeries
    C. Provider services and visits
    D. Medical necessity for services and procedures

32. In the ICD-9 coding system, a late effect is:

    A. A separately identifiable condition that is present during treatment of an acute illness or injury
    B. A symptom or condition arising from an acute illness that is still being treated after the acute illness has passed
    C. Always found by looking up "late effect" in the alphabetical index
    D. Left off of the CMS-1500 universal claim form after the acute illness is no longer being treated

33. The money owed to a physician for items such as rent, utilities, and payroll is referred to as what?

    A. Accounts receivable
    B. Business expenses
    C. Fixed accounts
    D. Accounts payable

34. What is the best way to ensure an accurate visual acuity exam?

    A. Provide adequate lighting
    B. Have the patient close one eye
    C. Ask the patient to speak up
    D. Allow the patient to sit down if necessary

35. At what age should children have their first MMR vaccination?

    A. Birth
    B. 12–15 months
    C. 2–3 months
    D. 12 months

36. At what age should children have their first hepatitis B vaccination?

    A. Birth
    B. 12–15 months
    C. 2–3 months
    D. 12 months

37. Which of the following is a normal rectal temperature?

    A. 99.6°F
    B. 98.6°F
    C. 97.6°F
    D. 95.6°F

38. Autoclaving is the only process that destroys all forms of living organisms, including:

    A. Spores
    B. Tuberculosis
    C. Viruses
    D. Bacteria

39. Following sterilization by autoclaving, the items remain sterile for how long?

    A. 21 days
    B. 2 weeks
    C. 30 days
    D. It depends on the item

40. In order to accomplish sterilization, the autoclave should reach what temperature?

    A. 250–270°F
    B. 260–270°F
    C. 35-37°C
    D. 150°F

41. What is the most effective way to break the infection cycle?

    A. Wash your hands often
    B. Use only antibacterial soap
    C. Wash hands in Clorox
    D. Stay at home

42. Cross-contamination can be prevented by:

    A. Washing your hands between patients
    B. Washing the examination table with Clorox and water
    C. Sterilizing and/or disinfecting instruments
    D. All of the above

43. The most accurate way to measure the length of an infant is to:

    A. Use the measuring device on the back of the infant scale
    B. Make a mark on the exam table paper at the baby's head and bottom of feet
    C. Use a yard stick
    D. Stand the infant up on the adult scale

44. Anaphylactic shock involves:

    A. Dysfunction of the nervous system following spinal injury
    B. General infection of the bloodstream
    C. Loss of blood and/or body fluids
    D. General allergic reaction to a foreign substance

45. In a physical examination, inspection refers to:

    A. Visual scanning of the patient
    B. Determining a patient's level of pain by his facial expression
    C. Feeling the patient's internal organs
    D. Looking over the patient's chart

46. Where is a Colles' fracture located?

    A. Ankle
    B. Wrist
    C. Elbow
    D. Leg

47. Hepatitis B and rubella are examples of disease caused by what?

    A. Yeasts
    B. Fungi
    C. Bacteria
    D. Viruses

48. Which of the following sutures does not usually require removal from the body?

    A. Catgut
    B. Silk
    C. Nylon
    D. Cotton

49. The first step performed to set up a sterile field is to do what?

    A. Open the sterile pack
    B. Wash your hands
    C. Prepare the local anesthetic in a syringe
    D. Put on gloves

50. In a standard EKG, lead V3 is located where?

    A. At the fourth intercostal space
    B. At the fifth intercostal space
    C. Midway between V2 and V4
    D. Anywhere on the right side of the chest

51. The EKG tracing is printed on graph paper at what standard speed?

    A. 10 cm/sec
    B. 50 mm/sec
    C. 35 cm/sec
    D. 25 mm/sec

52. A subcutaneous injection is given using which of the following techniques?

    A. A 45-degree angle with a 25-gauge needle
    B. A 15-degree angle with a 21-gauge needle
    C. A 90-degree angle with a 25-gauge needle
    D. A 45-degree angle with any size needle

53. The reason you must aspirate before injecting a medication is to be sure:

    A. The patient receives all of the medication
    B. The needle is not in a blood vessel
    C. The injection is less painful
    D. The needle is in the muscle

54. An iron preparation is administered by which of the following methods?

    A. Subcutaneous
    B. Z-track
    C. Intravenous
    D. Sublingual

55. The five phases of Korotkoff sounds may be heard when auscultating what?

    A. The pulse
    B. The carotid arteries
    C. The blood pressure
    D. The heart

56. Which classification of drugs prevents or decreases clotting?

    A. Anticoagulant
    B. Antiemetic
    C. Antineoplastic
    D. Antipyretic

57. The physician orders 500 mg of a medication tid for 10 days. The medication is available only in 250-mg capsules. How many capsules will the patient need to complete the course of medication?

   A. 60
   B. 120
   C. 45
   D. 30

58. Which organization developed guidelines to help people in making healthy diet decisions?

   A. FDA
   B. USDA
   C. CDC
   D. DEA

59. Which type of cholesterol is referred to as the "good cholesterol"?

   A. Unsaturated fats
   B. High-density lipoproteins
   C. Low-density lipoproteins
   D. Saturated fats

60. A clear liquid diet includes all of the following, except:

   A. Chicken broth
   B. Apple juice
   C. Tea
   D. Milk

61. Exercises performed with assistance are called what?

   A. Passive exercises
   B. Active exercises
   C. Range-of-motion exercises
   D. Aerobic exercises

62. Reasons a physician might order a 24-hour urine collection for a test include all of the following, except:

   A. Because of diurnal variation
   B. To compare the 24-hour value with the serum value
   C. For a culture and sensitivity
   D. To aid in diagnosis of glomerular disease

63. Which of the following is the white blood cell count useful in determining?

   A. Anemia
   B. Coagulation factors
   C. Infection
   D. Platelet count

64. What information does a hemoglobin result provide about the patient?

   A. Helps to diagnose heart and liver diseases
   B. The amount of sugar in the blood
   C. The oxygen-carrying capacity of the blood
   D. The count of the number of cells that participate in blood clotting

65. A 9-year-old child falls off his skateboard going down a flight of concrete stairs. The child comes running home, where his mother notes some blood over the child's right knee and takes him to the emergency room. The ER doctor notes that the skin just below the knee has been scraped and irregularly broken to reveal underlying soft tissue over an area of 1×3 cm. This injury is best described as a/an:

   A. Abrasion
   B. Contusion
   C. Incision
   D. Laceration

66. A 54-year-old male has a long history of diabetes mellitus. Most of the time, his blood sugar was really high, causing damage to his kidneys. What laboratory result is most likely to be elevated?

   A. Blood urea nitrogen
   B. Rheumatoid factor
   C. Calcium
   D. Prothrombin

67. The ability to repeatedly run a lab test and get the same result is called what?

   A. Accuracy
   B. Acceptability
   C. Calibration
   D. Precision

68. What action do you take if you have a critical value result on a patient?

   A. Get the information to the physician as soon as possible
   B. Record the information in the patient's chart
   C. Repeat the quality control before reporting the result
   D. Repeat the test

69. Two levels of quality control material must be analyzed:

   A. Annually
   B. By the policy you learned at school
   C. Following the manufacturer's instructions
   D. With each unknown specimen

70. The purpose of OSHA is:

    A. To protect all workers from occupational injury
    B. To identify epidemiology and track public health
    C. To establish policies on total quality management
    D. To provide tax relief for all laboratories

71. Anyone who has been thoroughly trained and demonstrates competency for the testing procedures regardless of educational background can perform which of the following?

    A. Complex tests
    B. Lab tests
    C. Waived tests
    D. Moderately complex tests

72. The first drop of a capillary puncture is removed with a clean gauze pad because it contains what?

    A. Bacteria
    B. Hemolysis
    C. Tissue thromboplastin
    D. Lipids

73. Bloodborne pathogens are:

    A. Human blood components and products made from human blood
    B. Disease-producing microorganisms transmitted by blood, body fluid, and tissue
    C. The presence of blood, body fluid, and tissue that can cause disease in humans
    D. Blood with potentially infectious materials that has soiled laundry

74. Why can latex gloves cause problems in providing patient care?

    A. They are easily perforated
    B. They may cause allergic reactions
    C. The powder frequently gets in workers' eyes
    D. Most manufacturers cannot keep up with demand

75. Which of the following vacuum tubes provides the least vacuum draw?

    A. 10 mL
    B. 7 mL
    C. 4.5 mL
    D. 2 mL

76. What is the reason why a 25-gauge needle is not recommended for blood collection?

    A. The red cells may be broken
    B. The needle will be too painful for the patient
    C. The bevel is too large
    D. The needle is too short to reach deeper veins

77. The fibrinogen-filled fluid that remains after centrifuging a tube of blood is:

    A. Plasma
    B. Anticoagulated blood
    C. Serum
    D. Whole blood

78. The primary veins located in the anticubital fossa are basilica, cephalic, and:

    A. Median cubital
    B. Brachial
    C. Median cephalic
    D. Median capital

79. All of the following are reasons for blood specimen rejection, except:

    A. Not enough blood collected
    B. Hemolysis
    C. Hematoma resulted
    D. Unlabeled tubes

80. What is the maximum time a tourniquet can be applied without jeopardizing the quality of the specimen?

    A. 2 minutes
    B. Two times
    C. 3 minutes with a difficult draw
    D. 1 minute

81. The process used to trace the direction of the vein and to hold it in place is called what?

    A. Pumping
    B. Locating
    C. Anchoring
    D. Palpating

82. Which of the following is a glucose procedure that is collected 2 hours after consuming a carbohydrate meal?

    A. Stat glucose
    B. GTT
    C. 2-hour postprandial
    D. 2-hour glucose tolerance

83. The chemical examination of urine includes measurements of what?

    A. Color
    B. Bilirubin
    C. Clarity
    D. Odor

84. Some noncellular components of plasma are:

    A. Fats and hormones
    B. RBCs and WBCs
    C. Hormones and RBCs
    D. WBCs and serum

85. Oxygen is distributed in the cells of the body by which of the following?

    A. Platelets
    B. Leukocytes
    C. Erythrocytes
    D. Plasma

86. Where are erythrocytes formed?

    A. Liver
    B. Bone marrow
    C. Kidney
    D. Blood

87. Lipid tests include all of the following, except:

    A. HDL
    B. Bilirubin
    C. LDL
    D. Triglycerides

88. What hormone are you looking for in a pregnancy test?

    A. IgG
    B. hCG
    C. Estrogen
    D. Testosterone

89. What must laboratories provide for their employees?

    A. Safety and protection
    B. Education and training
    C. Health and welfare
    D. Retirement and health insurance

90. A patient's urine is yellow-orange. Which of the following substances would be found in the urine?

    A. Protein
    B. Glucose
    C. Nitrate
    D. Bilirubin

91. In the process of containing a blood sample by Vacutainer, a hematoma begins to form. Which is the most likely scenario?

    A. The bevel is inserted above the vein
    B. The bevel is only partially inserted in the vein
    C. The bevel is against the wall of the vein
    D. The bevel is in the middle of the vein

92. Which of the following tubes is used for RBC and WBC counts?

    A. Lavender
    B. Light blue
    C. Green
    D. Gray

93. What test is done by the Westergren method?

    A. CBC
    B. Sedimentation rate
    C. Coagulation test
    D. Hemoglobin

94. What is the best description of low-density lipoprotein?

    A. A complex molecule consisting of protein and a fat such as cholesterol
    B. The form in which carbohydrates are stored in the body
    C. A lipoprotein consisting of protein and cholesterol that removes excess cholesterol from blood vessel walls
    D. A lipoprotein consisting of protein and cholesterol that adheres to blood vessel walls, forming plaque

95. Which of the following is the causative agent of infectious mononucleosis?

    A. Variola major
    B. Epstein-Barr virus
    C. Cytomegalovirus
    D. Human immunodeficiency virus

96. The major purpose of an MSDS is:

    A. To provide information to clean up spills
    B. To provide information to protect employees and patients
    C. To complete all OSHA regulations
    D. To guide PPE use, identifying hazardous chemicals and procedures to follow for chemical exposure

97. Which laboratory department deals with disease-producing eggs present in specimens taken from the body?

    A. Parasitology
    B. Hematology
    C. Virology
    D. Chemistry

98. The presence of sugar in the urine is called what?

    A. Glycogen
    B. Hypoglycemia
    C. Glycosuria
    D. Hyperglycemia

99. What is the BEST way to avoid cross-contaminating patients who receive instillation of eyedrops from the same bottle?

    A. Wash your hands after instillation
    B. Wipe the tip of the dropper with a paper towel before and after each use

C. Avoid touching the tip of the dropper to the patient's eye

D. Have each patient bring their own bottle

100. Which laboratory department deals with the identification of pathogens?

A. Chemistry
B. Hematology
C. Microbiology
D. Immunohematology

Appendix A

Health Insurance Portability and Accountability Act (HIPAA)

Throughout the text, The Health Insurance Portability and Accountability Act of 1996, known as HIPAA, is discussed. Chapters 2 and 8 discuss HIPAA's Privacy Ruling The 104th US Congress had six goals in passing Public Law 104-191.

- To improve the portability of group and individual insurance companies by regulating such issues as refusal of coverage for pre-existing conditions and continuing coverage when changing jobs
- To fight against fraud, abuse, and waste in the health care industry.
- To promote the use of Medical Savings Accounts
- To improve access to long-term care services and coverage
- To promote efficiency by simplifying the business of filing claims and processing of health insurance
- To provide funds for reforms and other related purposes.

In keeping with the focus of this textbook, the discussion of HIPAA has been limited to issues related to the outpatient health care arena. Two areas directly influencing the medical office are found in Title II: Preventing Health Care Fraud and Abuse; Administrative Simplification; Medical Liability Reform. The Privacy Ruling from Title II addresses the issues of the rights of patients to protect their personally identifiable health information (PIHI). Information revealing physical and/or mental conditions and treatments that can be **directly linked** to a particular patient is considered personally identifiable health information (PIHI). Your goal is to protect the patient's privacy.

Following are some scenarios you might encounter in a typical day in a physician's office. An explanation follows.

1. A new patient refuses to sign the acknowledgment of receipt of a Notification of Privacy Practices (NOPP), the form requested by HIPAA's Privacy Ruling. Do we turn the patient away?

    No. You are only required to make a "good faith effort" to received acknowledgment of an NOPP. Document the patient's refusal to sign.

2. One of your duties is to call patients to remind them of their appointments. Would leaving a message with the time and location of the appointment be a violation of the Privacy Ruling?

    No. "This is Terri at Dr. Smith's office calling to remind you of your appointment tomorrow at 10:00" does not disclose personal health information.

3. You have been asked to notify a patient with his test results? Can you leave a message?

    Maybe. Sensitive information should be treated as such. Patients should sign an authorization that gives you permission to leave any message on their voicemail. In the absence of that documentation, you would not leave test results on voicemail.

4. A hospital admissions representative calls and asks for a patient's insurance information. Is it okay to give her the patient's subscriber number, etc.?

    HIPAA was never meant to limit the sharing of information to the point that it interferes with the patient care or the financial issues involved. Only the minimum amount of information should be shared with only those who need to know. Giving the representative the information helps the patient in the long run.

5. A patient requests copies of her records. The chart contains letters and reports from other physicians and facilities. Should she be given these documents also, or would she need to request these from the physicians or facilities that generated them?

    Once the medical information becomes a part of a patient's chart in your office, it is okay to release it with proper authorization. Since all of the documents were used in the care and management of the patient in your office, all documents are now part of the record.

6. You need to request a radiology report on a patient coming in this afternoon. Is it okay to have it faxed over?

    Yes, it is okay as long as the fax machine is out of the view of patients and other visitors. The fax

should have a cover sheet with the name of the person who should receive the fax. It should be delivered to that person by anyone who retrieves it.

7. You receive an operative report addressed to Dr. Richard Adams on your fax machine, but your physician is Dr. Robert Adams. As soon as you see the cover sheet, you realize you received it by mistake. What should you do?

Since you do not have a need to know, do not read the report. Call the number on the cover sheet, and tell them that you received the report in error. This alerts them to send another one to the correct Dr. Adams. Then shred the copy you received by mistake.

8. What if the last scenario was reversed? You sent a fax to the wrong number. You realize it just as you push the "Send" button.

Call the party who received the information and ask them to shred it. Document the error in the patient's chart. If you do not know who received the misdirected fax, you should notify the patient of the possible breach.

9. Your boss asks you to check on the condition of his next door neighbor who is in the hospital. He tells you to let them know that he is the one requesting the information. Is this possible?

Yes. A patient being admitted to a hospital may choose to be excluded from the hospital directory, and no information can be given out by the hospital. If the neighbor did not opt out of the directory, you will be given the patient's room number and general condition. Unless involved in the patient's care, your physician has no special privileges to protected health information.

10. You work in a busy pediatric office. You are the PA as he examines a 2-year-old boy with a possible concussion. He tells you that he suspects abuse. Can you report this without authorization?

Not only can you report it, but you MUST report it. The Child Abuse Prevention and Treatment Act of 1974 (CAPTA) made reporting possible child abuse mandatory.

Adapted from Krager D, Krager C. HIPAA for Medical Office Personnel. New York: Thomson Delmar Learning; 2005.

Appendix B

Key English-to-Spanish Health Care Phrases

Although English is the major language spoken in North America, a variety of languages are used in certain areas. Prominent among them is Spanish, representing Spain, the Caribbean Islands, Central and South America, and the Philippines. Rapport can be more easily established, and the patient and family will be at ease and feel more relaxed, if someone on the staff speaks their language. Some health care facilities, especially in areas with a large population of Spanish-speaking people, provide interpreters. In smaller hospitals or smaller communities this may not be possible.

It is to your advantage to learn the second most prominent language in your community. For this reason, the following table of English-to-Spanish phrases has been prepared. Instructions for using it are simple. Look for the phrase in English in the first column of the table. The second colulmn gives the phrase in Spanish. You can write this or point to it. The third column gives a phonetic pronunciation. The syllable in each word to be accented is printed in italic type. Even if you are not proficient in English-to-Spanish, your Spanish-speaking patients will appreciate your trying to converse in their language. Begin with "Buenos días. ¿Cómo se siente?" And remember "por favor."[a]

Introductory Phrases

English	Spanish	Pronunciation
please[a]	por favor	por fah-*vor*
thank you	gracias	*grah*-see-ahs
good morning	buenos días	*bway*-nos *dee*-ahs
good afternoon	buenas tárdes	*bway*-nas *tar*-days
good evening	buenas noches	*bway*-nas *noh*-chays
my name is	mi nombre es	me *nohm*-bray ays
yes/no	si/no	see/no
What is your name?	¿Cómo se llama?	¿Koh-moh say *jah*-mah?
How old are you?	¿Cuántos años tienes?	¿*Kwan*-tohs ahn-yos tee-*aynj*ays?
Do you understand me?	¿Me entiende?	¿Me ayn-tee-*ayn*-day?
Speak slower.	Habla más despacio.	*Ah*-blah mahs days-*pah*-see-oh
Say it once again.	Repítalo, por favor.	Ray-*pee*-tah-loh, por fah-*vor*
How do you feel?	¿Cómo se siente?	¿*Koh*-moh say see-*ayn*-tay?
good	bien	bee-ayn
bad	mal	*mah*l
physician	médico	*may*-dee-koh
hospital	hospital	*ooh*-spee-tall
midwife	comadre	koh-*mah*-dray
native healer	curandero	ku-ren-*day*-roh

From Rosdahl, C.B. [1995]. Textbook of Basic Nursing, 6th ed. Philadelphia: J.B. Lippincott.
[a] You should begin or end any request with the word PLEASE (POR FAVOR).

General

zero	cero	*se*-roh
one	uno	*oo*-noh
two	dos	dohs
three	tres	trays
four	cuatro	*kwah*-troh
five	cinco	*sin*-koh
six	seis	says
seven	siete	see-*ay*-tay
eight	ocho	oh-choh
nine	nueve	new-*ay*-vay
ten	diez	*dee*-ays
hundred	ciento, cien	see-*en*-toh, see-*en*
hundred and one	ciento uno	see-*en*-toh oo-noh
Sunday	domingo	doh-*ming*-goh
Monday	lunes	*loo*-nays
Tuesday	martes	*mar*-tays
Wednesday	miércoles	mee-*er*-cohl-ays
Thursday	jueves	*hway*-vays
Friday	viernes	vee-*ayr*-nays
Saturday	sábado	*sah*-bah-doh
right	derecho	day-*ray*-choh
left	izqierdo	ees-kee-*ayr*-doh
early in the morning	temprano por la mañana	tehm-*prah*-noh por lah mah-*nyah*-na
in the daytime	en el dìa	ayn el *dee*-ah
at noon	a mediodía	ah meh-dee-oh-*dee*-ah
at bedtime	al acostarse	al ah-kos-*tar*-say
at night	por la noche	por la *noh*-chay
today	ñoy	oy
tomorrow	mañana	mah-*nyah*-nah
yesterday	ayer	ai-*yer*
week	semana	say-*may*-nah
month	mes	mace

Parts of the Body

the head	la cabeza	la kah-*bay*-sah
the eye	el ojo	el o-hoh
the ears	los oídos	lohs o-*ee*-dohs
the nose	la nariz	la nah-*reez*
the mouth	la boca	lah *boh*-kah
the tongue	la lengua	la *len*-gwah
the neck	el cuello	el koo-*eh*-joh
the throat	la garganta	lah gar-*gan*-tah
the skin	la piel	la pee-el
the bones	los huesos	lohs hoo-*ay*-sos
the muscles	los músculos	lohs *moos*-koo-lohs
the nerves	los nervios	lohs *nayhr*-vee-ohs
the shoulder blades	las paletillas	lahs pah-lay-*tee*-jahs
the arm	el brazo	el *brah*-soh
the elbow	el codo	el *koh*-doh
the wrist	la muñeca	lah moon-*yeh*-kah
the hand	la mano	lah *mah*-noh
the chest	el pecho	el *pay*-choh

the lungs	los pulmones	lohs puhl-*moh*-nays
the heart	el corazón	el koh-rah-*son*
the ribs	las costillas	lahs kohs-*tee*-jahs
the side	el flanco	el *flahn*-koh
the back	la espalda	lay ays-*pahl*-dah
the abdomen	el abdomen	el ahb-*doh*-men
the stomach	el estómago	el ays-*toh*-mah-goh
the leg	la pierna	lah pee-ehr-nah
the thigh	el muslo	el *moos*-loh
the ankle	el tobillo	el toh-*bee*-joh
the foot	el pie	el *pee*-ay
urine	urino	u-*re*-noh

Diseases

allergy	alergia	ah-*layr*-hee-ah
anemia	anemia	ah-*nay*-mee-ah
cancer	cancer	kahn-sayr
chickenpox	varicela	vah-ree-*say*-lah
diabetes	diabetes	dee-ah-bay-tees
diphtheria	difteria	deef-*tay*-ree-ah
German measles	rubéola	roo-*bay*-oh-lah
gonorrhea	gonorrea	gun-noh-*ree*-ah
heart disease	enfermedad del corazón	ayn-*fayr*-may-*dahd* dayl koh-rah-*sohn*
high blood pressure	presión alta	pray-see-*ohn* *al*-ta
influenza	gripe	*gree*-pay
lead poisoning	envenenamiento con plomo	ayn-vay-nay-nah-mee-*ayn*-toh kohn *ploh*-moh
liver disease	enfermedad del hígado	ayn-*fayr*-may-dahd del *ee*-gah-doh
measles	sarampión	sah-rahm-pee-*ohn*
mumps	paperas	pah-*pay*-rahs
nervous disease	enfermedades nerviosa	ayn-fayr-may-*dahd*-days nayr-vee-oh-sah
pleurisy	pleuresía	play-oo-ray-*see*-ah
pneumonia	pulmonía	pool-moh-*nee*-ah
rheumatic fever	reumatismo (fiebre reumatica)	ray-oo-mah-*tees*-moh (fee-*ay*-bray ray-oo-*mah*-tee-kah)
scarlet fever	escarlatina	ays-kahr-lah-*tee*-nah
syphilis	sífilis	*see*-fee-lees
tuberculosis	tuberculosis	too-*bayr*-koo-lohs-sees

Signs and Symptoms

Do you have stomach cramps?	¿Tiene calambres en el estómago?	¿Tee-*ay*-nay kah-*lahm*-brays ayn el ays-*toh*-mah-goh?
chills?	escalofrios?	ays-kah-loh-*free*-ohs?
an attack of fever	un ataque de fiebre?	oon ah-*tah*-kay day fee-*ay*-bray?
hemorrhage?	hemoragia?	ay-moh-*rah*-hee-ah?
nosebleeds?	hemoragia por la nariz?	ay-moh-*rah*-hee-ah por-lah nah-*rees*?
unusual vaginal bleeding?	hemoragia vaginal fuera de los periodos?	ay-moh-*rah*-hee-ah *vah*-hee-nahl foo-*ay*-rah day lohs pay-ree-*oh*-dohs?
hoarseness?	ronquera?	rohn-*kay*-rah?
a sore throat?	le duele la garganta?	lay doo-*ay*-lay lah gahr-*gahn*-tah?

Does it hurt to swallow?	¿Le duele al tragar?	¿Lay doo-ay-lay ahl trah-gar?
Have you any difficulty in breathing?	¿Tiene difficultad al respirar?	¿Tee-ay-nay dee-fee-kool-tahd ahl rays-pee-rahr?
Does it pain you to breathe?	¿Le duele al respirar?	¿Lay doo-ay-lay ahl rays-pee-rahr?
How does your head feel?	¿Cómo siente la cabeza?	¿Koh-moh see-ayn-tay lah kah-bay-sah?
Is your memory good?	¿Es buena su memoria?	¿Ays bway-nah soo may-moh-ree-ah?
Have you any pain the head?	¿Le duele la cabeza?	¿Lay doo-ay-lay lah Kah-bay-sah?
Do you feel dizzy?	¿Tiene usted vértigo?	¿Tee-ay-nay ood-stayd vehr-tee-goh?
Are you tired?	¿Está usted cansado?	¿Ay-stah ood-stayd kahn-sah-doh?
Can you eat?	¿Puede comer?	¿Pway-day koh-mer?
Have you a good appetite?	¿Tiene usted buen apetito?	¿Tee-ay-nay ood-stayd bwayn ah-pay-tee-toh?
How are your stools?	¿Cómo son sus heces fecales?	¿Kog-moh sohn soos bay-says fay-kal-ays?
Are they regular?	¿Son regulares?	¿Sohn ray-goo-lah-rays?
Are you constipated?	¿Está estreñido?	¿Ay-stah ays-trayn-yee-do?
Do you have diarrhea?	¿Tiene diarrea?	¿Tee-ay-nay dee-ah-ray-ah?
Have you any difficulty passing water?	¿Tiene dificultad en orinar?	¿Tee-ay-nay dee-fee-kool-tahd ayn oh-ree-nahr?
Do you pass water involuntarily?	¿Orina sin querer?	¿Oh-ree-nah seen kay-rayr?
How long have you felt this way?	¿Desde cuándo se siente asi?	¿Days-day Kwan-doh say see-ayn-tay ah-see?
What diseases have you had?	¿Qué enfermedades ha tenido?	¿Kay ayn-fer-may-dah-days hah tay-nee-doh?
Do you hear voices?	¿Tiene los voces?	¿Tee-ay-nay los vo-ses?

Examination

Remove your clothing.	Quítese su ropa.	Key-tay-say soo roh-pah.
Put on this gown.	Pongáse la bata.	Phon-gah-say lah bah-tah.
We need a urine specimen.	Es necesário una muestra de su orina.	Ays nay-say-sar-ee-oh oo-nah moo-ay-strah day oh-ree-nah.
Be seated.	Siéntese.	See-ayn-tay-say.
Recline.	Acuestése.	Ah-cways-tay-say.
Sit up.	Siéntese.	See-ayn-tay-say.
Stand.	Parése.	Pah-ray-say.
Bend your knees.	Doble las rodíllas.	Doh-blay lahs roh-dee-yahs.
Relax your muscles.	Reláje los músculos.	Ray-lah-hay lohs moos-koo-lohs.
Try to . . .	Atente . . .	Ah-tayn-tay . . .
Try again.	Atente ótra vez.	Ah-tayn-tay oh-tra vays.
Do not move.	No se múeva.	Noh say moo-ay-vah.
Turn on (or to) your left side.	Voltese a su lado izquierdo.	Vohl-tay-say ah soo lah-doh is-key-ayr-doh.
Turn on (or to) your right side.	Voltése a su ládo derécho.	Vohl-tay-say ah soo lah-doh day-ray-choh.
Take a deep breath.	Respíra profúndo.	Ray-speer-rah pro-foon-doh.
Hold your breath.	Deténga su respiración.	Day-tayn-gah soo ray-speer-ah-see-ohn.
Don't hold your breath.	No deténga su respiración.	Noh day-tayn-gah soo ray-speer-ah-see-ohn.
Cough.	Tosa.	Toh-sah.
Open your mouth.	Abra la boca.	Ah-brah lah boh-kah.

Show me . . .	Enséñeme . . .	Ayn-*sayn*-yay-may . . .
Here?	¿Aqui?	¿Ah-*kee*?
There?	¿Allí?	¿Ah-*jee*?
Which side?	¿En qué lado?	¿Ayn kay *lah*-doh?
Let me see your hand.	Enséñeme la mano.	Ayn-*sehn*-yay-may lah *mah*-noh.
Grasp my hand.	Apriete mi mano.	Ah-*pree*-it-tay mee *mah*-noh.
Raise your arm.	Levante el brazo.	Lay-*vahn*-tay el *brah*-soh.
Raise it more.	Más alto.	Mahs *ahl*-toh.
Now the other.	Ahora el otro.	Ah-*oh*-rah el *oh*-troh.

Treatment

It is necessary.	Es necessario.	Ays neh-say-*sah*-ree-oh.
An operation is necessary.	Una operación es necesaria.	Oo-nah oh-peh-rah-see-*ohn* ays neh-say-*sah*-ree-ah.
a prescription	una receta	*oo*-na ray-say-tah
Use it regularly.	Tómelo con regularidad.	*Toh*-may-loh kohn ray-goo-*lah*-ree-dad.
Take one teaspoonful three times daily (in water).	Toma una cucharadita tres veces al dia, con agua.	*Toh*-may oo-na koo-chah-rah-*dee*-tah trays *vay*-says ahl *dee*-ah, kohn ah-gwah.
Gargle.	Haga gargaras.	*Ah*-gah gar-*gah*-rahs.
Use injection.	Use una inyección.	*Oo*-say *oo*-nah in-*yek*-see-ohn.
oral contraceptives	una pildora	*oo*-nah peel-*doh*-rah
a pill	una pastilla	*oo*-nah pahs-*tee*-yah
a powder	un polvo	oon *pohl*-voh
before meals	antes de las comidas	*ahn*-tays day lahs koh-*mee*-dahs
after meals	despues de las comidas	*days*-poo-ehs day lahs koh-mee-dahs
every day	todos los día	*toh*-dohs lohs *dee*-ah
every hour	cada hora	*kah*-dah *oh*-rah
Breathe slowly—like this (in this manner).	Respire despacio—asi.	Rays-*pee*-ray days-*pah*-see-oh—ah-*see*.
Remain on a diet.	Estar a dieta.	Ays-*tar* a dee-*ay*-tah.

General

How do you feel?	¿Cómo se siénte?	¿*Koh*-moh say see-*ayn*-tay?
Do you have pain?	¿Tiéne dolor?	¿Tee-*ay*-nay doh-*lorh*?
Where is the pain?	¿Adónde es el dolor?	¿Ah-*dohn*-day ays ayl doh-*lorh*?
Do you want medication for your pain?	¿Quiére medicación para su dolor?	¿Kay-*ay*-ray may-dee-kah see-*ohn* *pak*-rah soo doh-*lorh*?
Are you comfortable?	¿Está confortáble?	¿Ay-*stah* kohn-for-*tah*-blay?
Are you thirsty?	¿Tiéne sed?	¿Tee-*ay*-nay sayd?
You may not eat/drink.	No cóma/béba.	Noh *koh*-mah/bay-*bah*.
You can only drink water.	Solo puede tomar agua.	Soh-loh *pway*-day toh-mar *ah*-gwah.
Apply bandage to . . .	Ponga una vendaje a . . .	*Pohn*-gah *oo*-nah vehn-*dah*-hay ah . . .
Apply ointment.	Aplíquese unguento.	Ah-*plee*-kay-say oon-goo-*ayn*-toh.
Keep very quiet.	Estese muy quieto.	Ays-*tay*-say moo-ay key-*ay*-toh.
You must not speak.	No debe hablar.	Noh *day*-bay ha-*blahr*
It will be uncomfortable.	Séra incomódo.	*Say*-rah een-koh-*moh*-doh.
It will sting.	Va ardér.	Vah ahr-*dayr*.
You will feel pressure.	Vá a sentír presión.	Vah ah sayn-*teer* pray-see-*ohn*.
I am going to . . .	Voy a . . .	Voy ah . . .
Count (take) your pulse.	Tomár su púlso.	Toh-*marh* soo *pool*-soh.

Take your temperature.	Tomár su temperatúra.	Toh-*marh* soo taym-pay-rah-*too*-rah.
Take your blood pressure.	Tomar su presión.	Toh-*mahr* soo pray-see-*ohn*.
Give you pain medicine.	Dárle medicación para dolór.	*Dahr*-lay may dee-kah-see-*ohn* pah-rah doh-*lohr*.
You should (try to) . . .	Trate de . . .	*Tray*-tay day . . .
Call for help/assistance.	Llamar para asisténcia.	Yah-*marh* pah-rah ah-sees-*tayn*-see-ah.
Empty your bladder.	Orinar.	Oh-ree-*narh*.
Do you still feel very weak?	¿Se siente muy débil todavía?	¿Say see-*ayn*-tay moo-ee *day*-beel toh-dah-*vee*-ah?
It is important to . . .	Es importánte que . . .	Ays eem-por-*tahn*-tay Kay . . .
Walk (ambulate).	Caminar.	Kah-mee-*narh*.
Drink fluids.	Beber líquidos.	Bay-*bayr lee*-kay-dohs.

Appendix C

Two-Letter Postal ZIP Code Abbreviations

Alabama	AL	Nebraska	NE
Alaska	AK	Nevada	NV
Arizona	AZ	New Hampshire	NH
Arkansas	AR	New Jersey	NJ
American Samoa	AS	New Mexico	NM
California	CA	New York	NY
Colorado	CO	North Carolina	NC
Connecticut	CT	North Dakota	ND
Delaware	DE	Northern Mariana Islands	MP
District of Columbia	DC	Ohio	OH
Federated States of Micronesia	FM	Oklahoma	OK
Florida	FL	Oregon	OR
Georgia	GA	Palau	PW
Guam	GU	Pennsylvania	PA
Hawaii	HI	Puerto Rico	PR
Idaho	ID	Rhode Island	RI
Illinois	IL	South Carolina	SC
Indiana	IN	South Dakota	SD
Iowa	IA	Tennessee	TN
Kansas	KS	Texas	TX
Kentucky	KY	Utah	UT
Louisiana	LA	Vermont	VT
Maine	ME	Virginia	VA
Marshall Islands	MH	Virgin Islands	VI
Maryland	MD	Washington	WA
Massachusetts	MA	West Virginia	WV
Michigan	MI	Wisconsin	WI
Minnesota	MN	Wyoming	WY
Mississippi	MS	Armed Forces of the Americas	AA
Missouri	MO	Armed Forces Europe	AE
Montana	MT	Armed Forces Pacific	AP

Abbreviations and symbols that appear in red font are considered "Dangerous Abbreviations" and should not be used.

Abbreviation or Symbol	Meaning
ā	before
A	anterior; assessment
A&P	auscultation and percussion
A&W	alive and well
AB	abortion
ABG	arterial blood gas
a.c.	before meals
ACE	angiotensin-converting enzyme
ACS	acute coronary syndrome
ACTH	adrenocorticotropic hormone
AD	right ear
ad lib.	as desired
ADH	antidiuretic hormone
ADHD	attention-deficit/hyperactivity disorder
AIDS	acquired immunodeficiency syndrome
AKA	above-knee amputation
alb	albumin
ALS	amyotrophic lateral sclerosis
ALT	alanine aminotransferase (enzyme)
a.m.	morning
amt	amount
ANS	autonomic nervous system
AP	anterior-posterior
APKD	adult polycystic kidney disease
Aq	water
AS	left ear
ASD	atrial septal defect
AST	aspartate aminotransferase (enzyme)
AU	both ears
AV	atrioventricular
Ⓑ	bilateral
BAEP	brainstem auditory evoked potential
BAER	brainstem auditory evoked response

Abbreviation or Symbol	Meaning
BCC	basal cell carcinoma
BD	bipolar disorder
b.i.d.	twice a day
BKA	below-knee amputation
BM	bowel movement
BMP	basic metabolic panel
BP	blood pressure
BPH	benign prostatic hypertrophy; benign prostatic hyperplasia
BRP	bathroom privileges
BS	blood sugar
BUN	blood urea nitrogen
Bx	biopsy
c̄	with
C	Celsius; centigrade
C&S	culture and sensitivity
CABG	coronary artery bypass graft
CAD	coronary artery disease
Cap	capsule
CAT	computed axial tomography
CBC	complete blood count
cc	cubic centimeter
CC	chief complaint
CCU	coronary (cardiac) care unit
CF	cystic fibrosis
CHF	congestive heart failure
CIN	cervical intraepithelial neoplasia
CIS	carcinoma in situ
cm	centimeter
CMP	comprehensive metabolic panel
CNS	central nervous system
c/o	complains of
CO	cardiac output
CO_2	carbon dioxide
COPD	chronic obstructive pulmonary disease
CP	cerebral palsy; chest pain
CPAP	continuous positive airway pressure

Abbreviation or Symbol	Meaning
CPD	cephalopelvic disproportion
CPR	cardiopulmonary resuscitation
CSF	cerebrospinal fluid
CSII	continuous subcutaneous insulin infusion
CT	computed tomography
CTA	computed tomographic angiography
cu mm or mm^3	cubic millimeter
CVA	cerebrovascular accident
CVS	chorionic villus sampling
CXR	chest x-ray
d	day
D&C	dilation and curettage
D&E	dilation and evacuation
DC	discharge; discontinue; doctor of chiropractic
DDS	doctor of dental surgery
DJD	degenerative joint disease
DKA	diabetic ketoacidosis
DO	doctor of osteopathy
DPM	doctor of podiatric medicine
dr	dram
DRE	digital rectal exam
DTR	deep tendon reflex
DVT	deep vein thrombosis
Dx	diagnosis
ECG	electrocardiogram
echo	echocardiogram
ECT	electroconvulsive therapy
ECU	emergency care unit
ED	erectile dysfunction
EDC	estimated date of confinement
EDD	estimated date of delivery
EEG	electroencephalogram
EGD	esophagogastroduodenoscopy
EKG	electrocardiogram
EMG	electromyogram
ENT	ear, nose, and throat
EPS	electrophysiologic study
ER	emergency room
ERCP	endoscopic retrograde cholangiopancreatography
ESR	erythrocyte sedimentation rate
ESWL	extracorporeal shock wave lithotripsy
ETOH	ethyl alcohol
EUS	endoscopic ultrasonography
F	Fahrenheit
FBS	fasting blood sugar
Fe	iron
FH	family history
fl oz	fluid ounce

Abbreviation or Symbol	Meaning
FS	frozen section
FSH	follicle-stimulating hormone
Fx	fracture
g	gram
GAD	generalized anxiety disorder
GERD	gastroesophageal reflux disease
GH	growth hormone
GI	gastrointestinal
gm	gram
gr	grain
gt	drop
gtt	drops
GTT	glucose tolerance test
GYN	gynecology
h	hour
H&H	hemoglobin and hematocrit
H&P	history and physical
HAV	hepatitis A virus
HBV	hepatitis B virus
HCT or Hct	hematocrit
HCV	hepatitis C virus
HD	Huntington disease
HEENT	head, eyes, ears, nose, and throat
HGB or Hgb	hemoglobin
HIV	human immunodeficiency virus
hpf	high-power field
HPI	history of present illness
HPV	human papillomavirus
HRT	hormone replacement therapy
h.s.	hour of sleep
HSV-1	herpes simplex virus type 1
HSV-2	herpes simplex virus type 2
Ht	height
HTN	hypertension
Hx	history
I&D	incision and drainage
ICD	implantable cardioverter defibrillator
ICU	intensive care unit
ID	intradermal
IM	intramuscular
IMP	impression
IOL	intraocular lens
IP	inpatient
IUD	intrauterine device
IV	intravenous
IVP	intravenous pyelogram
IVU	intravenous urogram
JCAHO	Joint Commission on Accreditation of Healthcare Organizations
kg	kilogram

Abbreviation or Symbol	Meaning
KUB	kidneys, ureters, bladder
L	liter
Ⓛ	left
L&W	living and well
LASIK	laser-assisted in situ keratomileusis
lb	pound
LEEP	loop electrosurgical excision procedure
LH	luteinizing hormone
LLETZ	large-loop excision of transformation zone
LLQ	left lower quadrant
LP	lumbar puncture
lpf	low-power field
LTB	laryngotracheobronchitis
LUQ	left upper quadrant
m	meter
ⓜ	murmur
MCH	mean corpuscular (cell) hemoglobin
MCHC	mean corpuscular (cell) hemoglobin concentration
MCV	mean corpuscular (cell) volume
MD	medical doctor; muscular dystrophy
mg	milligram
MI	myocardial infarction
ml or mL	milliliter
mm	millimeter
mm³ or cu mm	cubic millimeter
MPI	myocardial perfusion image
MRA	magnetic resonance angiography
MRI	magnetic resonance imaging
MS	multiple sclerosis; musculoskeletal
MSH	melanocyte-stimulating hormone
MUGA	multiple-gated acquisition (scan)
MVP	mitral valve prolapse
NAD	no acute distress
NCV	nerve conduction velocity
NG	nasogastric
NK	natural killer (cell)
NKA	no known allergy
NKDA	no known drug allergy
noc.	night
NPO	nothing by mouth
NSAID	nonsteroidal antiinflammatory drug
NSR	normal sinus rhythm

Abbreviation or Symbol	Meaning
O	objective
O_2	oxygen
OA	osteoarthritis
OB	obstetrics
OCD	obsessive-compulsive disorder
OCP	oral contraceptive pill
OD	right eye; doctor of optometry
OH	occupational history
OP	outpatient
OR	operating room
ORIF	open reduction, internal fixation
OS	left eye
OU	both eyes
oz	ounce
p̄	after
P	plan; posterior; pulse
PA	posterior-anterior
PACU	postanesthetic care unit
$PaCO_2$	partial pressure of carbon dioxide
PaO_2	partial pressure of oxygen
Pap	Papanicolaou (smear)
PAR	postanesthetic recovery
p.c.	after meals
PCI	percutaneous coronary intervention
PD	panic disorder
PDA	patent ductus arteriosus
PE	physical examination; pulmonary embolism; polyethylene
PEFR	peak expiratory flow rate
per	by or through
PERRLA	pupils equal, round, and reactive to light and accommodation
PET	positron emission tomography
PF	peak flow
PFT	pulmonary function testing
pH	potential of hydrogen
PH	past history
PI	present illness
PID	pelvic inflammatory disease
PIH	pregnancy-induced hypertension
p.m.	after noon
PLT	platelet
PMH	past medical history
PMN	polymorphonuclear (leukocyte)
PNS	peripheral nervous system
p.o.	by mouth
post-op or postop	postoperative
PPBS	postprandial blood sugar

Abbreviation or Symbol	Meaning
PR	per rectum
pre-op or preop	preoperative
p.r.n. or prn	as needed
PSA	prostate-specific antigen
PSG	polysomnography
pt	patient
PT	physical therapy; prothrombin time
PTCA	percutaneous transluminal coronary angioplasty
PTH	parathyroid hormone
PTSD	posttraumatic stress disorder
PTT	partial thromboplastin time
PUD	peptic ulcer disease
PV	per vagina
PVC	premature ventricular contraction
Px	physical examination
q	every
q.d.	every day, daily
qh	every hour
q2h	every 2 hours
q.i.d.	four times a day
q.o.d.	every other day
qt	quart
R	respiration
Ⓡ	right
RA	rheumatoid arthritis
RBC	red blood cell; red blood count
RLQ	right lower quadrant
R/O	rule out
ROM	range of motion
ROS	review of symptoms
RP	retrograde pyelogram
RRR	regular rate and rhythm
RTC	return to clinic
RTO	return to office
RUQ	right upper quadrant
Rx	recipe; prescription
$\bar{s}$	without
S	subjective
SA	sinoatrial
SAB	spontaneous abortion
SAD	seasonal affective disorder
SC	subcutaneous
SCA	sudden cardiac arrest
SCC	squamous cell carcinoma
SH	social history
Sig:	instruction to patient
SLE	systemic lupus erythematosus
SOB	shortness of breath
SPECT	single-photon emission computed tomography

Abbreviation or Symbol	Meaning
SpGr	specific gravity
SQ	subcutaneous
SR	systems review
$\overline{\overline{ss}}$	one-half
STAT	immediately
STD	sexually transmitted disease
SUI	stress urinary incontinence
suppos	suppository
SV	stroke volume
Sx	symptom
T	temperature
T_3	triiodothyronine
T_4	thyroxine
T&A	tonsillectomy and adenoidectomy
tab	tablet
TAB	therapeutic abortion
TB	tuberculosis
TEDS	thromboembolic disease stockings
TEE	transesophageal echocardiogram
TIA	transient ischemic attack
t.i.d.	three times a day
TM	tympanic membrane
TMR	transmyocardial revascularization
tPA or TPA	tissue plasminogen activator
Tr	treatment
TSH	thyroid-stimulating hormone
TURP	transurethral resection of the prostate
TV	tidal volume
Tx	treatment; traction
UA	urinalysis
UCHD	usual childhood diseases
URI	upper respiratory infection
US or U/S	ultrasound
UTI	urinary tract infection
VC	vital capacity
VCU or VCUG	voiding cystourethrogram
V/Q	ventilation/perfusion
VS	vital signs
VSD	ventricular septal defect
VT	tidal volume
w.a.	while awake
WBC	white blood cell; white blood count
WDWN	well developed, well nourished
wk	week
WNL	within normal limits
Wt	weight
x	times; for

Abbreviation or Symbol	Meaning	Abbreviation or Symbol	Meaning
x-ray	radiography	♀ (sitting symbol)	sitting
y.o. or y/o	year old	♀ (lying symbol)	lying
yr	year	×	times; for
♀	female	>	greater than
♂	male	<	less than
#	number; pound	♱	one
°	degree; hour	♱♱	two
↑	increase; above	♱♱♱	three
↓	decrease; below	♱v	four
✓	check	I, II, III, IV, V,	uppercase Roman numerals
∅	none; negative	VI, VII, VIII,	1–10
♀ (standing symbol)	standing	IX, and X	

From Willis MC. Medical Terminology: The Language of Health Care. 2nd ed. Baltimore: Lippincott Williams & Wilkins; 2006.

Appendix E

Commonly Misused Words

Because these words have similar spellings and pronunciation, they can easily be confused or misused. Watch your spelling carefully! Always proofread all business letters for accuracy and grammar.

Word	Example of Correct Use
adverse (harmful) averse (opposed to)	Some adverse reactions can be life threatening. I am not averse to working on Mondays.
affect (verb, to influence, change) effect (noun, result)	The protesters will not affect the outcome. The effect of the antibiotics has been beneficial.
already (previously) all ready (prepared, all set)	We already tried that approach. Are we all ready to go?
anoxia (without oxygen) anorexia (without appetite)	Anoxia will cause the brain cells to die quickly. Anorexia is a serious illness that affects teenagers.
aphagia (without swallowing) aphasia (without speech)	A feeding tube is needed because of her aphagia. Her stroke caused aphasia.
appendices (end of book) appendicitis (inflammation of appendix)	There are five appendices at the end of the book. The patient was treated for appendicitis.
biannual (twice a year) biennial (occurring every 2 years)	Productivity reports are printed on a biannual basis. Staff contracts are renewed on a biennial basis.
bite (grip with teeth) byte (character)	The patient's bite is poorly aligned. Buy a computer with enough bytes for future growth.
bowl (container) bowel (intestines, colon)	The jelly beans are in the bowl. Instruct the patient to complete the bowel preparation.
emphysema (chronic lung disease) empyema (accumulation of pus)	Smoking causes emphysema. Empyema most commonly occurs in the pleural cavity.
ensure (be certain) insure (protect against risk) assure (provide confidence)	Call the patient to ensure that he comprehends the instructions. Please insure this package for $200. I assure you that he is getting the correct treatment.
everyday (adjective, routine, ordinary) every day (adverbial phrase, each day)	Quality checks are an everyday procedure. There can be legal ramifications if this is not done every day.
except (exclude) expect (anticipate) accept (agree)	All antibiotics except penicillin will work. I expect this work to be completed by noon. I accept this challenge.
farther (greater distance) further (greater degree)	It is 1 mile farther down the road. The process needs further refinement.
fundus (pertains to hollow organ) fungus (organism that can lead to infection)	The fundus was firm after the baby's delivery. A fungus was growing under her nails.
its (possessive pronoun) it's (contraction of it and is)	The pharmacy must protect its supply of opioids. It's time to take a break.

Word	Example of Correct Use
lactose (type of sugar in milk)	I have a lactose allergy.
lactase (enzyme)	Lactase is responsible for dissolving lactose.
libel (written defamatory statement)	The statements about John Roberts were libel.
liable (legally responsible)	You are liable for your actions.
may be (compound verb)	Dr. Rogers may be in surgery this afternoon.
maybe (adverb, perhaps)	Maybe it will snow tomorrow.
metatarsals (bones in foot)	Crutches are often needed when the metatarsals are fractured.
metacarpals (bones in palm)	Typing is difficult for patients with a metacarpal fracture.
mucus (substance that is secreted)	The patient had a mucus plug.
mucous (membrane that secretes)	The mucous membrane secretes the mucus.
parental (pertaining to parent)	Follow parental guidelines for TV use.
parenteral (not by mouth)	Parenteral feedings will start on Monday.
postnatal (after birth)	Complications can occur in the postnatal period.
postnasal (behind nose)	Postnasal drainage can be uncomfortable.
principle (noun, law)	A key principle of economics is understanding cash flow.
principal (noun, leader; adjective, most important)	The principal's name is Tina Sefferin; her experience is the principal reason she was hired.
rubella (German measles)	You need a rubella vaccination.
rubeola (14-day measles)	There is a outbreak of rubeola at the middle school.
serum (watery component of blood)	The patient's serum is used for various tests.
sebum (oily substance secreted by the sebaceous glands)	Sebum helps to lubricate the skin surface.
tact (behavior)	He handled his child with great tact.
tack (different direction)	A new tack may be needed for us to win that bid.
than (to show comparison)	Salaries are higher now than they were a year ago.
then (next)	Clean room 2; then go to lunch.
there (place, point)	You need to be there at 2:00 PM.
their (possessive pronoun)	Leaving their bikes on the road caused the accident.
they're (pronoun plus verb)	They're going to be late.
uvula (soft tissue at back of palate)	The patient's uvula was swollen.
vulva (external female organ)	A laceration of the vulva was noted during the gynecologic examination.
weather (climate)	The weather is unpredictable.
whether (indicating a possibility)	I wonder whether it will rain or snow.

Sample Medical Reports

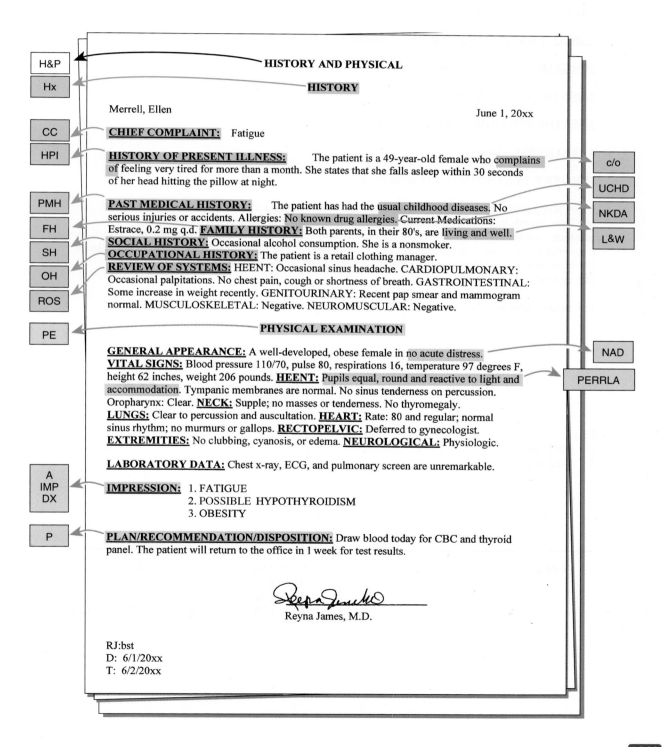

H&P		HISTORY AND PHYSICAL
Hx		HISTORY

Merrell, Ellen   June 1, 20xx

CHIEF COMPLAINT: Fatigue — CC

HISTORY OF PRESENT ILLNESS: The patient is a 49-year-old female who complains of feeling very tired for more than a month. She states that she falls asleep within 30 seconds of her head hitting the pillow at night. — HPI / c/o

PAST MEDICAL HISTORY: The patient has had the usual childhood diseases. No serious injuries or accidents. Allergies: No known drug allergies. Current Medications: Estrace, 0.2 mg q.d. **FAMILY HISTORY:** Both parents, in their 80's, are living and well. — PMH / FH / UCHD / NKDA / L&W

SOCIAL HISTORY: Occasional alcohol consumption. She is a nonsmoker. — SH

OCCUPATIONAL HISTORY: The patient is a retail clothing manager. — OH

REVIEW OF SYSTEMS: HEENT: Occasional sinus headache. CARDIOPULMONARY: Occasional palpitations. No chest pain, cough or shortness of breath. GASTROINTESTINAL: Some increase in weight recently. GENITOURINARY: Recent pap smear and mammogram normal. MUSCULOSKELETAL: Negative. NEUROMUSCULAR: Negative. — ROS

PE — **PHYSICAL EXAMINATION**

GENERAL APPEARANCE: A well-developed, obese female in no acute distress. — NAD
VITAL SIGNS: Blood pressure 110/70, pulse 80, respirations 16, temperature 97 degrees F, height 62 inches, weight 206 pounds. **HEENT:** Pupils equal, round and reactive to light and accommodation. Tympanic membranes are normal. No sinus tenderness on percussion. — PERRLA
Oropharynx: Clear. **NECK:** Supple; no masses or tenderness. No thyromegaly.
LUNGS: Clear to percussion and auscultation. **HEART:** Rate: 80 and regular; normal sinus rhythm; no murmurs or gallops. **RECTOPELVIC:** Deferred to gynecologist.
EXTREMITIES: No clubbing, cyanosis, or edema. **NEUROLOGICAL:** Physiologic.

LABORATORY DATA: Chest x-ray, ECG, and pulmonary screen are unremarkable.

A / IMP / DX — **IMPRESSION:** 1. FATIGUE
                 2. POSSIBLE HYPOTHYROIDISM
                 3. OBESITY

P — **PLAN/RECOMMENDATION/DISPOSITION:** Draw blood today for CBC and thyroid panel. The patient will return to the office in 1 week for test results.

Reyna James, M.D.

RJ:bst
D: 6/1/20xx
T: 6/2/20xx

CENTRAL MEDICAL CENTER

211 Medical Center Drive • Central City, US 90000-1234 • PHONE: (012) 125-6784 • FAX: (012) 125-9999

OPERATIVE REPORT

DATE OF OPERATION: June 3, 20xx.

PREOPERATIVE DIAGNOSIS: Chronic tonsillitis.

POSTOPERATIVE DIAGNOSIS: Frequent, recurrent tonsillitis.

SURGEON: Patrick Rodden, M.D.

ASSISTANT SURGEON: None

ANESTHESIOLOGIST: Robert Jung, M.D.

ANESTHESIA: General.

SURGERY PERFORMED: Tonsillectomy.

DESCRIPTION OF OPERATION: After general anesthesia induction, with intubation, the McGivor mouth gag and tongue retractor were utilized for exposure of the oropharynx. Local anesthetic consisting of 6 mL of 0.5% Xylocaine with 1:100,000 epinephrine was utilized. Tonsillectomy was carried out using dissection and air technique. The right tonsillectomy electrocoagulation Bovie suction was utilized for hemostasis. Examination of the nasopharynx was normal.

The patient tolerated the procedure well and went to the recovery room in good condition.

P. Rodden MD
PATRICK RODDEN, M.D.

JR:as
D: 6/3/20xx
T: 6/4/20xx

OPERATIVE REPORT	PT. NAME:	PERRON, CARLEEN
	ID NO:	672894017
	ROOM NO:	312
	ATT. PHYS:	PATRICK RODDEN, M.D.

CENTRAL MEDICAL CENTER

211 Medical Center Drive • Central City, US 90000-1234 • PHONE: (012) 125-6784 • FAX: (012) 125-9999

PATHOLOGY REPORT

PATIENT: PERRON, CARLEEN
                  28 Y (FEMALE)

DATE RECEIVED: June 3, 20xx.   DATE REPORTED: June 4, 20xx

GROSS:

Received are two tonsils each 2.5 cm in greatest diameter.

MICROSCOPIC:

The sections show deep tonsilar crypts associated with follicular lymphoid hyperplasia. No bacterial granules are seen.

DIAGNOSIS:

CHRONIC LYMPHOID HYPERPLASIA OF RIGHT AND LEFT TONSILS.

Mary Needham MD
MARY NEEDHAM, M.D.

MN:gds

D: 6/4/20xx
T: 6/5/20xx

CENTRAL MEDICAL CENTER

211 Medical Center Drive • Central City, US 90000-1234 • PHONE: (012) 125-6784 • FAX: (012) 125-9999

DISCHARGE SUMMARY

DATE OF ADMISSION: 10/25/20xx   DATE OF DISCHARGE: 10/29/20xx

ADMITTING DIAGNOSIS:
Left ureteropelvic junction obstruction.

DISCHARGE DIAGNOSIS:
Left ureteropelvic junction obstruction.

PROCEDURE PERFORMED:
Left dismembered pyeloplasty and placement of stent.

BRIEF SUMMARY:
The patient is a 19-year-old male who was admitted to the hospital a month ago with left pyelonephritis. He was found to have a left ureteropelvic junction obstruction. The patient was brought to the hospital at this time for repair of the moderately to severely obstructed left kidney. A preoperative urine culture was sterile. The patient underwent the procedure without complication. A double-J stent was placed. The Jackson-Pratt drain was removed on the second postoperative day because of minimal drainage. The patient initially had urinary retention, but this resolved by the third postoperative day. He was doing fine at the time of discharge. His condition on discharge is good.

INSTRUCTIONS TO THE PATIENT:
1) Regular diet. 2) No heavy lifting, straining, or driving an automobile for six weeks from the day of surgery. He should also keep the incision relatively dry this week. 3) Follow up in my office in three weeks. 4) It is anticipated the stent will remain indwelling for six weeks and then will be removed cystoscopically at that time. 5) Discharge medication is Tylenol #3, 1-2 q 4 h p.r.n. pain.

L. Zlatkin, M.D.

LZ:mr

D: 10/29/20xx
T: 10/30/20xx

DISCHARGE SUMMARY

PT. NAME: MERCIER, CHARLES F.
ID NO: IP-392689
ROOM NO: 444
ATT. PHYS: L.ZLATKIN, M.D.

CENTRAL MEDICAL CENTER

211 Medical Center Drive • Central City, US 90000-1234 • PHONE: (012) 125-6784 • FAX: (012) 125-9999

OPERATIVE REPORT

DATE: December 7, 20xx

PREOPERATIVE DIAGNOSIS: Congenital left ureteropelvic junction obstruction status post pyeloplasty. Indwelling left ureteral stent.

POSTOPERATIVE DIAGNOSIS: Congenital left ureteropelvic junction obstruction status post pyeloplasty. Indwelling left ureteral stent, removed

OPERATION: Cystoscopy, removal of left ureteral stent, and left retrograde pyelogram.

PROCEDURE: The patient was identified, was placed on the operating table, and was administered a general anesthetic. He was placed in the lithotomy position, and a KUB was obtained. The genitalia were prepped and draped in a sterile fashion. After reviewing the KUB, it was noted at this time that the position of the stent was normal. Cystoscopy was performed with a #22 French cystoscope. The stent was identified coming from the left ureteral orifice, and the end was grasped with forceps and removed through the cystoscope. A #8 French cone-tipped ureteral catheter was then placed in the left ureteral orifice and passed to 10 cm. Then, 20 cm^3 of contrast was injected into a left collecting system. A film was exposed, and this showed patency without extravasation at the left ureteropelvic junction. There was some filling of calyces and partial filling of the dilated renal pelvis. A drainage film was subsequently obtained showing complete emptying of the pelvis and partial emptying of the mid and distal ureters. Dilated calyces were noted in the kidney. The patient was allowed to awaken and was returned to the recovery room in satisfactory condition. There were no intraoperative complications. He had no bleeding. The patient did receive 1 gm Ancef one-half hour prior to the onset of the procedure.

L. Zlatkin, M.D.

LZ:mr
D: 12/07/20xx
T: 12/08/20xx

OPERATIVE REPORT	PT. NAME:	MERCIER, CHARLES F.
	ID NO:	OP-912689
	ROOM NO:	ASC
	ATT. PHYS:	L.ZLATKIN, M.D.

CENTRAL MEDICAL GROUP, INC.

Department of Internal Medicine

201 Medical Center Drive • Central City, US 90000-1234 • PHONE: (012) 125-8888 • FAX: (012) 125-3434

PATIENT: COHEN, SARA E.   DATE: April 8, 20xx

HISTORY

CHIEF COMPLAINT: Epigastric distress

HISTORY OF PRESENT ILLNESS: This 33-year-old Caucasian female comes in because of excessive burping, epigastric distress and nausea for several weeks. Coffee makes it worse. She complains that it is worse at night when lying down. She gets an acid-like taste in her mouth. She has tried antacids, to no avail.

PAST MEDICAL HISTORY: The patient states that she had the usual childhood diseases. She has had no serious medical illnesses and has been involved in no accidents. Family History: There is some diabetes on her mother's side. Her mother is 52 and has hypertension. Her father, age 56, is living and well. She has a sister who is anemic and a brother who has ulcers. Social History: The patient discontinued smoking ten years ago. Drinks alcohol socially. Allergies: NKDA. Current Medications: Medications at this time consist of Entex, Guaifed, birth control pills, iron and vitamin supplements.

REVIEW OF SYSTEMS: HEENT: Chronic sinusitis. She sees an ENT specialist and an allergist. Respiratory: Negative. Cardiac: Occasional flutters. Gastrointestinal: As stated above. Genitourinary: Occasional infections. Pap smear is up-to-date and negative. She has had no mammogram at this point. Neuromuscular: Negative.

PHYSICAL EXAMINATION

GENERAL APPEARANCE: Reveals a well-developed, well-nourished female in no acute distress.

VITAL SIGNS: Blood Pressure: 120/80. Pulse: 76 and regular.

HEENT: Head normocephalic. Eyes: Pupils are equal, round, and reactive to light and accommodation. Fundi are benign. Ears, nose and throat are negative. NECK: No thyromegaly. No carotid bruits.

CHEST: Clear to percussion and auscultation. BREASTS: Reveal no masses. HEART: Normal sinus rhythm. No murmurs.

ABDOMEN: Liver, spleen and kidneys could not be felt. Femorals pulsate well, no bruits.

EXTREMITIES: No edema. Pulses are good and equal.

PELVIC & RECTAL EXAMS: Deferred to gynecologist.

NEUROLOGIC EXAM: Physiologic.

IMPRESSION: 1. PROBABLE PEPTIC ULCER DISEASE WITH GASTROESOPHAGEAL REFLUX.
                  2. POSSIBLE GALLBLADDER DISEASE.

PLAN: Patient started on Pepcid 40 mg, 1 at night. She is given Gaviscon tablets so she can carry them with her. Schedule routine lab work and upper GI series. If negative, schedule ultrasound of the gallbladder.

D. Everley, M.D.

DE:mc
D: 4/8/20xx
T: 4/9/20xx

©2006, Lippincott Williams & Wilkins, Medical Terminology: The Language of Health Care, 2nd edition, by Marjorie Canfield Willis.

CENTRAL MEDICAL GROUP, INC.

Department of Otorhinolaryngology

201 Medical Center Drive • Central City, US 90000-1234 • PHONE: (012) 125-8888 • FAX: (012) 125-3434

Patient: Perron, Carleen　　　　　　　　　　　　　　　　　　　　　DATE: February 17, 20xx

Referring Physician: C. Camarillo, M.D.

CONSULTATION

REASON FOR CONSULTATION: This 28-year-old white female presents with a one week history of upper respiratory infection (URI), sinusitis, and some periorbital headaches in recent weeks. She also has expectorated yellow-green mucus occasionally and has had a history of tonsillitis.

MEDICATIONS: None. **ALLERGIES:** No known allergies (NKA). **SURGERIES:** None. **HOSPITALIZATIONS:** None.

PAST MEDICAL HISTORY/REVIEW OF SYSTEMS: Cardiopulmonary: There is no history of angina, dyspnea, hemoptysis, emphysema, asthma, chronic obstructive pulmonary disease (COPD), hypertension, or heart murmurs. Cardiovascular: There is no history of high blood pressure. Renal: There is no history of dysuria, polyuria, nocturia, hematuria, or cystoliths. Gastrointestinal: There is no history of gallbladder disease, hepatitis, pancreatitis, or colitis. Musculoskeletal: There is no history of arthritis. Endocrine: There is no history of diabetes. Hematologic: There is no history of anemia, blood transfusion, or easy bruising. Gynecological: The patient states her menses are regular, and the start of her last menstrual cycle occurred 15 days ago.

FAMILY HISTORY: The patient states her maternal grandmother has diabetes.

SOCIAL HISTORY: The patient is single and has no children. She denies smoking tobacco. She denies drinking alcoholic beverages. She denies taking drugs.

CHILDHOOD DISEASES: The patient has had the usual childhood diseases.

OTOLARYNGOLOGIC EXAMINATION: Otoscopy: Tympanic membranes (TMs) are dull and slightly congested. Sinuses: There is maxillary fullness. Rhinoscopic examination reveals mild nasoseptal deviation (NSD). Pharynx: There is moderate inflammation; no exudates. Oropharynx: No masses. Nasopharynx: No masses. Larynx: Clear. Neck: Supple. Cervical Adenopathy: There is mild adenopathy.

IMPRESSION:
1. MAXILLARY SINUSITIS.
2. PHARYNGITIS.
3. CHRONIC TONSILLITIS.

DISPOSITION:
1. Warm salt water gargle (WSWG).
2. Ery-Tab 333, #24, 1 t.i.d. p.c.
3. Robitussin.
4. Return to office (RTO) in one week.

P. Rodden MD

PATRICK RODDEN, M.D.

JR:ti
D:　2/17/20xx
T:　2/18/20xx　9:50 a.m.

©2006, Lippincott Williams & Wilkins, Medical Terminology: The Language of Health Care, 2nd edition, by Marjorie Canfield Willis.

CENTRAL MEDICAL GROUP, INC.

Department of Otorhinolaryngology

201 Medical Center Drive • Central City, US 90000-1234 • PHONE: (012) 125-8888 • FAX: (012) 125-3434

PROGRESS NOTES

Patient: PERRON, CARLEEN

03/30/20xx

S: The patient presents with a sore throat × 2 weeks.

O: Sinus exam: Maxillary and frontal congestion. Hypopharynx/adenoids: No inflammation.

A: Recurrent pharyngitis/sinusitis × 2 weeks.

P: 1)   Ceftin 250 mg, #21, 1 t.i.d. p.o. p.c.

2)   Entex LA, #30, 1 b.i.d. p.o.

3)   Warm salt water gargle.

P Rodden MD
PATRICK RODDEN, M.D.

05/25/20xx

S: Recurrent sore throat every month.

O: Recurrent tonsillitis, cryptic tonsillitis. Sinus exam: Maxillary and frontal congestion.
Neck: Supple; no masses. Hypopharynx/Adenoids: No inflammation. Paranasal Sinus X-ray: Bilateral frontal and maxillary sinusitis.

A: Recurrent tonsillitis, 8-10 times per year. Chronic maxillary and frontal sinusitis.

P: 1)   Tonsillectomy discussed with the patient. The risks of general and local anesthesia, as well as the surgical procedure, were discussed with the patient. The consent form was signed.

2)   An admitting order was given to the patient for CBC, UA, and basic metabolic panel to be done one day prior to being admitted.

3)   Ceftin 250 mg, #21, 1 t.i.d. p.o. p.c.

4)   Entex LA, #30, 1 b.i.d. p.o.

5)   Flonase nasal inhaler, 2 sprays each nostril b.i.d.

6)   Warm salt water gargle.

P Rodden MD
PATRICK RODDEN, M.D.

©2006, Lippincott Williams & Wilkins, Medical Terminology: The Language of
Health Care, 2nd edition, by Marjorie Canfield Willis.

CENTRAL MEDICAL CENTER

211 Medical Center Drive • Central City, US 90000-1234 • PHONE: (012) 125-6784 • FAX: (012) 125-9999

X-RAY REPORT

LUMBOSACRAL SPINE:
Multiple views reveal no evidence of fracture. There is slight lumbar spondylosis with slight lipping and minimal bridging. The disc spaces appear maintained except for slight narrowing at L4-L5 and L5-S1. There is also a Grade I spondylolisthesis of L5 on S1 and evidence of spondylolysis at L5 on the left. There is also slight dextroscoliosis in the lumbar region and slight increased lordosis in the lumbosacral region. The bony architecture is unremarkable except for eburnation between the articulating facets at L5-S1. The SI joints appear unremarkable. Incidentally noted are slight osteoarthritic changes involving both hips.

CONCLUSION:

1. Slight lumbar spondylosis with hypertrophic lipping and slight narrowing of the L4-L5 and L5-S1 disc spaces, rule out discogenic disease. If clinically indicated, CT of the lumbosacral spine may prove helpful in further evaluation.

2. Grade I spondylolisthesis of L5 on S1 with evidence of spondylolysis at L5 on the left.

3. Slight dextroscoliosis in the lumbar region and slight increased lordosis in the lumbosacral region.

M. Volz MD
M. Volz, M.D.

MV:ti

D: 10/19/20xx
T: 10/20/20xx

X-RAY REPORT	PT. NAME:	DORN, JAY F.
	ID NO:	RL-483091
	ATT. PHYS:	T. LIGHT, M.D.

Medical reports courtesy of Willis M. Medical Terminology: A Programmed Learning Approach to the Language of Health Care. 2nd ed. Baltimore: Lippincott Williams & Wilkins, 2007; and Willis MC. Medical Terminology: The Language of Health Care. 2nd ed. Baltimore: Lippincott Williams & Wilkins; 2006.

Appendix G

Metric Measurements

Unit	Abbreviation	Metric Equivalent	U.S. Equivalent
Units of Length			
kilometer	km	1000 meters	0.62 miles; 1.6 km/mile
meter*	m	100 cm; 1000 mm	39.4 inches; 1.1 yards
centimeter	cm	1/100 m; 0.01 m	0.39 inches; 2.5 cm/inch
millimeter	mm	1/1000 m; 0.001 m	0.039 inches; 25 mm/inch
micrometer	μm	1/1000 mm; 0.001 mm	
Units of Weight			
kilogram	kg	1000 g	2.2 lb
gram*	g	1000 mg	0.035 oz; 28.5 g/oz
milligram	mg	1/1000 g; 0.001 g	
microgram	μg, mcg	1/1000 mg; 0.001 mg	
Units of Volume			
liter*	L	1000 mL	1.06 qt
deciliter	dL	1/10 L; 0.1 L	
milliliter	mL	1/1000 L; 0.001 L	0.034 oz; 29.4 mL/oz
microliter	μL	1/1000 mL; 0.001 mL	

*Basic unit.

Appendix H

Celsius–Fahrenheit Temperature Conversion Scale

Celsius to Fahrenheit

Use the following formula to convert Celsius readings to Farenheit readings:

$$°F = 9/5 × °C + 32$$

For example, if the Celsius reading is 37°:

$$°F = (9/5 × 37) + 32$$
$$= 66.6 + 32$$
$$= 98.6°F \text{ (normal body temperature)}$$

Fahrenheit to Celsius

Use the following formula to convert Fahrenheit readings to Celsius readings:

$$°C = 5/9(°F − 32)$$

For example, if the Fahrenheit reading is 68°:

$$°C = 5/9(68 − 32)$$
$$= 5/9 × 36$$
$$= 20°C \text{ (a nice spring day)}$$

temperature
conversion
scale

From Memmler RL, Cohen BJ, Wood, DL. The Human Body in Health and Disease. 10th ed. Baltimore: Lippincott Williams & Wilkins; 2005.

Appendix I

Laboratory Tests

TABLE 1	Routine Urinalysis	
Test	**Normal Value**	**Clinical Significance**
General characteristics and measurements		
Color	Pale yellow to amber	Color change can be due to concentration or dilution, drugs, metabolic or inflammatory disorders
Odor	Slightly aromatic	Foul odor typical of urinary tract infection; fruity odor in uncontrolled diabetes mellitus
Appearance (clarity)	Clear to slightly hazy	Cloudy urine occurs with infection or after refrigeration; may indicate presence of bacteria, cells, mucus, or crystals
Specific gravity	1.003–1.030 (first morning catch; routine is random)	Decreased in diabetes insipidus, acute renal failure, water intoxication; increased in liver disorders, heart failure, dehydration
pH	4.5–8.0	Acid urine accompanies acidosis, fever, high protein diet; alkaline urine in urinary tract infection, metabolic alkalosis, vegetarian diet
Chemical determinations		
Glucose	Negative	Glucose present in uncontrolled diabetes mellitus, steroid excess
Ketones	Negative	Present in diabetes mellitus and in starvation
Protein	Negative	Present in kidney disorders, such as glomerulonephritis, acute kidney failure
Bilirubin	Negative	Breakdown product of hemoglobin; present in liver disease or in bile blockage
Urobilinogen	0.2–1.0 Ehrlich units/dL	Breakdown product of bilirubin; increased in hemolytic anemias and in liver disease; remains negative in bile obstruction
Blood (occult)	Negative	Detects small amounts of blood cells, hemoglobin, or myoglobin; present in severe trauma, metabolic disorders, bladder infections
Nitrite	Negative	Product of bacterial breakdown of urine; positive result suggests urinary tract infection and needs to be followed up with a culture of the urine
Microscopic		
Red blood cells	0–3 per high-power field	Increased because of bleeding within the urinary tract from trauma, tumors, inflammation, or damage within the kidney
White blood cells	0–4 per high-power field	Increased in infection of the kidney or bladder

(continued)

TABLE 1	Routine Urinalysis *(continued)*	
Test	**Normal Value**	**Clinical Significance**
Renal epithelial cells	Occasional	Increased number indicates damage to kidney tubules
Casts	None	Hyaline casts normal; large number of abnormal casts indicates inflammation or a systemic disorder
Crystals	Present	Most are normal; may be acid or alkaline
Bacteria	Few	Increased in infection of urinary tract or contamination from infected genitalia
Others	Any yeasts, parasites, mucus, spermatozoa, or other microscopic findings would be reported here	

TABLE 2	Complete Blood Count (CBC)	
Test	**Normal Value***	**Clinical Significance**
Red blood cell (RBC) count	Men: 4.6–6.2 million/µL Women: 4.2–5.4 million/µL	Decreased in anemia; increased in dehydration, poly cythemia
Hemoglobin (Hb)	Men: 13.–18 g/dL Women: 12–16 g/dL	Decreased in anemia, hemorrhage, hemolytic reactions; increased in dehydration, heart and lung disease
Hematocrit (Hct) or packed cell volume (PCV)	Men: 45%–52% Women: 37%–48%	Decreased in anemia; increased in polycythemia, dehydration
Red blood cell (RBC) indices (examples)		These values, calculated from the RBC count, HGB, and HCT, give information valuable in the diagnosis and classification of anemia
Mean corpuscular volume (MCV)	80–95 µL/red cell	Measures the average size or volume of each RBC: small size (microcytic) in iron-deficiency anemia; large size (macrocytic) typical of pernicious anemia
Mean corpuscular hemoglobin (MCH)	27–31 pg/red cell	Measures the weight of hemoglobin per RBC; useful in differentiating types of anemia in a severely anemic patient
Mean corpuscular hemoglobin concentration (MCHC)	32–36 g/dL	Defines the volume of hemoglobin per RBC; used to determine the color or concentration of hemoglobin per RBC
White blood cell (WBC) count	4300–10,800µL	Increased in leukemia and in response to infection, inflammation, and dehydration; decreased in bone marrow suppression
Platelets	200,000–400,000/µL	Increased in many malignant disorders; decreased in disseminated intravascular coagulation (DIC) or toxic drug effects; spontaneous bleeding may occur at platelet counts below 20,000 µL
Differential (peripheral blood smear)		A stained slide of the blood is needed to perform the differential. The percentages of the different WBCs are estimated, and the slide is microscopically checked for abnormal characteristics in WBCs, RBCs, and platelets.

(continued)

TABLE 2   Complete Blood Count (CBC) *(continued)*

Test	Normal Value*	Clinical Significance
WBCs		
Segmented neutrophils (SEGs, POLYs)	40%–74%	Increased in bacterial infections; low numbers leave person very susceptible to infection
Immature neutrophils (BANDs)	0%–5%	Increased when neutrophil count increases
Lymphocytes (LYMPHs)	20%–40%	Increased in viral infections; low numbers leave person dangerously susceptible to infection
Monocytes (MONOs)	3%–8%	Increased in specific infections
Eosinophils (EOs)	0%–6%	Increased in allergic disorders
Basophils (BASOs)	0%–1%	Increased in allergic disorders

*Values vary depending on instrumentation and type of test.

TABLE 3   Blood Chemistry Tests

Test	Normal Value	Clinical Significance
Basic panel: An overview of electrolytes, waste product management, and metabolism		
Blood urea nitrogen (BUN)	7–18 mg/dL	Increased in renal disease and dehydration; decreased in liver damage and malnutrition
Carbon dioxide (CO_2) (includes bicarbonate)	22–29 mmol/L	Useful to evaluate acid-base balance by measuring total carbon dioxide in the blood; elevated in vomiting and pulmonary disease; decreased in diabetic acidosis, acute renal failure, and hyperventilation
Chloride (Cl)	98–107 mmol/L	Increased in dehydration, hyperventilation, and congestive heart failure; decreased in vomiting, diarrhea, and fever
Creatinine	0.5–1.2 mg/dL	Produced at a constant rate and excreted by the kidney; increased in kidney disease
Glucose	Fasting: 70–100 mg/dL Random: 85–125 mg/dL	Increased in diabetes and severe illness; decreased in insulin overdose or hypoglycemia
Potassium (K)	3.4–5.0 mmol/L	Increased in renal failure, extensive cell damage, and acidosis; decreased in vomiting, diarrhea, and excess administration of diuretics or IV fluids
Sodium (Na)	135–145 mmol/L	Increased in dehydration and diabetes insipidus; decreased in overload of IV fluids, burns, diarrhea, or vomiting
Additional blood chemistry tests		
Alanine aminotransferase (ALT)	6–47 U/L*	Used to diagnose and monitor treatment of liver disease and to monitor the effects of drugs on the liver; increased in myocardial infarction

(continued)

A1-C = Glycated Hemoglobin test for diabetes.

TABLE 3	Blood Chemistry Tests (continued)	
Test	**Normal Value**	**Clinical Significance**
Albumin	2.5–5.7 g/dL	Albumin holds water in blood; decreased in liver disease and kidney disease
Albumin–globulin ratio (A/G ratio)	>1	Low A/G ratio signifies a tendency for edema because globulin is less effective than albumin at holding water in the blood
Alkaline phosphatase (ALP)	30–95 U/L*	Enzyme of bone metabolism; increased in liver disease and metastatic bone disease
Amylase	<180 U/L*	Used to diagnose and monitor treatment of acute pancreatitis and to detect inflammation of the salivary glands
Aspartate aminotransferase (AST)	5–30 U/L*	Enzyme present in tissues with high metabolic activity; increased in myocardial infarction and liver disease
Bilirubin, total	<1.5 mg/dL	Breakdown product of hemoglobin from red blood cells; increased when excessive red blood cells are being destroyed or in liver disease
Calcium (Ca)	8.6–10.0 mg/dL	Increased in excess parathyroid hormone production and in cancer; decreased in alkalosis, elevated phosphate in renal failure, and excess IV fluids
Cholesterol	<200 mg/dL	Screening test used to evaluate risk of heart disease; levels of 200 mg/dL or above indicate increased risk of heart disease and warrant further investigation
Creatine phosphokinase (CPK or CK)	130–250 U/L*	Elevated enzyme level indicates myocardial infarction or damage to skeletal muscle; when elevated, specific fractions (isoenzymes) are tested for
Gamma-glutamyltransferase (GGT)	Men: 6–26 U/L Women: 4–18 U/L*	Used to diagnose liver disease and to test for chronic alcoholism
Globulins	2.3–3.5 g/dL	Proteins active in immunity; help albumin keep water in blood
Iron, serum (Fe)	40–60 µg/dL	Decreased in iron deficiency and anemia; increased in hemolytic conditions
High-density lipoproteins (HDLs)	>40 mg/dL	Used to evaluate the risk of heart disease
Lactate dehydrogenase (LDH or LD)	95–200 U/L*	Enzyme released in many kinds of tissue damage, including myocardial infarction, pulmonary infarction, and liver disease
Lipase	<60 U/L*	Enzyme used to diagnose pancreatitis
Low-density lipoproteins (LDLs)	<130 mg/dL	Used to evaluate the risk of heart disease
Magnesium (Mg)	1.2–2.1 mEq/L	Vital in neuromuscular function; decreased levels may occur in malnutrition, alcoholism, pancreatitis, diarrhea
Phosphorus (inorganic)	2.7–4.5 mg/dL	Evaluated in response to calcium; main store is in bone; elevated in kidney disease; decreased in excess parathyroid hormone
Protein, total	6–8 g/dL	Increased in dehydration, multiple myeloma; decreased in kidney disease, liver disease, poor nutrition, severe burns, excessive bleeding

(continued)

TABLE 3	Blood Chemistry Tests (continued)	
Test	**Normal Value**	**Clinical Significance**
Serum glutamic oxalacetic transaminase (SGOT)		See Aspartate aminotransferase (AST)
Serum glutamic pyruvic trans-aminase (SGPT)		See Alanine aminotransferase (ALT)
Thyroxin (T4)	4.0–12.0 µg/dL (may vary by test method)	Screening test of thyroid function; increased in hyperthyroidism; decreased in myxedema and hypothyroidism
Thyroid-stimulating hormone (TSH)	0.5–5.0 mU/L	Produced by pituitary to promote thyroid gland function; elevated when thyroid gland is not functioning
Triglycerides	<150 mg/dL	An indication of ability to metabolize fats; increased triglycerides and cholesterol indicate high risk of atherosclerosis
Uric acid	Men: 3.5–7.2 mg/dL Women: 2.6–6.0 mg/dL	Produced by breakdown of ingested purines in food and nucleic acids; elevated in kidney disease, gout, leukemia

* Varies significantly by test method.

Compare patient results to normal range printed on laboratory report.

Adapted from Memmler RL, Cohen BJ, Wood DL. The Human Body in Health and Disease. 10th ed. Baltimore: Lippincott Williams & Wilkins; 2005.

Glossary

A

abandonment withdrawal by a physician from a contractual relationship with a patient without proper notification while the patient still needs treatment.

abdominal regions divisions of the abdomen into nine regions by two horizontal and two vertical lines; used to identify specific locations.

ablation removal or excision of a part; laser ablation is destruction/removal of tissue by use of laser.

abortion termination of pregnancy or products of conception prior to fetal viability and/or 20 weeks of gestation.

accounting cycle a consecutive 12-month period for financial record keeping following either a fiscal year (starting on a specified date) or the calendar year (January to December).

accounts payable a record of all monies owed.

accounts receivable a record of all monies due.

accreditation a nongovernmental professional peer review process that provides technical assistance and evaluates educational programs for quality based on pre-established academic and administrative standards.

acquired immunodeficiency syndrome (AIDS) a cluster of disorders caused by HIV that specifically destroys cell-mediated immunity.

acromegaly a disorder marked by progressive enlargement of the head, face, hands, and feet, due to excessive secretion of growth hormone after puberty.

acrosome the superior surface of the head of the spermatozoon.

activities of daily living (ADL) activities usually performed in the course of the day, i.e., bathing, dressing, feeding oneself.

acute abrupt in onset.

Addison's disease partial or complete failure of the adrenal cortex functions, causing general physical deterioration.

adenosine triphosphate (ATP) the energy currency used by the body; breaking down the phosphate bond of the compound releases high energy potential.

adipose of or pertaining to fat.

adjustment a change in a posted account.

administrative pertaining to administration (e.g., office procedures and nonclinical tasks that a medical assistant will perform).

adnexa any part added to a main structure; an accessory part.

advance beneficiary notice document that informs covered patients that Medicare may not cover a certain service and the patient will be responsible for the bill.

advance directive a statement of a patient's wishes regarding health care prior to a critical medical event.

aerobe microorganism that requires oxygen to live and reproduce.

aerosol suspended particles in gas or air.

afebrile body temperature not elevated above normal.

afferent carrying impulses towards the center.

affiliation to connect or associate with, as a medical site would associate with a school to assist in completion of student training.

agar a type of seaweed or algae that helps solidify culture media; the media may be referred to as agar.

agenda a brief outline of the topics to be discussed at a meeting.

agglutination clumping of cells due to the presence of antibodies called agglutinins.

aging schedule a form used to track outstanding balances.

aliquots portions of the original patient specimen that have been placed into a separate container to be routed to the appropriate laboratory work station for testing

allergen any substance that causes manifestations of an allergy, usually a protein to which the body has built antibodies.

allergy acquired abnormal response to a substance (allergen) that does not ordinarily cause a reaction.

alopecia baldness.

alphabetic filing arranging of names or titles according to the sequence of letters in the alphabet.

alpha-fetoprotein substance produced by the embryonic yolk sac.

alternative an option or substitute to the standard medical treatment plan, e.g. herbal therapies, acupuncture, hypnosis.

alveolar-capillary membrane the structure in the lung fields through which oxygen and carbon dioxide diffuse during the respiratory process.

amenorrhea condition of not menstruating, without menses.

American Association of Medical Assistants (AAMA) professional organization for medical assistants.

Americans With Disabilities Act (ADA) a law designed to meet the needs of people with physical and mental challenges.

amniocentesis puncture of the amniotic sac in order to remove fluid for testing.

amphiarthroses slightly movable joints.

ampule small glass container that must be broken at the neck to aspirate the solution into the syringe.

amylase an enzyme secreted by the pancreas and the salivary glands into the intestines to aid in digestion.

anabolism the constructive phase of metabolism, when smaller molecules are converted to large ones.

anacusis complete hearing loss.

anaerobe bacterium that does not require oxygen for growth and reproduction.

anaphylactic shock severe allergic reaction within minutes to hours after exposure to a foreign substance.

anaphylaxis severe allergic reaction that may result in death.

anatomic position a position used for reference in which the subject is standing erect, facing forward, feet are slightly apart and pointing forward, and the hands are down at the sides with palms forward and thumbs outward.

anatomy the study of the structure of the body.

anencephaly a neural tube defect in developing fetuses.

aneroid sphygmomanometer that measures blood pressure without using mercury.

aneurysm local dilation in a blood vessel wall.

angina pectoris paroxysmal chest pain usually caused by a decrease in blood flow to the heart muscle due to coronary artery occlusion.

angiotensin a substance occurring in the blood that works with renin to affect the blood pressure, usually increasing the pressure by vasoconstriction.

anions chemicals that carry a negative charge.

anisocytosis blood abnormality in which red blood cells are not equal in size (aniso = unequal).

ankylosing spondylitis stiffening of the spine with inflammation.

annotation the process of reading, highlighting, and summarizing a document for another person.

anorexia loss of appetite.

anovulation condition of not ovulating.

antagonism mutual opposition or contrary action with something else; opposite of synergism.

antagonist any muscle that opposes the action of the prime mover to balance movement. (Example: When the biceps contract and pull the forearm upward, the triceps oppose the motion and relax.)

antecubital space inner surface of the bend of the elbow where the major veins for venipuncture are located.

antepartum period of time prior to labor.

anthropometric pertaining to measurements of the human body.

antibiotic a drug that inhibits or destroys pathogenic microorganisms.

antibody a complex glycoprotein produced by B lymphocytes in response to an antigen.

anticoagulant a chemical compound introduced to the blood or blood sample to prevent clotting. Anticoagulants suppress the function of clotting factors normally present in blood.

antigen protein markers on cells that cause formation of antibodies and react specifically with those antibodies.

antihistamine medication that opposes the action of a histamine.

antiseptic any substance that inhibits the growth of bacteria; used on skin before any procedure that breaks the integumentary barrier.

anuria failure of the kidneys to produce urine.

apnea the absence of respirations.

apothecary system of measurement old system that uses grains, minims, and drams.

appeal process by which a higher court reviews the decision of a lower court.

appendicular skeleton the parts of the skeleton added to the axial skeleton, including the shoulder and pelvic girdles and all of the bones of the upper and lower extremities.

applicator device for applying local treatments and tests.

approximate bring tissue surfaces as close as possible to their original positions.

arachnoid web-like membrane covering the brain and spinal cord.

arrector pili involuntary muscle attached to the hair follicle that, when contracted, causes "goose bumps."

arteriole a small arterial branch that joins a capillary to an artery.

arthrogram x-ray of a joint.

arthroplasty surgical repair of a joint.

arthroscopy examination of the inside of a joint through an arthroscope.

artifact activity recorded in an electrocardiogram caused by extraneous activity such as patient movement, loose lead, or electrical interference.

artifactual something added to a substance or structure, not belonging to it; in medicine, generally implies a negative connotation.

ascites accumulation of serous fluid in the peritoneal cavity.

asepsis a state of being sterile; a condition free from germs, infection, and any form of life, including spore forms.

aspiration drawing in or out by suction; as in breathing objects into the respiratory tract or suctioning substances from a site.

assault an attempt or threat to touch another person without his or her consent.

assessment process of gathering information about the patient and the presenting condition.

assignment of benefits transfer of the patient's legal right to collect third-party benefits for medical expenses to the provider of the services.

astigmatism unfocused refraction of light rays on the retina.

asymmetry lack or absence of symmetry; inequality of size or shape on opposite sides of the body.

asymptomatic without any symptoms.

atelectasis collapsed lung fields; incomplete expansion of the lungs, either partial or complete.

atherosclerosis buildup of fatty plaque on the interior lining of arteries.

atraumatic without injury; may pertain to treatments or instruments that are not likely to cause further damage.

atria (plural) the upper chamber of each half of the heart; the atria receive blood from the great vessels (singular: atrium).

atrioventricular (AV) node located on the floor of the right atrium on or close to the septum; receives the electrical impulse from the SA node after it is transmitted through the upper half of the heart; transmits the impulse to the bundle of His.

attenuated diluted or weakened; pertaining to reduced virulence of a pathogenic microorganism.

attitude a state of mind; how a person feels about a given subject or at a given time.

attribute a characteristic or quality of a person; usually considered a positive feature.

audit a review of an account; inspection of records to determine compliance and to detect fraud.

auscultation act of listening for sounds within the body, usually with a stethoscope, such as to evaluate the heart, lungs, intestines, or fetal heart tones.

autoclave appliance used to sterilize medical instruments with steam under pressure.

autonomic self-controlling, spontaneous.

autonomous existing or functioning independently.

axial skeleton the bones forming the main skeleton around which the appendicular skeleton moves, including bones of the head, thorax, and trunk.

axon part of the neuron that transmits impulses away from the cell body.

azidothymidine (AZT) a drug used to treat AIDS by blocking the growth of the virus after it enters the T-cell lymphocyte.

azotemia from the Latin *azote* meaning nitrogen, plus -emia, meaning blood; the condition of having excessive amounts of nitrogen in the blood.

B

Babinski reflex reflex (dorsiflexion of the great toe and extension and fanning of the other toes upon stroking the sole of the foot) exhibited normally by infants. This reflex is abnormal in children and adults.

bacilli rod-shaped or cylindrical organisms.

back-up *noun*, a duplicate file made to a separate disk to protect information; *verb*, to make a duplicate file.

bactericidal substance that kills or destroys bacteria.

bacteriology the science and study of bacteria.

balance equality between the debit and credit sides of an accounting equation; that which is left over after additions and subtractions have been made to an account; remainder; amount due.

balance billing billing the patient for the balance or difference between the physician's charges and the Medicare-approved charges; prohibited by most managed care contracts.

bandage *noun*, a soft material applied to a body part to hold a dressing in place, immobilize a body part, or aid in controlling bleeding; *verb*, to apply a wrapping material for treatment.

barrier precautions any device including PPE that provides an obstacle to minimize the risk of infection with blood-borne pathogens.

Bartholin's glands small mucous glands bilaterally in the vaginal vestibule.

basal ganglia pertaining to the gray matter in the cerebral hemispheres.

basal metabolic rate the amount of energy used in a unit of time to maintain vital functions by a fasting, resting subject.

baseline original or initial measure with which other measurements will be compared.

basophil a type of leukocyte.

battery actual touching of a person without his or her consent.

B-cells lymphoid stem cells from the bone marrow that migrate to and become mature antigen-specific cells in the spleen and lymph nodes.

beliefs ideas that are held to be true.

bench trial trial in which the judge hears the case and renders a verdict; no jury is present.

benign not cancerous or malignant.

bevel the angled point of the needle cut on a slant to ease skin penetration.

bias formation of an opinion without foundation or reason; prejudice.

BiCaps words or phrases with unusual capitalization.

bicarbonate the dissolved form of carbon dioxide; it combines with water to make carbonic acid, H_2CO_3. Carbonic acid loses one of its hydrogen (H) ions to then form bicarbonate, HCO_3^-.

bile a bitter, yellow-green secretion of the liver stored by the gallbladder; derived from bilirubin, cholesterol, and other substances. Emulsifies fats in the small intestine so they can be further digested and absorbed.

biliary obstruction blockage of one of the bile ducts (the tubes leading from liver and gallbladder into duodenum); common causes include cysts, tumors, and stones.

bilirubinuria bilirubin in the urine.

bimanual pertaining to the use of both hands; an examination performed with both hands.

bioethics moral issues and concerns that affect a person's life.

biohazardous describing a substance that is a risk to the health of living organisms.

biotransform convert the molecules of a substance from one form to another, as in medications within the body.

birthday rule determination of which policyholder's insurance is the first to pay when a patient is covered by two policies. The policyholder whose birth month and day comes first in the calendar is primary.

blister a collection of fluid in or beneath the epidermis; a vesicle.

block a type of letter format in which the date, subject line, closing, and signature are justified to the right margin; all other lines are justified left.

blood-borne pathogens viruses that can be spread through direct contact with blood or body fluids from an infected person.

blood urea nitrogen (BUN) blood test to determine the amount of nitrogen in blood in the form of urea, a waste product normally excreted in urine.

body fluids any of the fluids that accumulate in the compartments of the body, such as the blood plasma, and the intracellular and extracellular spaces.

body mass index a measurement of an individual's ratio of fat to lean body mass. It is calculated by using the following formula: [weight (pounds) $\div$ height (inches)^2] $\times$ 703. A BMI over 30 is considered obese.

boil an abscess of the subcutaneous tissues of the skin; a furuncle.

bolus a mobile mass, for instance, a mass of food that passes into the upper gastrointestinal tract in one swallow, or a dose of medication injected intravenously.

bookkeeping organized and accurate record keeping for financial transactions.

boot to start up the computer.

bradycardia heart rate of less than 60 beats per minute.

bradykinesia abnormally slow voluntary movements.

Braxton-Hicks contractions uterine contractions during pregnancy.

breach an infraction, such as breach of contract, in which the agreed-on terms are violated.

bruit abnormal sound or murmur in the blood vessels during auscultation.

buccal describing medication administered between the cheek and gum of the mouth.

budget financial planning tool that helps an organization estimate its anticipated expenditures and revenues.

buffer extra time to accommodate emergencies, walk-ins, and other demands on the provider's daily time schedule that are not considered direct patient care.

bulla large blister or vesicle.

BUN *see* blood urea nitrogen.

bundle of His a band of specialized cardiac muscle fibers that receives the electrical impulse from the AV node and transmits it through right and left branches to the Purkinje fibers.

bursae small sacs filled with clear synovial fluid that surround some joints.

byte a unit of symbolic transfer; each character equals one byte.

C

caduceus a symbol using a wand or staff with two serpents coiled around it; sometimes used as the sign of the medical profession (the more appropriate symbol has only one snake).

calibrated marked in units of measurement, as a thermometer calibrated in Celsius.

calibration the standardization of any measuring instrument or testing procedure.

callus in the musculoskeletal system, a deposit of new bone tissue that forms between the healing ends of broken bones; in the integumentary system, a thickened area of the epidermis caused by pressure or friction.

calorie A unit of heat content or energy. The amount of heat necessary to raise 1 g of water from 14.5 to 15.5°C (small calorie).

calyx (plural, calyces) a cup-like collecting structure of the kidney.

cancellous porous, spongy bone inside the medulla of the bone, usually filled with marrow.

capitation managed care plan that pays a certain amount to a provider over a specific time for caring for the patients in the plan regardless of what or how many services are performed.

carbohydrates chemical elements in food that convert to sugar, providing energy.

carbuncle infection of interconnected group of hair follicles or several furuncles forming a mass.

cardiac cycle period from the beginning of one heartbeat to the beginning of the next; includes systole and diastole.

cardiac output the amount of blood ejected from either ventricle per minute, either to the pulmonary or to the systemic circulation.

cardinal signs usually, vital signs; signifies their importance in assessment.

cardiogenic shock type of shock in which the left ventricle fails to pump enough blood for the body to function.

cardiomegaly enlarged heart muscle.

cardiomyopathy any disease affecting the myocardium.

carina a ridge-like structure; that part of the trachea that projects from the lower end of the trachea.

carrier person infected with a microorganism but without signs of disease; a company that assumes the risk of an insurance company.

cassette light-proof holder in which x-ray film is exposed.

catabolize to break down fats.

cataracts progressive loss of transparency of the lens of the eye, resulting in opacity and loss of sight.

catheterization procedure for introducing a flexible tube into the body; urinary catheterization is for removal of urine from the bladder.

cations chemicals that carry a positive charge.

cautery means, device, or agent that destroys or coagulates tissue; may be electrical current, freezing or burning agent, or chemical solution (caustic).

cell the most basic unit of all living organisms.

cellulitis inflammation or infection of the skin and deeper tissues that may result in tissue destruction if not treated properly.

Celsius, centigrade (C) a temperature scale on which 0 degrees is the freezing point of water and 100 degrees is the boiling point of water at sea level.

centesis surgical puncture made into a cavity.

central processing unit (CPU) circuitry imprinted on a silicon chip that processes information; the "brain" of the computer.

cephalalgia headache.

cerebellum located in the posterior part of the brain, responsible for balance and muscle coordination.

cerebrovascular accident (CVA) ischemia of the brain due to an occlusion of the blood vessels supplying the brain, resulting in varying degrees of debilitation.

cerebrum largest part of the brain, divided into two hemispheres; responsible for thought processes, sensory and motor functions, speech, writing, memory, and emotions.

certification voluntary process that involves a testing procedure to prove an individual's baseline competency in a particular area.

cerumen yellowish or brownish wax-like secretion in the external ear canal; earwax.

Chadwick's sign sign of early pregnancy in which the vaginal, cervical, and vulvar tissues develop a bluish-violet color.

challenge a method of testing a patient's sensitivity or response to a substance by introducing it into the body and watching its effects.

chancre a hard ulcer that appears 2 to 3 weeks after exposure to syphilis, near the site of infection.

charge slip a preprinted three-part form that can be placed on a daysheet to record the patient's charges and payments along with other information in an encounter form.

check register place to record checks that have been written.

check stub indicates to whom a check was issued, in what amount, and on what date.

Chemical Hygiene Plan (CHP) a part of OSHA's HazCom standard.

chemical name exact chemical descriptor of a drug.

chief complaint main reason for the visit to the medical office.

chlamydia a parasitic microorganism with properties common to bacteria but unable to sustain life without a host, in the manner of a virus.

chronic long-standing.

chronic obstructive pulmonary disease (COPD) progressive, irreversible condition with diminished respiratory capacity.

chronological order placing in the order of time; usually the most recent is placed foremost.

chyle milky, fatty product of digestion absorbed through the small intestines and returned to circulation by the lymphatics.

chyme the thick, semi-liquid mass of ingested food mixed with gastric juices as it passes from the stomach.

cilia hair-like projections on cells that either propel the cell or objects that come in contact with the cell.

circumcision surgical removal of the prepuce.

civil law a branch of law that focuses on issues between private citizens.

claims requests to an insurance company for reimbursement of costs.

claims administrator an individual who manages the third-party reimbursement policies for a medical practice.

clarification explanation; removal of confusion or uncertainty.

clearinghouse a company that receives, reviews, sends, and manages insurance claims for physicians.

climacteric period menopause; developmental phase in which a woman's reproductive ability ceases.

clinical pertaining to direct patient care (e.g., nonadministrative tasks that a medical assistant will perform).

clinical chemistry the study of the presence and measurement of substances in blood.

clinical diagnosis a diagnosis based only on the patient's clinical symptoms.

Clinical Laboratory Improvement Amendments (CLIA) guidelines established by Congress in 1988 to standardize and improve laboratory testing.

Clinical and Laboratory Standards Institute (CLSI) a committee appointed to establish rules to ensure the safety, standards, and integrity of all testing performed on human specimens.

cloning genetically identical replication of cells, an organ, or an organism in the laboratory.

closed captioning printed words displayed on a television screen to help people with hearing disabilities or impairments.

closing a one- to two-word phrase that precedes the sender's signature and indicates the end of the letter.

clustering grouping patients with similar problems or needs.

coagulate change from a liquid to a solid or semi-solid mass.

coagulation the study of the blood's ability to clot.

cocci spherical bacteria.

coinsurance the agreed-upon amount paid to the provider by a policyholder. Also called co-payment.

collagen protein substance that gives structure to the connective tissue.

collection a process of acquiring funds that are due.

colpocleisis surgery to occlude the vagina.

colporrhaphy suturing of the vagina.

colposcopy visual examination of the vagina and cervix under magnification.

common law traditional laws that were established by the English legal system.

comparative negligence a percentage of damage awards based on the contribution of negligence between two parties.

complete blood count (CBC) the CBC is a frequently ordered laboratory test consisting of white blood cell count and differential, red blood cell count, hemoglobin, hematocrit, erythrocyte indices, and platelet count.

compliance willingness of a patient to follow a prescribed course of treatment.

compliance officer person charged with ensuring that a facility follows laws, policies, and protocols.

concussion injury to the brain due to trauma.

confidentiality protection of patient data from unauthorized personnel.

congenital anomaly abnormality, either structural or functional, present at birth.

congestive heart failure condition in which the heart cannot pump effectively.

consent an agreement between a patient and physician to do a given medical procedure.

constellation of symptoms a group of clinical signs indicating a particular disease process.

consultation request for assistance from one physician to another.

continuing education units (CEUs) credits awarded for attendance at approved local and state AAMA meetings and seminars, completion of guided study courses, and journal articles designed to submit a posttest for CEU credit.

contract an agreement between two or more parties for a given act.

contracture abnormal shortening of muscles around a joint caused by atrophy of the muscles and resulting in flexion and fixation.

contraindication situation or condition that prohibits the prescribing or administering of a drug or medication.

contrast medium substance ingested or injected into the body to facilitate imaging of internal structures.

contributory negligence a defense strategy in which the defendant admits to negligence but claims that the plaintiff assisted in promoting the damages.

contusion collection of blood in tissues after an injury; a bruise.

conventions general notes, symbols, typeface, format, and punctuation that direct and guide the coder to the most complete and accurate ICD-9 code.

convoluted tubules the twisted portion of the nephron that connects the glomerulus to the collecting tubules; consists of a proximal and a distal portion connected by the loop of Henle.

convulsion sudden, involuntary muscle contraction of a voluntary muscle group.

cookies tiny files that are left on your computer's hard drive by a website without your permission.

coordination of benefits the method of designating the order in which multiple carriers pay benefits to avoid duplication of payment.

co-payments that part of an insured service the patient must pay.

coping mechanisms unconscious methods of alleviating intense stressors.

coronary artery bypass graft surgical procedure that increases the blood flow to the heart by bypassing the occluded or blocked vessel with a graft.

corpora cavernosa the erectile bodies of the penis or clitoris.

corpus spongiosum erectile tissue around the male urethra.

corticoid any of the hormonal steroid substances obtained from the adrenal cortex.

cortisol a naturally occurring steroidal hormone that regulates metabolism and acts as an anti-inflammatory agent.

coumarin an anticoagulant prescribed for persons likely to form blood clots, such as valve replacement recipients; also called Coumadin (trade name) or warfarin.

covered entity anyone required to follow HIPAA's requirements. Health care providers, insurance companies, and insurance clearinghouses are covered entities.

cranium the portion of the skull that encloses the brain.

creatinine a breakdown product of creatine that aids in delivering energy to cells.

credit balance in one's favor on an account; promise to pay a bill at a later date; record of a payment received.

cretinism severe congenital hypothyroidism; signs include dwarfism, low intelligence, puffy features, dry skin, macroglossia, and poor muscle tone.

criteria the standard, rule, or test by which something or someone can be judged.

crossover claim a claim that crosses over automatically from one coverage to another for payment.

cross-reference notation in a file telling that a record is stored elsewhere and giving the reference; verification to another source; checking the tabular list against the alphabetic list in ICD-9 coding.

cryosurgery the surgical destruction of tissue using freezing temperature with liquid nitrogen or carbon dioxide.

cul-de-sac blind pouch or cavity, as in the cul-de-sac that lies between the rectum and the posterior uterus.

culdocentesis surgical puncture and aspiration of fluid from the vaginal cul-de-sac for diagnosis or therapy.

culture a laboratory process whereby microorganisms are grown in a special medium often for the purpose of identifying a causative agent in an infectious disease; also means the way of life, including commonly held beliefs, of a group of people.

curettage scraping of a body cavity, such as the uterus.

Current Procedural Terminology a comprehensive list of codes used by physicians to bill for procedures and services.

cursor flashing line on the monitor indicating where data input will occur.

Cushing's syndrome a disorder resulting from increased adrenocortical secretion of cortisol.

cyanotic a bluish discoloration of the skin due to the lack of oxygen.

cystocele herniation of the urinary bladder into the vagina.

cystoscopy direct visualization of the urinary bladder through a cystoscope inserted through the urethra.

cytogenetics a type of cytology in which the genetic structure of the cells obtained from tissue, blood, or body fluids, such as amniotic fluid, are examined or tested for chromosome deficiencies related to genetic disease.

cytology Study of the microscopic structure of cells.

D

DACUM a code of educational standards for medical assisting students developed by the American Association of Medical Assistants.

damages the resulting injury or suffering that resulted from negligence.

data information that is stored and processed by the computer.

database accumulation of files on the computer

daysheet/daily journal a daily business record of charges and payments.

debit a charge or money owed on an account.

decibel (db) unit of intensity of sound.

deciduous to fall or shed; deciduous teeth: the set of 20 teeth appearing during infancy and shedding during childhood.

decongestant substance that reduces congestion or swelling.

deductible a specified amount paid by the policyholder before the carrier begins paying.

defamation of character making false or malicious statements about a person's character or reputation.

defendant the party that is accused.

degenerative joint disease (DJD) also known as osteoarthritis; arthritis characterized by degeneration of the bony structure of the joints, usually noninflammatory.

deglutition the act of swallowing.

dehiscence separation or opening of the edges of a wound.

demeanor the way a person looks, behaves, and conducts himself or herself.

dementia progressive organic mental deterioration with loss of intellectual function.

demographic relating to the statistical characteristics of populations.

dendrite part of the neuron that transmits impulses toward the cell body.

denial saying that something is not true; refusing to acknowledge.

dental cavities holes in the teeth.

dentin the main component of the tooth structure, surrounds the inner pulp and lies just below the enamel.

dependent spouse, children, and sometimes other individuals designated by the insured who are covered under a health care plan.

depolarization progressive wave of stimulation causing contraction of the myocardium.

deposition a process in which one party questions another party under oath.

dermatophytosis fungal infection of the skin.

dermis layer of skin under the epidermis.

descriptor description of a service listed with its code number.

detoxification clearing of drugs from the body and treating the withdrawal symptoms.

dextrocardia the condition of having the heart in the right side of the thoracic cavity.

diabetes insipidus a disorder of metabolism characterized by polyuria and polydipsia; caused by a deficiency in ADH or an inability of the kidneys to respond to ADH.

diagnosis identification of a disease or condition by evaluating physical signs and symptoms, health history, and laboratory tests; a disease or condition identified in a person.

diagnostic related group (DRG) categories used to determine hospital and physician reimbursement for Medicare patients' inpatient services.

dialysis removal of waste in blood not filtered by kidneys by passing fluid through a semipermeable barrier that allows normal electrolytes to remain, either with a machine with circulatory access or by passing a balanced fluid through the peritoneal cavity.

diaphoresis profuse sweating.

diaphragmatic excursion the movement of the diaphragm during respiration.

diarthroses freely movable joints; also called synovial joints.

diastole relaxation phase of the cardiac cycle.

diction the style of speaking and enunciating words.

dideoxycytidine (ddC) a drug used to treat AIDS by blocking the growth of the virus after it enters the T-cell lymphocytes.

dideoxyinosine (ddI) a drug used to treat AIDS by blocking the growth of the virus after it enters the T-cell lymphocytes.

diencephalon part of the brain lying beneath the hemispheres, containing the thalamus and hypothalamus.

differential diagnosis a diagnosis made by comparing the patient's symptoms to two or more diseases that have similar symptoms.

diluent specified liquid used to reconstitute powder medications for injection

diplomacy the art of handling people with tact and genuine concern.

directory a "table of contents" of a file system.

discrimination making a difference in favor of or against someone.

disease definite pathologic process having a distinctive set of symptoms and course of progression.

disinfectant a chemical that can be applied to objects to destroy microorganisms; will not destroy bacterial spores.

disinfection killing or rendering inert most but not all pathogenic microorganisms.

disk drive a device that gets information on and off a floppy disk.

dissemination the process of distributing information on community resources.

diuretics substances that promote the formation and excretion of urine.

diurnal variation variation over a 24-hour period.

documentation the process of recording patient information.

donor one who contributes something to another.

double booking the practice of booking two patients for the same period with the same physician

dowager's hump exaggerated cervical curve with prominence of the top thoracic vertebrae found in some osteoporotic elderly women; a type of kyphosis.

downloading transferring information from an outside location to your computer.

dressing a covering applied directly to a wound to apply pressure, give support, absorb secretions, protect from trauma or microorganisms, stop or slow bleeding, or hide disfigurement.

drug any substance that may modify one or more of the functions of an organism.

due process a formal proceeding in which the accused is considered not guilty until a verdict is reached.

dura mater the outer covering of the brain.

durable power of attorney a legal document giving another person the authority to act on one's behalf.

duress the act of compelling or forcing someone to do something that they do not want to do.

dwarfism (endocrine or pituitary) abnormal underdevelopment of the body with extreme shortness but normal proportions; achondroplastic dwarfism is an inherited growth disorder characterized by shortened limbs and a large head but almost normal trunk proportions.

dysmenorrhea painful menstruation.

dyspareunia painful coitus or sexual intercourse.

dysphagia inability to swallow or difficulty in swallowing.

dysphasia difficulty speaking.

dysphonia impairment of voice; hoarseness.

dyspnea difficulty breathing.

dysuria painful or difficult urination.

E

E-codes codes indicating the external cause or reason for an injury or illness.

ecchymosis characteristic black and blue mark that results from blood as it accumulates under the skin.

eczema superficial dermatitis.

edema an accumulation of fluid within the tissues.

efferent carrying impulses away from the center.

elastin protein substance that gives elasticity and flexibility to the connective tissues.

electrocardiography procedure that produces a record of the electrical activity of the heart.

electrode medium for conducting or detecting electrical current.

electroencephalogram (EEG) tracing of the electrical activity of the brain.

electrolytes certain chemical substances dissolved in the blood and having numerous basic functions such as conducting electrical currents; the principal electrolytes are sodium, potassium, chloride, and bicarbonate.

electromyography recording of electrical nerve transmission in skeletal muscles.

electronic health records information about patients that is recorded and stored on computer.

element a substance that cannot be separated or broken down into substances with properties other than its own; a primary substance.

eligibility the determination of an insured's right to receive benefits from a third-party payer based on such criteria as payment of premiums and date of start of coverage.

emancipated minor a patient under the age of majority but who is legally considered to be an adult.

embolus mass of matter (thrombus, air, fat globule) freely floating in the circulatory system.

emergency medical service (EMS) a group of health care providers working as a team to care for sick or injured patients before they arrive at the hospital.

empathy the ability to understand or to some extent share what someone else is feeling.

employee a person hired to perform given duties in return for financial compensation.

enclosure indication for the reader that an item is accompanying the letter.

encounter form a preprinted statement that lists codes for basic office charges and has sections to record charges incurred in an office visit, the patient's current balance, and next appointment.

encryption scrambling E-mail messages as they leave one site and unscrambling them when they arrive at the designated address.

endemic a disease that occurs continuously in a particular population but has a low mortality; used in contrast to epidemic.

endocarditis inflammation of the inner lining of the heart.

endocardium the innermost part of the heart wall; it lines the heart chamber and covers the connective tissue skeleton of the heart valves.

endocrinologist a physician who specializes in disorders of the endocrine system.

endogenous having its origin within an organism.

endorphins chemicals that are often called the body's "natural painkillers" that tend to produce a euphoria, or "good feeling." Release of endorphins is often caused by physical movement or exercise.

endotracheal tube a large instrument usually inserted through the mouth (may use the nose) and into the trachea to the point of the tracheal division to deliver oxygen under pressure.

enumerated counted.

enuresis bed wetting.

enzyme a protein that begins (catalyzes) a chemical reaction.

eosinophil a type of leukocyte increased in allergic reactions and parasitic infections.

epicardium the inner or visceral layer of the pericardium that forms the outermost layer of the heart wall.

epidermis outer layer of the skin.

epiglottis the leaf-like flap that closes down over the glottis during swallowing.

epiphyseal end plate a thin layer of cartilage at the end of long bones where new growth takes place.

episiotomy incision of the perineum to accommodate vaginal delivery of fetus.

eponym word derived from a personal name, e.g., *Alzheimer's* disease.

ergonomic describes a workstation designed to prevent work-related injuries and to promote work efficiency.

erythema redness of the skin.

erythematous characterized by redness (erythema).

erythrocyte a red blood cell.

erythrocyte indices three measurements (mean cell volume, mean cell hemoglobin, and mean cell hemoglobin concentration) that indicate the size of the red blood cell and how much hemoglobin the red blood cell holds.

erythrocyte sedimentation rate measures the rate in millimeters per hour at which red blood cells settle out in a tube.

erythropoietin a hormone produced mainly by the kidney in response to lowered oxygen levels; stimulates the production of red blood cells to increase blood oxygen levels.

essential amino acids amino acids nutritionally required by an organism and that must be supplied in its diet (i.e., cannot be synthesized by the organism).

ethernet system that allows the computer to be connected to a cable or DSL system.

ethics guidelines for moral behavior that are enforced by peer groups.

ethylene oxide gas used to sterilize surgical instruments and other supplies.

etiology cause of disease.

eunuchoidism deficient production of male hormone by the testes, resulting in loss of the secondary male characteristics.

euphoria a feeling of well-being.

eustachian tubes a mucous membrane-lined tube between the nasopharynx and the middle ear bilaterally that equalizes the internal and external otic air pressure.

euthanasia allowing a patient to die with minimal medical interventions.

evacuated tube a type of blood collection tube that is sealed with a premeasured, partial vacuum by rubber stoppers. The tube receives the patient's blood during venipuncture.

evaluation the process of indicating how well the patient or person is progressing toward a particular goal; to appraise; to determine the worth or quality of something or someone.

exogenous having its origin outside of the organism; its opposite is endogenous.

exophthalmia abnormal protrusion of the eyeballs.

exophthalmic goiter abnormal protrusion of the eyeballs accompanied by goiter.

expected threshold a numerical goal.

expert witness a professional who testifies on the standard of care in a trial.

explanation of benefits (EOB) a statement that accompanies a payment from an insurance carrier and outlines which dates and services are being paid.

exposure control plan written plan required by the Occupational Safety and Health Administration that outlines an employer's system for preventing infection.

exposure risk factors conditions that tend to put employees at risk for contact with biohazardous agents such as blood-borne pathogens.

expressed consent a statement of approval from the patient for the physician to perform a given procedure after the patient has been educated about the risks and benefits of the particular procedure; also referred to as informed consent.

expressed contracts formal agreements between two or more people.

expulsion formal discharge from a professional organization.

externship an educational course that allows the student to obtain hands-on experience.

extracellular outside of the cell.

extraocular outside the eye, as in extraocular eye movement.

F

familial referring to a disorder that tends to occur more often in a family than would be anticipated solely by chance.

Family and Medical Leave Act a law designed to allow an employee up to 12 weeks of unpaid leave from his or her job to meet family needs.

fascia fibrous membrane tissue that covers and supports the muscles and joins the skin with underlying tissue.

fast to abstain from eating or drinking anything but water; often done before a medical test or procedure.

febrile having an above-normal body temperature.

federal unemployment tax tax used to finance all administrative expenses of the federal/state unemployment insurance system and the federal costs involved in extended benefits.

fee-for-service an established set of fees charged for specific services and paid by the patient or insurance carrier.

fee schedule a list of pre-established fee allowances set for specific services and procedures performed by a provider.

fee-splitting sharing of fees between physicians for patient referrals.

feedback in communication, the response to input from another.

FICA Federal Insurance Contributions Act; the law that established Social Security and that mandates Social Security tax payments and benefits.

file grouping of data that is given a name for easy access.

filing system a method for organizing records so that they can be found when needed.

film raw material on which x-rays are projected through the body; prior to processing, it does not contain a visible image (similar to photographic film).

fixative a chemical substance used to bind, fix, or stabilize specimens of tissue to slides for later examination.

flagella hair-like extremity of a bacterium or protozoan; used to facilitate movement.

floppy disk thin magnetic film on which to store data.

flow sheet color-coded sheets that allow information to be recorded in graphic or tabular form for easy retrieval.

fluorescein angiography intravenous injection of fluorescent dye; photographing blood vessels of the eye as dye moves through them.

fluoroscopy special x-ray technique for examining a body part by immediate projection onto a fluorescent screen.

folate a salt of folic acid; it acts to help enzymes that build structures such as blood cells.

folliculitis inflammation of hair follicles.

font a typeface; affects the way written messages look.

forced expiratory volume (FEV) volume of air forced out of the lungs.

forceps surgical instrument used to grasp, handle, compress, pull, or join tissues, equipment, or supplies.

fraud a deceitful act with the intention to conceal the truth.

fulgurate destroy tissue by electrodessication.

full block a type of letter format in which all letter components are justified left.

full-thickness burn burn that has destroyed all skin layers.

furuncle infection in a hair follicle or gland; characterized by pain, redness, and swelling with necrosis of tissue in the center.

G

gait manner or style of walking.

galactosuria condition in newborns lacking an enzyme that metabolizes galactose; increased levels of galactose appear in the blood and urine (if proper therapy is not initiated, mental retardation and other difficulties will occur).

gastroenteritis inflammation of the gastrointestinal tract caused by bacteria or viruses.

gauge diameter of a needle lumen

gel separator a nonreacting substance located in an evacuated tube that forms a physical barrier between the cells and serum or plasma after the specimen has been centrifuged.

generic name official name given to a drug whose patent has expired.

germicide chemical that kills most pathogenic microorganisms; disinfectant.

gerontologist specialist who studies aging.

gestation period of time from conception to birth; usually 37–41 weeks.

gestational diabetes a disorder characterized by an impaired ability to metabolize carbohydrates, usually due to insulin deficiency, occurring in pregnancy and usually disappearing after delivery.

gigantism excessive size and stature caused most frequently by hypersecretion of the human growth hormone (HGH).

gingiva the gums; the mucous membrane–covered tissues that support the teeth.

glaucoma abnormal increase in the fluid in the eye, usually as a result of obstructed outflow, resulting in degeneration of the intraocular components and blindness.

glomerulus a small cluster of blood vessels within the Bowman's capsule.

glycosuria the presence of glucose in the urine.

goiter an enlargement of the thyroid gland.

gonads a generic term referring to the sex glands of both sexes, either ovaries or testes.

goniometer instrument used to measure the angle of joints for range of motion.

Goodell's sign softening of the cervix early in pregnancy.

granulocytes white blood cells that have visible granules when stained.

Graves' disease pronounced hyperthyroidism with signs of enlarged thyroid and exophthalmos.

gravid pregnant.

gravida pregnant woman.

gravidity pregnancy.

grief great sadness caused by loss.

gross income the amount of money earned by an employee before taxes are withheld.

group member a policyholder who is a member of a group and covered by the group's insurance carrier.

guaiac substance used in laboratory tests for occult blood in the stool.

gyri the convolutions of the brain tissue.

H

hard drive a place where the computer stores programs and data files.

hardware equipment on the computer system, e.g., keyboard, disk drive, monitor, printer.

Hashimoto's thyroiditis Diffuse infiltration of the thyroid gland with lymphocytes, resulting in diffuse goiter and hypothyroidism.

HCFA *see* Health Care Financing Administration.

HCPCS *see* Health Care Financing Administration Common Procedures Coding System.

Healthcare Common Procedure Coding System AMA's coding system based on CPT-4. Assigns alphabetic and numeric codes to items such as ambulance service, wheelchairs, and injections.

Health Care Financing Administration (HCFA) a federal agency that regulates health care financing and the procedural classification (Volume 3 of the ICD-9-CM coding book).

Health Care Financing Administration Common Procedures Coding System (HCPCS) a numerical system used by HCFA for services not covered by the CPT coding system.

health care savings accounts (HSAs) a benefit offered by some employers that allows employees to save money through payroll deduction to accounts that can only be used for medical care.

health insurance a policy that promises to pay some or all of a customer's medical bills.

Health Insurance Portability and Accountability Act (HIPAA) federal law, originally passed as the Kassebaum-Kennedy Act, that requires all health care settings to ensure privacy and security of patient information. Also requires health insurance to be accessible for working Americans and available when changing employment.

health maintenance organization (HMO) an organization that provides a wide range of services through a contract with a specified group at a predetermined payment.

heat cramps type of hyperthermia that causes muscle cramping resulting from high-sodium heat exhaustion; hyperthermia resulting from physical exertion in heat without adequate fluid replacement.

heat exhaustion a type of hyperthermia that causes an altered mental status due to inadequate fluid replacement.

heat stroke most serious type of hyperthermia; body is no longer able to compensate for elevated temperature.

hematemesis vomiting blood or bloody vomitus.

hematocrit the percentage of red blood cells in whole blood.

hematology the study of blood and blood-forming tissues.

hematoma blood clot that forms at an injury site.

hematopoiesis blood cell production.

hematuria blood in the urine.

hemoconcentration decrease in the volume of plasma in blood causing an increase in blood components. Can be caused by excessive application of the tourniquet.

hemoglobin the functioning unit of the red blood cell.

hemoglobinuria presence of free hemoglobin in urine.

hemolysis rupture of erythrocytes with the release of hemoglobin into the plasma or serum causing the specimen to appear pink or red in color.

hemolytic anemia a disorder characterized by premature destruction of the red cells; this may be brought on by an infectious process, inherited red cell disorders, or as a response to certain drugs or toxins.

hemoptysis coughing up blood from the respiratory tract.

hemostasis process that results in control of bleeding after an injury.

hemostat surgical instrument with slender jaws used for grasping blood vessels.

heparin a naturally occurring anticoagulant given to prevent clot formation.

hepatomegaly enlarged liver.

hepatotoxin substance that can damage the liver.

hereditary referring to traits or disorders that are transmitted from parent to offspring.

hernia protrusion of an organ through the muscle wall of the cavity that normally surrounds it.

herpes simplex infection caused by the herpes simplex virus.

herpes zoster infection caused by reactivation of varicella zoster virus, which causes chickenpox.

hiatus an opening or gap; hiatal hernia: a protrusion of part of the stomach upward through the diaphragm.

HIPAA *see* Health Insurance Portability and Accountability Act.

Hippocratic Oath a code of ethics written by Hippocrates.

hirsutism abnormal or excessive growth of hair in women.

histamine substance found normally in the body in response to injured cells, producing the inflammatory process: dilation of capillaries, increased gastric secretions, and contraction of smooth muscles.

histology study of the microscopic structure of tissue.

homeopathic referring to an alternative type of medicine in which patients are treated with small doses of substances that produce similar symptoms and use the body's own healing abilities.

homeostasis maintaining a constant internal environment by balancing positive and negative feedback.

hormone a substance that is produced by an endocrine gland and travels through the blood to a distant organ or gland where it acts to modify the structure or function of that gland or organ.

human chorionic gonadotropin (hCG) hormone secreted by the placenta and found in the urine and blood of a pregnant female.

humidifier appliance that increases the moisture content in the air.

hydrogen ion hydrogen that is missing an electron and therefore readily binds with substances having extra electrons; it is an important constituent of acids.

hypercalcemia an excessive amount of calcium in the blood.

hyperglycemia an increase in blood sugar, as in diabetes mellitus.

hyperopia farsightedness.

hyperosmolarity a condition of having increased numbers of dissolved substances in the plasma.

hyperplasia excessive proliferation of normal cells in the normal tissue arrangement of an organism.

hyperpnea abnormally deep, gasping breaths.

hyperpyrexia dangerously high temperature, 105° to 106°F.

hypertension morbidly high blood pressure.

hyperthermia general condition of excessive body heat.

hyperventilation a respiratory rate that greatly exceeds the body's oxygen demands.

hypoglycemia deficiency of sugar (glucose) in the blood.

hypopnea shallow respirations.

hypothalamus part of the diencephalon; activates and controls the peripheral nervous system, endocrine system, and certain involuntary functions.

hypothermia below-normal body temperature.

hypovolemic shock shock caused by loss of blood or other body fluids.

hysterosalpingogram radiograph of the uterus and fallopian tubes after injection with a contrast medium.

hysteroscopy visual examination with magnification of the uterus.

I

iatrogenic a condition caused by treatment or medical procedures.

idiopathic unknown etiology.

immune globulins proteins produced by plasma cells in response to foreign antigens; provide immediate antibody protection for a few weeks to a few months.

immunity lack of susceptibility to a disease.

immunization act or process of rendering an individual immune to specific disease.

immunohematology the study of blood typing and compatibility testing for transfusion.

immunology the study of antigen–antibody reactions.

impetigo highly infectious skin infection causing erythema and progressing to honey-colored crusts.

implementation the process of initiating and carrying out an action such as a teaching plan or patient treatment.

implied consent an informal agreement of approval from the patient to perform a given task.

implied contracts contracts between physician and patient not written but assumed by the actions of the parties.

impotence inability to achieve or maintain an erection.

incident report a form used by an organization to document an unusual occurrence to a patient, visitor, or employee.

incontinence inability to control elimination, either urine or feces or both.

independent practice association (IPA) several independently practicing physicians contracted with a health maintenance organization to provide services to HMO members.

indices (singular, index) numbers expressing a property or ratio.

induration hardened area at the injection site after an intradermal screening test for tuberculosis.

infarction death of tissues due to lack of oxygen.

infection invasion by disease-producing microorganisms.

infiltration leakage of intravenous fluids into surrounding tissues.

informed consent a statement of approval from the patient for the physician to perform a given procedure after the patient has been educated about the risks and benefits of the procedure; also referred to as expressed consent.

inguinal pertaining to the regions of the groin.

inpatient a medical setting in which patients are admitted for diagnostic, radiographic, or treatment purposes.

insertion a place of attachment, usually the freely movable portion of a muscle.

inspection visual examination.

installment partial payment of a bill.

institutional review board internal committee that reviews ethical issues.

insufflator device for blowing air, gas, or powder into a body cavity.

insula fifth lobe of the cerebrum.

insulin-dependent diabetes mellitus a deficiency in insulin production that leads to an inability to metabolize carbohydrates.

insured an individual who owns a policy that promises to pay some or all of his or her medical bills.

interaction effects, positive or negative, of two or more drugs taken by a patient.

intercaps words or phrases with unusual capitalization.

interferon group of proteins released by white blood cells and fibroblasts when the invading microorganism is a virus.

intermittent occurring at intervals.

Internal Revenue Service (IRS) a federal agency that regulates and enforces various taxes.

International Classification of Diseases, Ninth Revision, Clinical Modification a system for transforming verbal descriptions of disease, injuries, conditions, and procedures to numeric codes.

Internet global system used to connect one computer to another.

interosseous between bones.

interstitial the spaces between the cells.

intracellular inside of the cell.

intranet a private network system of computers.

intraocular pressure pressure within the eyeball.

intrauterine pregnancy (IUP) pregnancy located in the uterus.

intravascular coagulation clot formation within the vessels; strands of fibrin may form from one wall of the vessel to the other and shear red cells as they pass by.

intravenous pyelogram (IVP) radiography using contrast medium to evaluate kidney function.

intrinsic found within a structure.

introitus vaginal orifice.

invoice a statement of debt owed; a bill.

iodine an element that is an essential micronutrient used in the thyroid gland to manufacture its hormones; present in seafood, foods grown in iodized soil, iodized salt, and some dairy products.

ion an atom or group of atoms that has become electrically charged by the loss or gain of one or more electrons.

iontophoresis introduction of various chemical ions into the skin by means of electrical current.

ischemia decrease in oxygen to tissues.

J

job description a statement that informs an employee about the duties and expectations for a given job.

Joint Commission on Accreditation of Health Care Organizations (JCAHO) a voluntary organization that sets and evaluates the standards of care for health care institutions; based on the JCAHO evaluation, an accreditation title will be given to the organization.

K

Kaposi sarcoma cancer of the skin that is extremely rare except in AIDS patients.

Kegel exercises isometric exercises in which the muscles of the pelvic floor are voluntarily contracted and relaxed while urinating.

keratin a tough, insoluble protein substance of the stratum corneum, hair, and nails.

keratoses (senile) premalignant overgrowth or thickening of the upper layer of epithelium or horny layer of the skin.

keratosis skin condition characterized by overgrowth and thickening.

ketoacidosis acidosis accompanied by an accumulation of ketones in the body.

ketones the end products of fat and protein metabolism.

key components the criteria or factors on which the selection of a CPT-4 evaluation and management is based.

kinesics a form of nonverbal communication including gestures, body movements, and facial expressions.

Krebs cycle a sequence of reactions within cells that metabolizes sugars and other energy sources, such as carbohydrates, proteins, and fats, into carbon dioxide, water, and ATP.

kyphosis (dowager's hump) abnormally deep dorsal curvature of the thoracic spine; also known as humpback or hunchback.

L

labor involuntary contractions of the uterine muscle resulting in cervical dilation and effacement (thinning) of the cervix; prelude to childbirth.

laboratory a place where research, investigation, or scientific testing takes place.

laboratory procedure manual CLIA regulations require each laboratory to have its own procedure manual describing how to perform every test in the laboratory.

laparoscopy process of viewing the internal abdominal cavity and its contents through a specialized endoscope.

laparotomy incision of the abdominal cavity.

laryngectomy surgical removal of the larynx.

laser ablation destruction or removal of tissue by use of laser.

late effects conditions that result from another condition. For example, left-sided paralysis may be a *late effect* of a stroke.

lead electrode or electrical connection attached to the body to record electrical impulses in the body, especially the heart or brain.

learning objectives steps that need to be achieved to accomplish the learning goal.

learning goal an agreed upon outcome of the teaching process.

ledger card a record of the patient's financial activities; a continuous record of business transactions with debits and credits.

legally required disclosure reporting of certain events to governmental agencies without the patient's consent.

lentigines brown skin macules occurring after exposure to the sun; freckle; tan or brown macules found on elderly skin after prolonged sun exposure; also known as liver spots.

leukocyte a white blood cell.

leukocyte esterase an enzyme present in leukocytes; a reagent strip test that is positive for leukocyte esterase can identify a urinary tract infection.

leukocytosis abnormal increase of leukocytes (white blood cells).

leukoplakia white, thickened patches on the oral mucosa or tongue that are often precancerous.

liabilities amounts the practice owes.

libel written statements that defame a person's reputation or character.

ligament a flexible band of tissue that holds joints together.

lightening the descent of the fetus in the pelvis.

lipase any of several enzymes that begin the breakdown of fats in the digestive tract.

lipids any of the free fatty acids (fats) in the body.

lipoproteins a substance made up of a lipid and a protein.

literary search finding professional journal articles on a given subject.

lithotripsy crushing of a stone with sound waves.

litigation process of filing or contesting a lawsuit.

lochia uterine discharge following childbirth, composed of some blood, mucus, and tissue.

locum tenens a substitute physician.

login use of a password to gain access to the computer.

loop of Henle a portion of the renal tubule that is shaped like a U and consisting of a thick ascending and thin descending vessels.

lordosis abnormally deep ventral curve at the lumbar flexure of the spine; also known as swayback.

lubricant agent that reduces friction.

Luer adapter a device for connecting a syringe or evacuated holder to the needle to promote a secure fit.

lymphocyte a type of leukocyte.

lyse to cause disintegration; i.e., destruction of adhesions or the breakdown of red blood cells.

M

macrophage a monocyte that has left the circulation and settled and matured in tissue; macrophages process antigens and present them to T cells, activating the immune specific response.

macule small, flat discoloration of the skin.

magnetic resonance imaging imaging technique that uses a strong magnetic field.

main terms words in a multiple-word diagnosis that a coder should locate in the alphabetic listing. They represent the condition (not the location) to be coded.

mainframe central computer to which individual computers are connected; used in large institutions.

malaise general feeling of illness without specific signs or symptoms.

malignant cancerous.

malocclusion abnormal contact between the teeth in the upper and lower jaw.

malpractice a tort in which the patient is harmed by the actions of a health care worker.

managed care the practice of third-party payers to control costs by requiring physicians to adhere to specific rules as a condition of payment.

manipulation skillful use of the hands in diagnostic procedures.

Mantoux intradermal injection screening test for tuberculosis.

margin the blank space around the edges of a piece of paper, such as a letter or page of a book.

masticate the act of chewing or grinding, as in chewing food.

material safety data sheet (MSDS) a detailed record of all hazardous substances kept within a site.

matrix a system for blocking off unavailable patient appointment times.

media a Petri plate containing a solid nutrient gel for growing bacteria from culture specimens.

mediastinum the mid-portion of the thoracic cavity containing the heart, the great vessels, the upper esophagus, and the trachea.

medical asepsis removal or destruction of microorganisms.

medical assistant a multiskilled health professional who performs a variety of clinical and administrative tasks in a medical setting.

medical history record containing information about a patient's past and present health status.

medical necessity a determination made by a third party that a certain service or procedure was necessary based on sound medical practice.

medical setting a place that is designed to meet the health care needs of patients; may be inpatient or outpatient.

Medicare Social Security–established health insurance for the elderly.

medulla oblongata part of the brain that controls breathing, heart rate, and blood pressure.

megabyte one million bytes; a way to measure the quantity of computer information that a particular device can hold.

meiosis the cell division specific to sperm and ova that results in 23 chromosomes rather than 46 (23 pairs).

melanin dark pigment that gives color to the skin, hair, and eyes.

melanocyte cell that produces melanin.

melena black, tarry stools caused by digested blood from the gastrointestinal tract.

memorandum a type of written documentation used for interoffice communication.

menarche onset of first menstruation.

meninges membranes of the spinal cord and brain.

meningocele meninges protruding though the spinal column.

meniscus the curved upper surface of a liquid in a container.

menorrhagia excessive bleeding during menstruation.

menses menstruation; bloody discharge monthly or cyclically in the female when fertilization has not occurred.

mensuration the act or process of measuring.

message words sent from one person to another; information sent through spoken, written, or body language.

metabolic acidosis an acidic condition of the body caused when excess acids are produced in the body's fluids (as in the metabolism of fats instead of glucose) or when the body's natural bicarbonates are lost or diminished.

metabolism sum of chemical processes that result in growth, energy production, elimination of waste, and body functions performed as digested nutrients are distributed.

metric system system of measurement that uses grams, liters, and meters.

metrorrhagia irregular uterine bleeding.

microbiology the study of pathogen identification and antibiotic susceptibility determination.

microfiche sheets of microfilm.

microfilm photographs of records in a reduced size.

microorganisms microscopic living organisms.

microprocessor a chip that allows the computer to function.

micturition also known as voiding or urination.

midbrain part of the brainstem, responsible for relaying messages.

migraine type of severe headache, usually unilateral; may appear in cluster.

minerals inorganic substances (such as sodium, potassium, calcium, phosphorus, magnesium, iron, iodine, fluorine, zinc, copper, cobalt, and chromium) used in the formation of hard and soft body tissue; necessary for muscle contraction, nerve conduction, and blood clotting.

mission statement a statement describing the goals of the medical office and those it serves.

modem (modulator/demodulator) a communication device that connects a computer to the standard telephone system, allowing information exchange with other computers off site.

modifiers letters or numbers added to a code to clarify the service or procedure.

monocyte a type of leukocyte.

monosaccharide a simple sugar that cannot be broken down further.

mordant a substance used to fix, or bind, dyes or stains.

morphology description of the structural characteristics of blood cells.

motherboard fiberglass board that contains the central processing unit (CPU), memory, and other pieces of circuitry.

mourning to demonstrate signs of grief; grieving.

multidisciplinary involving many disciplines; a group of health care professionals from various specialties brought together to meet the patient's needs.

multimedia various forms of communication available on the computer, e.g., stereophonic sound, animation, full-motion video, photographs.

multipara woman who has given birth to more than one viable fetus.

multisample needle used with the evacuated tube method of blood collection, because multiple tubes of blood can be drawn during a multitube draw without removing the needle from the vein. The end of the needle that penetrates the stopper of the tube has a retractable rubber sleeve that covers it when the tube is removed and prevents leaks during tube changes.

multiskilled health professional an individual with versatile training in the health care field.

muscular dystrophies a group of genetically transmitted diseases characterized by progressive atrophy of skeletal muscles.

mycology the science and study of fungi.

myelofibrosis a disorder in which bone marrow tissue develops in abnormal sites such as the liver and spleen; signs include immature cells in the circulation, anemia, and splenomegaly.

myelogram invasive radiologic test in which dye is injected into the spinal fluid.

myelomeningocele protrusion of the spinal cord through the spinal defect; spina bifida.

myocardial infarction (MI) death of cardiac muscle due to lack of blood flow to the muscle; also known as heart attack.

myocarditis inflammation of the myocardial layer of the heart.

myocardium the middle layer of the walls of the heart, composed of cardiac muscle.

myofibrils a slender light/dark strand of muscle tissue in striated muscle.

myopia nearsightedness.

myringotomy incision into the tympanic membrane to relieve pressure.

myxedema the most severe form of hypothyroidism; signs include edema of the extremities and the face.

N

narrative a paragraph indicating the contact with the patient, what was done for the patient, and the outcome of any action.

nasal septum wall or partition dividing the nostrils.

nebulizer device for administering respiratory medications as a fine inhaled spray.

needle holder type of surgical forceps used to hold and pass suture through tissue.

negative feedback a decrease in function in response to a stimulus.

negative stress stress that does not allow for relaxation periods.

negligence performance of an act that a reasonable health care worker would not have done or the omission of an act that a reasonable person would have done.

neonatologist physician who specializes in the care and treatment of newborns.

neoplasm abnormal growth of new tissue; tumor.

nephron the portion of the kidney responsible for the production of urine.

nephrostomy placement of a catheter in the kidney pelvis to drain urine from an obstructed kidney.

net pay the amount of money an employee is paid after all taxes are withheld.

networking a system of personal and professional relationships through which to share information.

neurogenic shock shock that results from dysfunction of nervous system following spinal cord injury.

neuron a nerve cell.

neurotransmitter chemical needed to transmit a message between synapses.

neutrophil the most abundant leukocyte and the main granulocyte.

nitrite a factor used to assess the presence of bacteria in urine.

nitrogenous pertaining to or containing nitrogen, usually the end-product of protein metabolism.

nocturia excessive urination at night.

non compos mentis mental incompetence.

noncompliance the patient's inability or refusal to follow prescribed orders.

non–insulin-dependent diabetes mellitus (NIDDM) a type of diabetes in which patients do not require insulin to control the blood sugar.

nonlanguage not expressed in spoken language, e.g., laughing, sobbing, grunting, sighing.

normal flora microorganisms normally found in the body; also known as resident flora.

normal value acceptable range as established for an age, a population, or a sex; variations usually indicate a disorder.

nosocomial infection infection acquired in a medical setting, generally presumed to be in a hospital setting but may also refer to the medical office.

nuclear medicine branch of medicine that uses radioactive isotopes to diagnose and treat disease.

nulligravida a woman who has never been pregnant.

nullipara a woman who has never given birth to a viable fetus.

numeric filing arranging files by a numbered order.

nutrition the study of food and how it is used for growth, nourishment, and repair.

O

obligate to require; a parasite that has no choice but to attach to a living organism.

obstipation extreme constipation.

obturator smooth, rounded, removable inner portion of a hollow tube, such as an anoscope, that allows for easier insertion.

occult hidden or concealed from observation.

Occupational Safety and Health Administration (OSHA) the federal agency that oversees working conditions, with the mission to protect employees from work-related hazards.

olecranon fossa the depression in the posterior surface of the humerus that allows the arm to extend by receiving the olecranon process.

olecranon process the proximal end of the ulna that becomes the point of the elbow that fits into the olecranon fossa.

oligomenorrhea scanty menstruation.

oliguria scanty urine production.

online direct link to off-site computers.

oophorectomy excision of an ovary.

operating system the program that tells the computer how to interface with hardware and software.

ophthalmic describing medication instilled into the eye.

ophthalmologist physician who specializes in treatment of disorders of the eyes.

ophthalmoscope lighted instrument used to examine the inner surfaces of the eye.

opportunistic infection infection resulting from a defective immune system that cannot defend against pathogens normally found in the environment.

optician specialist who grinds lenses to correct errors of refraction according to prescriptions written by optometrists or ophthalmologists.

optometrist specialist who can measure for errors of refraction and prescribe lenses but who cannot treat diseases of the eye or perform surgery.

order of draw guidelines for proper tube sequence to reduce cross-contamination from one tube to the next and to prevent tissue thromboplastin contamination on specimens for coagulation testing. Carryover of additives and/or tissue thromboplastin can cause erroneous test results.

organ the source or starting point; (muscle) any part that is made up of cells and tissues that cause it to perform its specified function in conjunction with a body system.

organizational chart a flow sheet depicting the members of a team in a structured or hierarchical manner.

origin the source or starting point; (muscle) the more fixed end of a muscle, usually the proximal end.

orthopnea inability to breathe lying down; the patient usually has to sit upright to breathe.

OSHA *see* Occupational Safety and Health Administration.

osteoporosis abnormal porosity of the bone, most often found in the elderly, predisposing the affected bony tissue to fracture.

otic describing medication instilled into the ear.

otolaryngologist physician who specializes in treatment of diseases and disorders of the ears, nose, and throat.

otoscope instrument used for visual examination of the ear canal and tympanic membrane.

outlier a patient whose hospital stay is longer than allowed by the DRG.

outpatient a medical setting in which patients receive care but are not admitted.

overdraft protection protection against having insufficient funds to cover checks.

over-the-counter available without a prescription; includes herbal and vitamin supplements.

ovulation the periodic rupture of the mature ovum from the ovary.

ovum (plural, ova) the female reproductive cell; sex cell or egg.

P

packing slip a document that accompanies a supply order and lists the enclosed items.

Paget's disease degenerative bone disease usually in older persons with bone destruction and poor repair.

palliative easing symptoms without curing.

palmar the palm surface of the hand.

palpate to examine by feel or pressing, used in diagnostic procedures such as vein location for phlebotomy.

palpation technique in which the examiner feels the texture, size, consistency, and location of parts of the body with the hands.

palpitations feeling of an increased heart rate or pounding heart that may be felt during an emotional response or a cardiac disorder.

panels laboratory tests organized into standard groups to effectively evaluate disease processes or organ systems.

panic value critical limits defining the boundaries of the life-threatening values of laboratory test results.

Papanicolaou (Pap) test or smear smear of tissue cells examined for abnormalities including cancer, especially of the cervix; named for George N. Papanicolaou, a physician, anatomist, and cytologist.

papilla (plural, papillae) a small nipple-shaped projection.

papillae lingua the taste buds.

paralanguage factors connected with, but not essentially part of, language, e.g., tone of voice, volume, pitch.

parameters values used to describe or measure a set of data representing a physiologic function or system.

paraphrasing restating what you heard using your own words.

parasitology the science and study of parasites.

parasympathetic the part of the autonomic nervous system involved in periods free from stress.

parenteral describing medication administered by any method other than orally.

parity pregnancy that resulted in a viable birth.

partial-thickness burn burn that involves epidermis and varying levels of the dermis.

participating providers those who agree to participate with managed care contracts and other third-party payers in exchange for building a solid patient base.

passive range of motion assisted range-of-motion movements.

pathogens disease-causing microorganisms.

patient co-payment the part of an insured service that the patient must pay.

patient education active participation of the patient in a process that will yield a change in behavior.

pediatrician physician who specializes in the care of infants, children, and adolescents.

pediatrics specialty of medicine that deals with the care of infants, children, and adolescents.

pediculosis infestation with parasitic lice.

peer review organization a group of physicians and specialists that conducts a review of a disputed case and makes a final recommendation.

percussion striking with the hands to evaluate the size, borders, consistency, and presence of fluid or air.

percutaneous transluminal coronary angioplasty (PTCA) procedure that improves blood flow through a coronary artery by pressing the plaque against the wall of the artery with a balloon on a catheter, allowing for more blood flow.

pericarditis inflammation of the sac that covers the heart.

pericardium the double-layered serous, membranous sac that encloses the heart and the origins of the great vessels.

peripheral pertaining to or situated away from the center.

peristalsis contraction and relaxation of involuntary muscles of the alimentary canal producing wavelike movement of products through the digestive system.

PERRLA abbreviation used in documentation to denote pupils equal, round, reactive to light, and accommodation if all findings are normal; refers to the size and shape of the pupils, their reaction to light, and their ability to adjust to distance.

personal protective equipment (PPE) equipment used to protect a person from exposure to blood or other body fluids.

pessary device that supports the uterus when inserted into the vagina.

petri plate a shallow glass or plastic dish with a lid to hold solid media for cultures.

pH abbreviation for potential hydrogen; pH is a scale representing the relative acidity or alkalinity of a substance in which 7.0 is neutral; numbers lower than 7.0 are acid, and numbers above 7.0 are basic.

phagocyte a cell that has the ability to ingest and destroy particular substances such as bacteria, protozoa, cells, and cell debris by ingesting them.

phagocytosis the process by which certain cells engulf and dispose of microorganisms; to eat or ingest.

pharmacodynamics study of how drugs act within the body.

pharmacokinetics study of the action of drugs within the body from administration to excretion.

pharmacology study of drugs and their origin, nature, properties, and effects upon living organisms.

phimosis narrowing or tightening of the prepuce that prevents retraction over the glans penis.

phonophoresis ultrasound treatment used to force medications into tissues.

phosphates compounds containing phosphorus and oxygen; they are very important in living organisms, especially for the transfer of genetic information.

physician hospital organization a coalition of physicians and a hospital contracting with large employers, insurance carriers, and other benefits groups to provide discounted health services.

physiology the study of the function of the body.

pia mater thin vascular covering that adheres to the surface of the brain.

placebo an inert substance given as a medicine for its suggestive effect; an inert compound identical in appearance to material being tested in experimental research, which may or may not be known to the physician and/or patient, administered to distinguish between drug action and suggestive effect of the material under study.

plaintiff the party who initiates a lawsuit.

plan maximum the highest amount paid by a third-party payer for any given service.

planes a point of reference made by a straight cut through the body at any given angle.

planning the process of using information gathered during the assessment phase to organize learning or patient care objectives in order to accomplish the specific learning or treatment goal.

pleura the serous membrane enclosing the lungs (visceral pleura: the layer that covers the lungs most closely; parietal pleura: the layer that follows the contours and lines the chest wall, the diaphragm, and the mediastinum).

poikilocytosis abnormal variations in the shapes of red blood cells (poikilo = variation).

policy a statement that reflects the organization's rules on a given topic.

polydipsia excessive thirst.

polymenorrhea abnormally frequent menstrual periods.

polyphagia abnormal hunger.

polyuria excessive excretion and elimination of urine.

pons part of the brainstem, responsible for communication with the central nervous system.

portfolio a portable case containing documents.

positive feedback an increase in function in response to a stimulus.

positive stress stress that allows a person to perform at peak levels and then relax afterward.

positron emission tomography (PET) computerized radiography using radioactive substances to assess metabolic or physiologic functions within the body rather than anatomic structures.

postexposure testing laboratory tests that may be performed after a person comes into contact with a biohazard.

posting listing financial transactions in a ledger.

postural hypotension sudden drop in blood pressure upon standing.

potentiation describes the action of two drugs taken together in which the combined effects are greater than the sum of the independent effects.

precedents the use of previous court decisions as a legal foundation.

preceptor a teacher; one who gives direction, as in a technical matter.

precertification approved documentation prior to referrals to specialists and other facilities.

pre-existing condition medical problem treated by a physician before an insurance plan's effective date. A third-party payer may exclude coverage for pre-existing conditions.

preferred provider organization (PPO) an organization whose purpose is to contract with providers and then lease this network of contracted providers to health care plans.

prepuce a fold of skin that forms a cover.

presbyacusis (also: presbycusis) loss of hearing associated with aging.

presbyopia vision change (farsightedness) associated with aging.

present illness a specific account of the chief complaint, including time frames and characteristics.

preservative substance that delays decomposition.

primary diagnosis the condition or chief complaint that brings a person to a medical facility for treatment.

primary survey an initial assessment of an emergency patient for life-threatening problems.

prime mover the muscle most responsible for the desired muscle action or movement.

primigravida a woman who is pregnant for the first time.

primipara a woman who has given birth to one viable infant.

problem-oriented medical record (POMR) a common method of compiling information that lists each problem of the patient, usually at the beginning of the folder, and references each problem with a number throughout the folder.

procedure a series of steps required to perform a given task; a medical service or test that is coded for reimbursement.

professional courtesy a discount fee given to health care professionals.

profit-and-loss statement statement of income and expenditures; shows whether, in a given period, a business made or lost money and how much.

proofreading the part of editing a document in which the writer reads the draft for accuracy and clarity and corrects errors.

prophylaxis prevention of development of a disease or condition.

proprietary private school with preset curricula.

prostate-specific antigen normal protein produced by the prostate that usually elevates in the presence of prostate cancer.

prosthesis any artificial replacement for a missing body part, such as false teeth or an artificial limb.

protected health information (PHI) individually identifiable personal health information as defined by HIPAA. Information that can be linked to a particular individual by name, code, or number is PHI.

proteinuria the presence of large quantities of protein in the urine; usually a sign of renal dysfunction.

protocol a code of proper conduct; a treatment plan.

provider a health care worker who delivers medical care.

proxemic having to do with the degree of physical closeness tolerated by humans.

pruritus itching.

psoriasis chronic skin disorder that appears as red patches covered by thick, dry, silvery scales.

psychogenic of psychological origin.

psychomotor describes a physical task.

psychosocial relating to mental and emotional aspects of social encounters.

puerperium period of time (about 6 weeks) from childbirth until reproductive structures return to normal.

purchase order a document that lists the required items to be purchased.

Purkinje fibers extensions of the bundle of His that branch through the myocardium to end the transmission of the electrical impulse and cause the ventricles to contract.

purulent describes drainage that is white, green, or yellow; characteristic of an infection.

pyosalpinx pus in the fallopian tube(s).

pyrexia body temperature of 102°F or higher rectally or 101°F or higher orally.

pyuria pus in the urine.

Q

quadrants a division of the abdomen into four equal parts by one horizontal and one vertical line dissecting at the umbilicus.

quality assurance (QA) an evaluation of health care services as compared to accepted standards.

quality control (QC) method to evaluate the proper performance of testing procedures, supplies, or equipment in a laboratory.

quality improvement a plan that allows an organization to scientifically measure the quality of its product and service.

quantification the process of ascertaining the amount of something.

quantitative the measuring of an amount.

Queckenstedt test test to determine presence of obstruction in the CSF flow performed during a lumbar puncture.

R

radiograph processed film that contains a visible image.

radiographer technical specialist who works to assist the radiologist in the performance of procedures and who is responsible for producing routine examination images for the radiologist to interpret.

radiography art and science of producing diagnostic images with x-rays.

radioimmunoassay (RIA) the introduction of radioactive substances into the body to determine the concentration of a substance in the serum, usually the concentration of antigens, antibodies, or proteins.

radiologist physician who specializes in radiology; performs some procedures and interprets images to provide diagnostic information.

radiology branch of medicine including diagnostic and therapeutic applications of x-rays.

radiolucent permitting the passage of x-rays.

radionuclide radioactive material with a short life that is used in small amounts in nuclear medicine studies.

radiopaque not permeable to passage of x-rays.

random access memory (RAM) temporary memory; data is lost when the computer is turned off if it is not backed up on disk.

range of motion (ROM) range in degrees of angle through which a joint can be extended and flexed.

ratchet notched mechanism, usually at the handle end of an instrument, that clicks into position to maintain tension on the opposing blades or tips of the instrument.

read only memory (ROM) permanent memory inside the computer.

reagent a substance used to react in a certain manner in the presence of specific chemicals to obtain a diagnosis.

receptionist a person who greets patients as they arrive at a medical office and performs various administrative tasks.

recertification certification renewed either by taking the examination again or by completing a specified number of continuing education units in a 5-year period.

rectocele herniation of the rectum into the vaginal area.

rectovaginal pertaining to the rectum and vagina.

reduction correcting a fracture by realigning the bones; may be closed (corrected by manipulation) or open (requires surgery).

reference value a range established for test results assumed to be typical for a population asymptomatic for disease processes.

referral instruction to transfer a patient's care to a specialist.

reflecting repeat what one heard using open-ended questions.

reflux a return or backward flow of fluid.

refraction bending of light rays that enter the pupil to reflect exactly on the fovea centralis, the area of greatest visual acuity.

relapsing fever fever that returns after extended periods of being within normal limits.

remittent fluctuating.

renal cortex the portion of the kidney that contains the structures that form urine.

renal medulla the inner portion of the kidney that contains the collecting structures.

renal pelvis the funnel-shaped upper portion of the ureters that collects urine from the kidneys.

renal pyramids situated in the renal medulla, part of the collecting structures.

renin enzyme formed in the kidney that works with angiotensin to affect the blood pressure.

repolarization the active process of restoring the cardiac fibers to the resting (polarized) state; re-establishment of the electrical polarized state in a muscle or nerve fiber following contraction or conduction of a nerve impulse.

reportable range the very lowest and highest value the manufacturer has documented the test can determine.

res ipsa loquitur "the thing speaks for itself."

res judicata "the thing has been decided."

resident flora microorganisms normally found in the body; also known as normal flora.

resistance body's immune response to prevent infections by invading pathogenic microorganisms.

Resource-Based Relative Value Scale (RBRVS) a value scale designed to decrease Medicare Part B costs and establish national standards for coding and payment.

respiration the exchange of oxygen and carbon dioxide (external respiration: the exchange between the alveoli and the bloodstream; internal respiration: the exchange between the cells and the bloodstream).

respondent superior "let the master answer."

restrain control or confine movement.

résumé document summarizing individual's work experience or professional qualifications.

retinal degeneration pathologic changes in the cell structure of the retina that impair or destroy its function, resulting in blindness.

retrograde pyelogram an x-ray of the urinary tract using contrast medium injected through the bladder and ureters; useful in diagnosing obstructions.

retroperitoneal the space behind the peritoneal cavity that contains the kidneys.

retrovirus virus containing reverse transcriptase, which allows the viral cell to replicate its DNA in the DNA of the host cell, thereby taking over the substance of the cell.

returned check fee amount of money a bank or business charges for a check written with insufficient funds.

reverse chronological order items placed with oldest first.

Rickettsia organism that is smaller than bacteria, larger than viruses.

ringworm lay term for tinea, a group of fungal diseases.

risk factors any issue that possesses a safety or liability concern for an organization.

role delineation chart a list of the areas of competence expected of the graduate.

Romberg test test for inability to maintain body balance when eyes are closed and feet are together; indication of spinal cord disease.

rugae ridges or folds in the skin or mucous membranes that allow for expansion of a part.

rule of nines the most common method of determining the extent of burn injury; the body surface is divided into sections of 9% or multiples of 9%.

S

salpingectomy excision of the fallopian tube.

salpingo-oophorectomy surgical excision of both the fallopian tube and the ovary.

salutation an introductory phrase that greets the reader of a letter.

sanitation maintenance of a healthful, disease-free environment.

sanitization processes used to lower the number of microorganisms on a surface by cleansing with soap or detergent, water, and manual friction.

sanitize reduce the number of microorganisms on a surface by use of low-level disinfectant practices.

scale a thin, dried flake of skin.

scalpel small, pointed knife with a convex edge for surgical procedures.

scanner a piece of office equipment that transfers a written document into a computer.

scissors sharp instrument composed of two opposing cutting blades, held together by a central pin on which the blades pivot.

sclera white fibrous tissue that covers the eye.

sclerotherapy use of chemical agents to treat esophageal varices to produce fibrosis and hardening of the tissue.

scoliosis lateral curve of the spine, usually in the thoracic area, with a corresponding curve in the lumbar region, causing uneven shoulders and hips.

screening a preliminary procedure, such as a test or exam, to detect the more characteristic signs of a disorder.

search engine program that allows you to find information on the Internet rapidly and effectively.

sebaceous gland oil gland.

seborrhea overproduction of sebum by the sebaceous glands.

sebum fatty secretion of the sebaceous gland.

secondary survey an assessment of an emergency victim for head to toe injuries.

sediment the cells and other particulate matter that collect in the bottom of the tube when a urine sample is centrifuged..

seizure abnormal discharge of electrical activity in the brain, resulting in involuntary contractions of voluntary muscles.

semi-block a type of letter format that is styled the same as block, except the first sentence of each paragraph is indented five spaces.

senility general mental deterioration associated with aging.

sensitivity susceptibility to a certain substance.

sensitivity testing testing to determine the antibiotic that will most effectively inhibit the pathogen.

sentinel event an unexpected death or serious physical or psychological injury to a patient in a health care facility.

septic shock shock that results from general infection in the bloodstream.

septicemia presence of pathogenic bacteria in the blood.

serration groove, either straight or crisscross, etched or cut into the blade or tip of an instrument to improve its bite or grasp.

service medical interventions completed by a provider.

service charge a charge by a bank for various services.

sesamoid resembling the shape of a sesame seed.

sharps container a rigid, leak-proof, plastic container used to discard disposable sharp devices in a manner to reduce needlesticks.

shift a situation where QC results make an obvious change in performance levels.

shock lack of oxygen to individual cells of the body.

sick-child visit a pediatric visit for the treatment of illness or injury.

sickle cell anemia a condition in which the patient has both copies of the gene for hemoglobin S; the red cells become sickle shaped and nonflexible causing obstruction of small vessels and capillaries. Necrosis due to tissue hypoxia occurs beyond the obstruction. Most commonly seen in African-Americans.

signs objective indications of disease or bodily dysfunction as observed or measured by the health care professional.

sinoatrial (SA) node considered the pacemaker of the heart, located in the upper portion of the right atrium; a specialized group of cells that initiate the electrical impulse of the heart.

slander oral statements that defame a person's reputation or character.

smegma a cheesy secretion of the sebaceous glands in either the labia or the prepuce.

SOAP a style of charting that includes subjective, objective, assessment, and planning notes.

software application programs that direct the hardware to perform given tasks.

sound long instrument for exploring or dilating body cavities or searching cavities for foreign bodies.

specialty a subcategory of medicine, such as pediatrics, studied after completion of medical school.

specific gravity density of a liquid, such as urine, compared with water.

specificity relating to a definite result.

specimen a small portion of anything used to evaluate the nature of the whole.

speculum instrument that enlarges and separates the opening of a cavity to expose its interior for examination.

sphygmomanometer device used to measure blood pressure.

spicules sharp points.

spina bifida occulta, spina bifida congenital defect in the spinal column caused by lack of union of the vertebrae.

spinal pertaining to the spine.

spirochete long, flexible, motile microorganisms.

splint device used to immobilize a sprain, strain, fracture, or dislocated limb.

spore bacterial life form that resists destruction by heat, drying, or chemicals. Spore-producing bacteria include botulism and tetanus.

staff privileges hospital approval for a physician to admit patients for treatment.

staghorn stone formation in the renal pelvis that fills the chamber and assumes the shape of the calyces.

standard precautions usual steps to prevent injury or disease.

staphylococci spherical microorganism found in grapelike clusters.

stare decisis "the previous decision stands."

STAT immediately.

status asthmaticus asthma attack that is not responsive to treatment.

statute of limitations a legal time limit; e.g., the length of time in which a patient may file a lawsuit.

statutes laws that are written by federal, state, or local legislators.

stereotyping to place in a fixed mold, without consideration of differences.

sterile field a specific area, such as within a tray or on a sterile towel, that is considered free of microorganisms.

sterilization process, act, or technique for destroying microorganisms using heat, water, chemicals, or gases.

stoma an opening to the surface; suggests that it is surgically created.

stomatitis inflammation of the mucous membranes of the mouth.

stratum corneum outer layer of the epidermis.

stratum germinativum innermost layer of the epidermis.

streaming a method of allotting time for appointments based on the needs of the individual patient to minimize gaps in time and backups.

Streptococcus genus of bacteria commonly implicated in infections of the skin.

stress a factor that induces body tension; can be positive or negative.

striated having a striped appearance with alternating light and dark bands.

subcutaneous beneath the skin.

subject filing arranging files according to their title, grouping similar subjects together.

sublingual describing medication administered under the tongue.

subpoena a court order requiring an individual to appear at court at a given date and time.

subpoena duces tecum a court order requiring medical records to be submitted to the court at a given date and time.

substrate an underlying layer; a substance acted upon, as by an enzyme or reagent.

sudoriferous gland sweat gland.

sulci a groove in the brain tissue.

sulfosalicylic acid an acid used to test for protein.

summarizing briefly reviewing the information discussed to determine the patient's comprehension.

summation report any report that provides a summary of activities, such as a payroll report or a profit-and-loss statement.

superbill preprinted patient bill that lists a variety of procedures.

superficial burn burn limited to the epidermis.

supernatant the urine that rises above the sediment when the tube of urine is centrifuged.

surfing navigating the Internet.

surgical asepsis destruction of organisms before they enter the body.

surrogate mother a woman who carries a baby to term for another female who is unable to carry a pregnancy to term.

suspension temporary removal of privileges.

sustained fever fever that is constant or not fluctuating.

swab *noun*, stick topped with cotton or other absorbent manmade fiber for cleaning areas, applying treatments, or obtaining specimens; *verb*, to wipe with a swab.

swaged needle metal needle fused to suture material.

symmetry equality in size or shape or position of parts on opposite sides of the body.

sympathetic the part of the autonomic nervous system involved in stress reaction.

sympathy feeling sorry for or pitying someone.

symptoms subjective indications of disease or bodily dysfunction as sensed by the patient.

synapse the junction of two neurons.

synarthroses immovable joints.

syncope sudden fall in blood pressure or cerebral hypoxia resulting in loss of consciousness.

synergism harmonious action of two agents, such as drugs or organs, producing an effect that neither could produce alone or that is greater than the total effects of each agent operating by itself.

synergist muscles that work together for more efficient movement.

system a collection of organs that perform a certain function.

systole contraction phase of the cardiac cycle.

T

T cells lymphoid cells from bone marrow that migrate to the thymus gland where they mature into differentiated lymphocytes that circulate between blood and lymph.

tachycardia heart rate of more than 100 beats per minute.

tactile pertaining to the sense of touch.

task force a group of employees that works together to solve a given problem.

tax withholding the amount of tax that is withheld from a paycheck.

teleradiology use of computed imaging and information systems to transmit diagnostic images to distant locations.

teletypewriter (TTY) a special machine that allows communication on a telephone with a hearing-impaired person.

template a skeleton of a letter or document with preset and prespaced elements.

tendons tough, flexible fibers that bind muscle to bone.

tetany severe cramping, convulsions, or muscle spasms due to an abnormality of calcium metabolism.

thalamus part of the diencephalon, responsible for sorting messages.

thalassemia a hemolytic anemia caused by deficient hemoglobin synthesis; more commonly found in those of Mediterranean heritage.

therapeutic having to do with treating or curing disease; curative.

third-party administrator administrator who processes claims for the sponsor of self-funded benefit planning.

thoracentesis surgical puncture into the pleural cavity for aspiration of serous fluid or for injection of medication.

thrombocytes platelets in the blood.

thromboplastin a complex substance found in blood and tissues that aids the clotting process.

thyrotoxicosis excess quantities of thyroid hormone in the tissues.

tickler file a file that provides a reminder to do a given task at a particular date and time.

tidal volume amount of air inhaled and exhaled during a normal respiration.

tine test skin test for exposure to tuberculosis, involves pricking the skin with sharp tines coated with the tuberculin bacillus.

tinnitus an extraneous noise heard in one or both ears, described as whirring, ringing, whistling, roaring, etc.; may be continuous or intermittent.

titer measure of the amount of an antibody in serum.

tomography procedure in which the x-ray tube and film move in relation to each other during exposure, blurring out all structures except those in the focal plane.

tonometry measurement of intraocular pressure using a tonometer.

tonsils a small mass of lymphoid tissue; includes the palatine, nasopharyngeal, and lingual tonsils.

tonus the steady, partial contraction of skeletal muscles that allows the body to remain upright.

topical describing medication applied directly to the skin or mucous membranes.

tort the righting of wrongs or injuries suffered by someone because of another person's wrongdoing.

toxicology the study of the presence and measurement of drugs in the blood.

toxoid toxin treated to destroy its toxicity but still capable of inducing formation of antibodies.

tracheostomy permanent surgical stoma in the neck with an indwelling tube.

tracheotomy incision into the trachea below the larynx to circumvent a blockage superior to this point; suggests an emergency situation and a reversible procedure.

trade name name given to a medication by the company that owns the patent.

transcription the process of typing a dictated message.

transient flora microorganisms that do not normally reside in a given area; transient flora may or may not produce disease.

transient ischemic attack (TIA) acute episode of cerebrovascular insufficiency, usually a result of narrowing of an artery by atherosclerotic plaques, emboli, or vasospasm; usually passes quickly but should be considered a warning for predisposition to cerebrovascular accidents.

transillumination passage of light through body tissues for the purpose of examination.

transition passing from one place or activity to another.

traumatic causing or relating to tissue damage.

trend when results progressively increase or decrease over time.

triage sorting of patients into categories based on their level of sickness or injury to ensure that life-threatening medical conditions are treated immediately.

trigone the triangle formed in the base of the bladder by the entrance of the two ureters and the exit of the urethra.

truss a device that presses against a hernia to keep it in place.

turbid cloudy.

turbinates mucous membrane–covered conchae, the three scroll-shaped bones that project into the nasal cavity bilaterally from the lateral walls; each covers a sinus meatus.

turgor normal tension in a cell or the skin; normal skin turgor resists deformation and will resume its former position after being grasped or pulled.

tympanic membrane thin, semitransparent membrane in the middle ear that transmits sound vibrations; the eardrum.

tympanic thermometer device for measuring the temperature using the blood flow through the tympanic membrane, or eardrum.

U

ultrasound imaging technique that uses sound waves to diagnose or monitor various body structures.

unbundling the practice of submitting a claim with several separate procedure codes rather than a single code that represents the services performed.

unemployment tax federal tax paid by the employer based on each employee's gross income.

unit each part of a name or title that is used in indexing; a quantity of a standard measurement.

upcoding billing more for a patient care service than it is worth by selecting a code that is higher on the coding scale; this is an illegal practice.

upper respiratory infection (URI) infection of the nasopharynx, throat, and bronchi.

urea the final product of protein metabolism in the body and the main nitrogenous component in the urine.

uremic frost a frost-like deposit of uremic compounds on the skin of patients whose kidneys are no longer functional.

ureterostomy surgical opening to the outside of the body from the ureter to facilitate drainage of urine from an obstructed kidney.

ureters the pair of tubes designed to carry urine from the kidneys to the bladder.

urethra the short tube that carries urine from the bladder to the outside of the body.

uric acid a byproduct of protein metabolism present in the blood and excreted by the kidneys.

urinalysis examination of the physical, chemical, and microscopic properties of urine.

urinary frequency the urge to urinate occurring more often than is required for normal bladder elimination.

urobilinogen the chemical that results when bacterial action converts bilirubin when it is secreted in the bile.

urticaria hives.

usual, customary, and reasonable (UCR) the basis of a physician's fee schedule, the usual and customary cost of the same service or procedure in a similar geographic area and under the same or similar circumstances.

utilization review an analysis of individual cases by a committee to make sure services and procedures being billed to a third-party payer are medically necessary and to ensure compliance with its rules and regulations regarding reimbursement.

V

V-codes codes assigned to patients who receive service but have no illness, injury, or disorder, e.g., a vaccination or a screening mammogram.

vaccine suspension of infectious agents or some part of them; given to establish resistance to an infectious disease.

values established ideals of life, conduct, customs, etc., of an individual person or members of a society.

varicella zoster viral infection manifested by characteristic rash of successive crops of vesicles that scab before resolution; also called chicken pox.

vasopressin a hormone formed in the hypothalamus and transported to the posterior lobe of the pituitary through the hypothalamo-hypophyseal tract. It has an antidiuretic and a pressor effect that elevates the blood pressure.

vector (biologic) a living, nonhuman carrier of disease, usually an arthropod; (mechanical) a carrier of disease that does not support growth; examples include contaminated inanimate objects.

ventricle either of the two lower chambers of the heart that, when filled with blood, contract to propel it into the arteries.

venule the small vessel that joins a capillary to a vein.

verruca wart.

vertigo sensation of whirling of oneself or the environment; dizziness.

vesicle skin lesion that appears as a small sac containing fluid; a blister.

viable capable of growing and living.

vial glass or plastic container sealed at the top by a rubber stopper.

villus (plural, villi) tiny, almost microscopic projections in the mucous membrane of the small intestines.

virology the science and study of viruses.

virtual a paperless system or chart on your computer.

virulent highly pathogenic and disease producing; describes a microorganism.

virus a harmful invader that can damage your computer.

visualization a relaxation technique that allows the mind to wander and the imagination to run free and focus on positive and relaxing situations.

W

wave scheduling system a flexible scheduling method that allows time for procedures of varying lengths and the addition of unscheduled patients, as needed.

well-child visit visit to the medical office for administration of immunizations and evaluation of growth and development.

Western blot specific confirmatory antibody test for presence of HIV in blood.

whorls a spiral arrangement, as in the ridges on the finger that make up a fingerprint.

withdrawing the act of terminating a medical treatment that has already been initiated.

withholding not initiating certain medical treatments.

workers' compensation employer insurance for treatment of an employee's injury or illness related to the job.

write-off cancellation of an unpaid debt.

X

x-rays invisible electromagnetic radiation waves used in diagnosis and treatment of various disorders.

Y

yolk sac a structure that develops in the inner zygotic cell mass and supplies nourishment for the embryo until the seventh week when the placenta takes over the function.

Index

Page numbers in *italics* denote figures; those followed by a t denote tables.

AAMA (*see* American Association of Medical Assistants)
AANP (American Academy of Nurse Practitioners), 12
AAOS (American Academy of Orthopaedic Surgeons), 75
AAP (*see* American Academy of Pediatrics)
AAPC (American Academy of Professional Coders), 17
AAPCC (American Association of Poison Control Centers), 559
ABA number, 241
Abandonment, 25
Abbreviations
　legal issues, 136, 166
　for medication administration, 494, 495t
　standardization of, 136–137
　table of, 1062t–1066t
　zip code, 1061
Abdomen
　assessing in emergency care, 552
　physical examination, 416
Abdominal hernia, 710–711
ABG (arterial blood gas), 667
ABHES (Accrediting Bureau of Health Education Schools), 15, 16
ABN (advance beneficiary notice), 277
ABO group, 978
Abortion
　physician-performed, 41
　spontaneous, 771, 778
Abrasion, 554
Abruptio placentae, 779
Absence seizures, 727
Abuse
　child, 822
　elder, 839–840, *840*
　reporting of, 29–30
Accounting, 232–259
　accounts payable, 245–247
　　ordering goods and services, 245
　　paying invoices, 246–247
　　receiving supplies, 245, 245–246
　adjustments
　　defined, 235
　　posting, 236, 238, 251
　audits, 244, 247
　banking (*see* Banking)
　cash basis, 234
　computerized, 238–239
　　overview, 238–239
　　paying invoices, 247
　　posting to accounts, 239
　　reports, 239
　corrections, 243
　cycle, 244
　manual, 234–238
　　balancing a daysheet, 254
　　charge slip, 234, *234*, 235–236, 237
　　credit balance, processing, 236, 250
　　daysheet, *234*, 234–235
　　deposit slip, 234
　　encounter form, 235–236, 237

　　ledger card, 234, *234, 235, 235*
　　NSF checks, processing, 238, 253
　　paying invoices, *246*, 246–247
　　pegboard bookkeeping system, *234*, 234–236, 246, *246*
　　posting a charge, 236, 248–249
　　posting a credit adjustment, 236, 251
　　posting a debit adjustment, 238
　　posting collection agency payments, 236, 252
　　posting proofs, 234, 235
　　posting to cash-paid-out section of daysheet, 238
　　refunds, processing, 236, 251
　　overview, 243
　　record-keeping components, 244–245
　　reports, 244–245, 247
　　Spanish terminology, 248
Accounting cycle, 244
Accounts
　aging, 226, 226–227, 227
　collections, 225–228, 230
Accounts payable, 234, 245–247
　ordering goods and services, 245
　paying invoices, 246–247
　receiving supplies, 245, 245–246
　writing checks for, 240–241
Accounts receivable, 234, 235
Accreditation, 14–15
Accrediting Bureau of Health Education Schools (ABHES), 15, 16
Accuracy
　in diagnostic coding, 304
　in written communication, 133, 135
Acetest, 952
Achilles reflex, *733*, 733t
Acne vulgaris, 582
ACOG (American College of Obstetricians and Gynecologists), 766
Acromegaly, 799, *799*
ACS (American Cancer Society), 417, 539
ACTH (adrenocorticotropic hormone), 795t, 798
Action words, 1036
Active listening, 52–53
Activities of daily living (ADL), 839, 847t
Actual (compensatory) damages, 32
Acupressure, 77
Acupuncture, 77
Acutely ill patient, adapting schedule for, 121
ADA (*see* Americans with Disabilities Act)
ADA (American Diabetes Association), 1009
Addiction, 60, 328–329
Addison's disease, 798, *798*
Address books, e-mail, 184
Addressing envelopes, 145–146, *146*
Addressing patients, 63
ADH (antidiuretic hormone), 795t, 799
ADHD (attention deficit hyperactivity disorder), 826
Adhesive capsulitis, 611
Adhesive skin closures, 453–454, *454*

Adjustment, accounting
　defined, 235
　posting credit, 236
　posting debit, 238
Adjustment, fee, 224
ADL (activities of daily living), 839, 847t
Administrative duties, of medical assistant, 9
Administrative law, 22, 23
Administrative software packages, 189–190
Adrenal gland disorders
　Addison's disease, 798, *798*
　Cushing's syndrome, 798, *798*
Adrenergic blocking agents, 482t
Adrenergics, 482t
Adrenocorticotropic hormone (ACTH), 795t, 798
Adson forceps, *433*
Advance beneficiary notice (ABN), 277
Advance directives, 42, *44*, 159, 187, 839
Adverse reactions, 489t
Advocacy, 39
AED (*see* automatic external defibrillator)
Aerobes, 336, 966
Aesculapius, 5, *5*
Afebrile, 373
Affection needs, 72
AFP (alpha-fetoprotein), 728, 779
Agar, 968–971
Age
　blood pressure and, 384
　body temperature and, 374
　effect on pharmacodynamics, 486–487
　patient education and, 74
　variations in pulse rate by, 380t
　variations in respiration by, 382t
Age Discrimination in Employment Act of 1967, 38
Agendas, 143, *144*
Aging (*see also* Geriatrics)
　concepts of, 835
　coping with, 838
　effects on body systems, 842t–845t
Aging accounts, 226, 226–227, 227
Aging schedule, 226, 226–227, 227
AHA (American Hospital Association), 278
AHFS (American Hospital Formulary Service), 282, 489
AHIMA (*see* American Health Information and Management Association)
AIDS prevention, 747, 766–767
Air pollution, 326
Airbags, 326–327
Airway
　assessing in emergency care, 549
　opening with head tilt-chin lift method, 549, *550*
　opening with jaw thrust method, 549, *550*
　procedure for managing foreign body obstruction, 568–569
Alanine aminotransferase (ALT), 1007
ALARA concept, 536
Albinism, 583, *584*

Albuterol, 662
Alcohol
    consumption, 320
    as disinfectant, 341t
Alcoholism, 60, 328, 838
Aldosterone, 795t
Alfalfa, 79t
Aliquots, 860
Alkaline phosphatase (ALP), 1006–1007
Allergens, 558
Allergic reactions, 557–558
Allergic rhinitis, 641
Allergies, drug, 488–489
Allied health professionals, 13–14
Alligator biopsy, 431t
Allis tissue forceps, 433
Allocation of resources, ethics of, 40–41
Alopecia, 580, 583
ALP (alkaline phosphatase), 1006–1007
Alpha-fetoprotein (AFP), 728, 779
Alphabetic filing, 169, 170
ALT (alanine aminotransferase), 1007
Alternative medicine
    acupressure, 77
    acupuncture, 77
    defined, 77
    herbal supplements, 78, 79t
    hypnosis, 77
    yoga, 77–78
Alzheimer's disease, 847–848, 847t
AMA (see American Medical Association)
Amenorrhea, 765
American Academy of Nurse Practitioners
        (AANP), 12
American Academy of Orthopaedic
        Surgeons (AAOS), 75
American Academy of Pediatrics (AAP), 75,
        99, 187, 807, 828
American Academy of Professional Coders
        (AAPC), 17
American Association of Medical Assistants
        (AAMA)
    certification (CMA), 14, 15, 16
    code of ethics, 40
    CPR certification, 547
    description of association, 17
    founding of, 14
    recertification, 1041
American Association of Physician
        Assistants, 12
American Association of Poison Control
        Centers (AAPCC), 559
American Cancer Society (ACS), 417, 539
American College of Emergency Physicians,
        187
American College of Obstetricians and
        Gynecologists (ACOG), 766
American Diabetes Association (ADA), 1009
American health care system, 7–8, 18
American Health Information and
        Management Association
        (AHIMA), 17, 187, 278
American Heart Association, CPR certifica-
        tion and training by, 547
American Hospital Association (AHA), 278
American Hospital Formulary Service
        (AHFS), 282, 489
American Medical Association (AMA)
    AAMA and, 14
    code of ethics, 38–39
    Council on Ethical and Judicial Affairs,
        40
    CPT-4 and, 294, 296
    ICD-9-CM coding resources, 279

laboratory test panels, 864, 866t
American Medical Technologists (AMT)
    certification (RMA), 15, 16
    description of association, 17
    recertification, 1041
American Red Cross, 547, 978
American Safety and Health Institute, CPR
        certification and training by, 547
American Sign Language, 59
American Society of Bariatric Surgery, 708
Americans with Disabilities Act (ADA),
        36–37, 38, 99, 100t
Amino acids, essential, 313
Amniocentesis, 41, 779
Amphetamines, 328–329
Ampules, 503, 503
Amputation injury, 554–555
AMT (see American Medical Technologists)
Amylase, 1008
Amyotrophic lateral sclerosis (ALS),
        726–727
Anabolism, 315
Anacusis, 58
Anaerobes, 336, 966
Analgesics, 482t
Anaphylactic reactions (anaphylaxis), 488,
        553, 557–558
Anatomic and surgical pathology depart-
        ment, 862
Anemia, 687–688
    folate deficiency, 931
    hemoglobin determination, 933
    iron deficiency, 932, 932
    sickle cell, 932
Anesthesia
    CPR-4 coding, 300
    local anesthetics, 451–452, 453
Aneurysm, 687, 688
Angina pectoris, 678, 679
Angiocatheter, 509 (see also IV catheter)
Angry patients, communicating with, 60–61
Anions, 1003
Anise, 79t
Anisocytosis, 932
Ankle reflex, 733
Ankylosing spondylitis, 607
Annotation, 148
Anorexia, 709
Anoscope, 410–411, 411, 431t
Anoscopy, 711, 716–717
ANS (autonomic nervous system), 723
Answering machines, leaving messages on,
        228
Answering service, 96
Antacids, 482t
Antagonism, 488
Antecubital space, 910
Antecubital vein, 911
Anthelmintics, 482t
Anthropometric measurements
    baseline, 372
    height, 373, 374, 388
    weight, 372–373, 373, 386–387
Anti-inflammatory agents, 483t
Antianginal agents, 482t
Antianxiety agents, 482t
Antiarrhythmics, 482t
Antibiotics
    action, 482t
    sensitivity testing, 974–975, 975
Antibodies, 975–976
Anticholinergics, for Parkinson's disease,
        846
Anticoagulants, 482t, 861–862, 902, 935

Anticonvulsants, 482t
Antidepressants, 482t
Antidiarrheals, 482t
Antidiuretic hormone (ADH), 795t, 799
Antiemetic agents, 482t
Antifungals, 482t
Antigens, 975
Antihistamines, 482t, 582, 846
Antihypertensives, 483t
Antineoplastic agents, 483t
Antipsychotics, 483t
Antipyretics, 483t
Antiseptics, 898
Antithyroid agents, 484t
Antitussives, 483t
Antivirals, 483t
Aortic stenosis, 683t
Apgar score, 817
Aplastic anemia, 688
Apnea, 382
Apostrophe, 134
Apothecary system of measurement,
        497–498, 498t
Appeal, 34
Appearance, personal, 93, 1028
Appendicitis, 711
Application, employment, 1037
Applicators, 406
Appointment book, 114, 114
Appointment reminder card, 101, 119, 119
Appointments
    adapting the schedule
        acutely ill patients, 121
        emergencies, 120, 121, 121
        late patients, 121–122
        missed appointments, 122
        physician delays, 122
        walk-in patients, 121
    admission to inpatient facility, 129
    cancellations, 122–123
    computer management of, 189
    consultations, 123, 124
    for diagnostic testing, 124
    missed, 122
    in other facilities, 123–124
    patient reminders, 119–120
        appointment cards, 119, 119
        mailed cards, 120, 120
        telephone, 119–120
        tickler file use, 120
    problems with scheduling, 124–125
    referrals, 123, 123–124, 128
    rescheduling, 106
    schedule preparation, 119
    scheduling, influences on
        patient needs, 117
        physical facilities, 118
        provider preferences and needs,
            117–118
    scheduling guidelines, 118–119
        established patients, 118–119, 127
        new patients, 118, 126
    scheduling systems, 113–115
        computerized, 114–115, 115
        manual, 114, 114
    Spanish terminology, 125
    for surgery, 124
    telephone calls requesting, 103
    time to allot, 116
    types of scheduling
        clustering, 116
        double booking, 116
        fixed, 116
        flexible hours, 116

open hours, 116–117
streaming, 116
structured appointments, 115
wave, 116
Approximating wound edges, 453
Arm sling, applying, 618–619
Arms, assessing in emergency care, 552
Arrhythmias (*see* Cardiac arrhythmia)
Arterial blood gas (ABG), 667
Arterial laceration, 554
Arteriosclerosis, 384
Artery, accidental puncture of, 912
Arthritis, 607
Arthrograms, 613
Arthroplasty, 612
Arthropods, 970
Arthroscopy, 612, *612*
Artifacts, ECG, 692, 694t
Artificial insemination, 42
Artificial pacemakers, 681
Artificial respiration, 549–550, *550*
Ascites, 712
ASD (atrial septal defect), 682, 683t
Asepsis (*see* Medical asepsis; Surgical asepsis)
Aseptic technique, 100
Aspartate aminotransferase (AST), 1007
Aspergillus, 968
Aspiration, 821
Aspiration, suprapubic, 947
Aspirin, Reye's syndrome and, 726, 823
Assault, 33
Assessment, in patient education process, 68–69
Assessment, patient, 362–363
chief complaint and present illness, 362–363, 366–369
putting patient at ease, 363
signs and symptoms, 362
Assignment of benefits, 265, 269, 272
Assisted living facilities, 839
Association membership, 16–17
Assumption of risk defense, 34
AST (aspartate aminotransferase), 1007
Asthma, 661–662, 824
Astigmatism, 633
Asymmetry, observing during physical examination, 411
Asymptomatic, 337
Atherosclerosis, 384, 683–685, *684*
Athlete's foot, 580
ATM (automated teller machine), 241
Atraumatic needle, 452
Atrial septal defect (ASD), 682, 683t
Attachments, e-mail, 184
Attendance, externship, 1028
Attention deficit hyperactivity disorder (ADHD), 826
Attitude, 93, 1028
Audiometer, 638, *639,* 641
Audiometry, 641, 652–653
Audioscope, 408
Audiovisual material, for patient education, 69
Audit, 244, 247, 289
Aura, 727
Auscultation
in cardiovascular examination, 689
in physical examination, 412
for respiratory system evaluation, 665–666, 666t
Auscultatory gap, 383–384
Authorization release form, 157, *157,* 158
Auto-attendant, 107

Autoclave
description, 427–428, *428*
loading, 429, *429*
maintenance, 429
operating, 429, 442–443
sterilization indicators, *428,* 428–429
wrapping instruments for sterilization, 440–441
Automated blood cell counters, 930
Automated teller machine (ATM), 241
Automatic external defibrillator (AED), 189, 550, *551, 557,* 565–567, 679, 682
Autonomic nervous system (ANS), 723
Autonomous child, 814
AVPU system, for assessing consciousness, 551
Avulsion, 554
Ayre spatula, 410, *410*

Babcock forceps, *433*
Babinski reflex, 407, 811t
Back, assessing in emergency care, 552
Back pain, 610
Back strain, 610
Backhaus towel clamp, *435*
Bacteria
bacilli, 966
categories, 966t
chlamydiae, 967
cocci, 966, *967*
morphology, 966, *967, 968*
rickettsias, 967
skin infections, 576–578, *579*
spirochaetes, 966
in urine sediment, 953
Bactericidal, 335
Bacteriology, 966
Bag-valve-mask device, for artificial respiration, 550
Bailey foreign body remover, 432t
Balance
account, 234
physical examination, 417
Balance billing, 272
Balancing a daysheet, 254
Baldness, 583 (*see also* Alopecia)
Ballenger sponge forceps, *433*
Bandage scissors, 433, *434*
Bandaging
application guidelines, 588
applying tubular gauze, 593–595
changing, 338
elastic bandages, 587, *587*
phlebotomy and, 899
roller bandages, 587, *587, 589*
techniques, *589*
tubular gauze bandages, 587, *588,* 593–595
Bands, *928,* 931
Banking
account types, 239
checking, 239
money market, 239
savings, 239
checks, types of, 240
fees
monthly service fee, 240
overdraft protection, 240
returned check fee, 240
responsibilities of the medical assistant, 240–242
receiving checks and making deposits, 241

reconciling bank statements, 241–242, 255–256
writing checks for accounts payable, 240–241
Barbiturates, 329
Bard Parker, 448
Barium studies, 534, 537, 538, *539, 542,* 715
Barrett's esophagus, 706
Barrier devices, 342
Barrier precautions, 897
Barton, Clara, 6
Basal cell carcinoma, 584, *585*
Basal metabolic rate, 324
Baseline data, 372
Baseline information, 406
Basophils, *928,* 931
Battery, 33
Battery backup, 181
Behavioral emergency, 561
Bench trial, 34
Benign prostatic hyperplasia, 745–746
Benzalkonium chloride, 898
Benzene hexachloride, 581
Benzoyl peroxide, 582
Berry aneurysm, 687
Bevel, needle, 900
Biases, 55, 58
BiCaps, 136
Biceps reflex, *733,* 733t
Bicuspid aortic valve, 683t
Bikram yoga, 78
Bile acids, 1010
Bilirubin, 951, 952, *953,* 1006
Bilirubinuria, 951
Billing
electronic health record, 160–161
ledger card copy use, 235
Billing inquiries, telephone calls concerning, 103
Bills, paying (*see* Invoices, paying)
Bimanual examination, 410, 417, *770, 770,* 787
Bioethics
AMA Council on Ethical and Judicial Affairs, 40
defined, 38
social policy issues, 40–42, *43, 44*
allocation of resources, 40–41
clinical investigations and research, 41
obstetric dilemmas, 41
organ transplantation, 42, *43*
stem cell research, 42
withholding or withdrawing treatment, 42, *44*
Biohazard waste containers, 344
Biohazardous materials, 35–346, 100, 342, 344, *346, 347,* 353–354
Biopsy
bone, 608
cervical, 788–789
endometrial, 771
muscle, 608
skin, 586
Biopsy forceps, 430t
Biotransformation, 840
Birth control, 779
Birthday rule, 269
Birthmark, 584
Black cohosh root, 79t
Blackwell, Elizabeth, 6
Bladder catheterization, 946–947
Blades, scalpel
disposal of, 434
types, 433–434, *435*

Blastomycosis, 968
Bleach, as disinfectant, 341t, 898, 899
Bleeding
    controlling, procedure for, 570
    epistaxis, 642
    management of, 554–555
Block letter format, 140
Blood
    collecting for culture, 973t, 987–988
    specimen handling, 973t
    in urine, 951
Blood, occult, 416, 711, 972–973, 989–990
Blood-borne pathogens, 37, 887, 897
Blood cell counters, automated, 930
Blood chemistry (*see* Clinical chemistry)
Blood collection systems
    evacuated tube system, *900, 900–902, 901, 902,* 903t–904t
    order of draw, 902, 905t
    syringe system, 902, *905*
    winged infusion set, *906, 906, 907*
Blood donation, 978
Blood drawing station, 898, *898*
Blood flow, *678*
Blood gas, arterial, 667
Blood pressure
    auscultatory gap, 383–384
    cuff size, 384, *384*
    of dialysis patient, 385
    errors in readings, causes of, 384
    factors influencing, 384
    hypertension, 383, 383t
    Korotkoff sounds, 383
    measurement, 382–385, 400–403
    pediatric, 820, 820t
    phases of, 383t
    postural hypotension, 382
    pulse pressure, 383
Blood smear
    appearance, *928*
    preparing, 936–937
    staining, 938
Blood urea nitrogen (BUN), 749, 1005, 1005t, 1012t
Blood vessel disorders
    anemia, 687–688
    aneurysm, 687, *688*
    atherosclerosis, 683–685, *684*
    cerebrovascular accident (CVA), 687
    hypertension, 685
    pulmonary embolism, 686
    transient ischemic attack (TIA), 687
    varicose veins, 685–686, *686*
    venous thrombosis, 686
BNDD (Bureau of Narcotics and Dangerous Drugs), 481
Body language, 51–52
Body mass index (BMI), 325, *325*
Body surface area (BSA), 500, *500,* 555, *555*
Body systems, effects of aging on, 842t–845t
Bone tumors, 608
Bookkeeping
    computerized, 238–239
    defined, 234
    pegboard system, *234,* 234–236
    single-entry system, 234
Books, waiting room, 99
Borrelia burgdorferi, 966, 967
Bozeman forceps, *433*
Brachial pulse, *379*
Brachioradialis reflex, 733t
Brackets, 236
Bradycardia, 679

Bradykinesia, 845
Brain
    traumatic brain injuries, 729, 730
    tumors, 730–731
Braxton-Hicks contractions, 771
Breach of legal duty, 23
Breast
    cancer, 766
    physical examination, 416
    self-examination, 417, 782–784
Breast cancer screening guidelines, 539
Breath sounds, abnormal, 666t
Breathing
    artificial respiration, 549–550, *550*
    assessing in emergency care, 549
    techniques, for relaxation, 80
Brochures, 206–207, *207*
Bronchitis, 661
Bronchodilators, 483t, 662, 824
Bronchoscopy, 666–667
Bruit, 415
BSA (body surface area), 500, *500,* 555, *555*
Buccal route of administration, 502
Buck ear curet, 431t
Buck neurologic hammer, 731, *732*
Budget, 207
Buffer time, in schedule, 115
Buffered caplet (oral medication form), 502t
Bulla, 576, *578*
Bulletin boards, 199
BUN (blood urea nitrogen), 749, 1005, 1005t, 1012t
Bupivacaine, 451
Bureau of Narcotics and Dangerous Drugs (BNDD), 481
Burns
    calculation of body surface area (BSA) burned, 555, *555*
    chemical, *555*
    classification of injury, *555*
    electrical, *555*
    management of burn patient, 556
    radiation, *555*
    thermal, *555*
Burr cells, 933t
Bursae, 606
Bursitis, 606
Business letter (*see* Letter)
Butterfly collection system, *906, 906, 907*

CAAHEP (Commission on Accreditation of Allied Health Education Programs), 15, 16
CABG (coronary artery bypass graft), 678
CAD (coronary artery disease), 556–557, *684,* 684–685
Caduceus, 5, *5*
Calcitonin, 795t
Calcium oxalate crystals, 953
Calculators, health-related, 186
Calculi, 742
Calibration
    instrumental, 883
    thermometer, 376, *377*
Callus, 582, 605
Calories, 315, 324–325
Cancellations
    by office, 122
    by patients, 123
Cancer
    brain tumors, 730–731
    breast, 766
    colorectal, 711, *711*
    esophageal, 706

    gallbladder, 714
    gastric, 707–708
    gynecologic, 765–766, 765t
    liver, 713
    oral cavity, 705
    pancreatic, 714
    patient education, 75
    prostate, 746
    reporting of, 30
    respiratory system, 664–665
    testicular, 746
    urinary system, 742
Candida albicans, 704–705, 768
Candidiasis, 968, *969*
Canes, 616, *616*
Canker sore, 704
Capillary puncture
    complications, 914
    error sources, 914
    procedure, 921–924
    site selection, 912, 914
Capillary puncture (microcollection) equipment, 906–908
    filter paper test requisitions, 908, *909*
    microcollection containers, 907–908
    microhematocrit tubes, 907, *908*
    puncture devices, 907, *908*
    warming devices, 908, *909*
Capitalization, 134, 136
Capitation, 266
Capsule (oral medication form), 502t
Carbohydrates, 312–313
Carbuncle, 577–578, *578*
Cardiac arrhythmia, 678–679
Cardiac calcium scoring, 685
Cardiac catheterization, 694–695
Cardiac cycle, 382
Cardiac function tests
    creatine kinase-MB, 1007
    troponin, 1007–1008
Cardiac stress test, 693, 695
Cardiac surgery, 680
Cardinal signs, 372 (*see also* Vital signs)
Cardiogenic shock, 553
Cardiologist, 676
Cardiology, 675–701
    blood vessel disorders
        anemia, 687–688
        aneurysm, 687, *688*
        atherosclerosis, 683–685, *684*
        cerebrovascular accident (CVA), 687
        hypertension, 685
        pulmonary embolism, 686
        transient ischemic attack (TIA), 687
        varicose veins, 685–686, *686*
        venous thrombosis, 686
    diagnostic and therapeutic procedures
        cardiac catheterization, 694–695
        cardiac stress test, 693
        chest radiography, 693
        coronary arteriography, 695
        echocardiography, 693
        electrocardiogram, 689–693, *690,* 691t, *692, 693,* 694t, *695,* 695–700
        physical examination, 688–689
    heart anatomy, 677
    heart disorders
        angina, 678, 679
        artificial pacemakers, 681
        cardiac arrhythmia, 678–679
        carditis, 677–678
        congenital disease, 682, 683t
        congestive heart failure (CHF), 678

myocardial infarction (MI), 677, 678, 679
  symptoms, 676
  valvular disease, 682, 683t
  Spanish terminology, 700
Cardiomegaly, 677
Cardiomyopathy, 693
Cardiopulmonary resuscitation (CPR)
  AED (automatic external defibrillator), 550, *551*
  cardiovascular emergency use, 557
  certification in, 547, 679
  chest compressions, 550, *551*
  classes, 209
  procedure for, 563–565
Cardiotonics, 483t
Cardiovascular emergencies, 556–557
Cardiovascular endurance exercises, 322, 324
Cardiovascular system
  benefits of exercise, 848t
  effects of aging on, 843t
Carditis, 677–678
Career (*see* Employment)
Caries, 703–704
Carotid pulse, *379*, 550, *550*
Carpal tunnel syndrome, 611, 612
Carpuject, 503
Carriers
  disease, 336
  Medicaid, 264
Cartridges, 503, *503*, *504*
Cash basis type of accounting, 234
Cashier's checks, 240
Cassette, x-ray film, 533
Cast cutter, 602, *605*
Cast saw, 430t
Casts
  application, 602, *604*
  care of, 605
  circulation, assessment of, 605
  fiberglass, 602
  plaster, 601–602
  removal, 602, *605*
  types, 604
Casts, in urine sediment, 954
Catabolism, 313
Cataract, 631, *632*, 844t
Catheterization, urinary
  bladder, 946–947
  principles of, 749
  procedures
    female catheterization, 752–753
    male catheterization, 754–755
  sizes of catheters, 748, *748*
  types of catheters, 748, *748*
Cations, 1003
Cautery, 454
CAUTION acronym, 418
CBC (*see* Complete blood count (CBC))
CCHIT (Certification Commission for Healthcare Information Technology), 159
CCS (certified coding specialist), 17
CCS-P (certified coding specialists-physician-based), 17
CDC (*see* Centers for Disease Control and Prevention)
Celiac sprue, 708
Cell counter, 864
Cellular telephone, 107
Cellulitis, 578, *579*
Celsius-Fahrenheit temperature conversion scale, 1079
Celsius scale, 376, 376t, *377*

Centers for Disease Control and Prevention (CDC)
  breast cancer screening guidelines, *539*
  fingernail recommendations, 93
  immunization recommendations, 417–418
  infection control guidelines, 337
  role of, 29
  standard precautions, 342
Centers for Medicare and Medicaid Services (CMS)
  billing criteria, 160–161
  CLIA, 874–876
  description, 8, 213, 264
  diagnostic coding, 278
  diagnostic guidelines, 284
  forms, 263
  hematologic testing, 928
  inspections, 155
  laboratory test panels, 864, 866t
  surgery package definition, 301
  urinalysis and, 945
Central nervous system (CNS), 723
Central processing unit (CPU), 180
Centrifuge, 868–869
Cephalagia, 731
Cerebral cortex, functional areas of, *724*
Cerebral palsy, 728, 824
Cerebrospinal fluid (CSF), 733–734
Cerebrovascular accident (CVA), 686, 687, 842t
Certification
  AAMA, 14, 15, 16
  AMT, 15, 16
  recertification, 15, 16, 1041
  regulation of, 31
Certification Commission for Healthcare Information Technology (CCHIT), 159
Certified checks, 240
Certified coding specialist (CCS), 17
Certified coding specialists—physician-based (CCS-P), 17
Certified mail, 146–147, *147*
Certified medical assistant (CMA)
  certification examination, 14, 15, 16
  CPR certification, 547
  recertification, 1041
Certified Nursing Assistant, 12
Certified professional coder (CPC), 17
Cerumen, 415, 638
Ceruminosis, 638
Cervical biopsy, 788–789
Cervical cancer, 766, 766t
Cervical fracture, 552
Cervical scraper, 410
Cervical spine injury, 552
Cesarean section, 776–777
CEUs (continuing education units), 16
Chadwick's sign, 771
Chamomile, 79t
Charge, posting on daysheet, 236, 248–249
Charge slip, 234, *234*, 235–236, *237*
Charting
  missed appointment, 123
  patient education, 71
  point-of-care, 160
Charts
  preparation by receptionist, 97
  virtual, 188
Check register, 244, 246, *246*
Check stub, 246
Checking accounts, 239

Checks
  bounced, 240
  endorsed, 241, *241*
  pegboard, 246, *246*
  receiving, 241
  returned check fees, 240
  stale, 241
  types of, 240
    cashiers, 240
    certified, 240
    travelers, 240
  writing, 240–241, 246, 258
Chemical burns, 555
Chemical hazards, 884–885, *886*, 887–888
Chemical Hygiene Officer, 888
Chemical Hygiene Plan (CHP), 888
Chemical name, 481
Chemical spill, 437
Chemistry analyzer, 867–868
Chest
  assessing in emergency care, 552
  physical examination, 416
  radiography, 666, 693
CHF (congestive heart failure), 678
Chickenpox, 579
Chickenpox vaccination, 418
Chief complaint, 158, 362–363, 366–369
Chief technologist, 863
Child abuse, 29–30
Children (*see also* Pediatrics)
  communicating with, *61*, 61–62
  injuries, 187
  Internet safety, 182
  medical records, 156
  patient education, 74, *74*
Chinese medicine, 5
Chlamydia, 767, 967
Chlorhexidine gluconate, 898
Chlorine, as disinfectant, 341t
Choking, 551
Cholecystitis, 713
Cholecystography, 714, 715
Cholelithiasis, 713–714, *714*
Cholestech analyzer, *1010*
Cholesterol
  lipoproteins, 314–315, 1011, 1011t
  patient education, 1011
  sources, 314
  testing, 1010, 1011t, 1012t, 1016
Cholestin, 79t
Cholinergic blocking agents, 483t
Cholinergics, 483t
Chondromalacia patellae, 612
CHP (Chemical Hygiene Plan), 888
Chronic obstructive pulmonary disease (COPD), 662–663
Chronological order, 167
CINAHL, 186
Circulation
  assessing after cast application, 605
  assessing in emergency care, 550, *550*
Cirrhosis, 713
Civil law, 22, 23
Civil Rights Act, 36, 38, 200
Claims, insurance
  denial, 271t
  filing, 269–272
Claims administrator, 262, 269, 271
Clarification, 50, 54
Clarity, urine, 948–949, 949t, 959
Clark's rule, 500
Clean Air Act of 1990, 326
Clean-catch midstream urine specimen, 946, 955–956

Clean technique, 338 (*see also* Medical asepsis)
Cleaning, examination table and operative area, 456, 458
Clearinghouses, 155
CLIA (*see* Clinical Laboratory Improvement Amendments)
CLIA Waiver Registration, 874
Clinical and Laboratory Standards Institute (CLSI), 879
Clinical chemistry, 1002–1017
  automation, 1003
  cardiac function, 1007–1008
    creatine kinase-MB, 1007
    troponin, 1007–1008
  glucose, 1008–1010–1013–1015
    fasting blood glucose (FBS), 1009, 1012t
    hemoglobin A1C, 1010
    maintenance of glucose meter, 1017
    obstetric patients, 1010
    oral glucose tolerance test, 1009–1010, *1010*
    patient education, 1009
    procedure for testing, 1013–1015
    random, 1009
    two-hour postprandial glucose, 1009
  lipids and lipoproteins, *1010,* 1010–1011, *1011,* 1011t
    cholesterol, 1010, 1011t, 1012t, 1016
    high-density lipoprotein (HDL), 1011, 1011t
    low-density lipoprotein (LDL), 1011, 1011t
    patient education, 1011
    triglycerides, 1011, 1011t, 1012t
  liver function, 1006–1007
    alanine aminotransferase (ALT), 1007
    alkaline phosphatase (ALP), 1006–1007
    aspartate aminotransferase (AST), 1007
    bilirubin, 1006
  normal values and clinical significance, 1082t–1084t
  pancreatic function
    amylase, 1008
    glucagon, 1008
    insulin, 1008
    lipase, 1008
  panel tests, 1012t
  renal function, 1003–1006
    creatinine, 1005–1006, 1012t
    electrolytes, 1003–1005
      bicarbonate, 1004–1005
      calcium, 1005, 1012t
      chloride, 1004, 1012t
      magnesium, 1005
      phosphorus, 1005, 1012t
      potassium, 1004, 1004t, 1012t
      sodium, 1004, 1004t, 1012t
    urea (BUN), 1005, 1005t, 1012t
    uric acid, 1006, 1012t
  thyroid function
    thyroid-stimulating hormone (TSH), 1007, *1007*
  usefulness of, 1003
Clinical chemistry department, 862
Clinical diagnosis, 406
Clinical duties, of medical assistant, 9
Clinical investigations and research, ethical issues, 41
Clinical laboratory (*see* Laboratory)

Clinical Laboratory Improvement Amendments (CLIA)
  description, 38, 213, 858
  laboratory standards, 876
  laws governing the clinical laboratory, 874
  levels of testing
    high-complexity, 875–876
    moderate-complexity tests, 11, 875
    waived tests, 874–875
  urinalysis and, 945
Clinical laboratory scientist, 863
Clinical laboratory technician, 863
Clinical trials, 748
Clinitest, for reducing sugars, 952, *952*
Closed captioning, 98
Closed records, 171
Closed wound, 553–554, *554*
Clostridium tetani, 725, 824
Clot formation, 935
Clothing, dress code, 93
Clotting time, 935
CLSI (Clinical and Laboratory Standards Institute), 879
Cluster headaches, 731
Clustering, appointment scheduling, 116
CMA (*see* Certified medical assistant)
CMS-1500 claim form, 269, *270, 271,* 274
  CPR-4 coding, 294, *295*
  diagnostic coding, 278, 284, *287*
CNS (central nervous system), 723
Co-payments, 223, 266
Coagulate, 454, 455
Coagulation tests
  description, 861
  partial thromboplastin time (PTT), 935
  prothrombin time (PT), 935
Coagulation tubes, 905t
Coarctation of the aorta, 683t
Coarse adjustment knob, microscope, 867
Cocaine, 328
Cocci, *966, 967*
Coccidioidmycosis, *968, 968*
Cochlear implants, 639
Code of ethics, laboratory, 877
Codeine, 329
CodeManager (software), 279
Coding, of electronic health record, 160–161
Coinsurance, 266
COLA (Commission on Office Laboratory Accreditation), 875–876
Cold applications
  compress, applying, 590–591
  for orthopedic conditions, 613–614, 614t, 620–621
Cold sores, 579, 704
Colectomy, 709
Colitis, ulcerative, 709
Collection agency, 236, 252
Collection analysis, 223
Collection letter, 227, *228,* 230
Collection percentage, 223
Collections
  aging accounts, 226, 226–227, 227
  alternatives, 228
  legal considerations, 225
  monthly billings, 225–226
  overdue accounts, 227–228
  from patient's estate, 226
  Spanish terminology, 229
  by telephone, 225, 227
Colon, 134
Colon polyps, 710

Colonoscopy, 417, 709, 710, 711
Color, of urine, 948, 949t, 959
Color deficit, 634
Color deficit testing, 635–636, *636,* 646–647
Colorectal cancers, 711
Colpocleisis, 764
Colporrhaphy, 764
Colposcopy, 766, 771, 788–789
Coma, diabetic, 797
Comedone extractor, 432t
Comma, 134
Commercial law, 23
Commission on Accreditation of Allied Health Education Programs (CAAHEP), 15, 16
Commission on Office Laboratory Accreditation (COLA), 875–876
Common cold, 814t
Common law, 22
Communicable diseases
  reporting of, 28–29
  waiting room environment and, 101
Communication, 49–66
  active listening, 52–53
  barriers to, 361
  barriers to patient education, 74
  basic flow, 50, *51*
  challenges
    angry or distressed patients, 60–61
    children, *61,* 61–62
    grieving patient or family member, 62–63
    hearing-impaired patients, 58–59, *59*
    mental health illnesses, 60
    sight-impaired patients, 59–60
    speech impairments, 60
    substance abuse, 60
  charting patient communications, 167
  confidentiality, 65
  defined, 49
  factors affecting, 55–58
    biased opinions, 55, 58
    cultural differences, 55, 56t–57t
    language barriers, 58
    stereotyping, 55, 58
  gestures, 51
  interview techniques, 53–54, 53t, *54*
  kinesics, 51
  by medical office manager
    with patients, 198–199
    with staff, 198–199, *199*
  miscommunication or misinterpretation, 55, 70
  nonlanguage sounds, 51
  nonverbal, 51–52
  paralanguage, 51
  patient education (*see* Patient education)
  positive patient relationships, establishing
    addressing patients, 63
    professional distance, 63
  professional communication
    peers, 64
    physicians, 64
    referrals, 64
  proxemics, 52
  Spanish terminology, 65
  staff
    bulletin boards, 199
    communication notebooks, 199
    electronic, 199
    staff meetings, 199, *199*
  teaching patients, 63–64

therapeutic touch, 52, *52*
verbal, 50–51
written (*see* Written communication)
Community resources, locating, 83, 84–85
Comparative negligence, 35
Compendium of Drug Therapy, 489
Complete blood count (CBC)
  erythrocyte indices, 933–934
    mean cell hemoglobin (MCH), 934
    mean cell hemoglobin concentration
      (MCHC), 934
    mean cell volume (MCV), 934
  hematocrit, 933
  hemoglobin, 932–933
  normal values and clinical significance,
    1081t–1082t
  platelet count, 934
  red blood cell morphology, 932, *932,*
    933t
  white blood cell count, 930
  white blood cell differential, 930–931
    basophils, 931
    eosinophils, 931
    lymphocytes, 931
    monocytes, 931
    neutrophils, 930–931
Compliance, in the elderly, 835, 836, 836f
Composition, business letter, 141
Compress, applying warm or cold, 590–591
Computed tomography (CT) scans, 7, 538,
    540, 685
Computer
  care and maintenance, 181, *181,* 193
  downloading information, 182
  ethics, 192
  handheld, 191
  hardware, 179–180, *180*
  Internet (*see* Internet)
  intranet, 187
  medical software applications, 188–191
    administrative applications, 189–190
    clinical applications, 188–190
    Meeting Maker, 191
    paging system software, 190
    PowerPoint, 190
    vendors, 188
  passwords, 183
  peripherals, 180–181
  purchasing, 191
  Spanish terminology, 192
  training, 191–192
  viruses, 182
Computerized accounting (*see* Accounting,
    computerized)
Computerized appointment scheduling,
    114–115, *115*
Condenser, microscope, 867
Conduction (heat transfer), 375t
Conduction system of the heart, *681*
Conductive hearing loss, 58
Condylomata acuminata, 767
Confidentiality
  breach, 117
  ethics of, 39
  of laboratory tests, 860
  sign-in sheets, 117
Confirmatory consultation, 301
Congenital anomalies, 806
Congestive heart failure (CHF), 678
Conjunctivitis, 632, *632*
Consciousness, assessing level of, 551
Consent
  defined, 25
  expressed, 26–27

form
  information on, 26
  sample, *26*
  signing of, 26–27
implied, 26
informed, 26–27
refusal of, 27
for surgery, 450, *451*
Constellation of symptoms, 120
Constipation, 711–712
Constitutional law, 23
Consultation
  confirmatory, 301
  description, 123
  referral compared to, 124
  reports, 159, 1075
  subcategories of, 301
Contact dermatitis, 888
Continuing education, 15, 16, 1039
Continuing education units (CEUs), 16, 209
Contraception, 779, 780t
Contract law, 23
Contraction stress test (CST), 779
Contracts
  acceptance, 24
  consideration, 24
  defined, 24
  expressed, 24
  implied, 24
  offer, 24
  termination, 24–25
    abandonment, 25
    patient-initiated, 25
    physician-initiated, 25
    protocol, 24
    sample letter, *25*
Contracture, 611
Contraindications, 489, 489t
Contrast medium, 534, 537–538, *539*
Contributory negligence, 35
Controlled substances
  abuse, reporting, 485
  DEA and, 481, 484–485
  disposal of, 486
  inventory of, 485, *486*
  schedule of, 484–485, 484t
Controlled Substances Act (1970), 31
Contusions, 553, *554,* 600, 602
Convection (heat transfer), 375t
Conventions, ICD-9-CM, 283
Convulsions, 727 (*see also* Seizure)
Coordination, in physical examination, 417
Coordination of benefits, 269
COPD (chronic obstructive pulmonary dis-
    ease), 662–663
Copper reduction test, 952, *952*
Corn, 582
Corneal reflex, 733t
Corneal ulcer, 632
Coronary arteriography, 695
Coronary artery bypass graft (CABG), 678,
    680
Coronary artery disease (CAD), 556–557,
    684, 684–685
Corrections, letter, 142
Correspondence, in medical record, 159
Corticosteroids, for asthma, 662
Cortisol, 795t
Coulter Ac-T diff2 Hematology Analyzer,
    932
Coumadin, 686, 861, 935
Counseling, CPT-4 E/M coding and, 299,
    300
Courtesy, 94, *102,* 102–103

Cover letter, 1035–1037
Covered entity, 155
CPC (certified professional coder), 17
CPR (*see* Cardiopulmonary resuscitation)
CPT-4 (*see* Current Procedural Terminology,
    fourth edition)
CPT (Current Procedural Terminology), 239
CPU (central processing unit), 180
Crack cocaine, 328
Cramps, heat, 560
Creatine kinase-MB, 1007
Creatinine, 749, 1005–1006, 1012t
Creatinine clearance test, 1006
Credit, 224–225, 234
Credit adjustment, posting, 236, 251
Credit balance, processing, 236, 250
Credit card authorization, 190
Credit card payment, 223–224
Credit score, 224
Credits
  overpayment, 236
  refunds, 236, 251
Creed for medical assistants, 40
Crile hemostat, *433*
Crile-Wood needle holder, *433*
Criminal law, 23
Crohn's disease, 709
Cross-reference, 170, 282
Crossover claim, 263
Croup, 824
Crush injuries, 553–554
Crutches
  gaits, 624–626
  measuring patient for axillary, 623–624
  tips for use, 615–616
  types, 615, *615*
Cryosurgery, 458
Cryptorchidism, 746, 746–747
Crystals, in urine sediment, 953
CSF (cerebrospinal fluid), 733–734
CST (contraction stress test), 779
Culdocentesis, 768
Cultural differences
  effect on communication, 55
  effect on patient care, 56t–57t
Culture
  blood, 973t, 987–988
  inoculation of, 974, 994–996
  sputum, 666
  stool, 973
  throat, 643
  wound, 586
Culture CATS, 972
Culture media
  caring for, 971, *971*
  types, 970–971, *971*
Culturette, 972, *972*
Curet, 430t, 431t
Curettage, 761
Curie, Marie, 6–7
Current Procedural Terminology, fourth edi-
    tion (CPT-4)
  alphabetic index, 294
  anesthesia section, 300
  categories, 296
  CMS-1500 claim form, 294, *295*
  descriptors, 294
  evaluation and management (E/M
    codes), 299–300, 299t
    counseling, 299, 300
    history, 298, 299t
    key components, 296, 298
    medical decision making, 298–299
    physical examination, 298, 299t

Current Procedural Terminology, fourth edition (CPT-4) *(con't)*
  time, 299–300
  layout of, 294
  locating a code, 306
  Medicare claims, 263–264
  medicine section, 303
  modifiers, 303
  overview, 294
  pathology and laboratory section, 302–303
  place of service codes, 295–296, 298t
  radiology section, 302
  sample page, 297
  section guidelines, 296
  surgery section, 300–302
  unlisted procedures and special reports, 296
Cushing's syndrome, 798, *798*
Customer service, 94
CVA (cerebrovascular accident), 686, 687, 842t
Cystic fibrosis, 824
Cystitis, 744
Cystocele, 764
Cystoscopy, 742, 749, *749*
Cystourethroscopy, 749
Cysts, ovarian, 765
Cytogenetics, 862
Cytologist, 863
Cytology, 862

Damage
  defined, 32
  jury awards for, 32–33
DASH (Dietary Approaches to Stop Hypertension), 322, 322t
Daysheet
  balancing, 254
  description, *234*, 234–235
  errors on, 235
  posting a charge, 236, 248–249
  posting a payment, 236, 249–250
  posting adjustments, 236, 238, 251–252
  posting to cash-paid-out section of, 238
D&C (dilation and curettage), 771
DEA (*see* Drug Enforcement Agency)
Death certificates, 28
DeBakey forceps, *433*
Debit, 234
Debit adjustment, posting, 238
Debit card, 241
Debt collector, 225
Decibel (dB), 641
Decimal point placement, 137
Decongestants, 483t
Decubitus ulcers, 582–583, 583t
Deductible
  insurance, 266
  Medicare, 263
Deep-brain stimulation, 846
Defamation of character, 33
Defendant, 32, 34
Defense mechanisms, 80, 81t
Defenses against disease, nonspecific, 335
Degenerative joint disease, 607, 842t
Dehiscence, 452
Delayed cutaneous hypersensitivity (type IV allergy), 888
Deltoid muscle, 506, *506*
Demeanor, 52
Dementia, 835, 847, 847t
Demographics, 160, 190, 357
Demonstration, in patient education, 69

Denial (defense mechanism), 81t
Dental caries (cavities), 327, 703–704
Denver Developmental Screening Test II, 807, *812, 813*
Department of Public Health, reportable diseases and, 878
Dependent, 262, 269
Deposit slip, 234
Depositions, 34
Deposits, making bank, 241, 254–255
Depressants, 329
Dereliction of duty, 32
Dermal medications, 508
Dermatology, 575–597
  alopecia, 583
  bacterial infections, 576–578, *579*
    carbuncle, 577–578, *578*
    cellulitis, 578, *579*
    folliculitis, 577, *578*
    furuncle, 577, *578*
    impetigo, 576–577
  bandaging, 587–588, *589*, 593–594
  diagnostic procedures
    physical examination, 586
    skin biopsy, 586
    urine melanin, 586
    Wood's light analysis, 587
    wound culture, 586
  fungal infections, 580, *580*
    tinea capitis, 580
    tinea corporis, 580, *580*
    tinea cruris, 580
    tinea pedis, 580
    tinea unguium, 580
    tinea versicolor, 580
  inflammatory reactions
    acne vulgaris, 582
    eczema, 581, *581*
    psoriasis, 582, *582*
    seborrhea dermatitis, 581
    urticaria, 581–582
  instruments and equipment, 432t
  parasitic infections
    pediculosis, 581
    scabies, 580–581
  pigmentation disorders
    albinism, 583, *584*
    leukoderma, 584
    nevus, 584
    vitiligo, 584
  pressure-associated disorders
    callus, 582
    corn, 582
    decubitus ulcers, 582–583, 583t
  procedures
    therapeutic soak, 592–593
    tubular gauze bandage application, 593–595
    warm or cold compresses, applying, 590–591
  skin anatomy, 576, *577*
  skin cancer
    basal cell carcinoma, 584, *585*
    malignant melanoma, 585, *585*
    squamous cell carcinoma, 585, *585*
  skin lesions, types of, 576, 578
  Spanish terminology, 596
  viral infections, 579, *579*
    herpes simplex, 579
    herpes zoster, 579, *579*
    verruca, 579
  wound healing disorders, 582
Dermatophytosis, 580, *580*
Descriptor, CPT-4, 294

Desmarres lid retractor, 432t
Diabetes insipidus, 799
Diabetes mellitus
  coma, 797
  controlling, 797
  description, 794–797, 950–951
  emergencies, 796–797, 801–803
  gestational, 796
  ketoacidosis, 797
  managing patient with, 801–803
  retinopathy, 797
  type 1 (insulin-dependent diabetes mellitus), 794
  type 2 (non-insulin-dependent diabetes mellitus), 795–796
Diabetic retinopathy, 632
Diagnosis, 159, 406
Diagnostic coding
  accuracy, 304
  Current Procedural Terminology, fourth edition (CPT-4)
    alphabetic index, 294
    anesthesia section, 300
    categories, 296
    CMS-1500 claim form, 294, *295*
    descriptors, 294
    evaluation and management (E/M codes), 296–300, 299t
    layout of, 294
    locating a code, 306
    medicine section, 303
    modifiers, 303
    overview, 294
    pathology and laboratory section, 302–303
    place of service codes, 295–296, 298t
    radiology section, 302
    sample page, 297
    section guidelines, 296
    surgery section, 300–302
    unlisted procedures and special reports, 296
  diagnostic related groups (DRGs), 304
  fraud, 305
  Healthcare Common Procedure Coding System (HCPCS)
    level I codes (CPT), 293–304
    level II codes, 293–294
    level III codes, 293–294
  hospital coding, 278–279
  ICD-9-CM
    CMS guidelines, 284
    conventions, 283, *285*
    documentation required, 289
    HIPAA mandate, 278
    late effects, 288, *288*
    locating appropriate code, 283–289, 290
    maintenance of classification system, 278
    multiple codes, 284–285, *287*
    overview, 277
    primary codes, 284
    privacy issues, 278
    suspected conditions, 289
    tenth revision, 289
    Volume 1: Tabular List of Diseases, 279–280, *280, 281*
    Volume 2: Alphabetic List of Diseases, 280, 282–283
    Volume 3: Tabular List and Alphabetic Index of Procedures, 283
  inpatient *versus* outpatient, 278–279

overview, 277
resource-based relative value scale
(RBRVS), 304
Spanish terminology, 290
usefulness of, 277
Diagnostic imaging, 532–545
diagnostic procedures, 536–540
computed tomography (CT), 538,
540
contrast medium examinations,
538–539, *539*
examination by body region, table of,
538t
fluoroscopy, 538
magnetic resonance imaging (MRI),
539, *540*
mammography, 537, 539, *539*
nuclear medicine, 539–540
sonography, 538–539, *540*
interventional procedures, 540
radiation therapy, 540–541
radiology principles, 533–536
contrast media, 534
examination sequencing, 534
outpatient x-rays, 534
patient positioning, 534, *535*, *536*
safety, 534–535, *537*, *538*
x-ray machine, 533–534
x-rays, 533–534
role of medical assistant, 541–542
assisting with examinations, 541–542
calming patient fears, 541
film storage and handling, 542, *542*
preparing patient for x-ray, 543
teleradiology, 542–543
transfer of information, 542–543
Diagnostic related groups (DRGs), 304
Diagnostic testing, making appointments for,
124
Diagonal, 134
Dialysis, 741–742
Dialysis shunt, 385
Diaphoresis, 378
Diaphragm, microscope, 867
Diaphragmatic hernia, *705*, 705–706
Diarrhea, 712
Diastole, 382
Diazo test, 952, *953*
Diction, 102
Diet
Dietary Approaches to Stop
Hypertension (DASH), 222t, 322
of elderly patients, 849
liquid supplements, 849
vegetarian, 321
Dietary Approaches to Stop Hypertension
(DASH), 322, 322t
Dietary Guidelines for Americans, 315, 320
Differential diagnosis, 406
Digestion, 315
Digital rectal examination, 417, 745
Digital subscriber line (DSL), 181
Digitalis, 4
Dilation and curettage (D&C), 771
Diluent, 503
Diplomacy, 94
Dipstick Reader, Bayer Clinitek, *950*
Direct cause, 32
Directors, 434, *435*
Discharge instructions, 52
Discharge summary, 1072
Disciplinary action, 202, *204*
Discrimination, 36, 55, 58, 200
Discussion, in patient education, 69

Disease
carriers, 336
communicable, 28–29, 101, 338t
genetic, 361
hereditary, 360
reportable, 878
Disease prevention
medical asepsis, 334, 338–339
nonspecific defenses against disease, 334
OSHA guidelines for the medical office,
340–348
biohazardous material, 342, 344,
345–346, *346*, 347, 353–354
blood-borne pathogen training, 341
disposal of infectious waste,
345–346, 347, 353–354
environmental contamination, 345
exposure control plan, 342
exposure risk factor, 341
hepatitis B, 346–348
human immunodeficiency virus
(HIV), 346–348
OSHA 300 log, 342, *343*
personal protective equipment, 341,
342, 344, *347*
standard precautions, 342
principles of infection control, 337–340
Disinfectants, 339–340
Disinfection, 339–340, 341t, 426, 438–439
Dislocations, 600
Displacement (defense mechanism), 81t
Disposing of infectious waste, 345–346,
347, 353–354
Dissecting aneurysm, 687
Disseminating information, 83
Distressed patients, communicating with,
60–61
Dittel urethral sound, 431t
Diuretics, 483t
Diurnal variation, 946
Diverticulitis, 710
Diverticulosis, 710
Documentation
electronic health record, 160
externship, 1029, *1030*
guidelines, 166–167
legal issues, 71
of medication administration, 496
of patient education, 70–71
Documents
guidelines for producing, 133–138
hospital, 133
medical office, 133t
Dopamine, 845, 846
Doppler device, for fetal heart tones, 775, *775*
Doppler ultrasonography, 684
Dorsal lithotomy position, 769
Dorsal recumbent position, *413*, 414t
Dorsalis pedis pulse, 379, 380, *380*
Dorsogluteal site, *507*, 821
Dosimeter, 536, *538*
Double booking, 116
Down syndrome, 728
Downloading, 182
Drainage, wound
incision and drainage, 456, 458
type, 456
Draping, 450, *452*
Dress code, office, 93
Dressings (*see* Sterile dressings)
DRGs (diagnostic related groups), 304
Drug abuse, 328–329
Drug and Alcohol Testing Industry
Association, 948

Drug Enforcement Agency (DEA), 31, 481,
484–485
Drug interactions, 488
Drug testing
chain of custody, 947, 948
legal guidelines, 947–948
patient preparation, 947
Drugs (*see also* Pharmacology)
classifications of, 482t–484t
defined, 481
generic equivalent, 481
names, 481
pharmacodynamics, 486–487
pharmacokinetics, 487–488
terminology, 489t
DSL (digital subscriber line), 181
Duodenal ulcers, 708
Duplay tenaculum forceps, 430t, *433*
Dupuytren contracture, *611*, 611–612
Durable power of attorney, 25–26
Duress, 33
Duty, 32
Dwarfism, 799
Dysfunctional uterine bleeding, 761
Dysmenorrhea, 763
Dyspareunia, 763
Dysphagia, 725, 843
Dysphasia, 60, 726
Dysphonia, 60
Dyspnea, 382, 661
Dysuria, 744

E-codes, 279
Ear
anatomy, 637, *638*
diagnostic studies
audiometry, 641, 652–653
tuning fork tests, 641
tympanometry, 641
visual examination, 641
disorders, 637–640
ceruminosis, 638
hearing loss, 638–639
Ménière's disease, 639
otitis externa, *639*, 639–640
otitis media, 640, *640*
otosclerosis, 640
patient education concerning, 640
effects of aging on, 844t
instilling medication, 641, 654–655
irrigations, 641, 650–652
physical examination, 415, *415*
Spanish terminology, 644
Ear medications, 641, 654–655
Ear tubes, 640
Ecchymosis, 553
Echinacea, 79t
Echocardiography, 684, 693
Eclampsia, 778
ECRP (endoscopic retrograde cholangiopancreatography), 714, 716, *716*
Ectopic pregnancy, 778
Eczema, 581, *581*
EDC (Estimated Date of Confinement), 773
EDD (expected date of delivery), 773
Editing letters, 142
EDTA (ethylenediaminetetraacetic acid)
tubes, 905t
Education
of office manager, 209
patient (*see* Patient education)
staff, 208
Educational background, effect on patient
education, 74–75

EEG (electroencephalogram), 727, 733
EEOC (Equal Employment Opportunity Commission), 36
Egyptians, ancient, 4
EHR (*see* Electronic health records)
Einthoven leads, 691
Elastic bandages, 587, *587*
Elbow, tennis, 611
Elder abuse, 839–840, *840*
Elderly patients (*see also* Geriatrics)
    abuse of, 30
    teaching, 74
Electrical burns, 555
Electrocardiogram (ECG)
    artifacts, 692, 694t
    baseline, 417
    on child, 690
    ECG leads, 689, 691, 691t
    graph paper, 689, *690*
    Holter monitor, 692, 693, *693*, 698–699
    interpretation, 691–692, *692*
        PR interval, 691
        PR segment, 692
        ST segment, 692
        ventricular activation time, 692
    myocardial infarction diagnosis, 678
    overview, 689
    procedure for 12-lead, 695–697
    rhythm strip, 692
Electrocautery, 454
Electrodes, electrosurgical unit, 454–455
Electrodesiccation, 454
Electroencephalogram (EEG), 727, 733
Electrolyte solution, oral, 560
Electrolytes, 1003–1005
    bicarbonate, 1004–1005
    calcium, 1005, 1012t
    chloride, 1004, 1012t
    magnesium, 1005
    phosphorus, 1005, 1012t
    potassium, 1004, 1004t, 1012t
    sodium, 1004, 1004t, 1012t
Electromyography, 608
Electronic data storage
    backup copy, 171
    off-site, 171
Electronic Doppler, 775, *775*
Electronic health records (EHR)
    billing and coding, 160–161
    choosing a vendor, 159
    description, 155, 159
    features, 160
    medical assistant's role, 161
    power failure and, 161
    security, 161–162
    standards, 159
    transition to, 159–160
Electronic mail (e-mail)
    access, 183
    address book, 184
    attachments, 184
    communicating electronically, 199
    composing messages, 183–184
    description, 96, 145
    encryption, 183
    ethical issues, 192
    in medical record, 167
    opening, 184
    tips for using, 145, 183
Electronic thermometers, 376, *378*, 395
Electrosection, 454
Electrosurgery, 454–455, *455*
Eligibility, health plan, 261–262
Elimite, 581

Elixir (oral medication form), 502t
Ellipsis, 134
Elliptocytes, 933t
Emancipated minor, 27, 814
Embolization, 540
Embolus, 684, 686
Embolus, fat, 606
Emergencies, 546–574
    action plan, 547–548
    documenting in medical record, 549
    Emergency Medical Services (EMS) system, 548–549
    medical kit, 548
    overview, 547
    patient assessment, 549–552
        physical examination, 552
        primary assessment, 549–550
            airway, 549, *550*
            breathing, 549–550, *550*
            circulation, 550, *550*
            responsiveness, 549
        recognition of emergency, 549
        secondary assessment, 551–552
            general appearance, 551
            level of consciousness, 551
            skin temperature, moisture, and color, 551–552
            vital signs, 551
    procedures
        AED (automatic external defibrillator) use, 565–567
        bleeding, control of, 570
        CPR (cardiopulmonary resuscitation), 562–563, *563*–565
        foreign body airway obstruction, management of, 568–569
        oxygen administration, 562–563
    schedule adaptation for, 120, 121, *121*
    Spanish terminology, 571
    types of emergencies, 553–561
        allergic and anaphylactic reactions, 557–558
        behavioral, 561
        bleeding, 553–555, *554*
        burns, 555, 555–556
        cardiovascular, 556–557
        frostbite, 561
        hyperthermia, 560
        hypothermia, 560–561
        musculoskeletal injuries, 556, *556*
        neurologic, 557, *557*
        poisoning, 558–560, *559*
        psychiatric, 561
        shock, 553
        soft tissue injuries, 553–555, *554*, *555*
Emergency action plan, 547–548
Emergency medical kit, 548
Emergency medical service (EMS), 106–107, 548–549
Emetics, 483t
Empathy, 62
Employees (*see also* Staff)
    disciplinary action, 202, *204*
    evaluating, 202, *203*
    health benefits, 261, 262
    interviewing and hiring, 200
    references for, 202
    terminating, 202
Employer surveys, 1030, *1032*
Employment
    applying for a job
        action words, 1036
        application, completing, 1037

calls from prospective employers, 1034
    cover letter, 1035–1037
    newspaper advertisements, 1033
    résumé preparation, 1033–1035, 1042–1043
    résumé samples, *1035*, *1036*
    finding a job, 1033
    goals, setting, 1031–1032
    interview
        follow-up, 1040
        foreign language, knowledge of, 1038
        importance of, 1037
        job skills, employer's interest in, 1037
        portfolio for, 1038
        preparing for, 1037–1038, *1038*
        questions, crucial, 1038–1040, 1039t–1040t
        thank you letter, 1040, *1040*
    job openings, information on, 1033
    leaving a job, 1041
    networking, 1033
    opportunities, 17–18, 1033
    professionalism, 1041
    self-analysis, 1032
    surveys, 1030, *1032*
Employment and safety laws
    Age Discrimination in Employment, 38
    Americans with Disabilities Act (ADA), 36–37, 38
    Civil Rights Act, 36, 38
    discrimination, 36
    Fair Labor Standards Act, 38
    Family and Medical Leave Act, 38
    Immigration Reform and control Act, 38
    Occupational Safety and Health Act, 37
    sexual harassment, 36
EMS (emergency medical service), 106–107, 548–549
Emulsion (oral medication form), 502t
Encephalitis, 724, 823–824
Enclosure, 140
Encounter, 235–236, *237*
Encryption, 183
Endocarditis, 677–678
Endocrine system
    benefits of exercise, 848t
    effects of aging on, 844t
Endocrinologists, 793
Endocrinology, 792–804
    adrenal gland disorders
        Addison's disease, 798, *798*
        Cushing's syndrome, 798, *798*
    anatomy, *794*
    diabetes mellitus, 794–797
        coma, 797
        controlling, 797
        emergencies, 796–797, 801–803
        gestational, 796
        ketoacidosis, 797
        managing patient with, 801–803
        retinopathy, 797
        type 2 (non-insulin-dependent diabetes mellitus), 795–796
        type I (insulin-dependent diabetes mellitus), 794
    diagnostic and therapeutic procedures, 799–800, 800t
    glands and hormones, table of, 795t
    overview, 793
    pituitary gland disorders
        acromegaly, 799, *799*
        diabetes insipidus, 799
        dwarfism, 799

gigantism, 798–799
Spanish terminology, 800
thyroid gland disorders
hyperthyroidism, 793–794, 796, *796*
hypothyroidism, 794
Endometriosis, 763–764
Endoscopic retrograde cholangiopancreatography (ECRP), 714, 716, *716*
Endoscopy
assisting with procedure, 718–720
bowel preparation for, 717
gastrointestinal, *716*, 716–717, *717*, 718–720
insufflator, 717
obturator, 717
English-to-Spanish health care phrases
body parts, 1056–1057
diseases, 1057
examination, 1058–1059
general phrases, 1059–1060
general words, 1056
introductory phrases, 1055
signs and symptoms, 1057–1058
treatment, 1059
Entamoeba, 969
Enteric coated tablet (oral medication form), 502t
Envelopes, addressing, 145–146, *146*
Environment, for learning, 72
Environmental Protection Agency (EPA), 326, 345–346
Enzymes, liver, 1006–1007
EOB (explanation of benefits), 224
Eosinophils, *928*, 931
Ephedrine, 78
Epididymitis, 747
Epiglottitis, 824
Epilepsy, 30, 727
Epinephrine, 451, 582, 795t
Epistaxis, 642
Epithelial cells, in urine sediment, 953
Eponym, 283
Epstein-Barr virus, 977
Equal Employment Opportunity Commission (EEOC), 36
Equipment
autoclave, 426–429, *428*, *429*
for patient education, 72
records, 436
sanitizing, 426, 438–439
sterilization, 426–429, 427t
Ergonomics, 97–98
Errors, in daysheet, 235
Erythema, 576
Erythrocyte indices, 933–934
mean cell hemoglobin (MCH), 934
mean cell hemoglobin concentration (MCHC), 934
mean cell volume (MCV), 934
Erythrocyte sedimentation rate (ESR), *934*, 934–935, 941–942
Erythropoiesis, 932
Erythropoietin, 932
Escherichia coli (E. coli), 335
Esophageal cancer, 706
Esophageal disorders
cancer, 706
gastroesophageal reflux disease (GERD), 706
hiatal hernia, *705*, 705–706
Esophageal varices, 706
ESR (erythrocyte sedimentation rate), *934*, 934–935, 941–942
Essential amino acids, 313

Essential fatty acids, 313
Essential hypertension, 685
Estate, collecting debt from, 226
Esteem, 72
Estimated Date of Confinement (EDC), 773
Estrogen, 781, 795t
Ethernet, 181
Ethics
accuracy in diagnostic coding, 304
bioethics
AMA Council on Ethical and Judicial Affairs, 40
defined, 38
social policy issues, 40–42, 43, *44*
allocation of resources, 40–41
clinical investigations and research, 41
obstetric dilemmas, 41
organ transplantation, 42, 43
stem cell research, 42
withholding or withdrawing treatment, 42, *44*
computer, 192
confidentiality, *65*, 117
defined, 22
diagnostic coding, 289
fees, 225
HIPAA and students, 1026
laboratory code of ethics, 877
medical
AAMA code, 40
AMA code, 38–39
defined, 38
honesty, 39
patient advocacy, 39
patient confidentiality, 39
minutes of meetings, 144
office management issues, 43, 45
patient rights, 156
petty cash use, 242
provider ethics, 268
support *versus* judgment, 76
withholding information, 202
Ethylene oxide, 426, 427t
Ethylenediaminetetraacetic acid (EDTA) tubes, 905t
Eustachian tubes, 825
Evacuated tube system
color code system, 903t–904t
multisample needles, 901, *901*
tube additives, 901–902
tube holder, *900, 901, 901, 902*
vacuum, 901
venipuncture using, 912
Evaluation
of employees, 202, *203*
externship, 1029–1030, *1031*
in patient education process, 70
Evaporation (heat transfer), 375
Examination, comprehensive final, 1045–1052
Examination light, *408*, 408–409
Excision of skin lesions, 458
Exercise
benefits of, 848t
for older patients, 848–849, *849*
as stress reliever, 80
Existing illnesses, effect on learning, 73
Exophthalmia, 794, *796*
Expected date of delivery (EDD), 773
Expected threshold, 214
Expectorants, 483t
Expenditures, categories of, 244
Expert witness, 32

Expiration, 381–382 (*see also* Respiration)
Explanation of benefits (EOB), 224, 239, 271–272, *273*
Exposure control plan, 342
Exposure risk factor, 341
Express mail, 146
Expressed consent, 26–27
Expressed contracts, 24
Expression, on telephone, 102
Externship
benefits
to externship site, 1026
to medical assisting program, 1026
to student, 1025–1026
description, 14
documentation, 1029, *1030*
evaluations, 1029–1030, *1031*
facilities, 1025
guidelines for success, 1027–1029
appearance, 1028
attendance, 1028
attitude, 1028
preparedness, 1027–1028
procedural performance, 1027
journal, 1026, 1029
preceptor, 1025, 1027, 1028
responsibilities
to externship site, 1027
to medical assisting program, 1027
to student, 1026
role of, 1025
sites, 1025, 1026, 1027
time sheet, *1030*
Extracellular fluid, 1004
Extract (oral medication form), 502t
Extraocular eye movement, 415
Eye loop, 432t
Eye medications, 647–648
Eye movements, as communication, 51
Eyes
anatomy, *631*
defenses against disease, 335
diagnostic studies
color deficit testing, 635–636, *636*, 646–647
gonioscopy, 636–637
tonometry, 636
visual acuity testing, 634–635, *636*, 644–645
disorders, 630–634
cataract, 631, *632*
color deficit, 634
conjunctivitis, 632, *632*
corneal ulcer, 632
glaucoma, 633
refractive errors, 633, 634, *634*
retinopathy, 632–633
strabismus, 633, *635*
sty (hordeolum), 632
effects of aging on, 844t
instilling eye medications, 637, 647–648
irrigation, 649–650
physical examination, 415
preventative eye care, 637
Spanish terminology, 644
Eyewash basin, 344, 889, *889*

Face mask with one-way valve, for artificial respiration, 550, *550*
Facial expressions, 51
Facsimile machines, 96, 144–145
Fahrenheit-Celsius temperature conversion scale, 1079
Fahrenheit scale, 373, 376, 376t, *377*

Fair Labor Standards Act of 1939, 38
Fall prevention, teaching, 75–76
False labor, 776
Falsifying medical credentials, 30
Falsifying medical records, 22
Familial diseases, 360
Family and Medical Leave Act of 1993, 38
Family history, 158, 360, 361
Farsightedness, 633, *634*
Fasting, 910
Fasting blood glucose (FBS), 799, 1009,
        1012t
Fat embolus, 606
Fats, 313, 313t
Fatty acids, essential, 313
FDA (*see* Food and Drug Administration)
Fears, calming the patient's, 541
Febrile seizures, 727, 728
Fecal occult blood, 972–973, 989–990
Fecal tests, 717
Federal Child Abuse Prevention and
        Treatment Act, 29, 822
Federal Food, Drug, and Cosmetic Act, 481
Federal Register, 875
Fee-for-service, 266
Fee schedules, 222–223, *223,* 266
Fee splitting, 30
Feedback, 50
Fees
    adjusting, 224
    bank, 240
    co-pays, 223
    collection, 225–228, 230
    collection analysis, 223
    discussing in advance, 223
    ethics, 225
    forms of payment, 223–224
    late payment, 225
    nonparticipating, 223
    participating, 223
    payment
        credit, 224–225
        forms of, 223–224
        by insurance company, 224
    setting, 222–223
    write-off, 224
Female reproductive system (*see also*
        Gynecology; Obstetrics)
    anatomy, *761*
    cancers, 765–766, 765t
    effects of aging on, 844t
    menstrual cycle, 760–761, *762*
    procedures
        breast self-examination, 782–784
        colposcopy and cervical biopsy,
            788–789
        pelvic examination and Pap smear,
            785–787
Femoral pulse, *379*
Fencing reflex, 811t
Fetal development, 774
Fetal ultrasonography, 779
Fetoscope, 775, *776*
Fetus, drugs dangerous to, 776
Fever
    intermittent, 375, 376t
    patient education, 377–378
    patterns, variations in, 376t
    processes, 374
    relapsing, 375, 376t
    remittent, 375, 376t
    stages of, 374–375
    sustained, 375, 376t
Fever blisters, 579, 704

Fiber, 315
Fibrin, 935
Fibromyalgia, 607
Fibrosis, liver, 713
Filing
    alphabetic, 169, 170
    drawer files, 171
    indexing rules, 169
    insurance claims, 269–272
    ledger cards, 235
    numeric, 169–170
    procedures, 168, 175
    rotary files, 171
    shelving units, 171, *171*
    subject, 170
Film, x-ray, 533, 534, 542
Filter paper test requisitions, 908, *909*
Final examination, comprehensive,
        1045–1052
Financial software programs, 190
Fine adjustment knob, microscope, 867
Fine-point splinter forceps, *433*
Fingernails, 93
First impressions, 94
Fixed scheduling, 116
Flashlight, 409
Fleming, Sir Alexander, 6
Flexibility, 322
Flow sheet, 164, *164, 165,* 878–879, *879*
Fluids, for intravenous administration, 509
Fluorescein angiography, 633
Fluorescein dye, 632
Fluoroscopy, 538
Folate deficiency, 930, 931, 934
Folic acid, 314, 772
Follicle-stimulating hormone, 795t
Folliculitis, 577, *578*
Food, thermic effect of, 324
Food and Drug Administration (FDA)
        food label regulation, 321, 324
        role in drug regulation, 481
Food-borne illness, preventing, 320
Food-drug interaction, 488
Food label, 321, *321,* 324, 330–331
Food programs, government, 324
Foot, plantar fasciitis, 612–613
Forced expiratory volume, 667
Forceps, 432, *433*
Foreign language, knowledge of, 1038
Form of address, 63
Formaldehyde, 341t, 427t, 428
Fowler's position, *413,* 414t
Fractures, 600–606
    casts, 601–602, 604, *604, 605*
    healing, 605
    hip, 606
    overview, 600–601
    reduction, 600–601
    types, 603t–604t
Fraud, 22, 30, 33, 200, 268, 305
Freezers, in clinical laboratory, 869
Fried's rule, 501
Frostbite, 561
Frozen shoulder, 611
Fruits, food group guidelines, 319
Fulguration, 454, 458
Full block letter format, 140
Full thickness (third degree) burns, 555
Fungi
    diseases, 968, *968, 969*
    molds, 968
    patient education, 580
    skin, 580, *580*
    yeasts, 968

Furniture, waiting room, 98
Furuncle, 577, *578*

Gait, in physical examination, 417
Galactosuria, 952
Galen, 5
Gallbladder disorders
    cancer, 713
    cholecystitis, 713
    cholelithiasis, 713–714, *714*
Gardnerella vaginitis, 768
Garlic, 79t
Gas, intestinal, 712
Gastric bypass surgery, 708
Gastric cancer, 707–708
Gastritis, 707
Gastroenteritis, 708, 814t, 823
Gastroenterology
    anatomy of gastrointestinal tract, *704*
    diagnostic and therapeutic procedures
        blood tests, 715
        endoscopy, *716,* 716–717, *717,*
            718–720
        fecal tests, 717
        nuclear imaging, 716
        physical examination, 715
        radiology studies, 715–716
        ultrasonography, 716
    esophageal disorders
        cancer, 706
        gastroesophageal reflux disease
            (GERD), 706
        hiatal hernia, *705,* 705–706
    gallbladder disorders
        cancer, 713
        cholecystitis, 713
        cholelithiasis, 713–714, *714*
    intestinal disorders
        appendicitis, 711
        cancer, 711, *711*
        constipation, 711–712
        Crohn's disease, 709
        diarrhea, 712
        diverticulosis, 710
        duodenal ulcers, 708
        functional disorders, 711–712
        gas, 712
        gastroenteritis, 708
        hemorrhoids, 711
        hernias, 710–711
        irritable bowel syndrome, 709–710
        malabsorption syndromes, 708
        polyps, 710
        ulcerative colitis, 709
    liver disorders, 712–713
        cancer, 713
        cirrhosis/fibrosis, 713
        diagnostic tests for, 712
        hepatitis, 712–713, 712t
    mouth disorders
        caries, 703–704
        gingivitis, 705
        oral cancers, 705
        stomatitis, 704–705
    overview, 701
    pancreatic disorders
        cancer, 714
        pancreatitis, 714
    Spanish terminology, 720
    stomach disorders
        cancer, 707–708
        gastritis, 707
        peptic ulcer, 707
Gastroesophageal reflux disease (GERD), 706

Gastrointestinal system
    defenses against disease, 335
    effects of aging on, 843t
Gatekeeper provision, managed care, 268
Gauge
    needle, 504, 900
    suture, 453
Gauze pads, 899
Gel (oral medication form), 502t
Gel separator, 902
Gelcap (oral medication form), 502t
Generic equivalent, 481
Generic name, 481
Genetic counseling, 361
Genetic diseases, 361
Genetic testing, 41–42
Genetics, effect on health, 327
Genital specimens, collecting for culture, 988–989
Genital warts, 767
Genitalia, physical examination, 417
Genitourinary tract, 335
Geographical practice cost index (GPCI), 304
GERD (gastroesophageal reflux disease), 706
Geriatrics, 834–853
    advanced directives, 839
    compliance, 835, 836
    coping with aging, 838
        alcoholism, 838
        suicide, 838
    diseases of the elderly
        Alzheimer's disease, 847–848, 847t
        Parkinson's disease, 841, 845–847, 846f
    elder abuse, 839–840, 840
    hard-of-hearing patient, communicating with, 841
    health maintenance
        diet, 849
        exercise, 848–849, 848t, 849
        safety, 849–850
    home care options, 839
    long-term care, 838–839
    medications, 840–841
    reinforcing mental health in elderly, 837
    Spanish terminology, 850
    stereotypes about the elderly, 835, 836
    systemic changes in elderly, 841
Germicides, 339–340
Gerontologists, 835
Gestational diabetes mellitus, 796
Gestational wheel, 773
Gestures, 51
Giardia, 969
Gingivitis, 705
Ginkgo, 79t, 837
Ginseng, 79t
Glass mercury thermometers, 375–376, 377, 392–393, 394
Glaucoma, 633, 844t
Glomerulonephritis, 743–744
Gloves
    applying sterile, 467–469
    latex allergy, 342
    patient offense at wearing of, 344
    as personal protective equipment, 344
    removing contaminated, 351–352
    types, 898
    use in phlebotomy, 898
    when to wear, 342
Glucagon, 795t, 1008
Glucosamine, 79t

Glucose
    testing, 1008–1010–1013–1015
        fasting blood glucose (FBS), 1009, 1012t
        hemoglobin A1C, 1010
        maintenance of glucose meter, 1017
        obstetric patients, 1010
        oral glucose tolerance test, 1009–1010, 1010
        patient education, 1009
        procedure for testing, 1013–1015
        random, 1009
        two-hour postprandial glucose, 1009
    urine, 950
Glucose meter, 1008, 1008, 1009
Glucose tolerance test (GTT), 799, 1009–1010, 1010
Glutaraldehyde, 341t, 427, 427t
Glycohemoglobin, 799
Glycosuria, 794, 950
Goals, employment, 1031–1032
Goiter, 794, 796
Goniometer, 613, 613
Gonioscopy, 636
Gonorrhea, 767–768
Good Samaritan acts, 31
Goodell's sign, 771
Gooseneck lamp, 408, 408, 417
Gout, 607, 1006, 1006
Government-sponsored health benefits, 263–265
GPCI (geographical practice cost index), 304
Graduate surveys, 1030, 1031
Grains, food group guidelines, 316, 318
Gram stain, 974, 975, 992–993
Grammar, 134
Grand mal seizures, 727
Granulocytes, 930
Grasp reflex, 811t
Graves' disease, 793–794, 796
Graves vaginal speculum, 430t
Gravid, 771
Gravida, 773
Gravidity, 773
Grief
    communicating with patient or family member, 62–63
    five stages of, 62
Griseofulvin, 580
Grooming, 93
Group A strep test, 977, 978, 999–1000
Group benefit plan, 261–262
Group homes, 839
Group member, health benefits plan, 261
Growth charts, 325, 818f, 819
Growth hormone, 795t, 798–799
GTT (glucose tolerance test), 1009–1010, 1010
Guaiac methods, 711, 972, 989–990
Guided imagery, 326
Gynecologic disorders, 761–768
    diagnostic and therapeutic procedures
        colposcopy, 771, 788–789
        dilation and curettage, 771
        gynecologic examination, 768–770, 769, 785–787
        hysterosalpingography, 771
    dysfunctional uterine bleeding, 761
    endometriosis, 763–764
    gynecologic cancers, 765–766, 765t, 766t
    infertility, 766
    leiomyomas, 764–765

ovarian cysts, 765
    premenstrual syndrome, 761–763
    sexually transmitted diseases, 766–768
        AIDS, 766–767
        chlamydia, 767
        condylomata acuminata, 767
        gonorrhea, 767–768
        herpes genitalis, 768
        pelvic inflammatory disease (PID), 768
        salpingitis, 768
        syphilis, 767
        vulvovaginitis, 768
    uterine prolapse and displacement, 764, 764
Gynecologic examination, 768–770, 769, 785–787
Gynecology
    defined, 760
    instruments and equipment, 430t

Haemophilus influenzae, 824
Hallucinogens, 329
Halsted mosquito hemostat, 433
Hammer, percussion, 407, 407
Hand, Dupuytren contracture of, 611, 611–612
Hand uterine dilator, 430t
Handheld computers, 191
Handwashing, 100, 101, 327, 338–339, 349–350
Hard drive, 180
Hard-of-hearing patient, 841
Harvey, William, 5–6
Hashimoto's thyroiditis, 794
Hashish, 328
Hazardous Communication (HazCom) Standard, 887–888
Hazardous materials
    biological hazards, 887
    chemical hazards, 884–885, 886, 887–888
    Chemical Hygiene Plan (CHP), 888
    classification system, 884–885, 886
    guidelines, 889–890
    incident reports, 890
    OSHA, 887–888, 890
    physical hazards, 884
    Right to Know law, 437
HCG (human chorionic gonadotropin), 771
HCG pregnancy test, 977, 977, 997–998
HCl (hydrochloric acid), 707
HCPCS (see Healthcare Common Procedure Coding System)
HDL (see High-density lipoprotein)
Head
    assessing in emergency care, 552
    physical examination of, 415
Head light, 409, 409
Head Start, 324
Head tilt-chin lift method for opening the airway, 549, 550
Headaches, 731
Healing process, 457–458
Health Care Financing Administration (HFCA), 8
Health Care Savings Accounts (HSAs), 262–263
Health care system, 18
Health care team
    allied health care professionals, 13–14
    nurse practitioners, 12
    nurses, 12–13
    physician assistants, 12
    physicians, 12

Health insurance
  balance billing, 272
  co-payments, 266
  coinsurance, 266
  deductible, 266
  filing claims, 269–272
    assignment of benefits, 265, 269, 272
    birthday rule, 269
    claim denial and corrective action, 271t
    CMS-1500 claim form, 269, 270, 271, 274
    coordination of benefits, 269
    dependent children, 269
    electronic submission, 271
    explanation of benefits, 271–272, 273
    signature on file, 271
  funding, 261, 262
  health benefits plans, 261–265
    CHAMPVA, 265
    dependents, 262, 269
    eligibility, 261–262
    government-sponsored health benefits, 263–265
    group health benefits, 261–262
    group member, 261
    health care savings accounts (HSAs), 262–263
    individual health benefits, 263
    insured benefits, 261
    Medicaid, 264
    Medicare, 263–264
    patient identification card, 262, 262, 269
    premium, 262
    self-funded benefits, 261
    third-party administrator (TPA), 262
    TRICARE, 264
  managed care, 265–268
    assignment of benefits, 265, 269, 272
    capitation, 266
    defined, 265
    gatekeeper provisions, 268
    HMO (health maintenance organization), 266
    independent practice association (IPA), 266
    overview, 265
    PHO (physician hospital organization), 268
    PPO (preferred provider organization), 267, 267–268
  practice policies, 272
  Spanish terminology, 272
  workers compensation, 269
Health Insurance Portability and Accountability Act of 1996 (HIPAA), 263
  administrative simplification, 155
  covered entities, 155
  description, 8
  goals, 154, 1053
  HCPCS and, 294
  ICD-9-CM and, 278
  officer, 155
  patient right, 156
  privacy rule, 23, 27, 93, 95–96, 156, 183, 228, 357
  sample office scenarios, 1053–1054
  security, 182
  student training and, 1026
  titles, 154, 154t
Health Level Seven (HL7), 159

Health maintenance organization (HMO), 8, 266
Healthcare Common Procedure Coding System (HCPCS)
  description, 264
  level I codes (CPT), 293–304
  level II codes, 293–294
  level III codes, 293–294
Hearing aids, 639
Hearing-impaired patients
  assisting, 638
  communicating with, 58–59, 59
Hearing loss, 638–639
Heart
  anatomy, 677
  cardiac surgery, 680
  conduction system, 681
  sounds, abnormal, 689
Heart disorders
  angina, 678, 679
  artificial pacemakers, 681
  cardiac arrhythmia, 678–679
  carditis, 677–678
  congenital disease, 682, 683t
  congestive heart failure (CHF), 678
  myocardial infarction (MI), 677, 678, 679
  patient with potential, 121, 121
  symptoms, 676
  valvular disease, 682, 683t
Heart rate, target, 323
Heartburn, 706
Heat, 373, 374, 375t
Heat applications
  for orthopedic conditions, 613–614, 614t, 615, 621–623
  patient education, 615
Heat cramps, 560
Heat exhaustion, 560
Heat stroke, 560
Heel puncture, 914
Hegar uterine dilator, 430t
Height, measuring, 374, 388
Helicobacter pylori, 335, 707
Helminths, 970
Hematemesis, 707
Hematocrit, 933, 940–941
Hematology, 926–943
  ABO group, 978
  blood cell formation, 927, 929
  coagulation tests, 935
    partial thromboplastin time (PTT), 935
    prothrombin time (PT), 935
  complete blood count (CBC), 928, 930–934
  erythrocyte indices, 933–934
    mean cell hemoglobin (MCH), 934
    mean cell hemoglobin concentration (MCHC), 934
    mean cell volume (MCV), 934
  erythrocyte sedimentation rate (ESR), 934, 934–935
  hematocrit, 933
  hemoglobin, 932–933
  laboratory department, 861
  platelet count, 934
  procedures
    blood smear preparation, 936–937
    blood smear staining, 938
    erythrocyte sedimentation rate, 941–942
    hemoglobin determination, 939
    microhematocrit determination, 940–941

red blood cell count, 931–932, 932
red blood cell morphology, 932, 932, 933t
Rh type, 978, 979
white blood cell count, 930
white blood cell differential, 930–931
  basophils, 931
  eosinophils, 931
  lymphocytes, 931
  monocytes, 931
  neutrophils, 930–931
Hematomas, 553, 912, 914
Hematopoiesis, 927, 929
Hematuria, 742, 743–744, 951
Hemiplegia, 730t
Hemoccult, 711
Hemoconcentration, 899
Hemodialysis, 741
Hemoglobin, 932–933
Hemoglobin A1C, 799, 800t, 1010
Hemoglobinuria, 951
Hemolysis, 899
Hemoptysis, 665
Hemorrhoidectomy, 711
Hemorrhoids, 711
Hemostasis, 927
Hemostat, 432, 433
Hennig plaster spreader, 430t
Heparin, 861, 935
Hepatitis, 712–713, 712t
Hepatitis A virus (HAV), 712
Hepatitis B virus (HBV), 341, 346–348, 352–353, 418, 712
Hepatitis C virus (HCV), 712–713
Hepatitis D virus (HDV), 713
Hepatitis E virus (HEV), 713
Hepatomegaly, 712
Hepatotoxins, 712
Herbal supplements, 78, 79t, 837
Hereditary diseases, 360
Hernia
  abdominal, 710–711
  hiatal, 705, 705–706
  inguinal, 711, 747
  physical examination and, 416
  umbilical, 711
Herniated intervertebral disc, 609–610
Herniorrhaphy, 711
Heroin, 329
Herpes genitalis, 768
Herpes simplex, 579, 704, 768
Herpes zoster, 579, 579, 725
HFCA (Health Care Financing Administration), 8
HGH (human growth hormone), 798–799
Hiatal hernia, 705, 705–706
High-density lipoprotein (HDL), 315, 1011, 1011t
Hip
  fractures in the elderly, 606
  total hip replacement, 605, 606
Hippocrates, 5
Hippocratic Oath, 5
Hirschman anoscope, 431t
Hirsutism, 765
Histamine H2 antagonists, 483t
Histobrush, 410, 410
Histologist, 863
Histology department, 862
Histoplasmosis, 968, 969
History
  cardiovascular examination, 688
  CPT-4 E/M codes, 298, 299t
  pediatric, 817
  sample report, 1069, 1074

History of medicine
ancient, 4–5
modern, 5–6
prevention of disease transmission, 6
recent, 7
women in medicine, 6–7
HIV (human immunodeficiency virus), 346–348, 767
Hives, 581–582
HL7 (Health Level Seven), 159
HMO (health management organization), 8, 266
Holter monitor, 692, 693, 698–699
Home oxygen therapy, 663
Homeopathic medications, 362
HON (Health on the Net) seal, 184
Honesty, 39
Hordeolum, 632
Hormonal replacement therapy (HRT), 781
Hormones, 483t, 793, 795t (see also specific hormones)
Hospice, 63
Hospital laboratory, 860
Host
reservoir, 336
susceptible, 337
Hours
flexible, 116
open, 116–117
Household system of measurement, 497–498, 498t
HPV (human papilloma virus), 767
HSAs (Health Care Savings Accounts), 262–263
Human chorionic gonadotropin (HCG), 771
Human genome, sequencing of, 7
Human growth hormone (HGH), 798–799
Human immunodeficiency virus (HIV), 346–348, 767
Human papilloma virus (HPV), 767
Human resources policy, 205, 206
Hunter, John, 6
Hydrocele, 746
Hydrocephalus, 728
Hydrochloric acid (HCl), 707
Hydrogen peroxide, as disinfectant, 341t
Hydronephrosis, 742
Hyerkalemia, 1004
Hygiene, personal, 93
Hyperadrenocorticalism, 798, 798
Hypercalcemia, 1005
Hyperchloremia, 1004
Hyperchromasia, 933t
Hyperemesis gravidarum, 778
Hyperglycemia, 794
Hypermagnesemia, 1005
Hypernatremia, 1004
Hyperopia, 633, 634
Hyperphosphatemia, 1005
Hyperpigmentation, 798, 798
Hyperpituitarism, 798–799
Hyperplasia of the adrenal cortex, 798
Hyperpnea, 382
Hyperpyrexia, 374
Hypersensitivity, 489t
Hypertension, 383, 383t, 685, 778
Hyperthermia, 560
Hyperthyroidism, 793–794, 796, 796
Hyperventilation, 382
Hypnosis, 77
Hypnotics, 484t
Hypoadrenocorticalism, 798, 798
Hypocalcemia, 1005
Hypochloremia, 1004

Hypochromasia, 932, 933t
Hypoglycemia, 797, 1009
Hypokalemia, 1004
Hypomagnesemia, 1005
Hyponatremia, 1004
Hypophosphatemia, 1005
Hypopituitarism, 799
Hypopnea, 382
Hypothalamus, 374
Hypothermia, 560–561
Hypothyroidism, 30, 794
Hypovolemic shock, 553
Hysterectomy, 761, 764
Hysterosalpingography, 771

ICD-9-CM
code book
appendices, 282t
updating, 279
Volume 1: Tabular List of Diseases, 279–280, 280, 281
Volume 2: Alphabetic List of Diseases, 280, 282–283
Volume 3: Tabular and Alphabetic Index of Procedures, 283
HIPAA mandate, 278
inpatient coding, 278–279, 283
locating appropriate code, 283–289, 290
CMS guidelines, 284
conventions, 283, 285
documentation requirements, 289
fourth and fifth digit codes, 283–284, 286
late effects, 288, 288
main term, 283
multiple codes, 284–285, 287
primary codes, 284
suspected conditions, 289
maintenance of classification system, 278
outpatient coding, 278
overview, 277
privacy issues, 278
supplementary classifications
E-codes, 279–280
V-codes, 279, 283
tenth revision, 289
Ictotest, 952, 953
Idiosyncratic reaction, 489t
Ileostomy, 709, 709
IM injections (see Intramuscular (IM) injections)
Immigration Reform and Control Act of 1986, 38
Immune system, effects of aging on, 844t
Immunization
hepatitis B, 341, 347–348
OSHA requirements, 344
recommendations for adults, 417–418
vaccine information statement (VIS), 807, 814
during well-child visits, 807
Immunization schedule
aged 0-6 years, 808
aged 7-18 years, 809
catch-up for aged 4 months-18 years, 810
Immunohematology department, 862
Immunologic agents, 483t
Immunology
antibodies, 975–976
antigens, 975
immunoassay
reagent and kit storage and handling, 976

tips for performing, 976
troubleshooting tips, 976
immunohematology
ABO group, 978
Rh type, 978, 979
testing principles, 976
tests
group A streptococcus, 977, 977, 999–1000
infectious mononucleosis, 977, 996
pregnancy, 977, 977, 997–998
Immunology department, 862
Impaled object, 555, 555
Impetigo, 576–577, 823, 823
Implementation, in patient education process, 69–70
Implied consent, 26
Implied contracts, 24
Impotence, 747–748
Inactive records, 171
Incident reports
description, 209, 890
guidelines for completing, 210
information in, 210, 890
medication error, documenting, 211
sample, 210
trending, 210–211
when to complete, 209–210
Income tax return, 244
Incompetence, 30
Incubator, 869, 971
Independent practice association (IPA), 266
Indexing rules for alphabetic filing, 169
Indications, 489t
Indicators, sterilization, 428, 428–429
Induration, 505
Infant heel puncture, 914
Infarction, 556
Infection, 335
Infection control
levels
disinfection, 339–340, 341t
sanitation, 339
sterilization, 339
medical asepsis, 338–339
policy manual, 206
Infection cycle, 336, 336–337
Infectious disease
reporting of, 28–29
waiting room environment and, 100–101
biohazard waste, 100
communicable disease exposure, 101
receptionist role in control, 100
Infectious disease prevention, 327–328
Infectious mononucleosis, 977, 996
Infertility, female, 766
Infiltration, 510
Inflammatory reactions, skin, 581, 581–582, 582
Influenza vaccine, 418
Informed consent, 26–27, 450, 451
Ingenix (publisher), 279
Inguinal hernia, 711, 747
Inguinal lymph nodes, 416
Inhalation, of medication, 508
Inhaler, 508, 662, 824
Injections
administering to children, 821, 822
angles of insertion, 505
equipment for, 503–505, 503–505
ampules, 503, 503
cartridges, 503, 503
diluent, 503
needles, 503–504, 504, 505

Injections *(con't)*
  syringes, 503–505, *504*
  vials, 503, *503*
  preparing, 514–516
  sterility, maintaining, 503
  types
    intradermal, 505, *505, 506,* 517–518
    intramuscular, *505–510, 506,* 521–524
    subcutaneous, *505, 506,* 519–520
Inoculating a culture, 974, 994–996
Inpatient, 278–279
INR (international normalized ratio), 935
Inspection, in physical examination, 411
Inspiration, 381–382 *(see also* Respiration)
Installment plan, 226
Instruments and supplies, 406–411,
    407–411
  anoscope, 410–411, *411*
  audioscope, 408
  calibration and maintenance, 882–884,
    883, 884, 885, 893
  examination light, *408,* 408–409
  gooseneck lamp, 408, *408*
  head light or mirror, 409, *409*
  histobrush, 410, *410*
  history record, *884*
  laryngeal mirror, 409
  laryngoscope, 409–410, *410*
  lubricant, 410
  nasal speculum, 407, *407*
  ophthalmoscope, 408, *408*
  otoscope, 407–408, *408*
  penlight or flashlight, 409, *409*
  percussion hammer, 407, *407*
  proctoscope, 411
  sigmoidoscope, 411, *411*
  for specialty examinations, 409–411,
    409–411
  stethoscope, 409, *409*
  tuning fork, 407, *407*
  vaginal speculum, 410, *410*
  wrapping for sterilization in an auto-
    clave, 440–441
Insufflator, 717
Insulin, 483t, 794–797, 795t, 1008
Insulin-dependent diabetes mellitus, 794
Insulin syringe, *504,* 504–505, 797
Insurance *(see also* Health Insurance)
  explanation of benefits (EOB), 271–272,
    273
  liability, 209
  malpractice, 36, 209, 1029
  pre-existing condition, 269
  software for claim submission and pa-
    tient eligibility, 190
  websites, 186
Insurance card, 224
Insurance company
  explanation of benefits (EOB), 224,
    239
  payment by, 224
  posting to cash-paid-out section of
    daysheet, 238
Insured benefits, defined, 262
Integumentary system, effects of aging on,
    842t
Intellectualization (defense mechanism),
    81t
Intentional torts, 33
Interactions, drug, 488
Intercaps, 136
Interest, bank account, 239
Intermittent fever, 375, 376t
Internal Revenue Service (IRS), 244

International Classification of Disease,
    Ninth Revision, Clinical
    Modification (ICD-9-CM) *(see*
    ICD-9-CM)
International law, 23
International normalized ratio (INR), 935
Internet
  child safety, 182
  connecting to, 181
  downloading information, 182
  e-mail, 183–184
  medical applications, 184–187
    calculators, health-related, 186
    HON (Health on the Net) seal, 184
    insurance-related sites, 186
    literary searches, 186
    professional medical sites, 185
    translation sites, 185–186
  patient teaching issues
    financial assistance for medications,
      187
    injury prevention, 187
    medical record forms, 187
    medical records, storing online, 187
    medication purchase, 186–187
  safe websites, 184–185
  search engines, 185, 194
  security, 182
  surfing, 184
  working offline, 183
Internet service provider (ISP), 181
Interpreter, 26, 27
Intertrigo, 583
Intervertebral disc herniation, 609–610
Interview, employment
  follow-up, 1040
  foreign language, knowledge of, 1038
  importance of, 1037
  job skills, employer's interest in, 1037
  portfolio for, 1038
  preparing for, 1037–1038, *1038*
  questions, crucial, 1038–1040,
    1039t–1040t
  thank you letter, 1040, *1040*
Interview, patient
  components of initial patient, 53t
  techniques, 53–54
    asking for examples or clarification,
      54
    open-ended questions, 54
    paraphrasing or restatement, 54
    reflecting, 54
    silences, allowing, 54
    summarizing, 54
Interviewing employees, 200
Intestinal disorders
  appendicitis, 711
  cancer, 711, *711*
  constipation, 711–712
  Crohn's disease, 709
  diarrhea, 712
  diverticulosis, 710
  duodenal ulcers, 708
  functional disorders, 711–712
  gas, 712
  gastroenteritis, 708
  hemorrhoids, 711
  hernias, 710–711
  irritable bowel syndrome, 709–710
  malabsorption syndromes, 708
  polyps, 710
  ulcerative colitis, 709
Intracellular fluid, 1004
Intradermal injections, 505, *505, 506,*

517–518
Intramuscular (IM) injections
  administering to children, 821, *822*
  administration procedure, 521–523
  angle of insertion, *505, 506*
  sites, 506, *506–508*
    deltoid muscle, 506, *506*
    dorsogluteal, *507*
    rectus femoris, *508*
    vastus lateralis, *508*
    ventrogluteal, *507*
  Z-track method, 506, *509,* 523–524
Intranet, 187
Intraocular pressure, 633
Intravenous pyelogram (IVP), 742, 749
Intravenous (IV) therapy
  description, 508–509
  equipment, 509–510, *511*
  fluids, 509–510, *511*
  site preparation, 526–529
  troubleshooting problems, 510–511
Invasion of privacy, 33
Inventory
  of controlled substances, 485, *486*
  of medications, 485–486
  office manager's role in management,
    208
Invoices, paying
  computer payment, 247
  manual payment, 246
  pegboard payment, 246
Iodinated contrast medium, 537
Iodine, as disinfectant, 341t
Iodophors, as disinfectant, 341t
Ions, 1003
Iontophoresis, 607
IPA (independent practice association),
    266
Irate patients, telephone calls from, 105
Iron deficiency, 932, *932,* 934
Irrigation
  ear, 641, 650–652
  eye, 649–650
Irritable bowel syndrome, 709
Irritant dermatitis, 888
IRS (Internal Revenue Service), 244
Ischemia, 556
Ishihara color plate, 635–636, *636,*
    646–647
Isopropyl alcohol, 898
ISP (Internet service provider), 181
IV catheter, 509–511
IV therapy *(see* Intravenous (IV) therapy)
Ives rectal speculum, 431t
IVP (intravenous pyelogram), 742
Iyengar yoga, 78

Jaundice, 712, 713, *713*
Jaw thrust method for opening airway, 549,
    550
JCAHO *(see* Joint Commission on
    Accreditation of Healthcare
    Organizations)
Jehovah's Witness, 27
Jenner, Edward, 6
Jewelry, 93
Job description, 199, 200, *201*
Jobs *(see* Employment)
Jock itch, 580
Joint
  arthritis, 607
  dislocation, 600
  prosthetic joint replacement, 605,
    606

Joint Commission on Accreditation of Healthcare Organizations (JCAHO), 136–137, 166
  accreditation process, 212–213
  COLA and, 875
  description, 38, 211–212
  goals, 212–213
  sample standard, 213
  sentinel event policy, 213
  type of facilities accredited, 212
Jones cross-action towel clamp, *435*
Journal, externship, 1026, 1029
Jury, 32, 34

Kaposi's sarcoma, 767
Kava, 79t
Keep-vein-open (KVO) rate, 510
Kegel exercises, 777, 844t
Keith needles, 452
Kelly clamp, 432, *433*
Keloids, 582
Keratoses, 842t
Ketoacidosis, 797
Ketones, 797, 950–951, *952*
Key components, E/M codes, 296, 298
Keyboard, 180
Keyes cutaneous punch, 432t
Kinesics, 51
Kit package inserts, 863–864
Knee
  arthroscopy of, 612, *612*
  chondromalacia patellae, 612–613
Knee-chest position, *413*, 414t
Knee replacement, 605, *606*
Knowledge, requirement for patient education, 72–73
Korotkoff sounds, 383
Kubler-Ross, Dr. Elisabeth, 62
KVO (keep-vein-open) rate, 510
Kyphosis, 608, *610*, 842t

Labor, 772, 776, 777
Laboratory
  code of ethics, 877
  departments
    anatomic and surgical pathology, 862
    clinical chemistry, 862
    coagulation, 861–862
    cytogenetics, 862
    cytology, 862
    hematology, 861
    histology, 862
    immunohematology, 862
    immunology, 862
    microbiology, 862
    toxicology, 862
    urinalysis, 862
  equipment
    cell counter, 864
    centrifuge, 868–869
    chemistry analyzer, 867–868
    incubator, 869
    instrument calibration and maintenance, 882–884, *883, 884, 885,* 893
    microscope, 867, *867, 868,* 869–871
    refrigerator and freezer, 869
  medical assistant's role in, 858–859
  personnel, 863
  quality assurance
    flow sheets, 878–879, *879*
    instrument calibration and maintenance, 882–884, 883f, *884, 885,* 893

laboratory procedure manual, 876–877
  patient test management, 876
  proficiency testing, 881
  quality control, 879–881, *880, 881, 882,* 892
  reagent management, 881–882
  test results, screening and follow-up, 877–878, 891
  testing
    kit package inserts, 863–864
    request forms, 864, *865*
  types
    hospital laboratory, 860
    physician office laboratory, 860
    reference laboratory, 859–860
Laboratory assistant, 863
Laboratory duties, of medical assistant, 11
Laboratory manager, 863
Laboratory procedure manual, 876–877
Laboratory result form, *861*
Laboratory results, in medical record, 159
Laboratory safety
  biological hazards, 887
  chemical hazards, 884–885, *886,* 887–888
  Chemical Hygiene Plan (CHP), 888
  guidelines, 889–890
  incident reports, 890
  OSHA, 887–888, 890
  physical hazards, 884
Laboratory standards, CLIA, 876
Laboratory tests
  common uses, 858
  CPT-4 coding, 302–303
  kit package inserts, 863–864
  normal values and clinical significance, tables of
    blood chemistry tests, 1082t–1084t
    complete blood count (CBC), 1081t–1082t
    urinalysis, 1080t–1081t
  request forms, 864, *865*
  telephone report
    from laboratory, 103–104
    to patients, 104
Laceration, 554, *554*
Lahey retractor, *436*
Lancets, *908*
Language barriers, 58
Laparoscopy, 763, *763,* 768
Laryngeal cancer, 664
Laryngeal mirror, 409, 416
Laryngectomy, 664
Laryngitis, 643
Laryngoscope, 409–410, *410*
Laryngotracheobronchitis, 824
Laser angioplasty, 540
Laser surgery, 455, 634
LASIK, 634
Last menstrual period, 761, 773
Late effects, 288, *288*
Late patients, adapting schedule for, 121–122
Lateral epicondylitis, 611
Latex allergy, 344
Latex reactions, 888
Law
  branches, 22–23
  civil, 22, 23
  common, 22
  public, 23
  sources of, 22
Law of agency, 35–36

Lawsuits, 22
LDL (*see* Low-density lipoprotein)
Leads, ECG, 689, 691, 691t
Learning (*see also* Patient education)
  conditions needed for patient education, 71–73
  hindering factors, 73–75
  patient motivation, 71
Learning goal, 81, 82t
Learning objectives, 69, 81, 82t
Ledger card, 234, *234, 235, 235*
Leeuwenhoek, Anton von, 6
Legal issues
  advanced directives, 839
  appeal, 34
  assessing circulation after a cast application, 605
  blood-borne pathogen standard training, 341
  branches of law, 22–23
  certification, 31
  child abuse, 822
  clinical trials, 748
  Controlled Substances Act, 31
  correcting financial documents, 243
  debt collection, 225
  defenses in liability suits
    assumption of risk, 34
    comparative, 35
    contributory negligence, 35
    medical records, 34
    res judicata, 34
    statute of limitations, 34
  diagnosing, 643
  diagnostic coding, 305
  drug screening, 947–948
  elder abuse, 840
  employment and safety laws
    Age Discrimination in Employment, 38
    Americans with Disabilities Act (ADA), 36–37, 38
    Civil Rights Act, 36, 38
    discrimination, 36
    Fair Labor Standards Act, 38
    Family and Medical Leave Act, 38
    Immigration Reform and control Act, 38
    Occupational Safety and Health Act, 37
    sexual harassment, 36
  of extending credit, 224
  fetal protection, 776
  Good Samaritan acts, 31
  ICD-9-CM coding, 282
  informed consent, 450
  interview questions, 200
  laboratory test confidentiality, 860
  licensure, 30–31
  litigation avoidance, 36
  litigation process, 34
  malpractice, 23, 1029
  medical practice acts, 30
  medical records, 157
  medication errors, 496
  messages on answering machines, 228
  minor patients, 814
  missed appointments, documenting, 122
  monitoring regulations, 46
  online forms, 187
  orders for laboratory tests, 864
  passwords, 183
  pharmacology
    abuse of controlled substances, 485

Legal issues *(con't)*
    Drug Enforcement Agency (DEA), 481, 484–485
    Food and Drug Administration (FDA), 481
    inventory, storage, dispensation, and disposal of medications, 485–486, *486*
    phlebotomy liability, 906
    physical examination, 414
    physician-patient relationship
        consent, 25–27, *26*
        contracts, 24–25, *25*
        legally required disclosures, 28–30
        medical record release, 27–28
        rights and responsibilities, 23–24
    privacy, 278, 361
    promises of care, 663
    protected health information, 456
    registration, 30, 31
    respondeat superior (law of agency), 35–36, 1029
    Right to Know law, 437
    risk management, 723
    signature on file, 271
    sources of law, 22
    Spanish terminology, 45
    subpoena duces tecum, 157
    tort law, 32–33
        intentional torts, 33
        unintentional torts, 32–33
    trial, 34
    worker's compensation, 168
Legal system
    branches of law, 22–23
    sources of law, 22
Legal tips
    litigation avoidance, 36
    prescription pad safety tips, 31
Legally required disclosures
    abuse, neglect, or maltreatment, 29–30
    cancer, 30
    defined, 28
    examples of, 157
    infectious/communicable diseases, 28–29
    medical examiner's reports, 28
    patient education, 29
    state requirements, 30
    vaccine side effects, 29
    violent injuries, 30
    vital statistics, 28
Legs
    assessing in emergency care, 552
    physical examination, 417
Leiomyomas, 764–765
Lentigines, 842t
Letter
    collection, 227, *228*, 230
    components of, 138, *139*, 140
        body, 140
        closing, 140
        copy, 140
        date, 138
        enclosure, 140
        identification, 140
        inside address, 138
        letterhead, 138
        salutation, 138, 140
        sample letter, *139*
        signature and typed name, 140
        spacing, 140
        subject line, 138
    composition, 141–142, 148–149
    editing, 142

formats, 140, *140, 141*
how to start writing, 141
organization, 141
preparation, 141
types of, 143
Letterhead, 138
Leukocyte esterase, 951
Leukocytes, in urine, 951
Leukoderma, 584
Leukoplakia, 705
Levodopa (L-dopa), 846
Liabilities, record-keeping, 244
Liability insurance, 209
Libel, 33
Lice, 581
Licensed Practice Nurse (LPN), 12
Licensure, 30–31
Licorice, 79t
Lid retractor, 432t
Lidocaine, 451
Lifestyle changes, 76
Light
    examination, *408*, 408–409
    head, 409, *409*
Lightening, 776
Limiting charge, 223
Linens, handling soiled, 345
Lipase, 1008
Lipids
    in diet, 313
    tests, *1010*, 1010–1011, *1011*, 1011t
        cholesterol, 1010, 1011t, 1012t, 1016
        high-density lipoprotein (HDL), 1011, 1011t
        low-density lipoprotein (LDL), 1011, 1011t
        patient education, 1011
        triglycerides, 1011, 1011t, 1012t
Lipoproteins
    high-density lipoprotein (HDL), 314, 1011, 1011t
    low-density lipoprotein (LDL), 315, 1011, 1011t
Liquid dietary supplements, 849
Listening
    active, 52–53
    on telephone, 102
Lister, Joseph, 6
Lister bandage scissors, *434*
Literary searches, 186
Lithotomy position, 413, *413*, 414t, 417
Lithotripsy, 742
Litigation, 22, 34, 36
Liver disorders
    cancer, 713
    cirrhosis/fibrosis, 713
    diagnostic tests for, 712
    hepatitis, 712–713, 712t
Liver function tests
    alanine aminotransferase (ALT), 1007
    alkaline phosphatase (ALP), 1006–1007
    aspartate aminotransferase (AST), 1007
    bilirubin, 1006
Local anesthetics, 451–452, *453*
Lochia, 777
Locum tenens, 25
Lofstrand crutches, 615, *615*
Long, Crawford Williamson, 6
Long-term care, 838–839
Long-term care facilities, 839
Lordosis, 608, *610*
Lou Gehrig's disease, 726–727
Lovenox, 686
Low-density lipoprotein (LDL), 314, 1011,

1011t
Lozenge (oral medication form), 502t
LPN (Licensed Practice Nurse), 12
LSD (lysergic acid diethylamide), 329
Lubricant, 410
Lucae bayonet forceps, 431t
Luer adapter, 906
Lumbar puncture, 733–734, *734, 735–737*
Lung cancer, 664–665
Luteinizing hormone, 795t
Luxation, 600
Lyme disease, 966–967, *967*
Lymphocytes, *928, 931*
Lymphogranuloma venereum, 767, 967
Lysergic acid diethylamide (LSD), 329
Lysozyme, 335

Macrocytosis, 933t, 934
Macule, 576, *578*
Magnetic resonance imaging (MRI), 7, 539, *540*
Mail
    addressing envelopes, 145–146, *146*
    electronic (*see* electronic mail)
    incoming, 147
    opening and sorting, 147–148, 150
    postage, 146
    United States Postal Service (USPS) options, 146–147, *147*
Main terms, ICD-9-CM, 282, 283
Maintenance, office, 208
Malabsorption syndromes, 708
Male reproductive disorders
    benign prostatic hyperplasia, 745–746
    cryptorchidism, 746, 746–747
    epididymitis, 747
    hydrocele, 746
    impotence, 747–748
    infections, 747
    inguinal hernia, 747
    orchitis, 747
    prostate cancer, 746
    prostatitis, 747
    testicular cancer, 746
Male reproductive system, effects of aging on, 845t
Malfeasance, 32
Malignant hypertension, 685
Malignant melanoma, 585, *585*, 586
Malocclusion, 703–704
Malpractice, 23, 32
Malpractice insurance, 36, 209
Maltreatment, reporting of, 29–30
Mammography, 417, 537, 539, *539*
Managed care
    assignment of benefits, 265, 269, 272
    capitation, 266
    defined, 8, 265
    elements
        approval referrals, 265
        assignment of benefits, 265
        network, 265
        precertification of hospital admissions, 265
    gatekeeper provisions, 268
    HMO (health maintenance organization), 266
    independent practice association (IPA), 266
    overview, 265
    PHO (physician hospital organization), 268
    PPO (preferred provider organization), *267*, 267–268

Mandatory Guidelines for Federal Workplace Testing Programs, 947
Mandl, Dr. M., 13–14
Manipulation, 411
Mantoux test, 505
Manual accounting (*see* Accounting, manual)
March of Dimes, 314
Marie-Strumpell disease, 607
Marijuana, 328
Maslow, Abraham, 71
Maslow's hierarchy of needs, *71,* 71–72
Material safety data sheets (MSDS), 37, 344, 437, 884, 888
Matrix, 114
MCH (mean cell hemoglobin), 934
MCHC (mean cell hemoglobin concentration), 934
MCV (mean cell volume), 933–934
Meales, mumps, rubella (MMR) vaccination, 418
Mean cell hemoglobin (MCH), 934
Mean cell hemoglobin concentration (MCHC), 934
Mean cell volume (MCV), 933–934
Measurement systems
    apothecary, 497–498, 498t
    converting between systems
        apothecary or household to metric, 497–498
        metric to metric, 498
    dosage calculation
        for adults, 498–499
        BSA (body surface area) method, 500
        Clark's rule, 500
        formula method, 499
        Fried's rule, 501
        for pediatrics, *500,* 500–501
        ratio and proportion method, 498–499
        Young's rule, 500
    household, 497–498, 498t
    metric, 497–498, 498t
    table of equivalents, 498t
Meat and beans, food group guidelines, 319–320
Media, culture, 970–971, *971*
Median cubital vein, 910–911
Medic alert bracelet, 682, 798
Medicaid
    carrier, 264
    electronic claims submission, 271
    government audits, 160
    online eligibility verification, 269
    overview, 264
Medical asepsis
    defined, 334, 338
    guidelines for maintaining, 339
    handwashing, 338–339, 349–350
    surgical asepsis compared, 427t
Medical assistant
    characteristics of professional, 11–12
    clothing and appearance, 11
    description of profession, 8–9
    duties
        administrative, 9
        clinical, 9
        laboratory, 11
    legal defense, 35–36
    representing yourself appropriately, 13
    role in ethics, 39, 40
Medical Assistants' Creed, 40
Medical assisting
    education, 14–15

history of, 13–14
    program accreditation, 14–15
Medical decision making, CPT-4 coding, 298–299
Medical emergencies, telephone calls
    incoming, 105
    outgoing, 106–107
Medical ethics, 38–40 (*see also* Ethics)
Medical examiner's reports, 28
Medical history
    collection methods, 357
    defined, 357
    elements of
        demographic information, 357, 360
        family history, 360
        past history, 360
        review of systems, 360
        social history, 360
    patient interview, 360–362, *362*
        barriers to communication, 361
        introducing yourself, 361
        preparation, 360–361
        procedure, 365
    privacy, 361
    sample form, *358–359*
Medical history forms, 164
Medical insurance card, 224
Medical laboratory technician, 863
Medical management software, 114–115
Medical necessity, 277
Medical office, 8
Medical Office Management Association, 209
Medical office manager
    communication, 198–199
        with patients, 198–199
        with staff, 199, *199*
    education
        of managers, 209
        of patients, 209
        of staff, 208
    financial issues
        budgets, 207
        payroll, 208
    office maintenance, 208
    policy and procedures manuals, 203–206
        administrative procedures, 206
        clinical procedures, 205–206
        creating, 217
        human resources policy, 205, *206*
        infection control, 206
        mission statement, 204–205, *205*
        organizational structure, 205
        quality improvement, 205
        tips for writing, 205
    promotional material development, 206–207, *207*
    responsibilities, 198–209
    staffing issues, 200–203, *201 203, 204*
    traits of successful, 198
Medical practice acts, 30
Medical records
    classification, 171
        active records, 171
        closed, 171
        inactive records, 171
    contents of, 158–159
    for defense, 34, 71
    documentation forms
        flow sheets, 164, *164, 165*
        medical history forms, 164
        progress notes, 164
    documenting emergency care, 549
    electronic health records, 159–162

billing and coding, 160–161
        choosing a vendor, 159
        features, 160
        medical assistant's role, 161
        power failure and, 161
        security, 161–162
        standards, 159
        transition to, 159–160
    entries, 164–167
        abbreviations, 166
        additions to records, 167
        charting communications with patients, 167
        charting example, *166*
        documentation guidelines, 166–167
        error correction, 167
    falsifying, 22
    filing
        alphabetic, 169, 170
        indexing rules, 169
        numeric, 169–170
        procedures, 168, 175
        subject, 170
    Health Insurance Portability and Accountability Act (HIPAA)
        administrative simplification, 155
        covered entities, 155
        goals, 154
        officer, 155
        patient right, 156
        privacy rule, 156
        titles, 154, 154t
    as legal document, 27, 166
    of medication administration, 496
    online forms, 187
    organization
        groupings, 162
        narrative format, 162
        POMR, 163, *163*
        SOAP, *162,* 162–163
    overview, 153
    patient storage online, 187
    preparation, 168, 173–174
    problem list, 69
    releasing, 27–28, 155–158
        authorization, 157, 158
        charging for copying, 156
        legally required disclosures, 157
        originals, 155, 157
        to patients, 156
        requests, 155–156
    required disclosures, 28–30
    retention of, 172
    Spanish terminology, 172
    statute of limitations, 156
    storing, 158
        backup copy, 171
        classification of records and, 171
        electronic data storage, 171
        filing procedures, 168, 175
        length of storage, 172
        microfilm/microfiche, 171–172
        preparation of records, 168, 173–174
        standard records, 171
    workers' compensation, 167
Medical reports
    guidelines for document preparation, 133–138
    hospital documents, 133t
    medical office documents, 133t
    sample reports
        consultation, 1075
        discharge summary, 1072

Medical reports *(con't)*
    history and physical examination, 1069, 1074
    operative report, 1070, 1073
    pathology report, 1071
    progress notes, 1076
    X-ray report, 1077
Medical specialties, 8, 9t, 10t
Medical technologist, 863
Medicare
    crossover claim, 263
    deductible, 263
    electronic claims submission, 271
    fee schedule, 223, *223*
    fraud, 305
    government audits, 160
    medically necessary procedures, 277
    overview, 263–264
    Part A, 263
    Part B, 263
    reimbursement
        diagnostic related groups (DRGs) and, 304
        resource-based relative value scale (RBRVS), 304
    secondary benefits, 263
    website, 186, 187
Medication administration, in medical record, 159
Medication management, electronic health record and, 160
Medication therapy teaching tool, 76–77, 77
Medications *(see also* Pharmacology)
    administration basics, 494–501
        abbreviations, 494, 495t
        calculating adult dosages, 498–499
        calculating pediatric dosages, *500,* 500–501
        errors, 496
        measurement systems, 497–498, 498t
        safety guidelines, 494, 496
        seven rights, 496
    administration routes, 501–508
        buccal, 502
        inhalation, 508
        injections, 503–507, *503–510,* 514–524
        oral, 501, *501,* 502t, 512–513
        parenteral, 502–507
        rectal, 507, *511*
        sublingual, 501–502
        transdermal, 508, 524–525
        vaginal, 507–508, *511*
    buying online, 186–187
    discussing with elderly patients, 836, *836*
    drug interactions, 488
    elderly and, 840–841
    errors, 211, 496
    financial assistance for, 187
    intravenous therapy, 508–511, 526–529
    inventory, storage, dispensation, and disposal of, 485–486
    medical software and, 188–189
    names, 481
    patient education, 76–77, 77
    reconstituting dry, 503
    side effects and allergies, 488–489
Medicine section, CPT-4 coding, 303
Medicode (publisher), 279
Meeting Maker, 191
Melanin, in urine, 586
Melanoma, 584, 585
Melena, 552, 707
Memorandum, 143, *143*

Memory loss, 835
Menarche, 760
Ménière's disease, 639
Meningitis, 724, 823
Meningocele, 728, 729
Menopause, 779, 781
Menorrhagia, 761, 771
Menses, 760
Menstrual cycle, 760–761, *762*
Mental health
    illnesses
        communication with patients, 60
        effect on learning, 73
    reinforcing in the elderly, 837
Mental outlook, positive, 327
Mepivacaine, 451
Meridians, 77
Mescaline, 329
Message retrieval
    answering service, 96
    electronic mail, 96
    facsimile machines, 96
    privacy and, 95–96
    voice mail systems, 96
Messages *(see also* Communication)
    on answering machines, 228
    e-mail, composing, 183–184
    handling, 50
    taking telephone, 106
Metabolism, 315, 703
Metastasis, 584
Metazoa, 970
Metric measurements, 1078
Metric system, 497–498, 498t
Metrorrhagia, 761
MI (myocardial infarction), 677, 678, 679
Microbiology
    aerobes, 966
    anaerobes, 966
    categories of life forms
        bacteria, 966–967, 966t, *967, 968*
        fungi, 968, *968, 969*
        metazoa, 970
        protozoa, 969
        viruses, 968–969
    inoculation, 974, 994–996
    microscopic examinations, 973–974
        Gram stain, 974, *975,* 992–993
        smear preparation, 990–991
        wet mount, 974
    normal flora, 966
    nosocomial infections, 966
    pathogens, 966
    sensitivity testing, 974–975, *975*
    specimen collection and handling
        blood, 973t, 987–988
        culture media, 970–971, *971*
        fecal occult blood, 972–973, 989–990
        genital specimens, 988–989
        guidelines, 970
        nasopharyngeal specimens, 982
        sputum specimens, 984–985
        stool specimens, 973, 973t, 985–986
        throat specimens, 980–981
        transporting specimens, 971–972, *972*
        types of specimens, 970
        urine, 973t
        wound specimens, 983–984
Microbiology department, 862
Microcollection containers, 907–908
Microcytosis, *932,* 933t, 934
Microfiche, 171–172

Microfilm, 171–172
Microhematocrit centrifuge, 869
Microhematocrit tubes, 907, *908*
Microorganisms
    aerobes, 336
    anaerobes, 336
    carriers and reservoirs of, 336
    defined, 334
    infection cycle, 336, 336–337
    nonspecific defenses against disease, 334
    normal flora, 335
    pathogens, 335–337
    transmission, modes of, 337
Microprocessor, 180
Microscope
    care of, 868–871
    components of, 867, *867*
    handling, 868
    provider-performed microscopy (PPM), 875
Migraine, 731
Military time, 138, *166*
Milk, food group guidelines, 319
Minerals, 314
Minor
    consent form, 27
    emancipated, 27, 814
    parental permission, 814
Minutes, 143–144
Mirror
    head, 409
    laryngeal, 409, 416
Miscarriage, 771, 778
Miscommunication, 55, 70
Misfeasance, 32
Misinterpretation, 70
Mission statement, 204–205, *205*
Misused words, common, 1067–1068
Mitral valve prolapse, 683t
Mitral valve stenosis, 682
MMR (meales, mumps, rubella) vaccination, 418
Modem, 181
Modifiers, CPT-4, 300, 303
Molds, 968
Mole, 584
Money market accounts, 239
Money orders, 240
Monitor, 180
Monocytes, *928, 931*
Mononucleosis, 977, 996
Monsel solution, 771
Monthly service fees, bank, 240
Morning sickness, 778
Moro reflex, 811t, 814
Morphine, 329
Morphology, of bactera, 966, *967, 968*
Moses, 5
Motivation, patient, 71
Motor vehicle deaths, 326–327
Mourning, 62
Mouse, 180–181
Mouth
    defenses against disease, 335
    physical examination, 416
Mouth disorders
    caries, 703–704
    gingivitis, 705
    oral cancers, 705
    stomatitis, 704–705
MRI (magnetic resonance imaging), 7, 539, *540*
MS (multiple sclerosis), 726
MSDS *(see* Material safety data sheets)

Mucolytics, 483t
Mucous plug, 771–772, 776
Mucus, in urine sediment, 954
Multidisciplinary, 12
Multipara, 773
Multiple sclerosis (MS), 726
Multisample needle, *900, 901, 901*
Multiskilled health professional, 4
Mummy restraint, 821
Murmurs, 689
Muscle strength, assessing in emergency care, 552
Muscular dystrophy, 607–608
Musculoskeletal injuries
    management of, 556
    splints, 556, *556*
Musculoskeletal system (*see also* Orthopedics)
    benefits of exercise, 848t
    bones, *600*
    diagnostic studies, 613, *613*
    disorders, 599–613
    effects of aging on, 842t
    overview, 599
    pain, 602
    physical exam, 613
    range of motion of joints, *601*
Mycobacterium tuberculosis, 350
Mycology, 968
Myelomeningocele, 728, *729*
Myocardial infarction (heart attack)
    symptoms, *557*
    treatment, *557*
Myocardial infarction (MI), 677, 678, 679
Myocarditis, 677
Myoglobin, 951, 953
Myopia, 633, *634*
Myringotomy, 640
Myths, about the elderly, 835, 836

Nails, 93
Narcotics, 329
Narrative, 162
Nasal polyps, 642
Nasal septum, 415
Nasal speculum, *407, 407,* 431t, 642, *642*
Nasopharyngeal specimen, collecting, 982
National Center for Complementary and Alternative Medicine (NCCAM), 77, 78
National Center for Health Statistics (NCHS), 278
National Childhood Vaccine Injury Act of 1986, 29
National Cholesterol Education Program (NCEP), 314
National Commission on Certification of PAs (NCCPA), 12
National Conference of Commissioners for Uniform State Laws, 43
National Council on Patient Information and Education (NCPIE), 77
National Fire Protection Association, 884
National Safe Kids foundation, 187
National Safety Council, CPR certification and training by, 547
NCCAM (National Center for Complementary and Alternative Medicine), 77, 78
NCCPA (National Commission on Certification of PAs), 12
NCEP (National Cholesterol Education Program), 314

NCHS (National Center for Health Statistics), 278
NCPIE (National Council on Patient Information and Education), 77
Nearsightedness, 633, *634*
Nebulized breathing treatment, 662, 670–672
Nebulizer, 508, 824
Neck
    assessing in emergency care, 552
    physical examination of, 415
Needle holder, 432
Needles
    bevel, 900
    choosing, 503–504
    gauge, 504, 900
    multisample, *900, 901, 901*
    parts, *504, 505*
    phlebotomy, 900
    positioning for venipuncture, 912, *913*
    stick from contaminated, 887
    surgical, 452–453, *453*
Needlestick injuries, 897, 898, 912
Needlestick Safety and Prevention Act, 460
Needs, Maslow's hierarchy of, *71,* 71–72
Negative stress, 79–80
Neglect
    of elderly, 839–840
    reporting of, 29–30
Negligence, 32, 35
Neisseria gonorrhoeae, 767
Nematodes, 970
Neonatologists, 806
Neoplasm, 585
Nephrostomy, 742
Nervous system
    benefits of exercise, 848t
    effects of aging on, 842t
Network, managed care, 265
Networking, 1033
Neural tube defects, 314, 728, 729
Neurogenic shock, 553
Neurologic emergencies, *557*
Neurologist, 723
Neurology, 722–738
    brain tumors, 730–731
    degenerative disorders
        amyotrophic lateral sclerosis (ALS), 726–727
        multiple sclerosis (MS), 726
        Parkinson's disease, 727
    developmental disorders
        cerebral palsy, 728
        hydrocephalus, 728
        neural tube defects, 728, 729
    diagnostic tests
        cranial nerve assessment, 731, 732t
        EEG, 733
        lumbar puncture, 733–734, *734,* 735–737
        physical examination, 731–732
        reflex testing, 731, *733,* 733t
        Romberg test, 731
    functional areas of cerebral cortex, *724*
    headaches, 731
    infectious disorders
        encephalitis, 724
        herpes zoster, 725
        meningitis, 724
        poliomyelitis, 725
        rabies, 726
        Reye's syndrome, 726
        tetanus, 725
    seizure disorders, 727–728

trauma, 729–730
    brain injuries, 729, 730
    paralysis, types of, 730t
    spinal cord injuries, 729–730, 730t
Neutrophils, *928,* 930–931
Nevus, 584
New patients, scheduling appointments for, 118, 126
Newspaper advertisements, answering, 1033
Nightingale, Florence, 6, 7
911 system, 548
Nitrite, in urine, 951
Nitroglycerin, 681–682
Nitroprusside test, 952
Nits, 581
NLEA (Nutritional Labeling and Education Act), 321
Nocturia, 745
Nomogram, 500, *500*
Non-insulin-dependent diabetes mellitus, 795–796
Noncompliance, 70
Nonfeasance, 32
Nonlanguage sounds, 51
Nonparticipating fee, 223
Nonstress test (NST), 779
Nonsufficient funds (NSF) check, 238, 240, 253
Nonverbal communication, 51–52
Norepinephrine, 795t
Normal flora, 335, 966
Normal values, 877
Nose
    disorders
        allergic rhinitis, 641
        epistaxis, 642
        nasal polyps, 642
        patient education concerning, 642
        sinusitis, 642
    physical examination, 415
    Spanish terminology, 644
    visual inspection, *642, 643*
Nosepiece, microscope, 867
Nosocomial infections, 966
Notebooks, communication, 199
Nothing by mouth (NPO), 538, 910
Notices, overdue, 227
NP (nurse practitioner), 12
NPO orders, 910
NSF (nonsufficient funds) check, 238, 240, 253
NST (nonstress test), 779
Nuclear imaging, of gastrointestinal system, 716
Nuclear medicine, 539–540
Nulligravida, 773
Nullipara, 773
Numbers, in written communications, 137–138
Numeric filing, 169–170
Nurse practitioners (NPs), 12
Nurses
    education levels, 12
    supervision by, 13
Nutrition
    cholesterol, 314–315
    Dietary Approaches to Stop Hypertension (DASH), 322, 322t
    digestion, 315
    fiber, 315
    healthy food preparation tips, 315
    metabolism, 315
    nutrients
        carbohydrates, 312–313

Nutrition (con't)
  fats, 313, 313t
  minerals, 314
  proteins, 313
  vitamins, 313–314
  Spanish terminology, 330
  therapeutic, 321
Nutritional guidelines
  food labels, 321, 321, 330–331
  MyPyramid
    for 2000-calorie diet, 317
    anatomy of pyramid, 316
    for children, 318
    fruits, 319
    grains, 316, 318
    meat and beans, 319–320
    milk, 319
    oils, 320
    overview, 315–316
    vegetables, 318–319
  patient education, 320
Nutritional Labeling and Education Act
    (NLEA), 321

Obesity
  in children, 826
  gastric bypass surgery for, 708
Obstetrics
  acronyms and abbreviations, 777
  cesarean section, 776–777
  contraception, 779, 780t
  defined, 760
  disorders
    abortion, 778
    abruptio placentae, 779
    eclampsia, 778
    ectopic pregnancy, 778
    hyperemesis gravidarum, 778
    placenta previa, 779
    preeclampsia, 778
  ethical issues
    abortion, 41
    artificial insemination, 42
    genetic testing, 41–42
  expected date of delivery (EDD), 773
  fetal development, 774
  instruments and equipment, 430t
  labor onset, 776
  menopause, 779, 781
  placenta previa
    eclampsia, 778
  postpartum care, 777
  pregnancy diagnosis, 771–772
  prenatal visits
    fetal heart tones (FHT), 775, 775, 776
    first, 772–773
    fundus height, 775, 775
    schedule, 775t
    subsequent, 773, 775
  signs and symptoms, 772t
  Spanish terminology, 781
  tests and procedures
    alpha-fetoprotein (AFP), 779
    amniocentesis, 779
    contraction stress test (CST), 779
    fetal ultrasound, 779
    nonstress test, 779
    pregnancy tests, 779
Obturator, 410–411, 411, 717
Occult blood, 417, 711, 972–973, 989–990
Occupational Exposure to Blood-borne
    Pathogens Standard, 887
Occupational Safety and Health Act (1970),
    37

Occupational Safety and Health
    Administration (OSHA)
  Blood-borne Pathogens standard, 887
  compliance, 890
  description, 37
  guidelines for the medical office, 37,
    340–348
    biohazardous material, 342, 344,
      345–346, 346, 347, 353–354
    blood-borne pathogen training, 341
    disposal of infectious waste,
      345–346, 347, 353–354
    environmental contamination, 345
    exposure control plan, 342
    exposure risk factor, 341
    hepatitis B, 346–348
    human immunodeficiency virus
      (HIV), 346–348
    OSHA 300 log, 342, 343
    personal protective equipment, 341,
      342, 344, 347
    standard precautions, 342
  Hazardous Communication (HazCom)
    standard, 887–888
  infection control guidelines, 337
  quality improvement (QI) programs, 211
  recommendations for injury prevention,
    97–98
  Right to Know law, 437
  surgical instrument handling, 434
OCR (optical character reader), 145–147
Office brochure, 223
Office management
  ethical issues in, 43, 45
  organizational chart, 197, 198
  overview, 197–198
  preparation by receptionist, 95
  quality improvement (QI) programs
    case review, 215, 215
    developing, 214–215, 218
    regulatory agencies, 211–214
    tracking incident reports, 210–211
  responsibilities of medical office man-
    ager, 198–209
    communication, 198–199
    education, 208–209
    financial, 207–208
    inventory management, 208
    office maintenance, 208
    policy and procedures manuals,
      203–206, 206, 217
    promotional material development,
      206–207, 207
    service contracts, 208
    staffing issues, 200–203
  risk management, 209–211
    incident reports, 209–211
    liability insurance, 209
  Spanish terminology, 216
Office of Management and Budget (OMB)
    Custody and Control Form
    (CCF), 948
Oils, food group guidelines, 320
Oligomenorrhea, 781
Oliguria, 741, 743
Online banking, 241
Onychomycosis, 580
Open-ended questions, asking, 54
Open wound, 554, 554
Operative report, 1070, 1073
Ophthalmic medications, 637
Ophthalmologist, 630
Ophthalmology, instruments and equipment,
    432t

Ophthalmoscope, 408, 408, 631, 634, 635
Opium, 4, 329
Optical character reader (OCR), 145–147
Optician, 633
Optometrist, 633
Oral cancers, 705
Oral communication, 51
Oral glucose tolerance test, 1009–1010,
    1010
Oral hygiene, 93
Oral hypoglycemics, 483t
Oral medications
  administering, 512–513
  administering to children, 821
Oral route of administration, 501, 501,
    502t, 512–513
Orchiopexy, 746
Orchitis, 747
Order of draw, 902, 905t
Ordering supplies, 245, 257
Organ transplantation
  ethical issues and, 42
  Uniform Anatomical Gift Act, 43
Organizational chart, 197, 198, 205
Orientation of patients, 97
Orthopedics, 598–628
  ambulatory assist devices, 614–617
    canes, 616, 616
    crutches, 615, 615–616, 623–626
    walker, 616, 616–617
  diagnostic studies, 613, 613
  disorders, common
    arthritis, 607
    bone tumors, 608
    bursitis, 606
    dislocation, 600
    fibromyalgia, 607
    fracture, 600–606, 603t–604t
    gout, 607
    muscular dystrophy, 607–608
    osteoporosis, 608
    sprains, 599–600
    strains, 600
    tendonitis, 607
  disorders, lower extremity, 612–613
    chondromalacia patellae, 612
    plantar fasciitis, 612–613
  disorders, spinal, 608–610
    curvature, abnormal, 608–609, 610
    herniated intervertebral disc,
      609–610
  disorders, upper extremity, 610–612
    adhesive capsulitis (frozen shoulder),
      611
    carpal tunnel syndrome, 611, 612
    Dupuytren contracture, 611,
      611–612
    lateral epicondylitis (tennis elbow),
      611
    rotator cuff injury, 611
  instruments and equipment, 430t
  physical examination, 613
  procedures
    arm sling application, 618–619
    cold pack application, 620–621
    crutch gaits, 624–626
    hot pack application, 621–623
    measuring for axillary crutches,
      623–624
  Spanish terminology, 617
  warm and cold applications, 613–614,
    614t, 620–623
Orthopnea, 382
Orthostatic hypotension, 382

Oscillating plaster saw, 430t
OSHA 300 Log, 342, *343*
Osteoarthritis, 607
Osteoporosis, 608, 842t
Other potentially infectious material (OPIM), 344
Otis-Dittel urethral sound, 431t
Otitis externa, *639*, 639–640
Otitis media, 52, 640, *640*, 814t, 824–825
Otolaryngologist, 630
Otology, instruments and equipment, 431t
Otosclerosis, 640
Otoscope, 407–408, 638, 641, *641*
Outlier, 304
Outpatient, 278
Outpatient medical facility, 8
Outpatient x-rays, 534
Ovalocytes, 933t
Ovarian cysts, 765
Over-the-counter medications, 362
Overdraft protection, 240
Overdue accounts, collecting, 227–228
Overpayment, 236
OVID, 186
Oxalate/fluoride tubes, 905t
Oxygen
    administration of, 562–563
    home therapy, 663
Oxytocin, 795t

PA (physician assistant), 12
PABA (para-aminobenzoic acid), 586
Pacemaker, artificial, 681
Packing slip, 245–246
PACS (picture archiving and communication system), 542–543
Pager systems, 107
Paging system software, 190
Pain
    back, 610
    musculoskeletal, 602
Palliative treatment
    for lung cancer, 665
    for multiple sclerosis, 726
Palpation
    bimanual, 411
    in cardiovascular examination, 689
    in physical examination, 411
    pulse, 378, *379*
    for respiratory system evaluation, 665
    venipuncture site, 911
Palpitations, 693
Pancreatic disorders
    cancer, 714
    pancreatitis, 714
Pancreatic function
    amylase, 1008
    glucagon, 1008
    insulin, 1008
    lipase, 1008
Pancreatitis, 714
Panels, laboratory test, 864, 866t
Panic values, 877–878
Papanicolaou (Pap) smear, 410, 417, 766, 766t, 768–769, 770, 785–787
Papilloma, 579
Paralanguage, 51
Paralysis, types of, 730t
Paranasal sinuses, 416
Paraphrasing (interview technique), 54
Paraplegia, 730t
Parasites, 973
Parasitic infections, skin, 580–581
Parasitology, 969

Parenteral administration, 502–507, 514–524 (*see also specific routes*)
Parentheses, 134
Parity, 773
Parkinson's disease, 727, 841, 845–847, *846*
Partial thickness (second degree) burns, *555*
Partial thromboplastin time (PTT), 935
Participating fee, 223
Participating providers, 222
Passwords, 183
Past history, in medical history, 360
Pasteur, Louis, 6
Patellar reflex, *733*, 733t
Patent ductus arteriosus (PDA), 682, 683t
Pathogens
    carriers and reservoirs of, 336
    conditions that favor the growth of pathogens, 335–336
        darkness, 335
        moisture, 335
        neutral pH, 336
        nutrients, 335
        oxygen, 336
        temperature, 335
    defined, 335, 966
    handwashing to prevent growth and spread, 338–339, 349–350
    infection cycle, *336*, 336–337
    susceptible host, 337
    transmission, modes of, 337
Pathologist, 863
Pathology
    CPT-4 coding, 302–303
    sample report, 1071
Patient advocacy, 39
Patient co-payment, 223
Patient confidentiality, 39, 65
Patient education, 67–87
    AIDS prevention, 747
    alpha-fetoprotein, 728
    anticoagulant therapy, 686–687
    asthma inhalers, 662
    basic aseptic technique, 338
    body's warning, 418
    brochures, 209
    carpal tunnel syndrome, 612
    charting example, 71
    choking, 551
    cholesterol, 1011
    claims filing process, 267
    conditions needed for, 71–73
        environment, 72
        knowledge, 72–73
        Maslow's hierarchy of needs, 71
        motivation of patient, 71
        resources, 73
    COPD, 663
    crutch walking, 615
    diabetes mellitus, controlling, 797
    dietary folate, 772, 931
    dietary restrictions, 910
    expectant mothers and RhoGAM, 979
    fecal occult blood testing, patient preparation for, 972–973
    fever, 377–378
    folic acid before and during pregnancy, 772
    food-drug interaction, 488
    fungal infections, 580
    gastric bypass surgery to treat obesity, 708
    genetic diseases, 361
    gestational diabetes mellitus, 796

glucose meter use, 1009
good bowel habits, 710
guidelines, 63–64
hearing-impaired patient, 83–84
heart rate, calculating target, 323
heating pads, 615
herbal supplements, 837
hindering factors, 73–75
    age, 74
    communication barriers, 74
    educational background, 74–75
    existing illnesses, 73
    physical impairments, 75
hip fractures, 606
hypertension, 383
iron deficiency anemia, 932
Kegel exercises, 777
learning objectives, 69
legally required disclosures, 29
liquid dietary supplements, 849
Lyme disease, 966–967
medical office manager role in, 209
medications, 412
memory improvement tips for the elderly, 837–838
middle ear infections, 825
miscommunication/misinterpretation, 70
nasal disorders, 642
nitroglycerin, 681–682
otologic disorders, 640
physician charges, 238
postoperative instructions, 459
posture and back pain, 610
premenstrual dysphoric disorder, 763
preventative eye care, 637
preventative medicine, 363
process, 68–71
    assessment, 68–69
    documentation, 70–71
    evaluation, 70
    implementation, 69–70
    planning, 69
rectal medications, administering at home, 507
renal calculi, 742
self-relaxation techniques, 80
sense of taste and smell, 416
signing authorization forms, 158
smoking, effects of, 659
Spanish terminology, 85
specific topics
    alternative medicine, 77–78, 79t
    lifestyle changes, 76
    medications, 76–77, 77
    preventive medicine, 75–76
    stress management, 79–80, 81t
specimen collection, 859
spinal cord and traumatic brain injuries, 730
sun safety, 585–586
surgical procedures, advancement in, 541
teaching plans, 81–83
    community resources, 83
    developing a plan, 81, 82
    developing material, 82–83
    disseminating information, 83
    selecting and adapting material, 82
television, 99
urinary tract health, 744–745
urine collection, instructions for 24-hour, 953
vegetarian diets, 321
vitamins, herbs, and natural remedies, 412

Patient education (con't)
  websites, guidelines for selecting safe,
    184–185
  while assessing patients, 362
  women and folic acid, 314
Patient ID card, 269
Patient identification card, health plan, 262,
  262
Patient information brochure, 206–207,
  207
Patient information sheet, 97
Patient interview, 360–362, 362
  barriers to communication, 361
  introducing yourself, 361
  preparation, 360–361
  procedure, 365
Patient preparation
  for drug testing, 947
  for phlebotomy, 910
  for physical examination, 412
Patient reminders, 119–120
  appointment cards, 119, 119
  mailed cards, 120, 120
  telephone, 119–120
  tickler file use, 120
Paying invoices
  computer payment, 247
  manual payment, 246
  pegboard payment, 246
Payment
  credit, 224–225
  forms of, 223–224
  by insurance companies, 224
  posting on daysheet, 236, 249–250
Payroll
  office manager and, 208
  record-keeping, 244
  software, 190
PCP (primary care physician), 268
PDA (patent ductus arteriosus), 682, 683t
PDA (personal digital assistant), 161–162,
  191
PDR (see Physician's Desk Reference)
Peak flowmeter, 661, 662
Pederson vaginal speculum, 430t
Pediatric waiting rooms, guidelines for, 99
Pediatrician, 806
Pediatrics, 805–833
  child abuse, 822
  defined, 806
  growth and developmental stages,
    815t–816t
  illnesses and disorders, 822–826
    asthma, 824
    attention deficit hyperactivity disor-
      der (ADHD), 826
    cerebral palsy, 824
    common cold, 814t
    croup, 824
    cystic fibrosis, 824
    encephalitis, 823–824
    epiglottitis, 824
    gastroenteritis, 814t, 823
    impetigo, 823, 823
    meningitis, 823
    obesity, 826
    otitis media, 814t, 824–825
    tetanus, 824
    tonsillitis, 825–826
  immunization schedule
    aged 0-6 years, 808
    aged 7-18 years, 809
    catch-up for aged 4 months-18 years,
      810

infant reflexes and responses, 807, 811t,
  814, 816
medication administration, 821
office safety, 806–807
office visits
  catch-up for aged 4 months-18 years,
    810
  Denver Development of Screening
    Test II, 807, 812–813, 814
  parental role, 814
  physiologic aspects of care, 811, 814
  psychological aspects of care, 811
  sick-child, 807
  well-child, 807
physical examination, 817–821
  Apgar, 817
  history, 817
  measurements, 817, 818, 819, 820,
    827–830
procedures
  applying urinary collection device,
    830–831
  head and chest circumference,
    829–830
  infant length and weight, 827–828
restraint, 814, 821
Spanish terminology, 826
urine specimen collection, 821–822,
  830–831
vital signs, 820, 820t
Pediculosis, 581
Peel-back packages, 448–449, 449
Peer review organization, 265
Peers, communicating with, 64
Pegboard bookkeeping system, 234–236,
  246, 246
Pelvic inflammatory disease, 768
Penicillin drug allergy, 558
Penlight, 409, 409
Peptic ulcers, 707
Percussion
  indirect, 411
  in physical examination, 411
  for respiratory system evaluation, 665
Percussion hammer, 407, 407
Percutaneous transluminal coronary angio-
  plasty (PTCA), 540, 678, 680
Pericarditis, 677
Perineal resection, 746
Peripheral nervous system (PNS), 723
Peripheral vision, 415
Peristalsis, 703, 712
Peritoneal dialysis, 741–742
Peritonitis, 707
Permiethrin, 581
PERRLA, 415
Personal digital assistant (PDA), 161–162,
  191
Personal health information (PHI), 182
Personal history, 158
Personal manual, 199
Personal protective equipment (PPE), 341,
  342, 344, 347, 887
Personnel manual, 204
Pessary, 764
PET (positron emission tomography), 7,
  539–540
Petit mal seizures, 727
Petri plates, 971, 971
Petty cash, 242–243, 243, 256–257
Peyote, 329
PH, urine, 950
Phalen's test, 611
Pharmacodynamics, 486–487

Pharmacokinetics, 487–488
Pharmacology, 480–492
  allergies, 488–489
  classification of drugs, 482t–484t
  controlled substances
    abuse, reporting, 485
    DEA and, 481, 484–485
    disposal of, 486
    inventory of, 485, 486
    schedule of, 484–485, 484t
  defined, 481
  drug interactions, 488
  information resources, 489, 489
  legal regulations
    abuse of controlled substances, 485
    Drug Enforcement Agency (DEA),
      481, 484–485
    Food and Drug Administration
      (FDA), 481
    inventory, storage, dispensation, and
      disposal of medications, 485–486,
      486
  medication names, 481
  pharmacodynamics, 486–487
  pharmacokinetics, 487–488
  prescriptions
    documentation in medical record,
      480, 490
    filling out, 489–490
    form, sample, 491
    refilling, 490
  side effects, 488–489
  sources of, 486, 487t
  terminology, 489t
Pharmacy, Internet, 187
Pharyngitis, 643, 643, 825–826
Phencyclidine, 329
Phenols, as disinfectant, 341t
Phenylalanine hydroxylase, 807
Phenylketonuria (PKU), 30, 807
PHI (protected health information), 154,
  156, 157, 182
Phlebitis, 511
Phlebotomists, 860, 863, 897
Phlebotomy, 896–925
  capillary puncture
    complications, 914
    error sources, 914
    procedure, 921–924
    site selection, 912, 914
  equipment, 898–908
    antiseptics, 898
    bandages, 899
    blood collection systems, 900–902,
      900–906, 903t–904t, 905t, 906,
      907
    blood drawing station, 898, 898
    capillary puncture (microcollection),
      906–908
    filter paper test requisitions, 908, 909
    gauze pads, 899
    gloves, 898
    microcollection containers, 907–908
    microhematocrit tubes, 907, 908
    needles, 900
    puncture devices, 907, 908
    sharps containers, 899
    spill kit, 898–899
    tourniquets, 899–900
    warming devices, 908, 909
  hemoconcentration, avoiding, 899
  hemolysis, avoiding, 899–900
  patient faintness during, 914–915
  patient preparation, 910

quality control, 908–910
safety, 897, 898
venipuncture
    complications, 912, 914
    error sources, 913
    evacuated tube, 912
    needle positioning, 912, *913*
    procedure, 916–920
    site selection, *911*, 911–912
    winged infusion system, 912
Phlebotomy chairs, 898
Phlebotomy liability, 906
PHO (physician hospital organization), 268
Phonophoresis, 611
Physical examination, 405–424
    cardiovascular system, 688–689
    CPR-4 E/M codes, 298, 299t
    emergency care, 552
    format, 415–417
        balance, 417
        chest, breasts, and abdomen, 416
        coordination, 417
        eyes and ears, 415, *415*
        gait, 417
        genitalia and rectum, 416–417
        head and neck, 415
        legs, 417
        mouth and throat, 416
        nose and sinuses, 415–416
        posture, 417
        reflexes, 417
        strength, 417
    frequency of, 417
    gastrointestinal system, 715
    general health guidelines, 417–418
    gynecologic, 768–770, *769*, 785–787
    instruments and supplies, 406–411,
            407–411
        anoscope, 410–411, *411*
        audioscope, 408
        examination light, *408*, 408–409
        gooseneck lamp, 408, *408*
        head light or mirror, 409, *409*
        histobrush, 410, *410*
        laryngeal mirror, 409
        laryngoscope, 409–410, *410*
        lubricant, 410
        nasal speculum, 407, *407*
        ophthalmoscope, 408, *408*
        otoscope, 407–408, *408*
        penlight or flashlight, 409, *409*
        percussion hammer, 407, *407*
        proctoscope, 411
        sigmoidoscope, 411, *411*
        for specialty examinations, 409–411,
            409–411
        stethoscope, 409, *409*
        tuning fork, 407, *407*
        vaginal speculum, 410, *410*
    legal issues, 414
    nervous system, 731–732
    orthopedic, 613
    patient positions, *413*, 414t
    pediatric, 817–821
    purpose, 406
    respiratory system, 665–666, 665t
    responsibilities of medical assistant,
            412–415
        assisting the physician, 412, 419–423
        patient preparation, 412
        postexamination duties, 413, 415
        room preparation, 412
    sample report, 1069, 1074
    skin, 586

Spanish terminology, 418
techniques, 411–412
    auscultation, 412
    inspection, 411
    palpation, 411
    percussion, 411
Physical facilities, effect on appointment
        scheduling, 118
Physical fitness (*see also* Exercise)
    components of, 322
    sample workout schedule, 324
    suggestions for patients, 323
    target heart rate, 323
Physical impairments, effect on patient edu-
        cation, 75
Physician assistant (PA), 12
Physician delays, adapting schedule for, 122
Physician hospital organization (PHO), 268
Physician office laboratory (POL)
    CLIA and, 875
    overview, 860
    quality assurance, 876
Physicians
    communicating with, 64
    licensure, 30
    medical practice acts, 30
    role in health care team, 12
Physician's Desk Reference (PDR), 489,
        489, 496, 501, 776
Physiologic needs, 72
Pictogram, 59, *59*
Picture archiving and communication system
        (PACS), 542–543
Pigmentation disorders
    albinism, 583, *584*
    leukoderma, 584
    nevus, 584
    vitiligo, 584
PIH (pregnancy-induced hypertension), 778
Pinworms, 973
Pituitary gland disorders
    acromegaly, 799, *799*
    diabetes insipidus, 799
    dwarfism, 799
    gigantism, 798–799
Pityriasis versicolor, 580
PKU (phenylketonuria), 30, 807
Place of service codes, 295–296, 298t
Placebo, 78
Placenta previa, 778
Placing reflex, 811t
Plaintiff, 32, 34
Plan maximum, 272
Planning, in patient education process,
        69
Plantar fasciitis, 612–613
Plasma separator gel tube (PST), 905t
Plasmodium, 969
Plaster casts, 601–602
Platelet count, 934
Platelets (thrombocytes), *928*, 934
Pluralization, 137
PMDD (premenstrual dysphoric disorder),
        763
PMS (premenstrual syndrome), 761–763
Pneumococcal vaccine, 418
Pneumocystis carinii, 767
Pneumonia, 661
PNS (peripheral nervous system), 723
Poikilocytosis, 932
Poison control center, 559
Poisoning
    management of emergencies, 559–560
    overview, 558–559, *559*

poison control center, 559
POL (*see* Physician office laboratory)
Policy
    defined, 204
    types of human resources, 205
Policy and procedures manuals, 203–206
    administrative procedures, 206
    clinical procedures, 205–206
    creating, 217
    human resources policy, 205, *206*
    infection control, 206
    laboratory, 876
    mission statement, 204–205, *205*
    organizational structure, 205
    quality improvement, 205
    tips for writing, 205
Polio, 7
Poliomyelitis, 725
Pollution, 326
Polychromasia, 933t
Polycystic ovary syndrome, 765
Polydipsia, 794
Polymenorrhea, 761
Polyphagia, 794
Polyps
    colon, 710
    nasal, 642
Polyuria, 794
POMR (problem-oriented medical record),
        163
Popliteal pulse, *379*
Portal of entry, in infection process,
        336–337
Portfolio, 1038
Positioning, of patient for surgery, 450
Positive attitude, transmission of, 93
Positive mental outlook, 327
Positive stress, 79
Positron emission tomography (PET), 7,
        539–540
Possessive, word form, 137
Postage, 146
Postal zip code abbreviations, 1061
Posterior tibial pulse, *379*
Postexamination duties, of medical assistant,
        413, 415
Postexposure testing, 342
Posting
    a charge, 236, 248–249
    collection agency payments, 236, 252
    to computer accounts, 239
    a payment, 236, 249–250
    proofs, 234, 235
Postpartum care, 777
Postpoliomyelitis muscular atrophy (PPMA)
        syndrome, 725
Postural hypotension, 382
Posture, 417, 610
Potentiation, 488, 838
Potts-Smith dressing forceps, *433*
Povidone iodine, 898
Powder (oral medication form), 502t
Power of attorney, 25–26
PowerPoint, 190
PPD (purified protein derivative), 505
PPE (personal protective equipment), 341,
        342, 344, *347*, 887
PPM (provider-performed microscopy), 875
PPMA (postpoliomyelitis muscular atrophy)
        syndrome, 725
PPO (preferred provider organization), *267*,
        267–268
PR interval, 691, 692
PR segment, 692, 692

Practicing medicine without a license, 23
Pratt rectal speculum, 431t
Pre-existing condition, 269
Precedents, 22
Preceptor, 1025, 1027, 1028
Precertification of hospital admissions, 265
Precipitation test, 952
Predisposition, 326
Preferred provider organization (PPO), 267, 267–268
Pregnancy
    acronyms and abbreviations, 777
    cesarean section, 776–777
    diagnosis, 771–772
    disorders
        abortion, 778
        abruptio placentae, 779
        eclampsia, 778
        ectopic pregnancy, 778
        hyperemesis gravidarum, 778
        placenta previa, 779
        preeclampsia, 778
    drugs dangerous to fetus, 776
    ectopic, 778
    expected date of delivery (EDD), 773
    fetal development, 774
    folic acid in diet, 314, 772
    labor onset, 776
    postpartum care, 777
    signs and symptoms, 772t
    tests and procedures
        alpha-fetoprotein (AFP), 779
        amniocentesis, 779
        contraction stress test (CST), 779
        fetal ultrasound, 779
        nonstress test, 779
        pregnancy tests, 779
Pregnancy-induced hypertension (PIH), 778
Pregnancy test, 779, 977, 977, 997–998
Premenstrual dysphoric disorder (PMDD), 763
Premenstrual syndrome (PMS), 761–763
Premium, health insurance, 262
Preparedness, for externship, 1027–1028
Presbyacusis, 58, 638, 844t
Presbyopia, 633, 844t
Prescription pads, 31
Prescriptions
    documentation in medical record, 480, 490
    filling out, 489–490
    form, sample, 491
    management software, 188–189
    refilling, 104, 490
Present illness, 158, 362–363, 366–369
Preservative, 454, 454
Presidential Physical Fitness Award, 324
Preventive medicine, patient education, 75–76, 363
Primary care physician (PCP), 268
Primary diagnosis, 284
Primary intention, 457
Primigravida, 773
Primipara, 773
Printed material, for patient education, 69
Printer, 180
Priority mail, 146
Privacy
    e-mail, 183
    electronically shared information, 96
    HIPAA and, 95–96, 156
    of ICD-9 codes, 278
    invasion of, 33
    medical history, 357

messages on answering machines, 228
    reception area and, 95, 96, 103
Private law, 23
Probes, 434, 435
Problem list, in medical records, 69
Problem-oriented medical record (POMR), 163
Procedure, 204, 294
Proctology, instruments and equipment, 431t
Proctoscope, 411, 431t
Proctoscopy, 711
Professional Association of Health Care—Office Managers, 209
Professional coder associations, 17
Professional courtesy, 224
Professional distance, 63
Professional image
    attitude, 93
    courtesy, 94
    diplomacy, 94
    first impressions, 94
    role model, 93
Professionalism, 1041
Proficiency testing, 881
Profit-and-loss statement, 244
Programmed instructions, for patient education, 69
Progress notes, 158, 164, 1076
Progress reports, telephone, 104
Projection (defense mechanism), 81t
Promotional materials, developing, 206–207, 207
Prone position, 413, 414t
Pronunciation, 102
Proofreading, 142
Prophylaxis, 897
Prostate cancer, 417, 746
Prostate gland
    benign prostate hyperplasia, 745
    cancer, 746
    infection, 747
    surgical intervention for hypertrophy, 745–746
Prostate-specific antigen (PSA), 417, 746
Prostatitis, 747
Prosthesis, 605
Protected health information (PHI), 154, 156, 157
Proteins
    diet, 313
    in urine, 951, 952
Proteinuria, 743, 778, 951
Prothrombin time (PT), 935
Protocol, legal, 24
Protozoa, 969
Provider-performed microscopy (PPM), 875
Providers, 113
Proxemics, 52
Pruritus, 581, 795
PSA (prostate-specific antigen), 417, 746
Psoriasis, 582, 582
PST (plasma separator gel tube), 905t
Psychiatric disorders
    communication with patients, 60
    emergencies, 561
Psychological defense mechanisms, 80, 81t
Psychomotor skill, 72
Psychosocial development, 806
PT (prothrombin time), 935
PTCA (percutaneous transluminal coronary angioplasty), 540, 678, 680
PTT (partial thromboplastin time), 935
Puberty, 760

Public law, 23
PubMed, 186
Puerperium, 777
Pulmonary embolism, 686
Pulmonary function tests, 667, 667, 672–673
Pulmonary medicine, 658–674
    anatomy of respiratory system, 660
    arterial blood gases, 667
    bronchoscopy, 666–667
    cancers
        laryngeal, 664
        lung, 664–665
    chest radiography, 666
    defense of respiratory system, 660t
    nebulized breathing treatment, 662, 670–672
    peak flowmeter, 661, 662, 669–670
    physical examination, 665–666, 665t
        abnormal breath sounds, 666t
        abnormal respiratory patterns, 665t
        auscultation, 665–666, 666t
        inspection, 665
        palpation, 665
        percussion, 665
    pulmonary function tests, 667, 667, 672–673
    pulse oximetry, 667, 667
    respiratory disorders, 661–664
        asthma, 661–662
        bronchitis, 661
        chronic obstructive pulmonary disease (COPD), 662–663
        pneumonia, 661
        tuberculosis, 663–664
        upper respiratory disorders, 661
    smoking, effects of, 659
    Spanish terminology, 668
    sputum culture and cytology, 668
Pulmonic stenosis, 683t
Pulse
    characteristics, 380
        rate, 380
        rhythm, 380
        volume, 380
    Doppler device, 378, 380, 388
    factors affecting rate, 380, 381t
    location
        apical, 380, 381
        brachial, 379
        carotid, 379
        dorsalis pedis, 379, 380, 380
        femoral, 379
        popliteal, 379
        posterior tibial, 379
        radial, 379, 380, 380, 398
    palpation, 378, 379
    pediatric, 820, 820t
    rate variations by age, 380t
Pulse oximetry, 667, 667
Pulse points, 378, 379
Pulse pressure, 383
Punch biopsy, 431t, 432t
Punctuation, 134
Puncture devices, 907, 908
Puncture wounds, 554
Punitive damages, 32–33
Pupils, 415, 552
Pure Food and Drug Act, 481
Purified protein derivative (PPD), 505
Purulent drainage, 456
Pustule, 576, 578
Pyelogram, 749

Pyelonephritis, 744
Pyloric stenosis, 823
Pyloroplasty, 823
Pyrexia, 374
Pyuria, 744

Quadriplegia, 730t
Qualitative test, 302–303
Quality assurance (QA)
    flow sheets, 878–879, *879*
    instrument calibration and maintenance,
        882–884, *883, 884, 885,* 893
    laboratory procedure manual, 876–877
    patient test management, 876
    proficiency testing, 881
    quality control, 879–881, *880, 881, 882,*
        892
    reagent management, 881–882
    role of medical assistant, 858
    test results, screening and follow-up,
        877–878, 891
Quality control (QC)
    log sheet, *880*
    overview, 879–880
    phlebotomy, 908–910
    physician office laboratory, 860
    QC charts, 880–881, *881, 882,* 892
    for qualitative methods, 880
    for quantitative methods, 880–881
    reference laboratory, 860
    role of medical assistant, 858
Quality improvement (QI) programs
    case review, 215, *215*
    developing, 214–215, 218
    policies and procedures manual, 205
    regulatory agencies, 211–214
        Centers for Medicare and Medicaid
            Services (CMS), 213
        Joint Commission on Accreditation
            of Healthcare Organizations
            (JCAHO), 211–213
        Occupational Safety and Health
            Administration (OSHA), 211
        state health departments, 213–214
        tracking incident reports, 210–211
Quantitative test, 302
Quechenstedt test, 733
Quotation marks, 134

Rabies, 726
Radial artery, pulse, *379, 380, 380,* 398
Radiation (heat transfer), *375t*
Radiation burns, 555
Radiation safety, 534–535, *537, 538*
Radiation therapy, 540–541
Radiographic reports, in medical record,
    158–159
Radiography, 533–534, 666, 693
Radioimmunoassay (RAI), 800
Radiologist, 534
Radiology
    CPT-4 coding, 302
    diagnostic procedures, 536–540
        computed tomography (CT), 538,
            540
        contrast medium examinations,
            538–539, *539*
        examination by body region, table of,
            538t
        fluoroscopy, 538
        mammography, *537, 539, 539*
    discussing results with patient, 541
    gastrointestinal studies, 715–716
    general principles, 533–536

    contrast media, 534
    examination sequencing, 534
    outpatient x-rays, 534
    patient positioning, 534, *535, 536*
    safety, 534–535, *537, 538*
    x-ray machine, 533–534
    x-rays, 533–534
    interventional procedures, 540
    radiation therapy, 540–541
    role of medical assistant, 541–542
        assisting with examinations, 541–542
        calming patient fears, 541
        film storage and handling, 542, *542*
        preparing patient for x-ray, 543
    teleradiology, 542–543
    transfer of information, 542–543
Radiolucent tissues, 534
Radionuclides, 539
Radiopaque tissues, 534
RAI (radioimmunoassay), 800
Range of motion (ROM), 411, *601*
Rapid group A strep testing, 977, *978,*
    999–1000
Ratchets, on forceps, 432
Rationalization (defense mechanism), 81t
RBRVS (resource-based relative value scale),
    222
Reagent management, 881–882
Receipt, petty cash, 243, *243, 257*
Reception
    duties and responsibilities, 94–97
        chart preparation, 97
        diplomatic solutions to common chal-
            lenges, 95t
        manage waiting time, 97
        message retrieval, 95–96
        office preparation, 95
        register and orient patients, 97
        welcoming patients and visitors, 97
    end of patient visit, 101
    ergonomics, 97–98
    privacy issues, 95, 96, 103
    role of receptionist, 94
    telephone (*see* Telephone)
    waiting room environment, 98–101
        Americans with Disabilities Act re-
            quirements, 99, 100t
        furniture, 98
        general guidelines, 98
        infection control issues, 100–101,
            101
        pediatric, 99
        reading material, 98
        television, 98, 99
Receptionist
    duties and responsibilities, 94–97
    ergonomic concerns, 97–98
    role, 94
Recertification, 15, 16, 1041
Reconciling bank statements, 241–242, *242,*
    255–256
Reconstituting dry medication, 503
Record keeping
    components, 244–245
    of sterilized items and equipment, 436
Recovery position, 557, *557*
Rectal administration, 507, *511*
Rectal cancers, 711
Rectal examination, 417, 750
    instruments, 410–411, *411*
Rectocele, 764
Rectovaginal examination, 417
Rectus femoris site for intramuscular injec-
    tions, *508*

Red blood cell count, 931–932, *932*
Red blood cell morphology, 932, *932,* 933t
Red blood cells (RBCs)
    appearance, *928*
    in urine sediment, 953
Reducing sugar, 952, *952*
Reduction, fracture, 600–601
Reference, for employee, 202
Reference laboratory, 859–860
Referral
    approved in managed care, 265
    consultation distinct from, 124
    defined, 301
    form, *123*
    making appointments for, 123–124,
        128
    types, 64
Reflecting (interview technique), 54
Reflex hammer, 407, *407*
Reflexes
    infant, 807, 811t
    physical examination, 417
    testing, 731, *733,* 733t
Reflux disease, 706
Refractive errors, 633, 634, *634*
Refractometer, 949
Refrigerators, in clinical laboratory, 869
Refunds, processing, 236, 251
Registered mail, 147
Registered Medical Assistant (RMA)
    certification examination, 15, 16
    recertification, 1041
Registered Nurse (RN), 12
Registering patients, 97
Registration, 30, 31
Regression (defense mechanism), 81t
Reimbursement
    diagnostic related groups (DRGs) and,
        304
    resource-based relative value scale and,
        304
Relapsing fever, 375, 376t
Relative value unit, 304
Relaxation techniques, 80
Reminders
    appointment cards, 119, *119*
    mailed cards, 120, *120*
    telephone, 119–120
    tickler file use, 120
Remittent fever, 375, 376t
Renaissance, 5
Renal epithelial cells, in urine sediment,
    953
Renal failure, 741–742
Renal function tests, 1003–1006
    creatinine, 1005–1006, 1012t
    electrolytes, 1003–1005
        bicarbonate, 1004–1005
        calcium, 1005, 1012t
        chloride, 1004, 1012t
        magnesium, 1005
        phosphorus, 1005, 1012t
        potassium, 1004, 1004t, 1012t
        sodium, 1004, 1004t, 1012t
        urea (BUN), 1005, 1005t, 1012t
        uric acid, 1006, 1012t
Reportable conditions, 28–29
Reportable diseases, 878
Reportable range, 878
Reports
    computer accounting, 239, 256
    medical (*see* Medical reports)
Repression (defense mechanism), 81t
Request forms, laboratory, 864, *865, 866*

Res ipsa loquitur, 32
Res judicata, 34
Research
  ethical issues, 41
  stem cell, 42
Reservoirs, 336
Resident flora, 335
Resistance, to infection, 335
Resource-based relative value scale
    (RBRVS), 222, 304
Resources
  allocation of, 40–41
  for patient education, 73
Respiration
  characteristics
    depth, 382
    rate, 381
    rhythm, 381
  factors affecting, 382
  measuring, 381, 399
  patterns, abnormal, 665t
  pediatric, 820, 820t
  physiology of, 381
  rate variation by age, 382t
Respiratory system, 658–674
  anatomy of respiratory system, 660
  arterial blood gases, 667
  bronchoscopy, 666–667
  cancers
    laryngeal, 664
    lung, 664–665
  chest radiography, 666
  defense of respiratory system, 660t
  effects of aging on, 843t
  nebulized breathing treatment, 662,
    670–672
  peak flowmeter, 661, 662, 669–670
  physical examination, 665–666, 665t
    abnormal breath sounds, 666t
    abnormal respiratory patterns,
      665t
    auscultation, 665–666, 666t
    inspection, 665
    palpation, 665
    percussion, 665
  pulmonary function tests, 667, 667,
    672–673
  pulse oximetry, 667, 667
  respiratory disorders, 661–664
    asthma, 661–662
    bronchitis, 661
    chronic obstructive pulmonary dis-
      ease (COPD), 662–663
    pneumonia, 661
    tuberculosis, 663–664
    upper respiratory disorders, 661
  smoking, effects of, 659
  Spanish terminology, 668
  sputum culture and cytology, 668
Respiratory tract, defenses against disease,
    335
Respondeat superior, 35–36, 1029
Responsiveness, assessing in emergency care,
    549
Restatement (interview technique), 54
Restraint, 814, 821
Résumé
  preparation, 1033–1035, 1042–1043
  samples, 1035, 1036
Retention enema, 507
Retinal degeneration, 632
Retinopathy, 632–633, 797
Retractors, 434, 436
Retrograde pyelogram, 749

Retropubic resection, 746
Returned check fee, 240
Review of systems
  in medical history, 360
  in medical record, 158
Reye's syndrome, 726, 823
Rh type, 978, 979
Rheumatic heart disease, 682
Rheumatoid arthritis, 607
Rhinitis, allergic, 641
RhoGAM, 978, 979
Rhythm strip, 692
Rickettsias, 967
Rider, insurance policy, 263
Right to Know, 437, 887
Ringworm, 580, 580
Rinne test, 641
Risk management, 209–211, 723
RMA (see Registered Medical Assistant)
RN (Registered Nurse), 12
Rochester-Ochsner forceps, 433
Rochester-Pean forceps, 433
Rocky Mountain spotted fever, 967
Roentgen, Wilhelm Konrad, 7
Role model, medical assistant as, 93
Role playing, 69
Roller bandages, 587, 587, 589
ROM (range of motion), 411
Roman Empire, medicine in, 5
Roman numerals, 137
Romberg test, 731
Room preparation, 412
Rooting reflex, 811t, 814
Rotator cuff injury, 611
Routes of administration, 501–508
  buccal, 502
  inhalation, 508
  injections, 503–507, 503–510, 514–524
  intravenous (IV), 508–511, 526–529
  oral, 501, 501, 502t, 512–513
  parenteral, 502–507
  rectal, 507, 511
  sublingual, 501–502
  transdermal, 508, 524–525
  vaginal, 507–508, 511
Rule of nines, 555, 555
Rush, Benjamin, 6

SA (sinoatrial) node, 679
Sabin, Albert, 7
Sacculated aneurysm, 687
Safety
  of elderly patients, 849–850
  laboratory, 884–890
  medication administration, 494, 496
  pediatric office, 806–807
  phlebotomy, 897, 898, 912
  radiation, 534–535, 537, 538
  tips, teaching, 75
Safety and security needs, 72
Saliva, 335
Salk, Jonas Edward, 7
Salpingitis, 767, 768
Salpingo-oophorectomy, 764
Salutation, letter, 138, 140
Sanitation, 338, 339, 426, 438–439
Sanitization, 339, 345
Savings accounts, 239
Scabies, 580–581
Scales, 372–373, 373, 386–387
Scalpels, 433–434, 435
Scanner, 180
Schamberg comedone extractor, 432t
Scheduling

adapting for
  acutely ill patients, 121
  emergencies, 120, 121, 121
  late patients, 121–122
  missed appointments, 122
  physician delays, 122
  walk-in patients, 121
employees, 202–203
factors affecting
  patients' needs, 117
  physical facilities, 118
  provider preferences and needs,
    117–118
guidelines
  established patients, 118–119, 127
  new patients, 118, 126
preparing daily or weekly, 119
problems with, 124–125
systems
  computerized, 114–115, 115
  manual, 114, 114
types
  clustering, 116
  double booking, 116
  fixed, 116
  flexible-hour, 116
  open-hour, 116–117
  streaming, 116
  structured appointments, 115
  waver, 116
Schiotz tonometer, 432t
Schistocytes, 933t
Schroeder tenaculum forceps, 430t
Scissors, 432–433, 434
Sclera, 415
Sclerotherapy, 706
Scoliosis, 608, 610
Scope of practice decision-making tree, 35,
    35
Scrotal examination, 750, 756–757
Search engines, 185, 194
Seat belt use, 326–327
Seborrhea, 581
Seborrheic dermatitis, 581
Secondary intention, 457
Security
  e-mail, 183
  electronic health record, 161–162
  of electronically shared personal health
    information, 182
  Health Insurance Portability and
    Accountability Act (HIPAA) and,
    182
  Internet, 182
  passwords, 183
Sedatives, 484t
Seizure
  aura, 727
  emergency management, 557
  epilepsy, 727
  febrile, 727, 728
  focal (Jacksonian), 728
  grand mal, 727
  petit mal, 727
Self-actualization, 72
Self-Determination Act, 42
Self-hypnosis, 77
Self-relaxation techniques, 80
Semi-Fowler position, 413
Semiblock letter format, 140
Semicolon, 134
Semmelweis, Ignaz, 6
Senility, 835
Senn retractor, 436

Sensation, assessing in emergency care, 552
Sensitivity testing, 974–975, *975*
Sensorineural hearing loss, 58
Sentence structure, 134
Sentinel event, 213
Septic shock, 553
Serrations, on forceps, 432
Serum separator gel tube (SST), 905t
Service charge, bank, 240
Service contracts, 208
Seven rights for correct medication adminis-
    tration, 496
Sexual harassment, 36
Sharps biohazard containers, 434
Sharps container, 345, 346, *346*, 899
Sharps injury log, 460
Shifts, in quality control charts, 880–881,
    882f
Shingles, 579, *579,* 725
Shingling, 167
Shock
    anaphylactic, 553, 558
    cardiogenic, 553
    EMS notification, 548
    hypovolemic, 553
    management of, 553
    neurogenic, 553
    septic, 553
    signs and symptoms, 553
Shoulder
    adhesive capsulitis, 611
    rotator cuff injury, 611
Sick-child office visit, 807
Sickle cell anemia, 932
Side effects, 488–489
Sight-impaired patients
    assisting, 631
    communicating with, 59–60
Sigmoidoscope, 411, *411,* 431t
Sigmoidoscopy, 711, 717, *717*
Sign-in sheets, 116–117
Sign language, 59
Signature on file, 271
Signs, 362
Silences, allow in an interview, 54
Silver nitrate, 771
Simpson uterine sound, 430t
Sims position, *413,* 414t, 416, 769
Sims uterine curet, 430t
Sims uterine sound, 430t
Single photon emission computed tomogra-
    phy (SPECT), 540
Sinoatrial (SA) node, 679
Sinus rhythm, 679
Sinuses, physical examination, 416
Sinusitis, 642
Sitting position, *413,* 414t
Sivananda yoga, 78
Skeleton, *600*
Skilled nursing facilities, 839
Skin
    biopsy, 586
    cancer
        basal cell carcinoma, 584, *585*
        malignant melanoma, 585, *585*
        squamous cell carcinoma, 585, *585*
    defenses against disease, 335
    effects of sunlight on the, 586
    evaluation in emergency care, 551–552
    infections
        bacterial, 576–578, *579*
        fungal, 580, *580*
        parasitic, 580–581
        viral, 579, *579*

lesions, *578*
    physical examination, 586
    preoperative preparation, 450–451,
        466
Skin staples
    description, 453
    removal, 477–478
Slander, 33
Smallpox, 6
Smear preparation, 990–991
Smell (sense), 416
Smoking
    cessation, 329
    effect on airways, 659
    lung cancer and, 664–665
Snellen eye chart, 634–635, *636*
Soak, therapeutic, 592–593
SOAP (subjective-objective-assessment-plan)
    format, *162,* 162–163
Social history, in medical history, 360
Social Security benefits, 263
Sodium hypochlorite, as disinfectant, 341t
Soft tissue injuries
    impaled object, 555, *555*
    management of, 554–555
    types, 553–554, *554*
Software
    medical management, 114–115
    medical software applications, 188–191
        administrative applications, 189–190
        clinical applications, 188–189
        Meeting Maker, 191
        paging system software, 190
        PowerPoint, 190
        vendors, 188
Sonography, 538–539, *540*
Sore throat, 825–826
Spanish health care phrases
    body parts, 1056–1057
    diseases, 1057
    examination, 1058–1059
    general phrases, 1059–1060
    general words, 1056
    introductory phrases, 1055
    signs and symptoms, 1057–1058
    treatment, 1059
Spansule (oral medication form), 502t
Speaker phones, 107
Specialties, medical, 8, 9t, 10t
Specialty examinations, instruments and
    supplies, 409–411, *409–411*
Specific gravity, 748, 949
Specificity, 283, 975
Specimen
    defined, 858
    transport containers, 859, *859*
Specimen collection
    patient education, 859
    surgical procedure, 454, *454*
Specimen processor/accessioner, 863
SPECT (single photon emission computed
    tomography), 540
Speculum
    nasal, 407, *407*
    vaginal, 410, *410*
Speech impairments, 60
Spell check, 133
Spelling, 133, 135
Spencer stitch scissors, *434*
Spherocytes, 933t
Sphygmomanometer, 382, *383,* 400–403
Spill kit, 898–899
Spills, cleaning biohazardous, 345, *346,*
    353–354, 889–890

Spina bifida, 779
Spina bifida occulta, 728, *729*
Spinal cord injuries, 729–730, 730t
Spine disorders
    curvature, abnormal, *310,* 608–609
    herniated intervertebral disc, 609–610
Spirochaetes, 966
Splash shield, 890
Splatter guard, 890
Splints, 556, *556*
Spores, 335
Spousal abuse, 30
Sprain, 599–600
Spring or thumb forceps, 432
Sputum
    culture and cytology, 666
    specimen collection, 984–985
SQ (subcutaneous) injections, *505,* 506,
    519–520
Squamous cell carcinoma, 585, *585*
Squamous epithelial cells, in urine sediment,
    953
SST (serum separator gel tube), 905t
St. John's wort, 79t
ST segment, 692, *692*
Staff
    education, 208
    meetings, 199, *199*
Staffing issues
    disciplinary action, 202, *204*
    evaluating employees, 202, *203*
    interviewing, 200
    references, 202
    scheduling, 202–203
    terminating employees, 202
    writing job descriptions, 200, *201*
Stage, microscope, 867
Staining
    microorganisms, 973–974, *975,* 992–993
    peripheral blood smear, 938
Stale check, 241
Standard precautions, 342
Standards of care, 32, 211–213
Stapedectomy, 639
Staphylococcus, 335, 576, 577, 632, 823
Staples, skin
    description, 453
    removal, 477–478
Stare decisis, 22
Startle reflex, 811t, 814
Stasis ulcer, 686
STAT, 120
State health departments, 213–214
Status asthmaticus, 662
Statute of limitations, 34, 156, 172
Statutes, 22
Steam under pressure, 426, 427t
Stein-Leventhal syndrome, 765
Stem cell research, 42
Stent, 680
STEP program, 16
Stepping reflex, 811t, 814
Stereotyping, 55, 58
Sterile dressings
    applying, 469–471
    changing existing, 472–473
    description, 455–456
    reasons for use, 456
Sterile gloves, applying, 467–469
Sterile solutions, pouring, 449, 464–465
Sterile technique, 426 (*see also* Surgical
    asepsis)
Sterilization
    cold, 427

Sterilization *(con't)*
  defined, 426
  equipment, 426–429
  indicators, *428*, 428–429, 448
  for infection control, 339, *340*
  methods, 426, 427t
  sanitizing equipment for, 438–439
  wrapping instruments for autoclaving, 440–441
Sterilizer forceps, 432
Steroids, for asthma, 662
Sterotypes, about the elderly, 835, 836
Stethoscope, 409, *409*
Stille plaster shears, 430t
Still's disease, 607
Stimulants, 328–329, 484t
Stomach disorders
  cancer, 707–708
  gastritis, 707
  peptic ulcer, 707
Stomatitis, 704–705
Stool
  culture, 973
  specimen
    collecting, 985–986
    handling, 973, 973t
    for occult blood, 417
Storage
  computer hardware, 180
  of medications, 485–486
  readiographic films, 542, *542*
  of sterilized items and equipment, 435–436
Storing medical records, 170–172, *171*
Strabismus, 633, *635*
Strain, 599
Streaming, appointment scheduling, 116
Strength, in physical examination, 417
Strength training, 322, 324
Streptococcus, 576, 823, 825–826, 977
Stress
  causes, 79
  indications, 326
  negative, 79–80
  physiologic responses, 79–80
  positive, 79
Stress management
  coping strategies, 80
  defense mechanisms, 80, 81t
  negative stress, 79–80
  positive stress, 79
  techniques, 80, 326
Stretching exercises, 322, 324
Stroke, 687
Stroke, heat, 560
Stuttering, 60
Sty, 632
Subcutaneous (SQ) injections, *505*, 506, 519–520
Subject filing, 170
Sublimation (defense mechanism), 81t
Sublingual route of administration, 501–502
Subpoena duces tecum, 157
Substance abuse, 328–329
  alcohol, 328
  communication with patients, 60
  drugs, 328–329
  smoking cessation, 329
Sucking reflex, 811t
Suicide, 838
Sulfosalicylic acid, *952*
Summarizing (interview technique), 54
Summation reports, 244
Sunscreen, 586

Superficial (first degree) burns, 555
Supernatant, 953
Supine position, *413*, 414t, 416
Supplements, herbal, 78, 79t
Supplies (*see also* Instruments and supplies)
  maintaining surgical, 436
  office manager's role in management, 208
  ordering, 245, 257
  peel-apart packages, 448–449, *449*
  receiving, 245, *245*
Support groups, 83
Suppository, 507, *511*
Suprapubic aspiration, 947
Suprapubic prostatectomy, 745–746
Surfing, 184
Surgery
  assisting the physician
    electrosurgery, 454–455, *455*
    laser surgery, 455
    local anesthetics, 451–452, *453*
    specimen collection, 454, *454*
    sterile glove, applying, 467–469
    wound closure, 452–454, *473*, *474*
  cleaning examination table and operative area, 456, 458
  CPT-4 coding, 300–302
  excision of skin lesion, 458, 474–475
  health information, protected, 456
  incision and drainage, 456, 458, 475
  Joint Commission on Accreditation of Healthcare Organizations (JCAHO) standards, 213
  making appointments for, 124
  minor office, 445–479
  patient preparation
    draping, 450, *452*
    informed consent, 450, *451*
    instructions, 450
    positioning, 450
    skin preparation, 450–451, 466
  responsibilities of medical assistant, 446–447
  Spanish terminology, 460
  sterile dressings
    applying, 469–471
    changing existing, 472–473
    description, 455–456
    reasons for use, 456
  sterile field
    adding peel-back packages to, 448–449, *449*
    guidelines to maintain, 447
    pouring sterile solutions, 449, 464–465
    sterile transfer forceps, 448, *448*, *449*, *463*
    surgical packs, 447, 447–448, 461–462
  suture and staple removal, 459, *459*, 476–478
  terminology, 302t
Surgical asepsis
  goal of, 426
  medical asepsis compared, 427t
  principles and practices of, 426–429
  role of medical assistant in, 426
Surgical instruments, 429–435
  care and handling, 434–435
  forceps, 432, *433*
  probes and directors, 434, *435*
  retractors, 434, *436*
  scalpels and blades, 433–434, *435*
  scissors, 432–433, *434*

specialty
  dermatology, 432t
  obstetrics and gynecology, 430t
  ophthalmology, 432t
  orthopedics, 430t
  otology, 431t
  proctology, 431t
  urology, 431t
sterilization, 426–429, 427t
storage and recordkeeping, 435–436
towel clamps, 434, *435*
wrapping for sterilization in an autoclave, 440–441
Surgical packs, sterile
  disposable, 447
  guidelines for, 448
  opening, 447–448, 461–462
  sterilization indicators, 448
Surgical specialties, 9t
Surgical supplies, maintaining, 436
Survey
  employer, 1030, *1032*
  graduate, 1030, *1031*
Susceptible host, 337
Suspension (oral medication form), 502t
Sustained fever, 375, 376t
Suture scissors, *434*
Sutures
  absorbable, 453
  gauge, 453
  nonabsorbable, 453
  packaging, 452, 453, *453*
  removal, 459, *459*, 476–477
Swaged needles, 452
Swimmer's ear, *639*, 639–640
Symbols, 136–137, 1062t–1066t
Symmetry, observing during physical examination, 411
Sympathy, 62
Symptoms, 362
Syncope, 560, 843, 910
Synergism, 488
Syphilis, 767
Syringe
  calibration, 504–505
  parts, 503, *504*
  for phlebotomy, 902, 905
  types, 503, *504*
Syrup (oral medication form), 502t
Syrup of ipecac, 560
Systemic changes, in the elderly, 841
Systole, 382

Tablet (oral medication form), 502t
Tachycardia, 679
Tape, autoclave, *428*, *428*
Target cells, 933t
Task force, 214, 215
Task manager, 188
Taste (sense), 416
Taste buds, 416
Tax return, 244
TB (tuberculin) syringe, 504, *504*
Teaching patients, 63–64 (*see also* Patient education)
Teaching plans, 81–83
  community resources, 83
  developing a plan, 81, *82*
  developing material, 82–83
  disseminating information, 83
  selecting and adapting material, 82
Telecommunication device for the deaf (TDD), 59

Telecommunication relay systems (TRS), 108
Telephone
 auto-attendant, 107
 cellular, 107
 collecting a debt, 225, 227
 equipment and services, 107, *107*
 etiquette, 104
 importance in medical office, 102
 incoming calls
  appointments, 103
  billing inquiries, 103
  challenging, 105
  irate patients, 105
  medical emergencies, 105
  from other physicians, 104
  personal calls, 104
  prescription refills, 104
  progress reports, 104
  taking messages, 106
  test results, reports from laboratories, 103–104
  test results request from patients, 104
  triaging, 105–106
  unidentified callers, 105
 medical record documentation of communications, 167
 multiple lines, 107
 outgoing calls
  emergency medical services, 106–107
  general guidelines, 106
  long distance, 106
 reminders, 119–120
 Spanish terminology, 108
 telecommunication relay system (TRS), 108
 triage, 189
 use guidelines
  courtesy, *102*, 102–103
  diction, 102
  expression, 102
  listening, 102
  pronunciation, 102
Telephone numbers, in written communication, 138
Teleradiology, 542–543
Teletypewriter (TTY), 108
Television
 closed captioning, 98
 as teaching tool, 99
 in waiting room, 98
Temperature
 axillary, 375, 376t, 394
 Celsius-Fahrenheit conversion scale, 1079
 factors influencing, 374
 fever patterns, variations in, 376t
 fever processes, 374
 fever stages, 374–375
 heat balance, 373, *374*
 heat transfer mechanisms, 375t
 hyperthermia, 560
 hypothermia, 560–561
 normal range, 374
 oral, 375, 376, 376t, 389–391
 pediatric, 820
 rectal, 375, 376t, 392–393
 temporal artery, 376, 377, 397–398
 tympanic, 376t, 377, 378, 396
Template, letterhead, 138
Temporal artery thermometer, *376, 377, 397–398*
Tenaculum, 430t
Tendonitis, 607

Tennis elbow, 611
Tension headaches, 731
Teratogenic, 489t
Terminally ill patients
 communicating with, 62
 hospice, 63
Terminating employees, 202
Termination or withdrawal of contract, 24–25, *25*
Tertiary intention, 457
Test
 flow chart for evaluation, *885*
 package inserts, 863–864
Test results
 normal values, 877
 panic (critical) values, 877–878
 reportable range, 878
 screening and followup, 877–878, 891
Testicular cancer, 746
Testicular self-examination, 750, 756–757
Testosterone, 795t
Tetanus, 725, 824
Tetanus booster vaccination, 418
Tetracycline, 582
Tetralogy of Fallot, 683t
Text messaging, 107
Text telephone (TTY), 59
Thank you letter, 1040, *1040*
Therapeutic, 489t
Therapeutic nutrition, 321
Therapeutic soaks, 592–593
Therapeutic touch, 52, *52*
Thermal burns, 555
Thermic effect of food, 324
Thermometer
 axillary, 394
 calibration, 376, *377*
 disposable, 377, *378*
 electronic, 376, *378*, 395
 glass mercury, 375–376, *377*, 389–391, 392–393, 394
 rectal, 375, *377*, 392–393
 sheath, 376
 temporal artery, 373, 376, 377, 397–398
 tympanic, 373, 377, *378*, 396
Third-party administrator (TPA), 262
Third-party payer, 262
Thomas uterine curet, 430t
Thoracentesis, 665
Threshold levels, glucose renal, 950
Throat
 culture, 643
 disorders
  laryngitis, 643
  pharyngitis, 643, *643*
  tonsillitis, 643
 physical examination, 416
 Spanish terminology, 644
 specimen, collecting, 980–981
 visual inspection, 643
Thrombocytopenia, 934
Thrombocytosis, 934
Thrombolytics, 482t
Thrombus, 683, *684*, 686
Thrush, 705
Thyroid agents, 484t
Thyroid function test, 799–800, 1007, *1007*
Thyroid gland disorders
 hyperthyroidism, 793–794, 796, *796*
 hypothyroidism, 794
Thyroid hormones, 793–794, 795t
Thyroid-stimulating hormone (TSH), 795t, 1007, *1007*
Thyroid storm, 796

Thyrotoxicosis, 793–794, 796
TIA (transient ischemic attack), 687, 842t
Tickler file, 120
Tidal volume, 667
Time, in written communication, 138
Time-release capsule (oral medication form), 502t
Time sheet, externship, *1030*
Tine test, 505, *506*
Tinea, 580, 968
Tinnitus, 638
Tissue, disposable, 338
To-keep-open (TKO) rate, 510
Tomography, 538, *540*
Tonic neck reflex, 811t
Tonometry, 432t, 633, 636
Tonsillitis, 643, 825–826
Tooth decay, 703–704
Topical medications, 508
Tort law, 23
Tort of outrage, 33
Torts
 defined, 32
 intentional
  assault and battery, 33
  defamation of character, 33
  duress, 33
  fraud, 33
  invasion of privacy, 33
  tort of outrage, 33
  undue influence, 33
 unintentional, 32–33
  damage, 32
  dereliction of duty, 32
  direct cause, 32
  duty, 32
  jury awards, 32–33
  malpractice, 32
  negligence, 32
Total hip replacement, 605, *606*
Touch, therapeutic, 52, *52*
Tourniquets, 899–900, 911
Towel clamps, 434, *435*
Toxicology department, 862
Toxoplasma, 969
Toys, waiting room, 99
TPA (third-party administrator), 262
Tracheostomy, 664, *664*
Trade name, 481
Training
 blood-borne pathogens, 341
 computer, 191–192
Transcription, computer software, 190
Transdermal administration, 508
Transdermal medications, 524–525
Transfer forceps, sterile, 448, *448, 449*, 463
Transient flora, 335
Transient ischemic attack (TIA), 687, 842t
Transillumination, 416
Transitional epithelial cells, in urine sediment, 953
Translation, Web sites for, 185–186
Transmission
 common communicable diseases, 338t
 direct, 337
 indirect, 337
 sources of, 337
Transport, specimen, 971–972, *972*
Transport containers, 859, *859*
Transurethral resection of the prostate, 745
Traumatic needle, 452
Traveler's checks, 240
Treadmill stress test, 693, *695*

Tremors, with Parkinson's disease, 845, 846
Trendelenburg position, *413*
Trends, in quality control charts, 880–881, 882f
Treponema pallidum, 767
Tretinoin, 582
Triage, 360
Trial, 34
TRICARE, 264
Triceps reflex, *733*, 733t
Trichomonas vaginalis, 768, 954, 969
Triglycerides, 1011, 1011t, 1012t
Triple phosphate crystals, 953
Troponin, 1007–1008
TRS (telecommunication relay systems), 108
Truth-in-lending statement, 224
TSH (thyroid-stimulating hormone), 795t, 1007, *1007*
TTY (teletypewriter), 108
Tube holder, *900*, 901, *901, 902*
Tuberculin (TB) syringe, 504, *504*
Tuberculosis screening, 505, *506*, 663–664
Tubex, 503
Tubular gauze bandages, 587, *588*, 593–595
Tumor, urinary system, 742
Tuning fork, 407, *407,* 641
Turgor, skin, 715
Tympanic membrane, 407–408, 415, *415, 825*
Tympanic method, for temperature, 373, 377, *378*, 396
Tympanic thermometers, 373, 377, *378,* 396
Tympanometry, 641
Type I allergy, 888

UB-92 (uniform bill), 278
UCR, 222
UCR (usual, customary, and reasonable) tables, 272
Ulcer
  corneal, 632
  decubitus, 582–583, 583t
  duodenal, 708
  peptic, 707
  stasis, 686
Ulcerative colitis, 709
Ultrasound
  fetal, 779
  gastrointestinal system, 716
  overview, 538–539, *540*
  urinary system, 750
Umbilical hernia, 711
Undescended testis, 746, 746–747
Undue influence, 33
Uniform Anatomical Gift Act, 43
Unintentional torts, 32–33
Unit dose packages, 501, *501*
United States Department of Agriculture (USDA), 315–320
United States Pharmacopeia Dispensing Information (USPD), 489
United States Postal Service (USPS), 145–147
Universal serial bus (USB), 180
Upcoding, 305
Upper respiratory infection, otits media and, 640
Urea (BUN), 1005, 1005t, 1012t
Ureterostomy, 742, *743*
Urethral sounds, 431t
Urethritis, 744
Uric acid, 607, 749, 1006, 1012t
Uric acid crystals, 953
Urinalysis, 748, 944–963

chemical properties, 949–951, 950t
  bilirubin, 951, *952, 953*
  blood, 951
  chemical reagent strip analysis, 960–961
  dipsticks, 950
  glucose, 950, 952
  ketones, 950–951, 952
  leukocyte esterase, 951
  nitrite, 951
  pH, 950
  proteins, 951, 952
  urobilinogen, 951
confirmatory testing, 951–952
  copper reduction test, 952
  diazo test, 952, *953*
  nitroprusside test, 952
  precipitation test, 952
diurnal variation, 946
normal values and clinical significance, 1080t–1081t
physical properties, 948–949, 948t
  clarity, 948–949, 949t
  color, 948, 949t, 959
  specific gravity, 949
specimen collection methods, 945–948
  24-hour collection, 946, 954, 956–958
  bladder catheterization, 946–947
  clean-catch midstream urine specimen, 854–855, 946
  container, 945, 946
  drug testing, 947–948
  first morning void, 946
  postprandial specimen, 946
  random specimen, 946
  refrigeration of specimen, 945
  suprapubic aspiration, 947
  timing of collection, 945
urine sediment, 952–954
  bacteria, 953
  casts, 954
  crystals, 953
  epithelial cells, 953
  preparation, 953, 962
  red blood cells, 953
  white blood cells, 953
Urinalysis department, 862
Urinary frequency, 744
Urinary system
  effects of aging on, 843t
  infections, 743–745
Urine
  melanin, 586
  specimen
    collecting from pediatrics, 821–822, 830–831
    handling, 973t
Urine Specimen Collection Handbook, 947–948
Urinometer, 949, *950*
Urobilinogen, 951
Urology, 739–758
  anatomy of urinary system, *741*
  diagnostic and therpeutic procedures
    blood tests, 749
    catheterization, 748, *748,* 749, 752–755
    cystoscopy, 749, *749*
    intravenous pyelogram (IVP), 749
    rectal examination, 750
    retrograde pyelogram, 749
    scrotal examination, 750, 756–757
    ultrasound, 750

urinalysis, 748
    vasectomy, 750
  instruments and equipment, 431t
  male reproductive disorders
    benign prostatic hyperplasia, 745–746
    cryptorchidism, 746, 746–747
    epididymitis, 747
    hydrocele, 746
    impotence, 747–748
    infections, 747
    inguinal hernia, 747
    orchitis, 747
    prostate cancer, 746
    prostatitis, 747
    testicular cancer, 746
  overview, 740
  procedures
    female urinary catheterization, 752–753
    male urinary catheterization, 754–755
    testicular self-examination, 756–757
  Spanish terminology, 751
  urinary disorders
    calculi, 742
    cystitis, 744
    glomerulonephritis, 743–744
    hydronephrosis, 742
    infections, 743–745
    pyelonephritis, 744
    renal failure, 741–742
    symptoms, 744t
    tumors, 742
    urethritis, 744
Urticaria, 581–582
USB (universal serial bus), 180
USDA (United States Department of Agriculture), 315–320
USP (United States Pharmacopeia) label, 78
USPD *(United States Pharmacopeia Dispensing Information),* 489
USPS (United States Postal Service), 145–147
Usual, customary, and reasonable (UCR) tables, 272
Uterine bleeding, dysfunctional, 761
Uterine dilator, 430t
Uterine prolapse and displacement, 764, *764*
Uterine sounds, 430t
Utilization management, 265
Utilization review, 265

V-codes, 279, 283
Vaccine information statement (VIS), 807, 814f
Vaccine side effects, 29
Vaginal administration, 507–508, *511*
Vaginal speculum, 410, *410,* 430t, 769, 769–770
Vagotomy, 707
Valvular disease, 682, 683t
Varicella vaccine, 418
Varicose veins, 685–686, *686,* 706
Varro, Marcus, 5
Vascular stent, 540
Vasectomy, 750
Vasodilators, 681–682
Vastus lateralis site, *508,* 821, 822f
Vector, 337
Vegetables, food group guidelines, 318–319
Vegetarian diets, 321

Vehicle, for transmitting microorganisms, 336
Veins
    arm, *911*
    rolling of, 911
Venipuncture
    complications, 912, 914
    equipment
        blood collection systems, *900–902,*
            900–906, 903t–904t, 905t, 906,
            907
        needles, 900
        tourniquets, 899–900
    error sources, 913
    evacuated tube, 912
    needle positioning, 912, *913*
    procedure, 916–920
    site selection, *911,* 911–912
    winged infusion system, 912
Venous thrombosis, 686
Ventricular activation time, 692
Ventricular fibrillation, 679
Ventricular septal defect (VSD), 682, 683t
Ventricular tachycardia (VT), 679
Ventrogluteal site, *507*
Verbal communication, 50–51
Verbal warnings, 202
Verified Internet Pharmacy Practice Site
    (VIPPS), 187
Verruca, 579
Vertebrae fractures, 552
Vertebral column, 608, *609*
Vertigo, 842t
Vesalius, Andreas, *5*
Vesicle, *576, 578*
Vials, 503, *503*
Vienna nasal speculum, 431t
Violent injuries, reporting of, 30
VIPPS (Verified Internet Pharmacy Practice
    Site), 187
Viral disease, 579, *579,* 968–969
Virology, 968
Virtual patient chart, 188
Virulent, 335
Virus, computer, 182
Visual acuity testing, 634–635, *636,*
    644–645
Visualization, 80
Vital signs
    assessing in emergency care, 551
    blood pressure, 382–385, *383,* 383t,
        384, 400–403, 820, 820t
    pediatric, 820, 820t
    pulse, 378–381, *379–381,* 380t, 381t,
        398, 820, 820t
    respiration, 381–382, 382t, 399, 820,
        820t
    Spanish terminology, 385
    temperature, 373–378, 375t, *376–378,*
        376t, 389–398, 820
Vital statistics, 28
Vitamin B$_{12}$ deficiency, 688, 930, 931,
    934
Vitamins, 313–314
Vitiligo, 584
Voice mail systems, 96
Volkman retractor, *436*

Vomiting, by children, 823
Voucher, petty cash, 243, 257
VSD (ventricular septal defect), 682, 683t
VT (ventricular tachycardia), 679
Vulvovaginitis, 768

Waiting time, managing, 97
Waived tests, 874–875
Walk-in patients, adapting schedule for, 121
Walkers, *616,* 616–617
Warm compress, applying, 590–591
Warming devices, 908, *909*
Wart, 579, 767
Waste disposal, 345–346, 347, 353–354
Wave scheduling system, 116
Web browser, 181
Weber test, 641
Weight, measuring, 372–373, *373,* 386–387
Weight management
    body mass index (BMI), 325, *325*
    overview, 323
    physiologic issues
        basal metabolic rate (BMR), 324
        calories, 324–325
        level of physical activity, 324
    sociologic and psychological issues, 325
Welcoming patients and visitors, 97
Well-child office visit, 807
Wellness, maintaining
    dental health, 327, *327*
    genetics, 327
    infectious disease prevention, 327–328
    overview, 325–326
    pollution, 326
    positive mental outlook, 327
    seat belt use and airbags, 326–327
    stress, 326
Westergren erythrocyte sedimentation rate,
    934, *934,* 941–942
Wet mounts, 973, 974
Wheals, *578,* 582
White blood cell differential, 930–931
    basophils, 931
    eosinophils, 931
    lymphocytes, 931
    monocytes, 931
    neutrophils, 930–931
White blood cells, in urine sediment, 953
White out, 243
Wilde ear forceps, 431t
Winged infusion set, 906, *906, 907,* 912
Withdrawal, 81t, 329
Withdrawing treatment, 42
Withholding treatment, 42
Witness, expert, 32
Women in medicine, 6–7
Wood's light, 587
Worker's compensation, 167–168, 269
Workout schedule, sample, 324
World Health Organization (WHO), 278
World Wide Web (WWW) (*see* Internet)
Wound
    cleaning, *458*
    closed, 553–554, *554*
    closure
        adhesive skin closures, 453–454, *454*
        needles and sutures, 452–453, *453*

    staples, 453
    cultures, 586
    drainage, 456
    open, 554, *554*
    specimen, collecting, 983–984
Wound healing
    phases, 458
    primary intention, 457
    secondary intention, 457
    tertiary intention, 457
Wrist, carpal tunnel syndrome of, 611, 612
Write off, 224, 236, 238
Written communication, 131–151
    agendas, 143, *144*
    annotation, 148
    guidelines for document production
        abbreviations and symbols, 136–137
        accuracy, 133, 135
        capitalization, 134, 136
        grammar and punctuation, 133, 134
        numbers, 137–138
        plural and possessive, 137
        spelling, 133, 135
    incoming mail, 147
    letters
        components of, 138, *139,* 140
        composition, 141–142, 148–149
        editing, 142
        formats, 140, *140, 141*
        how to start writing, 141
        preparation, 141
        types of, 143
    memorandum, 143, *143*
    minutes, 143–144
    opening and sorting, 147–148, 150
    overview, 132
    sending, 144–147
        addressing envelopes, 145–146
        electronic mail, 145
        facsimile machine, 144–145, *145*
        mailing options, 146–147, *147*
        postage, 146
        United States Postal Service, 145–147
        via delivery services, 147
    Spanish terminology, 148
Written notice, 202

X-ray envelope, 542, *542*
X-ray machines, 533–534
X-ray report, 1077
X-rays (*see also* Radiology)
    discovery of, 7, 533
    outpatient, 534
    patient positioning, 534, *535, 536*
    preparing a patient for, 543
    safety, 534–535, *537, 538*

Yanagimachi, Ryuzo, 7
Yeasts, 968
Yoga, 77–78
Young's rule, 500

Z-track method of intramuscular injections,
    506, *509,* 523–524
Zip code abbreviations, 1061

CCacksm

CCS0409